All Your Health Questions Answered Naturally

by
Maureen Kennedy Salaman

MKS, Inc.

All Your Health Questions Answered Naturally
by Maureen Kennedy Salaman

This Edition 1998
by Maureen Kennedy Salaman
Original Hardcover Edition 1998
by Maureen Kennedy Salaman

Library of Congress No.97-93409

ISBN:0-913087-21-1

Original Hardcover Edition, July 1998
First Paperback Edition, July 1998

Published by
MKS, Inc.
(650) 854-3922

Distributed by:
BAY TO BAY DISTRIBUTION, INC.
453 Ravendale Drive, Suite A
Mountain View, California 94043
(650) 691-0108

Printed in the United States of America

Cover Photo by Harry Langdon
Cover Design by Carla Radosta @
Design Visual Communications

IMPORTANT NOTICE

This book is neither a medical guide nor a manual for self-treatment. It is instead intended as a reference work only. The information in this book is meant to help you make informed choices about your health, but is not intended as a substitute for any treatment that may be prescribed or recommended by your doctor or health care practitioner. If you should suspect that you suffer from a medical condition or problem, you should seek competent medical care without delay.

DEDICATION

A book is not mere pieces of paper held between two covers. It is one mind touching another mind.

It is a relationship, and I have enjoyed a healing love affair with my readers for three decades.

For this reason I dedicate this book to you my many readers – my friends – who have inspired me through my 30-year search for truth, answers and hope.

I truly love you, all of you. From my heart to yours.

ACKNOWLEDGEMENTS

My acknowledgements start with special thanks to Hope P. Daly for every one of life's little drudgeries that you bear cheerfully for me and for your insistence on excellence in every task. To Bette Steesy, who helps her carry the load.

My life's work would not be complete without the incredibly talented, capable and unflappable Jim Rezoski. He is one of a kind, and I am blessed to know him.

To my incomparable friend and researcher Julia Bauer – the brilliance of your mind lights my path and illuminates the lives of so many. My heartfelt thanks also goes out to Gina Chiotti-Hovey and Shirley Osward for your years of help, support and devotion. To Carol Frates, whose expertise and experience proves invaluable time and time again.

I point with pride to the commitment, loyalty and assiduousness of my staff. For them, selfishness and personal glory are subordinate to team effort and team glory. The success I have achieved as an individual has been because I am part of this dedicated team.

To the officers, board members, staff and membership of the National Health Federation: I have served them with passion and dedication for over two decades and for the last 16 years as their President. May God continue to make them brave and keep them true. To Patrick von Mauck, a splendid, tireless soldier in the battle for health freedom.

To my brother Major Thomas C. Gillespie, USMC, for carrying on the legacy of love of God, country and selfless dedication to cause; Jackie Gillespie, an angelic presence, and Alexandra Helen and Christopher Thomas Gillespie, who carry on the beautiful character of their parents. I am duly proud of you both.

The Alonzo family, my adopted family, Alan, Holly, Jamie, Mathew, Rachael, Renaldo, Sara and Sharon, all close to my heart, who give me hope for tomorrow and hope for America in tomorrow.

To my truest friend, Karl H. Rolfes, that one in ten thousand who has stuck with me closer than a brother.

To Heide Van Doren Betz, whose integrity, beauty and heart make it more than a privilege to call her my friend.

To Bella Farrow, whose personal power, grace and hard work have brought both joy and provision into the lives of thousands, including my own.

To my son Sean who started me on my search for truth.

Many think of fulfillment as something to be found in money, wealth, success and applause; and don't learn until it's too late that the greatest gift God gives is loving friends. In this I am the wealthiest of people. My true wealth is manifest in the following people. To my friends who bless my life so richly: Julia "Cori" Haskett Abbruszzese and Stefan Abbruszzese, Elaine Becker, Joe Betz, Norma and Russ Bixler, Susan Blais, Freda and Claud Bowers, Theodore and Ellie Brown, Helen Gurley Brown, The Coonce Family, Tony and Bobby Cortesese, David and Linda Swan/Detert, Betsy Dohrman, Donna Douglas, Terri Shaffer-Douglas and family, Judd Dunning, Oleen Eagle, Dehlia Ehrlich, Eddie and Betty Fisher, Bonnie Fleming, Shirley and Kenny Foreman, Kurt and Dawn Foreman, Kenny and Alisa Foreman, Jr., Charlie Fox, Carol Gentry, Blackie andAngie Gonzales, Mary Kay Gonzales, Dr. Garry Gordon, Annette Gozales, Kathryn Grayson, Jeffrey Harsh, Connie and Ronn Haus and family, Fred Hirth, Tim Hodley and family, William Holloway, Nancy and Jack Horton, Wendy and Frank Jordon, Cristabel Kerr, Evelyn Kean, Alan Konce, Dr. Hans Kugler, Nick Lampros and family, Dave McAllister, Ruth and Merl McAnich, Michael McKenna and Laurie Miller, Vonda Haus Montgomery, Vincent Narayan, Becky Niven, The Nolan Family, The Carlton Pearson Family, The Glen Plummer Family, Dr. Henry and Mary Ritter, Jerry Roberts and family, Jerry Rose, Fran Sanchez, Dave Scott, Patricia Sinclair, Peter and Sue Sumrall, JoAnn and Jim Thompson, Karen and Scott Tips, Princess Paul of Romania (Lia Triff), John Trowbridge, M.D., Alan and Barbara Virchow, Kimberly and Arie Volger, Vladimir and Tatiana von Witte, and Greg West.

Dr. Ross Gordon deserves my gratitude and praise for the rare and real healing genius which he shared so brilliantly in this book.

TABLE OF CONTENTS

CHAPTER LIST

Introduction

Allow me to introduce the book you are about to meet. *All Your Health Questions Answered Naturally* not only contains 56 more chapters than my bestselling book, *Foods That Heal*, but encompasses more personal experiences, more research and more fascinating information than any book you'll find on the market today.

Since my ground-breaking book, *Foods That Heal*, in 1988 there have been a blizzard of imitators. *All Your Health Questions Answered Naturally* is also a leader. This is not just a book, it is an exhaustively researched, all-encompassing manual on optimizing health and reversing disease through nutrition.

I combined my worldwide personal experiences with what amounts to a library full of national and international journal-published studies, all scientifically based, to bring you the most extensively-researched, fact-based anthology of nutritional therapies and solutions to the most common afflictions, diseases and syndromes offered anywhere today. More than just scientific research from journal articles, mine is a personal search for answers. I personally sought and reached those who healed themselves, finding cures for the "incurable."

The information contained in this volume was pursued with an infatigable passion for solutions to your problems. I am well aware of the concerns faced by you because I hear from you by the thousands through my television appearances. Whether in person as I travel the world, or through your hundreds of thousands of letters sent to my offices; as you seek me out for answers, I seek out solutions. Since I live in front of the television camera, I am not only accessible, I am accountable. During my appearances I frequently ask people to call back during my next scheduled appearance so the viewing audience might hear with me the results of the information and research I have shared.

I also find that nothing compares with 30 years being on the cutting edge of this new frontier. Having been at the forefront of pushing this paradigm shift (if not into center stage) I feel I've been in an understudy position, so that when the old lead player finally falters for the last time (which it does daily), the new medicine will be there forgetting old insults.

The solutions, treatments and therapies outlined in this book will enable you to take charge and control of your ailments, from the smallest annoyance to the most heart-wrenching tragedy you'll ever have to face. They really work! And you'll meet the people who know that firsthand. Don't take it from me, take it from them.

In Your Best Interest

Because everyone is different, protocols have to be individualized. I recommend that you seek out a health practitioner who is versed in nutritional and alternative medicine before you attempt to reverse an unhealthy body. Certain tests can evaluate your blood levels of nutrients, your ability to assimilate them and indicate of which nutrients you may be deficient. These are all factors that must first be taken into account before taking therapeutic doses of nutritional supplements.

Call 1-800-445-4325 to obtain information about doctor referral organizations.

Uncovering the Cause by Understanding The Problem

Thanks to conventional medicine, you have nothing to lose! The therapies or nutrients described in this book are derived from natural sources. They are not dangerous chemicals that might cure the original problem but leave you disabled, blind or dead! They are principles and practices that use the body's inherent defense mechanisms to work against disease–a concept completely ignored by conventional medicine.

How many times have you heard the excuse "we don't know what causes it," or "there is no cure." People are left to die because alternatives are not acknowledged or considered. Consider the term "syndrome." It is typically used to describe a pattern of symptoms in which a cause is unknown. You'll see this term throughout this book. Alzheimer's is a syndrome. So is Tourette's. Most of our diseases are syndromes. Since doctors readily admit they don't know what causes them, anything can be the cause. Instead of investigating all the possibilities, they discount those that haven't been included in their realm of education and industry, choosing instead to prescribe drugs that mask the symptoms, not cure the cause. As you read this book–read all of it, you'll be amazed at what you'll learn–you will see where causes and solutions have been swept under the rug, denying the afflicted of valid, scientific therapies that could have saved them.

If your doctor, friends or loved ones use that old excuse, "It isn't curable," then do your own investigating into the pages of this book. Find the research-supported answers contained within and talk your doctor into trying them. The alternatives are natural substances, therefore the risk is minimal. Certainly less risky than the dangerous pharmaceuticals they're experimenting with on adults and even children today.

Let's say your uncle is in a mental hospital and his doctors won't tell you anything, so you insist on seeing his medical records. But the medical records don't help because physicians use such specific jargon you can't understand a word of it! Don't despair. You may recognize some of the terms here in this volume. In the table of contents, I've listed ailments by symptoms when possible. If you don't recognize a term, write it down, then consult a medical dictionary. Don't stop until you fully understand what doctors *think* is your son's problem.

Unfortunately, when doctors don't have a clue as to what is causing symptoms, or what to do about it, they give the collection of symptoms a fancy Latin name–calling it a syndrome, or name it after the doctor who first identified it, or after a celebrity who suffered from it. Without the fancy name, you wouldn't be impressed enough to shell out the big bucks required to attempt trial and error treatments.

In order to be fully instrumental in the healing of yourself and/or loved ones, you have to know the jargon used by conventional medicine. That's why I included technical terms. How can you be sure the problem isn't a result of the drug given if you can't read the medical chart? The medical industry is fraught with confusing terms and descriptions that when understood, can hold the key to understanding, and dealing with the affliction.

Use What You Learn

My staff tells me that more and more of you are passing the information I give you on to your physicians, and I am encouraged by reports that your doctors are listening to you and in some cases want to see the studies. All the information in all the chapters comes from valid scientific study accessible by your physician. Remember, it is his job to do the research, not yours. The discipline of medicine involves more than utilizing textbooks. It is and should be a constant learning process, requiring investigation, research and an open mind by all parties involved, whether they be MDs, medical technicians or therapists. Your health practitioner has the best tools and background to understand and apply complicated scientific research to your particular problem.

The information is what I am emphasizing here, not the physicians. In some cases–alas–the doctors who conducted the study or applied the protocol are either no longer alive, or have been put out of business by the government. It's a very difficult thing to keep treating people when you have the FDA breaking down your doors at gunpoint and confiscating records, taking years to give them back, without making any formal charges. This happened to my good friends Dr. Jonathan Wright, a licensed M.D. in Kent, Washington, and Dr. Cal Streeter of Highland, Indiana. In Texas, Stanislaw R. Burzynski, M.D., Ph.D. has been helping cancer patients with the blessing (and funding) of the federal government–all while the state of Texas tries to shut him down. (See my book *Nutrition: The Cancer Answer II* for details.)

You are the senior partner in your health care. Your doctor is only the junior partner. You are the one who has to live with your affliction. God didn't make us sheep. He made us intelligent, thinking human beings capable of making good and bad decisions. Nobody is more responsible than you are for your health. If the doctor you trust recommends a drug, you should still make sure that drug is safe–for you and your loved one. Side effects are not always given. Always ask, and demand literature. Doctors do not know everything about the drugs–the pharmacists do.

One of my goals for this book is to arm the public with the information they need to help prevent one of life's greatest tragedies: the medical misdiagnosis. As you read through these chapters, something might stick in your mind: a plan, an option, an idea, that when followed through with your physician could make all the difference.

Information is empowering. Anyone can tell you what to do, asking you to blindly follow them. That's what doctors do! In your best interest, I am giving you everything you need to know about your bodies, your illnesses, and your ailments, so that you can make the best decision for yourself, about yourself. And while you're at it, perhaps inform your doctor so he or she may help as well.

This research is valid, scientific and accurate. If a piece of information isn't backed by at least two sources, I don't include it. You can trust this data and you can use it to your benefit. Don't blindly follow me. Take this information and be your own guide to good health and recovery.

Conventional Excuses

It's fascinating what happens when you tell members of the conventional medical industry that you plan to inform the public of natural solutions to disease. They get very alarmed. They don't want to know what you know, no matter how conventional the source (much of my research came from conventional medical journals), they only want you to tell people it can't be true. Regardless how valid the information or compelling the study, it is disregarded as patently impossible.

They tell you this not because they know firsthand, but because they are taught to tell you this by the pharmaceutical companies who fund their research, give them scholarships for their education, and essentially pay, or are responsible for, every aspect of their training and education, including the medicines they use. Even when a nutrient is reported to help; even when it has been *proven* to help, we are told not to take it seriously. Don't let them put you off. Their motivations are political, and not in the best interest of their patients.

The Genetic Lie

How many times have you read about a faulty gene being the cause of a disease? All the illnesses that befall us are caused or influenced by genes. They recently discovered the gene for being overweight. It was found at the bottom of a container of Haagen Daz ice cream!

Just because you are born with faulty genes, doesn't mean you have to live with them. We tolerate more defects in our jeans than our genes. The fact is, the body has enzymatic machinery designed to destroy and repair faulty nuclear DNA (genes). This offensive line depends on good nutrition for optimum performance. Emanual Cheraskin, M.D., D.M.D. says, "Think of the gene as the seed, the environment as the soil. You can grow a healthy plant in good soil even if you start out with a weak seed."

Hope isn't dependent upon questionable gene therapy–not when defects can be corrected with nutrition. The correction of genes and DNA through nutrition is being done today for children with Down's syndrome, which is the result of an extra chromosome. Parents and doctors are seeing children grow up without mental retardation, and in some cases are seeing the typical facial features disappear.

Ultimately, every state of health or sickness is influenced or dependent upon the nutrients that make up our bodies. To deny this influence is like saying you don't need wood, stucco, drywall or concrete to build and maintain a house. Just one missing roof tile can cause a plethora of problems that will only get worse over time.

Eating For Your Good Health

This is not just a book, it's a user's guide, a workbook, a reference source. Look at the food chart to determine which foods you should eat to target which nutrients. It is compiled based on the most accurate scientific data, which of course varies depending upon where grown and with what. If you want to eat meat or organs for nutrients, make sure they were raised on chemically-free grasslands with no added hormones or chemicals. Make sure all the meats and produce you eat are organically grown on naturally-nourished soils.

Unfortunately, our soils have been depleted of most minerals by modern agriculture. Farming companies primarily replenish only the nitrogen, phosphorous, and potassium necessary for maximum crop yields. This leaves the foods we eat void of some 60 minerals vital to our good health. As far back as 1936, U.S. Senate Document 264, 74th Congress, 2nd Session reported: "Farm soils are depleted of minerals...Crops grown in these soils are minerally deficient and people who eat them get mineral deficiency diseases...The only prevention or cure is with mineral supplements...". Is it any wonder that 60 years later we are such a disease-ridden society? The U.S. Surgeon General has reported that 68 percent of all disease is diet related.

Likewise, I don't recommend eating shellfish. Shellfish can be hazardous to your health because they nourish themselves with sewer-water loaded with industrial pollutants, bacteria and viruses. Outbreaks of gastroenteritis, infectious hepatitis, meningitis, polio, strep throat and typhoid fever have been traced to shellfish. Some authorities refer to the lobster as the cockroach of the sea.

Choose recipes that, for the most part, feature raw or lightly cooked natural foods. Cooking rearranges atoms and molecules, loses certain nutrients and denatures protein. Raw food contains essential digestive enzymes and therefore is absorbed most efficiently. Maximum absorption of foods means maximum assimilation of nutrients.

I stress natural, whole foods, not man-made foods such as margarine, egg substitutes (eggs laid by chemists), flours with no grain or B vitamins left in them, refined sugar, hydrogenated oils and baked goods made from white flour and refined sugar.

Man-made, imitation foods are fine for imitation people. God-given, real foods are made for real people. I do not favor processed foods–canned and packaged–because they have lost too many needed ingredients, and they are embalmed with additives to give them greater shelf life–or shelf death–however you want to look at it.

Further, they have many hidden ingredients which can bring on food sensitivities and allergies. Illness is your body's typical response to man-made foods.

Cooperate with your body and it will cooperate with you, making your visits to the doctor and hospital fewer and farther between. Norman Cousins said it best: "A hospital is no place for a person who is seriously ill." Or anyone else, Norman!

I feel truly blessed for the opportunity to write this volume for you. I hope it will both entertain and heal you. Writing is a relationship, and I have enjoyed a healing love affair with my readers for 30 years. I am so grateful that after three decades of painstakingly searching for this information, you, my readers, have given me a platform for spreading this vital message.

Now it is your turn to get to work on your and your loved ones' bodies and their ailments to make them better. It's been said that if you get to work at making something better it heals you in a deeper place than you cry from.

– Maureen Kennedy Salaman

FOREWORD

Maureen Kennedy Salaman delivers another prophetic blockbuster. Like her other masterpieces, this one delivers bleeding edge information which catapults our health and healing 20 years ahead of our time.

As a physician whose life work is devoted to restoring health, I am embarrassed and disappointed that my profession has not taken the leading role in delivering these wonderful discoveries to our patients before millions have suffered and died (usually with their bank accounts depleted). But I am thrilled that Maureen did. And you will be grateful to her forever for sharing these lifesaving facts with you.

In a reader-warm manner, Maureen shows you how you can overcome chronic diseases and general maladies. Just look at the Table of Contents. You or someone close to you (family, friends, neighbors) is suffering with some of these problems and need help NOW! The time is right for you to begin the journey back toward better health.

You're healthy – not really "suffering" with anything, except this or that recurring problem, or constant nuisance or bothersome limitation. You're "getting through" like the rest of us, trying to make up here and there for problems that are getting you down.

Here is where Maureen's work really shines. She has taken most of the symptoms and complaints – the "stuff" you "suffer with" – and outlined effective ways to relieve and even reverse them. The solutions are simple *and* available.

Maureen has created a manual that will be enormously useful to you – not just right now, but even more as the years go by. You'll find yourself turning the pages just for the pleasure of learning that something real, something wonderful can be done to help so many people who are needlessly suffering. You'll be calling friends and family on the phone, sharing practical pointers. Weeks later, they'll be calling you, excitedly sharing their success stories.

Take this book with you to your doctor. He or she will enjoy the fact that Maureen never fails to entertain while she educates, and her reader-friendly style makes it easy for them to begin to catch up with you.

Wishing you WELL –

John Parks Trowbridge, M.D., FACAM
Do What You Want to Do, Appleday Press, Houston, TX, 1996.

CHAPTER 1:

Abscesses: Boils, Carbuncles

As a result of editing three magazines in this field for thirty years, plus television shows on nutrition for well over a decade, and my books on the subject, people seek me out when they are in pain and trouble. For instance, I was squeezing fruit at my local farmer's market when a voice called out my name:

"It *is* you! Maureen Salaman! God must have brought you to me!"

The voice came from a woman who introduced herself as Mary. Around a swollen chin she had tied an herbal compress, and it made me remember how, as a child, my grandmother made me wear a necklace of garlic if I had a sore throat.

"I hope I can help you," I replied.

Last summer she developed an abscess in her gums and was told she had to have a root canal. One month later she developed another abscess. An oral surgeon told her it was hopeless and that she would lose the tooth in five years. She got a second opinion and was told she should have another root canal to clean out the infection, but there was still only a 50/50 chance of saving the tooth, even though she was taking antibiotics.

"I'm in such pain, I can't concentrate on anything!" Mary's eyes filled with tears and she motioned for me to join her away from the crowd.

After a long hug so she could compose herself, I told her about the vitamin C studies – the ones you'll read as you continue. I told

Mary to give it a month, taking vitamin C with bioflavonoids, minerals in solution, an antioxidant formula and liquid garlic extract. I made a note to myself to come back to the market as soon as I could, to see how she was doing.

The Preventative Magic of Vitamin C

You brush and floss your teeth every day to prevent cavities and gum disease. If you don't you should. What you should also do to protect those pearly whites is take vitamin C. Studies have shown that vitamin C prevents periodontal abscesses by lowering the amount of plaque and bacteria in the mouth.

The *New York Journal of Dentistry* reported on a study in which plaque accumulation was measured among subjects all brushing well, some supplementing with vitamin C, some not. The findings determined that those supplementing with vitamin C actually had less tartar and bacteria than those only brushing. The study found that when the subjects took vitamin C inflammation of their gums from concentrations of bacteria was reduced 58 percent![1]

How does vitamin C perform its magic? By increasing the numbers of the antibody warriors that come to our defense when infection sets in. In one study, University of Witwatersrand, South Africa, medical students were given one gram a day (1,000 mg) of ascorbic acid (vitamin C) and monitored for blood immunologic levels. Unlike the control group who did not get the vitamin C, the ones who did experienced a marked increase in their defense antibodies, IgA and IgM. Vitamin C is renowned for alleviating the symptoms of colds and flues, and studies have shown it to be of benefit for tuberculosis, herpes, tetanus and diphtheria. Any type of infection can be helped with vitamin C.[2]

Dr. Robert Cathcart, a California physician, has successfully treated over 15,000 patients with massive doses of vitamin C; curing viral pneumonia, mononucleosis, influenza, colds, hepatitis, shingles, and cold sores with this method. He has developed a guideline for practical application of vitamin C which he refers to as "bowel tolerance."

The individual's own body will determine how much vitamin C it requires. The cutoff point is determined by the onset of diarrhea. The tolerance level in each individual differs. Some days you can tolerate more, some days less, but from general experience I label a cold as a 20-to-30-gram cold, or 60-gram flu, according to how much a person can take before he reaches the bowel tolerance level.

To achieve bowel tolerance, I always recommend taking a vitamin C formula that includes bioflavonoids to boost the vitamin's therapeutic value. Your vitamin C formula should contain 500 mg of vitamin C, 50 mg bioflavonoids, 25 mg of the bioflavonoid rutin and 25 mg of green tea per capsule. To achieve bowel tolerance, take five capsules in the first two hours, then one every half hour after that. The vitamin C will permeate every cell of the body before it reaches the bowel. These massive doses are justified because viruses within the sick cells excrete toxins, rendering them scorbutic (with scurvy).

In short, if you have not reached bowel tolerance (diarrhea), you have not taken enough vitamin C.

When you target vitamin C as a supplement, choose a formulation that includes bioflavonoids. Bioflavonoids are potent anti-inflammatories. They reduce swelling while they act on the immune system, and they enhance the healing properties of vitamin C.

Supportive Nutrients

Target certain nutrients to relieve abscesses. Zinc, for example, is a notable wound-healer and exceptionally valuable for acne abscesses. A clinical trial reported in the *American Journal of Clinical Nutrition* found that zinc was effective in the treatment of recurrent boils.[3] Zinc must be balanced with a number of other minerals, especially copper, to be effective, and is found in sesame seeds, pumpkin seeds, torula yeast, blackstrap molasses, maple syrup and brewer's yeast.

Look for a good, easily absorbable, derived-from-nature mineral blend in solution. Liquid formulations provide the maximum absorption ratios.

Vitamin E is not only a potent antioxidant, working to cleanse the system of toxins, but increases the strength of tissues, protecting them against invading microorganisms. Vitamin E is found in nuts, oils and cabbage

Vitamin A is touted as an eye enhancer. The reasons why also work in favor of abscesses. The eyes contain probably the most delicate cellular tissue of the body. Not only are they counted on for sight, but are clobbered by the multitude of airborne pollutants that assail us daily. Anything that protects our eyes as well as vitamin A can, surely works just as well on the delicate tissues of the gums, intestines and inner ear. Vitamin A works by strengthening the cell walls, protecting them from bacterial invasion. Orange and yellow foods contain vitamin A, most especially carrots and carrot juice, and sweet potatoes.

Garlic – An Herbal Antibiotic

Another nutrient I advocate for all sorts of infections is liquid aged garlic extract, a powerful and effective detoxifier and immune system booster. The garlic is aged to reduce the toxic effects of large amounts of fresh garlic. If you crush fresh garlic and put it on your arm, you may get a burn. When garlic is aged, it no longer burns. Aged liquid garlic is odorless too, so you don't have to worry that you'll lose your friends and acquaintances. Garlic is recommended for afflictions from AIDS to cancer because of its ability to pull toxic time bombs out of the body.

If garlic were a pharmaceutical, you would see advertisements in all the magazines, and the lucky company with the patent would earn hundreds of millions of dollars a year. Everyone would learn of garlic's vast power and flock to their doctors for a prescription. Fortunately for those of us in the know, garlic is easily available and inexpensively obtained.

Unfortunately, because it's not patentable, few are aware of the many benefits they can derive from raw garlic and, especially liquid aged garlic extract.

Why is *aged* garlic so important? To get the kind of benefit that kills diseases, large amounts of garlic is needed. Excessive amounts of raw garlic can be toxic, but when it is aged, it enters the body's cells and stimulates immune response.

Dr. Tariq Abdullah, of the Akbar Clinic and Research Foundation in Panama City, Florida, conducted studies showing that raw and supplemental garlic enhances T-cell activity, the body's warriors of defense. He says, "No other substance, either natural or synthetic, can match garlic's proven therapeutic versatility and effectiveness."[4]

As for Mary, her pain, inflammation and abscess is gone. She got a third opinion and was told the tooth had remarkably healed and would need no further treatment.

Abscess-Fighting Nutrients
For maximum absorption, take supplements with meals.

Nutrient	Suggested Dosage	Formulation
Aged garlic extract	1 teaspoon three times daily	Liquid
Echinacea	100 mg daily	
Fiber	4-8 tablets daily	Psyllium, with herbhyssop
Multi-mineral	1-4 ounces daily	In liquid solution, with vitamin B12, biotin
Multi-vitamin/mineral	3-6 caplets daily	Freeze-dried plant sources
Vitamin A	25,000 IU daily*	
Vitamin C	Individual bowel tolerance**	With bioflavonoids (quercetin, proanthocyanidins)
Vitamin E	2 capsules (800 IU) daily	d-alpha tocopherol

* The FDA recommends pregnant women not exceed 10,000 IU of vitamin A daily.

** To determine individual dosage, on the first day take 1,000 mg hourly until diarrhea occurs, then reduce dosage to just below that for individual daily dosage. Vitamin C is not toxic in large doses but must be taken throughout the day to benefit. Divide dosage to three or four times a day.

CHAPTER 2:

Acne

The multitude of tear-stained grateful letters I've received on this subject have convinced me that whether the sufferers are teenagers or middle-agers, acne is not just a disruption of the skin but an affront to self-esteem and a shaker of confidence. I'm told by the multitude of on-air questions and letters on the subject that adult acne is actually quite common. I can only imagine the frustration at suffering through teen acne, looking forward to seeing it end, then going through the next twenty years battling it as an adult.

A friend tells me she often gets acne on her neck. The pimples become so pronounced she's been asked: "What's that on your neck?" I can only imagine the embarrassment of having to address that question as a 38-year-old woman. Via the message boards of a computer on-line service, here are the heartfelt comments of acne sufferers, reaching out to each other to share information and troubles.

Gregg: "OK! I have had enough! For a long time I've been washing, and applying, and torturing myself to stay just mildly clear. I give! I have a sort of mild case."

Jake: "I'm male, 36 years old and have been plagued with cystic pustules on my forehead for about two years now. They look more like boils that won't erupt yet leave marks when in their non-active stage. Does anybody know what I might have? I don't have the money to see a dermatologist but maybe that's my only hope!"

Joan: "Over the past three months I started having frequent breakouts along my jaw line and neck. The pimples are large and painful. What could be causing this? My diet hasn't changed and my stress level is down. I'm 35 and now feel like I'm an adolescent again!"

Hubert: "We are our own worst critics. Something on our face that someone else may not even notice may seem as large as a mountain to us. If it is of any comfort, next time you feel bad about your arms or legs, think of that poor boy at school none of the girls like, not because he is a jerk or mean or ugly in any other way. He might be the nicest boy in the school, but he is also called "pizza face," "zit face," etc. I know how that boy feels because I went through that in one of my high school years when the acne hit bad. Be thankful that is not you.

Zinc, Healer of Wounds

When it comes to curing acne, I wish I could take the credit, but my gospel is zinc. Let me explain by relating just one of the many success stories I've had the pleasure of seeing for myself.

While doing a live TV healthathon in Florida, I had the chance to see a talented young man perform a short violin concert. I had noticed his acne problem, but it wasn't as pronounced as when the studio lights fell on him and perspiration bathed his forehead. Then, as though he was aware of the effect, he bent his head down, letting his longish hair fall over his otherwise attractive face. He stayed that way throughout the performance. I thought, "What a shame he feels the need to hide his handsome face!"

After the show I talked to him about his complexion.
"I'm 25 years old, Maureen, and I still have acne! Shouldn't it be gone by now?" he pleaded.

"Unfortunately, many adults have acne," I told him. "It's not quite the same as teenage acne, but certainly causes the same embarrassment. The basic problem is that your skin produces too much oil, or sebum. The oil clogs the pores, causing whiteheads. If bacteria develop, the pores get infected, making them red and inflamed." I continued, watching him look more and more depressed. "Lots of things cause this, from too many male hormones, to food allergies, to stress, that reduces the body's ability to fend off infection. First of all, if you are drinking milk, I would suggest you stop for a while and see what happens."

I looked into his sad eyes and gave him a big smile. "But there is also a natural supplement you can take, and I've seen it work with many, many people."

"Really?" he exclaimed. "Can I really get rid of these awful zits?!" I almost laughed with joy seeing his face light up. Next to actually seeing the results of nutritional therapy, this is the part I enjoy the most: seeing people's reaction when hope brightens their day.

Whether you are a teenager afflicted with ongoing outbreaks, or a middle-aged woman pestered by premenstrual pimples, you can turn your pores to satin simply by taking zinc. I've seen hundreds of people who have tried everything over and behind the counter for their acne, and within months, had it cleared up with the zinc regimen first told to me by Dr. Robert Cathcart III.

Dr. Cathcart first learned of this acne antagonist from Dr. Michaelson of Sweden's Upsala University Hospital, who prescribed 50 milligrams of elemental zinc three times a day with meals, and was astounded to note excellent results.[1]

A renowned medical and alternative physician, Dr. Cathcart tried it on his patients and discovered that if the dosage were increased to 100-150 mg with each meal, patients got better results. He found that within 12 weeks, his patients taking the zinc improved their acne by a whopping 87 percent![2]

The next time I was back in Florida, I had the pleasure of seeing my young violinist friend and was delighted to note how much his face had cleared up. He was standing straighter, too, and held up his head proudly. I was amused that he didn't wince when the director called for close-ups. When he saw me standing there, he could hardly wait to greet me.

"Maureen! You're a miracle messenger!" he said, nearly knock-ing me out of my seat with a big embrace. "At first I thought the zinc wasn't working, but decided to at least finish off the bottle. By the time it was gone, so was my acne. I even have a girlfriend now," he proudly announced.

You can't know how heartwarming it is to make such a difference in people's lives. The credit goes to the wonderful physicians out there willing to forego convention and try new therapies, such as Dr. Cathcart.

More Winks for Zinc

Why does zinc work so well? The reasons are twofold. First, zinc is a wound-healer. A deficiency of zinc can actually cause skin lesions and dermatitis. Teens often develop acne as a result of marginal deficiencies of the mineral. [3] It probably has something to do with the way they eat. Have you ever known a teenager who eats well? When my grandfather was a boy, "fast food" meant the ones you couldn't catch. Today, a teenager's idea of vigorous exercise is counting the number of hamburgers they can wolf down in 15 minutes. In any case, it's a good bet most teenagers are nutrient deficient.

An important point to keep in mind whenever targeting a particular nutrient, is to include a multi-mineral *or* multi-vitamin formula (either or, not both – skip the mineral *and* vitamin formulations). Zinc must be balanced with a number of other minerals, especially copper, to be effective. Look for a good, easily absorbable, derived-from-nature mineral blend in solution.

Something I find absolutely fascinating is photo testimony from census workers in Alaska. Back in 1938, in order to keep a record of native Alaskan Eskimos, who couldn't speak English, census workers would photograph them. The old photos show their skin clear of acne. When you examine photos taken in recent years, you see that most Alaskan teenagers now have acne. This has been attributed to their adoption of the Western "civilized" low-nutritional, high-fat diet.

The second reason zinc works so well on acne is that it acts as an antibacterial. Teenagers are commonly prescribed tetracycline for their acne. Did you know that one percent of people who take tetracycline lose their sight? Antibiotics work because they kill bacteria. Unfortunately, antibiotics don't discriminate between good and bad bacteria.

Have you heard the news? Some bad bacteria are becoming immune to pharmaceutical antibiotics. What happens when the good bacteria are killed but the bad aren't? Something called flesh-eating syndrome – that's what. Using antibiotics makes no sense at all. At least not when you have zinc, vitamin A and garlic, which do the same thing, *and* nourish the body.

Research abounds with zinc testimonials.

An article in *Pediatric Clinics of North America*, an esteemed and well-referenced medical journal, related one study of young acne patients and concluded that "both oral and topical zinc were highly effective against severe cases of acne." Sound testimony if I ever heard it.

In another study, 27 patients with severe acne were given a placebo, while 29 received zinc sulfate daily. After 12 weeks, none of the placebo patients showed improvement, while 58 percent of the zinc-treated patients experienced noticeable improvement in their acne.[4]

Watch for things that deplete your body of zinc. Stress reduces the amount of this vital mineral stored in the body. One study of volunteers found that, although they had more than adequate zinc to begin with, the amount was reduced by an incredible 33 percent when they were under stress.[5]

Fats: The Good, The Bad, The Ugly

You hear all the time about the evils of fat. Everything on the supermarket shelves says No Fat, Nonfat or Lowfat. The question still remains, however, just how much nutritious food is included. Saturated fat can deplete your body of its storehouse of nutrients and/or reduce your body's ability to extract nutrients from your food. I'm talking about the saturated fat in dairy products, meat and especially the transfatty acids in hydrogenated oils, found in margarine and most processed foods. If you value your health, and your skin, reduce your intake of saturated fat and avoid hydrogenated anything!

Sixty percent of all fats consumed in this country are hydrogenated, which may explain the increasing number of acne sufferers. Margarine, red meat, fried food and most processed food contain hydrogenated fats or oils.[6]

Meat promoters will tell you fat is essential for health. This is true, but what they don't tell you is what *kind* of fat. You need to know about essential fatty acids, or EFAs, which are the good kind of fats. Essential means the body doesn't make it, and it must be received from food. The key term here is essential. Transfatty acids are not essential, they are just bad for you. I would bore you by listing all the essential fatty acids. The only one you need to concern yourself with here is linoleic acid.

A study published in the *Journal of the American Academy of Dermatology*, found acne sufferers have a deficiency of linoleic acid (or linolenic acid) in their skin. Not surprisingly, researchers suspect the deficiency may be due to an excess of hydrogenated fat in the diet. When test animals were fed a diet containing 10 percent of calories from hydrogenated fat, they developed a deficiency of linoleic acid.[7] Borage and evening primrose oil both contain this EFA, but I suggest you look for borage oil supplements because it delivers more bang for the buck and has higher EFAs for less cost. Use these oils high in linoleic acid in your cooking and salads: safflower oil, olive oil, cottonseed and sunflower. Incidentally, linoleic acid is recommended for other skin afflictions like dermatitis and eczema.

Some people, as was the case with the young violinist, have an allergy to milk products. Acne can be made worse by food allergies. For more on this culprit, see the chapter Allergies.

Other Clear Skin Nutrients

Another important acne fighter is vitamin A, found in carrots and other orange vegetables. Since the skin cells are among the more rapidly dividing of all body cells, nutrients, particularly vitamin A, are critical for new cell growth. In a study published in the *British Journal of Dermatology*, researchers reported that blood levels of vitamin A was significantly lower in all patients with severe cases of acne. Researchers have found high doses of vitamin A – 300,000 to 500,000 IU a day taken for a short period of time – can correct extremely bad cases of acne in a few weeks. However, high doses can cause side effects. For debilitating acne, consult a nutrition-oriented or alternative medicine physician. Signs of vitamin A toxicity are lips cracking, palms peeling or a small pounding headache at the front of your forehead.

There is a phytochemical contained in the herb <u>comfrey</u> that has been shown to be beneficial for the treatment of acne. The active ingredient is called <u>allantoin</u> and is contained in some skin care formulas. Allantoin works by speeding formation of epithelial cells, those that fill in and heal wounds, like the craters formed after a pimple erupts.[9] At least one pharmaceutical company uses allantoin in its acne medication. If you can't get to Samil Pharmaceuticals in Italy for their anti-acne product, look for comfrey or allantoin in your skin care line.

Chromium is often recommended for diabetics, and with good reason. It is all-important to maintaining healthy blood sugar levels. In an interesting connection, a study in *Medical Hypotheses* reported that patients with unstable blood sugar levels also had severe acne. When nine patients were given two teaspoons daily of high-chromium yeast containing 400 micrograms of chromium, their acne improved quickly.[10] Chromium is also found in whole grains, mushrooms and molasses.

A smart move for any affliction is to avoid all processed foods. Not only are they high in bad fats, but contribute to diabetes and blood sugar problems. When I was in Russia some years ago (before they discovered McDonald's) the people subsisted mostly on fresh foods from their gardens. They were so poor they couldn't afford the luxuries of life: soda pop, hamburgers and sugar snacks. I didn't see one case of acne until the face of the cabin boy on my ship, who earned his pay with free luxurious meals.

Flushing Away Your Acne

Never underestimate the benefits of water. A viewer wrote me to say all it took for her – after suffering from 15 years of adult acne – was drinking lots of water. Not just the usual 8-10 daily glasses. If your urine is very yellow, then you're not drinking enough. Drink, drink, drink until your urine turns clear – like water – and keep it clear. If your urine is yellow the body is eliminating waste that is too highly concentrated. You need more water to flush it out. Most people don't drink nearly enough water. The water you drink should be purified – free of chemicals. If you can't afford a fancy purification system, try one of those inexpensive carafe water filters.

It makes perfect sense. Your sweat glands excrete water through your pores, and help eliminate waste, just like urine. If your urine contains too much waste, your pores probably do too. And if there isn't enough water to flush your pores out, the toxins stay in the pores, they clog up, and clogged pores means pimples. You can't flush out your pores with anything applied from the outside. You have to do it from the inside.

The amount of extra water needed to drink differs from person to person. It depends on your genetics, your diet, your lifestyle, and how much exercise you get. It's so simple! I wonder why doctors don't ever mention it. Of course, they can't charge for a water prescription, can they?

Acne-Fighting Nutrients
For maximum absorption, take supplements with meals.

Nutrient	Suggested Dosage	Formulation
Aged garlic extract	1 teaspoon three times daily	Liquid
Fiber	4-8 tablets daily	Psyllium, with herb hyssop
Multi-mineral	1-4 ounces daily	In liquid solution, with vitamin B12, biotin
Multi-vitamin/mineral	3-6 caplets daily	Freeze-dried plant sources
Vitamin A	25,000 IU daily*	
Vitamin C	Individual bowel tolerance**	With bioflavonoids (quercetin, proanthocyanidins)
Vitamin E	2 capsules (800 IU) daily	d-alpha tocopherol
Zinc sulfate***	50 mg three times daily	

Wash with cleansing lotion containing alpha hydroxy acids, sage and papaya, followed with a toner containing witch hazel, licorice extract and aloe vera.

* The FDA recommends pregnant women not exceed 10,000 IU of vitamin A daily.

** To determine individual dosage, on the first day take 1,000 mg hourly until diarrhea occurs, then reduce dosage to just below that for individual daily dosage. Vitamin C is not toxic in large doses but must be taken throughout the day to benefit. Divide dosage to three or four times a day.

***Take with meals and lower dosage if stomach upset occurs.

CHAPTER 3:

AIDS

During a media tour of Australia I met a charming Italian man, Francois Ferrari, of the famous Ferrari family, who drove me anywhere, at any hour. I hadn't asked him for help, he was just there. Every time I needed a ride somewhere, even if it meant a middle of the night radio show, I could count on him. I assumed my hosts had hired him, but when I discovered he was doing it on his own, I asked him why. He replied, "Because, Mrs. Salaman, you saved my life!"

He had the most beautiful thick, curly black hair and I remember as he said this he was nervously combing it with his hand, pulling it back from his wide, dark eyes.

"It was your wonderful books that gave me the information I needed to save myself from AIDS," he said, sweeping his arm in a typically expressive flourish. "I was stricken blind," he started, making me gasp at the thought of it. "I had full blown AIDS and it had blinded me. I couldn't eat and I was so weak it took 20 minutes to get to the bathroom and 20 minutes back." The doctors gave him no hope of life beyond a few weeks.

Knowing his immune system needed help, Francois decided to take charge. My books told him what he needed to do. He started by drinking 1/4 bottle of liquid garlic a day, following it up with 1/2 bottle a day for three months. He ate only 100 percent organic raw food and purified water. Unable to find local fruits and vegetables that hadn't been either grown in pesticide-laden soils or sprayed with chemicals, he had his produce delivered from Japan. Even when traveling, he had his food sent to him. He was absolutely diligent that no chemicals touched his lips. His sight and strength returned, and he was cured of AIDS for 12 years before dying of a heart attack in 1996.

Alan Francis, the piano player at my church, is now HIV negative. Using the protocol in this book, he has gained back 60 pounds and is healthier than before.

AIDS: A Product Of Our Civilization

Evidence is accumulating that the HIV virus is an immune system defect aggravated and worsened by modern habits and a sedentary lifestyle. Some people exposed never get it. Others contract the virus but remain healthy. This is because they have strong immune systems, and are able to fight it off. It is my belief, based on numerous research findings, that what we call AIDS is actually the result of massive nutrient deficiencies caused by the HIV virus. Research has shown that while malnutrition is a hallmark of full blown AIDS, nutritional abnormalities also occur early in HIV disease. Dr. Marianna K. Baum, together with colleagues from the University of Miami School of Medicine, and the University of Alabama at Birmingham examined blood levels of vitamins A, E, B6, B12 and zinc in early-diagnosed HIV-positive patients. The researchers discovered that when the patients were given recommended daily allowances (government-recommended dosages) of these nutrients, they were still found to be deficient. It wasn't until after they received six to ten times the RDA did the majority have normal levels.[1]

Without essential nutrients, a complete breakdown of the immune system is imminent, and the body succumbs to opportunistic cancers and infections. Like a crack in the sidewalk that is widened and worsened by weather and pollutants, the HIV virus takes advantage of environmental and dietary pollutants that weaken the body's ability to fight back. As long as deficiencies are present, the patient cannot heal.

Numerous factors contribute to AIDS. The problem begins with vitamin and mineral deficiencies, legal and illegal drugs, "fast lane" living, vaccinations, steroids, birth control pills and recurrent sexually transmitted diseases that allow usually harmless bacteria to multiply into toxic amounts. All beat down the immune system so that exposure to HIV can mean a death sentence.[2]

The Deficiency Connection

The evidence that connects HIV and nutrition has not gone unnoticed. Many, many studies show that people with the HIV virus are dangerously deficient in the nutrients needed to keep their bodies and immune systems intact and healthy. When the levels get low enough, symptoms start occurring. Doctors choose to label this stage AIDS-Related Complex (ARC).

During a conference at the New York Academy of Sciences, attendees discussed the effects of HIV on the immune system and evaluated nutritional studies. One of the studies discussed was conducted by John D. Bogden, Ph.D., and colleagues at the New Jersey Medical School, Newark. They reported that their test subjects had below-normal blood levels of zinc, calcium, magnesium, beta carotene, choline, and vitamin C, even though some were taking megadoses of supplements. He found an appalling ninety-three percent of the patients were deficient in at least one nutrient.[3]

The amount of zinc and vitamin D available in the body appears to increase the resistance of laboratory animals to tuberculosis. TB is on the rise among AIDS patients. Vitamin D is largely obtained from sunlight, and is a powerful immune booster. Don't make the mistake of assuming that milk provides this vital vitamin. The so-called vitamin D in milk is merely a hormone, and less than nutritive. Fifteen minutes of sunlight a day is sufficient to obtain adequate amounts of vitamin D in healthy subjects. For AIDS patients, I would recommend applying a skin cream containing vitamins A, C and E and getting as much sunlight, fresh air and exercise as can be tolerated.

A deficiency in zinc, copper, selenium and vitamin A can also compromise the HIV-infected immune system.[4] Approximately two-thirds of AIDs patients may be deficient in vitamin B12 or folic acid.[5] A deficiency of zinc can lead to cell loss and infections. A deficiency of selenium is common in AIDS patients and is associated with not only heart disease but diarrhea and malabsorption.[6]

Malabsorption is a very important issue in the HIV patient, as it can literally mean the difference between life and death. If a person has this problem, he or she will be unable to fully absorb nutrients from food and even from supplements. There are many different causes of malabsorption, from inadequate stomach acid (possibly caused by antacids) needed to break down food, to a yeast overgrowth in the intestinal tract (candidiasis). By the way, you can battle any internal yeast infection by taking acidophilus bacillus supplementally or in yogurt with active cultures. Malabsorption leads to malnutrition. When we think of malnutrition, we think of people who do not eat the right foods, but we could all be malnourished and not know it.

Sally J. Sato, R.Ph., and Jay M. Mirtallo, M.S., R.Ph., believe malnutrition in the AIDS patient may be one of the reasons many succumb to the disease. Of the 30 AIDS patients they studied, 20 were malnourished.[7] Malnutrition is very common among people who have problems absorbing nutrients, whether from age, intestinal disorders or from the HIV virus. If people are dying from AIDS in part because they cannot absorb nutrients, and there is a solution at hand, it should be considered criminal that physicians don't use it.

Supplementing with a hydrochloric acid formula such as Betaine, available in health food stores, will help the body absorb nutrients, but studies show minerals dissolved in water before ingestion are considerably more bioavailable to the body than those even present in food. Look for a good, easily absorbable, derived-from-nature mineral blend in solution.

Warning: No AZT

Because the drug AZT is so widely recommended and used, I feel the need to warn the reader not to fall into this trap. Even the prestigious *New England Journal of Medicine* proclaims that AZT is not the best treatment for HIV. AZT is highly toxic and experts believe it is just as likely to kill the user as is the virus. The reasoning behind using this hazardous waste is that AZT kills T-cells infected with the HIV virus. However, for every one HIV cell killed, AZT kills 499 healthy T-cells, thus actually weakening the already-damaged immune system. What they don't tell you is that nine percent of patients who use AZT will get lymphatic cancer from the drug itself. Other side effects include acute hepatitis, dementia seizures and muscle wasting.[8] Is it worth it? Not on your life!

The only reason the medical establishment chooses to use AZT versus massive nutritional therapy is because AZT puts money in the pockets of the research institutions who depend on pharmaceutical companies for grants, and because they ignore the compelling research that shows nutritional deficiencies, not the virus itself, cause AIDS-related death and disease. Fortunately, not all physicians are willing to sacrifice their patients' lives in order to protect the sanctity of the almighty pharmaceutical dollar.

The Miracle Workers

Thankfully, there are doctors out there determined to show the world HIV and AIDS do not have to be death sentences. They are the ones who have read the research, stepped out of the pack and used mega-nutrients and lifestyle recommendations to treat their patients. If you need to find a physician knowledgeable in nutrient therapy, call 1-800-445-HEAL.

In one study conducted by Ian Brighthope, M.D., of Melbourne, Australia, the lives of 18 out of 20 AIDS patients and all 100 Aids-Related Complex patients he treated were prolonged. Dr. Brighthope prescribes massive intravenous doses of vitamin C initially, plus various other vitamins, minerals and herbs, as well as exercise to achieve these results.[9]

A man suffering from AIDS for five years came to Joan Priestley, M.D., a practicing physician in Los Angeles, California. The man's doctors told him his case was terminal and he had five months to live. He was suffering from severe weight loss and diarrhea and was ravaged by infections and an intestinal ailment. Today, over one year after beginning aggressive treatment with Dr. Priestley, the man is symptom-free and has regained forty pounds.[10]

Dr. Robert Cathcart III of Los Altos, California, was approached by a man suffering from night sweats and fever. His low T-cell count alerted Dr. Cathcart to test for the HIV virus. Dr. Cathcart is a pioneer in the use of vitamin C therapy for illness. Fifteen months after beginning intravenous vitamin C treatments, the patient's T-cell count rose from under 300 to 600. He was elated, and celebrated when he went a year without having a cold or flu.

My point here is to demonstrate that a growing number of doctors are successfully treating AIDS. Don't settle for questionable conventional treatments when you could increase your chances of survival by looking outside of orthodoxy.

Garlic, the Body Purifier

I explained how good garlic works against infections in the abscess chapter. Because of the loss of immune function, AIDS patients suffer from many infections, making this nutrient very important.

Garlic is the best example of the philosophy, "Let your medicine be your food, and your food your medicine." What will help in AIDS therapy, is supplementing with garlic and the active ingredients contained in it. Garlic contains germanium, magnesium, selenium, 17 amino acids, 33 sulfur compounds, vitamins B1, A and C. Organic germanium is a dramatic immunostimulant. In controlled studies, Dr. Stephen A. Levine, Ph.D., found organic germanium restores immune function in immune-depressed animals.[11] Studies of human subjects have shown that it enhances natural killer cell activity. Garlic is one of the richest sources of organic selenium and germanium.[12]

I advocate supplementing with Kyolic® brand garlic, manufactured by the Wakunaga Company of Japan. Their scientists have spent decades researching the health benefits of garlic, and use what they've learned to make their products. The quality of their garlic is impeccable, their standards unquestionable.

Immune-Energizing Nutrients
For maximum absorption, take supplements with meals.

Nutrient	Suggested Dosage	Formulation
Acidophilus	At least four billion flora daily on an empty stomach, three times daily	
Aged garlic extract	1 teaspoon three times daily	Liquid
Amino acids	4-6 capsules daily	Multiple formula from natural sources
Antioxidants	4 capsules daily*	With selenium and grapeseed extract
Borage oil	2 capsules daily	
Coenzyme Q10	2 capsules daily	With vitamin E, phospholipids and selenium
Flaxseed oil	1 tablespoon daily	
Melatonin (adults only)	3 mg daily at bedtime	With B vitamins
Multi-mineral	3-4 ounces daily	In liquid solution, with vitamin B12, biotin
Multi-vitamin/mineral	6 caplets daily	Freeze-dried plant sources
Vitamin B6	100 mg daily	
Vitamin C	Individual bowel tolerance**	With bioflavonoids (quercetin, rutin proanthocyanidins)
Vitamin E	2 capsules (800 IU)	d-alpha tocopherol

* The FDA recommends pregnant women not exceed 10,000 IU of vitamin A daily.

** To determine individual dosage, on the first day take 1,000 mg hourly until diarrhea occurs, then reduce dosage to just below that for individual daily dosage. Vitamin C is not toxic in large doses but must be taken throughout the day to benefit. Divide dosage to three or four times a day.

CHAPTER 4:

Alcoholism

I was busy autographing my book *Foods That Heal* for the throng of people lined up in front of me in Orlando, Florida, when a woman who approached caught my attention.

Her eyes were circled with fatigue, her hands were shaking, and she had an unmistakable desperation about her that made me reach out with one hand and place it over hers.

"What can I do for you?" I asked her, looking into her sad eyes.

"Oh, Maureen, I'm at the end of my rope," she told me. "My husband just cannot stop drinking! He's gone to three alcohol treatment programs, lost his driver's license twice, uses me as a verbal whipping post and I can't take his rages much longer. He wants to quit, he really does, but just can't seem to help himself! I don't know what to do!"

I explained to her what I have learned from much innovative research and the experience of my physician friends: that alcoholism can be a chemical imbalance brought on by nutritional deficiencies and/or low thyroid.

"Have you talked to an alternative physician about nutritional therapy?" I asked. She looked surprised. "You mean he can be cured with vitamins?"

"It's not as simple as that, but nutrition can help," I answered.

As I explain in the thyroid chapter, low thyroid function can cause depression. For some, alcohol is a way to alleviate the depression. For others, the depression or alcoholism is a result of chemical imbalances traced to poor nutrition.

What is most important to me, in writing this chapter, is that you feel empowered. For sufferers and their loved ones, alcoholism takes away control of their lives. If you drink, or have a loved one who drinks, I have news that will save you a broken heart and/or a broken life. Through nutrition, you can take charge of your health and become clean and sober for the rest of your life.

The Nutrition Answer

Good nutrition is all-important in getting off the bottle. In fact, I was amazed to discover that even the American Dietetic Association (ADA) has determined alcoholics can benefit from nutrient therapy and that most hospitals now incorporate improved nutrition in their alcohol programs. The ADA even performed its own study to see if nutrition would help the alcohol rehabilitation success rate.

This bottle-breaking study compared two groups of alcoholics, each on the standard AA 12-step therapy. The only difference was one group was put on a special diet of complex carbohydrates (beans, peas and whole grains), low sugar and no caffeine. Those on the special diet said they experienced less craving for alcohol and were more successful in kicking the addiction.[1]

Researchers at Loma Linda University School of Public Health demonstrated that a diet of mostly simple carbohydrates and junk food – white bread products and sugar – can increase the craving for alcohol. In their experiment, rats placed on a junk food diet drank a weekly average of what would be a quart of 100 proof whiskey a day for a man. Rats on the same diet but with the addition of vitamin and mineral supplements drank a third less, and rats fed a balanced human diet drank one-seventh the original amount. The addition of nutrients and food to their diets in truth made them want/need less alcohol. Now, here's a staggering observation: in a previous study, 20 percent of the rats on a complex carbohdrate diet developed no taste for alcohol – until sugar was added to it. Then they became the heaviest drinkers of all, drinking in a week what would be 1-1/2 quarts a day for a man.[2]

The connection between nutrients and cravings and the brain is very interesting. I don't think we quite realize, or fully comprehend, the effect our diet has on our mental health. It appears nutritional imbalances can actually alter brain function to such a degree that it causes cravings, depression and even psychosis!

What came first, the chicken or the egg? Do nutritional imbalances create the craving for alcohol or does the alcohol create the imbalances, and an addiction? I think the answer is **both**. Many alcoholics started with a depression problem. They seek a way out, and the craving for alcohol becomes a secondary problem.

Dr. Ross Gordon, M.D. told me about a patient of his who came to him with depression. The poor man barely made it through each day. Dr. Gordon put him on a regimen of B12 injections and folic acid, with instructions that he lay off coffee and sugar, and eat more whole grains, fruits and vegetables. The regimen worked, and the patient reported that he had a new lease on life. But what fascinated me was a revelation from the man's wife. Some time after his therapy had ended, she came to Dr. Gordon's office.

"I hope you'll excuse me for interrupting your work, doctor," she said, barely containing her enthusiasm. "But there's something you have got to know. My husband has been an alcoholic for the last 15 years, and only now, after his treatment for depression has he been able to stop drinking." Doctor Gordon says he'll never forget the look on her face, or the squeeze she gave his arm as she shyly confided, "Instead of a divorce, I'm giving him a second honeymoon!"

Award-winning actress Patty Duke made public the fact that she battled with depression as a youngster and went on to abuse drugs and alcohol.

Massachusetts Governor Michael Dukakis blamed his wife Kitty's alcohol problem on his 1988 presidential election loss to then Vice President Bush. He said the stress, coupled with physical exhaustion, caused a depression she tried to alleviate with alcohol. What wasn't widely publicized was that Kitty started abusing diet pills at the age of 19 and for 20 years had an amphetamine habit. More than likely the post campaign stresses revived a pre-existing nutritional imbalance. She probably turned to alcohol to relieve both the physical symptoms and the mental anguish.

The Serotonin Factor

Many of the same imbalances and nutritional deficiencies that cause depression create an inner "need" for alcohol. Why do people turn to mind-altering substances? What is physically missing that they have a need to replace? Many researchers believe it is serotonin, a brain chemical that is needed to regulate sleep, secrete pituitary hormones and alleviate pain.

Serotonin levels in the brain are influenced by tryptophan, an amino acid that your body needs, but doesn't produce. This is why diet is so important. Ever notice how certain big meals make you drowsy? If you recall what you were eating, you'll realize it was mostly carbohydrates and proteins. Protein food – meat, milk and eggs – contain tryptophan. And carbohydrates – bread, beans, natural sugars and pasta – allow more tryptophan to enter the bloodstream. It is the amount of tryptophan that has entered your brain that causes you to want a siesta after lunch. That is why, when I have much work to do, I eat salads for lunch.

The trouble with alcohol is it provides the wrong kind of carbohydrates to increase serotonin, not to mention depleting the body's store of nutrients, most especially the B vitamins. Most alcohol contains grain and sugar in a refined state. Refined carbohydrates provide the body with almost instant energy because they cause a sudden rise in blood sugar. However, the blood sugar level drops again quickly, creating a craving for more. It is this pseudo serotonin and blood sugar rush that doctors believe makes a person addicted to alcohol. Many alcoholics binge on refined sugar products, like pastry and candy to further achieve this state. Eating these foods will not only perpetuate the alcohol craving but create dangerous nutritional deficiencies.

The first thing to do is eat right. These are the YES foods: brown rice instead of white rice, beans and lentils, whole grain bread, whole grains and whole grain cereals, and lots of fruits and vegetables –

preferably raw. Foods high in complex carbohydrates and brain-healthy B vitamins are barley, millet, bulgur, wheat, pinto beans, lima beans and lentils. Try a lentil soup breakfast for a pick me up that will last all day.

No-no foods include salt and sugar, coffee and caffeinated tea, and all sodas, especially the ones with caffeine. The idea is to strengthen the body while strengthening the willpower. If you or someone you know is serious about staying on the wagon, a program of good eating will be the best start possible.

Saved by Amino Acids

There's another connection as well – the amino acid connection. Carbohydrates can be manufactured in the body from certain amino acids.

Kenneth Blum, Ph.D., chief of the Division of Addictive Diseases and director of the Laboratory of Pharmacogenetics, University of Texas Health Sciences Center at San Antonio, has been successfully treating alcoholism with amino acid formulas.[3]

What is interesting is that studies have shown some of the amino acids contained in these formulas work to alleviate depression as well. Dirk Pearson and Sandy Shaw, in their fascinating volume *Life Extension*, describe a study in which the amino acids tyrosine and L-phenylalanine, given in doses of 500 to 1000 mgs daily for two weeks, alleviated depression. Look for formulas that contain these brain-healthy amino acids: taurine, arginine, cysteine, acetyl-L-carnitine, phenylalanine, leucine, isoleucine, tryptophan, valine, methionine, histidine and tyrosine. They are essential to healthy communication between brain and body, and can be found in health food and vitamin stores.

Missing in Action

Whether it is the alcohol that is causing a dangerous deficiency of nutrients, or something else, it could be your mental health that suffers.

These nutrients are most commonly deficient among alcoholics:

folic acid, vitamins A and D, thiamine (B1), vitamin B6, zinc, potassium, calcium and magnesium.[4]

Let's start with magnesium. Magnesium is essential to proper glucose, or blood sugar balance. Do you ever feel light-headed when you haven't eaten in a while? This is because your blood sugar is low, and your energy along with it. There is a direct relationship between blood sugar and energy levels.

All the B vitamins are important to healthy brain cells. Listen to what *The Mount Sinai School of Medicine Complete Book of Nutrition*, a conventional medical textbook, says about B vitamin deficiencies:

"Serious deficiencies of thiamine (B1), vitamin B6, vitamin B12, vitamin C and folic acid can provoke psychiatric symptoms...A thiamine deficiency, most often seen in alcoholics, can cause Korsakoff's psychosis, a condition that affects recent memory and causes emotional changes. It can also cause Wernicke's syndrome, a condition that reduces blood flow to the brain and can lead to coma and eventually death. A deficiency of B6 can cause mental retardation in infants...In adults, B6 deficiency...can result in mood changes, and in some cases, psychosis.."[5] The list goes on. Suffice it to say, never take your nutritional, or mental, health for granted. And the next time a neighbor laments that her husband is a different man when he drinks, tell her why!

Not coincidentally, all the nutrients found to be deficient in alcoholics are in some way important to mental health.

Not enough vitamin A can result in insomnia, fatigue and depression.

Zinc is needed for all tissue repair, including a damaged liver. Since zinc is necessary for wound healing, heavy drinkers recover slower from everything from a cut finger to major surgery. Zinc supplementation is paramount to alcoholics. If you find yourself hosting a party, instead of serving dip, offer liver pate, which is high in zinc and copper, both important to the other. Zinc is also essential in a number of major biochemical processes that affect brain function. An imbalance of copper and zinc can cause nervous system disorders.[6]

Calcium is essential for the normal functioning of neurons, the "electrical wires" of the nervous system. A deficiency of calcium and vitamin D can cause mental symptoms.

Alcohol, coffee and sugar causes the body to lose potassium and magnesium. What happens then? Have you ever noticed how alcoholics look bloated and puffy? This is because when they lose potassium, but not sodium, their body retains water. Potassium and sodium must be on equal footing in your body to balance moisture loss and gain. A potassium deficiency also causes poor reflexes, soft, sagging and weak muscles, and compulsive disorders.

Remember, all the nutrients must be balanced against each other. Look for a good, easily absorbable, derived-from-nature mineral blend in solution. Formulations in solution provide the maximum absorption ratios. Don't depend on the common multi-vitamin and mineral formulas. Minerals work best together, and vitamins work best together. Instead choose formulas that are minerals *only* or vitamins *only*.

Success Comes to Those Who Don't Give Up

You might have been wondering about my friend from Orlando. The poor woman who came to me with tears in her eyes and heart. Well, the next time I was in the Florida city, guess who came to visit?! I had hoped to see her again, but this time she brought her husband. She had gone to an alternative physician in her area who had helped them both with nutrition and lifestyle advice.

"Hi, Maureen, do you remember me?" she asked. It took me a second to place her since she was a changed woman. At that moment I realized how important inner health really is. She looked incredibly healthy! Love truly does heal.

"And this is my recovered-husband." When I looked straight ahead, all I saw was a smartly fashionable suit. He was so big I had to follow his tie upward. But the effort was worth it because when I got to his face he had a grin that lit him up like a Christmas tree.

"Maureen, I have to shake your hand," he said. "If it wasn't for you, I'd have given up. We saw an alternative doctor and he showed me my problem was mostly physical. I had been blaming myself and my wife for my weakness. Tests showed I was severely malnourished, causing both my depression and craving for alcohol. Just knowing it was not entirely my fault and that I could do something about it was a tremendous relief! I took charge of my life and my health, and here I am! God bless you Maureen, over and over again."

With those words he reached out over the table, drew my arms toward him, and gave me the biggest bear hug I'd ever received. The rest of the day my arms were numb but my heart was happy. This is why I'm doing this: for all of you.

Alcoholism-Alleviating Nutrients
For maximum absorption, take supplements with meals

Nutrient	Suggested Dosage	Formulation
Amino acids	4-6 capsules daily	Multiple formula from natural sources
Antioxidants	4 capsules daily	With selenium and grapeseed extract
Borage oil	2 capsules daily	
Coenzyme Q10	2 capsules daily	With vitamin E, phospholipids and selenium
Fiber	4-8 tablets daily	Psyllium, with herb hyssop
Flaxseed oil	1 tablespoon daily	
L-Glutamine	500 mg three times daily	
Magnesium	200 mg daily	
Melatonin	3 mg at bedtime	With B vitamins
Multi-mineral	1-4 ounces daily	In liquid solution, with vitamin B12, biotin
Multi-vitamin/mineral	3-6 caplets daily	Freeze-dried plant sources
Milk thistle	150 mg twice daily	
Vitamin C	Individual bowel tolerance*	With bioflavonoids (quercetin, proanthocyanidins)
Vitamin E	2 capsules (800 IU) daily	d-alpha tocopherol

* To determine individual dosage, on the first day take 1,000 mg hourly until diarrhea occurs, then reduce dosage to just below that for individual daily dosage. Vitamin C is not toxic in large doses but must be taken throughout the day to benefit. Divide dosage to three or four times a day.

CHAPTER 5:

Alcohol's Mental Effects

Richard's grandfather had been drinking for years, and everybody knew it. But he was a stubborn old coot and his family members decided there would be no harm in letting him have his way. He lived alone, didn't drive, and as long as Richard kept his liquor and food cabinets supplied, the old man was happy and didn't ask for a thing. What the family didn't figure on was the expense of a mental institution when his poor diet resulted in irreversible brain damage.

"Wernicke's what?" asked a perplexed and frightened Richard, when confronted with the news that his grandfather was going to be institutionalized.

"Your grandfather has Wernicke-Korsakoff psychosis," answered the doctor.

Unable to get much more out of his grandfather's physician, Richard came to me for help, information and advice.

"Its early stages are known as Wernicke's reaction, Wernicke's syndrome, Wernicke's encephalopathy (encephalopathy means brain damaged), Wernicke's disease, and in its advanced stages, Wernicke-Korsakoff psychosis," I told him. "Wernicke is the name for the part of the brain that is affected."

"It was the alcohol, wasn't it?" Richard asked me.

"Actually, we believe it's more a result of malnutrition. Did anyone prepare your grandfather's meals?"

"He didn't eat much, so nobody bothered. His meals came out of the bottle."

Shaking my head, I told him, "Your grandfather has irreversible brain damage probably due to a long-term deficiency of thiamine and alcohol toxicity. A chronic deficiency of thiamine causes brain lesions, swelling and eventually destruction of the brain itself. This condition is most commonly found in chronic alcoholics but has been diagnosed in nonalcoholics as well. The symptoms are similar to those of senile dementia, with memory problems being the first to appear. Classic signs include massive confusion, paralysis of the muscles that move the eyes, involuntary eye movements and an inability to walk.[1]

"These were your grandfather's early symptoms. If he had received help earlier, it wouldn't have gotten this far. Researchers are thinking now that a thiamine deficiency is what causes alcoholics to drink to the point of death because a thiamine deficiency affects judgement and emotions."

Not Just in Alcoholics

Thiamine is needed to produce and use the vital brain chemical acetylcholine, and to avoid emotional excesses. People who indulge in refined sugar, milled flour and processed foods, who drink alcohol regularly, or are addicted to coffee, literally drain thiamine, or vitamin B1, from their system. We should remember that sugar and fats, which make up a high percentage of processed foods and supply over 35 percent of our calories, give us no thiamine or other B vitamins. The chronic use of tea and the eating of raw fish has also been linked to thiamine deficiency.

The symptoms of a thiamine deficiency are listed officially as anorexia, confusion, depression, irritability and memory loss.[2]

In an experimental study reported in the *American Journal of Clinical Nutrition*, five of nine normal volunteers placed on a thiamine-deficient diet developed depression and irritability.[3]

Vitamin B1 is involved in the conversion of blood sugar to caloric energy in the body. During stressful periods it can give a boost to your energy level. Thiamine deficiency, or beriberi, is known to produce psychiatric and neurological symptoms.

In one experiment, rats trained to get through a maze were divided into two groups, one given a nutritionally complete diet and the other a diet totally lacking in B1. When the rats were tested 20 days later, the group on the good diet sped through in an average of 22 seconds, while the B1-deprived rats took 55 seconds, almost three times as long. However, putting the deprived rats on a diet rich in B1 induced a remarkable memory recovery and ability to run through the maze.

Anything that causes malnutrition, from poor eating habits to alcoholism, can cause a thiamine deficiency. I find it interesting that anorexia is considered a symptom of a thiamine deficiency. If a lack of thiamine causes depression and nervous system disorders, it stands to reason that a young person who diets consistently could first become thiamine deficient, causing the kind of obsessive behavior that leads to anorexia.

Even a moderate thiamine deficiency can cause anxiety or neuroses. In one study, subjects deprived of thiamine complained of poor mental alertness, fatigue and nervousness.[4] Since psychiatrists are the least likely to inquire about diet, I have to wonder how many of their anxiety patients are being treated with drugs when they are simply thiamine-deficient. Studies of autopsies show that Wernicke's encephalopathy is much more prevalent than recognized during life.[5]

Consider these symptoms: inattention, disorientation, sleepiness, apathy, indifference, impaired memory, stupor.[6] How many people living on the streets show these symptoms of thiamine deficiency? How well do you think they are eating? Wouldn't it be incredible if we could turn a population of dependents into a population of gainfully-employed, intelligent and aware citizens simply by offering them nutritional supplementation? It's definitely something to think about. Here's more food for thought!

Shockingly Overlooked

Sometimes I come across case histories so unnecessarily tragic, they beg uncovering. Such is the case of a 3-1/2 year old little girl who had been chemically treated for leukemia. Six months after receiving chemotherapy she developed vomiting and diarrhea. Hospitalized, she was put on parenteral nutrition (tube feeding). She had eye disturbances after four weeks and died three days later. The autopsy revealed she died of Wernicke's encephalopathy.[7]

Inadequate amounts of thiamine reduces blood flow to the brain, and if it continues it can cause death. The *Clinical Neuropathology* article that reported this case didn't attempt to explain how someone receiving nutritional supplementation in a hospital managed to become thiamine deficient to the point of death, but I have one hypothesis. Many vitamin supplements do not contain proper amounts of thiamine. The RDAs (recommended daily allowances) are notoriously low, since they are calculated to maintain health, not to improve it, and aren't designed to overcome situations that result in depleted nutrients, like the stress of illness. Pharmaceutical companies often use RDA amounts to formulate their supplementals – the same supplementals used in hospitals for very sick people. It is quite likely that in this case the chemotherapy effectively jeopardized the child's intestinal system to such a degree that the low doses of thiamine present in the hospital's supplementation wasn't enough to fully nourish her body. It wasn't until she was postmortem that they discovered what caused her death – death that could have been prevented. Even more telling, the author of the article suggests that "thiamine supplementation should be considered in all patients who have persistent malnutrition and malabsorption," insinuating that in the case of this little girl, she was not given thiamine at all!

The Australian Discovery

Thiamine deficiencies in people who drink are so prevalent that the Australian medical establishment has been considering supplementing alcohol with thiamine. A symposium held October 21, 1988 at the University of New South Wales had participants discussing the possibility of enriching beer and other alcohol with thiamine in order to prevent Wernicke's encephalopathy and Korsakoff's psychosis.[8]

There was general agreement that the Australian diet is deficient in thiamine compared to other western countries. It is attributed to the complete extraction of thiamine in the preparation of Australian white flour products. Most participants thought that thiamine enrichment of the Australian diet would be beneficial. Others believed thiamine enrichment would reduce the incidence of beriberi-related heart disease and peripheral neuropathy. The cost benefit was considered and, on the whole, was found to be economically beneficial. Incredibly, opponents thought that thiamine enrichment would increase the consumption of alcohol since it would be perceived as being safer or even a "health drink." Others thought of thiamine in alcohol as a form of "mass medication."[9] No policy decisions were made.

Recommended Protocol

Gunter R. Haase, M.D., and colleagues at the Department of Neurology, University of Pennsylvania School of Medicine in Philadelphia write in *Patient Care* that Wernicke's encephalopathy requires immediate intravenous thiamine at 50 mgs given in an IV piggyback fashion. In severe cases he says vitamin therapy is usually slow and may take weeks or perhaps months to see results.[10]

Michael C. Lindberg, M.D., of the Department of Internal Medicine, University of Alabama School of Medicine in Tuscaloosa, Alabama reports in *American Family Physician* that if left untreated, 17 percent of patients with acute Wernicke's encephalopathy will die. Because thiamine has no reported side effects, and because as many as 80 percent of people with Wernicke's encephalopathy will develop Korsakoff's psychosis, Dr. Lindberg takes a preventive approach, recommending patients with certain symptoms, even before a diagnosis is made, be given high doses of thiamine intravenously. He also recommends thiamine levels be evaluated in patients receiving tube feedings or other fluid diets.[11]

He recommends that 100 mg IV immediately be given for all

comatose or hypothermic patients, and for those who have classic thiamine deficient symptoms: confusion, involuntary eye movements and incoordination *before* they are given glucose. His treatment recommendations are 100 mgs of intravenous thiamine which can be given daily for three days and possibly up to 1000 mgs of thiamine during the first 12 hours. He also suggests parenteral administration of magnesium. A deficiency of magnesium is frequently found in alcoholism and magnesium is needed for thiamine to be absorbed. Dr. Lindberg contents that supplemental thiamine is more effective when magnesium levels are adequate.[12]

Wernicke-Whipping Nutrients
For maximum absorption, take nutrients with meals.

Nutrient	Suggested Dosage	Formulation
Acetyl L-Carnitine	500 mg three times daily	
Aged garlic extract	1 teaspoon three times daily	Liquid
Amino acids	4-6 capsules daily	Multiple formula from natural sources
Antioxidants	4 capsules daily*	With selenium and grapeseed extract
Borage oil	2 capsules daily	
Coenzyme Q1 (NADH)	2.5 mg daily	
Coenzyme Q10	2 capsules daily	With vitamin E, phospholipids and selenium
Flaxseed oil	1 tablespoon daily	
Ginkgo biloba	60 mg three times daily	
Multi-mineral	3-4 ounces daily	In liquid solution, with vitamin B12, biotin
Multi-vitamin/mineral	6 caplets daily	Freeze-dried plant sources
Niacin	200 mg three times daily	
Vitamin B6	100 mg daily	
Vitamin C	Individual bowel tolerance**	With bioflavonoids (quercetin, proanthocyanidins)

* The FDA recommends pregnant women not exceed 10,000 IU of vitamin A daily.

** To determine individual dosage, on the first day take 1,000 mg hourly until diarrhea occurs, then reduce dosage to just below that for individual daily dosage. Vitamin C is not toxic in large doses but must be taken throughout the day to benefit. Divide dosage to three or four times a day.

CHAPTER 6:

Allergies: Chemical, Food, Hay Fever & Pet

Two young people are running through a glorious field of vivid yellow flowers. As the couple run toward each other, arms outstretched, the soft breeze gently ripples the flowers, gathering up its shimmering pollen dust and dropping it on them like a silken waterfall. They stop, seemingly caught up in the sight of each other, an arms embrace away.

Suddenly they throw their heads back and erupt with ferocious sneezes. Eyes watering and red-rimmed, they gasp for breath, falling in a heap among nature's glory. Another precious moment destroyed by allergies.

Those of us fortunate enough not to suffer from hay fever sympathize with the red eyes, stuffy noses and omnipresent tissues our friends have to deal with during the pollen season. We thank the Lord we are fortunate enough not to have this problem.

Signs and Symptoms

When it comes to allergies, it's often what you don't know that hurts you. You don't need a doctor to tell you you have allergies. Just look for these signs. Black circles under the eyes can indicate a food allergy, as can multiple horizontal wrinkles under the lower eyelid caused by allergic swelling.

Do you "salute" without knowing it? A telltale sign is the allergic salute – rubbing an itchy nose. A scalloped tongue results when allergies cause itching and the individual "scratches" his or her tongue against the teeth. An over three pound weight gain from morning to evening can indicate a food allergy. Take milk, for example. The body says, "Hey! What's this cow doing here?! We'd better hold water in every cell to wash out the foreign invader." Then you gain three to five pounds of water and get symptoms like a runny nose, sneezing, wheezing and itchy eyes.

Do you suffer from migraines, indigestion, ulcers, itchy nose, heartburn, hives, skin blemishes, menstrual cramps or painful urination? All of these symptoms can be caused by allergies.

Your behavior could even be linked to your diet. I'm not talking about your neighbor, who would cross Lake Erie in a kayak for a Snickers bar, although there is a connection. I'm talking about hyperactivity and attention deficit disorder in kids, depression, headaches, mood swings, and even PMS. All are symptoms of allergies. Food allergens are documented as causing gallbladder problems, and even Alzheimer's has been linked to food allergies and chemical sensitivities.

Seasonal Sneezes – Minimizing the Misery of Hay Fever

For many, hay fever season is synonymous with asthma. Emergency room physicians report an increase in patients admitted with breathing problems during the spring when blossoms are blooming. Fortunately, there is help. British researchers have found eating the right foods can make a difference. Researchers at the University of Nottingham's Division of Respiratory Medicine found that of 2,633 asthmatics, those whose dietary magnesium intake was above the average 380 milligrams a day, showed significantly improved lung function and less wheezing. Low blood levels of magnesium, the researchers suspect, could be a factor in causing allergies and asthma in the first place.[1] Foods maximum in magnesium include seafood, whole grains, dark-green vegetables, molasses and nuts.

Vitamin C may offer relief of asthma. In three experiments, reduced ability to breathe was controlled for three or four hours by taking 500 mg of vitamin C.[2]

In a double-blind study of 49 Nigerian asthma patients over 14 weeks during the rainy season when asthma attacks are more severe, 22 were given 1000 mg of vitamin C daily and 19 were given a look-alike pill (placebo).

Those who took the vitamin C had fewer than one-fourth asthma attacks than those on placebos and they were not as serious. Thirteen of those taking vitamin C experienced no attacks during the 14 weeks, but suffered at least one in the eight week span after quitting the vitamin.

A Hot Solution

Have you ever heard someone say, "that'll clear the sinuses" when discussing the effect of chili peppers? Cayenne pepper, or capsicum, is an expectorant, say alternative doctors and numerous grandmothers. Not only does it sting the sinuses and bring tears to the eyes, it temporarily irritates the stomach and sets up a sympathetic reaction in the bronchial tubes and lungs to increase fluids and discharge mucus, making the lungs and tubes less thick and sticky and more open for breathing. Important, however, is drinking lots of water to make it easier for the mucus to thin out and be discharged.

It turns out spicy foods for colds, asthma and sinus problems have been used for centuries by early civilizations. Ancient Egyptian medical writings recommended mustard for respiratory therapy. Hippocrates prescribed vinegar and pepper as respiratory medicines; and Oriental medicine still uses hot peppers, black pepper, mustard, garlic, tumeric and other spices to treat colds and asthma.

In more modern times, researchers at Montreal General Hospital found that the active ingredient in tumeric – curcumin – acts as an antihistamine in reducing the symptoms of allergies and asthma.[3]

Chemical Sensitivities – A Product of Our "Civilized" Environment

What's in that loaf of bread you just bought at the market? Have you read the label? It's crammed with synthetic chemicals designed to make the bread look appealing and stay soft on the grocer's shelf until you buy it. Many studies have shown children with behavioral disorders often have chemical sensitivities. All processed foods, whether bottled, bagged, canned or packaged have hidden dangers. Monosodium glutamate (MSG) is only one of the identified dangers lurking in the plethora of chemicals contained in processed food. A very good friend of mine has migraines for days after ingesting MSG. Unfortunately, he eats out often, and forgets to ask the waitress to "hold the MSG."

Sulfites are preservatives found in many processed foods – and in most U.S. wines. They may preserve food, but in the body they deplete it of thiamine, an essential nutrient that when deficient, can cause its own host of symptoms. Many chemicals can also drain the body of essential nutrients, compounding the problem.

If there is any chance at all that you are chemically sensitive, stay away from processed foods. Some supermarkets are proclaiming their produce is free from pesticide residues. What they don't tell you is the food is often grown in chemically-fertilized or chemically-sterilized soil.

Symptoms of chemical sensitivity include: tension, memory loss, fatigue, insomnia, headaches, confusion, depression, and hyperactivity in children.

Carol Channing's friends joke that the musical-comedy star is almost as famous for her offstage eating habits as for her public performances. Channing has suffered for many years from an allergic reaction to chemicals used in food production and preparation. When on tour, she travels everywhere with special organic foods packed in silver *Tiffany* containers, and additional supplies are shipped to her by airmail – even if she's invited by the Queen of England to dinner at Buckingham Palace.

It's Time to Detoxify

Some people are allergic to latex, the rubber used in surgical and food handling gloves. Whenever they eat out, they mysteriously get allergic symptoms because the food preparers used latex gloves.

Chemically-sensitive people are literally poisoned by chemicals, and their bodies need to be detoxified to remove the heavy metals that have accumulated.

Researchers have discovered that garlic is a powerful detoxifier and body cleanser. In one pilot study, Honolulu dentist Dr. Samuel Wong used garlic to treat 14 patients with silver-mercury amalgam fillings. He found that garlic helped take mercury out of his patients' systems.

Detoxification is normally accomplished by the liver – the largest organ in the human body. Besides regulating sugars and metabolizing proteins, the liver detoxifies alcohol, drugs and other poisonous chemicals that enter the body. When liver cells break down, the liver loses this function and the body becomes poisoned.

In one detoxifying study, researchers headed by Dr. Tohru Fuwa at the Central Research Laboratories of Wakunaga Pharmaceutical Company in Japan reported in the *Hiroshima Journal of Medical Sciences* that four of the six sulfur-containing compounds isolated from garlic protected liver cells from damage caused by a toxic chemical, carbon tetrachloride. This finding was confirmed by Dr. Hiroshi Hikino and associates at the Pharmaceutical Institute of Tohoku University.

The best source is not fresh garlic, because it has the tendency to burn. Instead look to aged garlic extract, which isolates the most effective ingredients of garlic and is odorless!

The common milk thistle is another ingredient from God's garden proven to be a curative. Not only do extracts (called silymarin) from this plant block allergic and inflammatory reactions, they are helpful when it comes to detoxifying and protecting the liver. The highest concentration of silymarin is found in the plant's fruit, but it is also contained in the plant's leaves and seeds.

Studies of patients taking anti-convulsants, mood-altering medications or receiving anesthesia show that silymarin can protect their livers from damage. Additional studies in Germany suggest it works for those whose exposure to pesticides results in liver disease. Others report success in the treatment of heavy metal poisoning.

Methylsulfonylmethane sounds like a chemical you should avoid. Not so. Actually, MSM is a dietary source of sulfur, necessary for production of valuable amino acids. Studies have shown it to be extremely helpful in not only building up the body's immune system, but in alleviating allergic symptoms, including those due to the environment. MSM can be purchased in health food stores and tests have proven it to be perfectly safe even in high doses.

Pet Allergies

Recently, a dear friend of mine came to visit me for a week. Unfortunately I hadn't realized she was allergic to cats. I put my cat, Happy Cat, in a back room, but it didn't help. I vacuumed and even cleaned the carpet but to no avail. The poor woman was miserable and went through three boxes of tissues in one day alone. Finally I called Dr. Ross Gordon and asked his advice.

He said it is a protein in the animal's saliva that causes the problem. Every hair on the animal is coated with saliva from the cat's cleaning efforts, which dries and floats around in the air, so no amount of cleaning or washing helps. The solution, according to Dr. Gordon, is to change the chemical composition of the animal's saliva. "And how might I do that?" I asked. "By giving the cat vitamin E," he responded.

Since it wasn't likely to harm the cat, I added one vitamin E capsule – 400 IU – to her food every day. The following month my friend planned to visit again. I told her I didn't think she would have the same problem with my cat. Despite my optimism, she arrived armed with several surgical masks. I am happy to report she didn't need any of them. The whole time she was there she had not one sniffle. And my cat's coat never looked better!

Food Allergies

In a healthy individual, food is partially broken down in the mouth by thorough chewing, then further broken down by stomach acid, then the vitamins, minerals and enzymes are absorbed in the intestines for distribution through the bloodstream into the body's cells. In many cases of food allergies, it is a problem in one of these areas that causes the food to remain whole in the intestine. When food enters the intestine without being broken down first the body considers it foreign. That's where the allergy symptoms come in, as the body tries to flush out the foreign substance with mucus and irritation.

Milk is a very common allergen. You've heard of lactose intolerance? Many children who are asthmatic are allergic to the lactose in milk. They don't have enough of the enzyme lactase to break it down.

When lactose escapes the stomach undigested, it meets intestinal bacteria which feed on it, causing fermentation. Then the small intestine becomes a war zone of cramps, diarrhea, gas and bloating. These are the symptoms of a milk allergy.

To make up for an insufficiency of lactase, drink milk or eat yogurt that contains lactobacillus acidophilus, a bacterial culture that makes the necessary lactase. Or you can buy milk that already contains lactase. Lactase enzymes can also be purchased at health food stores and taken as a supplement.

The system's reaction to a food allergy can be severe and long-term. In a study reported in the *European Journal of Pediatrics*, researchers tested infants from parents with a family history of milk allergy. After only one dose of cow's milk, "before" and "after" pictures showed the stomach lining was turned to mush. A zinc supplement, a notorious wound-healer, and vitamin B12, can help restore the stomach lining.

Narrow your list down to the following foods suspect for most allergy sufferers: beef, sugar, chocolate, eggs, citrus fruits, coffee, corn, malt, milk, pork, potatoes, soybeans, spices, tomatoes, wheat and yeast.

Food Allergy Self-Tests

Foods which a person is sensitive or allergic to increase the heart rate considerably. If your heartbeat soars after you eat a certain food – say 20 or so beats a minute above normal – that food is suspect. Here's a test to determine if you are allergic to certain foods:

Find the area on the underside of the wrist where you can feel the pulse of blood pumped by your heart. It will be under your thumb. Touch lightly, or you won't feel it. Use your index and middle fingers. Then, count your pulse for six seconds and multiply by ten to find your resting pulse.

First, take your pulse after waking up in the morning, while still in bed. Repeat just before eating. Eat just one food at a time. Then take the test thirty minutes later, then sixty minutes later.

Food allergies can make a heartbeat skyrocket from 72 to 92 or even as high as 180 beats per minute. One or more of the aforementioned symptoms could follow within minutes or hours. Once a food turns out to be an allergen, just omit it from your diet. Results are not always obvious. Sometimes it takes 14 to 16 hours to notice a marked reaction. If you make it a habit to check your pulse throughout the day you may hit it at just the right time.

Another, more accurate test, has you eating only one food at a time. Then you avoid it for four days before eating it again. At this point, if you're sensitive or allergic to it, you will sense a heightened flare-up.

Repeat the process with other foods – suspected and unsuspected – until you develop a broad range of tolerable foods. It is unwise to repeat even unsuspected foods more than every five days because, by repetition, you could develop new sensitivities or allergies.

Treating the Symptoms After Discovering the Cause

Ignorance is not bliss, knowledge is. Knowing how to identify allergic symptoms is the first step. Using natural, God-given nutrients to help the body overcome the effects is the second.

Recent advances by nutritionally-oriented doctors have dramatically changed the picture for people with allergies. The regimen is two-fold: boosting the body's natural ability to withstand the onslaught of chemicals and allergens, and cleansing the body of offending substances. This can be done by you through food, specialized supplements and common nutrients, all found in your health food store.

Quercetin, a bioflavonoid, is valued for its anti-inflammatory properties. Quercetin is the most effective nutritional antihistamine I have seen yet. It also acts to protect vitamin C from getting broken down in the body.[4] Quercetin is so powerful, it is compared to cromolyn, a prescription antihistamine. Quercetin is found in yellow and red onions. Interestingly, applying a cut onion to an insect bite is a folk remedy.

Leukotrienes are immune system chemicals believed to contribute to allergic swelling, such as from insect bites. Quercetin, combined with bromelain extracted from pineapple for increased absorption, has been shown in studies to effectively inhibit the formation of leukotrienes.[5]

Bromelain is a digestive enzyme helpful for increasing absorption and assimilation of nutrients and food. Both bromelain and papain are digestive enzymes, called proteolytic enzymes, which break down protein. You've heard that you should use meat tenderizer on bee stings? Well, bromelain from pineapple and papain from papaya are proteolytic enzymes, meaning they break down protein, and are essentially meat tenderizers. The reason they work on bee stings is because bees inject a protein to break down blood. If applied soon enough, they will neutralize the protein before the body has a chance to recognize it as a foreign substance. Papaya is also high in vitamin C, so you can't go wrong there!

Forget over-the-counter remedies! Choosing a vitamin C formula that contains bioflavonoids will work better than any antihistamine you can buy. You cannot overdose on vitamin C and bioflavonoids. To combat colds and allergy symptoms, alternative doctors recommend taking 2-3 grams of vitamin C and bioflavonoids in divided doses up to the point where you get diarrhea – called bowel tolerance. Then just cut down on the dosage, and increase slowly. This occurs because the vitamin C is flushing toxins. You'll notice when you are sick you can tolerate more vitamin C. Drink as much water as possible to further flush the body.

Watercress is an old folk remedy for sneezing, a stuffy head and watery eyes.

For many people, allergies mean skin rashes. To tame your hives place the inside of a banana skin right where it itches. It will cool and soothe the inflammation. Eat the fruit too – it contains nutrients healthy for your skin. I watched elephants in Africa gorge on bananas and watercress – their favorite foods. Can you imagine an elephant with a runny nose?

Medicated greases and lotions, especially those containing perfumes and colorings, may make a skin rash worse. To moisturize the skin without irritating it, rub in a little olive oil or lanolin-based cream containing vitamins A, C and E, aloe vera gel or calendula lotion.

After bathing, rub cucumber juice on the skin or dab apple-cider vinegar, calendula ointment, or cooled teas of elder flower, blackberry leaf, goldenseal or yellow dock on the areas of the rash. Oatmeal, moistened and wrapped in a cloth that is held on the irritated areas, will help soothe the itching.

For more on dealing with the symptoms of allergies, see my chapter Inflammation.

Using what I've learned through my years of research and experience, you can avoid the shots, avoid the drugs and avoid the allergies as well. The next time you take a drive in the country, stop and smell the daisies!

Allergy-Fighting Nutrients
For maximum absorption, take supplements with meals.

Nutrient	Suggested Dosage	Formulation
Aged garlic extract	1 teaspoon three times daily	Liquid
Antioxidants	4 capsules daily*	With selenium and grapeseed extract
Borage oil	2 capsules daily	
Enzymes	2 capsules twice daily	Multiple formula
Bromelain	200 mg twice daily	
Deglycyrrhizinated licorice	1-2 tablets before meals	Chewable
Flaxseed oil	1 tablespoon daily	
Magnesium	200 mg daily	
MSM (methylsulfonylmethane)	500 mg three times daily	
Multi-mineral	3-4 ounces daily	In liquid solution, with vitamin B12, biotin
Multi-vitamin/mineral	6 caplets daily	Freeze-dried plant sources
Niacinamide	1,000 mg twice daily	
Quercetin	400 mg twice daily	With vitamin C
Taurine	3 grams daily	
Vitamin B6	200 mg daily	
Vitamin C	Individual bowel tolerance**	With bioflavonoids (quercetin, rutin proanthocyanidins)

* The FDA recommends pregnant women not exceed 10,000 IU of vitamin A daily.

** To determine individual dosage, on the first day take 1,000 mg hourly until diarrhea occurs, then reduce dosage to just below that for individual daily dosage. Vitamin C is not toxic in large doses but must be taken throughout the day to benefit. Divide dosage to three or four times a day.

CHAPTER 7:

Alzheimer's

Actors are fond of the adage, all the world's a stage. Actually, all the world's a movie and each day is the sequel. I fiercely believe in living life to its fullest, and that you don't stop living until you stop learning. Alzheimer's is no exception. Too many people are led to believe Alzheimer's is a prison sentence – trapped in a body that has lost its mind.

I'm here to say Alzheimer's is not a death sentence! There are people who have cured themselves and others of this life-destroying disease. I've talked to them, and I've seen their successes. I know firsthand it can be done, and now you will too!

Alzheimer's is not an incurable, degenerative disease. It's not even a true disease! Alzheimer's is a physical reaction to poisons present in the environment and the body. Not only is Alzheimer's preventable, but it is reversible.

The Alzheimer's Difference

Most medical volumes dump memory loss, dementia and Alzheimer's together. What authors and physicians apparently fail to understand is that aging does not necessarily mean forgetfulness, and that Alzheimer's is a serious disease, not a product of aging cells. The fact is, memory loss can occur to anyone, at any age, for many reasons. Chemical imbalances and reactions don't occur only in the aged, it just takes that many years for them to affect the brain. Comparing memory loss to Alzheimer's is like comparing a stubbed toe to gangrene. I'll let the experts explain the devastating effects.

The September 17, 1994 medical journal *The Lancet* documented the striking differences in brain cell loss experienced by mentally alert elderly compared to those with Alzheimer's. The study headed by Warren J. Strittmatter of Duke University Medical Center found that Alzheimer's patients autopsied after death lost brain cells in a much greater number and in more areas of the brain than in their elderly subjects. A certain amount of brain cell loss is accepted by conventional medicine to be a normal process of aging (not in *my* opinion – see my chapter on Memory Loss), but among Alzheimer's patients, the loss is much greater. In two Alzheimer's victims, they literally found no brain cells.[1] In the early '70s, a research team led by Dr. D. Crapper at the University of Toronto autopsied Alzheimer's victims and each time found isolated aluminum accumulated in localized brain areas and incredible tangles of nerve fibers (neurofibrils; nerve conductors inside brain cells). If nothing is done, Alzheimer's is quite literally capable of turning a thinking, living human being into a brain-dead zombie.

The Fantastic Story of Tom Warren

Tom Warren is living proof that Alzheimer's can be reversed. Tom experienced a "comeback" to normal life after doctors told him he had incurable Alzheimer's disease and would be dead within seven years. Fortunately for him, he didn't take their word for it.

His full story is told, much of it by him, in my audiotapes and in his book *Beating Alzheimer's* (Avery Publishing Group, New York, 1991). Tom describes how he went to specialist after specialist; scouring libraries, books and health food stores to read everything he could find on the subject. My books were of great help to him. His wife, Louise, a pharmacist by trade, helped when his memory failed him. A statement he made to me that will stick in my heart forever was his regret that if he wasn't successful, he would no longer be able to make a positive contribution to the world. He also says, in the many papers he has written about his discoveries, that "the Alzheimer's sufferer is in a fight for his life and sanity – and frankly, sanity is more important than life."

I'm happy to report that Tom Warren won his battle. Four years after the original diagnosis, a CAT scan showed the disease had reversed. He says he had it checked and re-checked by various specialists, and that one doctor's hand shook as he related the findings. Most neurologists, he says, refuse to believe he had Alzheimer's, a disease they consider incurable. This is a sad state of affairs when you consider all the people who are diagnosed and left to die.

Incurable should be stricken from a physician's vocabulary. Medical science must necessarily be in a constant state of discovery and inherently never will be absolute or perfect. To make someone believe there is no hope has to be at the very least unethical. The real problem is that the doctor making such a statement has simply reached the limits of his knowledge.

The Mercury Menace

Tom talks about how, after he discovered his fillings could be pur-veyors of deadly mercury poison, he had them all replaced. When the new fillings caused a reaction, he had all his teeth removed. He figured he could live without his teeth, but not without his mind.

His discovery of research done by Patrick Stortebecker, M.D., Ph.D., former professor of neurology at the Karolinska Institute, Stockholm, Sweden convinced him. Dr. Stortebecker wrote a book entitled *Mercury Poisoning from Mercury Amalgam – a Hazard to the Human Brain*. Dr. Stortebecker states that mercury vapor, released from dental fill-ings, is absorbed from the upper nasal area and passes directly to the brain.

Other medical researchers have made the connection between sil-ver-amalgam dental fillings and mercury poisoning. A Swedish report by Jaro Pleva, Ph.D., suggests that silver amalgams should be more accurately called *mercury* amalgams since they contain 52 percent mercury. When Dr. Pleva found that five-year-old fillings contain 27 percent mercury, he concluded that the mercury evaporated slowly from the dental fillings.

As a result, your mouth may be a toxic waste dump. The environ-mental protection agency considers silver amalgam a toxic waste and has strict guidelines for its storage and disposal. The minute the dentist removes it from a patient's mouth, he is required by law to deal with it as hazardous waste.

Tom also talks about the dangers of processed food causing food allergies. He found, after a doctor gave him the Heidelberg stomach acid test, that he had no stomach acid, and therefore was not assimilat-ing much of the food he was eating. He was not getting enough nutri-ents to keep his brain healthy. After eliminating processed junk food, particularly coffee, sugar and white flour products, his stomach acid returned to normal. Supplementing with Betaine, available from health food stores, can also help in restoring stomach acid.

I believe Tom's primary problem was his chemical sensitivities. There are some people who are literally so sensitive to chemicals they have to live in a completely organic home, free of even the most hypoallergenic products. Something is missing for these people, something that allows the rest of us to drive in smog and apply perfume without becoming deathly ill. It turned out Tom was sensitive enough for the mercury in his fillings and the aluminum in his environment to affect his brain. His immune system was so burned out he put himself on a super-nutritional program, which also helped the imbalance that caused the sensitivities in the first place.

The Aluminum Association

If you found suspicious clues at the scene of a crime which pointed directly toward a particular suspect, wouldn't you at least take him in for questioning? Isolated aluminum is just such a suspect in brain deterioration, but orthodox medicine refuses to even admit to the evidence and research. The studies are there, for those who wish to find them.

Researchers at the University of Kentucky, headed by Robert A Yokel, found in their studies that animals with aluminum toxicity had the same nerve fiber tangles as Alzheimer's patients.[2] Their conclusion? There is a relationship between aluminum toxicity and Alzheimer's disease. This study is interesting because it comes from the University's Division of Pharmacology and Experimental Therapeutics. In other words, a conventional institution that investigates alternative therapies! For them to find this evidence is telling indeed!

Further evidence that increased exposure to aluminum may be linked to Alzheimer's disease comes from kidney patients. Researchers in the United Kingdom found that kidney dialysis patients receiving aluminum supplements to control their blood phosphate levels showed brain changes similar to those that occur in Alzheimer's disease.[3]

In clinics offering kidney dialysis treatment, where the isolated aluminum content of the water used in treatments is high, dementia is also found to be high. Where it is low, dementia is low. There is a good reason for this. Our kidneys are charged with filtering out toxins that invade our bodies. If too many toxins enter, the kidneys are overloaded. If we have kidney problems from whatever source, we become more susceptible to heavy metal toxicity. It is obvious to me that kidney patients shouldn't be given isolated aluminum or any other heavy metal.

Sources of Isolated Aluminum

The time of battle is at hand. How can you wage war against criminal isolated aluminum? Start by avoiding the following non-food products that stealthily implant isolated aluminum into the body and mind. They are: most acne medications and antacids (health food stores carry isolated aluminum-free alternatives), anti-diarrhea products, antiperspirants and deodorants, many cosmetics, douches, feminine hygiene products, some hemorrhoid preparations, lipstick, skin creams and lotions, and toothpaste. Read the labels!

Watch for aluminum in processed food and food items. For example, sodium aluminum phosphate is used in some cake mixes, frozen dough, pancake batter and self-rising flour to cause the rising action. Alkaline aluminum phosphates are used in processed cheeses to make them soft and melt easily. Sodium aluminum sulfate is found in baking powder. Aluminum ammonium sulfate is used as a firming agent in pickled fruits and vegetables and appears on the product labels as "alum." A dill pickle of medium size that has been soaked in a 0.1 percent alum solution may contain between five and 10 milligrams of isolated aluminum. This may explain, in part, why some commercially prepared pickles have a metallic taste.

Some nonprescription drugs contain high levels of isolated aluminum. Many over-the-counter antacids contain aluminum hydroxide, an aluminum salt. The maximum daily dosage of these antacids, as recommended on their product labels, can deliver between 1,000 and 7,000 milligrams of isolated aluminum per day. Isolated aluminum intoxication has been shown in some elderly patients who take maintenance doses of such antacids.

Aluminum hydroxide is also found in buffered aspirin. If you use buffered aspirin to avoid the stomach upset caused by regular aspirin, you should be aware that you may be consuming between 200 and 1,000 milligrams of isolated aluminum a day.

The use of aluminum cookware can add isolated aluminum to the foods cooked in them, especially acidic foods such as tomatoes, rhu-barb, cabbage, apricots, cranberries and sauerkraut. Also, avoid storing foods in aluminum containers and aluminum foil. Ever notice how aluminum foil turns black and develops holes when it is placed over acidic foods? Imagine what it does to your body!

Your tap water could be another isolated aluminum culprit. Municipal water often contains fluoride, which increases the amount of isolated aluminum leached from cookware and absorbed in foods cooked in it. Another problem is the possibility your drinking water contains dissolved isolated aluminum, or alum. Some studies have shown that fluoride in the water actually increases the body's absorption of aluminum. Call your local water district to find out the concentration of aluminum in your drinking water. If it is above 0.01 milligrams (10 micrograms) per liter, some home filtering system might be warranted. In addition, municipal water treatment systems might be encouraged to use less aluminum in the treatment process.

Are you singing the blues because the list seems impossibly prohibitive? Cheer up! Once started, you'll find it easier to eat everything you like and you'll find you don't miss the convenience of processed foods. You can eat your fill of fish, poultry and other lean meats (non-chemicalized meats can be purchased from health food stores), fresh fruits and vegetables, and whole grain products.

Aluminum Detoxifiers

The battle against Alzheimer's can be stacked in your favor by setting an ambush against isolated aluminum absorption in your body. Your soldiers of protection can include supplements of vitamin C – 1,000 mg daily – calcium and magnesium. The brain's memory center, the hippocampus, has a special affinity for magnesium. If your memory is like a sieve, you may be lacking this mineral.

Adequate calcium limits the accumulation of isolated aluminum in the brain, according to a study by Judith Marquis of the Department of Pharmacology at Boston University.[4]

Concentrate on spinach for all three aluminum antagonizers. Dark green leafy vegetables contain both calcium and magnesium, as do nuts and soybeans.

Studies have found that malic acid – naturally found in apples, cherries and other fruits – is very effective in removing isolated aluminum from the brains of isolated aluminum-poisoned mice. It can also be taken orally from supplements. In fact, it has shown to be more effective than the prescription drug of choice, deferoxamine, which is injected and can have dangerous side effects.

I learned of a pair of identical twins who did not follow the usual rule for Alzheimer's. Normally, if one identical twin develops Alzheimer's disease, the other does too, at about the same time. One twin developed Alzheimer's in her early 50s, but 10 years later the other twin had no trace of the disease – and she was reported to have been thoroughly and repeatedly tested. They lived near each other for their entire lives, and had been exposed to the same drinking water and other environmental factors. The scientist who described this case found that the only lifestyle difference he could identify was that the healthy twin had a long standing habit of drinking half a bottle of wine per day, while the twin with Alzheimer's did not. This could be coincidental, but it was pointed out that malic acid is among the most common of many compounds found in wine. Half a bottle of wine per day would typically provide about 1-1/2 grams of malic acid per day, which would be an effective aluminum chelating dose based on the mouse experiments already discussed. Of course, there's no telling what the woman's liver looked like. I wouldn't recommend that you drink half a bottle of wine every day; grape juice is just as effective.

Foods containing sulfur and the amino acids cysteine and methionine naturally chelate heavy metals. When sulfur is combined with hydrogen, they form sulfhydryl groups, which are very effective in removing toxins and poisons.

Fish, onions, garlic, horseradish, chives, red hot peppers and egg yolks contain relatively large amounts of sulfur compounds and are natural chelators of toxic metals. Have you noticed how asparagus changes the odor of your urine, often soon after the vegetable is eaten? This is due to the sulfur-bearing compounds contained in this desirable vegetable.

Another excellent dietary source of sulfhydryl groups are beans such as peas, limas, pintos, kidneys, soybeans and other legumes, all of which remove isolated aluminum and are advised for your risk-reduction program. Sesame, pumpkin and sunflower seeds as well as English walnuts all contain ample methionine and should be eaten regularly as snack foods.

Ok, so you've spent a lifetime breaking all the aluminum rules. How can you tell if you're being affected by it all? There is a hair test available which can be useful for indicating any increase of isolated aluminum in your system over what would be considered "normal." The test is known as "flameless atomic absorption analysis of acid-digested hair samples" and can be ordered through your natural healing physician or health practitioner.

Hopeful Treatments

You say you think you may be experiencing symptoms of Alzheimer's or have been diagnosed with it? Don't despair! As I've been saying all along, there is hope. Treatments and therapies do exist to stop Alzheimer's.

Richard Casdorph, M.D., Ph.D., of Long Beach, California, told participants of a National Health Federation convention that his patients in the early or mid-stages of Alzheimer's disease had marked improvement when isolated aluminum was removed by means of chelation treatment with an amino acid formulation called EDTA. In the case of Alzheimer's disease, EDTA may remove isolated aluminum from brain tissue as well as restoring elasticity to cerebral arteries, increasing brain blood flow. Incidentally, scientists have discovered a connection between artery plaque build up and Alzheimer's.

Dr. Casdorph, formerly assistant clinical professor of medicine at the University of California Medical School, Irvine, California, is a key proponent of chelation treatment. Dr. Casdorph looked at the effects of EDTA chelation therapy in brain disorders, including Alzheimer's disease, and reported a significant increase in the flow of blood to the cerebrums in all but one of 15 patients treated. This improvement generally took approximately 20 chelation treatments. And while he stated that all 15 patients showed clinical improvement, one improved without any increased blood flow to the brain. He ascribes this clinical improvement to the fact that EDTA chelates and removes isolated aluminum.

What *is* chelation? Medically, the term means an agent with the ability to "grab" another compound and remove it. Progressive physicians, albeit few, are utilizing this technique in which a protein-like material is introduced that binds with or "chelates" calcium and other metals in the bloodstream, and is excreted from the body through the urinary system.

A study from Geneva, Switzerland reports that preliminary trials treating Alzheimer's disease with zinc aspartate shows promise. The researchers from University Psychiatric Institutes started with the knowledge that the hippocampus is the area of the brain with the highest zinc concentration. They put two and two together when they realized that Alzheimer's primarily effects the hippocampus, its memory center. Sure enough, they found that there was a displacement of zinc in that area with heavy metals such as aluminum and mercury, and that enzymes essential to brain cells were becoming non-functional. They found improvement when they put back the missing zinc.[5]

The Missing Links

In a nutshell, Alzheimer's is basically heavy metal poisoning, caused by toxins such as mercury and aluminum, resulting in brain damage. Why this occurs in some people and not others probably has a lot to do with their nutritional health. Healthy individuals don't have accumulations of aluminum in their brains, no matter how old they are. Yet, people who die of Alzheimer's do. Healthy people don't get mercury poisoning from their fillings, yet people with Alzheimer's do. Why does this happen? More to the question, what is missing that causes it to happen?

I believe it has something to do with a breakdown of the blood-brain barrier. This barrier is the body's way of keeping compounds like mercury and aluminum from traveling from the bloodstream to the brain, causing damage. It seems logical that among people who aren't exposed to large amounts of chemicals, yet are being poisoned by them, this barrier has somehow become defective. We know that oil-soluble compounds such as nicotine, cocaine and alcohol slip through, as do certain medicines.[6] For most of us, however, the amounts of toxic chemicals and metals we eat, inhale and absorb do not slip through and effect us mentally, even over long periods of exposure.

Clues to solving this mystery will be found when we can isolate those nutrients which are necessary to a strong blood-brain barrier, and that are missing among those with Alzheimer's. Unfortunately, instead of looking for ways to make it stronger, conventional medicine's goals are to find drugs that will break the barrier down, so drugs can be introduced directly into the brain, bypassing the bloodstream. This is not the healthy nor best way to solve the problems of neurological disease. Every time we alter our God-given bodies, whether through legal or illegal chemicals, we jeopardize our health. It is always better to work with nature, rather than fighting against it.

In the meantime, the clues to a healthy blood-brain barrier lie in the nutrients we know effect, restore and boost our mental capabilities.

In studies at the University of North Carolina, researchers discovered that deficiencies of the B vitamin choline can effect the severity of Alzheimer's Disease.[7] Choline is a basic constituent of lecithin, a common dietary supplement, but is also found in egg yolk, liver, brewer's yeast and wheat germ. Interestingly, choline is important to the utilization of fats and cholesterol in the body, as well as the myelin sheath that protects nerves. Since the blood-brain barrier is composed of lipids (fats), perhaps a deficiency of choline lowers the barrier's resistance.

In another study, four of six patients with familial Alzheimer's disease had low blood levels of vitamin B12.[8] Vitamin B12 is necessary for healthy nerve tissue and is involved in protein, fat and carbohydrate metabolism. It also helps iron function better and helps folic acid synthesize choline. Severe B12 deficiency has been found to cause a type of brain damage resembling schizophrenia.[9]

These studies aren't surprising because anyone versed in nutrition will tell you that the B vitamins are central to the nervous system. In fact, the whole body communication system can break down with a B vitamin deficiency. They are so important as a whole, that they must be taken or eaten together.

Numerous studies have traced one amino acid, acetyl-L-carnitine, with improvements in Alzheimer's symptoms.[10] One double-blind study found a beneficial effect on short-term memory.[11] Not coincidentally, this nutrient is important to the synthesis of choline.

Studies in Japan have shown that daily supplements of coenzyme Q10 and vitamin B6 returned some Alzheimer's-diagnosed patients to "normal" mental capacity.[12] Coenzyme Q10 is a marvelous nutrient for heart disease because it restores tissues and circulation. It is also a powerful antioxidant, breaking up free radicals that may contribute to age-related memory loss. I would give most of the credit of this study to the B6. Vitamin B6, like B12, is necessary for carbohydrate, fat and protein metabolism.

For more details on the benefits of nutrients on memory, see the chapter on Memory Loss. Adding these nutrients to your arsenal can only help in a battle against Alzheimer's.

Alzheimer's Axing Nutrients
For maximum absorption, take supplements with meals.

Nutrient	Suggested Dosage	Formulation
Acetyl L-Carnitine	500 mg three times daily	
Aged garlic extract	1 teaspoon three times daily	Liquid
Amino acids	4-6 capsules daily	Multiple formula from natural sources
Antioxidants	4 capsules daily*	With selenium and grapeseed extract
Borage oil	2 capsules daily	
Coenzyme Q1 (NADH)	2.5 mg daily	
Coenzyme Q10	2 capsules daily	With vitamin E, phospholipids and selenium
Flaxseed oil	1 tablespoon daily	
Ginkgo biloba	60 mg three times daily	
Multi-mineral	3-4 ounces daily	In liquid solution, with vitamin B12, biotin
Multi-vitamin/mineral	6 caplets daily	Freeze-dried plant sources
Niacin	200 mg three times daily	
Vitamin B6	100 mg daily	
Vitamin C	Individual bowel tolerance**	With bioflavonoids (quercetin, rutin proanthocyanidins)

* The FDA recommends pregnant women not exceed 10,000 IU of vitamin A daily.

** To determine individual dosage, on the first day take 1,000 mg hourly until diarrhea occurs, then reduce dosage to just below that for individual daily dosage. Vitamin C is not toxic in large doses but must be taken throughout the day to benefit. Divide dosage to three or four times a day.

CHAPTER 8:

Anemia

A very dear friend of mine found out the hard way that curing anemia is not as simple as taking iron supplements. She went to her doctor complaining that she was tired all the time and felt weak. Her physician ordered a blood test, diagnosed her as having iron-deficiency anemia and prescribed iron supplements.

After a couple of weeks she was concerned that she didn't feel better. After a month of taking iron supplements, she was sure something was wrong. She had an upset stomach all the time, even when she wasn't eating, and diarrhea when she was. She took my advice and went to see my doctor, a physician versed in the intricacies of nutrition.

Tests showed her anemia was a result of a B12 deficiency coupled with too little stomach acid, and that if she had continued taking the iron supplements, she could have had serious liver damage.

The Over-Diagnosis of Iron Poor Blood

Iron-deficiency anemia has been over-diagnosed in the U.S. In fact, a 1988 survey of people with iron overload revealed that one in three had met with more than 11 doctors before getting a correct diagnosis![1]

How can you tell if you have too much stored iron? Only certain blood tests, such as the serum ferritin test and transferrin saturation test, provide the answer. The reason for this common mistake goes back to the definition of anemia. Simply put, anemia is a reduction in the number of hemoglobin molecules and/or in the number or size of red blood cells. However, this condition can result from many things that have nothing to do with whether the body is taking in or storing enough iron. Anemia can be caused by deficiencies of folic acid, vitamin B6, vitamin B12 and copper, and by anything that reduces stomach acid. Trauma and illnesses that cause internal bleeding can lead to anemia as well.

Churchill's Medical Dictionary lists over one hundred different kinds of anemias. Among them are iron deficiency, folic acid deficiency and pernicious anemia. What it comes down to is that anemia is not a problem unto itself, but rather a red blood cell/hemoglobin disorder that can be caused by any number of factors, especially a deficiency of B vitamins and iron. Only through extensive testing that evaluates the body's stores of nutrients, can the cause be isolated.

Pernicious Anemia and B12

Churchill's defines pernicious anemia (PA) as "anemia resulting from impaired intestinal absorption of vitamin B12." It is called pernicious because it is fatal if left untreated. It has been estimated that the majority of elderly people with symptoms of senility are actually suffering from pernicious anemia. This occurs because they have two strikes against them: they don't eat well and they often lack stomach acid.

This is how B12 causes anemia. Think of our bone marrow as a maternity ward. In it, baby blood cells are born and cared for so they grow big and strong enough to leave the nest and enter the bloodstream. Without enough nurses – vitamin B12 – the babies aren't nurtured and fed. Some die, others are malformed or obese. The red blood cells are too few in number, are incompletely developed, or too large.

The symptoms of pernicious anemia range from early signs of paleness, fatigue, diarrhea, heart palpitations and numbness in fingers and toes, to delusions, senility and schizophrenia in later stages.

No treatment for pernicious anemia was available until 1926, when Drs. George Minot and William Murphy discovered that feeding patients enormous amounts of liver could reverse PA symptoms. It was discovered that when animal liver was fed to PA patients, their bone marrow started producing normal red cells again, and patients recovered completely. To obtain such an effect and to maintain it, however, one pound of almost raw liver had to be eaten. I don't know about you, but my idea of fun is definitely not eating raw liver. After years more of research, however, scientists isolated the element in liver that cured pernicious anemia. We now know it is vitamin B12, or cobalamin.

During one of my many excursions throughout the country, an Indiana University neurology professor told me of a tragic case in which a patient with pernicious anemia was confined for several years in an Illinois state hospital with psychoses. Eventually the B12 link was discovered and he was restored to good mental health with supplements. He was able to resume his interrupted career as a schoolteacher, but because of the irreversible neurological damage, he was confined to a wheelchair.

Important to all this is the knowledge that B12 is only absorbed in two places of the body: the stomach and the end of the small intestine. If the stomach has too little acid, whether from illness, stress or age, this absorption is compromised. However, some doctors, like Dr. Christian Jansen, believe that it only takes one milligram of B12 – 500 times the RDA – to overcome the stomach acid limitation and be absorbed in the intestine. Dr. Jansen takes exception to the RDA's minuscule recommendation of two micrograms (one thousandth of a milligram), pointing out that raising the recommendation could effectively prevent pernicious anemia.

Dr. Jansen has been trying for more than 33 years to convince the FDA, as well as colleagues who edit medical journals, that oral B12 is the preferred way to treat PA patients. He believes doctors have a responsibility to prevent pernicious anemia from developing at all. He continues to insist that the FDA authorize the marketing of oral B12 for the treatment of pernicious anemia.

Important to note is the fact that B12 is primed for active duty by other B vitamins, namely niacin, riboflavin and folic acid, and the mineral manganese.[2]

The absorption of vitamin B12 is also dependent on something called intrinsic factor. It is a chemical or enzyme generated by the stomach that combines with chemicals in the intestine to make B12 available to the body. Research shows that low levels of intrinsic factor, common among the elderly, is associated with low blood levels of B12. People who suffer from atrophic gastritis, in which the stomach lining is impaired, have low levels of intrinsic factor and suffer from pernicious anemia. Low levels of B12 are also associated with atrophic gastritis.

The bottom line is that between the stomach and the intestine, there are so many factors that can inhibit absorption of vitamin B12, we are best served if we supplement this vital vitamin in solution form. Look for a good, easily absorbable, derived-from-nature mineral blend in solution that contains B12 and manganese.

When supplementing with any one B vitamin, include a B-complex formula. All the B vitamins are dependent upon one another, and without one, you may have a deficiency of another.

Anemia-Fighting Nutrients
For maximum absorption, take supplements with meals.

Nutrient	Suggested Dosage	Formulation
Aged garlic extract	1 teaspoon three times daily	Liquid
Fiber	4-8 tablets daily	Psyllium, with herb hyssop
Multi-mineral	1-4 ounces daily	In liquid solution, with vitamin B12, biotin
Multi-vitamin/mineral	3-6 caplets	Freeze-dried plant sources
Milk thistle	150 mg twice daily	
Vitamin C	Individual bowel tolerance*	With bioflavonoids (quercetin, rutin proanthocyanidins)
Vitamin E	2 capsules (800 IU)	d-alpha tocopherol

* To determine individual dosage, on the first day take 1,000 mg hourly until diarrhea occurs, then reduce dosage to just below that for individual daily dosage. Vitamin C is not toxic in large doses but must be taken throughout the day to benefit. Divide dosage to three or four times a day.

CHAPTER 9:

Ankylosing Spondylitis

Why must the medical community use these hard-to-pronounce words to describe our afflictions? I have to wonder if early physicians came up with their medical vocabulary to sanctify and mystify the medical profession. Whatever the purpose, ankylosing spondylitis (AS) sounds like something that grows in deep, dark forests and is dug up by wild hogs. In human terms, it is a chronic progressive disease of the spine that can cause excruciating pain, stiffness and if the spinal joints become fused together, a curved spine and humped back.

Early symptoms are low back pain, pain along the sciatic nerve from buttocks to leg and foot, and stiffness upon rising in the morning. As the affliction progresses, pain and stiffness spread to the neck, arms and the muscles. Its cause, as usual, is subject to debate.

Once again, we're forced to put on our Sherlock Holmes hat, grab the magnifying glass and search for clues.

Osteoporosis of Men

Some researchers believe that osteoporosis may lead to AS. Whatever causes the bones to become brittle and weak, seems to also cause this horrible effect on the spine. What is interesting, however, is that while osteoporosis primarily affects women, ankylosing spondylitis primarily affects men. Ninety percent of cases occur in males from age 20 to 40.[1]

In one study, summarized in *The Lancet*, researchers evaluated bone mineral density, a measurement of bone strength, in 25 healthy men versus 25 men with early stages of AS. They found that not only was the average reduction of bone minerals greater in the AS patients than in the control group, but that they even exceeded levels recorded in postmenopausal women. In other words, men with AS were found to be losing more bone than even postmenopausal women.[2]

The logical course of action, based on this information, is to target bone strengthening nutrients. Here are the nutrients to keep in mind: calcium, vitamin B6, folic acid, silica, vitamins A, C, D and K, manganese, copper and zinc.

Calcium of course is first, although not foremost. There are many reasons dairy foods are not ideal sources of calcium, including their high saturated fat.

Instead of dairy foods, eat high-calcium, low phosphorous foods such as kale, sesame seeds, maple syrup and seaweed.

Too much phosphorous can cause you to lose too much calcium, and vice versa. Avoid soft drinks, they contain too much phosphorous. Instead, eat foods that have the ideal calcium/phosphorous ratio of close to one to one: radishes, apples and pears.

Too much meat protein can also drain off needed calcium. That's because meat is high in sulfur and phosphorous, upsetting the delicate bone balance. To get your daily allowance of complete protein combine whole grains with legumes.

Add a little brewer's yeast to your diet for calcium, zinc, folic acid and vitamin B6, also important to bone formation.

What is probably foremost is silica – a relatively unknown source nutrient necessary for calcium absorption. Green peppers have both vitamin C and silica, both bone enhancers. Best sources of silica are brown rice bran, bell peppers, leafy green vegetables and the herb horsetail.

Cherries and other berries are high in both vitamin C and two flavonoids proven to be osteoporosis-preventives. Concentrate on eating berries when they are in season for help with your skeleton. Rose hip tea is also a tasty source of vitamin C.

If you're home-bound and don't often get out in the sun, consider a food source of vitamin D. Best foods for vitamin D are sardines,

salmon, tuna, egg yolk, sunflower seeds, liver and bee pollen. Vitamin A is also important. A daily dose of cod liver oil will help make
sure you get both of these important nutrients.

A warning about milk. The milk carton says it is fortified with
vitamin D. However, this vitamin D is a hormone, not a nutrient. It
has been shown to actually *decrease* magnesium. And your bones
need magnesium. So lay off the fortified milk or purchase certified
raw milk, which is perfectly safe and much healthier.

Foods For Strong Bones

I've isolated five foods that contain most of the nutrients important to bone formation. They are:

1. Blackstrap molasses. This kind of molasses contains all the
    nutrients left after sugar cane is processed into white table
    sugar. The list is impressive: calcium, copper, manganese,
    vitamin K, and vitamin B6.
2. Soybeans contain vitamin K and zinc. Look for soymeal and
    soy milk too. Tofu is soybean curd, so try it instead of meat
    in salads or stir fries.
3. Eating unsalted raw nuts instead of potato chips will give
    you copper and manganese.
4. When mom said "Eat your vegetables," she more than likely
    was talking about green leafy vegetables. She was right. They
    contain calcium, manganese, vitamin B6 and folic acid.
5. Look to legumes. Beans, peas and lentils contain copper, man-
    ganese, vitamin B6 and folic acid.

Also important in any healthy diet is plenty of fiber and water.
Always eat whole grains and drink at least two quarts of water a day.
Eating whole grains including the bran and germ will help keep toxins moving through your system, and the water will keep nutrients
going where they're supposed to.

Lifestyle is always important. Staying involved in life will encourage you to take care of yourself, and do what it takes to stay
happy and healthy. Part of that lifestyle should include exercise. It is
accepted by both alternative and conventional doctors that exercise

is essential to health and well-being. Studies have shown weight-bearing exercise, where the weight of the body is concentrated on the bones, can actually increase bone density and strength.

AS and Allergy to Dairy Products

Knowing that milk is one of the most common food allergens, researchers in Belgium decided to see if AS patients would improve if they stopped eating dairy products. Twenty-five outpatients were told to exclude milk, cheese, ice cream and butter from their diet.

The researchers found that more than half of the patients with AS noted a subjective improvement of their symptoms within six weeks. They felt better, had less pain and morning stiffness, their joint and spine symptoms decreased and they were able to take less pain medication. A large number of these patients were so satisfied they continued on the diet past the study period for months and even years.[3]

Alan R. Gaby, M.D., has been successfully treating AS patients by identifying their allergies and recommending food allergy nutrients.[4]

For more on allergies and how to identify them, see my ALLERGIES chapter.

AS and Candida

There is a reason dairy products may be causing problems among AS sufferers: they encourage the overgrowth of Candida albicans, a naturally-occurring fungus in the body. Fungus, or yeast, infections caused by Candida, can lead to problems ranging from itching and burning to infertility, immune system problems, rheumatoid arthritis and, apparently, ankylosing spondylitis.

Researchers at King College Hospital in London discovered that when they put AS patients on a low-starch diet, their symptoms subsided. They attributed this to the fact that starch, and starchy food products (like white bread and white rice) encourage the overgrowth of klebsiella bacteria in the bowel, something they found in these patients.[5]

An overgrowth of Candida fungus can allow the klebsiella bacteria to become a problem. Battle the bad with the body's good bacteria to prevent and reduce overgrowth of fungus.[6]

If you suspect yeast infections may be contributing to your AS, see a doctor versed in nutrition. Also read the chapter Fungus Infections in this book. In the meantime, there are many things you can do. Avoid foods high in yeast such as beer and risen breads. Avoid sugar, including honey, fruit juice and jams, and supplement with acidophilus, bifidobacteria and lactobacillus bulgaricus. These are your body's good-buddy bacteria and will help kill the bad guys. You can find these supplements in health food stores. Aged garlic extract will also help cleanse the colon of fungus and bacteria bad guys. Also avoid high fat foods, especially dairy products and fatty meat.[7]

Bone-Boosting Nutrients
For maximum absorption, take supplements with meals.

Nutrient	Suggested Dosage	Formulation
Borage oil	2 capsules daily	
Fiber	4-8 tablets daily	Psyllium, with herb hyssop
Flaxseed oil	1 tablespoon daily	
Glucosamine sulfate	500 mg three times daily	
MSM (Methylsulfonylmethane)	500 mg three times daily	
Multi-mineral	1-4 ounces daily	In liquid solution, with vitamin B12, biotin
Multi-vitamin/mineral	3-6 caplets daily	Freeze-dried plant sources
Niacinamide	1,000 mg twice daily	
Vitamin C	Individual bowel tolerance*	With bioflavonoids (quercetin, rutin proanthocyanidins)
Vitamin E	2 capsules (800 IU)	d-alpha tocopherol
Yucca	300 mg three times daily	

* To determine individual dosage, on the first day take 1,000 mg hourly until diarrhea occurs, then reduce dosage to just below that for individual daily dosage. Vitamin C is not toxic in large doses but must be taken throughout the day to benefit. Divide dosage to three or four times a day.

CHAPTER 10:

Appendicitis

The late British medical surgeon Denis Burkitt liked to use humor to make a point. "Countries with large stools are the ones with small hospitals. And countries with small stools have large hospitals. When compared with world standards, America and England are, you might say, constipated nations."[1]

I met this most enlightened man in Africa, when I was doing my own research on the health benefits of fiber. He spent many years in his native country as a medical-missionary-researcher-clinician noting the lack of digestive maladies, most especially appendicitis, among the high-fiber eating rural Africans. He observed they had a lower incidence of not only appendicitis, but hemorrhoids, diverticular disease, cardiovascular disease, and cancer of the colon compared to industrialized societies where diets are low in fiber.

"Transit time in the nursing homes in Britain takes a fortnight!" he joked, comparing the two-week passage of typical English refined food through the digestive tract to the seven-hour transit time for food in his beloved Africa.

Burkitt bragged about how African kids would run as far as seven miles to school, just for the joy of running. His point was that on their complex carbohydrate and fiber diets, they had plenty of energy to run instead of walk. This was long before our society caught up with the notion that we shouldn't feed our athletes steak, but teach them to "carb up" with carbohydrates for sustained energy.

What is the Appendix?

The appendix is a two to six inch long tube, a bit thicker than a pencil, that dead-ends off the upward turn of the large intestine. When a lack of fiber and water makes waste matter hard to move it backs up, eventually finding its way into the appendix. Once there, how is it going to get out? It's a dead end, remember? It sits until it putrefies, inviting bacteria that produces gas and poisons. These bacteria multiply, increasing the amount of gas and poisons. The appendix swells, getting bigger and bigger until it gets tender, painful and threatens to burst.

The pain may feel like a simple stomachache at first, but if it worsens over time, and seems to center on the lower right area of the stomach, see a doctor at once. When the pain becomes acute, and worsens with movement, the body basically goes into shock. Symptoms include nausea, vomiting, rapid pulse and a mild fever. Muscles over the appendix may tighten in what's called a protective spasm. A rigid stomach is the sign of acute appendicitis and the signal to call the ambulance for a siren-screaming, tire-squealing race to the hospital. If the appendix should burst, the toxins released into the body can kill.

Well-intentioned individuals sometimes try to relieve the victim's pain with a laxative or purgative. This only increases the risk of the appendix bursting, making it more hazardous for the patient and more difficult for the surgeon. No pain medication should be taken.

A Fiber-Healthy Appendix

Obviously, the key to avoiding appendicitis is not to allow waste matter to back up. In other words, avoid chronic constipation.

One study that analyzed the diets of 135 children with appendicitis and 212 without it showed that children who consumed low-fiber diets were twice as likely to develop appendicitis. A brother and sister who basically ate the same foods as they grew up are a case in point. At the age of 14 the boy developed acute appendicitis. The girl never did. The difference in their diets? She enjoyed eating carrots as a snack food, while he preferred potato chips.

Fiber and water are necessary to move waste through smoothly and easily, without stretching or damaging delicate tissues, and without accumulating long enough for bacteria to grow.

Burkitt offers a common sense approach for telling whether or not the diet contains enough fiber and whether or not one is in danger of developing appendicitis.

Typical of his sense of humor, he coins the words "floaters" and "sinkers" to describe healthy versus unhealthy stool consistency. Floaters are stools with enough fiber to make them float in the toilet bowl. Sinkers are heavy and hard and indicate that a person may be headed for problems. Watch, also, how much fiber floats out when you flush the toilet.

Fruits high in moisture, and those which have seeds, are good sources of fiber. Look to watermelon, strawberries and kiwifruit for high-moisture, high fiber food. Fiber is activated by water. Whenever fiber intake increases, the need for fluids increases. Anyone who takes a fiber supplement should drink at least six 10-ounce glasses of water a day, in addition to any other beverages. Without the water, bran cannot move, and you risk getting constipated.

Good sources of vegetable fiber are carrots, celery, radishes, beans, lentils, peas and whole grains. It's the bran part of whole grains that contain fiber. For concentrated fiber, eat just the bran. It is also high in B vitamins, which are essential to the nervous system.

So far as fiber is concerned, seven tablespoons of oat bran daily have been found to keep bowel movements regular and to guard against appendicitis.

An experimental controlled study revealed that eating bran increased the number of bowel movements and reduced intestinal transit time. A report in the *American Journal of Gastroenterology* claims that corn bran is superior to wheat bran.

In another controlled study, 10 grams (less than a tablespoon) of wheat bran two times daily proved markedly superior to a bulk laxative in 10 constipated elderly patients. The bran reduced bowel transit time from 126 hours to 89 hours.

Some top sources of fiber include psyllium, hyssop, oat bran, alfalfa leaves and seeds, bentonite, whey, rhubarb, buckthorn, goldenseal, gentian, ground flax seed, kelp, rice bran, corn bran and wheat bran.

There are some good colon cleansing supplemental formulas on health food store shelves. I "spring clean" using a formula that contains hyssop as a primary ingredient. It was used in biblical times to cleanse the colon and is historically proven to be of excellent benefit to the intestine.

Purge me with hyssop, and I shall be clean... –Psalms 51:7

For more on constipation combatants, see the chapter Constipation.

Do we need our Appendix?

You may think it wise to get rid of this so-called unnecessary intestinal appendage, since it has no real purpose in your life. Aah, but that's where you might be wrong.

It pays to keep your appendix, if possible, say some authorities. Several epidemiological studies indicate that it may protect against cancer, although researchers can't prove it.

A study conducted at the Medical College of (Toledo) Ohio revealed that 67 percent of 1,165 patients who had developed bowel cancer before the age of 50 had their appendixes taken out.[2]

George Padanilam, M.D., one of the researchers, suggests that the appendix may produce antibodies which keep cancer-causing viruses from attacking the colon. He advises against permitting doctors performing other surgery to remove a normal appendix.

Howard R. Bierman, M.D., of the Institute for Cancer and Blood Research, warned a meeting of the American College of Surgeons against removing the appendix prematurely, stating that it may function immunologically such as in protecting against leukemia.[3]

Dr. Bierman's study of 549 persons who died of some kind of

cancer showed that 34.8 percent of them had their appendixes surgically removed, compared with 23.4 percent for the group which didn't develop cancer. Nearly half the people who died of colon or rectal cancer had their appendixes removed. Dr. Bierman, too, cautioned surgeons against taking out normal appendixes while doing other surgery.

`Other researchers have found the incidence of colon cancer lower among those who have retained their healthy appendixes. Vegetarians have a super-low rate of colon cancer, mainly because they get so much fiber from their diets.

Appendicitis-Fighting Nutrients
For maximum absorption, take supplements with meals.

Nutrient	Suggested Dosage	Formulation
Acidophilus	At least four billion flora daily on an empty stomach, three times daily	
Aged garlic extract	1 teaspoon three times daily	Liquid
Amino acids	4-6 capsules daily	Multiple formula from natural sources
Borage oil	2 capsules daily	
Coenzyme Q10	2 capsules daily	With vitamin E, phospholipids and selenium
Flaxseed oil	1 tablespoon daily	
Multi-mineral	3-4 ounces daily	In liquid solution, with vitamin B12, biotin
Multi-vitamin/mineral	6 caplets daily	Freeze-dried plant sources
Vitamin B6	100 mg daily	
Vitamin C	Individual bowel tolerance*	With bioflavonoids (quercetin, rutin proanthocyanidins)

* To determine individual dosage, on the first day take 1,000 mg hourly until diarrhea occurs, then reduce dosage to just below that for individual daily dosage. Vitamin C is not toxic in large doses but must be taken throughout the day to benefit. Divide dosage to three or four times a day.

CHAPTER 11:

Arteriosclerosis

"As the arteries grow hard, the heart grows soft."
–H. L. Mencken

You probably think arteriosclerosis has something to do with the heart. What it means, literally, is hardening, or blockages, of the *arteries*. What it *does*, literally, is stop the blood from flowing. It doesn't take much of an imagination to realize what can happen when blood stops flowing to the brain, the legs or to the heart. Symptoms include excruciatingly painful walking, strokes, heart attacks and brain damage.

What is important to realize is that hardening of the arteries can not only be prevented, but reversed – *without* dangerous surgery.

Chelation Therapy

On my television show, *Maximize Your Life*, I had the opportunity to interview Dr. Ross Gordon, founder and past president of the American College of Advancement in Medicine, and an M.D. practicing in Albany, California. During this interview, I met a man who had his limbs restored to him by Dr. Gordon through chelation therapy.

Dr. Gordon, his patient Virgil Young and Virgil's wife Arvilla appeared together to tell their story. Virgil had intermittent claudication – the arterial blood flow in his lower extremities was being cut off. He couldn't walk without pain, and all the doctors could do was talk of amputating his legs.

"We had no choice, we had to try anything," said Arvilla, sitting in front of me in the television studio, her hands wringing a handkerchief. Virgil continued. "I was very frightened. The big toe on my left leg was dark blue. One doctor callously said to me 'Well, it ain't dead yet!' Arvilla's chiropractor told us about Dr. Gordon."

By the time they turned to Dr. Gordon, Virgil's big toe was on the verge of gangrene. Dr. Gordon started him at once on chelation therapy.

Chelation therapy, simply stated, consists of intravenously administering a solution commonly referred to as EDTA. This compound has the ability to attract fatty deposits (cholesterol plaque) in the veins or arteries, much as a magnet attracts metal filings. As the EDTA passes through the veins and arteries, it absorbs this plaque, which is then excreted in the urine.

By the time the couple got to the end of their story, tears were streaming down their cheeks. I couldn't help but join them as the emotions of their ordeal were relived.

"I saw a miracle happen!" said Virgil. "Before, I ate and ate but was never satisfied. I went from 172 pounds to 149 pounds. Now I'm back to my old weight. I'm healthier, and can walk again! Every chance I get, I tell people about Dr. Gordon."

The amount of time it takes for chelation therapy to work depends on the extent of the damage. It took one man three years to overcome a very bad case of arteriosclerosis. To prevent artery problems, it is important you eat less saturated fat and more plant food: vegetables and fruits.

Garlic – Nature's Chelator

Garlic acts as a natural chelator, thinning the blood and pushing fats and toxins out of the bloodstream. The ancient Greeks used garlic to keep the arteries open. This may be why people living in the Mediterranean have such a low incidence of heart disease.

Studies show that garlic eaten with a fatty meal will dramatically reduce cholesterol and fat levels in the blood. When taken for a couple of months, garlic can drop the level of cholesterol in the blood by 15 percent. A healthy diet can further reduce this hardened-artery risk by 30 percent. A study at Medical Research Council Laboratory in

Oxford, U.K., demonstrated that just half a clove of garlic a day thins the blood and reduces the stickiness that can contribute to plaque buildup.[1] If you must have that pizza, get it with lots of garlic!

The active compounds of aged garlic extract actually inhibit the growth and multiplication of artery lining cells that contribute to arteriosclerotic blockages.[2]

I personally take, and recommend you take, Kyolic® liquid aged garlic extract every day. I've been to the Wakunaga Pharmaceutical Company in Japan, the manufacturer of Kyolic®, and am confident of its quality. To their credit, the Wakunaga scientists have done much valid, scientific research on the health benefits of garlic. I am convinced the science of garlic is truly the science of Kyolic®.

Bioflavonoids

Bioflavonoids, found in citrus fruits and berries, are active in the fight against arterial insufficiency. They act as antioxidants to prevent the deterioration of blood vessels by free radicals, retard inflammation resulting from cellular damage that can contribute to narrowing, and they smooth the artery walls.

Probably the most potent bioflavonoid discovered by researchers is ginkgo biloba. When extracted from the plant and concentrated, it has been shown in studies to be far superior to pentoxifylline, the pharmaceutical treatment of choice for people suffering from intermittent claudication.

Out of nine double-blind randomized clinical trials of ginkgo biloba versus a placebo in patients with diminished leg circulation, all found it to be of significant benefit. Ginkgo biloba, while being poo-pooed by the FDA in the United States, is now among the leading prescription medicines in both Germany and France. The extracts account for one percent and 1.5 percent of total prescription sales in Germany and France respectively. Fortunately, those in need in the U.S. can get it anywhere health food items are sold.[3]

The Importance of B Vitamins

Researchers have shown that up to 20 percent of those with clogged arteries have too much homocysteine in their blood, an amino acid believed to be caused by deficiencies of folic acid and vitamin B6.[4]

In the *Physicians' Health Study*, researchers compared homocysteine levels of the five percent of people having the highest levels of homocysteine with those who had lower levels. Those in the top five percent were linked to a dramatic 3.4-fold greater risk of heart attack.[5]

Dr. Robert Superko, medical director of the Cholesterol Research Center at the Lawrence Berkeley Laboratory University of California screens all his coronary patients for this abnormality and has found that five mg or less per day of folic acid works for 80 percent of his patients. In the event the folic acid doesn't work, he turns to vitamin B6. If that doesn't cause improvement, he tries B6 and folic acid together.[6]

Researchers in the Netherlands found that the aforementioned homocysteine defect, called homocysteinemia, is corrected by a combination of vitamin B6 at 250 mg per day, folic acid of five mg per day and trimethylglycine at six grams per day by themselves or in combination.[7]

When supplementing with any B vitamin, always include a B-complex formula. All the B vitamins are dependent upon one another, and without one, you may have a deficiency of another. The B vitamins are found in whole grains, legumes and blackstrap molasses. For foods that contain the individual B vitamins, see the Food Chart in this book.

Artery-Smart Vitamin E

Anything that lowers the oxidation of cholesterol (called lipid peroxidation) helps guard against hardening of the arteries. What happens is the LDL, or bad cholesterol, combined with the oxygen we breathe, literally becomes rancid in our bloodstreams. The more bad cholesterol there is, the better the chance of damage. Here's what happens: acids from the rancid cholesterol damage the walls of the arteries and make it easier and more likely for plaque to build up. One of the most potent preventives of this process is vitamin E, an antioxidant that counters this oxidative aging process.

Vitamin E is the heart- and vascular-smart vitamin, touted by most doctors and researchers to be beneficial for the circulatory system. It works by not only preventing the oxidation of bad cholesterol, but increasing the good cholesterol. It acts like aspirin in thinning the blood so platelets don't stick together. And in dosages ranging from 300 to 1,600 IU/day, has been shown in studies to help patients suffering from intermittent claudication.

In a recent study, surgeons created a heart attack in rabbits by tying off one of their coronary arteries. If the animals were given extra vitamin E, the seriousness of the attack was reduced by 71 percent![8]

Vitamin E appears so important, in fact, that K. Fred Gey, M.D., and colleagues in Switzerland believe low blood levels of vitamin E place a person more at risk of a heart attack than any other factors including high cholesterol and high blood pressure. Researchers at Harvard School of Public Health recently reported that daily supplements of vitamin E appear to reduce the risk of heart disease by an incredible one-third to one-half.[9]

The artery-clogging effect of cigarette smoking has been found to be helped by vitamin E intake. Undisputed among doctors is the fact that cigarette smoking increases lipid peroxidation, and thus increases the chances of circulation blockages. In one study, reported in the *American Journal of Clinical Nutrition*, 50 men who smoked more than 15 cigarettes a day for 10 years were compared with men who had never smoked. It was found that when either group increased their dietary vitamin E, they had less lipid peroxidation.[10] There is hope out there for all you smokers. Quit if you can, but if you can't, by all means take vitamin E!

Other antioxidants of benefit to blood vessels are vitamin C, selenium and coenzyme Q10, all available at health food stores or through mail order. Selenium has been found to amplify the antioxidant properties of vitamin E and should always be included. For more see the chapters Circulation Problems, Hypertension and Heart Problems.

Arteriosclerosis-Fighting Nutrients
For maximum absorption, take supplements with meals.

Nutrient	Suggested Dosage	Formulation
Aged garlic extract	1 teaspoon three times daily	Liquid
Amino acids	4-6 capsules daily with exercise	Multiple formula from natural sources
Antioxidants	6 capsules daily*	With selenium and grapeseed extract
Borage oil	2 capsules daily	
Coenzyme Q10	4 capsules daily	With vitamin E, phospholipids and selenium
Flaxseed oil	1 tablespoon daily	
Folic acid	5-10 mg daily	
L-Carnitine	500 mg twice daily	
Magnesium	200 mg daily	
Multi-mineral	3-4 ounces daily	In liquid solution, with vitamin B12, biotin
Multi-vitamin/mineral	6 caplets daily	Freeze-dried plant sources
Niacin	500 mg four times daily	
Taurine	500 mg twice daily	
Vitamin B6	100 mg daily	
Vitamin C	Individual bowel tolerance**	With citrus bioflavonoids (quercetin, proanthocyanidins)
Vitamin E	2 capsules (800 IU) daily	d-alpha tocopherol

* The FDA recommends pregnant women not exceed 10,000 IU of vitamin A daily.

** To determine individual dosage, on the first day take 1,000 mg hourly until diarrhea occurs, then reduce dosage to just below that for individual daily dosage. Vitamin C is not toxic in large doses but must be taken throughout the day to benefit. Divide dosage to three or four times a day.

CHAPTER 12:

Arthritis

I once asked the late, great George Burns if he had arthritis. He replied, "I had it when it first came out!"

Your doctor tells you you have arthritis. Can he or she tell you what kind of arthritis you have or what is causing it? These are not unreasonable questions, yet you'll rarely get answers. This is because arthritis is largely a disorder of symptoms – a *syndrome*, to be more accurate. As long as physicians lump symptoms into one category, and don't examine the causes of the symptoms, there can be no hope or cure. All is not lost, however, or you wouldn't be reading this chapter!

Causes of arthritis are: digestive problems, malnutrition, a high-fat diet, chemical sensitivity, food allergies, and even a little organism known as the limax amoeba.

The Allergy Connection

Your body can be its own worst enemy, if you don't treat it right. Researchers consider arthritis an autoimmune disease because the symptoms are caused by the body's immune system attacking its own tissues. Just as we have come to identify red, itchy eyes as an allergic symptom, arthritis must be accepted as another. In getting to the cause of arthritis, we have to look at the possible allergens responsible.

When arthritis patients had their food allergies identified and eliminated, their symptoms ended or were improved.

When it comes to identifying allergens, scratch the conventional tests. The food elimination diet and Coca Pulse Test are much more reliable. Because allergens can cause the heart rate to soar, taking your pulse in the morning upon rising, and comparing it to your rate after eating certain foods will help you target offending foods.

Narrow your list down to the following foods suspect for most allergy sufferers: beef, sugar, chocolate, eggs, citrus fruits, coffee, corn, malt, milk, pork, potatoes, soybeans, spices, tomatoes, wheat and yeast.

Consider also eliminating nightshade foods, which many are allergic to. Approximately one-third of those who suffer from rheumatoid arthritis are sensitive to nightshade plants.[1]

Tobacco is a nightshade. Can you imagine rolling up a leaf of poison ivy and smoking it? That's what people who are allergic to nightshades do when they smoke. Other nightshades are potatoes, tomatoes, eggplant, and peppers. Read your labels! Nightshades can be hidden ingredients in processed foods. Better yet, avoid processed foods altogether. Researchers have found those with allergic symptoms are often sensitive to the 3,000 chemical additives we ingest, plus 10,000 environmental chemical contaminants assaulting our bodies every day.

A lack of hydrochloric acid and digestive enzymes in the stomach, common among people over forty, can also contribute toward food allergies. This slowdown of digestion will also create over-large food molecules which end up in the bloodstream. The defensive reaction by the body to these molecules create the allergic response that leads to arthritis symptoms.

It may sound hopeless, considering the sheer volume of chemical antagonists present in our environment today. But I wouldn't be here if there weren't answers and solutions to the arthritis dilemma.

Nutritional Considerations

As with any ailment, disorder or disease, good nutrition is essential. For such an extreme symptom as arthritis, supplementation is the best way to go.

An imbalance of prostaglandins – too much or too many – can be a source of many common diseases, arthritis for one. Borage oil is a good source of prostaglandins and early tests have shown it to be not only a valuable treatment for arthritis, but a substitute for commonly-used non-steroidal anti-inflammatory drugs (NSAIDs). NSAIDs have dangerous side effects. Frequent use causes stomach ulcers and liver and kidney disease. Deaths have even been associated with NSAID use.

Gamma linolenic acid, or GLA, present in borage oil, evening primrose oil or black currant seed oil, is one of the natural components of the prostaglandin chain disturbed by NSAIDs.

Researchers from the Arthritis and Metabolic Bone Disease Research Unit in Pellenberg, Belgium studied 90 patients with rheumatoid arthritis who were treated with three supplementations: 2.6 gm of omega-3 fatty acids, 1.3 gm of omega-3 fatty acids plus 3 gm of olive oil or six grams of olive oil. There was significant improvement only in those taking 2.6 gm of omega-3 fatty acids per day. Patients taking this daily dosage improved markedly, and were able to reduce their medications. This improvement was apparent after three months of supplementation and tended to increase throughout the 12-month study.[2]

It can get very confusing when talking about the different kinds of fatty acids, which are the kinds of fats we need for energy and health – **not** saturated fat from meat and dairy products and certainly **not** transfatty acids from hydrogenated margarine and foods. Suffice it to say that omega-3 fatty acids are found in fish oil and omega-6 fatty acids are found in vegetable and seed oils. The best source of omega-6 is borage oil, and is rich in gamma linolenic acid (GLA). GLA is a notoriously excellent anti-inflammatory. Take borage oil, obtained in health food stores or through mail order, while reducing NSAID dosage, and continue afterwards.

While copper bracelets for arthritis have been ridiculed by conventional doctors, researchers have found it is the copper absorbed through the skin that helps arthritis by restoring a common deficiency and boosting the immune system. However, zinc also must be taken to maintain an essential balance of the two.[3]

A zinc and copper balance may be particularly aggravated if there is also an overload of iron. Iron can accumulate in certain joints of the body, cause the joints to swell and inflame, and throw off the immune system.

Because of impaired absorption of nutrients, I recommend arthritics take their minerals in solution. I take one that has precipitated out the iron. Never take just one mineral without supplementing with a multi-mineral formula first!

Other arthritis nutritionals are the B vitamins, vitamin C, vitamin E, calcium and the amino acid histidine.

Researchers at Tufts University in Boston evaluated vitamin B6 levels in 23 adults with rheumatoid arthritis and compared them to 23 healthy control subjects. They found blood levels of B6 were lower in the rheumatoid arthritic patients.[4]

Stress, coupled with a deficiency of pantothenic acid (B5) and pyridoxine (B6), has shown in studies to bring on arthritis symptoms. Whenever you are in stressful situations, be sure and supplement with a B vitamin complex. The B vitamins all work together to make sure your nervous system stays healthy. They are found in whole grains, legumes and blackstrap molasses. For foods that contain the individual B vitamins, see the Food Chart in this book.

Vitamin C is another arthritis essential. Studies have shown vitamin C, enhanced with bioflavonoids, reduces inflammation and thins synovial joint fluid, contributing to easier and greater range of motion. There are many foods that contain more vitamin C than oranges. They include papaya, guava, black currants, cantaloupe, strawberries, chili peppers, parsley, broccoli and kale.

Check Your Calcium

A calcium deficiency can actually cause arthritis symptoms. But if you think just taking calcium supplements will help, think again. There are many, many factors that can block calcium from going where it is needed. Magnesium, for example. Magnesium is the traffic cop that tells calcium where to go. Without enough magnesium, calcium accumulates in the joints. Because of the high absorption rate of minerals in solution, and deficiency of magnesium in the diet, the ratio of magnesium and calcium in solution should be four to one, respectively. For more on the importance of the calcium/magnesium ratio, see the Heart chapter.

Instead of dairy foods, which are high in saturated fat and can be allergens, eat high-calcium, low phosphorous foods such as kale, sesame seeds, maple syrup and seaweed.

Too much phosphorous can cause you to lose too much calcium, and vice versa. Avoid soft drinks, they contain too much phosphorous. Instead, eat foods that have the ideal calcium/phosphorous ratio of close to one to one: radishes, apples and pears.

Too much meat protein can also drain off needed calcium. That's because meat is high in sulfur and phosphorous, upsetting the delicate balance. To get your daily allowance of complete protein combine whole grains with legumes.

Add a little brewer's yeast in your diet for calcium, zinc, folic acid and vitamin B6, each essential to bones and tissues.

Ultraviolet light from the sun is important in calcium metabolism. It converts skin oil to vitamin D which transports calcium from the stomach to the blood. Essential fatty acids – already discussed in relation to prostaglandins – are vital in the transport of calcium from the blood to the tissues.

A lack of the amino acid histidine, a vital building block protein in the body, has been linked to arthritis. Although the jury is still out on exactly how much is needed, eating foods rich in histidine can only help. They are: whole eggs, corn germ, fish, wheat germ, soybean meal, brown rice, whole wheat, brewer's yeast, peas and beans.

Niacin has been shown in studies to help with range of motion. Foods rich in niacin – vitamin B3 – include fish, brewer's yeast, peanuts, rice bran and cheese.

Doctors at an Israeli hospital discovered vitamin E helps arthritis symptoms. Foods high in vitamin E include liver, eggs, cold-pressed oil, wheat germ and molasses.

The potential benefits of exercise in treating arthritis is well known. Once arthritis patients get into a regular exercise program, their joints feel better. Moderate exercise helps shed the extra pounds that put weight on sore joints, it helps preserve good muscle tone, good bone formation, and increases range of movement. Exercise keeps us fit – physically, as well as mentally.

Natural Anti-Inflammatories

Just as there are foods to avoid, there are foods to target in an arthritis-avoidance diet. Researchers and others have discovered the benefits of pineapple, specifically its healing enzyme bromelain, known for its potent anti-inflammatory (pain-killing) effect.

Cherries and cherry juice, because of the bioflavonoids they contain, have been found to alleviate gout. Black currants are high in vitamin C and bioflavonoids, and touted for arthritis. Other foods recommended for arthritis are: yucca, raw potato juice, apple cider vinegar and honey, goat's milk, ginger, licorice extract, the spice tumeric, alfalfa tea, and couch grass tea.

Yucca, a southwest desert plant, can sometimes be found in supermarkets. Its juice has been used for centuries by Native Americans for arthritis.

According to a researcher from the Institute of Odense in Denmark, rheumatoid arthritis sufferers were relieved of joint pain after consuming either five grams of fresh ginger root or 1/2 to 1-1/2 grams of ginger powder every day for three months.

Licorice, specifically Glycyrrhiza, has valuable anti-inflammatory properties. Licorice contains a remarkable chemical called glycyrrhetinic acid or GA, which is effective for treating arthritis.

Clinical trials in New Zealand, as well as double-blind trials in Paris, Glasgow, Toronto, and other parts of the world, have proved that green-lipped mussel extract, encapsulated, is particularly effective for arthritic and rheumatic conditions.[5]

The shark is a unique creature in that it is apparently immune to cancer and arthritis. Scientists have found shark cartilage contains a protein substance that strongly inhibits development of new blood networks. Called an anti-angiogenic factor, the property works to not only inhibit the production of cancerous cells, but has been found in research studies to reduce pain and increase mobility in people with arthritis.[6]

Green mussel extract and shark cartilage powder are available in health food stores or through mail order.

Turmeric is also a renowned anti-inflammatory. To be more exact, it is the curcumin, that which gives tumeric its yellow color, that has been found in studies to work better than even ibuprofen, a popular over-the-counter pain medicine. In one study on rats, researchers found 20 mg of curcumin worked as well as 200 mg of ibuprofen.[7]

Another study compared this active ingredient to hydrocortisone acetate and phenylbutazone, other potent pharmaceuticals used for arthritis symptoms. Researchers found that in rats, the curcumin worked just as well as the drugs. No toxic effects from curcumin have been reported.[8] Curcumin and tumeric are available on your supermarket spice shelves but for more exact dosages, look for anti-inflammatory formulas in your health food store.

The Crab and Osteoarthritis

What does the crab have to do with osteoarthritis? Its shell is used to create a treatment that has been shown in experiments to regenerate damaged cartilage and even reverse the disease process. What is this amazing medicine? It is glucosamine sulfate, derived from chitin, that which is found in the exoskeleton of arthropods like the crab.

Glucosamine naturally occurs in the joint cartilage of humans and has been shown to both inhibit cartilage breakdown and promote cartilage repair. Sulfate is added because it enhances the healing effect of glucosamine. In one study, patients receiving glucosamine sulfate had a 71 percent improvement compared to a placebo group.[9]

In another study, 40 patients being treated for osteoarthritis of the knee received 500 mg three times a day of glucosamine sulfate or 1.2 gm a day of ibuprofen. By the eighth week the glucosamine sulfate was pronounced more effective than ibuprofen.[10]

While it takes longer for benefits to be noted with glucosamine sulfate, it does seem to reverse the disease process and results are longer lasting and more pronounced than standard therapy. Currently, glucosamine is considered a nutritional supplement and is therefore available in health food stores.

Arthritis-Fighting Nutrients
For maximum absorption, take supplements with meals.

Nutrient	Suggested Dosage	Formulation
Aged garlic extract	1 teaspoon three times daily	Liquid
Amino acids	4-6 capsules daily	Multiple formula from natural sources
Antioxidants	4 capsules daily*	With selenium and grapeseed extract
Borage oil	2 capsules daily	
Bromelain	200 mg twice daily	
Flaxseed oil	1 tablespoon daily	
Ginger	500 mg after meals daily	
Glucosamine sulfate	500 mg three times daily with yucca	
Magnesium	200 mg daily	
Melatonin (adults only)	3 mg daily at bedtime	With B vitamins
MSM (methylsulfonylmethane)	500 mg three times daily	
Multi-mineral	3-4 ounces daily	In liquid solution, with vitamin B12, biotin
Multi-vitamin/mineral	6 caplets daily	Freeze-dried plant sources
Niacinamide	1,000 mg twice daily	
Quercetin	400 mg twice daily	With vitamin C
Taurine	3 grams daily	
Vitamin B6	200 mg daily	
Vitamin C	Individual bowel tolerance**	With bioflavonoids (quercetin, rutin proanthocyanidins)
Yucca	300 mg three times daily	

* The FDA recommends pregnant women not exceed 10,000 IU of vitamin A daily.

** To determine individual dosage, on the first day take 1,000 mg hourly until diarrhea occurs, then reduce dosage to just below that for individual daily dosage. Vitamin C is not toxic in large doses but must be taken throughout the day to benefit. Divide dosage to three or four times a day.

CHAPTER 13:

Asthma

"We have an emergency here, doctor!"

I was in Dr. Ross Gordon's waiting room, when I overheard these disturbing words from his receptionist. A very frightened woman had her five year old son in her arms, and he was wheezing and gasping horribly for breath. The door slammed open and in walked Dr. Gordon. He quickly surveyed the situation and scooped up the child, marching back into the examining area, the distraught mother trailing behind.

I waited with bated breath, along with the others who had witnessed the crisis situation, for word on the boy's fate. We exhaled audibly when the boy and his mother stepped into the room, beaming happily.

"Thank you so much, doctor," she was saying. "I feel confident now that this will never happen again."

Later, when I saw Dr. Gordon, I asked him what happened. He told me the boy had been playing when he suddenly suffered an asthma attack. I asked him what he did for it.

"I gave him magnesium," was his answer.

"That's all?"

"That's all," he responded.

Magnanimous Magnesium

A deficiency of magnesium can cause asthma and an intravenous shot of magnesium can stop even the most acute asthmatic attack. Researchers at the University of Nottingham's Division of Respiratory Medicine found that of 2,633 asthmatics, those whose dietary magnesium intake was above the average 380 mg a day showed significantly improved lung function and less wheezing. Low blood levels of magnesium is a factor in causing allergies and asthma in the first place.[1] *The American Journal of Medicine* cites numerous clinical trials that showed the benefit of magnesium in treating asthma.[2] A study in *The Lancet*, a well-respected British medical journal, found that magnesium has an independent, beneficial influence on lung function, airway responsiveness, and wheezing in a general population.[3] This means that getting enough magnesium in the diet can prevent the symptoms that lead to asthma and keep an attack from being life-threatening. Apparently, magnesium helps the body control muscle spasms and is able to smooth the bronchial muscles so they don't contract and close off air.

It is ironic that some of the drugs used to treat asthma can cause magnesium depletion. Dr. Alan Gaby recommends asthmatics on medication take 200-600 mg of supplemental magnesium a day.[4]

One of the recommendations Dr. Gordon made to his patient was that his mother increase the amount of magnesium-rich foods in his diet and give him magnesium in solution. Foods high in magnesium are whole wheat, pumpkin seeds, millet, almonds, Brazil nuts and hazel nuts, dark-green vegetables and molasses.

Because there are so few areas in the body where magnesium is absorbed, a deficiency of stomach acid can cause a magnesium deficiency. Digestive enzyme supplements and a teaspoon of vinegar after eating are ways to help this problem, but to be sure you get your magnesium, take a good, easily absorbable, derived-from-nature magnesium blend in solution.

Asthma as an Allergic Response

Children with asthma haven't changed much since 1931, or for that matter since 31 B.C. What has changed is our understanding of the problem. Asthma is largely due to allergies.

One of the key categories of foods to avoid are dairy products. Israeli researchers found that when 22 asthma sufferers were taken off milk and related products, 15 responded with dramatic improvement. Then the fortunate 15 were challenged again with dairy products, and five experienced severe asthma attacks.[5]

It is now commonly recommended babies do not drink cow's milk before the age of one, until their immature digestive systems have had a chance to fully develop.

Asthma can be brought on by many causes: food and beverages, and the sulfites in them, or environmental allergens: fresh paint, perfumes, spray deodorants, cigarette smoke, gasoline or car exhaust fumes; hay, wood, coal or chalk dust; various chemicals such as cleaning solvents, household cleaners and insecticides; pollens and molds. Home humidifiers and air conditioners have been identified as harbors of bronchial-constricting molds. When eliminating offending allergens, leave no filter unchanged.

Obviously, the hardest part can be just finding out what caused the asthma. Yellow No. 5, a food coloring also known as tartrazine, has been reported to cause severe asthma. This is just one of many food additives contained in processed foods. If you or someone you know has asthma or breathing problems, and can't identify the cause, try to abstain from processed foods for a while and see if it doesn't get better. Consider investing in a food dehydrator or buy unprocessed dried fruit from a health food store during the winter when fresh food may be scarce.

The chronic use of antibiotics at an early age may be associated with asthma and allergies in children.

An Overlooked Cause

A little-known contributor to asthma is a high intake of polyunsaturated fatty acids (PUFAs), present in various vegetable and nut oils: corn, safflower, soy, sunflower seed, peanut and walnut, among others.[6]

The cholesterol craze and frenzied promotion of polyunsaturated fats over saturated fats have caused many individuals to overdo it a bit – like taking four tablespoons of vegetable oil, once recommended by the American Heart Association. Without added vitamin E, PUFAs can destroy cells, including those of the lung tissue.

Animal experiments show that in such circumstances, red blood cells tend to accumulate in arteries and reduce or block blood flow and oxygen delivery, a serious occurrence when coupled with air pollution found in most metropolitan areas, and stress.

Alleviating Symptoms the Natural Way

Vitamin C may offer relief of asthma. In three experiments, an inability to breathe was controlled for three or four hours by ingestion of 500 mg of vitamin C.

Yale University researchers exposed six healthy young male subjects to methacholine, a drug which tightens the bronchi and decreases breathing ability. When they took 1,000 mg of vitamin C an hour before exposure, their airflow was reduced by just nine percent – a more than four-fold improvement than what would have been expected.[7]

In experimental studies the bioflavonoid quercetin was found to prevent the wheezing symptoms associated with allergies. Bioflavonoids are notorious anti-inflammatories and help keep the bronchial tubes from swelling, a common asthma symptom. This bioflavonoid has also been found to benefit asthmatics, as it blocks formation of leukotrienes – vicious little compounds that cause the bronchial tissue in the lungs to constrict, making breathing difficult.

Honey with pollen has its followers among asthma sufferers. Dr. U. Wahn, M.D., a researcher at Heidelberg University Children's Clinic in Germany, studied 70 children with hay fever and allergy-related asthma who drank a solution of bee pollen and honey each day during the yearly hay fever period and three days per week in winter. Most of them showed fewer symptoms after this regime, indicating to Dr. Wahn that the pollen somehow made it into the bloodstream.[8] Probably the reason this regimen worked is that the bees were taking the pollen from the actual plants the children were allergic to. Others who have tried it say it is essential that the honey be taken from the same area where the allergic person resides. If you live in the country and find yourself sneezing in the spring, try to find a local beekeeper from whom you can get honey.

Cayenne pepper, or capsicum, acts as an expectorant. Not only does it sting the sinuses and bring tears to the eyes, it temporarily irritates the stomach and sets up a sympathetic reaction in the bronchial tubes and lungs to increase fluids and discharge mucus, making the lungs and tubes less thick and sticky and more open for breathing. Important, however, is drinking lots of water to make it easier for the mucus to thin out and be discharged.

More Solutions

When it comes to allergic asthma, you can't go wrong with chili peppers. Not only do they break up mucus, but they contain lots of vitamin C. Half a cup of hot chili peppers added to your omelet or in a recipe will give you 182 milligrams of vitamin C.

It turns out spicy foods for colds, asthma and sinus problems have been used for centuries by early civilizations. Ancient Egyptian medical writings recommended mustard for respiratory therapy. Hippocrates prescribed vinegar and pepper as respiratory medicines; and Oriental medicine still uses hot peppers, black pepper, mustard, garlic, tumeric and other spices to treat colds and asthma.

In more modern times, researchers at Montreal General Hospital found that the active ingredient in tumeric, curcumin, acts as an antihistamine in reducing the symptoms of allergies and asthma.[9]

If you have hay fever, eat a spicy meal at least once a day, or down a glass of water sprinkled with ten or twenty drops of Tabasco sauce, or chew on chili peppers. Also try a teaspoon of ground horseradish, add a glass of warm water and a little honey and drink it. Or mix up some garlicky-rich chicken soup with a hefty dash of red or black pepper.

Sometimes honey, chili peppers and other folk remedies don't do the job so reinforcements have to be brought in – vitamins with a higher potency than natural foods can provide, when we consider the limitation of stomach capacity.

Stress-less Nutrition

Eight out of 10 asthmatic children respond favorably to vitamin therapy. Injections of vitamin B12 are impressively effective in eliminating asthma. Not coincidentally, B vitamins get depleted in a body wracked by stress. I can't think of anything more stressful than the inability to breathe!

Early studies revealed that many asthma patients are dependent on vitamin B6 (pyridoxine). They do not have a deficiency as such, but an exaggerated need, due to an error in metabolism.

On this basis, five New York physicians designed a five-month, double-blind experiment with 76 youthful patients with moderate to severe asthma. Half of the patients were given two 100 mg tablets of vitamin B6. The other half received placebos.[10]

One month passed, and there was almost no difference between the two groups. However, with the start of the second month, the patients receiving the vitamin B6 had fewer asthma attacks and less breathing difficulty, wheezing and coughing.

The differences continued to be even more marked between the second and fifth months, with the researchers concluding that vitamin B6 reduces the severity of asthma attacks with no side effects, compared with the devastating side effects of prednisone, a steroid drug frequently used to manage asthma.

Even smaller amounts of B6 – 50 mg daily – appear to lessen the duration, frequency, and severity of asthma attacks. Dr. Robert Reynolds, a U.S. Department of Agriculture biochemist, reported that the symptoms of every asthmatic on this daily regime were relieved.[11]

Asthma-Fighting Nutrients
For maximum absorption, take supplements with meals.

Nutrient	Suggested Dosage	Formulation
Aged garlic extract	1 teaspoon three times daily	Liquid
Antioxidants	4 capsules daily*	With selenium and grapeseed extract
Borage oil	2 capsules daily	
Flaxseed oil	1 tablespoon daily	
Magnesium	200 mg daily	
MSM (methylsulfonylmethane)	500 mg three times daily	
Multi-mineral	3-4 ounces daily	In liquid solution, with vitamin B12, biotin
Multi-vitamin/mineral	6 caplets daily	Freeze-dried plant sources
Niacinamide	1,000 mg twice daily	
Quercetin	400 mg twice daily	With vitamin C
Taurine	3 grams daily	
Vitamin B6	200 mg daily	
Vitamin C	Individual bowel tolerance**	With bioflavonoids (quercetin, rutin proanthocyanidins)

* The FDA recommends pregnant women not exceed 10,000 IU of vitamin A daily.

** To determine individual dosage, on the first day take 1,000 mg hourly until diarrhea occurs, then reduce dosage to just below that for individual daily dosage. Vitamin C is not toxic in large doses but must be taken throughout the day to benefit. Divide dosage to three or four times a day.

CHAPTER 14:

Athlete's Foot

Non-athletes seem to have the monopoly on athlete's foot; fungus-caused reddish, cracked and itchy skin between the toes–mainly between the little toe and its too-close neighbor.

This is because athletes know how to protect themselves from the fungus among us, like wearing sandals when walking on the damp floors of athletic club shower and steam rooms, public swimming pools or on the much-traveled carpeting of motel and hotel rooms.

The husband of a dear friend of mine developed complications from his athlete's foot. He proved to be allergic to the salve given to him by the doctor, and his feet swelled up to almost twice their size. The cracks between his reddened and puffy toes migrated to the top of his feet, and fungus worked its way under his toenails.

His faith lost in orthodox medicine, he tried a folk remedy. We told him about an apple cider vinegar and water foot soak. When I told him about it, he was afraid the fiery burn of the vinegar would launch him through the roof. But he had to see if it worked.

He poured a cup of apple cider vinegar and a few quarts of warm water into a white enameled basin, sat on a chair, and gingerly lowered his feet into the basin. Somehow, he was able to stand it for 15 minutes. Strangely, his feet felt better.

That night, he repeated the process, and the swelling began to subside. He did the same thing every morning and night for a week. Apparently the warm water opened the pores and let the vinegar penetrate. Each time he would blot his feet dry with a clean Turkish towel. After another week of self-medication, he was healed. The fungus was gone – even from under his toenails.

I found out later that his problem had started when he was prescribed a lengthy series of antibiotic injections to combat a persistent infection. The antibiotics had eventually killed the harmful bacteria, and with it the intestinal organisms which synthesize B vitamins.

Without those B vitamins his immunity was lowered and his body had no resistance to the fungus. To restore the natural flora in his digestive tract, I had him eat a quart of quality yogurt daily (live cultures of acidophilus) and take supplements including minerals in solution, and a formula that uses freeze dried sprouts and vegetables, combined in such a way as to provide all the essential vitamins and minerals, as well as adding odorless garlic, acidophilus and green tea extract for immune-system boosting.

Other victims of athlete's foot have found dabbing diluted vinegar between their toes morning and night works to clear it up. Open sandals help keep feet dry, and one man I know walked around with cotton balls between his toes to keep them dry.

Tea tree oil is the best treatment I know for fungal infections of the skin. It will also clear up fungal infections of the toenails and fingernails, a condition notoriously resistant to treatment, even by strong systemic antibiotics. You just paint the oil on affected areas two or three times a day. To cleanse infected wounds, apply a 10 percent solution of the oil, or about one and a half teaspoons to a cup of warm water.

As with so many human disorders, prevention is easier than the cure. Less than Ten Commandments can help you avoid athlete's foot for a lifetime.

Thou Shalt Not:
1. Walk barefoot in public places.
2. Wear shoes made partially or wholly from synthetic (man-made) materials.
   Since leather works for the cow, it'll work for your feet.
3. Wear wet shoes or socks.

4. Wear socks made of synthetic fabrics. Wool or cotton are best.
5. Fail to dry feet thoroughly after bath or swimming.

Common sense will tell you how to avoid athlete's foot. And if you find you're prone to it, be especially careful and use cornstarch to powder your feet. Cornstarch is good at absorbing moisture, and it's cheaper than expensive powders with unknown additives. For more on fighting the fungus that infiltrate your feet, read my chapter Fungus Infections.

Fungus-Fighting Nutrients
For maximum absorption, take supplements with meals.

Nutrient	Suggested Dosage	Formulation
Acidophilus	At least four billion flora daily on an empty stomach, three times daily	
Aged garlic extract	1 teaspoon three times daily	Liquid
Borage oil	2 capsules daily	
Caprylic acid	100 mg three times daily	
Fiber	4-8 tablets daily	Psyllium, with herb hyssop
Flaxseed oil	1 tablespoon daily	
Grapefruit seed extract	100 mg three times daily	
Multi-mineral	1-4 ounces daily	In liquid solution, with vitamin B12, biotin
Multi-vitamin/mineral	3-6 caplets daily	Freeze-dried plant sources
Vitamin C	Individual bowel tolerance*	With bioflavonoids (quercetin, rutin proanthocyanidins)

* To determine individual dosage, on the first day take 1,000 mg hourly until diarrhea occurs, then reduce dosage to just below that for individual daily dosage. Vitamin C is not toxic in large doses but must be taken throughout the day to benefit. Divide dosage to three or four times a day.

CHAPTER 15:

Attention Deficit Disorder/ Hyperactivity/Autism

My friend was sure her three-year-old daughter Jane was hyperactive. The young child cried over everything, couldn't sit still for five minutes, talked incessantly, and couldn't concentrate long enough to even brush her teeth. Frustrated, her mother took Jane to the physician. Her doctor told her the child had attention deficit disorder (ADD) and prescribed the pharmaceutical drug Ritalin.

"Jane went from bad to worse," said her concerned mother. "She went from being energetic and enthusiastic to having no emotions whatsoever. I didn't want a tranquilized child, I wanted a normal child!"

After I talked to her, Jane took her daughter off the Ritalin, eliminated all processed foods from her diet and supplemented with magnesium and vitamin B6. Jane is back to being enthusiastic and energetic, but has a lot more self-control and is less prone to hysterics.

When supplementing with any B vitamin, always include a B-complex formula. All the B vitamins are dependent upon one another, and without one, you may have a deficiency of another. The B vitamins are found in whole grains, legumes and blackstrap molasses. For foods that contain the individual B vitamins, see the Food Chart in this book.

What's the difference between attention deficit disorder and hyperactivity? The nineties. It was in the '90s that doctors elevated the definition of hyperactivity to include ADD. Now they call it "attention-deficit hyperactivity disorder" (ADHD).

Conventional medicine considers it the most common

neurobehavioral disorder of childhood. An article in *Postgraduate Medicine* sums up the prevailing attitude. The authors estimate that from one to ten percent of school-aged children have it, "depending on the criteria used for diagnosis."[1] In other words, who your doctor is has more to do with whether your child has ADHD, than his biology.

Even more shocking is how they propose doctors treat it. The authors say, "The use of stimulant medication (Ritalin, Dexedrine and Cylert) is the most effective intervention for ADHD. Doses should begin at the low end of the range and be increased every two weeks until either an effective response is obtained or significant side effects are noted." In other words, treat it with useless drugs until the side effects become worse than the original problem. And they call this medicine? Their list of side effects include loss of appetite, insomnia, stomachache, headache, dizziness, drowsiness, dry mouth, constipation, sadness, oversensitivity, irritability, euphoria, anxiety, nightmares, a fast heart rate and hypertension. As if the side effects weren't enough, the use of pharmaceuticals to treat childhood hyperactivity can lead to adult schizophrenia. This is because children grow so rapidly, heavy chemicals or metals can actually become integrated in the tissues, causing permanent imbalances or metabolic dysfunctions. Think very seriously before you allow your children to take pharmaceuticals.

According to Eric Jones, N.D., the Dean of Academic Affairs at Bastyr College in Seattle, at least 50 percent of ADD children have been misdiagnosed. He has personally found in his practice that 80 to 85 percent have been misdiagnosed.[2]

What is probably safe to say is that any diagnosis of ADD, hyperactivity and even autism is a misdiagnosis. Why? Because they are not diseases, they are symptoms. A true diagnosis would be allergies, magnesium deficiency or a B vitamin deficiency.

Allergies and Behavioral Disorders

According to the FDA, approximately 5,000 food additives are used in food products in the United States. Food additives are just one of many chemicals ingested by children that have been linked to

ADD and autism.

Dr. Ben Feingold, a prominent allergist at San Francisco's Kaiser-Permanente Group Medical Center, investigated hyperactivity in children for 40 years. Within a ten year span, Dr. Feingold noted the number of hyperactive children in California skyrocketed from two to 25 percent, while the use of artificial colorings, flavorings and preservatives in foods soared even higher percentage-wise. Feingold saw a connection, took his young hyperactive patients off junk foods, and many of them recovered dramatically.

Feingold once said he could switch his patients on or off merely by regulating their diet. The major culprits were soft drinks, baked goods and bottled, canned and packaged foods heavy in refined carbohydrates, and chemicalized with additives.

The evidence is so compelling, even the government has conceded the possibility. Officials at the 1982 National Institutes of Health Consensus Development Conference on Defined Diets and Childhood Hyperactivity decided that further investigation into the role food additives play in ADD is warranted.

Bonnie J.Kaplan, Ph.D. and her colleagues at the University of Calgary in Alberta hypothesized that younger children and those with somatic symptoms (sleep disorders, allergic symptoms, etc.) as well as a diagnosis of hyperactivity would be most vulnerable to the effects of diet. They selected 24 boys aged three and a half to six years diagnosed with hyperactivity. The researchers prepared all the food for the boys during a four-week experimental phase and a three-week control phase. The experimental diet broadly eliminated food dyes, flavorings, preservatives, chocolate, caffeine, and any additional substances the parents felt might adversely affect their child. Ten of the 24 had significant improvement in their behavior, according to their parents.

Food dyes may play a role in autism. Autistic individuals should eat a diet of whole, unprocessed alkalinizing foods such as vegetables because many autistics' blood is overly acidic. Foods with yellow, red and green dyes should be eliminated, as well as aspartame, an artificial sweetener, and anything with processed sugar.[3]

Food allergies have been linked to behavioral symptoms, especially dairy products, wheat and processed sugar.

Doris J. Rapp, M.D., has done numerous fascinating studies on children and allergies which she discusses in her book, *The Impossible Child*. Through handwriting samples, the changes a child undergoes when exposed to an allergen are vividly portrayed, along with the samples that show when the reaction has been neutralized. You can try this at home if your child exhibits sudden personality changes or mood swings. She notes that hyperactive kids are often unable to confine their writing to a regular size piece of paper, or may suddenly switch from the right to the left side of the paper during schoolwork.

Other allergic-related characteristics that often accompany ADD are being very ticklish or overly sensitive (like the child who absolutely refuses to wear a certain shirt because it "feels scratchy") and more obvious signs like constant sniffles or stuffiness, circles under the eyes, eczema and food cravings.[4] See the chapter on Allergies for more.

Vitamin and Mineral Deficiencies

It is well-known that a deficiency of vitamin B6 can cause behavioral symptoms from senile dementia to schizophrenia. Now we can add hyperactivity and autism to that list.

Researchers both in the United States and abroad have demonstrated very clearly that 30 to 60 percent of autistic children and adults show significant behavioral and other benefits from administration of large amounts of vitamin B6 and magnesium.[5] Magnesium is important because the body cannot use vitamin B6 without it. A magnesium deficiency has been shown to cause both hypersensitivity and hyperirritability, symptoms associated with both autism and attention deficit disorder.[6]

A study published in a 1979 issue of *Biological Psychiatry* compared the effectiveness of Ritalin and vitamin B6 in a group of hyperactive boys. The B6 was found to work better and the benefits lasted longer than the Ritalin.[7]

Calcium is very important to the growth of brain transmitters, and a deficiency is associated with seizures. For this reason researchers at the Autism Research Institute in San Diego decided to study it. They found that four patients with autism who were hitting or poking their eyes had hypocalcinuria, a fancy name for a calcium deficiency. Three of these patients reduced or stopped their self-injury when they took calcium supplements.[8]

Vital to note is the importance of magnesium with calcium. Calcium will not travel where it should without magnesium as a crossing guard. When supplementing with one, always target the other. Better yet, look for a mineral blend in solution so they all work together for the best benefit to the brain. Because of the high absorption rate of minerals in solution, and deficiency of magnesium in the diet, the ratio of magnesium and calcium in solution should be four to one, respectively.

ADHD/Autism-Fighting Nutrients
For maximum absorption, take supplements with meals.

Nutrient	Suggested Dosage	Formulation
Antioxidants	2 capsules daily*	With selenium and grapeseed extract
Borage oil	2 capsules daily	
Flaxseed oil	1 tablespoon daily	
Aged garlic extract	1 teaspoon daily	Liquid
Magnesium	50 mg daily	
Multi-mineral	1 ounce daily	In liquid solution, with vitamin B12, biotin
Multi-vitamin/mineral	2 caplets daily	Freeze-dried plant sources
Niacinamide	100 mg three times daily	
Quercetin	50 mg twice daily	With vitamin C
Taurine	500 mg daily	
Vitamin B6	200 mg daily	
Vitamin C	Individual bowel tolerance**	With bioflavonoids (quercetin, proanthocyanidins)

Herbal teas from chamomile, passion flower and valerian.

* The FDA recommends pregnant women not exceed 10,000 IU of vitamin A daily.

** To determine individual dosage, on the first day take 1,000 mg hourly until diarrhea occurs, then reduce dosage to just below that for individual daily dosage. Vitamin C is not toxic in large doses but must be taken throughout the day to benefit. Divide dosage to three or four times a day.

CHAPTER 16:

Back Pain and Sciatica

When you get aches and pains, it's because your body is trying to tell you something. As you get older, your body becomes more talkative.

Dr. Jonathan Wright, M.D., writes in his book, *Dr. Wright's Book of Nutritional Therapy*, about a patient who had a degenerative spinal disk. The patient had seen Dr. Wright for his sciatica and now was left with only the back pain he'd had for the last three years to which he had resigned himself.

"Have you tried taking any vitamin C for your back pain?" asked Dr. Wright. "Vitamin C? For back pain? I thought that was for colds," responded the patient.

"It's for that too," replied the doctor. " It also helps in many cases of back pain from slight disk deterioration. Dr. James Greenwood, a neurosurgeon from Houston, Texas, discovered that it helped many of his patients. Your x-ray doesn't look extremely bad. It might work for you. Frequently the required amount is 2,000 to 3,000 mg daily. You can obtain 500 or 1,000 mg tablets. Split the dosage over the course of a day."

The patient returned in several months to report the pain was gone. "The sciatica never came back," he reported. "That's the first time it's been gone this long since the accident. My lower spine pain doesn't bother me any at all. Two weeks after I started that extra vitamin C, it went away and hasn't returned. I've been pain-free for the first time since 1968." Observed the patient's wife: "He's less grouchy than he's been since 1967, too."[1]

When You Overdo It

My husband liked to demonstrate his prowess on the football play-ing field by hurting his back. He'd come home moaning and groaning, bent over like an old man. I'd head to the nutritional-medicine cabinet and come back with vitamin C plus bioflavonoids.

Bioflavonoids, a group of substances related to vitamin C, has been shown in studies to speed the healing of bruised muscles, not surprising considering they are powerful anti-inflammatories. A report in *Medical Times* reported that athletes taking citrus bioflavonoids and vitamin C healed twice as fast as athletes who took either vitamin C alone or no supplements whatsoever. Another study found that injured football play-ers who took 200 to 600 mg daily of citrus bioflavonoids returned to the game in one-fourth the time of those not taking the supplements.[2]

Dr. Emanuel Cheraskin has done hundreds of scientific studies that he funded himself in order not to rely on either industrial or govern-ment money. In one of his most compelling studies done at Louisiana University, he gave half the football team vitamin C with bioflavonoids and the other half plain vitamin C. Those who had vitamin C plus bioflavonoids had 87 percent fewer injuries than the group who received vitamin C alone. Think about that for a moment. A baseball player on bioflavonoids and vitamin C is 87 percent safer if he runs into a cement wall when he's trying to catch a ball. According to Dr. Cheraskin, "taking vitamin C without bioflavonoids is like clapping with only one hand."

If you're thinking about starting a new exercise regimen, consider this: a study by Mark Kaminski, M.S., an associate professor at West-ern States Chiropractic College in Portland, Oregon, found that one gram of vitamin C taken three times daily dramatically reduces muscle soreness after strenuous and infrequent exercise.[3]

Vitamin E, too, has been found in studies to help alleviate the pain of sore back muscles. A study at the Human Nutrition Research Center on Aging at Tufts University, Boston, found vitamin E may reduce some of the muscle damage that occurs during vigorous exercise. Research-ers examined 21 sedentary men, half of whom were given 800 IU of vitamin E for seven days prior to running downhill on a treadmill for 45 minutes. The other half were given placebos. After both groups exercised, the group taking the vitamin E had less damage to muscle tissue.[4] High amounts of vitamin E are found in wheat germ, seeds, nuts, oils and cabbage.

A deficiency of manganese can cause low back pain. Add that to the fact that one third of the American population probably don't eat a balanced diet. Manganese is a tissue maker, and because we have muscles and bones we need at least five milligrams every day.

The importance of foods containing this mineral of life cannot be overstressed. A rule of thumb is that fruits and vegetables containing edible seeds will be rich in this precious mineral – such as green beans, squash, cucumbers, green peppers, dried beans, english peas, cranberries, eggplant, onions, nuts, berries and raisins. Manganese plays a vital part in so many body functions that I recommend everyone have a few ounces of cranberry juice daily as an insurance.

Dr. Trowbridge specializes in sports injuries and arthritis conditions, using an orthopedic technique called reconstructive therapy, or RT for short. Scientific studies – not to mention all the people I've sent to Dr. Trowbridge – have shown that 88 percent of patients receiving this therapy improve. Reconstructive therapy shows results by turning on the natural healing processes already found within your body, without surgery or drugs.[5] For your consultation, call John Parks Trowbridge, M.D. at (800) FIX-PAIN. His address is: 9816 Memorial Blvd., Suite 205, Humble, TX 77338.

Robert Cathcart, III, a former orthopedic surgeon and graduate of Stanford University, has found that a daily dose of the mineral manganese (50 mg) and one teaspoon of cod liver oil can prevent most back problems from occurring. For acute bouts of back pain, he ups the dosage to 50 mg. of manganese three times daily and as much as 15 tablespoons of cod liver oil, but advises that these larger doses be taken under physician supervision.

Some years ago my dear cousin Karl Rolfes, who is from Germany, broke his back surfing in East Africa and was paralyzed from the waist down. Out of sheer determination, he gained access to his toes and fingers, and eventually overcame his paralysis. But 18 long years later, he was still in constant pain. I recommended that he supplement his diet with a full complement of minerals. A few months later, Karl was watching a television show I had done in Pittsburgh, and there was a man who came on and said, "I've had back pain for seven years and nothing helped. I started taking minerals in solution, and within three months, I've never had a back pain. It's completely gone."

Karl said, "Oh my Gosh! Now I know what I've been missing – my back pain. I didn't realize it, but it's gone." Karl is now exercising again after 18 years of being held prisoner by his spine. In fact, he's just taken up rollerblading.

Look for a Cause

Obviously, the best way to stop back pain is to prevent it in the first place. Exercises that strengthen the stomach muscles also work for the back because if the stomach is strong, the back will not need to work as hard. Proper posture and lifting techniques will prevent injury as well. Remember when lifting, bend your knees, not your back! Don't sleep on your stomach. When sitting, walking or standing, keep your shoulders over your hips as much as possible. There should be a straight line from the base of the neck to the tailbone.

If back pain is chronic, find out why. A broken leg in childhood can cause one leg to be shorter than the other, causing back pain. Over-large breasts or belly can throw off alignment resulting in back pain, as can curvature of the spine. Get posture lessons and practice!

Douglas Lewis, N.D., chairperson of the Physical Medicine Department of Bastyr College in Seattle, recalls an interesting case of back pain. He treated his female patient for the pain, which would go away for two or three days. The following week the pain would return with exactly the same intensity. Finally he told her to see a gynecologist. She had an exam, and it was discovered she had a grapefruit-sized cyst on her right ovary. When it was removed, her back pain went away. Dr. Lewis sees a lot of back pain in smokers, which he attributes to the destruction of vitamin C in the body.[6] For more on these possible causes see the chapters Ovarian Cysts and Smoking.

A friend of mine tragically lost valuable time when a malignant tumor on her kidney went undiagnosed because her only symptom was back pain.

Don't Let it Stop You

If you are a back patient, don't let the pain stop you from going about your daily routine. It might just be therapeutic, as a group of Finnish researchers discovered.

The *New England Journal of Medicine* reported on a study in which back patients were given three different prescriptions for chronic, non-specific low back pain. Sixty-seven patients were given bed rest for two days, 52 patients were given back-mobilizing exercises and another 67 were told to continue their ordinary, everyday activities. After three and 12 weeks, the patients who resumed their everyday activities had better recovery than those prescribed either bed rest or exercises. The authors concluded that among patients with acute low back pain, continuing ordinary activities within the limits permitted by the pain leads to more rapid recovery than either bed rest or back-mobilizing exercises.[7]

Backache-Fighting Nutrients
For maximum absorption, take supplements with meals.

Nutrient	Suggested Dosage	Formulation
Amino acids	4-6 capsules daily	Multiple formula from natural sources
Borage oil	2 capsules daily	
Flaxseed oil	1 tablespoon daily	
Magnesium	200 mg daily	
Melatonin (adults only)	3 mg daily at bedtime	With B vitamins
MSM (Methylsulfonylmethane)	500 mg three times daily	
Multi-mineral	3-4 ounces daily	In liquid solution, with vitamin B12, biotin
Multi-vitamin/mineral	6 caplets daily	Freeze-dried plant sources
Vitamin B6	100 mg daily	
Vitamin C	Individual bowel tolerance*	With citrus bioflavonoids (quercetin, proanthocyanidins)

*To determine individual dosage, on the first day take 1,000 mg hourly until diarrhea occurs, then reduce dosage to just below that for individual daily dosage. Vitamin C is not toxic in large doses but must be taken throughout the day to benefit. Divide dosage to three or four times a day.

CHAPTER 17:

Bad Breath/Halitosis

My late-Great Dane dog Fred had breath that could wake the dead. He was such a friendly fellow, I felt bad when my otherwise dog-loving friends had to turn away from him as he greeted them, his big head perched on their laps. Finally I took him to my naturopathic veterinarian. The vet said that despite the dog biscuits and bones, Fred needed regular teeth cleaning to remove the build up of odoriferous plaque that clings to his teeth. The vet also suggested I brush and floss his teeth! Even the smallest amount of food particles in Fred's big mouth will eventually rot, the vet said, giving off odors and tooth-decaying acids.

Humans aren't in the habit of gnawing on bones to scrape off dental plaque, so it is important we brush and floss regularly. Run your tongue across your teeth. Do you feel rough surfaces? Everywhere you feel a rough surface, food has stuck to your teeth, depositing acids and bacteria-laden plaque. Enough of this stuff and people are going to smell it.

Try this: lick your hand, give it a second and smell it. Yuch! This is the best way to tell if, like Fred, your breath could reincarnate the dead.

Flossing is important because there are hundreds of tiny crevices between your teeth and at the gumline where food collects. Floss at least once a day. When you notice food is stuck between your teeth, brush at least twice a day, in the morning and at night. You may think there's no need to brush in the morning since you haven't eaten anything in your sleep, but that's where you'd be wrong. Think about it. Where does morning breath come from? As food digests, gases rise from the stomach and intestines. These gases contain bacteria which settle in your mouth and tongue. With your mouth closed all night and very little saliva being generated, it's even more important to brush in the morning. Oh, and brush your tongue as well. The tongue's taste buds collect even more bacteria than your teeth. To prevent gagging, stick your tongue out as far as you can when you brush.

Dentists recommend you replace your toothbrush at least once a month, or when the bristles get ragged. Between replacements soak it in bleach water once a week. Bleach kills bacterial germs as well as viral germs. A few drops in a cup of water is all it takes, then rinse well.

Fresh Breath from a Fresh Colon

Brushing and flossing can help, but that is not all you have to do. You also have to make sure your digestive system is healthy. You could have a mini car wash in your mouth and if your stomach acid is inadequate or you don't drink enough water or eat enough fiber, the smells of trapped, decaying food will rise from the depths, assailing all who get close.

What happens is this. When there's not enough hydrochloric acid and digestive enzymes in the stomach for complete digestion, undigested food passes into the intestines and putrefies. It might as well be your neglected refrigerator. The decaying food gives off foul gases which rise up as bad breath. Nutrition-oriented doctors suggest patients deficient in hydrochloric acid take a tablespoon of apple cider vinegar just before each meal. Adding lemon juice to a bedtime cup of water will help too. For a diagnosed deficiency, health food stores carry Betaine HCl or multiple enzyme formulas as digestive aids.

One of the body's reactions to stress is a reduction in stomach acid. B vitamins are important in keeping the body stabilized during periods of stress. One study showed that patients deficient in vitamin B6 often have offensive breath.[1]

Water is important not only to wash food and bacteria from the mouth, but help move waste through the bowels quickly. I recommend everybody drink at least two quarts of water a day, more when exercising or sweating. Bad breath can be caused by build ups of heavy metals so make sure your water is free from unnecessary ingredients.

Would you believe garlic can cure bad breath? Garlic, and especially liquid aged odorless garlic extract will help cleanse the colon of the kind of bacteria that causes infections and fouls the air.

If I were to pick one food to recommend for bad breath it would have to be parsley. Parsley contains vitamins A, B6 and chlorophyll. One cup of fresh parsley contains a whopping 5,100 IUs of vitamin A, important to healthy teeth and gums. When I eat out, which is often, I save the parsley garnish for last. Chewing it releases the chlorophyll so I can be assured my dinner partner isn't offended by my taste for garlic. Another tip is to drink green tea after a meal. If you can do it inconspicuously, gargle and swish with green tea before swallowing it. It kills the bacteria that causes bad breath and blocks the attachment of bacteria to the teeth.

Constipation contributes to bad breath. A viewer of my national television program wrote to tell me about her husband's problem with halitosis. "His breath is so bad it would curl the armorplate on a battleship," she testified. "I can't sleep in the same room with him, and nobody at the shipyard wants to work with him – even outdoors. I'm afraid he'll lose his job!"

It turned out that her husband had a bad case of constipation, caused by a low fiber diet, not drinking enough water, and an army of putrefactive bacteria at work on the accumulated waste matter in him.

A daily bowel cleanser that includes psyllium, hyssop and oat bran, with his whole wheat cereal, taken with cranberry or aloe vera juice, plus three glasses of water more than he habitually drank soon regularized him. A two-times daily supplement of intestinal and digestive enzymes quickly implanted friendly bacteria (lactobacillus acidophilus) in his intestines to colonize and take over. Within ten days, his breath "was as sweet as he is," his wife wrote.

For more on cleansing your colon, see the chapters Colon Problems and Constipation. In the meantime, here are nutrients in clinical setting dosages to beautify your breath.

Halitosis-Fighting Nutrients
For maximum absorption, take supplements with meals.

Nutrient	Suggested Dosage	Formulation
Acidophilus	At least four billion flora daily on an empty stomach, three times daily	
Aged garlic extract	1 teaspoon three times daily	Liquid
Enzymes	2 capsules twice daily	Multiple formula
Fiber	4-8 tablets daily	Psyllium, with herb hyssop
Multi-mineral	1-4 ounces daily	In liquid solution, with vitamin B12, biotin
Multi-vitamin/mineral	3-6 caplets daily	Freeze-dried plant sources
Vitamin C	Individual bowel tolerance*	With bioflavonoids (quercetin, rutin proanthocyanidins)

* To determine individual dosage, on the first day take 1,000 mg hourly until diarrhea occurs, then reduce dosage to just below that for individual daily dosage. Vitamin C is not toxic in large doses but must be taken throughout the day to benefit. Divide dosage to three or four times a day.

CHAPTER 18:

Bell's Palsy

Bill thought he was having a stroke. First he found he couldn't puff one of his cheeks out to shave. Then he couldn't close an eye. Then people started noticing one side of his face looked funny. The only thing he could think of that would cause half his face to be weak and numb was a stroke. The good news was that it wasn't a stroke, it was Bell's palsy. He was further heartened by the proclamation that full, spontaneous recovery occurs in 75 percent of people who get it.[1] While you wait out the weeks to recover, there are things you can do to minimize the problem, and perhaps speed up the recovery time.

Caused by Viruses, Alleviated with Antioxidants

In a controlled study, Japanese researchers concluded that a herpes simplex infection (the virus that causes cold sores) is the most likely cause of Bell's palsy and that the disease may benefit from treatment with antiviral agents. The triggers for Bell's palsy such as colds, fever, tooth extraction, menstruation or exposure to cold are also known to stimulate the herpes simplex virus.[2] Bell's palsy is also associated with Lyme disease, ear infections and the virus that causes shingles.

What is assumed is that as the body reacts to the virus, stress or infection, the facial nerve swells then becomes compressed. Ever been told your back pain is a result of a pinched nerve? Well, it can happen to your face too. When it becomes pinched due to swelling, it causes weakness, pain and paralysis.[3]

You can combat Bell's palsy, or at least limit its visit, by targeting antiviral/anti-infection nutrients such as vitamin C with bioflavonoids, liquid aged garlic extract, vitamin A, zinc and copper. Vitamin A, not beta carotene, must be taken because viruses can prevent beta carotene from being converted into vitamin A. Complete your antioxidant program with vitamin E and selenium, to minimize the free radical (cell) damage that occurs whenever the immune system is battling viral infections.

For colds and flu, and other viral infections, on the first day take 5,000 mg in the first two hours, then take 1,000 mg every half hour to bowel tolerance. Because vitamin C is water soluble, whatever the body uses is excreted. To get the most benefit, vitamin C has to be retained in the body. The only way to do this is to take it – lots of it – regularly throughout the day. Bioflavonoids – especially quercetin – are potent anti-inflammatories and work with vitamin C to battle infection. Food helps assimilate vitamins so take them with meals. Zinc needs B6, so include a B vitamin formula as well.

For more treatment options, see the chapters on Infections, Herpes, Inflammation, Shingles, Colds and Flu, Fever and Stress.

Physical Therapy at Home May Help

Hands-on therapy has been shown to help loosen tense muscles and relax pinched nerves. Try applying heat in the morning and evening for five minutes, followed by a five-minute rotating massage with a vitamin- and antioxidant-packed moisturizer from the angle of the jaw upward. Massaging helps prevent the skin stretching that slack muscles can produce. Exercises such as trying to raise the eyebrow, close the eye, wrinkle the nose, whistle, blow out the cheeks, and grin while looking in the mirror, complete the program.[4]

Bell's Palsy Beating Nutrients
For maximum absorption, take supplements with meals.

Nutrient	Suggested Dosage	Formulation
Acidophilus	At least four billion flora daily on an empty stomach, three times daily	
Aged garlic extract	1 teaspoon three times daily	Liquid
Antioxidants	4 capsules daily*	
Fiber	4-8 tablets daily	Psyllium, with herb hyssop
Multi-mineral	1-4 ounces daily	In liquid solution, with vitamin B12, biotin
Multi-vitamin/mineral	3-6 caplets daily	Freeze-dried plant sources
Vitamin C	Individual bowel tolerance**	With bioflavonoids (quercetin, proanthocyanidins)
Vitamin E	2 capsules (800 IU) daily	d-alpha tocopherol

* The FDA recommends pregnant women not exceed 10,000 IU of vitamin A daily.

** To determine individual dosage, on the first day take 1,000 mg hourly until diarrhea occurs, then reduce dosage to just below that for individual daily dosage. Vitamin C is not toxic in large doses but must be taken throughout the day to benefit. Divide dosage to three or four times a day.

CHAPTER 19:

Beriberi, A Thiamine Deficiency Disease

Have you ever wondered why we have "enriched" bread and cereal? What's the point, you have to wonder, if, as conventional doctors contend, we get all our vitamins and minerals from food and don't need to supplement? Over 50 years ago we discovered we weren't getting enough B vitamins from our foods. Through milling, grinding and processing, food processors were taking all the B vitamins out of our grains. The solution? Put it back by "enriching" bread and cereal with low grade supplemental vitamins. In the '40s, it was thiamine, or B1, to prevent beriberi, and in the '50s it was iron for anemia. In the '90s it is folic acid, another B vitamin, to prevent birth defects. The bottom line is we are not getting essential nutrients from food. Instead of informing the public, food processors add supplemental vitamins to cereal and bread. *Now* doctors figure they are telling the truth when they say we are getting all our essential nutrients from the food we eat.

I find it terribly ironic that food producers advertise their products as being so nutritious and good for you simply because they have added vitamins and minerals. Have you ever seen that television commercial that compares bowls of one cereal brand to another cereal brand? "You have to eat this many bowls of the other brand to get the vitamins and minerals in our brand." What's wrong with this picture? If you eat just one bowl of whole grain brown rice, you'll top both brands!

The History of Beriberi

For thousands of years, beriberi was a major disease in the Far East and other areas with high consumption of polished rice. The food given to Japanese sailors was not an exception to this dietary standard. On one naval voyage there were 169 cases of beriberi out of a total crew of 376, of which no fewer than 25 died. In 1882, a Japanese Navy doctor, Takaki, empirically determined beriberi to be a dietary deficiency. On the next training ship voyage, Takaki substituted a high-protein diet, accidentally containing sufficient vitamin B1 to eliminate beriberi. In 1878, 1,485 cases of beriberi were reported in the Japanese Navy. By 1888, it was completely eliminated. Similar results were reported from the Dutch East Indies, the Philippines and even the United States. It was found in 1897 that beriberi could be induced by feeding polished rice to chickens, and in 1911 that pigeons could be cured of beriberi by feeding them rice polishings (the part removed in rice processing).

In 1927, vitamin B was isolated by two Dutch researchers, Jansen and Dunath, and in 1936, vitamin B1 was synthesized. As in the case of vitamin C and rickets, we find that the cure for beriberi was determined empirically and then the substance was isolated and synthesized in the laboratory–but not until many years had passed.

The Many Faces of Beriberi Today

The symptoms of a thiamine deficiency are anorexia, confusion, constipation, coordination impairment, depression, digestive disturbances, fatigue, irritability, memory loss, muscular atrophy, nervousness, numbness of hands and feet, pain sensitivity, shortness of breath and weakness.[1]

In an experimental study reported in the *American Journal of Clinical Nutrition*, five of nine normal volunteers placed on a thiamine-deficient diet developed depression and irritability.[2]

Conventional medical journals claim beriberi only exists in polished rice-eating countries with poor nutritional standards and among refugees coming from these countries. Not so. Beriberi exists in our country today, and is probably far more common than convention believes.

Anything that causes malnutrition, from poor eating habits to alcoholism, can cause beriberi and its related disorders. I find it interesting that anorexia is a symptom of a thiamine deficiency. If a lack of thiamine causes depression and nervous system disorders, it stands to reason that a young person who diets constantly could first become thiamine deficient, causing the kind of obsessive behavior that leads to anorexia.

Even subclinical (moderate) thiamine deficiency can cause anxiety or neuroses. In one study, subjects deprived of thiamine complained of poor mental alertness, fatigue and nervousness.[3] Since psychiatrists are the least likely to inquire about diet, I have to wonder how many of their mental patients are being treated with drugs when they are simply thiamine-deficient.

A diet high in empty calories and junk foods has been linked to "neurotic behavior." In one study 20 patients with a thiamine deficiency reported symptoms including aggressiveness and hostility. Of the 20, 12 reported a diet high in carbonated and other sweet beverages, candy, and typical snack foods. Blood tests indicated that all 20 had low thiamine levels. After the patients were given thiamine supplements, all 20 had marked improvement or lost their symptoms completely.[4]

In 1962, a researcher by the name of Sebrell wrote: "The thought still seems to persist that severe thiamine deficiency is a disease of rice-eating people and does not occur in the United States. This leads to a situation where many physicians fail to consider the possibility of beriberi when they are faced with a puzzling diagnostic problem. However, in the past, severe clinical beriberi was widely found in the United States...New England, Arkansas, Texas and California." This was written about 20 years after enrichment of flour with thiamine was started. It is likely Sebrell would be as pessimistic today, as our food supply has deteriorated even more since then.[5]

Patients in modern hospitals are probably at risk of beriberi, and this is why:

Patients in hospitals are sometimes fed intravenously – often called tube feeding. Doctors refer to it as total parenteral nutrition, or TPN. This is done whenever the patient cannot eat or digest food the usual way. The problem is, this "liquid food" can be deficient in nutrients, most especially the B vitamins.

In 1988, three patients receiving intravenous feedings in a hospital died because the intravenous solution was deficient in thiamine, according to *The New York Times*. A B1 deficiency can develop within a week with these deficient feedings, which are 70 percent glucose, since the vitamin is necessary for metabolizing glucose.[6]

The Food and Drug Administration reported these patients died of refractory lactic acidosis. Autopsies performed on two of the patients revealed brain abnormalities.[7]

If you are anxious, depressed or suffer from neuroses, consider the possibility that you have beriberi. In the meantime, target foods high in thiamine: brewer's yeast, wheat germ, rice bran, whole grains, beans, peas and nuts.

A thiamine deficiency can be more than just a lack of B1. Minerals and all the B vitamins are necessary for its assimilation into the body. If you or someone you know has undiagnosed symptoms and you suspect a thiamine deficiency, your health has been compromised already. Just as important as restoring thiamine levels, is adding all the B vitamins. Each B vitamin has its own role in body function, centered on the nervous system. Since nerves bring messages to all the organs and stimulate glands to secrete their important biochemicals, the entire body communication system can break down with a B vitamin deficiency, hence the need for a good B complex formula. Since a thiamine deficiency can cause digestive problems, getting your B vitamins in solution or another method that eases assimilation is essential.

Beriberi-Fighting Nutrients
For maximum absorption, take supplements with meals.

Nutrient	Suggested Dosage	Formulation
Fiber	4-8 tablets daily	Psyllium, with herb hyssop
Multi-mineral	1-4 ounces daily	In liquid solution, with vitamin B12, biotin
Multi-vitamin/mineral	3-6 caplets daily	Freeze-dried plant sources
Thiamine	50 mg 3 times daily	
Vitamin C	Individual bowel tolerance*	With bioflavonoids (quercetin, rutin proanthocyanidins)

* To determine individual dosage, on the first day take 1,000 mg hourly until diarrhea occurs, then reduce dosage to just below that for individual daily dosage. Vitamin C is not toxic in large doses but must be taken throughout the day to benefit. Divide dosage to three or four times a day.

CHAPTER 20:

Body Odor

If you believe you or someone you know has the worst case of foot odor, think again. Every year the world celebrates foot odor with the Annual Odor-Eaters International Rotten Sneaker Contest. Kids from Alaska to Florida go toes to nose in a fiendish frenzy of foul and fetid footwear, with the champion rotten sneakers permanently enshrined in the Odor-Eaters Hall of Fumes. Really! I had to laugh when I first heard about this event, held every Spring in Montpelier, Vermont. Kids all over the country enter statewide events, with the winners going to Montpelier. With mothers smirking and judges wincing, a final smell-off eliminates the competition to identify the rankest, most rotten sneakers in the world.

The 1995 champion, eight-year-old Michael Moore of White Sands Missile Range, New Mexico boasted, "I knew I was going to win! I don't wear socks and my feet smell as bad as my Dad's!" He says his sneakers have never been washed – not even wiped. Michael's foot odor may be his claim to fame, but for those of us who like taking off our shoes after a hard day's work without complaints from the peanut gallery, we prefer solutions, not an odor that can qualify as chemical warfare.

There Is No Such Thing as Foot Odor

In a 1991 poll of 1,000 people conducted by Dr. Scholl's (admittedly, not the most disinterested source), 51 percent of the men and 38 percent of the women surveyed confessed to having stinky feet. Even more – 70 percent of women and 63 percent of men – said they'd been disturbed by someone else's foot odor.[1]

There's no such thing as foot odor. There's only shoe odor. Just look at societies in which people go unshod. You never hear of foot odor problems with them.

Yes, it's civilization that is to blame – never mind the fact that there are more than a quarter of a million sweat glands in a pair of feet. That's more than in any other part of the human body, including the underarms. The glands release about one gallon of moisture every week, but there's no problem so long as you're roaming around barefoot. Most of the sweat simply evaporates when your feet go through the world au naturel.

All that changes when you confine a foot in a shoe. Just ask any coach or mother who's ever encountered a well-loved pair of Pumas. The buildup of sweat creates a nearly unlimited food supply for hungry bacteria, with salt, vitamins, glucose, fatty acids, and lactic acid – exciting edibles for the nearly six trillion bacteria that thrive on our feet. Sweat also can corrode the lining, stitching, insole, and leather of shoes, creating small nooks and crannies that are perfect hideaways for microorganisms. With so much food and housing available, the organisms are fruitful and multiply. The food is digested, and what's not used is broken down and excreted.

There used to be an expression, "Smells as bad as a motorman's glove." That's because bacteria thrive in any dark, moist, warm environment, whether it be a pair of shoes or a pair of gloves.

Of course, that doesn't mean that all parts of the body were created to smell equally. It all depends on which bacteria are thriving. You don't have to be a connoisseur to tell the difference between underarm and foot odor, for instance. That's because one type of bacterium – staphylococcus – dominates in the armpit and produces its characteristic aroma, while the foot is a veritable melting pot of different bacteria and their odors. If you don't want to put up with foot odor – all right, shoe odor – your shoes should be your target.

Shoe Sense for Fetid Footwear

Before you make that trip to the drugstore, though, there are some simpler, and usually more effective, solutions to try. First, the Imelda Marcos approach. Avoid wearing the same shoes over and over again. If Marcos wore each of her 2,000 pairs of shoes on successive days, the microflora that accumulated with each wearing would have starved by the time she served them their next meal. No food, no digestion, no bacterial by-products, no smell.

Even if you don't have a roomful of shoes to choose from, rotate the ones you do wear. Each pair should air out for at least 24 hours between uses. This partly explains why I don't have stinky feet: I simply change shoes more often to match different outfits. Men and boys tend to wear the same clodhoppers over and over again. Yet researchers say it's particularly important for men to rotate their shoes, because – silly as it sounds – they have larger toes that stick together, making it harder for sweat to evaporate.

While you're choosing your shoes for the day, take note of any that need repairs. You can get rid of a sizable portion of an older shoe's bacterial population simply by replacing the lining. And watch what goes between you and your shoes as well. Microbial creatures especially delight in synthetic material, which retain heat better, increase sweating, and limit evaporation – so stick to porous natural fabrics, such as cotton or silk, or to particularly porous synthetics like rayon. This can apply to clothes as well, to avoid body odor.

If a favorite pair of shoes is excessively odiferous, try this tip before you toss them out: sterilization. Roll some blotting paper into a cylinder to make a wick, and insert it partway into a small jar of formaldehyde (available at any pharmacy). Then place the jar and the shoes inside a cardboard box, tape the box shut, and put it into a closet or garage for a day or two. After taking the shoes out, be sure to let them dry overnight before you wear them again. The shoes should be unharmed, and the smell of both the formaldehyde and the bacteria should be gone – at least for a while.

Nutritional Help for B.O.

Apply the foot odor principles to body odor. Natural-fabric clothes, frequent bathing and frequent change of clothes mean you have no body odor, right? Not always. I know someone who smells worse coming out of the shower than when she went in. Just the effort of bathing invokes her offensive odor.

Ross Gordon, an M.D. practicing out of Albany, California, uses a nutritional program for those bothered by B.O. He recommends 220 mg of magnesium, 30 mg of zinc, 100 mg of para-amino benzoic acid (PABA – one of the B vitamins) and 100 mg of vitamin B6 (pyridoxine).

Never supplement with an individual mineral unless you include a multi-mineral formula. For example, copper is important to balance out your zinc supplements. Be sure and include 2-4 mg. of copper with any zinc.

Any case of body odor can be lessened with magnesium. Dr. Alan Gaby says he can detect a magnesium deficiency in a patient based on the way he or she smells. And he usually gets it right.[2]

Calcium is important for magnesium and vice versa. For all your mineral needs target a mineral in solution supplement that includes calcium with magnesium. Without both, you can become deficient in either. Minerals in solution are easily assimilated into the body, and are not compromised by allergies, digestive problems or a lack of stomach acid. Because of the high absorption rate of minerals in solution, and deficiency of magnesium in the diet, the ratio of magnesium and calcium in solution should be four to one, respectively.

Like all of the B vitamins, PABA needs others of its kind to function, which is why whenever I recommend one B vitamin, I recommend all of them. Folic acid is also important for PABA synthesis.

Body Odor-Fighting Nutrients
For maximum absorption, take supplements with meals.

Nutrient	Suggested Dosage	Formulation
Acidophilus	At least four billion flora daily on an empty stomach, three times daily	
Aged garlic extract	1 teaspoon three times daily	Liquid
Fiber	4-8 tablets daily	Psyllium, with herb hyssop
Multi-mineral	1-4 ounces daily	In liquid solution, with vitamin B12, biotin
Multi-vitamin/mineral	3-6 caplets daily	Freeze-dried plant sources
Vitamin C	Individual bowel tolerance*	With bioflavonoids (quercetin, rutin proanthocyanidins)

* To determine individual dosage, on the first day take 1,000 mg hourly until diarrhea occurs, then reduce dosage to just below that for individual daily dosage. Vitamin C is not toxic in large doses but must be taken throughout the day to benefit. Divide dosage to three or four times a day.

CHAPTER 21:

Breastfeeding

When you consider the long range benefits of breastfeeding and the long range detriments of bottle feeding to the baby, it should then be considered indecent to bottle feed babies in public.

If you are thinking about breastfeeding, DO IT! If you are currently breastfeeding, DON'T STOP! No matter how uncomfortable breastfeeding is at the start, if you value the life and health of your baby, do whatever it takes to start and continue. It is my sincere hope that the information you derive from this chapter will not only convince you that breastfeeding is the right choice, but help you overcome any problems that might make you want to stop.

The following reasons you should breastfeed have been born out in numerous studies. Even formula manufacturers agree that breastfeeding is best.

- Infant formulas are potentially hazardous to your baby's health. There is at least one nutrient: linolenic acid, vital to a baby's well-being, that is not added to formula.[1] Other nutrients are omitted out of ignorance.

- Breastfeeding boosts the baby's immune system, increasing resistance to all types of infections and digestive disorders.

- Breastfeeding increases the survival rate for low birth weight newborns.

- Breastfeeding decreases the chances of infection via dirty or contaminated bottles.

- Breastfeeding lowers the chances for colic, food allergies and ear infections.[2]

- Breastfeeding is less costly than expensive bottles and formula.

- Breastfeeding may even increase a child's intelligence.[3]

Formula cannot supply colostrum, the first milk from the mother's breast, produced for three to five days after childbirth. Colostrum, rich in immunoglobulins (antibodies), guards the suckling infant from a host of human ailments, among them colds, flues, polio, staph infections and viruses.

A little known fact about colostrum is that it contains protective white blood cells in as high a concentration as in the blood of a healthy adult. These white cells protect against enterocolitis, a common and often fatal intestinal infection in infants.

Beatrice Trum Hunter in *The Great Nutrition Robbery* (Charles Scribner and Sons) cites a study done in Liverpool, England, in which two times as many formula-fed infants suffered illnesses compared to breastfed infants. Incredibly, almost six times as many formula-fed babies died!

What most likely comes into play here is the fact that mother's milk contains 200 known nutritive substances. Formulas average less than 30 nutrients. Not only are many essential nutrients missing from formulas, but many that are aren't absorbed as efficiently. Take zinc for example. Zinc is absorbed much more readily and at higher rates from mother's milk than from infant formulas. The mineral zinc is a key nutrient for a strong immune system, for repelling illness, sexual development and for wound healing. This fact alone means breastfeeding will help deter painful diaper rash.

Breastfed babies have been shown in studies to be smarter than formula-fed babies. Some of the reasons are the nutrients that are low or lacking in formulas. Lactose is directly related to brain growth. The species with the largest brains have the highest levels of lactose in their milk. Human milk has 50 percent more lactose than cow's milk. The many essential fatty acids contained in human milk but rare in formulas are essential to brain and nervous system growth and development. Taurine, an amino acid essential to infantile brain growth, is plentiful in human milk. Prior to 1984, however, it was all but absent from some infant formulas. Premature babies fed taurine-deficient formulas have experienced learning disabilities. Linolenic acid, important for healthy skin, blood, arteries and nerves, is still absent from formulas.

The biggest issue for me regarding infant formulas is the sheer volume of ignorance about nutrition that influences the formula manufacturers. Look at a multi-mineral and vitamin formula sometime and see how many of the nutrients do not have recommended daily allowances (RDAs). Most don't. The ones that do, are much, much too low. Formulas are based on the FDA's RDAs, and as a result are probably inaccurate and incomplete.

Dr. Mattie Crumpton Hardy and Carolyn Hoefer at Elizabeth McCormick Memorial Fund found in their studies that children breastfed for four to nine months had IQs four times higher than formula fed children. None of the formula-fed children they measured had IQs higher than 130, whereas nine percent of breastfed children qualified as geniuses.

Have Faith, It Gets Better

The first month of breastfeeding is probably the hardest. Both mother and baby are learning. The baby is learning how to find the nipple and suckle most effectively, and the mother is learning how to best position her baby and remember which breast was used last. This difficult period of adjustment is the time when most mothers quit trying. The nipples may be sore even to the point of blood blisters; the breasts may get hot, hard and engorged with milk since the baby may be sleeping more than eating at first; and milk ducts may get clogged, resulting in soreness or infection (mastitis). Don't expect to have all of these problems. Some lucky mothers have no difficulties at all. But if you realize they are normal, *temporary* problems, you may not be so inclined to quit.

It gets better, I promise. Eventually you'll learn how to position yourself and your baby so you're both comfortable, your nipples will get "broken in," and as your baby settles down to the most rewarding way to suckle, the milk flow will become predictable. You can breastfeed as long as your baby wants to, even after age one. In some countries, especially those with poor nutritional standards, mothers wisely breastfeed past the age of five. There is no better food than breastmilk, no matter what age. Milk flow continues as long as it is expressed or suckled.

A dear friend of mine went to work four weeks after her baby was born. She was away from her baby nine hours a day and manually expressed her milk into disposable plastic bottle bags, storing them in the freezer, to be delivered to the day care provider the following day. This way she was able to continue feeding her daughter breastmilk even while working.

Insufficient Milk

Many women have written me asking for information on milk insufficiency. After contacting experts on lactation, including members of the valuable La Leche League – people devoted to teaching new mothers about breastfeeding – it would appear that very few women have a physical reason for a lack of milk. Breast size has nothing to do with it. Skin is elastic; it will stretch to contain whatever amount of milk is needed. Too much time between feedings, ignoring a full breast of milk and not emptying a breast fully are the main reasons a woman can't produce enough milk.

The important thing to keep in mind is that the body produces milk based on the demand for it. If you don't empty a full breast, the next time it won't produce as much. If you need more milk, you need to express or nurse more. A nurse practitioner told me about a woman who bottle fed her first two children, then was dismayed to find she couldn't nurse the third. Because she never breastfed before, her body was led to believe it didn't need to produce milk the next time around.

Fear of insufficient breastmilk can, in itself, be a self-fulfilling prophecy. A baby who fusses or seems unsettled after a feeding may lead a mother to worry that she doesn't have enough milk. If she then gives the baby a bottle of formula, and the baby takes an ounce or two and falls asleep, she might feel that her theory is confirmed. Repeating this process quickly carries a woman who merely thinks her breastmilk is insufficient to a state where the decrease in demand causes her breasts to actually start producing less milk. What was only a perceived insufficiency then becomes a true insufficiency.

Healing Sore Nipples

Blood blisters can scare you into thinking about quitting but they may be avoidable. Sore nipples can result from poor positioning. If you grind your teeth in pain as your baby clamps down, try changing breasts and positions until they feel better. If nothing seems to help, try going without a bra to allow them to air out. Apply some of your milk to the nipple and let it dry. The same nutrients that are good for the baby are good for your skin. The inside of a banana peel can be applied to soothe sore nipples between feedings, and even slipped into the bra. Aloe vera straight from a plant (squeeze the gel out of a broken leaf) can also soothe sore skin. Coat the nipple and let it dry. If the baby suckles after, it won't harm him or her. People drink aloe vera juice for internal ulcers.

Since people learning to play the violin or guitar have to develop calluses on their fingertips to press down on the strings, it's not surprising our nipples go through a similar painful period. Limiting the amount of feeding only prolongs the soreness period.

Feed your baby on demand rather than on a schedule. Babies who are hungry feed harder. A nipple-toughening trick is exposure to warm dry air. Use the low setting of a hair dryer or a 60-watt bulb for 20 minutes a few times a day.[4] Remember, nipple soreness is temporary so just hang in there and eventually you won't even notice when baby feeds.

Plugged Milk Ducts and Mastitis

My friend believes she never got mastitis or plugged ducts because she expressed her milk manually. This is likely since experts recommend massaging the breasts with firm pressure to stimulate milk flow out of a previously clogged milk duct. While still pregnant, practice massaging fluid out of the nipples. Don't do this if there is any chance of premature labor, as you could incite uterine contractions. You may feel like you're milking a cow, but learning this technique will make your breastfeeding life a lot easier, especially if you plan to express and save your milk. Before you buy that expensive breast pump, try it with your hands. My friend claims she could express eight ounces of milk in ten minutes just using her hands – and she had small breasts.

Wearing a bra that is too tight can cause plugged ducts, as can interrupted or incomplete feeding. Express any milk left after feedings. Look for soreness or a lump in one area of the breast to identify a plugged duct. Check the nipple very carefully for a tiny dot of dried milk. If your breast doesn't feel completely empty (flaccid) after a feeding, express the rest of the milk. Attach a safety pin to the bra on the side of the breast last used so you don't inadvertently ignore one. Eventually, you'll know from the pressure which breast to offer first.

Mastitis occurs when bacteria breeds infection in plugged milk ducts. Cooked, warm cabbage leaves are wonderful for taking the heat out of an infected breast. Treat mastitis by drinking lots of spring water (not tap water), getting rest and avoiding stress if possible. Stress causes muscles to contract, which can restrict milk circulation. Apply warm compresses to the infected breast. B vitamins are special stress reducers. Folic acid, one of the B vitamins, is currently in the works to be added to commercial bread to prevent birth defects. It is especially important to the developing brain of a baby. Brewer's yeast is packed with B vitamins and is highly recommended for breastfeeding mothers. Add it to a fruit smoothie for a nutritious pick-me-up.

Herbs steeped and warmed can be made into soothing and healing compresses to treat mastitis. Try warm compresses of the herbs mallow or saniculae. Interestingly, saniculae is found in Tussiflorin, a German cough remedy, used for chest congestion. Mallow leaves and flowers are active ingredients in over a dozen European pharmaceuticals used to treat a variety of ailments including urinary tract infections, bronchitis and constipation. All of these ailments involve congestion and impediment of normal circulation, factors found in mastitis.[5]

I know from personal experience and the testimonials of others that liquid garlic extract combined with vitamin C and bioflavonoids are remarkably effective natural, nontoxic antibiotics, and are available in most food stores. Use as directed to combat any infection. Consult with a physician versed in nutrition for dosages and treatment protocols before attempting to treat yourself for an infection while breastfeeding. There's too much at stake when a newborn is involved to self-medicate.

In severe cases, the bacteria in milk ducts can proliferate to a point where abscesses form and fill with pus. If this happens, the breast milk should be expressed and discarded. For more, see the chapters Abscesses, Infections and Inflammations.

Keeping Your Baby and YOU Healthy

Eating can be difficult when meeting the constant demands of a baby. On the other hand, the best foods are those eaten in the raw state. Buy a good fruit and raw nut trail mix at your health food store or market and snack on it all day. Make sure it includes sunflower seeds, which are high in bone-building calcium, phosphorous, potassium and magnesium, not to mention muscle-building amino acids. Emphasize raw fruits and vegetables for all your vitamins and minerals and to ward away the constipation common to pregnant women and new mothers. Eating well will not only nourish yourself and your baby, but help to heal your body faster too. Nutritional supplements will ensure you achieve an optimal state of health.

Important to realize is that your breastmilk will be only as good as the state of your nutritional health. Your vitamin and mineral utilization is at peak now, and certain nutrients will be depleted if you don't have enough to share. You have enough to worry about without getting chronically fatigued and weak. It is essential that you supplement with three kinds of formulas: a B-complex formula with at least ten times the RDA (the RDA is low even for most healthy people), a multiple vitamin formula using natural ingredients as much as possible, and a mineral in solution formula. These formulas need to be taken separately because they work best that way, and some nutrients contradict each other.

Watch out for iron supplements. You may not really need them, and they could cause harm to you and your baby. See the chapter on Anemia for more on this.

Remember, you have many times the mineral needs now than you'll ever have. You need a mineral formula in solution because your organs and digestive system are out of whack and may not be assimilating your nutrients well enough. You're not what you put into your mouth, you're what you absorb and digest and deliver to cells. A tablet is only one to five percent absorbable. Since the process of digestion is a process of liquefaction, your body has to take a hard rock tablet and turn it into solution. This may not be possible due to a number of factors, such as inadequate stomach acid, food allergies and intestinal problems. This is why it is so important that when you decide to supplement, you target minerals in solution. Look for a good, easily absorbable, derived-from-nature mineral blend in solution. Formulations in solution provide the maximum absorption ratios.

Breastfeeding Support Nutrients
For maximum absorption, take supplements with meals.

Nutrient	Suggested Dosage	Formulation
Acidophilus	At least four billion flora daily on an empty stomach, three times daily	
Aged garlic extract	1 teaspoon three times daily	Liquid
Amino acids	4-6 capsules daily	Multiple formula from natural sources
Antioxidants	2 capsules daily	With selenium and grapeseed extract
Borage oil	2 capsules daily	
Fiber	4-8 tablets daily	Psyllium, with herb hyssop
Flaxseed oil	1 tablespoon daily	
Multi-mineral	1-4 ounces daily	In liquid solution,with vitamin B12, biotin
Multi-vitamin/mineral	3-6 caplets daily	Freeze-dried plant sources
Vitamin C	Individual bowel tolerance*	With bioflavonoids (quercetin, rutin proanthocyanidins)
Vitamin E	2 capsules (800 IU) daily	d-alpha tocopherol

* To determine individual dosage, on the first day take 1,000 mg hourly until diarrhea occurs, then reduce dosage to just below that for individual daily dosage. Vitamin C is not toxic in large doses but must be taken throughout the day to benefit. Divide dosage to three or four times a day.

CHAPTER 22:

Bronchitis and Pneumonia

Get a case of bronchitis, get antibiotics, get cured, right? Wrong! Studies are showing that our increasing dependence on antibiotics may be killing us. By the time doctors determine they aren't working, it's too late.

More than half of the 60,000 to 80,000 patients in the United States who die each year of bacterial infections they get in hospitals are probably caused by antibiotic-resistant strains of bacteria, according to the Centers for Disease Control (CDC).[1]

Since 1990, strains of tuberculosis resistant to many drugs have emerged around the country, including in New York City, spurred on by the HIV epidemic and by high transmission rates in prisons.[2]

Researchers are also concerned about rising drug resistance among the pneumococci, a family of bacteria that kill about 40,000 Americans a year through infections like pneumonia and meningitis. Pneumococci are also a leading cause of childhood ear infections. According to a study published in 1995 by researchers at the CDC and Emory University, one in four pneumococci samples taken in Atlanta were resistant to penicillin, a sharp increase on the rate of eight years prior.[3]

Ralph Gonzales, M.D. and Merle Sande, Department of Medicine at San Francisco General Hospital, wrote in *The Lancet* that antibiotics are never warranted in cases of acute bronchitis.[4]

They believe viral-caused bronchitis will take its own course, with or without antibiotics, and cite seven randomized, double-blind trials showing "no major clinical role for antibiotics in uncomplicated acute bronchitis." Despite this, conventional doctors continue to prescribe these drugs at an alarming rate. Physician surveys indicate that 50 to 70 percent of acute bronchitis patients leave their physicians' office with a prescription for antibiotics in hand. This despite the prevalence of antibiotic-resistant strains of common bacteria.

Antibiotics are often erroneously prescribed when phlegm has changed color, when fever or smoking history is reported, or in the hope of preventing a progression to pneumonia. The combination of patient expectation, along with pressures on the physician to limit appointment times, has encouraged prescribing antibiotics as the path of least resistance.

Antibiotics have their own dangers, the least of which is the fact they kill your good armies of immune-boosting bacteria, which protect you against yeast and other infections.

Bronchitis and Pneumonia Defined

The term bronchitis refers to an inflammation or infection of the bronchial tubes, as opposed to either the lung tissue itself, as in pneumonia, or the upper respiratory tract, as in the common cold. If you find yourself searching through medical journals, you'll see chronic bronchitis and emphysema defined as a "chronic obstructive pulmonary disease" (COPD), with studies referring to it. They call them COPD because they can eventually obstruct the airway, causing death by asphyxiation.

In otherwise healthy people, the common cold is caused by any of several viruses, and is confined to the upper respiratory tract. The body's response to the common cold is to create large rivers of mucus, designed to flush out the offending virus cells. If cough medicines or other factors inhibit the escape of mucus, it builds up, becomes thick and enters the bronchial tubes. An overgrowth of bacteria creates infection and the bronchi respond with an outpouring of mucus, pus, and fluid. This state is what is called acute bronchitis.

Typically, the patient develops what appears to be a routine cold with runny nose and perhaps a sore throat. Instead of running its course in a few days, however, a cough develops which starts out "dry" but quickly becomes congested with mucus. When the amount increases and becomes green, yellow, or gray, bronchitis may be present. Occasionally the irritation may rupture a small blood vessel, causing small amounts of blood to appear.

However, in the cases of people who smoke or have poor immune systems, the infection may spread downward into the lung, causing pneumonia. Pneumonia is defined as a severe inflammation of the lungs and ranks as the fifth leading cause of death in the United States, leading all other infectious diseases.[5]

Death By Smoking

Every year, 60,000 American smokers die from bronchitis and emphysema. Put simply, they destroy their lungs by smoking.

Some are deaths from chronic bronchitis. One of the ways the lungs clean themselves is by producing mucus, which traps dirt and then is swept out of the lungs by the cilia. With the cilia destroyed by smoking, only coughing can expel the mucus. Infection sets in. The lungs are inflamed and great quantities of mucus are produced, providing a good place for bacteria to grow. The passageways of the lungs narrow and breathing becomes difficult. Serious, even life-threatening infection can be the result.[6]

Smoking can cause bronchitis.[7] With or without a virus, smoking is so damaging that it creates lung problems.

Nothing is so tragic as the epidemic of teenage smoking. A 1994 study found that in 1991 2.7 million teenagers smoked 516 million packs of cigarettes, more than half of which were sold illegally.[8]

There are 70 million children now living in the United States. If 20 million of them become smokers (the percentage of today's adults who smoke), five million may eventually die of smoking-related diseases.[9] That's one out of four who may die because of their addiction!

According to a 1986 Center for Chronic Disease Prevention and Health Promotion report, an estimated 82 percent of deaths from emphysema and bronchitis are due to smoking.[10]

There is good news for those of you who have tried, but cannot quit smoking: my chapter on the topic in this book. Until you are able to quit, there are nutrients which have been shown to protect against getting bronchitis and pneumonia.

Vitamin C in Your Chicken?

Vitamin C has been found in many studies to be of benefit in protecting the lungs from damage by smoking and environmental factors, and from getting bronchitis or pneumonia.

In the early part of this century, before the advent of antibiotics, many controlled and uncontrolled studies demonstrated the positive effects of large doses of vitamin C in the treatment of pneumonia when started on the first or second day of infection. If started later, vitamin C was still found to lessen the severity of the disease. Researchers also demonstrated that in pneumonia, as well as other infections, white blood cells take up large amounts of vitamin C.[11]

Researchers in the Netherlands used vitamin C, in the form of ascorbic acid, to protect chickens against infectious bronchitis. It was found that 300 to 330 milligrams of ascorbic acid per kilogram in broiler feed was able to protect the chickens from the negative effects of IBV (infectious bronchitis virus) infections.[12]

If vitamin C can be used instead of antibiotics and vaccine drugs, we may end up with healthier chicken, in more ways than one!

In the First National Health and Nutrition Examination Survey (NHANES I) conducted by Brigham and Women's Hospital and Harvard Medical School, researchers evaluated vitamin C intake and lung function in 2,526 adults between 1971 and 1974. After adjusting for variables, the researchers determined that, in part due to its antioxidant capabilities, vitamin C appears to improve immune function, increase lung capacity, and protect against the development of infection in smokers and non-smokers, with increased benefit among patients with bronchitis and asthma. The researchers also found that lower dietary intakes of vitamin C were so significantly associated with poor lung function, that it could be a factor in developing chronic lung disease.[13]

More Evidence

California physician Dr. Robert Cathcart has successfully treated over 15,000 patients with massive doses of vitamin C; curing viral pneumonia, mononucleosis, influenza, colds, hepatitis, shingles, and cold sores with this method. He has developed a guideline for practical application of vitamin C which he refers to as "bowel tolerance."

Dr. Cathcart found that the individual's own body will determine how much vitamin C it requires. The cutoff point is determined by the onset of diarrhea. In short, if you have not reached bowel tolerance (diarrhea), you have not taken enough vitamin C.

It turns out there's even more you can do. You can make sure your vitamin C includes bioflavonoids.

At the Creighton University School of Medicine, Omaha, Nebraska, a group of nurses was given tablets containing the two substances. The nurses were checked for one year, as was another group which received a placebo. The nurses receiving the vitamin C and bioflavonoids had 55 percent fewer colds than the placebo group, and their infections lasted an average of 3.9 days, compared to 6.7 days for the placebo group.[14] That's a significant difference.

Another study reported that 20 of 22 patients with respiratory infections of varying intensity recovered in an 8- to 48-hour period after treatment with bioflavonoids and vitamin C. The patients received 600 mg of each of the two substances every day.

Quercetin, a particularly potent bioflavonoid, acts as an antihistamine, allowing you to clear your medicine chest of all the dangerous over-the-counter remedies you used to take.[15]

Some European studies have found that bioflavonoids slow bacterial and viral infections.[16] Quercetin has been shown to be effective against many viruses, including viruses that cause bronchitis.[17]

To prevent cell damage to your lungs in the event of a viral infection, instead of antibiotics, target naturally-derived antioxidant vitamins, minerals and herbals.

Relieving Bronchial Spasms with Magnesium

History keeps repeating itself when it comes to treating bronchial problems with magnesium. In 1993, Emil M. Skobeloff, M.D., of the Department of Emergency Medicine/Division of Research, The Medical College of Pennsylvania in Philadelphia, reported in the *Annals of Emergency Medicine* on a young pregnant woman who was relieved of her life-threatening bronchitis by magnesium – after everything else failed.

The woman was 28 years old and had a history of asthma. But it wasn't asthma that brought her to the emergency room; it was acute bronchitis. Unable to breathe due to heavy wheezing, the ER doctors gave her all the usual medicines, including a commonly used albuterol inhaler. After no relief, she was given three grams of magnesium sulfate in an IV over 20 minutes, resulting in a reduction of her symptoms. After an hour, she reported she was able to breathe normally again.[18]

Asthma and bronchitis are similar in that they both cause acute respiratory distress when the bronchial tubes become inflamed, cutting off air.

Researchers at the University of Nottingham's Division of Respiratory Medicine found that of 2,633 asthmatics, those whose dietary magnesium intake was above the average 380 mg a day showed significantly improved lung function and less wheezing. Low blood levels of magnesium, the researchers suspect, could be a factor in causing bronchial constriction in the first place.[19] *The American Journal of Medicine* cites numerous clinical trials that showed the benefit of magnesium in treating asthma.[20] A study in *The Lancet*, a well-respected British medical journal, found that magnesium has an independent, beneficial influence on lung function, airway responsiveness, and wheezing in a general population.[21] Apparently, magnesium helps the body control muscle spasms and is able to smooth and expand the bronchial muscles so they don't contract and close off air (referred to as a bronchodilating effect).

Following up these studies, in 1994 researchers gave 72 COPD patients either 1.2 grams of magnesium intravenously or a placebo over a 20 minute period, following an acute attack. They found that the magnesium exerted a bronchodilator effect that was greater than albuterol and lasted at least 25 minutes beyond the period of magnesium administration. With the magnesium, the number of patients able to forego hospitalization following a breathing crisis was reduced by 23 percent.[22]

Spicy Solutions

Irwin Ziment, M.D., professor of medicine at the University of California School of Medicine, Los Angeles, and chief of medicine and director of respiratory therapy at Olive View Medical Center, also in Los Angeles, comes from Great Britain where the diet is usually bland. Just the kind of thing the English don't need, he says, because they also have a damp climate. This fact, and the prevalence of smoking, contribute to a high incidence of bronchitis in that country. He says bronchitis was so rampant that for many years it was called "the English disease." He believes more Brits should try Tabasco with their fish and chips.

Spicy foods for colds, asthma and sinus problems have been used for centuries by early civilizations. Ancient Egyptian medical writings recommended mustard for respiratory therapy. Hippocrates prescribed vinegar and pepper as respiratory medicines; and Oriental medicine still uses capsicum peppers, black pepper, mustard, garlic, tumeric and other spices to treat colds and asthma.

You've heard of mustard plasters for colds? The idea isn't so farfetched. Naturopaths Michael Murray and Joseph Pizzorno offer the recipe: Mix one part dry mustard with three parts flour and add enough water to make a paste. Spread the paste on thin cotton (an old pillowcase works well) or cheesecloth. Fold it so the paste isn't against the skin and place it on the chest. Leave on for up to 20 minutes. Check periodically because it may cause blisters.[23]

A cough syrup can be made from six chopped white onions cooked in a double boiler with half a cup of honey or molasses. Cook slowly over low heat for two hours and strain. Take at regular intervals, preferably warm.[24]

To loosen tight bronchials eat a hot spicy meal at least once a day, or down a glass of water sprinkled with ten or twenty drops of Tabasco sauce, or chew on chili peppers. And if you have a cold, sore throat, or allergies, try a teaspoon of ground horseradish, add a glass of warm water and a little honey and drink it. Or mix up some garlicky-rich chicken soup with a hefty dash of red or black pepper.

Lung-Loving Nutrients
For maximum absorption, take supplements with meals.

Nutrient	Suggested Dosage	Formulation
Acidophilus	At least four billion flora daily on an empty stomach, three times daily	
Aged garlic extract	1 teaspoon three times daily	Liquid
Antioxidants	2 capsules daily	With selenium and grapeseed extract
Borage oil	2 capsules daily	
Echinacea	400 mg daily	
Fiber	4-8 tablets daily	Psyllium, with herb hyssop
Flaxseed oil	1 tablespoon daily	
Multi-mineral	1-4 ounces daily	In liquid solution, with vitamin B12, biotin
Multi-vitamin/mineral	3-6 caplets daily	Freeze-dried plant sources
Vitamin A	25,000 IU daily*	
Vitamin C	Individual bowel tolerance**	With bioflavonoids (quercetin, rutin proanthocyanidins)
Vitamin E	2 capsules (800 IU) daily	d-alpha tocopherol
Zinc Gluconate	25 mg three times daily	Lozenges

* The FDA recommends pregnant women not exceed 10,000 IU of vitamin A daily.

** To determine individual dosage, on the first day take 1,000 mg hourly until diarrhea occurs, then reduce dosage to just below that for individual daily dosage. Vitamin C is not toxic in large doses but must be taken throughout the day to benefit. Divide dosage to three or four times a day.

CHAPTER 23:

Bruises

I recall a television viewer who came to me with a variety of symptoms: muscle cramps, constipation, unusual body odor and easy bruising. The man was a logger, so he was used to a bruise here and there, in the course of his work. But when he counted 16 leg bruises in one day, he figured something wasn't right. He also complained he was more tired than usual.

My suggestion? More green leafy vegetables. The man was constipated because he wasn't eating enough fiber, a magnesium deficiency was causing his body odor and muscle cramps, and a lack of vitamin K was causing his bruising. Green leafy vegetables contain vitamin K and magnesium, and it was just what the logger needed to combat all his problems.

If your taste for green leafies is limited to mowing the lawn, you might consider supplementing with alfalfa tablets, available in health food stores. Vitamin K is highest in alfalfa, and with supplemental tablets, you won't have to join your kid's rabbit for lunch. Today's health food and vitamin market offers a plethora of food supplements. If bruising has got you blue–and black–look for formulas that contain both high fiber and skin strengthening vitamins: alfalfa, rhubarb, hyssop, oat bran, buckthorn and psyllium.

Those of you who are getting on in years should think about increasing your input of green leafy vegetables because as we get older, our skin gets thinner. Bruising occurs when something ruptures the small blood vessels or platelets (blood cells essential to clotting) underlying the surface of the skin. The purple color occurs from the minor bleeding that results. Thinner skin means less protection for blood vessels and platelets. If you don't have time to eat as well as you should, target supplements that offer freeze-dried sprouts for your greens in easy-to-take capsules.

Bruising Without Injury

Problems with excessive bleeding and blood clotting can cause bruises without external injury. Hemophiliacs, those who lack factors that clot blood, have problems with bruising, as do those taking anti-clotting drugs. Without the clot factor, bruises cannot stop bleeding and heal. If your bruises take longer than a week to diminish, please see your health care provider.

Obese people also have problems with bruising because the pounds weigh heavily against blood vessels, causing them to rupture. Then when they lose weight they can bruise easily as the tiny capillaries, once supported by fat, are on their own and rupture. Vitamin C and bioflavonoids can help here.

Bleeding disorders are just one reason bruises develop without external injury. A deficiency of vitamin C or bioflavonoids can compromise blood vessel integrity, leaving them weak and prone to breakage, bleeding and bruises.[1]

Bioflavonoids are the natural chemicals that color citrus rind, cherries, grapes, plums, black currants, apricots, buckwheat, blackberries and rose hips, and help strengthen connective tissue. Highest vitamin C foods are papaya, guava, parsley and kale.

Chill a Shiner

A so-called black eye is really a bruise of the cheek, eyelids and eyebrow. Skip the raw steak and instead apply a cold compress to constrict blood vessels and help prevent further bleeding/blackening. Because an injury to the eye area can mean injury to the actual eyeball, always have a physician check the eyeball and optic nerves. There is more cause for concern if your vision is blurred or you see double. Do not attempt to force open an eye that has been swollen shut.

The bioflavonoids, a group of substances related to vitamin C, can speed the healing of bruises. A report in *Medical Times* stated that athletes taking citrus bioflavonoids and vitamin C healed twice as fast as athletes who took either vitamin C alone or no supplements at all.[2]

A salve of tumeric and honey has been shown to remedy the swelling that sometimes accompanies bruising. Tumeric is a notable anti-inflammatory and honey guards against bacteria and speeds healing.

Try cabbage leaf poultices. If these prove to be too strong, alternate with a clay pack. Alternating the poultices from one day to the next is beneficial because clay reduces swelling and cabbage leaves contain healing properties that also draw out toxins.[3] Cabbage contains the skin-smart vitamins E and K. Another option is horsetail extract, a raw form of the mineral silica. Work from the inside to heal bruised tissues by supplementing with silica in a mineral in solution formula.

Bruise-Fighting Nutrients
For maximum absorption, take supplements with meals.

Nutrient	Suggested Dosage	Formulation
Aged garlic extract	1 teaspoon three times daily	Liquid
Bilberry	80 mg three times daily	
Bromelain	200 mg twice daily	
Fiber	4-8 tablets daily	Psyllium, with herb hyssop
Multi-mineral	1-4 ounces daily	In liquid solution, with vitamin B12, biotin
Multi-vitamin/mineral	3-6 caplets daily	Freeze-dried plant sources
Vitamin C	Individual bowel tolerance*	With bioflavonoids (quercetin, proanthocyanidins)
Vitamin E	2 capsules (800 IU) daily	d-alpha tocopherol

* To determine individual dosage, on the first day take 1,000 mg hourly until diarrhea occurs, then reduce dosage to just below that for individual daily dosage. Vitamin C is not toxic in large doses but must be taken throughout the day to benefit. Divide dosage to three or four times a day.

CHAPTER 24:

Bunions and Corns

No matter how attractive your shoes are, if you are limping in pain, nobody is going to notice. That's what I told an acquaintance during a social gathering in San Francisco recently. "Jean," I said, "Your shoes are beautiful, but what they are doing to your feet is not." She took her right shoe off, wincing in pain. I gasped in horror when I peeked at her poor peds. Her big toe was squeezed over the little ones by a huge, angry bump at the side where the ball of the foot meets the big toe. She told me that's where the pain was.

I put my hand on hers and said, "Honey, this is serious. If you let this go on, you'll never walk normally again." What this woman didn't realize was that a combination of her genetics (her mother had bunions) and wearing shoes that were too tight were creating bursitis of the foot, which had the potential of permanently disabling her.

Bursitis of the Feet

Bunions are actually big toe joints that have become misaligned. The technical name is hallux valgus – hallux being the Latin name for *the great toe* and valgus, another Latin word meaning *bent outward*. Normally the bones of the big toe lie more or less in a straight line with the large metatarsal bone of the foot. When a bunion develops, the large metatarsal bone angles outward, away from the toes, and the big toe bones are forced in the opposite direction. Prolonged pressure over this joint causes swelling of the bursa, a fluid-filled sac that prevents friction between two bones of a joint.[1] Hence, bunions are actually bursitis of the feet. Imagine how it would feel if you had to walk on a tennis elbow. It's bad enough trying to pick up a half gallon of milk. Anyone with bursitis can tell you the pain is acute and can take years to heal. As with most afflictions, prevention – and knowledge – is the key.

Peruse the chapter on Bursitis for complete and effective treatments of bursa bunions. In the meantime, soothe sore joints with hot epsom foot baths, walk barefoot whenever possible, exercise the balls of the feet by rolling them back and forth over a bottle and, for heaven's sake, get bigger shoes!

Sacrificing Your Big Toe for Beauty

Like Cinderella's wicked stepsisters, almost nine of 10 American women squeeze their feet into shoes that are too small. Eighty percent of American women have foot pain and disabling foot problems, according to a survey of more than 350 women reported by the American Orthopaedic Foot and Ankle Society (AOFAS). Are tight shoes to blame? Dr. Michael Coughlin, an orthopedic surgeon in Boise, Idaho, says he's gathered "overwhelming evidence" that they are.[2]

After reviewing more than 2,100 foot operations he performed between 1979 and 1993, Coughlin presented his findings at a meeting of the American Academy of Orthopaedic Surgeons. Incredibly, he found that nearly all these operations were on women. For example, of the 813 operations to correct bunions, 94 percent were done on women. Some experts contend that women are simply predisposed to agonies of de-feet. But Coughlin points to several studies of barefoot cultures in Africa and New Zealand that found no bunions among men or women.[3]

I'm willing to bet in states like Texas and Colorado, where men commonly wear cowboy boots, the cases of bunions increase. I've scratched my head in wonder, when looking at these boots with their almost triangular toes, amazed that men can even get their feet into them. But overall, women's toes have it worse. High-heeled shoes tilt the foot forward, cramming the toes against the front of the shoes, which are usually pointy and narrow to begin with. Even without heels, it's painfully hard to find a woman's shoe in a comfortable width.

Coughlin says the common practice of wearing constricting shoes over a long period of time is a huge public health risk in America, estimating that ill-fitting shoes cost a minimum of $3.5 billion a year in medical care and time lost from work.[4]

The obstacles to healthy feet include not just fashion and vanity – tight shoes make the foot look desirably narrow and high heels accentuate calf muscles – but ignorance about proper shoe size. "Nothing else on the body stays the same size after age 18, but everyone expects that their shoe size will," says Tom Brunick, director of The Athlete's Foot Wear Test Center in Naperville, Illinois. Over time, Brunick says, most people's feet become as much as a full size longer and wider.[5]

The AOFAS survey found most women judged their feet to be a full size narrower than they really were. Whether from choice or lack of it, nearly 9 out of 10 women wore shoes that were at least one size too small or too narrow.[6]

One Step Ahead – Buying Safe Shoes

To avoid buying shoes that are too tight in the toes, both men and women first need to know some basic shoe-shopping principles:

- As you age, your feet tend to spread and enlarge. Don't assume that your foot size is he same as it was the last time you had it measured.

- Your feet expand when you put weight on them. Stand up when the clerk measures your feet and when you're trying on the shoes.

- Over the course of a day, your feet swell as much as a full size. Shop in the afternoon or evening.

- Most people have one foot that's longer than the other. Select a pair that accommodates the longer foot. To tighten the fit on the shorter foot, slip an insole or heel saver into that shoe.

- Don't fall for the pitch that a shoe "just needs to be broken in." While shoes do stretch, they seldom stretch enough to make an uncomfortable shoe safe to wear.

The shoes you buy should:

- Leave about one-half inch of space between the longest toe and the tip of the shoe.

- Let your toes point straight ahead, not inward. To check, place your heel into the   shoe, leaving the rest of your foot outside, on top of the shoe. If your toes extendbeyond the outer edges of the shoe, they'll be squashed when you put it on.

- Give your toes enough room to wiggle upward.

- Be wide enough for the widest part of your foot, between the bases of the big and little toes. As you run your finger across the top of the shoe at that widest point, feel for a ripple in the material; that shows your foot hasn't stretched the shoe tight.

- Keep heels to a moderate one inch in height.

- Have rubber heels, which absorb shock better than leather or synthetic heels.

Shucking Corns

My acquaintance also had numerous corns on the top of her toes. Corns and calluses are pretty much the same. Both have a marked thickening of the top layer of the skin, and are caused by long periods of pressure or friction. Calluses can develop anywhere on weight-bearing areas, such as the sides and soles of the feet. They are usually raised, off-white in color, and have a normal pattern of skin ridges on the surface.

Corns come in two major varieties – hard and soft. Hard corns are the more common, usually occurring on the surfaces of the toes. They look shiny and polished. Soft corns are whitish in color and are most often found on the web between the fourth and little toe. Corns are more painful than calluses. This is because they are thicker at one point and create more pressure on the underlying nerve endings in the skin.

Corns will disappear when the pressure and friction of poor-fitting shoes is eliminated, but the process can be accelerated with the help of certain nutrients and botanicals.

A good home remedy is to soak the corn, and while it is still wet rub firmly with a pumice stone or other abrasive foot care product. The skin should scrape away readily. Stop if you have pain or bleeding. Wait until the break in the skin heals then repeat the process. This may be repeated daily until symptoms are gone, then done periodically as necessary.

Corns are more painful when they are hard because they press down on the underlying nerves. To keep them soft and pain-free, apply a salve of calendula (marigold) ointment. The anti-inflammatory properties of the botanical will reduce the swelling of the underlying tissues. Castor oil rubbed twice daily on corns is said to help, as is hot epsom foot and whirlpool baths.

Corn-Shucking and Bunion-Busting Nutrients

Healthy skin is protective skin. If your nutritional health is optimum, your skin will be better able to protect itself without resorting to calluses and corns.

Here's a news flash: vitamin A – found in orange and yellow fruits and vegetables – is a supreme skin nutrient! Not only is it extra essential to your epidermis, but it can actually reverse damage to your derma.

Just to give you an idea of the value of vitamin A, Retin-A, prescribed for acne but touted as a skin rejuvinator, is actually Tretinoin, a form of vitamin A. Skin-care companies, it seems, have been adding chemical cousins of vitamin A to moisturizers for years. Called retinoids, these vitamin A cousins work like drill sergeants, ordering wayward cells in line and sloughing off clumps of dead cells. Now, I don't advocate Retin-A to slough off corns and calluses, but internally, vitamin A helps speed up the shedding process so corns will disappear faster.

Unsaturated fatty acids are essential for all cell formation, including skin cells. A deficiency of these nutrients can undermine your skin's health, encouraging corns and calluses.

The best sources of unsaturated fatty acids, often coined "essential fatty acids" or EFAs, are contained in borage oil. It has such a reputation for skin care that the French put borage oil in their skin care products. It can be found in health food stores.

Pantothenic acid, one of the B vitamins, is required for the proper balance of fats and oils in the body, and is essential for proper skin function. Without it, the skin loses the ability to produce the sebum needed to moisten it. Sebum is the oil created by the body to make the skin waterproof and lubricated. It's also what helps keep the skin from becoming irritated by chafing.

Bunion-busting nutrients are those that beef up the bones and joints. Calcium of course is first, although not foremost. And remember all the reasons dairy foods are not ideal sources of calcium.

Instead of dairy foods, eat high-calcium, low phosphorous foods such as kale, sesame seeds, maple syrup and seaweed.

Too much phosphorous can cause you to lose too much calcium, and vice versa. Avoid soft drinks, they contain too much phosphorous. Instead, eat foods that have the ideal calcium/phosphorous ratio of close to one to one: radishes, apples and pears.

Include magnesium with calcium. Magnesium is the green light that tells calcium where to go, and where not to go. Foods that contain potassium, calcium and magnesium are items to keep in mind. They are: wheat germ, sunflower seeds, soybeans, almonds, brazil nuts, pistachios and pecans. Each of these foods can be added to salads, cereal and snack foods. Conveniently, they have a pretty decent shelf life as well.

Too much meat protein can also drain off needed calcium. That's because meat is high in sulfur and phosphorous, upsetting the delicate bone balance. To get your daily allowance of complete protein combine whole grains with legumes.

Add a little brewer's yeast in your diet for calcium, zinc, folic acid and vitamin B6, also important to bone formation.

What is probably foremost is silica – a relatively unknown source nutrient necessary for calcium absorption. Green peppers have both vitamin C and silica, both bone enhancers. For more on nutrition and healthy bones, read the chapters Osteoporosis and Ankylosing Spondylitis.

Bunion-Busting Nutrients
For maximum absorption, take supplements with meals.

Nutrient	Suggested Dosage	Formulation
Aged garlic extract	1 teaspoon three times daily	Liquid
Borage oil	2 capsules daily	
Bromelain	250 mg three times a day	
Flaxseed oil	1 tablespoon daily	
Magnesium: 200 mg daily		
MSM		
(Methylsulfonylmethane):	500 mg three times daily	
Multi-mineral	3-4 ounces daily	In liquid solution, with vitamin B12, biotin
Multi-vitamin/mineral	6 caplets daily	Freeze-dried plant sources
Tumeric	100 mg three times daily	
Vitamin B6	200 mg daily	
Vitamin C	Individual bowel tolerance*	With bioflavonoids (quercetin, proanthocyanidins)

* To determine individual dosage, on the first day take 1,000 mg hourly until diarrhea occurs, then reduce dosage to just below that for individual daily dosage. Vitamin C is not toxic in large doses but must be taken throughout the day to benefit. Divide dosage to three or four times a day.

CHAPTER 25:

Burning Mouth Syndrome

For my *Maximize Your Life* television shows, we ask the studio audience to write down personal questions for addressing on the air. Every once in a while, someone stands up to share what might be called epidemiological evidence. In other words, they had a problem and found a solution through unscientific means. I don't know about you, but when I hear someone speak of this double-blind study or that control-group study, I'm not as convinced as when my neighbor tells me he consistently controls his heartburn, for example, by eating a vinegar and oil salad before every meal. The studies are fine and dandy, but I relate to and am more impressed with real life experiences.

Anyway, during one of my shows, we had just finished talking about how capsaicin – a component of hot peppers – helps shingles, or burning skin, when this woman – her name was Martha – excitedly stood up and told us about her burning mouth. She said she had perplexing burning mouth pain nearly every day, which lasted all day. Martha spoke with her family doctor about the burning sensation, which sometimes extended to her throat, and received a response that made her even more red hot.

"He told me it was psychogenic and tried to refer me to a psychiatrist!" she proclaimed angrily. The studio audience obviously related to her experience, as they burst out chattering excitedly to themselves. After the studio became quiet again, Martha told her story.

"Thinking I would make the problem worse, I avoided spicy foods, concentrating on soft, bland food and dairy products. I swear that made it worse! Finally, figuring I had nothing to lose, I ate a hot pepper. At least the burning felt familiar. I fully expected the burning to continue, but was I amazed when it stopped! A few hours later it started up again, so I ate another hot pepper, and it went away for good this time. Every once in a while I need one when my mouth starts burning. Now I keep a jar of peppers in the fridge and when the pain starts, I pop one in!"

The Heat Source

Called Burning Mouth Syndrome, or BMS for short, the problem is characterized by a chronic spicy-hot burning sensation in the mouth and on the tongue. It is estimated to afflict 1.3 million U.S. adults, mostly postmenopausal women. It's called a syndrome because doctors don't know precisely what causes it. It could be caused by any number of things, including B vitamin deficiencies, pernicious anemia (B12 deficiency) or iron deficiency, diabetes, hormonal imbalances, the use of medications that contain heavy metals and Sjogren's syndrome, which is a lack of bodily fluids and dry mouth.[1]

More than 430 medications – many of them common – may be linked to burning-mouth pain by causing mouth dryness.[2]

Another possible cause is thrush, an overgrowth of the candida albicans fungus in the mouth. Candida is caused by a diet high in refined carbohydrates (white flour and sugar-laden fast/junk food), and a lowered immune system, which can be caused by illness or stress. Antibiotics can also cause thrush because it eliminates the natural bacteria that keep the fungus from multiplying.[3]

Studies by Steven S. Witkin, Ph.D., of Cornell University Medical College, show that candida overgrowth often follows the use of antibiotics, and that candida lowers the immune system which may relate to hormonal problems. Perhaps this is a reason postmenopausal women get BMS.[4]

In one study, researchers tested two groups, one healthy and one with BMS for the presence of candida fungus and coliform bacteria. They discovered that the BMS group had higher levels of candida albicans.[5]

When Finnish researchers looked at a random group of 431 middle-aged adults, they found 15 percent had burning mouth syndrome. Half of these were discovered to have thrush.[6]

For solutions to beating candida, see my chapter Fungus Infections.

Zinc and B Vitamins

Zinc has been shown in studies to help burning mouth. In a study conducted by British researchers, 30 patients with burning mouth syndrome compared to 30 controls were found to have significantly lower blood levels of zinc – 30 percent less. Dr. L. Ivanyi, Ph.D., head of the Department of Clinical Pathology and Immunology at London's prestigious Institute of Dental Surgery believes that some burning mouth sufferers could be helped with zinc.[7]

Two nutrients must be considered along with zinc: vitamin B6 and copper. Too much copper will deplete zinc stores; they must be equal for optimum usage. Include 2-4 mg of copper with any zinc supplement. Vitamin B6 enhances zinc absorption.

The possibility that a B vitamin deficiency can cause burning mouth isn't surprising considering the importance of the B vitamins to the nervous system.

The whole B complex family includes B1 (thiamine), B2 (riboflavin), B3 (niacin), B5 (pantothenic acid), B6 (pyridoxine), B12 (cobalamin), B15 (pangamic acid), biotin, choline, folic acid, inositol and PABA (para-aminobenzoic acid). Each B vitamin has its own role in body function, centered on the nervous system, and must be taken together. Since nerves bring messages to all the organs and stimulate glands to secrete their important biochemicals, the whole body communication system can break down with a B vitamin deficiency.

Stop Pain with Peppers

That hot peppers helped Martha's burning mouth didn't surprise me. An article in the *Journal of the American Academy of Dermatology* reported that capsaicin, the chemical which makes cayenne pepper, jalapenos and other hot peppers taste hot, has been found to benefit burning mouth syndrome.[8]

There have been over 600 studies of capsaicin, including more than 100 human clinical trials. Several research institutions nationwide have studied the safety and efficacy of capsaicin, and the chemical has become one of the most intensively researched plant compounds for treating external pain.

Capsaicin relieves burning pain because it affects certain types of nerve fibers. It thwarts a natural body chemical known as substance P that the body uses to send certain pain messages to the brain. When applied, capsaicin stops substance P from sending its impulses.[9]

In a double-blind study of 40 patients with shingles-related pain, 69 percent who were treated with capsaicin showed improvement. Preliminary data also indicate that it relieves similar burning pain in some patients with diabetic neuropathy, where damage to the peripheral nerves due to diabetes causes feelings of numbness and pain.[10]

Not only does capsaicin reduce the transmission of pain by altering the production and release of Substance P, but it also increases DNA synthesis and the production of collagenase and prostaglandins, which reduce both pain and inflammation.[11]

Chili peppers are a popular new treatment for mouth pain after cancer treatment. Capsaicin is shown to reduce the pain from mouth sores that result from chemotherapy and radiation therapy. In a Yale study, all of 11 patients had their mouth pain decreased and in two cases entirely stopped after eating capsaicin-laced taffy.[12]

Burn Be Gone Nutrients
For maximum absorption, take supplements with meals.

Nutrient	Suggested Dosage	Formulation
Acidophilus	At least four billion flora daily on an empty stomach, three times daily	
Aloe vera juice	Swish in mouth three times daily	
Aged garlic extract	1 teaspoon three times daily	Liquid
Borage oil	2 capsules daily	
Caprylic acid	100 mg three times daily	
Fiber	4-8 tablets daily	Psyllium, with herb hyssop
Flaxseed oil	1 tablespoon daily	
Multi-mineral	1-4 ounces daily	In liquid solution, with vitamin B12, biotin
Multi-vitamin/mineral	3-6 caplets daily	Freeze-dried plant sources
Vitamin A	25,000 IU daily*	
Vitamin C	Individual bowel tolerance**	With bioflavonoids (quercetin, rutin proanthocyanidins)

* The FDA recommends pregnant women not exceed 10,000 IU of vitamin A daily.

** To determine individual dosage, on the first day take 1,000 mg hourly until diarrhea occurs, then reduce dosage to just below that for individual daily dosage. Vitamin C is not toxic in large doses but must be taken throughout the day to benefit. Divide dosage to three or four times a day.

CHAPTER 26:

Burns

We called her the garden lady. She was my childhood friend, and seemed like the oldest person in the world. Her eyes were the deepest blue, set off by solid brown skin that wrinkled when she smiled, which was all the time. I loved her the minute she introduced me to her backyard. She had the most spectacular garden. Her orchard boasted plump, juicy peaches, pears, plums and cherries; huge luscious vegetables burgeoned under her care; tantalizing herbs flourished; and flowers blossomed in an unbelievable array of color. She even coaxed almonds, walnuts and grapes to take root and offer their rewards.

Even the weeds were lovingly cultivated, though kept in one place. I used to sit on the marble bench in her backyard, taking in the fragrant jasmine blossoms of summer, watching her while she meticulously harvested her riches. She called her garden her "pharmacy."

I didn't fully understand how her plants could be medicinal until one day I was given an unexpected demonstration. A little boy in the neighborhood had been playing with matches and had caught his pants on fire. He was near the garden lady's house when it happened and came running to her first. The fire was out, but it had left a very nasty-looking burn on his leg. He came screaming into the yard, tears streaming down his cheeks. As she examined the red skin, she talked to him in a quiet, calm voice.

Moving quicker than I knew she could, she went to some small trees and clipped off a few of its large, saucer-shaped yellow flowers. Then she hustled around to her "weed" garden and clipped flowers from it, all the while grinding them together in a bowl. She went into her kitchen and returned with the now-wet flowers wrapped in cheesecloth, and wrapped it around the boy's leg. "This will ease the pain and heal the burn," she said. The next day the boy returned with a gooseberry pie baked by his mother. I was surprised to see the burn had not blistered and was covered with only a bandaid.

Years later I would learn she was the last of the local "healers." When she was a child, neighbors far and wide came to her mother for extracts, dried herbs and plant combinations for various afflictions. Unfortunately for all of us, much of the garden lady's legacy of natural healing was lost as organized medicine took over, becoming the highest profit industry in the world.

First Aid

Over the years, many of the good burn treatments gave way to bad advice. Never put butter on a burn. The salt content will increase the heat and the fat will invite bacteria. Never put ice on a burn. The skin cells are already damaged. The contrast between extreme hot and extreme cold will damage the tissues further. However, moving quickly to cover a burn with cold water will lower the skin temperature before any further damage can be done.

For all burns (including sunburn) the best course of action is to run the burned area under cold water for about fifteen minutes. In the event of a chemical burn, run cold water over the skin for at least five minutes and then call for help.

The most common type of burn is a superficial, or first-degree, burn that occurs when skin is briefly exposed to a hot surface or to the sun. A first-degree burn is characterized by redness and possibly blisters. With a second-degree burn you may also experience swelling, and in the case of sunburn, fluid-filled blisters may form. Third-degree burns are very serious–initial lack of pain and white or charred skin are the symptoms. If you suspect that you have a third-degree burn, or if a first- or second-degree burn covers a large area of skin, seek medical help. If you received the burn from some type of chemical or radiation, seek medical attention immediately.

Think Zinc

Research abounds with evidence that zinc is a major player in the health and healing of the skin. Zinc was used topically as calamine lotion as far back as 1500 B.C. by the Egyptians. When you are deficient in zinc, burns do not heal as well and your chances of them getting infected is increased. A zinc deficiency also affects the immune system by causing a reduction in natural killer cells and the size of the thymus gland, an extremely important immune system organ.

A topical administration of zinc chloride as a spray or ointment reduces the size of burn wounds, shortens healing time, and produces less splitting of the skin as it heals. Zinc oxide is an effective wound healer. Zinc oxide is available as an over-the-counter ointment for skin rashes and sunburn. Remember seeing all those white noses at the pool and on the beach? That's zinc oxide. Every first aid kit should have some.[1]

Zinc is well-known in medical circles and well-used in pharmaceutical circles for wound and burn healing. Zinc oxide is incorporated into fillings by dentists to stave off infection and in *Martindale, The Extra Pharmacopoeia* I count over 100 skin pharmaceuticals worldwide that contain zinc oxide.[2]

More importantly, researchers have noted that burn patients have strongly depressed blood levels of zinc and copper. Burn patients typically lose zinc and copper as they lose fluids. A study of 10 burn patients reported in the journal *Burns* showed that of patients who had burns covering 33 percent or more of their body, blood levels of zinc and copper were very low during the first seven days. The authors concluded that these losses may be enough to induce a deficiency state and compromise the patients' immune system and ability to heal and recover.[3]

Try trail mix for your zinc and copper. Make sure it includes sesame seeds, pumpkin seeds and blackstrap molasses for zinc; and raisins and nuts for copper.

Nutritional Support for the Burn Patient

One of the first reactions by the burn patient is what physicians call hypermetabolism. The metabolic rate, or rate by which the body utilizes food to create energy, is increased, resulting in a need for higher amounts of food and nutrients by the burn patient. Researchers have found that this increase in the rate of metabolism is directly proportional to the severity of the burn. Therefore, the more severe or extensive the burn, the higher the need for added nutrients. In one study, two groups of 10 burn patients each were compared. One group received nutritional support beginning immediately after hospitalization, which was an average of four hours after the burn injury, while the other group began getting nutritional support an average of 58 hours after injury. The support was in the form of blenderized foods given through a tube entering the nose and extending into the stomach. Patients who were supplemented early were hospitalized for 20 fewer days than patients supplemented later. The researchers concluded that nutritional support in the critical 24 hours following a burn can significantly influence patient recovery.[4]

Doctors at Shriners Burn Institute in Cincinnati, realizing the importance of nutrition, created their own modular tube feeding formula for burn patients which included various vitamins and minerals such as vitamins A and C, and zinc. Also added were the usual carbodydrates and proteins, as well as essential fatty acids and amino acids. In their studies they had very impressive results. The patients using their nutritional supplementation had less hospitalization, less infection and less scarring.[5]

The concept of nutritional supplementation for burn patients seemed so obvious to me, I decided to find out for myself if medical institutions have embraced it. I talked to Pam Cornwell, Case Manager of the Burn Unit at University of California Davis Medical Center (UCDMC), in Sacramento, California, who said that she has seen nutritional supplementation used for burn patients for the past 18 years, and believes it is standard practice in the "burn world." The formula used at UCDMC includes multiple vitamins, emphasizing vitamins C and A, and zinc.

Vital Vitamins

When it comes to wound healing, if zinc is number one, vitamin A has to be number two. Retinoids – vitamin A derivatives – are used in a myriad of skin care products for skin problems from acne to wrinkles. Vitamin A – found in orange fruits and vegetables – can increase skin collagen, reduce inflammation, decrease postoperative immune suppression, improve healing and improve the appearance of scars. Vitamin A is sometimes applied directly to wounds with sponge implants.[6]

Vitamin C is needed to build strong collagen, the underlying support of skin. Poor wound healing is one of the symptoms of scurvy, caused by a deficiency of vitamin C. A vitamin C deficiency can actually cause a breakdown of already-healed wounds. Plasma vitamin C levels decrease during times of stress, bone fractures, burns, or major surgeries. The conventional recommended daily allowance (RDA) of vitamin C increases from 60-100 mg to 500-1500 mg per day in burn victims. Physicians versed in nutrition would increase that to 3,000-4,000 mg. Vitamin C in combination with the B vitamin pantothenic acid has been shown to increase skin strength and fibroblastic content of scar tissue. A deficiency of both causes wounds to take longer to heal. Megadoses of vitamin C, even when given to patients with normal vitamin C levels, can accelerate collagen formation above the degeneration rate of damaged collagen.[7]

Some years ago, David H. Klasson, M.D., at Greenpoint Hospital in Brooklyn, NY, brought pain relief and quicker healing to serious burn patients by spraying burns with a one percent solution of ascorbic acid (vitamin C). He also had patients take more oral vitamin C than they could possibly derive from food: 200-500 mg four times a day.[8]

B vitamins in the body are reduced during times of stress, and I can't think of anything more stressful than the excruciating pain of a burn. Therefore, burn patients should also supplement with a vitamin B complex in addition to pantothenic acid. We get our B vitamins from whole grains and legumes.

Vitamin E – isolated from nuts and seeds – is another nutrient essential to the skin and helpful in healing burns. At health food conventions in the 1960s and '70s, Drs. Evan and Wilfrid Shute of the Shute Clinic in Canada presented incredible "before" and "after" color photos illustrating how vitamin E had successfully treated patients with gangrene and severe burns.[9]

Vitamin E acts by reducing the inflammation of burned tissues, thus reducing damage to them. This antioxidant also helps stabilize skin membranes so healing can occur. In one study, injured tendons healed in the presence of vitamin E were stronger than those healed without it. It was also noted that with the vitamin E, there were smaller and less scars. Vitamin E is notorious for boosting the immune system, essential in any major injury.[10]

Plant Remedies

Tea tree oil, derived from Australia's Melaleuca alternifolia tree, is my first choice for a minor-burn ointment. My cousin burned his arm in my kitchen a week after I brought home my first bottle of tea tree oil. We applied the pure oil to the burned skin and were amazed at its effectiveness – the pain began to dissipate immediately, and the burn quickly healed. I have used it since on other burns with similar success.

You can also apply the homeopathic remedy calendula (pot marigold) tincture or cream to soothe a first-degree burn. I use calendula for all types of skin problems. Homeopath Dana Ullman recommends Hypericum (St. John's Wort) in tincture form for second-degree burns. He suggests using a medicine dropper so that the liquid will run over the burn without breaking the blisters. Hypericum, taken internally, is used to heal nerve damage caused by burns.[11]

To alleviate pain from any type of burn, raise the burned area above the level of the heart to slow circulation, and take the homeopathic remedy Urtica Urens (stinging nettle) every few hours.[12]

Elder flowers and berries contain various substances that ease the inflammation and pain associated with minor burns. The flowers can be mashed and wrapped in several layers of cheesecloth to make poultices, or incorporated into an oil-based salve for direct application on the skin. A number of herbal salves, available at health food stores, blend elder flowers with other skin-healing herbs such as comfrey, plantain and calendula.[13]

Aloe Vera

Aloe vera is a well-known burn remedy and is used in trauma centers in California, Illinois, New York, Texas and other states. One reason aloe has a range of beneficial effects, is its ability to very quickly penetrate the skin and reach injured tissue. It relieves pain, reduces inflammation, and dilates capillaries, increasing blood supply to the injured area so healing can occur.

Research conducted by Ivan E. Danhof, Ph.D., M.D., retired professor of clinical pharmacology and physiology at the University of Texas, found that aloe vera penetrates human skin almost four times faster than water.[14]

Aloe vera is an effective oral and topical agent for healing any skin wound. In an experiment involving wounded mice, Robert H. Davis, Ph.D., reported that when their drinking water included aloe vera, the size of their wounds were 62.5 percent smaller than those not given the aloe. When a topical 25 percent aloe vera preparation was applied to their wounds, they were further reduced by 50 percent.[15]

Master herbalist Debra Nuzzi recommends applying the juice of the aloe vera plant to a burn, but naturopathic physician Cathy Rogers, N.D., warns against using aloe on sunburn because of its drying effect. Either keep a plant in the house (break open a leaf and squeeze out the pulp when needed) or buy a bottle of pure aloe gel to keep on hand, especially if you're traveling.[16]

A Honey of a Healer

The newest buzz for burns is honey. Three million old wives can't be wrong. Over the centuries, honey has been used as a burn folk remedy to control bacterial infection and promote healing. But only recently has medical research investigated the historical evidence. An article in the research journal *Burns* reported on a study in which 64 burn patients received either a conventional burn dressing or a gauze dressing soaked in honey. The authors reported that of the patients treated with conventional dressing, 16.6 percent had residual scars. In the honey-treated burns, only eight percent had scarring. It was also reported that the burns treated with honey healed on average six days faster.[17]

Honey provides the optimal environment for burn healing: moistness, and a barrier that prevents fluid loss and bacterial invasion. Dr. Alan Gaby tells the fascinating story of a progressive surgeon who used honey for a patient's stomach incision that kept getting infected. "The doctor poured some honey into the wound and sutured it up, after which the patient had no further trouble. The only person who had trouble was the doctor, who was censured by the hospital peer review committee."[18]

Skin-Healing Nutrients

For maximum absorption, take supplements with meals.

Nutrient	Suggested Dosage	Formulation
Acetyl L-Carnitine	500 mg three times daily	
Aged garlic extract	1 teaspoon three times daily	Liquid
Antioxidants	4 capsules daily	With selenium and grape seed extract
Borage oil	2 capsules daily	
Flaxseed oil	1 tablespoon daily	
Multi-mineral	3-4 ounces daily	In liquid solution, with vitamin B12, biotin
Multi-vitamin/mineral	6 caplets daily	Freeze-dried plant sources
Vitamin A	25,000 IU daily*	
Vitamin C	Individual bowel tolerance**	With bioflavonoids (quercetin, rutin proanthocyanidins)

For minor burns, nourish skin with a therapeutic moisturizer that contains aloe vera gel, chamomile, vitamins A and C, and avocado oil.

* The FDA recommends pregnant women not exceed 10,000 IU of vitamin A daily.

** To determine individual dosage, on the first day take 1,000 mg hourly until diarrhea occurs, then reduce dosage to just below that for individual daily dosage. Vitamin C is not toxic in large doses but must be taken throughout the day to benefit. Divide dosage to three or four times a day.

CHAPTER 27:

Bursitis

What do the following people: Los Angeles Dodgers baseball starter pitcher Bob Welch, Cincinnati Reds star Mario Soto, marathon runner Paul Pilkington, Pittsburgh Steeler quarterback Mark Malone, Washington Redskins running back John Riggins and Denver Broncos quarterback John Elway have in common? All had successful sports careers jeopardized by bouts of bursitis. Elway's 1989 season performance was compromised by his elbow bursitis and Dynasty's Emma Samms became an actress when bursitis of the hip at age 16 halted a promising ballet career.[1-7]

Where Does It Hurt?

Bursitis, that dull misery in the shoulder, elbow or knee, can strike anybody, from sedentary people to highly-trained athletes. And though the shoulder is a common locale for bursitis, any of the bursae in the human body – there are around 150 – can become irritated.

What are bursae and why do they become inflamed? Bursae (from the Greek word for wine-skin, and related to the English word purse) are small, enclosed, fluid-filled sacs that protect muscles and tendons from irritation produced by contact with bones. Their normal function is to keep the movement of muscles and tendons smooth and painless. Though bursitis may hurt as much as arthritis, it isn't a joint disease.[8]

Bursitis results from nutritional deficiencies coupled with chronic pressure, overuse or injury. "Housemaid's knee" or "nun's knee" are clever terms to describe the reaction of the patellar bursa, which lies just beneath the kneecap and swells when subjected to repeated pressure from housekeeping, kneeling in prayer, laying carpet, gardening or playing baseball.

Today's computer age is lending itself to bursitis. A friend of mine injured her elbow while moving, but it was her deficiency of magnesium and the constant repetition of using her computer mouse that caused the olecranon bursa in her elbow to inflame. Pushing wrists onto the desk while using the computer keyboard or while holding the mouse can cause inflammation of the wrist bursa. "Writer's wrist" can afflict students as they spend hours intensely scribbling notes on hard desks in classrooms. Anywhere there is a "bone bump"–on the thumb, big toe, wrist, knee, elbow–there is a risk of bursitis. Watch that you don't overly depend on that convenient bump to rest your head, arms, hands or legs.

Poorly fitting shoes can cause the dreaded "pump bump" brought on by excessive pressure and friction where the shoe rubs the calcaneal bursa on the back of the heel. One of the most common foot ailments, the bunion, is a form of bursitis caused when a tight-fitting shoe causes a sac on the joint of the big toe to become inflamed. See the chapter Bunions for more.

That exercise guru on the floor, her hand and elbow supporting her head, looks healthy as she lifts her leg to a jazz beat. But what you don't see is the pain behind her eyes as the trochanteric bursa in her hip and the olecranon bursa in her elbow revolt against the daily workouts.

By far the most commonly affected bursa is the subacromial–the shoulder bursa. No other joint in the body has the astonishing range of motion as does the shoulder. It can rotate through 360 degrees and traverse any arc within that orbit. It moves forward, backward, and up and down.

This marvelous creation allows you to wave to your acquaintances, salute your flag and throw a frisbee. It also helps you wash your car, paint your kitchen, pull weeds, and hoe a garden.

This abundance of opportunity also serves as your undoing. As with a fan belt approaching 60,000 miles, a shoulder nearing forty years of use can wear out. Of course, you needn't be a middle-aged weekend athlete or handyman to have the problem. Doctors see it in anyone whose occupation or hobby involves moving the shoulder a certain way over and over again. I bet even the Pope has some pain.

Preventing the Problem

Preventing bursitis is possible. All it takes is paying attention to your body. Remember the body bumps. Don't rest your elbow or wrist against a hard desk, don't wear tight shoes, don't overdo it! Don't be macho. If you're in pain, quit! Check your posture. Sometimes just the way you hold yourself can make a difference in your health and your golf game. If a task calls for lots of kneeling, cushion your knees, change position frequently, and take breaks.

We all experience sudden blows, bumps or falls, so what makes the difference between those who get bursitis and those who don't? Nutrition! As our bodies lose their ability to absorb minerals, imbalances occur. Hypocalcemia is one, and probably contributes toward the onset of bursitis. It occurs as the body receives too little magnesium, the traffic cop of calcium, and calcium accumulates in the soft body tissues, such as the bursa. Because of the high absorption rate of minerals in solution, and deficiency of magnesium in the diet, the ratio of magnesium and calcium in solution should be four to one, respectively.

A Protocol That Worked

A friend came to me with shoulder bursitis. "It's just my old bursitis acting up again," he told me. It's amazing how we accept pain as a natural part of life, when it is not natural nor should be accepted at all. He said he usually got rid of the pain by taking aspirin and a couple of days off work. When that didn't work, he got a prescription for pain pills.

I warned him that long-term use of the phenylbutazone he had been taking could cause stomach bleeding and blood cell problems. I suggested shots of vitamin B12 instead, and gave him the name and number of my doctor. I also recommended minerals in solution for magnesium and calcium, and vitamin C – lots of it. My doctor did an analysis of my friend's mineral state and found he was deficient in magnesium and calcium. Then he added natural vitamin D to the man's nutritional program.

When I saw my friend again, a week later, he reported the pain started going away almost overnight, and was completely gone in five days. He could swing his arm in a circle without a wince of pain. I told him the use of vitamin B12 was nothing new. It was originally described by I.S. Klemes, M.D., in 1953 and later in 1957, in *Industrial Medicine and Surgery*. Dr. Klemes' reports covered nearly 60 cases, and it worked in all but three.[9]

Non-steroidal Anti-Inflammatory Nutrients (NSAINs)

Try the sane approach to inflammation–N-SAIN. Instead of gut-busting, cell-wrenching NSAID pharmaceuticals, target safe and effective natural nutrients instead.

Researchers and others have discovered the benefits of pineapple, specifically its healing enzyme bromelain, known for its potent anti-inflammatory effect.

Licorice, specifically glycyrrhiza, has valuable bursitis-busting properties. Licorice contains a remarkable chemical called glycyrrhetinic acid or GA, which is effective for treating inflammation.

Turmeric is also a renowned anti-inflammatory. To be more exact, it is curcumin, the ingredient which gives tumeric its yellow color, that has been found in studies to work better than even ibuprofen, a popular over-the-counter pain medicine. In one study on rats, researchers found 20 mg of curcumin worked as well as 200 mg of ibuprofen.[10]

Another study compared curcumin to the aforementioned phenylbutazone. Researchers found that in rats, the active ingredient worked just as well as the drugs. No toxic effects from curcumin have been reported.[11] Curcumin and tumeric are available on your supermarket spice shelves but for more exact dosages, look for anti-inflammatory formulas in your health food store.

Vitamin C alone helps repair damaged bursa tissues, especially in doses more than 1,000 mg. To increase its effect, add bioflavonoids. One of them, quercetin, has been shown in studies to be particularly effective.[12] Foods high in vitamin C and bioflavonoids include guava, papaya, black currants, parsley, broccoli and kale.

Bursitis-Busting Nutrients
For maximum absorption, take supplements with meals.

Nutrient	Suggested Dosage	Formulation
Aged garlic extract	1 teaspoon three times daily	Liquid
Antioxidants	4 capsules daily*	With selenium and grapeseed extract
Borage oil	2 capsules daily	
Bromelain	250 mg three times a day between meals	
Flaxseed oil	1 tablespoon daily	
Glucosamine sulfate	500 mg three times daily with yucca	
Magnesium	200 mg daily	
MSM (methylsulfonylmethane)	500 mg three times daily	
Multi-mineral	3-4 ounces daily	In liquid solution, with vitamin B12, biotin
Multi-vitamin/mineral	6 caplets daily	Freeze-dried plant sources
Niacinamide	1,000 mg twice daily	
Quercetin	400 mg twice daily	With vitamin C and bioflavonoids
Tumeric	100 mg three times daily	
Vitamin B6	200 mg daily	
Vitamin C	Individual bowel tolerance**	With bioflavonoids (quercetin, rutin proanthocyanidins)
Yucca	300 mg three times daily	

*The FDA recommends pregnant women not exceed 10,000 IU of vitamin A daily.

**To determine individual dosage, on the first day take 1,000 mg hourly until diarrhea occurs, then reduce dosage to just below that for individual daily dosage. Vitamin C is not toxic in large doses but must be taken throughout the day to benefit. Divide dosage to three or four times a day.

CHAPTER 28:

Cancer, Bladder

"It is with disease of the mind, as with those of the body; we are half dead before we understand our disorder, and half cured when we do."
                                    –Charles Caleb Colton

Consuming Carcinogens

Chlorine a carcinogen? Who says? After all, we've lived with chlorinated water since the birth of the 20th century, and it has wiped out typhoid fever and cholera.

A clue to chlorine's cancer contribution came originally from statistics showing New Orleans had the nation's highest rate of bladder cancer – 15 percent higher than the national average. Its water comes from the Mississippi River which ends its long downhill trip to the Gulf of Mexico at New Orleans.

A study by the Environmental Defense Fund found "a significant relationship between the incidence of certain types of cancer" in New Orleans and the drinking water.

The Environmental Protection Agency (EPA), in announcing 66 possible carcinogens in New Orleans water, theorized it was not the chlorine alone that caused bladder cancer but its blending with industrial and agricultural wastes. The EPA announced 79 other U.S. cities, including New York City; Boston; Los Angeles; Seattle; Evansville, Indiana; Cincinnati, Ohio and Duluth, Minnesota had carcinogens in their water supplies.

Nobel-Prize winning Dr. Joshua Lederber of Stanford University then announced chlorine had never been properly checked for safety. He said chlorine's incredible ability to annihilate bacteria comes from undermining the microbes' DNA, the nucleic acid that contains the genetic instructions for cells.

Inasmuch as DNA is a basic unit for cell replication and the continuity of life, the fact that chlorine damages DNA is frightening!

Almost a generation ago, University of Tokyo researchers discovered chlorinated water can cause red blood cells to clump. The National Cancer Research Institute in Tokyo referred to chlorine as a "co-carcinogen."

Dr. K.P. Cantor and colleagues at the National Institutes of Health believe that at least 12 percent of bladder cancers are attributable to drinking chlorinated tap water.

Robert D. Morris of the Medical College of Wisconsin in Milwaukee directed a study that found people who drink chlorinated water run a 21 percent greater risk of bladder cancer and a 38 percent greater risk of rectal cancer than people who drink water with little or no chlorine. An article in *Science News* estimated that at least 4200 cases of bladder cancer and 6500 cases of rectal cancer in the United States each year may be traced to the consumption of chlorinated water.[1]

It's not just chlorine that puts you at risk for bladder cancer. Daily, long-term exposure to chemicals in the workplace can make you more susceptible. The National Bladder Cancer Study found that as much as 11 percent of bladder cancers diagnosed among white women in the United States can be attributed to their work environment. Among white men it is much higher: 21-25 percent. The study found an increased risk among women employed in metal working and fabrication occupations. Punch and stamping press operators had a particularly increased risk depending upon how long they had been working. Chemical processing workers also were found to have an increased risk.[2]

Lifestyle Risks – How to Lower Them

You're addicted and you know it. But do you fully realize what it is doing to your health? If you smoke or drink coffee on a regular basis, you are increasing your risk of bladder cancer. In a study reported in *Annuals of Epidemiology*, John E.Vena, Ph.D., found heavy coffee drinking associated with an increased risk for this cancer.[3] Most know smoking is related to lung cancer. But did you know it also increases your risk of getting bladder cancer? Statistics over the years have shown that bladder cancer is twice as prevalent in smokers as in non-smokers.

A pair of Tulane University researchers scored a stunning victory over bladder cancer some decades ago. A victory, of course, that mainstream medicine ignored. However, ignoring it did not make it go away, particularly for cancer victims desperate for a successful solution.

Dr. Jorgen U. Schlegel, then head of the Urology Department of Tulane University, New Orleans and biologist George Pipkin made the exciting breakthrough. They discovered that vitamin C (ascorbic acid) can destroy cancer-producing substances that precede bladder cancer in smokers.[4]

Schlegel and Pipkin administered 1,500 mg of vitamin C in three time-spaced doses of 500 mg each.

The success rate was so phenomenal that Schlegel recommended such a regimen for "individuals who, due to age, cigarette smoking or other factors, may be prone to bladder cancer formation."

Because your body excretes any vitamin C it does not immediately use, take supplements at regular intervals. For 1,000 mg total, take 250 mg four times a day. Take vitamin C just after eating, when stomach acid is optimum for absorption. If this isn't possible, chewable tablets can be used.

Vitamin C is found in highest amounts in guava, papaya, black currants, parsley, broccoli and kale.

Treating Bladder Cancer with Nutritionals

Researchers state large doses of vitamins may provide protection against the high recurrence rates observed in bladder cancer. In one study, high doses of vitamins A, B6 (pyridoxine), C and E doubled the survival rate of patients with bladder cancer compared to those who weren't given vitamins. There were no side effects reported from these megadoses. An article in *Medical Tribune* quoted Dr. Michael Jewett, chairman of urology at the University of Toronto, as saying, "For now, I would certainly tell any bladder cancer patient who wants to try high doses of vitamins that there do not seem to be any harmful effects and there may be some benefit."[5]

Another study treated one group of bladder cancer patients with vitamins in recommended daily allowance (RDA) dosages and compared it to another group given RDA-dosage multivitamins plus 4,000 IU of vitamin A, 100 mg of vitamin B6, 2,000 mg of vitamin C, 400 IU of vitamin E and 90 mg of zinc. They found that after 10 months patients given megadoses of vitamins and zinc had a recurrence rate half that of the RDA group. The researchers concluded that bladder cancer patients can increase their chances of recovery by including megadoses of vitamins A, B6, C and E plus zinc in their therapies.[6]

Researchers at Loma Linda University School of Medicine in California successfully used aged garlic extract to treat bladder cancer patients. They compared it with Bacillus Calmette Guerin (BCG), a bacterial vaccine, and found that five consecutive treatments with the garlic extract completely inhibited tumor growth, and was more effective than BCG.[7] This doesn't surprise me. I take liquid aged garlic extract every day. Garlic is a renowned digestive tract cleanser. I travel from one end of the country to the other, and all over the world, and find the garlic spares me the indigestion and other digestive problems common to frequent travelers.

For more on the benefits of garlic and other nutritionals in preventing and treating bladder cancer, read my book *Nutrition: The Cancer Answer II.*

Bladder Cancer-Fighting Nutrients

For maximum absorption, supplements should be taken with meals.

Nutrient	Suggested Dosage	Formulation
Acidophilus	At least four billion flora daily on an empty stomach, three times daily	
Aged garlic extract	2 teaspoons three times daily	Liquid
Amino acids	4-6 capsules daily	Multiple formula from natural sources
Antioxidants	4 capsules daily*	With selenium and grape seed extract
Borage oil	2 capsules daily	
Coenzyme Q10	2 capsules daily	With vitamin E, phospholipids and selenium
Enzymes	2 capsules twice daily	Multiple formula
Flaxseed oil	1 tablespoon daily	
Fresh cranberry juice	As tolerated	
Fiber	8 tablets daily	Psyllium, with herb hyssop
Multi-vitamin/mineral	6 caplets daily	Freeze-dried plant sources
Multi-mineral	2-4 ounces daily	In liquid solution, with vitamin B12, biotin
Pancreatic enzymes	1 capsule after each meal	
Purified water	2 gallons daily	
Vitamin C	Individual bowel tolerance**	With bioflavonoids (quercetin, rutin proanthocyanidins)

* The FDA recommends that pregnant women not exceed 10,000 IU of vitamin A daily.

** To determine individual dosage, on the first day take 1,000 mg hourly until diarrhea occurs, then reduce dosage to just below that for individual daily dosage. Vitamin C is not toxic in large doses but must be taken throughout the day to benefit. Divide dosage to three or four times a day.

CHAPTER 29:

Cancer, Breast

The Cure for Breast Cancer is Political Action.
–Susan Love, National Breast Cancer Coalition

First the bad news. You can't depend on conventional, so-called modern medicine to keep you from getting breast cancer, or becoming your cure. A study by The Physician Insurers Association of America found that breast cancer accounted for 2,448 of the 117,000 malpractice claims filed since 1985 – more than any other disease. It analyzed 487 completed claims where a delay in diagnosis was proved, and found an average delay of 14 months. That's 2,448 women who dutifully performed breast self-exams, found a lump, reported it to her doctor, had a checkup, was told she was OK, then 14 months later discovered she had breast cancer. So much for early detection

All of the malpractice claimants were under age 50. Many doctors have the misguided belief that only women over 50 get breast cancer and when a younger woman approaches her doctor with a suspicious lump, the doctor proclaims it a cyst and sends her on her way. In 35 percent of the claimants, the physician was initially not impressed enough by the symptoms to either order a mammogram or schedule a follow-up exam. What I find most appalling is that an incredible 80 percent of these women had mammograms that were either negative or inconclusive. Failure to follow up with both the physical exams and inconclusive mammograms was the second leading cause of delay in diagnosing breast cancer. If you think mammograms are pretty accurate, the study *boasts* that routine screening mammograms *did* identify tumors in "almost 11 percent of the women. Up from *four* percent in 1990."[1]

Keep this in mind the next time you're scheduled for a mammogram: 89 percent of these women left their doctors' office with a cancerous tumor that went undetected by their mammogram test.

Have They Lost Their Way?

When it comes to curing breast cancer, conventional medicine is way off the success scale. A 1986 article in the *New England Journal of Medicine* written by Elaine M. Smith and John C. Bailar III, a former editor-in-chief of the National Cancer Institute, used the NCI's own statistics to proclaim that "we are losing the war against cancer." Among the many stunning observations made was that "There has been no apparent change in mortality from breast cancer since 1950." In fact, according to the American Cancer Society, the number of deaths among women attributed to breast cancer have doubled in the last thirty years from 22,871 in 1959 to 42,837 in 1989 (*Cancer Facts & Figures 1993*, ACS).

In 1989, the U.S. General Accounting Office studied the use of chemotherapy for breast cancer. They concluded that despite a three-fold increase in the use of chemotherapy since 1975, there has been no detectable increase in survival.[2]

An article in the February 6, 1993 issue of *The Lancet*, Britain's most respected medical journal, follows up these proclamations with its own conclusion. Written by *The Lancet* editors themselves, they observed that "mortality from breast cancer has remained the same for decades despite advances in early diagnosis and treatment," adding that "there is no reliable data to suggest that screening reduces mortality in the youngest (under 40) or oldest (over 50) age groups." The only claim to fame for early screening is a "30 percent reduction in breast cancer deaths for the middle group." That is, only 30 percent of all women between 40 and 50 benefit from early breast cancer screening tests. *The Lancet* editors announced a breast cancer conference to be held in Belgium in April 1994. Called *The Challenge of Breast Cancer*, the conference hosted researchers from all over the world in order to "challenge dogma and redirect research efforts along more fruitful lines."[3]

An April 1994 article in *The Lancet* reported on the conference. The conclusion of the world's imminent researchers? The good news was that exactly half the researchers believe "chemotherapy in the management of breast cancer has a dim future," with the authors of the article concluding that "the testing of new approaches has a better scientific foundation" than ever before.[4]

The Chemical Connection

Now that researchers have given the green light to explore new approaches, what exactly are they? First we need to discuss what scientists *do* know about breast cancer. Doctors have long known that excess estrogen, a hormone essential for reproduction, causes cells to mutate and increases the risk for breast cancer. But what they didn't discover until recently is that man-made estrogens can stack the deck against women and increase their estrogen levels by hundreds of times. Devra Lee Davis, Ph.D., a senior advisor to the U.S. Department of Health and Human Services pinpoints pesticides, household chemicals and common plastics as some of these man-made estrogens. That statisticians evaluate breast cancer mortality from 1950 on, is not incidental. Before 1950, a lot of pesticides, like DDT, were not so prevalent in the environment.[5]

Eliminating The Failsafe

The Delaney Clause of the Food, Drug and Cosmetic Act mandated that any food additive found to induce cancer cannot be deemed safe. It was in effect for two decades, since the early '70s, when one of my icons, Gloria Swanson, and I helped Congressman Delaney word the amendment. It did not, however, specify *how* cancerous, and this is the loophole the FDA, and eventually Congressional representatives, used to get out of it.

The whole story of the battle to get carcinogenic dyes out of our food supply is outlined in chapter 36 of my book, *Nutrition: The Cancer Answer II*. It's too lengthy to go into here. All you need to be concerned about is that ultimately, despite court rulings against them, private lawsuits and government mandates, the FDA won out. First the specific dyes in question were allowed, using a "negligible risk" standard. Then the Delaney clause was completely thrown out, and now our food supply can legally contain dangerous carcinogens and synthetic estrogens without being labeled as such.

Lower the Fat to Lower the Risk

I've been saying for decades that a high-fat, animal protein diet increases the risk of breast cancer, since it substantially increases a woman's estrogen load. Asian women who immigrate to the U.S. experience a fourfold increase in their breast cancer death rate – in just one generation! In my book *Nutrition: The Cancer Answer II*, I recommend a 25 percent fat-calorie diet for breast cancer prevention and a 15 percent fat diet as part of breast cancer therapy.[6]

Fighting with Flavonoids

Another anti-estrogen plan of action involves the use of bioflavonoids, also called flavonoids. They are potentially therapeutic because they may prevent man-made estrogens from entering cells. Flavonoids are substances found in brightly-colored fruits and vegetables, and have been credited with reducing breast tumors.

Michael Gould, Ph.D., of the University of Wisconsin used limonene, a flavonoid found in citrus peel, dill weed oil and caraway oil, to reduce mouse tumors. He found 60 percent of the mice receiving limonene had a complete disappearance of tumors.[7]

Researchers at *The Lancet* conference reported success with three other kinds of flavonoids: deltanoids, retinoids and terpenoids. Terpenoids are found in abundance in rosemary and citrus oil (the oil you squeeze out of the pores of citrus fruits); retinoids are precursors of vitamin A and are found in orange fruits and vegetables; and deltanoids are found in egg yolks. Michael Sporn, a researcher in Bethesda, Maryland, reported that these flavonoids have the same properties as tamoxifen, a pharmaceutical drug (with major side effects) that keeps breast cells from absorbing estrogen.[8]

On November 13, 1993, bioflavonoids stepped onto center stage when *The Lancet* reported that the low incidence of prostatic cancer in Japan was due to their high intake of bioflavonoids in their heavily vegetarian diet. Another *Lancet* study on the effectiveness of flavonoids in osteoporosis reported, "Flavonoids seem a very safe and rational alternative to estrogen replacement therapy in preventing bone loss without side effects."

Carotenoids and retinoids together have proven to be double trouble for breast tumors, according to Clinton J. Grubbs, Ph.D., director of Nutrition and Carcinogenesis Laboratories, University of Alabama at Birmingham. Carotenoids appear to protect the cells against cancer-causing chemicals, while retinoids help prevent cancer cells from growing.[9] Beta carotene is a retinoid.

Legumes – peas, beans and certain roots – are isoflavonoids, which act as a non-steroidal estrogen. Soybeans, a fabulous cancer fighter, is eaten in great quantities in Japan and China, and are one of the reasons researchers believe these countries have low rates of breast cancer.[10] Tofu, soybean curd, is not as bad tasting as it sounds. It has the unique ability to absorb the flavors it is cooked in.

In the early 1980s, nutrition educator Carlton Fredericks, Ph.D., reported that a high intake of the B complex vitamins, plus extra choline and inositol, helped the liver break down estrogen into estriol, a non-carcinogenic form of the hormone. In experiments, he demonstrated that B vitamins also reduced many symptoms of premenstrual syndrome – itself caused by excessive estrogen.[11]

Aged garlic extract has been found in studies to target breast tumors. Dr. John Pinto, director of nutrition research at Memorial Sloan Kettering Cancer Center in New York, reported on new research that found two organic sulfur compounds in aged garlic extract can fight breast cancer cells. Dr. John Milner, Pennsylvania State University, found that garlic extract inhibited breast cancer in an experimental model. Dr. Milner's research was the first to document how garlic extract was even more effective in preventing breast cancer tumors than fresh garlic or garlic powder.[12]

Natural progesterone cream, derived from wild yams, has been shown to help alleviate the carcinogenic effects of too much estrogen. Not only that, but progesterone is implicated in cancer protection. The *American Journal of Epidemiology* reports on a study in which premenopausal women with low progesterone levels were found to have 5.4 times the risk of developing breast cancer and a 10-fold increase in deaths from all malignant tumors compared to those with normal progesterone levels.[13]

Breast Cancer-Crushing Nutrients

For maximum absorption, supplements should be taken with meals.

Nutrient	Suggested Dosage	Formulation
Aged garlic extract	2 teaspoons three times daily	Liquid
Amino acids	4-6 capsules daily	Multiple formula from natural sources
Antioxidants	4 capsules daily*	With selenium and grape seed extract
Borage oil	2 capsules daily	
Enzymes	2 capsules twice daily	Multiple formula
Flaxseed oil	1 tablespoon daily	
Fiber	8 tablets daily	Psyllium, with herb hyssop
Lecithin	2 tablespoons with meals	
Multi-vitamin/mineral	6 caplets daily	Freeze-dried plant sources
Multi-mineral	2-4 ounces daily	In liquid solution, with vitamin B12, biotin
Natural progesterone cream	1/3 teaspoon daily	With pregnenolone, DHEA
Vitamin C	Individual bowel tolerance**	With bioflavonoids (quercetin, rutin proanthocyanidins)

* The FDA recommends that pregnant women not exceed 10,000 IU of vitamin A daily.

** To determine individual dosage, on the first day take 1,000 mg hourly until diarrhea occurs, then reduce dosage to just below that for individual daily dosage. Vitamin C is not toxic in large doses but must be taken throughout the day to benefit. Divide dosage to three or four times a day.

CHAPTER 30:

Cancer, Cervical

*"Every great advance in natural knowledge has in-
volved the absolute rejection of authority."*
                                        –Thomas Huxley

What is cancer, exactly? *Churchill's Medical Dictionary*
(Churchill/Livingstone, 1989) defines it as "uncontrolled proliferation of cells which usually destroys and invades adjacent tissues,
metastasizes and follows a fatal course if untreated..." A cancerous
tumor is a community of cancer cells that "convert" others in order
to increase their size.

The question remains: what causes otherwise normal, healthy cells
to change into cancer cells? Even orthodox medicine finally agrees
carcinogens are merely the irritant that determines the location of the
lump or bump the medical establishment recognizes as cancer. In
reality, lumps and bumps are only the symptom or final manifestation of an underlying metabolic imbalance or weakness in our body's
intrinsic defense against disease. Carcinogens change the body's
normal trophoblast cells into rapidly-proliferating cancer cells that it
either has not protected itself from or cannot.[1]

In the case of cervical cancer, the body's defenses are lowered by
the human papilloma virus, a name to describe the virus that causes
warts and herpes simplex II. In a recent study directed by M. Michele
Manos, Ph.D., and Dr. F. Xavier Bosch of the World Health Organization, scientists examining cervical tumors from 22 countries found
viral evidence in 93 percent of them.[2] These viruses are believed to
be transmitted through sexual relations.

Cervical Dysplasia and Cervical Cancer

Since the term dysplasia is so important to understanding cervical cancer, especially when your gynecologist comes to you to report your pap smear results showed cervical dysplasia, let me clarify it. The pap smear is used to detect abnormal cells on the cervix. The doctor scrapes off some cells, then the laboratory checks them for abnormalities. Just because they find dysplasia doesn't mean you have cancer, or will get cancer. All it means is that for some reason or another your cells have mutated, so to speak. What they think is dysplasia leads to cancer. This is because when they find cervical cancer cells, the outlying cells are in this dysplasia stage. That's why your doctor will recommend you have the abnormal cells removed. It's a precautionary measure, and shouldn't be thought of as cancer surgery. Preventing and treating dysplasia is believed to be the key to preventing cervical cancer. No dysplasia? No cervical cancer. At least that's the theory.

How long does it take to go from cervical dysplasia to cervical cancer? The average time for progression from cervical dysplasia to cancer cells in untreated women ranges from 86 months for patients with very mild dysplasia, to 12 months for patients with severe dysplasia.[3] This makes that annual pap smear important. For nutritional prevention options read my book *Nutrition: The Cancer Answer II.*

Other than the already-mentioned viruses, there are reasons doctors believe your cells mutate: smoking for one, birth control pills for another and toxic chemicals, like DES. Even douching too frequently has been associated with dysplasia.

Risk Factors

Studies at Emory University School of Medicine and at the Centers for Disease Control in Atlanta reveal cancers and other tumorous conditions of the cervix develop more readily in smokers than non-smokers. The more smoking the woman does, the greater the hazard.[4]

Studies have shown that women who use birth control pills run a higher risk of cervical dysplasia than non-users.[5] Why this happens can be explained. Women on birth control pills often are deficient in the B vitamin folic acid. A University of Alabama research team headed by medical doctors Charles E. Butterworth and Kenneth Hatch, discovered ten milligrams a day of folic acid may stop or even reverse early dysplasia.

They performed a study in which twenty-two women on birth control pills who had dysplasia were placed on this regimen for three months. Twenty were given placebos. Eighteen of the twenty-two on folic acid found their condition arrested. The remaining four were rewarded with total reversal of their condition.[6] The RDA for folic acid is a mere 400 micrograms (mcg). Since 1,000 micrograms is one milligram (mg); to get ten milligrams, you'd need to increase this dosage by 25 times. When buying any supplement, look at the label.

Inasmuch as folic acid is essential to proper cell division, some researchers think that a deficiency of this vitamin might cause abnormal cell division. In a study reported by the California State Department of Health's *The Nutrition Report,* 102 women with cervical dysplasia were compared to 102 women with normal pap smears. It was found that the odds of having dysplasia were 10 times higher for those with the lowest blood levels of folic acid, compared to those with the highest levels. Folic acid deficiency is a major problem worldwide. It is so prevalent in this country that the FDA has just mandated it be added to all commercial breads. This is an exercise in futility since folic acid is destroyed through food processing.

Anytime you decide to supplement with folic acid, be sure you include B12. A B-complex formula plus extra folic acid is probably the best way to go. Most of the B vitamins are dependent upon one another. B12 and folic acid are no exception.

The DES Threat

A generation ago, cervical cancer was a rarity. Now, next to breast cancer, it is the second most common cancer among women. One of the reasons is the presence of diethylstilbestrol (DES), a synthetic hormone, currently given to meat-source animals, and, in the '50s, commonly prescribed to pregnant women to prevent miscarriage. Now experts agree the drug can be traced to a high incidence of vaginal and cervical cancer among the daughters of these women.

The first reported connection came in the spring of 1971 from gynecologist Dr. Arthur L. Herbst and associates at Harvard Medical School.[7] While researching an unusual incidence of seven cases of cervical cancer, they found each had mothers who were administered DES in the '50s. Prior to these cases, the occurrence of this type of cancer was extremely rare. In the '70s, a registry was developed to track DES-exposed women and cases of cervical cancer.

According to Herbst, "As of June 1992, 589 cases had been reported to the registry and 60 percent of the investigated cases have a positive DES history."[8]

Unfortunately, we can't do a retake of the past, Hollywood-style, so we have to deal with what preventive measures can be taken. It is a sad fact that many pregnant women may still be ingesting synthetic estrogen unknowingly.

DES is used to increase the weight of cattle and chickens before being marketed. It is illegal to include it in animal or poultry feed, but the U.S. Department of Agriculture would need an army of agents to monitor the more than 50 million cattle and many times that quantity of chickens to determine residues of DES in meat and chicken.

Implants of DES are permitted in cattle and chickens, and supposedly the residues vanish prior to marketing time. However, who knows how much DES a pregnant woman, any of us for that matter, is ingesting along with that juicy hamburger?

Does such a small amount of DES amount to anything? Researchers have shown this hormone is so potent just two parts per billion is poisonous to mice. Only an infinitesimal amount daily – .07 millionths of a gram – is needed to cause cancer in mice.[9]

Whenever the DES issue rears it hideous head, agricultural economists use the threadbare argument that meat and poultry would cost a fortune if it weren't for diethylstilbestrol. Are they saying cancer doesn't cost our medical system a fortune in treatments and hospitalization, not to mention the pain and anguish to cancer patients and loved ones?

The tempered "good news" is an estimated 25 percent of market cattle is raised without DES. Such wholesome beef – poultry as well – is sold by health food stores that have the appropriate refrigeration. Yes, it costs more. But isn't it worth the price?

The Issue of Nutritional Status

Many conventional doctors don't take into account the numerous studies linking cervical cancer with vitamin and mineral deficiencies. Up to 67 percent of patients with cervical cancer have been found to be deficient in one or more nutrients.[10]

The evidence – and there is reams of it – shows that low levels of many important nutrients could be the reason why cervical cells mutate and eventually progress into cervical cancer. Antioxidants, like vitamins C and E and the mineral selenium protect from DES and smoking-incurred free radical damage. Vitamin A and beta carotene protect the skin cells from being affected by viruses.

One study, reported in the *Mt. Sinai School of Medicine Complete Book of Nutrition*, showed that a deficiency of vitamin C, that is, blood levels less than the recommended daily allowance (RDA), has been associated with cervical dysplasia.[11] This is a very conventional book, so for them to include this study is telling indeed.

The California State Department of Health reported that women with the highest levels of dietary vitamin C, compared to the lowest, were 4-5 times more likely *not* to have cervical dysplasia.[12]

Beta carotene, an antioxidant and vitamin A precursor, is also a factor in cervical dysplasia. Researchers have found that as a group, women with dysplasia have a level of beta carotene only one-half of normal women.[13]

A study by Dr. Sylvia Wassertheil-Smoller and associates at Albert Einstein College of Medicine disclosed healthy women ingest more beta carotene and vitamin C than women with abnormal pap smears.[14]

Vitamin E, a powerful antioxidant, has been linked with beta carotene in studies showing that these nutrients can reduce cell abnormalities. This determination was made by researchers headed by Prabhudas R. Palan, of the Department of Obstetrics and Gynecology, Albert Einstein College of Medicine in Bronx, New York. Palan and colleagues evaluated 116 women for blood levels of vitamin E and beta carotene, and found that women with dysplasia had severe deficiencies of both these nutrients. They concluded that the two nutrients are very important to cervical health.[15]

Other nutrients found in studies to be deficient in cervical dysplasia patients are selenium and vitamin B6 (pyridoxine). Selenium is important to all mucous membranes, including those found in the cervix, and vitamin B6 was found in a study to be decreased in one-third of the women tested who had cervical cancer.[16]

For the whole story of nutrition and cancer, read my book *Nutrition: The Cancer Answer II.*

Dysplasia Defeating-Nutrients

For maximum absorption, supplements should be taken with meals.

Nutrient	Suggested Dosage	Formulation
Aged garlic extract	2 teaspoons three times daily	Liquid
Amino acids	4-6 capsules daily	Multiple formula from natural sources
Antioxidants	4 capsules daily*	With selenium and grape seed extract
Borage oil	2 capsules daily	
Enzymes	2 capsules twice daily	Multiple formula
Flaxseed oil	1 tablespoon daily	
Fiber	8 tablets daily	Psyllium, with herb hyssop
Folic acid	10 mg daily	
L-lysine	500-1,200 mg daily	
Multi-vitamin/mineral	6 caplets daily	Freeze-dried plant sources
Multi-mineral	2-4 ounces daily	In liquid solution, with vitamin B12, biotin
Natural progesterone cream	1/3 teaspoon daily	With pregnenolone, DHEA
Vitamin C	Individual bowel tolerance**	With bioflavonoids (quercetin, rutin proanthocyanidins)

* The FDA recommends that pregnant women not exceed 10,000 IU of vitamin A daily.

** To determine individual dosage, on the first day take 1,000 mg hourly until diarrhea occurs, then reduce dosage to just below that for individual daily dosage. Vitamin C is not toxic in large doses but must be taken throughout the day to benefit. Divide dosage to three or four times a day.

CHAPTER 31:

Cancer, Colon

According to the book of records, the fattest man was buried in a piano crate. It must have been quite an undertaking!

Fat is dangerous. Not only when you eat it, but when you wear it. Measure the fat around your waist, and you'll have a good idea of the amount of fat surrounding your heart and clogging your colon. The trouble with overeating is that it usually means over-eating fatty foods. When was the last time you ate a full plate of vegetables? More than likely the last big meal you ate included mashed potatoes with butter, gravy and meat.

Several research studies reveal individuals on a high fat diet double their chances of developing colon cancer. Fat promotes cancer by stimulating production of anaerobic bacteria – those that need no oxygen to exist. One experiment revealed those who consume a great deal of fat have a 100 times increase in anaerobic bacteria. These bacteria are capable of changing the bile acids in fecal matter into chemicals that can cause cancer and also converting bile into estrogen, which also triggers tumor growth.[1]

If you think cancer is in the genes, you'd be wrong. A recent six-year study of Chinese individuals found those living in the U.S. who ate an average of only 100 more calories of saturated fat per day than participants living in China had colon cancer risks nearly double that of their counterparts.[2]

Fat is the dietary component most often linked to cancer. Diets of patients with colon cancer contain significantly more fat and sugars and far less fiber compared to diets of healthy individuals. Frequent consumption of high fat foods among blacks, especially, is directly associated with the incidence of colon cancer.[3]

If you find yourself eating more fat than you know is good for you, there are actions you can take. Studies have shown that aged garlic extract will not only stimulate growth of friendly intestinal bacteria, but the organosulfur compounds detoxify carcinogens. Onion oil has this benefit also. Both have been found to be beneficial in preventing colon cancer.[4,5] I highly recommend Kyolic® liquid aged garlic extract. I take it every day. The Wakunaga people, who manufacture Kyolic®, have had the integrity to do 90 percent of the scientific research available on garlic.

Increasing your dietary fiber will also make a significant difference. Fat intake is very high in Finland, where the incidence of coronary heart disease is one of the highest in the world. The occurence of colon cancer, however, is less than one third that of the United States. These lower colon cancer statistics have been attributed to consumption of a popular coarse, whole-grain rye bread. The bread has huge amounts of fiber and increases fecal bulk to three times that found in most Western nations.

Waste matter in the large bowel contains potential cancer-causing substances. The longer it presses on the colon wall, the greater the threat of colon cancer.[6] Insoluble fiber and roughage, present most abundantly in vegetables and whole grains, moves these substances through quickly, before they can carcinogize – so-to-speak – your colon.

Pass the Possum, Please

We can blame the progress of civilization for colon cancer. Our early ancestors had few of the problems we experience today since they ate a myriad of foods including nuts, seeds, roots and wild plants, mammals, rodents, bugs and reptiles. One can only wonder at the magnificence of the human body when we realize our ancestors were capable of not only eating lizards, but digesting them. Ugh! No doubt salamanders contain a lot of insoluble fiber – the stuff we don't absorb that rotor-rooters our intestines clean.

Early man used to eat so much roughage, his teeth were reduced to stubs by the age of 40. As we lived longer, we developed ways to save our teeth, but sacrificed our bowels. "Civilized" (wo)man invented grain mills and food processing. As a result we reduced and lost the natural roughage vital to our vitals. Whole foods became conveniently chopped, pressed and formed, like some packaged sliced meats, and the fiber in fruits became soft, sweet and denatured in cans.

Basic Foods for a Robust Bowel

Vegetables contain quality fiber, although not at whole grain bran level, and offer special protection against colon cancer. This is underscored by a significant study made by Dr. Saxon Graham, chairman of Social and Preventive Medicine at The State University of New York at Buffalo, and co-workers.[7]

The Graham team compared the diets of 256 male colon cancer patients at Roswell Park Memorial Institute and 783 non-cancer patients of the same age. They focused mainly on how frequently they ate 19 vegetables, including the now well-known cruciferous cancer fighters: cabbage, broccoli, Brussels sprouts, cauliflower and turnips, and other veggies such as beta carotene-rich carrots, yams, watercress, squash, peppers and tomatoes.

Colon cancer patients ate few vegetables regularly, compared with the others. Those who consumed the most vegetables ran the least risk of cancer. The more frequently they ate them, the less likely they were to develop colon cancer.

Consumption of tomatoes and strawberries are strongly associated with low cancer risk. A 20-year study found the higher the consumption of these vegetables, the lower the risk of colon cancer.

It's a lot more than fiber that make fruits and vegetables so important. Fruits and vegetables contain a plethora of cancer preventive and curative substances including carotenoids, vitamins C and E, selenium, flavonoids, polyphenols and other tongue-twisting compounds. Some work better than others for colon cancer.

Tomatoes contain lycopene, a carotenoid flavonoid. To evaluate the role of lycopene as a colon-cancer preventive, a study was conducted in Northern Italy, where the residents eat large amounts of tomatoes. The researchers found a 50 percent reduced rate for colon cancer among those who ate only one serving of raw tomatoes a week.[8] Other foods high in lycopene are apricots, grapefruit, guava juice and watermelon.[9]

Beta carotene, found in yellow and green leafy vegetables, like carrots, sweet potatoes, squash, cantaloupe, spinach and broccoli, has the potential of reducing the recurrence of colon cancer. Walter Reed Army Hospital Medical Center researchers led by James Walter Kikendall discovered that 30 mg of beta carotene – about a carrot a day – given to 20 males with colon cancer reduced their colonic carcinogens by 44 percent after two weeks and 57 percent after nine weeks of supplementation. The researchers reported that, incredibly, the reduction lasted six months after the beta carotene supplementation was discontinued.[10]

Just as some foods prevent colon cancer, a lack of others can increase your chances of getting colon cancer. Any program of good eating should include avocados, brown rice, wheat bran, soybeans, bean sprouts, artichokes, beets, cauliflower and corn. These are foods high in folic acid. Researchers have come to realize that a deficiency of folic acid is associated with colon cancer. It is a fact that without enough folic acid, cell division is impaired, leading to the kind of abnormalities that precede cancer. Even minor deficiencies have been associated with cell mutation. Researchers led by Joel B. Mason, M.D., USDA Human Nutrition Research Center, in an article in the *Journal of Nutritional Biochemistry* said that not only does a folic acid deficiency increase the chances of colon cancer, but that the B vitamin can actually reverse the DNA damage that occurs in patients with colon cancer.[11]

Tofutti Anyone?

Do you remember when food retailers tried to sell us on a frozen concoction made out of tofu? They called it tofutti, and since you don't see it anymore we have to assume it failed. It probably tasted like sweetened soybean curd. Fortunately, you can still find tofu in the refrigerated section of most supermarkets. It is packed in water, in small square boxes, usually by the milk and yogurt. You can even get cookbooks on how to use it deliciously in recipes. I won't go into detail on exactly how processors go from soybeans to soybean curd – suffice it to say it is probably the most effective colon-cancer preventive available in your supermarket today.

When I looked at colon cancer research I kept coming across *genistein*. Everywhere I looked, it seemed some researcher was talking about the wonders of genistein. Then I discovered it was none other than the bioflavonoid found in soybeans! Why don't they just use English?! Anyway, one study sought out the best source of genistein and it turned out to be tofu.

The researchers were from Tufts Medical School and New England Medical Center in Boston. They compared four brands of tofu with a soy drink and three soy-based baby formulas. Apparently, soybeans don't translate very well into liquid form because the researchers found important nutrients missing from the soy baby formulas, including genistein. The soy drink had the nutrients, but in very low amounts. They concluded that tofu soy products contain the most genistein.[12]

The National Cancer Institute, Chemoprevention Branch, performed their own study on the benefits of genistein to colon cancer. In animal experiments, when they gave the subjects genistein before dosing them with a known carcinogen, they found the genistein protected the colon from the cancer-causing agent. They added in their report that genistein had no side effects.[13]

If the idea of eating curd anything doesn't appeal to you, try it anyway. It is similar to scrambled eggs in texture and has the marvelous ability to absorb whatever flavors it is cooked in. Cut it in cubes and add it to your soup, or slice it and add it to your spaghetti sauce.

For the complete story of nutrition and cancer, read my book *Nutrition: The Cancer Answer II.*

Colon Cancer-Crushing Nutrients
For maximum absorption, supplements should be taken with meals.

Nutrient	Suggested Dosage	Formulation
Acidophilus	At least four billion flora daily on an empty stomach, three times daily	
Aged garlic extract	2 teaspoons three times daily	Liquid
Amino acids	4-6 capsules daily	Multiple formula from natural sources
Antioxidants	4 capsules daily*	With selenium and grape seed extract
Borage oil	2 capsules daily	
Coenzyme Q10	2 capsules daily	With vitamin E, phospholipids and selenium
Enzymes	2 capsules twice daily	Multiple formula
Flaxseed oil	1 tablespoon daily	
Fiber	8 tablets daily	Psyllium, with herb hyssop
Folic acid	10 mg daily	
L-Glutamine	500 mg three times daily	
Multi-vitamin/mineral	6 caplets daily	Freeze-dried plant sources
Multi-mineral	2-4 ounces daily	In liquid solution, with vitamin B12, biotin
Vitamin C	Individual bowel tolerance**	With bioflavonoids (quercetin, rutin proanthcyanidins)

* The FDA recommends that pregnant women not exceed 10,000 IU of vitamin A daily.

** To determine individual dosage, on the first day take 1,000 mg hourly until diarrhea occurs, then reduce dosage to just below that for individual daily dosage. Vitamin C is not toxic in large doses but must be taken throughout the day to benefit. Divide dosage to three or four times a day.

CHAPTER 32:

Cancer, Liver

If you are afraid all your years of living in the fast lane might get you run over, consider this: the liver is an incredibly resilient organ. It has to be, considering all it is required to do. The liver filters over a liter of blood a minute, effectively removing bacteria and toxins. It manufactures bile, which also helps remove dangerous chemicals, and is necessary for the absorption and storage of fats, vitamins and minerals. When the liver breaks down, the body follows. But it doesn't break down easily, and it has the capability of regenerating itself, when given the proper nutrients and a little time.

What you need to know to protect your liver are nutrients needed to prevent and overcome liver cancer. Liver protecting substances have been identified as the amino acids methionine and betaine and the B vitamins choline, folic acid and B12.[1]

Helping Your Liver Help Itself

Liver cancer does not just appear. It occurs after the liver's defense system has been reduced enough by deficiencies and disease to halt its ability to regenerate itself. Liver diseases such as hepatitis and mononucleosis wear down the liver's defenses. A high fat diet overloads it with fatty deposits and deficiencies. Poor diet, smoking and alcoholism coupled with the incredible toxic load of the average modern environment can make liver cancer a likelihood.

Fortunately for us, our health food stores offer us a cornucopia of nutrients to enliven your liver and keep cancer from invading your insides.

Researchers at the University of North Carolina, Chapel Hill, have found in animal experiments that a choline and lecithin deficiency may cause enough of a liver dysfunction to eventually result in liver cancer.[2]

Basically, all you have to know is that choline is a constituent of lecithin and if you take lecithin, you'll be getting your choline. Scientists separate them because the body does. Lecithin is available as a dietary supplement with food sources of choline identified as egg yolk, liver, brewer's yeast and wheat germ. Choline is manufactured in the body by the combination of – guess what? – folic acid, B12 and the amino acid methionine. Betaine is a digestive enzyme that helps unlock the body's absorption of these nutrients. All these nutrients must be taken as a group and are absolutely essential to the health and well-being of your liver.

Risk Factors Within Your Control

In some instances we invite environmental enemies into our body, even though we know they harm or even may kill us. These preventable factors include birth control pills, alcohol and, of course, cigarettes, which University of Southern California researchers have discovered are major risk factors for liver cancer.

Women who use birth control pills for more than five years have 5.5 times a greater risk of developing liver cancer than women who have never used the pill, found Mimi C. Yu, Ph.D., a professor of preventive medicine at the USC School of Medicine. Cigarette smokers have 2.1 times the risk of non-smokers, and heavy drinkers have a 4.3 better chance of developing cancer than teetotalers or light drinkers.[3]

Liver cancer is a rapidly-fatal disease that is common among Asian populations but relatively rare in non-Asians. The major cause of this degenerative disease is infection with hepatitis B virus, an ailment prevalent in Asian populations.

Yu and fellow USC researchers conducted a study with non-Asians to limit the confounding role of hepatitis infection. Blood samples of all subjects were taken to make sure they were hepatitis free.

The study sample consisted of 74 cases of liver cancer occurring in white and black residents of Los Angeles county, aged 18 to 74, and 162 healthy controls of comparable age, sex and race.

Results of the study showed that use of birth control pills increased the risk of liver cancer threefold and use for five or more years increased the risk 5.5 times.

These findings are indeed alarming. However, the risks may be even greater, because the research included women who were too old to need birth control when oral contraceptives became available. When the statistics were limited to women ages 64 and younger – women in their reproductive years when birth control pills were introduced (the 1960s) – the risk for more than five years of use jumped to almost 30 times that of women who had never used birth control pills.

Several other studies implicate birth control pills too, and tests with animals show that estrogen contained in birth control pills promote liver cancer. See my book *Nutrition: The Cancer Answer II* for more on reducing the risk of synthetic estrogens.

Dr. Yu warns against stacking the odds with more than one risk factor. For example, if a woman smokes cigarettes and has been infected with hepatitis B or C, she may not want to push her luck by taking birth control pills.

The data on alcohol consumption implicated only heavy drinkers. Moderate drinkers showed no increased risk. The greatest risk (4.7 fold) was for men who drank more than nine cans of beer, nine glasses of wine or nine shots of spirits daily. Men slightly below that had a 2.6-fold increased risk.

The female subjects drank relatively little and thus provided an opportunity to demonstrate the independent effect of cigarette smoking, inasmuch as drinking and smoking often go hand in hand. The data for both non-smoking women and men clearly indicate that cigarette smoking alone is a definite risk factor for liver cancer, states Yu.

A careful analysis shows that among non-Asians, 54 percent of the liver cases in women can be attributed to cigarettes and birth control pills, and 56 percent of these cases in men can be attributed to alcohol and/or cigarettes.

A magnesium deficiency may be one of the factors leading to an increased risk of liver cancer in alcoholics. Magnesium is essential to healthy tissues and the combination of a deficiency and the damaging effects of alcohol may be enough to restrict the liver's ability to heal itself.[4]

A deficiency of magnesium is common among alcoholics and is often unrecognized by health professionals. I suggest anyone with alcohol problems supplement with magnesium and include magnesium-rich foods in the diet.

Because of the host of problems associated with smoking and drinking, and because a damaged liver compromises the absorption of nutrients, it is a good idea to supplement with B12 and minerals in solution. Minerals in solution provide the optimum rate of absorption into the body.

Overcoming The Risk Factors

I've already covered the ways you can prevent cancer in general. There are also ways you can quench that risk for liver cancer specifically.

In 1993 Columbia University researchers evaluated the use of various vitamins to reduce the risk of liver cancer among people with high risk lifestyles. They found that the major antioxidant vitamins: A, C, E and beta carotene, worked particularly well to protect the liver *(Cancer, 1994)*.

In 1994, Hiroshi Nishida of the Gifu University School of Medicine, Japan, and colleagues found that a chemical component of green tea, which is a potent antioxidant, statistically reduced the chances of liver cancer developing in mice, with no toxic side effects.[5] The researchers say it's not the tea that does it, but the leaves. Therefore, look for supplements that use green tea leaves in its preparation.

Read my book *Nutrition: The Cancer Answer II* for proven liver cancer treatments and therapies.

Liver-Loving Nutrients
For maximum absorption, supplements should be taken with meals.

Nutrient	Suggested Dosage	Formulation
Aged garlic extract	2 teaspoons three times daily	Liquid
Amino acids	4-6 capsules daily	Multiple formula from natural sources
Antioxidants	4 capsules daily*	With selenium and grape seed extract
Borage oil	2 capsules daily	
Coenzyme Q10	2 capsules daily	With vitamin E, phospholipids and selenium
Enzymes	2 capsules twice daily	Multiple formula
Flaxseed oil	1 tablespoon daily	
Fiber	8 tablets daily	Psyllium, with herb hyssop
Folic acid	10 mg daily	
Multi-vitamin/mineral	6 caplets daily	Freeze-dried plant sources
Multi-mineral	2-4 ounces daily	In liquid solution, with vitamin B12, biotin
Milk thistle	150 mg twice daily	
Vitamin C	Individual bowel tolerance**	With bioflavonoids (quercetin, rutin proanthocyanidins)

* The FDA recommends that pregnant women not exceed 10,000 IU of vitamin A daily.

** To determine individual dosage, on the first day take 1,000 mg hourly until diarrhea occurs, then reduce dosage to just below that for individual daily dosage. Vitamin C is not toxic in large doses but must be taken throughout the day to benefit. Divide dosage to three or four times a day.

CHAPTER 33:

Cancer, Lung

*To cease smoking is the easiest thing I ever did, I ought
to know because I've done it a thousand times.*
                                                    –Mark Twain

As long as experts can say that approximately 85 percent of all lung cancer deaths in the U.S. may be directly attributable to active cigarette smoking, no discussion of lung cancer would be complete without warning against it.[1]

I remember a full page ad in *Life* magazine that said, "More doctors smoke Camels than any other cigarettes." In a May 1953 CMA journal MacDonald Garland reported, "A cigarette a day keeps the doctor away." Those days are long gone.

Smokers Beware

If you think it is just the tobacco that endangers our lungs, think again. Cigarettes contain more than just tobacco – a lot more. National Public Radio (NPR) obtained a list of 13 additives that tobacco companies add to their cigarettes. The chemicals are on a secret list of about 700 additives that tobacco companies report to the government each year. Federal law prohibits government officials from releasing information contained in the list.

As reported in an *Associated Press* article (April 9, 1994), these chemicals are so bad, the FDA doesn't allow any of them to be used in food and five are designated as hazardous substances by the Environmental Protection Agency. Among them are ammonia, which irritates the skin, eyes and respiratory tract, and freon, a chlorofluorocarbon used in refrigerator and automobile cooling systems. Add up even minute amounts in each cigarette and multiply that by the millions of people who smoke packs a day and it amounts to a major environmental problem.

An independent toxicologist, Dr. Barry Rumack, a professor at the University of Colorado, was consulted by NPR. He said the two chemicals that most concern him are ethyl furoid and sclareol. Ethyl furoid is a chemical in the family of notorious liver toxins, he stated. Little is known about it except that it causes liver damage when tested on animals, and it was discussed as a possible chemical warfare agent in the 1930s.

Sclareol causes convulsions in laboratory rats, Rumack said. When used in combination with other chemicals, "it lowers the threshold at which a human being can convulse."

I've always suspected it was more than just tobacco. People have been smoking tobacco for centuries, and only since it became commercialized has lung cancer become so epidemic. Now we know why.

Secondhand Smoke is Dangerous Too

As of this writing, the tobacco lobby is actively trying to convince the public that one of our constitutional inalienable rights is the right to subject others to tobacco smoke. They deny that secondhand smoke is dangerous. The facts tell a different story.

In 1986 the Surgeon General of the United States reported that involuntary smoking can cause lung cancer in nonsmokers. According to the American Lung Association, secondhand smoke actually has higher concentrations of some harmful compounds than the mainstream smoke inhaled by the smoker. Some studies show there is twice as much tar and nicotine in secondhand smoke as compared to mainstream. There is also three times as much carbon monoxide, which robs the blood of oxygen, as well as several suspected cancer-causing substances.[2]

Researchers at Louisiana State University Medical Center in New Orleans examined 653 cases of lung cancer and compared them to 1,253 controls for women age 65 years and older. They found that lifetime tobacco exposure by the spouse was associated with a 30 percent increase in lung cancers in these women, and that the highest level of exposure resulted in a 75 percent increased risk of lung cancer.[3] Do you remember when smoking was allowed in crowded movie theaters? I can remember watching the smoke trails as they were blown through the projector lights, thinking I might as well put my head over a smoking chimney. It wasn't that long ago that eight-hour airline flights included cigarette smoke. We have come a long way in understanding the dangers. Tobacco lobby or not, clean air must be the prevailing consideration!

Other Sources of Airway Pollution

Where we live can be just as much a factor of lung health as *how* we live. A shocking six out of every 10 people in the United States today reside in areas which fail to meet air quality standards set to protect human health.[4] This situation exists despite two decades of efforts to control air pollution in this country. The Environmental Protection Agency, recognizing the danger, enacted the Clean Air Act of 1970, establishing national standards for six pollutants: ozone, carbon monoxide, sulfur dioxide, nitrogen dioxide, lead and particulates.

An April 1993 report by the American Lung Association estimated that more than 31 million children and over 18 million elderly people in the U.S. are at risk for lung disease or respiratory irritation because they are exposed to unhealthful levels of air pollutants. The report added that 55 percent of Americans live in areas that do not meet current health standards for air quality (estimated by many to be too low).

In 1959, when the American Cancer Society started keeping track, they recorded 29,335 men died from lung cancer. Thirty years later, the number was 89,052. The number of women who died of lung cancer increased most alarmingly from less than 5,000 in 1959 to a little over 48,000 in 1989. Since 1987, more women have died of lung cancer than breast cancer, which, for over 40 years, was the major cause of death in women. An estimated 56,000 women and 93,000 men were estimated to succumb to lung cancer in 1993 (*Cancer Facts & Figures*, 1993).

Lung cancer among males has gone up nearly 2,000 percent since 1914. Dr. Eugene Houdry, a petroleum chemistry expert, reported that this increase corresponds exactly with the increase of gasoline consumption. He also noted that lung cancer declined 35 percent during the war years 1941-1945 when gas consumption was rationed.[5]

Researchers led by Douglas Dockery of the Harvard School of Public Health in Boston, Massachusetts have found prolonged exposure to microscopic pollutants, especially high in cities where transportation is dependent upon gasoline-powered engines, increases their mortality rates from lung cancer and heart disease.

The Dockery study tracked more than 8,000 adults over a 14- to 16-year period and measured air pollution levels in the six American cities where they lived. The researchers found those who breathed air with the highest concentration of fine particles such as smoke and soot had a 26 percent higher death rate than those who inhaled the least polluted air.[6]

They found high levels of fossil fuel pollutants (gasoline is a fossil fuel) were associated with elevated rates of lung cancer and cardiopulmonary disorders such as heart attacks, emphysema and pneumonia.

While past studies have linked air pollution to higher death rates, the Dockery study went one step further by taking into account individual differences such as smoking, diabetes, obesity, education and occupational hazards. After controlling for these factors, they still saw an association between air pollution and increased deaths.

The most significant aspect of the study is that the particles the investigators measured are smaller than those currently used by the EPA to set air quality standards.

The EPA evaluates larger particulates. These "not only have a different chemical composition, but are effectively removed by your nose and upper airways before they get to your lungs," Dockery said. "But the microscopic particles the study gauged are more toxic, as well as more likely to reach lung tissue."

The American Lung Association believes the current standards for two pollutants, ozone (smog) and sulfur dioxide, are too low and fail to protect the health of many Americans, said ALA President Lee B. Reichman, M.D.[7]

Fight Back with Antioxidants

Whether you smoke or don't, there are foods and nutrients that will protect you from the ravages of air pollution. Scientists have found that one of the ways airborne chemicals induce lung cancer are by creating free radicals, those marauding molecules you've heard about that wrinkle our skin and mutate our cells.

A combination of antioxidant nutrients protect the lungs against cancer, whatever its source.[8]

Several studies reveal that on a diet deficient in vitamin A – even without inordinate exposure to tobacco smoke, radon or concentrated city air pollution – lung tissues change their character and become more vulnerable to cancer. One study confirmed that smokers released from the ravages of lung cancer were best protected from cancer recurrences by taking high doses of vitamin A. In this study, almost half of 307 surgically-cured lung cancer patients receiving 300,000 IU of vitamin A daily for 12 months went cancer-free longer than those without the vitamin. The researchers concluded that long-term supplementation of vitamin A is beneficial in follow-up cancer therapy.[9]

Beta carotene is perhaps the greatest defender against lung cancer. It can destroy the dangerous, cell-damaging "singlet oxygen" found in tobacco smoke and polluted air. Researchers at the University of Melbourne found that deficiencies of beta carotene has also been directly associated with the development of human lung cancer.[10]

Yale researcher Susan Taylor Mayne, Ph.D., and associates, decided to study certain foods and their lung cancer protective effect among nonsmokers. They found that dietary beta carotene, raw fruits and vegetables and vitamin E supplements reduce the risk of lung cancer in nonsmokers.[11]

High amounts of air pollutants tend to use up large quantities of vitamin A. Then the liver produces reinforcing vitamin A from beta carotene. So that vitamin A is not destroyed by oxidation enroute to the lungs, vitamin E and selenium let themselves be destroyed to assure safe delivery of vitamin A to the lungs. Selenium, because of this role, and because it is a highly potent antioxidant, is another valuable lung cancer fighter. Scientists at the American Association of Cancer Research in Philadelphia found that among more than 120,000 men and women studied, 55 to 69 years of age, subjects with the highest blood levels of selenium had half the rate of lung cancer compared to those with the lowest levels.[12]

Foods And Prevention

By now you may have come to realize the importance of fresh fruits and vegetables in any course of cancer prevention. But there is more to it. You must also restrict the amount of saturated fat in your diet. Researchers at the National Cancer Institute and the Missouri Department of Health in Columbia discovered in surveying 1,450 female nonsmokers, 30 to 84 years of age, that 429 had been diagnosed with lung cancer between 1986 and 1991. Their eating habits four years prior to that were evaluated. The researchers found that the women who ate the most saturated fat had more than six times the risk of developing lung cancer as those who ate the least. What I find most fascinating is that women who ate the most beans and peas (legumes) had a 40 percent lower lung-cancer risk than those who ate the least of those foods.[13] Legumes are credited with helping to control blood sugar and lower cholesterol, one side effect of a high fat diet.

The European School of Oncology Task Force on Diet, Nutrition and Cancer estimates that 76 percent of lung cancers are potentially preventable by eliminating smoking, reducing the intake of saturated fat, and eating more vegetables.[14]

What exactly am I talking about when I say "saturated fat?" I mean red meat, whole milk and processed foods that contain high amounts of saturated fat. After seeing all the studies on hydrogenated foods, I will add hydrogenated oils in processed food to this to the list of fat no-nos. Margarine is the worst culprit. Saturated fat increases the bad cholesterol in your body, and is associated with heart disease and cancer. The transfatty acids in hydrogenated oils not only increase bad cholesterol, but lower the body's good cholesterol. This double whammy is why hydrogenated oils and margarine are being credited with Western civilization's epidemic of heart disease and cancer.

For the complete story of nutrition and lung cancer, read my book *Nutrition: The Cancer Answer II.*

Lung Cancer Crushing Nutrients

For maximum absorption, supplements should be taken with meals.

Nutrient	Suggested Dosage	Formulation
Aged garlic extract	2 teaspoons three times daily	Liquid
Amino acids	4-6 capsules daily	Multiple formula from natural sources
Antioxidants	4 capsules daily*	With selenium and grape seed extract
Borage oil	2 capsules daily	
Coenzyme Q10	2 capsules daily	With vitamin E, phospholipids and selenium
Enzymes	2 capsules twice daily	Multiple formula
Flaxseed oil	1 tablespoon daily	
Fiber	8 tablets daily	Psyllium, with herb hyssop
Folic acid	10 mg daily	
Multi-vitamin/mineral	6 caplets daily	Freeze-dried plant sources
Multi-mineral	2-4 ounces daily	In liquid solution, with vitamin B12, biotin
Vitamin A	25,000 IU daily*	
Vitamin C	Individual bowel tolerance**	With bioflavonoids (quercetin, rutin proanthcyanidins)
Vitamin E	2 capsules (800 IU) daily	d-alpha tocopherol

* The FDA recommends that pregnant women not exceed 10,000 IU of vitamin A daily.

** To determine individual dosage, on the first day take 1,000 mg hourly until diarrhea occurs, then reduce dosage to just below that for individual daily dosage. Vitamin C is not toxic in large doses but must be taken throughout the day to benefit. Divide dosage to three or four times a day.

CHAPTER 34:

Cancer, Ovarian

Gilda Radner, best known for her years of comedic work on Saturday Night Live, brought laughter and love to millions of fans. Her characters included Rhonda Weiss, the Jewish American Princess who was up in arms over the banning of saccharin. "I'm sorry about the lab animals," sniffed Rhonda, "but statistics prove that most guys prefer skinny girls with cancer over healthy girls with bulging thighs."

She didn't know then that she was destined to be that skinny girl with cancer. In 1986, she endured ten months of excruciating symptoms, including fainting spells, severe pain and bloating, and nervous legs. Desperate, she and her husband, comedian Gene Wilder, turned to doctor after doctor. They told her she had Epstein-Barr virus, ovulation problems, nerves, stomach problems or even no problem at all. By the time physicians believed what she had been telling them – that she was really sick – she had a grapefruit-sized tumor on one of her ovaries. It was advanced ovarian cancer, Stage IV, and the prognosis was dim. After enduring 2-1/2 years of painful and invasive conventional treatments, Gilda Radner died in the arms of her beloved husband.[1,2]

Wilder and others believe Gilda would have lived if the cancer had been detected earlier. Gilda had a family history of ovarian cancer, which she did not realize, since her doctors never asked. And if a certain test had been given to Gilda when the symptoms were first reported, a CA 125 blood test, she would have had more time to read my book *Nutrition: The Cancer Answer*, and exercise her freedom of medical choice with nutritional alternatives to the deadly therapies prescribed for her.

Pinpointing Causes to Prevent Cancer

Women desperate for pregnancy may be setting themselves up for cancer if they take fertility drugs. Mary Anne Rossing, Ph.D., and colleagues at the University of Washington and Fred Hutchinson Cancer Research Center found that women taking fertility drugs had 2-1/2 times the normal risk of developing ovarian cancer, especially long-term use of the drug clomiphene. Alice Whittemore, Ph.D., at Stanford University School of Medicine found a threefold greater risk of ovarian cancer among women using fertility drugs.

Ovarian cancer is thought to stem from genetic mistakes that occur as cells divide to repair the ovary after it ruptures to release an egg. Since pregnancy, which stops ovulation for months at a time, has been shown to greatly reduce the chances of a woman developing ovarian cancer, it stands to reason that anything that stimulates ovulation will have the opposite effect.[3]

This genetic defect, by the way, may be corrected through good nutrition. All the illnesses that befall us are caused or influenced by genes. Just because you are born with faulty genes, doesn't mean you have to live with them. The fact is, the body has enzymatic machinery designed to destroy and repair faulty nuclear DNA (genes). This offensive line depends on good nutrition for optimum performance. Emanuel Cheraskin, M.D., D.M.D, says "Think of the gene as the seed, the environment as the soil. You can grow a healthy plant in good soil even if you start out with a weak seed."

A friend told me they recently discovered the gene for being overweight. "It was discovered at the bottom of a container of Haagen Daz ice cream," she laughed.

The consumption of dairy products has been connected to a higher-than-normal incidence of ovarian cancer. In 1989, gynecologist Daniel W. Kramer at Harvard Medical School in Boston linked galactose consumption with an increased risk of ovarian cancer. Galactose is the sugar contained in milk and other dairy products. Since galactose has been found to be toxic to human eggs, it may be that it somehow interferes with our enzymatic offensive line.[4]

If you want to avoid ovarian cancer, don't eat fatty foods, and concentrate on fresh, whole vegetables. Harvey Risch, M.D., Ph.D., Department of Epidemiology and Public Health, Yale University School of Medicine found that the bad cholesterol-raising properties of transfatty acids (hydrogenated oils), saturated fat and eggs increased a woman's chances of getting ovarian cancer. He found eating vegetable fiber decreased the risk as it decreased the cholesterol. He concluded that reducing the intake of saturated fat and consuming more vegetables appears to lower the risk of ovarian cancer.[5] If your cholesterol is high and you are concerned about ovarian cancer, take aged garlic extract and read the chapter Cholesterol.

Insidious Asbestos

By now, most of us are familiar with the long-term dangers of inhaling asbestos. We've read about schools being closed while hazardous materials specialists carefully remove asbestos ceilings. Sources of asbestos abound. It wears off automobile brake linings and clutch facings, and is contained in such household items as ironing board covers and some pot holders. Asbestos, once inhaled, continues to react in the lungs for a lifetime, and is associated with lung cancer.

Talcum powder has been shown to be as potentially deadly as asbestos. Asbestos and talcum are naturally occurring minerals, and are chemically and geologically related. They are often found in the same geological sites. A well-known brand of talcum powder in England was withdrawn from the market after it was discovered to be laced with asbestos. Talc and asbestos are similar in the effect they have on the human body. It is known that older talc workers die of lung cancer at a rate four times higher than would be expected. Talc workers are also subject to talcosis, a disease that scars the lungs.[6]

Researchers have found particles of talc in approximately 75 percent of ovarian tumors and 50 percent of cervical tumors examined.[7] How does talc find its way into ovaries and cervixes? Doctors used to apply talcum to preserve their rubber gloves during surgery. For the same reason, it is common for women to dust talc on their diaphragms to keep them dry and extend their shelf life. Any product that contains talc can be a potential killer, including some feminine hygiene sprays.

Dr. Langer, a mineralogist with New York's Mount Sinai Hospital believes it may be asbestos particles hidden within the talcum that causes these cases of cancer. He and his associates examined ovarian biopsy slides and found asbestos fibers and talc.

After discovering talcum gave them skin lesions, doctors started using natural cornstarch instead. Cornstarch is an excellent non-toxic alternative to talcum.

Women whose partners use condoms may be facing an increased risk of damage to the reproductive organs. Researchers found that most condoms in the study had a few talc particles on the surface. They may be a contaminant of other lubricant powders also found on condoms, such as starch or lycopodium. Studies also found that women who dusted with talc containing powders for many years had an increased risk of ovarian cancer. Doctors have found talc in ovarian tumors as well as in normal ovarian tissue. It is speculated that these particles get trapped in the fallopian tubes and may contribute to scarring and infertility. All the condoms tested contained at least some particles of talc.[8]

Least expected is talcum on your vitamins. Many vitamin manufacturers use talc to keep pills from sticking together, and to increase their shelf life. Some vitamins are even coated with shellac, which is highly cancer causing. How can you tell if your supplements have talc? Watch carefully when you put a vitamin in a glass of water. If it contains talc, a small puff of white will kick up. Know your purveyor. I take a natural vitamin line that doesn't have unnecessary additives.

A Nutritional Alternative to Deadly Therapies

The fact is, many of the chemicals commonly used in conventional chemotherapies are themselves carcinogenic. Even doctors aren't sure if new cancerous tumors are caused by these chemicals. They are so toxic technicians have to wear masks and gloves to inject it into your veins. It is possible our late friend Gilda Radner died not from her original cancer, but from the toxic effect of the chemicals and radiation her body was too weakened to defend itself from. It is also possible that early detection is important, not so much for keeping the cancer from spreading, but so the body can be made healthy enough to defend itself from both the cancer and toxic therapies.

Physicians versed in nutrition believe, and have seen, that cancer can be overcome with super-nutrition. They know the body can fight off cancer – or we'd all have it. It is when the body has been overcome by both malnutrition and toxic forces, that cancer sets in. Super-nutrition reverses the process by detoxifying the tissues and boosting the body's own defenses.

Abram Hoffer, M.D., Ph.D., of Victoria B.C., Canada regularly treats cancer patients with vitamin therapy. In 1991, Hoffer asked Nobel laureate Linus Pauling, Ph.D., founder of the Linus Pauling Institute and discoverer of the benefits of vitamin C, to statistically compare the survival rates of 101 advanced cancer patients who followed Hoffer's specially-prescribed vitamin regimen with 34 who did not.

Pauling's analysis found patients with cancers of the breast, ovaries, uterus and cervix had a life expectancy 20 times longer when they adhered to Hoffer's regimen. A second study, published in the *Journal of Orthomolecular Medicine*, confirmed the benefits. A third study followed up the first cancer survivors. Pauling and Hoffer found half the patients with breast, ovarian, uterine and cervical cancer lived at least five years longer and some 15 years longer after being referred to Hoffer. The American Cancer Society considers five years or more of life after cancer as "cured."

For the complete story of nutrition and ovarian cancer, read my book *Nutrition: The Cancer Answer II*.

Ovarian Cancer-Cancelling Nutrients

For maximum absorption, supplements should be taken with meals.

Nutrient	Suggested Dosage	Formulation
Aged garlic extract	2 teaspoons three times daily	Liquid
Amino acids	4-6 capsules daily	Multiple formula from natural sources
Antioxidants	4 capsules daily*	With selenium and grape seed extract
Borage oil	2 capsules daily	
Enzymes	2 capsules twice daily	Multiple formula
Flaxseed oil	1 tablespoon daily	
Fiber	8 tablets daily	Psyllium, with herb hyssop
Folic acid	10 mg daily	
Multi-vitamin/mineral	6 caplets daily	Freeze-dried plant sources
Multi-mineral	2-4 ounces daily	In liquid solution, with vitamin B12, biotin
Natural progesterone cream	1/3 teaspoon daily	With pregnenolone, DHEA
Vitamin C	Individual bowel tolerance**	With bioflavonoids (quercetin, rutin proanthcyanidins)

* The FDA recommends that pregnant women not exceed 10,000 IU of vitamin A daily.

** To determine individual dosage, on the first day take 1,000 mg hourly until diarrhea occurs, then reduce dosage to just below that for individual daily dosage. Vitamin C is not toxic in large doses but must be taken throughout the day to benefit. Divide dosage to three or four times a day.

CHAPTER 35:

Cancer, Pancreatic

It is with pancreatic cancer that conventional medicine fails most miserably. The American Cancer Society reports that a mere three percent of patients live more than five years after diagnosis. They also report no progress in treatments or mortality rate since the early '70s claiming that "very little is known about what causes it or how to prevent it" (*Cancer Facts & Figures 1994*). Somebody hasn't been reading their medical journals. There is an abundance of information on why it occurs, what causes it, how it can be prevented, and even a treatment program developed by medical professionals that has greatly increased the odds of beating it.

First, what is the pancreas? Before I became an ostrich on the beaches of medical literature, I used to confuse the organs. What's the difference between the gallbladder, the bladder, the pancreas and the liver? What happens when the pancreas becomes diseased? I won't confuse you by trying to explain how each of the organs work together to keep you healthy, since we *are* talking about the pancreas here. Suffice it to say that each day the pancreas, when functioning at full capacity, secretes about 2-1/2 pints of pancreatic enzymes in the small intestine. This "juice" digests and breaks down carbohydrates, fats and protein.[1] Without adequate pancreatic enzymes, you can get food allergies, intestinal infections and cancer. The pancreas also produces insulin. A lack of insulin causes diabetes mellitus, a common but potentially fatal ailment. What does the pancreas need to remain healthy? Nothing. I mean it! Like the liver and other organs, the pancreas is fully capable of healing itself – provided we don't pummel it with poisons and overload it with fats.

Healing with Enzymes

Let's say you do all the no-nos. You smoke, are overweight, eat a lot of transfatty acids (hydrogenated oils), sugar and meat, drink too much alcohol, and don't exercise. Your pancreas is so overloaded your stools are pale and greasy, and the intense pain that goes from your stomach to your back makes you wish you were dead. You have pancreatitis, and you are lucky because if you fix it now, you might not get cancer.

Your pancreas will heal itself if you let it. But you need to quit those bad habits and give it some assistance. The best way to help it heal itself is by supporting it with its own digestive enzymes so it doesn't have to work so hard. Give it a ticket to Hawaii by adding a supplemental enzyme formula to your diet. You know how you reach for antacids when you have a stomachache? Try digestive enzymes instead. I know from personal experience that they work better and faster than antacids, which don't really deal with the problem – pancreatic overload – in the first place.

Enzymes fight cancer by exposing antigens on the surface of cancer cells so the body's natural killer cells recognize them for what they are and destroy them. They also stimulate the body's anti-cancer army of T-cells, natural killer cells and other anti-cancer agents that keep us from getting malignancies.

Hector Solorzano del Rio, M.D., D.Sc., Coordinator of the Program for Studies of Alternative Medicine and Professor of Pharmacology of the University of Guadalajara in Mexico uses pancreatic enzymes to treat degenerative and autoimmune diseases including pancreatic cancer. According to Solorzano, pancreatic enzymes remove the sticky coating that allows cancer cells to stick to the body, thus preventing cancer from metastasizing. Pancreatic enzymes also have the ability to enter cancer cells when they are at their most vulnerable. In Germany, pancreatic enzymes have been injected directly into tumors, causing them to dissolve. Vitamin A is important to these processes, and is given in conjunction with pancreatic enzyme therapy.[2]

Eat the following enzyme and vitamin A rich food raw and as fresh as possible: dandelion greens, carrots, yams, kale, parsley, turnip greens, collard greens, chard, watercress, red peppers, cantaloupe, persimmons, apricots, broccoli, mangoes, pumpkin and peaches. About 15 minutes before digging into that greasy hamburger, eat some pineapple off the salad bar. Pineapple contains bromelain, a protein-digesting enzyme. Unripe papaya contains high amounts of papain, another digestive enzyme, used in some digestive formulas. All raw foods contain enzymes. Enzymes are the first to go when foods are cooked or processed. We eat cold-pressed oils because the enzymes haven't been cooked out, and we eat raw fruits and vegetables because we know they are full of enzymes which make them easier to digest.

Zinc is a mineral, but it might as well be an enzyme considering how important it is to them. It is a constituent of at least 25 enzymes involved in digestion and metabolism, and is a component of insulin.[3] Studies have shown a deficiency of zinc compromises the ability of pancreatic enzymes to function. Add vitamin B6 because it enhances zinc absorption. Always, when supplementing one B vitamin, take a B vitamin complex.

A Healthy Diet for a Healthy Pancreas

As I've said through the decades, and in my book *Nutrition: The Cancer Answer II*, certain foods, and the nutrients contained in them, have been shown in studies to influence whether or not we get pancreatic cancer.

George Comstock of the Training Center for Public Health Research in Hagerstown, Maryland found that in evaluating over 25,000 volunteers from 1974 to 1975, low levels of lycopene were strongly associated with pancreatic cancer. Lycopene is a bioflavonoid found in tomatoes, apricots, grapefruit, guava juice and watermelon.[4]

Dr. W. Zatonski, of the Maria Sklodowski-Curi Memorial Cancer Center and Institute of Oncology in Warsaw, Poland, evaluated 110 cases of pancreatic cancer compared to 195 controls and found the risk of cancer was reduced among those who ate a lot of vitamin C foods and unsaturated fats.[5] Vitamin C is a notorious antioxidant and helpful in any cancer-preventive plan.

Unsaturated fats, or fatty acids, are basically oils, fresh and unhydrogenated. While the Polish study did not target exactly which unsaturated fats work against pancreatic cancer, David F. Horrobin, of the Efamol Research Institute in Nova Scotia, Canada did. He found that in over 30 patients with inoperable pancreatic cancer, and in smaller numbers with terminal breast and colon cancer, gamma-linolenic acid (GLA) dramatically increased their survival rates three-fold, without side effects.[6]

GLA is found in evening primrose oil, black currant oil, borage oil and spirulina. Borage oil is the best source. Independent clinical tests show it contains up to 26 percent GLA. Compare this to evening primrose oil and black currant oil, which contain no more than 18 percent. Not only that, borage oil costs less because the borage seed is three times larger than black currant or evening primrose seeds. Finally, borage is more bioavailable. In other words, the body more readily accepts it.

Pummeling Pancreatic Cancer with Nutrients

For maximum absorption, supplements should be taken with meals.

Nutrient	Suggested Dosage	Formulation
Aged garlic extract	2 teaspoons three times daily	Liquid
Amino acids	4-6 capsules daily	Multiple formula from natural sources
Antioxidants	4 capsules daily*	With selenium and grape seed extract
Borage oil	2 capsules daily	
Coenzyme Q10	2 capsules daily	With vitamin E, phospholipids and selenium
Enzymes	2 capsules twice daily	Multiple formula
Flaxseed oil	1 tablespoon daily	
Folic acid	10 mg daily	
Fiber	8 tablets daily	Psyllium, with herb hyssop
Multi-vitamin/mineral	6 caplets daily	Freeze-dried plant sources
Multi-mineral	2-4 ounces daily	In liquid solution, with vitamin B12, biotin
Pancreatin	160 mg daily after each meal	
Vitamin C	Individual bowel tolerance**	With bioflavonoids (quercetin, rutin proanthcyanidins)

* The FDA recommends that pregnant women not exceed 10,000 IU of vitamin A daily.

** To determine individual dosage, on the first day take 1,000 mg hourly until diarrhea occurs, then reduce dosage to just below that for individual daily dosage. Vitamin C is not toxic in large doses but must be taken throughout the day to benefit. Divide dosage to three or four times a day.

CHAPTER 36:

Cancer Prevention

My friend Carol is 55 years old and does not have breast cancer. This fact is not remarkable until you consider her background. Her mother died of breast cancer at the age of 41. Her sister is currently undergoing therapy for breast cancer, and her aunt is in remission after getting breast cancer at 61 years of age. Carol knows the odds are against her, but she also knows she is increasing the odds in her favor by eating right and living healthy.

Before I get into the whys and wherefores of cancer-preventive food and nutrients, I will tell you exactly what Carol does to guard her body against cancer. She buys only whole, organic foods from either her local farmer's market, the health food store, or she visits privately-owned, non-commercial orchards and buys from them. She eats no cow dairy products or processed foods, especially cured meats like hot dogs, sausage and bologna (she knows the nitrates are cancer-causing). She doesn't have a garden because she doesn't know what's in the soil. She knows her neighbors spray with pesticides and herbicides and she doesn't want to eat food nourished with water that has run off from their yards.

Carol starts out every day with a breakfast of whole hulled millet that has been cooked the night before in purified water, raisins and apples, then lightly heated, sprinkled with raw sesame seeds and drizzled with local raw honey, or a bowl of lentils flavored with herbs from her window box garden. She particularly likes the combination of mint and anise. For lunch she enjoys a hearty salad. It might be organic pasta flavored with lemon and dill, full of chopped green onions, hard-boiled egg, red pepper, celery and sesame seeds; or her "leafie-beanie" salad made with whatever beans she has, plus peas, spinach, Romaine lettuce, chopped fresh parsley, goat cheese, and her special homemade tarragon/walnut oil/vinegar dressing. For dinner she has vegetable soup, a different kind every day. For desserts she likes fruit sweetened with honey or a slice of carob millet cake topped with honey-sweetened pureed fruit. She drinks a gallon of spring water a day, supplementing with hot or cold herbal teas depending upon the time of year. To supplement her diet, as good as it is, she takes an antioxidant formula, vitamin C with bioflavonoids, liquid aged garlic extract, a borage oil supplement, a liquid mineral supplement and a multi-mineral and vitamin formula that uses dehydrated sprouts and vegetables for its nutrients.

Carol goes out of her way to avoid ingesting or inhaling chemicals, using natural, chemical-free alternatives for her cleaning solutions, face and hand cream, deodorant, soap and shampoo. She even stays out of chlorinated pools. Oh, and she takes a brisk hour-long walk every day. Her nutrition-oriented medical doctor tells her she has the health of an 18-year-old.

Your Antioxidant Armory

The antioxidants vitamins C, E and beta carotene in vegetables and fruits protect cells from damage by free radicals, wayward molecules which nutrition writer Patrick Quillin, Ph.D., calls "Great white sharks in the biochemical sea of life." These cell saboteurs have long been suspected of triggering various cancers.

Vegetable and fruit antioxidants are staunch defenders against numerous types of cancer. Even the conservative National Cancer Institute recommends eating five servings of fruits and vegetables a day to help prevent cancer.

University of California nutrition researcher Dr. Gladys Block, Ph.D., conducted an in-depth analysis of 99 studies to see whether there is actually a connection between diet and cancer. Eighty-nine of the studies disclosed vegetables and fruit, indeed, are a first line of defense against many types of cancer.

Thirty-three of the studies show vitamin C and flavonoids in berries, cantaloupes, citrus fruits and green leafy vegetables protect us against cancers of the cervix, the esophagus and stomach.[1]

Other research reveals vitamin E in wheat germ, nuts and whole grains guard us against cancers of the breast, pancreas and stomach.

A Japanese researcher, T. Harayama, conducted a 10-year study of 265,118 subjects who answered questions about their dietary intake. Harayama discovered that people who ate liberal amounts of vegetables containing beta carotene had a lower risk of lung, stomach and prostate cancer.

Selenium is an antioxidant mineral essential to any program of cancer preventive care. Add it to your arsenal. Other potent free-radical fighting supplements are coenzyme Q10 and SOD (superoxide dismutase).

Stay away from booze, which is notorious for depleting nutrients. Volunteers who had two alcoholic drinks daily turned out to have an 85 percent higher risk of developing tumors than non-drinkers.

Forearmed with Folic Acid

Now biochemists know it's more than just beta carotene and vitamins C and E in vegetables and fruits that help prevent cancer. Folic acid, one of the B vitamins, is a powerful nutrient, and often deficient in those who need it the most.

Researcher Edward Giovannucci, Harvard Medical School, thinks folic acid may help turn off cancer genes. Giovannucci's team discovered a high intake of folic acid, gotten from fresh vegetables and fruit and vitamin supplements, lowered the risk of tumor development.

Other research shows folic acid directs the growth of new cells in the body. A shortage or lack of this nutrient may contribute to improper or abnormal cell formation. We now know that a lack of folic acid in early stages of pregnancy increases the chances of birth defects.

It is a well-established fact few individuals eat enough fresh fruits and vegetables to obtain sufficient folic acid. Furthermore, use of birth control pills increases the requirement for this nutrient. There is such an unmet need for folic acid, in fact, that the FDA has authorized food processors to add it to all bread products in the U.S.

Quenching Cancer with Quercetin

One of the newer superstar anti-cancer nutrients in health food stores is quercetin, a bioflavonoid. Quercetin is one of the strongest anti-cancer agents known.

Various lab studies reveal that quercetin unleashes a one-two punch against cancer. It blocks cell changes that invite cancer and, if a tumor has already started, stops the spread of malignant cells.

Red and yellow onions contain an incredible amount of quercetin – 10 percent or more of their dry weight. Not so white onions or, for that matter, garlic, the onion's odoriferous cousin. It can also be obtained from supple-ment formulas.

Cancer-Fighting Phytochemicals

Adding to what we know about cancer and nutrients, scientists have isolated and identified the many healing chemicals contained in fruits and vegetables. They are collectively called phytochemicals ("phyto" is derived from the Greek word for plant).

Phytochemicals are neither vitamins nor minerals, yet they are equally potent and vital to the healthy functioning of our bodies. They are isolated from plants and are known technically as anthocyanosides, limonoids, glucarates, phenolic acids, flavonoids, coumarins, polyacetylenes and carotenoids.

Many of mainstream medicine's pharmaceuticals are derived or synthesized from phytochemicals, including aspirin from willow bark and an anti-cancer medication from the Pacific Yew tree.

Some naturally-occurring phytochemicals throw a biochemical wrench into one or more of the mechanisms leading to a tumor. At almost every one of the steps along the pathway leading to cancer, there are one or more compounds in vegetables or fruits that slow or reverse the process.[2]

Broccoli, cauliflower, Brussels sprouts, turnips, kale, turnip greens and bok choy are the most highly-regarded anti-cancer foods. Researchers have isolated a chemical in them called sulforaphane as responsible for their cancer preventive properties.

"The results are quite dramatic," says Dr. Paul Talalay of Johns

Hopkins Medical Institutions. In his initial studies he found that among lab animals exposed to carcinogens and given sulforaphane, few developed tumors.

Talalay added sulforaphane to human cells growing in a lab dish and reported that it boosted the growth of anti-cancer enzymes. In the April 1994 *Proceedings of the National Academy of Sciences*, his team reported conclusively that the compound protects living animals against cancer.

Anti-cancer enzymes are what make the difference between people who get cancer and those who don't. You need enough free-floating enzymes in your system to conquer cancer every day!

Enzymes are catalysts, specifically proteins. More than two thousand varieties play vital roles in every human physical function. Historically, enzyme therapy has been used in cancer treatment many times.

The most important role of enzymes is their ability to digest the cancer cell's protein coat-camouflage, leaving it open to attack by the body's natural white cell defenses. This is why using vitamin A in conjunction with enzymes has a greater anti-tumor effect.

Because enzymes are destroyed when cooked, the best way to prevent cancer is to eat lots of raw fruits and vegetables, which contain many cancer-fighting enzymes. Choose papaya for papain; pineapple for bromelain, and other fruits and vegetables for trypsin, protease, cellulase, amylase and lipase. Look for these in a digestive enzyme formula if you aren't eating as much fruits and vegetables as you wish.

Phytochemicals in the whole tomato have also been identified in a first line of cancer defense. Scientists at Cornell University reported that two of tomatoes' estimated 10,000 phytochemicals: p-coumaric acid and chlorogenic acid, stop the formation of cancer-causing substances.

During digestion, the body routinely makes compounds capable of causing cancer, called nitrosamines. Certain foods help. Tomato acids remove the nitrosamines before they can do any damage. Cornell's Joseph Hotchkiss gave volunteers tomato juice and found less nitrosamines in their bodies.

Cabbage and turnips contain another anti-cancer ingredient, acronymed PEITC. Reports Gary Stoner of Ohio State University, PEITC inhibits lung cancer in mice and rats. Ellagic acid in strawberries, grapes and raspberries also neutralizes carcinogens before they can invade DNA.

In 1993, German researchers announced they had isolated a chemical in soybeans that prevents tumors from growing. Called genistein, it might be why Japanese men who relocate to the West and adopt a soy-poor diet for even a few years have a greatly elevated risk of prostate cancer.

Onions and garlic contain cancer-countering chemicals, as does the capsaicin in hot peppers and the spices turmeric and cumin. And almost every fruit and vegetable, from berries to yams to citrus and cucumbers, contain flavonoids. In a cellular version of musical chairs, flavonoids race to sites on the cell where cancer-causing hormones, including estrogen, attach themselves. When the music stops, the flavonoids keep the hormones from sitting down on the cell's surface.

Cassava, bitter almonds, apricot pits, lentils, millet, beans and sweet potatoes all contain a tremendously beneficial chemical, amygdalin. Amygdalin – coined vitamin B17 – is the crown jewel in the extrinsic nutritional defense mechanism against cancer. Amygdalin was first used by a Chinese herbalist (Pen T'Sao) in the year 2800 B.C. and has been in use since that time. It is used to make laetrile, a successful but maligned alternative cancer treatment.

The Pueblo Indians of Taos, New Mexico traditionally eat many foods rich in amygdalin. Not coincidentally, cancer is rare among this population. I was given a recipe by them as I researched my book on cancer prevention, *Nutrition: The Cancer Answer*. It goes like this: In a glass of milk or juice mix a tablespoon of honey with a quarter ounce or two dozen freshly ground apricot kernels, or one kernel for every ten pounds of body weight. The drink was so delicious I had it daily. On the third day a funny thing happened. Two little benign skin growths on my arm, which were formerly pink, turned brown. By the seventh day, they were gone.[3]

For more on the therapeutic benefits of B17, read my second book *Nutrition: The Cancer Answer II*.

Garlic and Green Tea, Guerrilla Warfare

Cancer's future is in prevention, and garlic plays a starring role. I whole-heartedly support the National Cancer Institute-backed research on garlic and other food products as more cost-effective than looking for new drugs. The vast number of drugs that fail government scrutiny and the delays in new drug approval have forced science and the government to see food as the preventive medicine of the future.

One reason garlic may protect against cancer is its ability to help the body inactivate, metabolize and eliminate cancer-causing substances without damage. Garlic is also believed to enhance the body's immune system.

Biologist Dr. Michael Wargovic and colleagues at the University of Texas, M.D. Anderson Cancer Center, report a series of studies testing the cancer prevention power of garlic. They discovered that a water-soluble organosulfur compound, S-allylcysteine (SAC), in aged garlic extract, significantly blocks the development of colon cancer in mice.

Additionally, they found SAC enhances the body's production of glutathione S-transferase, a powerful enzyme that detoxifies many carcinogens. Because SAC is considered safe and causes fewer side effects than raw garlic, Dr. Hiromichi Sumiyoshi, a prominent researcher, considers it a "prime candidate" for further cancer-prevention study.

At The First World Conference on the Health Significance of Garlic and Garlic Constituents in 1990, sponsored by Nutrition International of Irvine, California, Pennsylvania State University, and the U.S. Department of Agriculture, Dr. John Pinto of Memorial Sloan Kettering Cancer Center, Dr. Raj Tiwari of Cornell Medical College and Dr. Lin demonstrated that aged garlic extract effectively inhibited the multiplication of cultured human breast cancer cells and human prostate cancer.[4]

At an annual meeting of the American Association of Cancer Research, April 10-13, 1994 in San Francisco, conventional researchers made the startling announcement that enough evidence has been found to proclaim that green tea (Camellia sinensis) does indeed appear to protect against cancer.[5] For many researchers following green tea and its epidemiological evidence, this is nothing new. Asian populations consume great quantities of green tea, and, not coincidentally, have one of the lowest cancer rates in the world. Even the Japanese, who have one of the highest populations of smokers, experience fewer cases of cancer than Americans.

Daily Cancer Preventive Protocol
For persons at high risk of getting cancer.
Recommended nutrients and amounts for prevention of cancer.

For maximum benefit, include a daily diet rich in organic whole fruits and vegetables, raw whenever possible, 30 minutes of moderate exercise, and prayer. For maximum absorption, supplements should be taken with meals.

Nutrient	Suggested Dosage	Formulation
Aged garlic extract	2 teaspoons three times daily	Liquid
Amino acids	4-6 capsules daily	Multiple formula from natural sources
Antioxidants	4 capsules daily*	With selenium and grape seed extract
Borage oil	2 capsules daily	
Enzymes	2 capsules twice daily	Multiple formula
Flaxseed oil	1 tablespoon daily	
Fiber	8 tablets daily	Psyllium, with herb hyssop
Multi-vitamin/mineral	6 caplets daily	Freeze-dried plant sources
Multi-mineral	2-4 ounces daily	In liquid solution, with vitamin B12, biotin
Vitamin C	Individual bowel tolerance**	With bioflavonoids (quercetin, rutin proanthocyanidins)
Vitamin E	2 capsules (800 IU) daily	d-alpha tocopherol

* The FDA recommends that pregnant women not exceed 10,000 IU of vitamin A daily.

** To determine individual dosage, on the first day take 1,000 mg hourly until diarrhea occurs, then reduce dosage to just below that for individual daily dosage. Vitamin C is not toxic in large doses but must be taken throughout the day to benefit. Divide dosage to three or four times a day.

CHAPTER 37:

Cancer, Prostate

What do these men have in common?: former President of France Francois Mitterand, ABC News President Roone Arledge, Supreme Court Justice John Paul Stevens, Two-time Nobel Prize winner Linus Pauling, former U.S. Senators Robert Dole and Alan Cranston, Time Warner Chairman Steven Ross, musician Frank Zappa, and actor Bill Bixby. They have all survived or succumbed to prostate cancer. A small consolation indeed, that even the rich and famous are stricken. Experts estimate that by the year 2,000 cancer of the prostate will be the number one killer of men.

Environmental Poisons

In 1993 an estimated 35,000 men died in America from prostate cancer, according to The American Cancer Society. It is the second leading cause of cancer deaths in men, behind lung cancer. The news doesn't get any better.

For people aged 50 to 60, compared to 30-40 years ago, the overall cancer rate has increased by 44 percent for breast cancer; 60 percent for male colon cancer; and for prostate cancer the rate has increased by as much as 100 percent. For malignant melanomas, malignant lymphoma, myeloma, non-Hodgkins lymphoma and some of the rarer cancers of this kind, the rates have increased by 150 percent. For testicular cancer, if you look for men between the ages of 28 and 35, the figures are almost 300 percent.[1]

To what do we attribute these findings? – to the ever-increasing numbers of dangerous chemicals present in our modern environment. In 1940 we manufactured and synthesized about a billion pounds of synthetic organic chemicals that year–new chemicals which never existed before in the world. By 1950 the figure had reached 50 billion pounds. By the late 1980s, this figure reached 500 billion pounds of synthetic chemicals including approximately 600 chemicals which have been clearly, in well-defined, validated experiments, shown to induce cancer in animals. Studies have identified about 25-26 chemicals which are known to cause cancer in humans. Some study findings have directly linked certain herbicides to prostate cancer. [2]

How Prostate Cancer Develops

Nearly 60 percent of men between the ages of 40 and 59 years of age have an enlarged prostate gland. Because of the often subtle symptoms, many don't even know it. Researchers found men with an enlarged prostate were four times more likely to develop cancer than those with normal prostates.[3]

If a cancerous tumor develops on the prostate, it usually grows on the outer portion and may not exhibit symptoms. By the time a tumor causes symptoms, it has grown so large it forces pressure on the urethra. An early-stage tumor can be detected during a regularly-scheduled rectal exam, a PSA blood test or by the use of ultrasound or x-ray.

Conventional therapy inadequacies make prevention the most solid bet. Pre-cancerous prostate problems, fortunately, can be managed with diet and nutrition. See the chapter Prostate Problems for these. Here, I will concentrate on prostate cancer.

Pass the Vegetables, Please

For a healthy prostate, pass on the pizza and red meat! This is because researchers are finding that a diet high in fat is linked to prostate cancer. Researchers estimate that 81 percent of prostate cancers are potentially preventable with a reduction of fat.[4]

A Japanese researcher, T. Harayama, conducted a 10-year study of 265,118 subjects who answered questions about their dietary intake. Harayama discovered that people who ate liberal amounts of vegetables containing beta carotene (carrots, sweet potatoes, yams, cantaloupe, apricots, spinach, squash and leafy green vegetables) had a lower risk of prostate cancer.

Some studies have shown vegetarians, who eat less fat, have a lower incidence of cancer of the prostate than men with high fat intake. The same studies show a vegetarian diet lowers circulating testosterone levels and a non-vegetarian diet raises them. Prostate cancer grows on testosterone and slows when testosterone is lowered. A study of Japanese men conducted in 1977 noted that the marked increase in mortality from prostate cancer paralleled the increase in fat intake in the Japanese diet since 1950.[5]

Eliminating most of the fat in men's diets would greatly reduce the number of prostatic maladies, according to Dr. Carl P. Schaffner, Ph.D., professor of microbial chemistry at Rutgers University. Dr. Schaffner discovered that by reducing cholesterol levels in aged dogs, he was also able to reduce the size of the animals' enlarged prostates. To reduce your cholesterol level naturally, read the chapter on Cholesterol.

Dr. Cammille Mallouh, M.D., Chief of Urology at Metropolitan Hospital in New York, examined 100 prostates from men of all ages and found an 80 percent increase in cholesterol content of enlarged prostates. Cholesterol has been shown to accumulate in an enlarged or cancerous human prostate (*Cancer Research*, December 1979).

Cancer of the prostate may be associated with our typical "civilized" Western diet. Peter Hill, Ph.D., of New York City's American Health Foundation, noted that rural black South Africans who typically ate a low-fat, whole-food diet had healthy prostates. He conducted a test to see if their diet was the reason. Dr. Hill and his associates put a group of South African volunteers on a typical Western diet of lots of meats and fats. At the same time, a group of North American volunteers, blacks and whites, were put on a low-fat diet. Dr. Hill and his colleagues then tested the subjects for the hormonal changes that are associated with prostatic cancer.

After three weeks, Dr. Hill found that the South Africans eating the Western diet excreted notably more hormones, while the reverse occurred with the North American subjects. Amazingly, all it took was a change in diet to increase the risk of prostate cancer among the

South Africans and decrease the risk among the North Americans. Dr. Hill stated, "This study is a preliminary indication that a low-fat diet is one of the factors which can lower the risk of prostatic cancer. By reducing total calorie intake, and substituting fruit and vegetable calories for animal calories, a high-risk prostatic cancer group has switched to a low-risk one."[6]

Researchers at Harvard Medical School found that in a study of 14,916 male physicians, those who ate red meat five or more times a week faced 2.5 times the risk of developing prostate cancer than those who ate red meat once a week or less.[7]

A Cancer-Fighting Bioflavonoid

Soy products have three times the benefit in fighting prostate cancer. Soy contains genistein, a bioflavonoid that works to reduce inflammation. Prostate cancer is similar to breast cancer in that it can be caused by excess hormones. In this case it is testosterone, the male hormone. Genistein is also a phytoestrogen, which lowers hormone levels, and is believed to inhibit the growth of prostate cancer.

High hormone levels can occur naturally, or unnaturally. The prevalence of all the aforementioned chemicals in our environment, especially pesticides, is said to increase hormone levels and contribute to male sex organ problems and infertility. Phytoestrogens – so named because of their influence on estrogen and other hormones – help combat the hormonal influence of chemicals.

Studies have found that among civilizations with a diet high in phytoestrogens, the incidence of cancer is lowered. This has been particularly true in the case of bioflavonoids. Sometimes referred to as bioflavonoids, they are substances found in brightly-colored fruits and vegetables, and have been credited with reducing tumors. See the chapter on Breast Cancer for more on phytoestrogens.

Dr. Herman Adlercreutz, M.D., and associates at the Department of Clinical Chemistry, University of Helsinki, Finland, did a study on Japanese men, who are notoriously free of prostate cancer. They found that the Japanese typically eat meals low in fat and high in soy products, and were found by Dr. Adlercreutz to have seven to 110 times more bioflavonoids in their blood than Finnish men with a high incidence of prostate cancer.[8]

Thomas B. Clarkson, M.D. agrees that bioflavonoids, particularly those derived from soybeans, protect against prostate cancer.[9]

Bioflavonoids work best with vitamin C in reducing prostate problems that can contribute to cancer. I tell my male friends to take vitamin C formula which includes all these flavonoids. For the best, target vitamin C and antioxidant formulas that include grape seed extract, green tea extract, rutin and citrus bioflavonoids.

Sunshine Sterilizes Cancer Cells

Researchers at Stanford University found in studies that vitamin D works to keep prostatic cancer cells from multiplying. D.M. Peehl and others applied vitamin D to both enlarged prostatic tissues and cancerous prostatic tissues and watched to see what would happen. They found even with limited exposure of less than two hours, the vitamin D severely inhibited the cancer cells' ability to proliferate – and the effect was permanent.[10]

Remember how Japanese men have low rates of prostate cancer? Here's one possible reason: UCSD epidemiologist Edward Gorham found the average intake of vitamin D in Japan is ten times that in the U.S. This is most likely due, he believes, to the popularity of fish that are rich in vitamin D. Anago, a type of eel favored by many Japanese, contains 5,000 international units of vitamin D per 100 grams. That's over ten times the U.S. RDA![11]

Vitamin D is a fat-soluble vitamin, and can be acquired either through food or exposure to sunlight. It is known as the "sunshine" vitamin because the sun's ultraviolet rays activate a form of cholesterol present in the skin, converting it to vitamin D. Air pollution, clouds and window glass inhibit the sun's action on the skin.

Let me warn you about the vitamin D in milk. An intake of dairy foods fortified with vitamin D, like milk, results in decreased magnesium absorption. This is because the so-called vitamin D added to milk is actually a hormone – and a synthetic one.

Beware of synthetic vitamin D because it can actually contribute to aging by depositing calcium in the soft tissue at the surface of the skin. Get your vitamin D from foods and sunlight instead. Foods containing high amounts of vitamin D are cod liver oil, salmon, sardines, herring, egg yolk, organ meats and bone meal. Too much sun is not recommended but Dr. Cedric Garland, director of the epidemiology program at the University of California, San Diego (UCSD) Cancer Center, believes 10-15 minutes a day will provide most individuals with the right amount of cancer-preventive vitamin D.[12]

For the complete story of nutrition and prostate cancer, and for proven alternative cancer therapies, read my book *Nutrition: The Cancer Answer II.*

Prostate-Healthy Nutrients

For maximum absorption, supplements should be taken with meals.

Nutrient	Suggested Dosage	Formulation
Aged garlic extract	2 teaspoons three times daily	Liquid
Amino acids	4-6 capsules daily	Multiple formula from natural sources
Antioxidants	4 capsules daily*	With selenium and grape seed extract
Borage oil	2 capsules daily	
Coenzyme Q10	2 capsules daily	With vitamin E, phospholipids and selenium
Enzymes	2 capsules twice daily	Multiple formula
Flaxseed oil	1 tablespoon daily	
Fiber	8 tablets daily	Psyllium, with herb hyssop
Folic acid	10 mg daily	
Multi-vitamin/mineral	6 caplets daily	Freeze-dried plant sources
Multi-mineral	2-4 ounces daily	In liquid solution, with vitamin B12, biotin
Pygeum	250 mg twice daily	
Saw palmetto	160 mg twice daily	
Vitamin B6	100 mg daily	
Vitamin C	Individual bowel tolerance**	With bioflavonoids (quercetin, rutin proanthocyanidins)
Vitamin E	2 capsules (800 IU) daily	d-alpha tocopherol

* The FDA recommends that pregnant women not exceed 10,000 IU of vitamin A daily.

** To determine individual dosage, on the first day take 1,000 mg hourly until diarrhea occurs, then reduce dosage to just below that for individual daily dosage. Vitamin C is not toxic in large doses but must be taken throughout the day to benefit. Divide dosage to three or four times a day.

CHAPTER 38:

Cancer, Skin

While it is true you don't expose the average 20 square feet of your skin to the sun, there is a lot you do expose on a hot summer day. It is this exposure, all experts warn, that increases your likelihood of getting skin cancer. What you probably don't realize is that there is more you can do to prevent skin cancer than using sunscreen and covering up.

The most common type of skin cancer is malignant melanoma, termed as such because it is the melanocytes – or pigmented skin cells in moles or freckles – that deform and turn cancerous. It is one of America's fastest-growing cancers, estimated to have struck 32,000 people in 1993, killing 9,100. Almost 75 percent of all skin cancer-related deaths will be from malignant melanoma. Since 1973, the incidence of skin cancer has increased a frightening four percent a year, according to the American Cancer Society. An additional 10,000 invasive non-melanoma skin cancers was estimated to have occurred in 1993, mostly sarcomas, including Kaposi's sarcoma, with 2,300 deaths from these types (*Cancer Facts & Figures*, 1993).

Protecting Yourself with Antioxidants

You know, of course, that sunscreens help protect your skin from ultraviolet radiation. But there is a lot they don't do. What is needed are nutrients that strengthen the skin against UV damage. If the skin is strong, and has essential nutrients, the cells aren't likely to mutate when exposed to radiation.

At a Gerontological Society of America meeting, Sheldon Pinnell, M.D., chief of dermatology at Duke University Medical

Center in Durham, NC reported on several studies on the protective effect of vitamin C on skin.

In one study, the skin of live pigs was treated with topical vitamin C, then exposed to ultraviolet light at one to five times the dose that produces sunburn. The topical vitamin C not only protected the pigs from sunburn, but protected the skin from cellular damage. The protective effect of the topical vitamin C lasted three days, even when the pigs were scrubbed with soap! Now, that's remarkable!

Vitamin C is found in the skin's collagen. Collagen is what gives skin elasticity, allowing it to bounce back after being damaged. One of the signs of scurvy, treated with vitamin C, is dry, rough skin and poor wound healing.

Vitamin C's ability to prevent UV damage in 15 participants produced impressive results that were reviewed by doctors at a Society of Investigative Dermatology meeting. Dermatologist James Leyden, who saw the study results remarked that treating skin with topical vitamin C "may influence the function of fibroblasts in a way that will make them produce more collagen."[1]

I have very sensitive skin, which burns at the slightest exposure to sunlight. After I read these impressive studies, I wanted to test them out. Taking a very great risk, I left my sunscreen in my hotel room and applied only a moisturizing lotion containing vitamin C when I went skiing at Lake Tahoe. I have to tell you, I was amazed! Not only did I not burn, after a full day of skiing in bright sunlight, but I actually tanned, probably for the first time in my life! Tanning is the body's way of protecting you against the sun. What this meant for me was that for the first time, my immune system was working to protect my skin. I am a believer!

Madhu Pathak, Ph.D., dermatology research professor at Harvard Medical School, believes there are various ways in which people can shield themselves from the sun. Dr. Pathak recommends using cosmetics and moisturizers that contain vitamins E and C and beta carotene, to counteract the skin oxidation caused by sunlight that damages cell membranes, DNA and skin proteins.[2]

"An antioxidant-enriched formulation will retard or minimize these damaging reactions both on the short term and long-term," said

Dr. Pathak. "Cosmetics and moisturizers might help minimize the damaging reactions, especially if used in conjunction with sunscreens."

Selenium is a power-packed antioxidant helpful for any disorder that involves damage or breakdown on the cellular level. Because "low plasma selenium levels have been linked to increased risk of non-melanoma skin cancer in human patients," E. Delver and B.C. Pence of Texas Technical University Health Sciences Center, Lubbock, Texas decided to see if increased selenium reduces the potential of skin cancer.[3]

Using hairless mice exposed to high doses of ultraviolet rays, the researchers supplemented the diets of three mice groups with varying amounts of selenium. Those fed the highest amount of selenium had the least number of tumors. Tests showed the mice produced high levels of glutathione, an enzyme essential for detoxification. Selenium helps the body produce glutathione.

In an abstract presented to members attending the 1993 Federation of American Societies for Experimental Biology (FASEB) conference, researchers concluded, "selenium has potential as a chemopreventive agent for human skin cancer."

When scientists surveyed the vitamin-taking habits of 131 people with skin cancer and 200 similar people without, they found that vitamin supplementation of any type was associated with a 60 percent reduction in skin cancer risk. More specifically, getting more than 100 international units (IU) of vitamin E (tocopherol) a day was linked to a 70 percent drop in risk; with more than 5,000 IU of vitamin A daily linked to a 90 percent reduction, according to a study presented at the American Society of Preventive Oncology. It's not the first time these antioxidants have been mentioned as possible skin-savers, but it is the first time average amounts of supplements have been linked to such a significant drop in risk (*Prevention*, February 1994).

A handful of studies show that some antioxidants, most notably vitamin E, act as a mild sunscreen – comparable to an SPF of about three – by blocking some of the sun's harmful ultraviolet rays. But more important, is topical antioxidant's potential for preventing free radical damage that happens when sunlight does get through the skin's top layers.

When it comes to cancer, take no chances. If you are at high risk, check with a qualified physician well-versed in nutritional therapy. In the meantime, there are issues to keep in mind regarding taking vitamins E and A.

Several substances interfere with, or even cause a depletion of vitamin E. When iron and vitamin E are taken together, they cancel out each other. Vitamin E should be taken in one dose. The best time to take it is before mealtime or bedtime. Chlorine in drinking water, ferric chloride, rancid oil or fat and inorganic iron compounds destroy vitamin E in the body. Large amounts of vegetable oil (polyunsaturated fats) in the diet increases the need for vitamin E. For optimal benefit, apply vitamin E to the skin as well as taking it internally.

Factors interfering with absorption of vitamin A and beta carotene include strenuous physical activity within four hours of consumption, intake of mineral oil, excessive consumption of alcohol and iron, and the use of cortisone and other drugs.

Tea Time

Green tea extracts possess a protective effect against skin cancer. Researchers found almost complete protection against tumor formation using green tea on the skin of mice subjected to cancer-causing substances. Green tea and extracts contain polyphenols, particularly powerful antioxidants.[4]

Important to realize when it comes to green tea, is that the active, anti-cancer ingredients are found in the leaves. Once they came to this realization, the Japanese started doing more than drinking their tea. Because much of the tea leaves' nourishment ended up matted to the bottoms of their tea cups, they started supplementing their foods with green tea powder and extract. Kazutami Kuwano, a researcher at Tokyo's Kasei Gakuin College, suggests a tablespoon of green tea leaves powder daily.[5]

For your fight against skin cancer, look for a food supplement that combines green tea extract and other herbal antioxidants like grape seed extract, ginkgo biloba and grass burdock extract with vitamins A, C, E and the minerals chromium and zinc.

Garlic is a detoxifying food that should be added to any cancer-preventive diet. Studies abound on the advantages of garlic in health. Japanese researchers found in clinical studies it suppressed the tendency of damaged skin cells to turn into cancerous cells.[6] The best source is liquid aged garlic extract, which leaves out the agricultural chemicals, odor and burn.

For the complete story of nutrition and skin cancer, and for proven alternative cancer therapies, read my book *Nutrition: The Cancer Answer II.*

Skin Cancer-Crushing Nutrients

For maximum absorption, supplements should be taken with meals.

Nutrient	Suggested Dosage	Formulation
Aged garlic extract	2 teaspoons three times daily	Liquid
Amino acids	4-6 capsules daily	Multiple formula from natural sources
Antioxidants	4 capsules daily*	With selenium and grape seed extract
Borage oil	2 capsules daily	
Coenzyme Q10	2 capsules daily	With vitamin E, phospholipids and selenium
Enzymes	2 capsules twice daily	Multiple formula
Flaxseed oil	1 tablespoon daily	
Fiber	8 tablets daily	Psyllium, with herb hyssop
Multi-vitamin/mineral	6 caplets daily	Freeze-dried plant sources
Multi-mineral	2-4 ounces daily	In liquid solution, with vitamin B12, biotin
Vitamin C	Individual bowel tolerance**	With bioflavonoids (quercetin, rutin proanthcyanidins)

Nourish with a moisturizing lotion containing vitamins A, C and E.

* The FDA recommends that pregnant women not exceed 10,000 IU of vitamin A daily.

** To determine individual dosage, on the first day take 1,000 mg hourly until diarrhea occurs, then reduce dosage to just below that for individual daily dosage. Vitamin C is not toxic in large doses but must be taken throughout the day to benefit. Divide dosage to three or four times a day.

CHAPTER 39:

Cancer, Stomach

"Cancer does not attack a healthy organ, but only one which has become weakened by abuse."
–J. H. Kellogg, M.D., 1895

J.H. Kellogg, M.D., founder of Kellogg cereals, and an early nutrition pioneer, wrote many books on nutrition and disease including *The Stomach: Its Disorders and How to Cure Them* (Modern Medicine Publishing Company, Battle Creek, Michigan, 1896). Dr. Kellogg believed people were not eating as well as they should. He invented the breakfast cereal as a digestive therapy for his Battle Creek Sanitarium clients. If you saw the movie *The Road to Wellville*, Kellogg's "sanitarium" advocated whole, healthy foods and a variety of interesting and natural, non-chemical therapies to induce health. Later, his Battle Creek Sanitarium Health Food Company distributed the cereal in stores so the public could benefit from a healthy breakfast.

There is a science – called salutogenesis – which strives to discover what causes health. It is the opposite of pathogenesis, which looks for a cause of disease. You could say Kellogg was an early pioneer of salutogenesis. He spent his life researching what it took to make people healthy and his practice and inventions were designed to maintain health and prevent illness.

Dr. Kellogg considered cancer a parasitic disease. He believed cancer cells take advantage of a weakened body, much like parasites do, and that the overuse of alcohol and chronic indigestion, not a cause and effect of malabsorption, are predisposing factors of stomach cancer.

Chronic Gastritis, Pernicious Anemia
Can Lead to Stomach Cancer

Gastritis can be caused by Helicobacter pylori, an organism that causes the stomach flu, which most of us, unfortunately, have experienced. The stomach lining becomes inflamed and irritated, causing diarrhea, vomiting and pain. If it lasts long enough, the intestinal lining is effected too. An impaired intestinal lining prevents absorption of vitamin B12, known to cause pernicious anemia.

Anything that damages the delicate tissues of the stomach lining can potentially mutate the cells, leading to cancer. This conclusion is backed by science.

An article in the medical journal *Cancer* cited a study in which researchers evaluating cancer patients in Mexico found 85 percent of them had Helicobacter pylori.[1]

Researchers looked at communities in Northeastern Italy when it was discovered they had a higher incidence of a rare type of stomach cancer than the general population. When they examined the people, they found 87 percent had Helicobacter pylori infections.[2]

A study of pernicious anemia patients, reported in *Cancer*, found that nine percent of them had stomach tumors. The researchers also found that nineteen out of 23 patients with gastritis had stomach tumors.[3]

Conventional Therapies Increase Stomach Cancer Risk

Before the dangers of radiation therapy were fully recognized, doctors treated ulcer patients with radiation therapy. Radiotherapy for peptic ulcer was used between 1937 and 1965 to control excess stomach acid. To determine if there were any health risks associated with this practice, Melvin L. Griem, M.D., and colleagues at the Department of Radiation Oncology, University of Chicago, evaluated the case histories of 3,609 patients, 1,831 of which were treated with radiation and 1,778 treated by other means. Dr. Griem and his colleagues found that not only did the radiation therapy increase the patients' risk of fatal cancer, but so did the surgical treatment of their peptic ulcers.

Nearly 70 percent of the patients were found to have died. Compared with the general population, patients treated with or without radiation were at significantly increased risk of dying of cancer and nonmalignant diseases of the digestive tract. Cancer of the stomach, pancreas, lung and prostate were increased in both irradiated and non-irradiated patients. Griem found that radiation therapy significantly increased the risk of these people dying of these cancers. More importantly, however, radiation combined with surgery increased the risk of stomach cancer by an incredible ten times! He also found that patients with stomach ulcers had a higher risk of developing stomach cancer than patients with intestinal ulcers. The death risk remained high for 50 years indicating that damage from radiation therapy may persist to the end of your life.[4]

Exactly how these therapies induce stomach cancer is not entirely known. However, there are clues to this puzzle. The fact that any disturbance in the stomach lining, whether from ulcers, gastritis or surgery, increases the risk of stomach cancer is one indicator. The other is the presence of alcohol. Studies have found a correlation between heavy alcohol consumption and stomach cancer. One researcher attributes this to alcohol's ability to change the acidity of stomach acid. This change in acidity is sure to disturb the stomach lining.

The important thing in preventing stomach cancer is to treat your stomach with care. Listen to what it is telling you. And stay away from the drug store! I believe it is possible that, because conventional therapies alter the natural state of our digestive system, they not only take away its ability to heal itself, but weakens it, leaving it susceptible to cancer. This is yet another reason to avoid standard conventional cancer therapies at all cost.

See my chapters on Gastritis and Ulcers for more.

Cured, Salted Foods = Stomach Cancer

A.B. Miller, Department of Preventive Medicine and Biostatistics, at the University of Toronto, Canada, reports that 74 percent of stomach cancer is potentially preventable with a reduction in the nitrites present in smoked and cured meats and salt-preserved foods.

He adds that stomach cancer is decreased with high fruit and vegetable consumption.[5]

Many studies of Asian populations back up Miller's contention. Stomach cancer is very high among the Japanese, Koreans and Chinese. So is their consumption of pickled food and salted and cured fish.

Dr. Shoichiro Tsugane and Dr. Shaw Watanabe, Epidemiology Division, National Cancer Center, Research Institute, Tokyo, Japan, examined the relationship between salt intake and the occurrence of stomach cancer. They found a strong correlation between the amount of salt consumed and death from stomach cancer. They estimated that a 40 percent reduction in salt intake could produce as much as a 65 percent reduction in stomach cancer mortality.[6]

Many cured meats, such as bacon, ham and sausage, contain nitrates and/or nitrites, chemical preservatives that link with amino acids and become nitrosamines, potent carcinogens.

Nitrosamines are a by-product of our "civilized" daily living. They are caused by chemicals in air pollution, cigarette smoke and processed foods. Nitrosamines are found anywhere you have chemical pollution, known or unknown.

In lab experiments with animals and people, Jinzhou Liu, a Chinese biochemist at Penn State University, has discovered that aged garlic extract can prevent nitrosamines from being formed.

Onions, too, apparently possess this cancer-preventive ability. Researchers at the Department of Laboratory Medicine, University of Minnesota, found four organosulfur compounds in garlic and onions that effectively prevent cancer cells from forming in the stomach.[7]

Antioxidants to the Rescue (Again)

In a host of research, scientists have found antioxidants, especially those in fresh fruits and vegetables, can reverse the effects of a bad diet and protect against stomach cancer.

Larry E. Johnson, M.D., Ph.D., Department of Family Medicine, at the University of Cincinnati Medical Center, Ohio, looked at antioxidants and how they effect stomach cancer. He examined the histories of 15,000 Chinese over a six year period and found that their rates of stomach cancer were considerably reduced with just minimal amounts of beta carotene (50 mg), vitamin E (30 mg) and selenium (50 mcg).[8]

The incidence of stomach cancer has decreased dramatically in Western Europe and North America in recent decades. It remains high in other parts of the world, particularly in Korea, where stomach cancer is the most common malignancy. A case control study conducted at two hospitals in Seoul, Korea, investigated the relationship between dietary factors and stomach cancer in both men and women. A total of 213 cases, matched with 213 hospital controls of the same age and sex, completed a 64-item food frequency questionnaire and provided other information about stomach cancer risk factors. The researchers found that the antioxidant nutrients in fruits and vegetables, especially carotenoids (beta carotene and vitamin A) and vitamin C, may be protective against stomach cancer. [9]

Green tea is a potent antioxidant and should be present in any antioxidant formula. In areas where green tea consumption is high, the incidence of stomach cancer is low. Shizuoka Prefecture and Kyushu are two Japanese communities found to have stomach cancer death rates lower than the national average. Studies confirmed they tended to drink green tea more frequently than did inhabitants in other areas.[10,11] Green tea and extracts contain polyphenols, particularly powerful antioxidants.

Important to realize when it comes to green tea, is that the active, anti-cancer ingredients are found in the leaves. Once they came to this realization, the Japanese started doing more than drinking their tea. Because much of the tea leaves' nourishment ended up matted to the bottoms of their tea cups, they started supplementing their foods with green tea powder and extract. Kazutami Kuwano, a researcher at Tokyo's Kasei Gakuin College, suggests a tablespoon of green tea leaves powder daily.[12]

For your fight against stomach cancer, look for a food supplement that combines green tea extract and other herbal antioxidants like grape seed extract, ginkgo biloba and grass burdock extract with vitamins A, C, E and the minerals chromium and zinc.

For more on nutrition and stomach cancer, read my book *Nutrition: The Cancer Answer II.*

Stomach Cancer-Crushing Nutrients

For maximum absorption, supplements should be taken with meals.

Nutrient	Suggested Dosage	Formulation
Aged garlic extract	2 teaspoons three times daily	Liquid
Amino acids	4-6 capsules daily	Multiple formula from natural sources
Antioxidants	4 capsules daily*	With selenium and grape seed extract
Borage oil	2 capsules daily	
Enzymes	2 capsules twice daily	Multiple formula
Flaxseed oil	1 tablespoon daily	
Fiber	8 tablets daily	Psyllium, with herb hyssop
Multi-vitamin/mineral	6 caplets daily	Freeze-dried plant sources
Multi-mineral	2 ounces daily	In liquid solution, with vitamin B12, biotin
Vitamin C	Individual bowel tolerance**	With bioflavonoids (quercetin, rutin proanthcyanidins)

* The FDA recommends that pregnant women not exceed 10,000 IU of vitamin A daily.

** To determine individual dosage, on the first day take 1,000 mg hourly until diarrhea occurs, then reduce dosage to just below that for individual daily dosage. Vitamin C is not toxic in large doses but must be taken throughout the day to benefit. Divide dosage to three or four times a day.

CHAPTER 40:

Carpal Tunnel Syndrome

Slam! I was startled out of my reverie by the sound of a book dropped in front of the table where I was signing my newest volume *Nutrition: The Cancer Answer II*. "I'm sorry, Maureen, I just can't seem to hold onto anything these days," came a small voice from under the table. As the voice's source straightened up I saw a tall brunette lady nervously massaging her hands as she spoke.

"Do you have numbness and tingling in your hands too?" I asked her. "Why, yes!" she responded. "It's not so bad when I first get up in the morning, but by the end of the day I have shooting pains from my wrist to my shoulder. I haven't been to a doctor yet, I'm hoping it's just temporary circulation problems."

I told her she needed to see a doctor because it sounded to me like carpal tunnel syndrome. I warned her not to see a conventional physician because their solution to the problem is to cut the wrist ligaments, a drastic and unnecessary solution to a problem that may be cured with vitamin B6.

The carpal tunnel is an anatomic area at the palm side of the wrist which is bordered by either bone or rigid ligaments. Through this "tunnel" passes, among other important structures, the median nerve. This nerve serves the thumb, index and middle fingers of the hand in both sensory as well as muscle functions. Because the tunnel is rigid, any swelling or compression in the area presses on the nerve and causes symptoms. The immediate cause of the compression is usually a thickening of the ligament that joins the two forearm bones at their further ends, just one to two inches from the palm. Dr. Ross Gordon diagnoses carpal tunnel syndrome when he finds three things: impaired feeling in the hand(s), a tingling sensation radiating out into the hands, and a worsening of the numbness and tingling when the wrist is flexed as hard as possible for 30 to 90 seconds.

Vitamin B6 Instead of Surgery

In his book, *Dr. Wright's Book of Nutritional Therapy* (Rodale Press, Emmaus, PA, 1979), Dr. Jonathan Wright describes how he treated a woman with a bad case of carpal tunnel in both hands. By the time she saw him, her grip strength was poor, she had a slight puffiness of both hands and the tendons on the back of her hands were not standing out as they should. Further clues were small, tender nodules over the furthest joints of three of her fingers. Last, she could not perform what he calls the "Ellis test." Keeping her palm straight, she was unable to curl her fingers inward so the fingertips touched the palm. He calls it the Ellis test because the B6/carpal tunnel connection was discovered by Dr. John Ellis and reported in his book *Vitamin B6, The Doctor's Report*. It is an excellent volume

Dr. Wright told his patient to take 200 milligrams of vitamin B6, along with a high dose B-complex formula three times daily. When she reported back in three weeks she said her symptoms were definitely improving, the numbness and tingling were gone and remained only in the center of her palms. She was no longer stiff in the mornings, and her hands didn't feel nearly as "tight." When her improvement seemed to slow, Dr. Wright added 250 mg of magnesium and one tablespoon of seed oils for fatty acids essential to healthy tissues and ligaments. The most complete way to get fatty acids are by taking both borage and flaxseed oils, which contain the most omega 3 and 6 fatty acids. A deficiency of magnesium can cause ligament and muscle cramping problems. In two months, Dr. Wright's patient was free of all symptoms.

Many other physicians report success using vitamin B6 for carpal tunnel syndrome. Louis S. Moore, M.D., of Naples, Florida reports that 100 mg of vitamin B6, three times daily may reduce the swelling from carpal tunnel syndrome.[1]

Robert D. Reynolds, Ph.D., Department of Nutrition and Medical Dietetics at the University of Illinois at Chicago, reports that 100 to 200 mg of vitamin B6 daily can relieve the symptoms of carpal tunnel syndrome in as little as 12 weeks.[2]

Even conventional medicine has to admit vitamin B6 works. Allan L. Berstein, M.D. at Kaiser Permanente Medical Center in Hayward, California discovered it relieved symptoms in all 20 of the carpal tunnel patients he examined. He determined B6 was safe at a 200 mg dose.[3]

Whenever you choose to supplement with one B vitamin, include an easily-absorbable B-complex formula since the B vitamins work together and are compromised by stress and intestinal disorders.

Caused by Our Modern Diet

When Dr. Wright questioned his patient about her diet, he wasn't surprised to note she subsisted mainly on white bread and processed foods, and had done so for years. There are several reasons why the modern diet makes us deficient in B vitamins. One reason is that whole grains are missing. White bread, and even many wheat breads do not contain the whole grains. B vitamins are contained in the outer portion of grains, which is usually left out of processed breads.

Certain drugs deplete our stores of B vitamins, like oral contraceptives. And yellow dye No. 5, allowed by the Food and Drug Administration to be added to processed foods, is also implicated in B vitamin deficiencies. Stress, another byproduct of our modern life, inhibits B6 metabolism in the body.[4] Certain pesticides, which you may or may not know you are ingesting, are also believed to drain your stores of B6.

Aiding the Healing Process

Eliminating the cause of carpal tunnel syndrome is the first step. But there are foods and nutrients that can be used to help reduce the inflammation that causes pressure on the median nerve and nourish the damaged tendon so healing can occur quickly.

Now, if I get sprains or stretch a ligament, I treat the pain and injury with vitamin C plus bioflavonoids.

Bioflavonoids, a group of substances related to vitamin C, have been shown in studies to speed the healing of bruised ligaments, not surprising considering they are powerful anti-inflammatories. A report in *Medical Times* stated that athletes taking citrus bioflavonoids and vitamin C healed twice as fast as athletes who took either vitamin C alone or no supplements whatsoever. Another study found that injured football players who took 200 to 600 mg daily of citrus bioflavonoids returned to the game in one-fourth the time of those not taking the supplements.[5]

A study by Mark Kaminski, M.S., an associate professor at Western States Chiropractic College in Portland, Oregon, found that one gram of vitamin C taken three times daily dramatically reduces pain following strenuous or infrequent exercise.[6]

Vitamin E, too, has been found in studies to help alleviate the pain of sore ligaments. A study at the Human Nutrition Research Center on Aging at Tufts University, Boston, found vitamin E may reduce some of the damage that occurs during vigorous exercise. Researchers studied 21 sedentary men, half of whom were given 800 IU of vitamin E for seven days prior to running downhill on a treadmill for 45 minutes. The other half were given placebos. After both groups exercised, the group taking the vitamin E had less injury.[7]

The spice turmeric has been used in both the Indian and Chinese systems of medicine for the treatment of many forms of inflammation. Its anti-inflammatory properties are likened to the pharmaceutical effects of hydrocortisone and phenylbutazone, only much safer. Curcumin is the active ingredient, and interestingly, contains a large amount of vitamin C. Vitamin C has been found to also act as an anti-inflammatory, and is recommended anytime we are under stress, since stress depletes our stores of C.[8]

Bromelain, the active phytochemical in pineapple is also recommended when joints, muscles or ligaments are swollen and inflamed. Since you would have to eat two whole pineapples a day to achieve this anti-inflammatory effect, it's good we have health stores that carry bromelain extract.[9]

Success Story

I don't often have the opportunity to learn the end of a story after passing information on. Many, many people come to me from the television studio audiences and personal appearances for help in diagnosing and treating their ailments with nutrition, commonsense and the assistance of an alternative-minded physician. I am always glad to help but even happier to learn they benefited.

Upon returning home from a long and arduous speaking tour, I opened my refrigerator to find a basket filled with health food goodies waiting for me. It was so large, there wasn't even room for a bottle of soy milk. Above the huge yellow ribbon was a short note from a woman thanking me for taking the time to help her. I didn't know who it was from until I read the card she had included. Then I realized it was the lady who asked me about the pain in her hands. She explained she had gone to her family doctor, who passed her on to an orthopedic surgeon, who ordered some x-rays, then told her he wasn't sure what her problem was and proposed exploratory surgery. It turns out this woman was a piano teacher.

While she was already finding it hard to work with the carpal tunnel syndrome, the surgeon told her she would lose all use of her hands for at least three weeks following the exploratory surgery. When she asked him if it could be carpal tunnel he said she could add another six weeks for recovery in the event she needed that surgical procedure. She told him she would have to think about it and on the way home stopped by a health food and vitamin store where she picked up my book *Foods That Heal*, and a nutritional food supplement that included B6, B12, and various health-giving nutrients derived from sprouts and vegetables. Her card said after ten weeks of taking the vitamins and being sure to include B6 foods in her diet, the pain was noticeably improved. In three months she had no pain at all. Now she tells all her friends to consider vitamin therapy before accepting their doctors' suggestions, especially where surgery is concerned.

Carpal Tunnel Syndrome-Smashing Nutrients
For maximum absorption, take supplements with meals.

Nutrient	Suggested Dosage	Formulation
Aged garlic extract	1 teaspoon three times daily	Liquid
Antioxidants	4 capsules daily*	With selenium and grapeseed extract
Borage oil	2 capsules daily	
Bromelain	250 mg three times a day between meals	
Curcumin	250 mg daily between meals	
Flaxseed oil	1 tablespoon daily	
Magnesium	200 mg daily	
MSM (methylsulfonylmethane)	500 mg three times daily	
Multi-mineral	3-4 ounces daily	In liquid solution, with vitamin B12, biotin
Multi-vitamin/mineral	6 caplets daily	Freeze-dried plant sources
Niacinamide	1,000 mg twice daily	
Quercetin	400 mg twice daily	With vitamin C and bioflavonoids
Tumeric	100 mg three times daily	
Vitamin B6	200 mg daily	
Vitamin C	Individual bowel tolerance**	With citrus bioflavonoids (quercetin, proanthocyanidins)

* The FDA recommends pregnant women not exceed 10,000 IU of vitamin A daily.

** To determine individual dosage, on first day take 1,000 mg hourly until diarrhea occurs, then reduce dosage to just below that for individual daily dosage. Vitamin C is not toxic in large doses but must be taken throughout the day to benefit. Divide dosage to three or four times a day.

CHAPTER 41:

Cataracts

When a former heavyweight champion began training for a return to the ring, he went on a special diet – a "see food" diet. He told the press, "Whenever I see food, I eat."

Believe me, there *is* such a thing as a see food diet. It's all contained here: better eating for better vision.

In the U.S., over 400,000 cases of cataracts are diagnosed yearly, and it has been estimated that there are about 40 million persons with cataract-related vision problems in the world.[1] That's a lot of people who could have been helped. If only they'd known!

This chapter is dedicated to those who, because of the condition of their eyes, need help reading this valuable information. What you'll learn here has the potential of halting your progressive eye disease.

First of all, cataracts are not an inevitable consequence of aging.

Don't be fooled by doctors and federal agencies who want you to believe nutritional solutions to medical problems do not exist. There are plenty of studies to prove that nutrition can help keep the cataract clouds off your corneas.

Just as what we eat affects our overall health and general performance, nutrition also impacts greatly on the eyes and visual system. Research from all fronts, alternative and conventional, reveals that cataracts can actually be prevented through the miracle of minerals and vitamins!

Free Radicals – Enemies of Eyesight

Paul Sternberg, M.D., associate professor of ophthalmology and director of retina service at Emory University School of Medicine, is one of several researchers throughout the country doing what they call the Age-Related Eye Disease Study, or AREDS. They're looking at how nutrients can control or stop cataracts and other eye problems. In his studies, Dr. Sternberg has found that sunlight plays an important role in the creation of cataracts.

What exactly are cataracts? They are a whitish film that covers the eye in places, eventually interfering with vision. You know how sunlight creates bubbles in water? It is actually creating oxygen and it is this oxygen that researchers believe contribute to cataracts.

The important thing to understand at this point is the role oxygen plays in eye disease. Exposure to ultraviolet rays can damage the sensitive tissues of the eye. The eyes are *living tissue* directly exposed to the damaging effects of the environment. They are the only part of the outer body that is actually living tissue. No wonder they are so easily damaged.

Although we cannot live without oxygen, the act of breathing in oxygen causes problems. In addition to using oxygen to generate greater amounts of energy, breathing produces unstable oxygen compounds known as oxygen free radicals that damage DNA, proteins, carbohydrates and fats.

We can see this process in everyday life in the form of rusting metal, browning fruit and rancid oils.

Highly charged with energy, and unstable and unpredictable as a madman who runs amuck in a crowd, scavenger molecules with unpaired electrons steal single electrons from other pairs and in the process break down our lawn furniture and shorten our lifespans. We call these boogie bombers "free radicals."

How do free radicals originate? In many ways. We encourage the production of free radicals in our bodies when we expose ourselves to toxic poisons. For example, when we spray insecticide on our gardens, eat rancid oil, inhale tobacco smoke, use strong cleaners with gloves and ventilation, and ingest drugs. Even stress can cause free radicals to form.

As if we need a reason not to smoke, here's a doosy: your eyesight.

One five-year study revealed that men who smoked a pack a day doubled their risk of developing cataracts. That's compared to men who never smoked. An eight-year study showed that women who smoked 30 cigarettes a day had about a 60 percent greater risk of cataracts.

There are two ways our bodies compensate for this problem: by replicating new cells and by creating antioxidant enzymes that snuff out the free radicals, changing them into harmless waste that's thrown off.

The Antioxidant Answer

Synthetic antioxidants were first used in the food service industry to keep lettuce from browning or keep vegetable oils from becoming rancid before being used by cooks. These undesirable color or flavor changes result from a reaction of food components with oxygen in the air.

The same chemical reactions that make food inedible ravage our immune systems, wrinkle our skin and invite illness and disease.

These chemical reactions may be a fact of life, but the impact on our body need not be.

Enter nature's wonder: antioxidants! They are super-duper nutrients that seek out and destroy the free radicals that seek out and destroy our skin, joints, tissues and bones—and we're discovering new ones all the time. Here's an experiment you can try at home. Peel and cut a banana in half. Mash up both halves separately. Now add some vitamin C powder (ascorbic acid) to one half. Which would you rather your eyes to be? The half that's turning brown or the half with the vitamin C that is staying white and fresh?

Vitamin C, vitamin E and beta carotene are the most well-known antioxidants. Most alternative doctors also recommend coenzyme Q10, selenium, superoxide dismutase (SOD) and the amino acids cysteine, glutathionine, methionine and taurine. Beta carotene is probably the most well-known to date. Everywhere you turn, someone's talking about beta carotene. Believe it or not, scientists have found another biologically-occurring nutrient with even more radical punching ability. Lycopene, a bioflavonoid in the carotenoid family that is found in the red pigment of the tomato, exhibits the highest oxygen-quenching rate of the antioxidants, as revealed in a German study.[2] It is also found in apricots, grapefruit, guavas and watermelon.

Do you want to prevent cataracts? Increase your intake of vitamin E. Among 660 people in a recent Baltimore Longitudinal Study, those with the most vitamin E in their bloodstreams were 50 percent less likely to develop the most common kind of cataracts.[3] The same study that revealed the benefit of lycopene also discovered that alpha tocopherol, or vitamin E is a highly-effective antioxidant.

What's good for the canine is good for the master. Selenium combined with vitamin E have been used successfully by veterinarians to treat cataracts in dogs. Dogs given these cataract-killers not only lost their cataracts but had improved vision as well. Now, what do you suppose they put on a dog eye chart? Bones and cats?

Allen Taylor, Ph.D., of the USDA Human Nutrition Research Center on Aging at Tufts University in Boston, believes cataracts are caused by the slow deterioration of lens proteins by oxidation, and that antioxidants help to prevent or retard this process.[4] Isn't that what I've been saying all along? Well, at least the government agrees with this one.

More Cataract Killers

Another testimonial for vegetarianism: a 1991 study found that older people who ate a diet of mostly fruits and vegetables were 37 percent less likely to develop cataracts. Many other studies have shown similar results. Look for foods with the crucial cataract-killers I'll tell you about shortly. These foods will work against the damaging effects of oxygen on the lenses of the eyes.

A large-scale study of more than 120,000 registered nurses, conducted at Brigham and Women's Hospital and Harvard Medical School, found a 40 percent lower rate of cataracts among nurses who consumed the most foods high in vitamin A, compared to nurses who ate the least.[5]

Eat your fruits and veggies! If the above information hasn't convinced you, this might. A 1991 report in the *American Journal of Clinical Nutrition* showed that people who eat 3-1/2 servings of fruits and vegetables every day have a substantially reduced risk of cataracts. Those who ate less than that are believed to be almost six times more at risk for cataracts.

The United States Department of Agriculture agrees. They said in a study that people who eat less than 1-1/2 servings of fruit or less than two servings of vegetables each day are roughly 3-1/2 times more likely to develop cataracts.

When researchers questioned the nurses participating in the study I just mentioned, they said most of their vitamin A foods were spinach, squash and sweet potatoes. Yum Yum!

In addition to its cataract prevention potential, vitamin A is important to the eyes and visual system in several ways. The ability of the eye to adapt to changes in light is dependent upon a chemical known as retinal purple, or rhodopsin. Retinal purple is comprised mainly of protein and a close relative of vitamin A, and is the army that keeps us seeing even in darkness. But the army has one enemy: light. When light hits the retina – such as when driving and being "blinded" by oncoming headlights – the retinal purple army splits up, temporarily fleeing. The next time you enter a dark room after being outside on a sunny day, see how long it takes for your vision to return. How long it takes depends upon two things: the amount of retinal purple present to begin with and the amount of light. Too much light and not enough vitamin A means the breakdown of night vision.

All orange and dark green vegetables and fruits as well as fish and cod liver oil are good food sources of vitamin A. One six-ounce glass of carrot juice contains 47,381 IU of vitamin A. However, the vitamin can be destroyed by poor liver function; alcohol; eating large amounts of mineral oil or ferrous sulphate, a common preservative; x-rays; and any kind of infection.

A word of caution: doctors like to scare people away from A by emphasizing that you can take too much. Vitamin A is a so-called fat soluble vitamin, meaning it doesn't dissolve well in water and as a result, our body stores excess A in the liver. Too much can cause liver and bone damage. However, toxic levels are considered to be above 100,000 IU, which is a lot, and more than anyone would expect you to take. Pregnant women should not exceed 10,000 IU a day. Signs of vitamin A toxicity includes cracked lips, peeling palms, and a small pounding headache at the front of the forehead. If you get these symptoms, eat something, and cut back on the dosage. Combining vitamin E with A boosts the benefit so lower amounts can be taken.

Vitamin E is another cataract-killer, and this too is backed by testimony from top medical authorities. Studies on vitamin E and cataracts have proven over and over again that it helps prevent them.

One eye-opening study involving 832 people showed that those with the highest blood levels of vitamin E had the fewest cataracts. According to Susan Vitale, assistant professor of ophthalmology at Johns Hopkins University, the risk of cataracts was cut in half in those people who had the highest blood levels of vitamin E.[6]

Canadian researchers James Robertson, John R.Trevithick and Allan P. Donner, of the University of Western Ontario in London, studied 175 middle-aged people with cataracts and 175 matched controls who did not have the disorder.[7]

The researchers reported that the cataract-free individuals had taken at least 400 IU of vitamin E and/or a minimum of 300 mg of vitamin C daily for five years. They also showed that diabetic and therefore cataract-prone rats given high dietary levels of vitamin E had less lens-protein leakage than did the non-diabetic rats.

The "See" Vitamins

See results with C! Vitamin C is a renowned free radical ravager as research has revealed.

Experiments with guinea pigs have demonstrated that vitamin C boosts the amount of ascorbic acid in the eye, helping to stop cataract formation. But there's more!

Researchers have found that the most detectable ascorbic acid (vitamin C) found in the body is in the eyes. D. Garland reported in the *American Journal of Clinical Nutrition* that low levels of vitamin C are associated with some forms of cataracts. The amount of C in the eye is 20 to 70 times higher than that of the blood and other tissues.[8] In eyes with cataracts, very little ascorbic acid is found. This isn't really surprising since vitamin C has been found to protect lens proteins and other components of the eye against damage by ultraviolet light.

In one sight-restoring study, 450 patients who were diagnosed with cataracts experienced a reduction in cataract formation only weeks after taking one gram of vitamin C daily.

Paul F. Jacques and colleagues at the USDA Human Nutrition Research Center on Aging at Tufts University in Boston, have observed that the highest protective effect was seen in people with unusually high blood levels of vitamin C, and recommend a daily intake of at least 500 mg of vitamin C to protect against cataracts.[9]

If you thought C and E were good, try them together! Vitamins C and E together provide even more protection against cataracts. Studies at John Hopkins University and the National Institute on Aging in Baltimore confirm this. Researchers there found that people who take only vitamin E supplements have about 50 percent less cataract risk than those who take no vitamins. Those taking vitamin C and E together show an incredible 70 percent risk reduction.[10]

Ask for whole wheat bread for your sandwich. Why? Because

the riboflavin in the wheat can also help fight cataracts.

Numerous studies have implicated a deficiency of riboflavin (vitamin B2) in cataract creation. In one study of 173 cataract patients, 20 percent of those under the age of 50 were deficient in riboflavin and 34 percent over 50 were deficient. None of the 16 controls over the age of 50 who did not have cataracts were deficient. In a study reported in the *Lancet*, eight of 22 cataract patients were found deficient in riboflavin. In another study, 81 percent of patients ages 48 to 80 with cataracts had a riboflavin deficiency.[11]

The riboflavin evidence is just the tip of the proverbial iceberg. The amino acid glutathione is found in high concentrations in the cornea and lens of the eye, and keeps the lens transparent, protecting against cataracts. Glutathione protects the lens from the destructive effects of ultraviolet light and – get this – is dependent on riboflavin for its production. Glutathione concentration also decreases when the body produces less of the amino acids necessary for its synthesis: cysteine and methionine. And, as I've already mentioned, they are antioxidants!

Another recommended antioxidant, selenium, was found to be only 15 percent of normal levels in the lenses of patients with cataracts. Not coincidentally, selenium also is required for the functioning of glutathione. Do you see a pattern here?

OK, you may have had trouble following all this impressive information, so let me summarize for you. If you aren't getting any younger, enjoy being out in the sunshine a lot – like if you're an avid golfer – and/or are concerned about cataracts, here are the nutrients you should consider: vitamin A, vitamin C, vitamin E, zinc, riboflavin, selenium, cysteine, methionine, glutathione, and, for good measure lycopene, taurine, coenzyme Q10 and superoxide dismutase (SOD).

Cataract-Quashing Nutrients
For maximum absorption, take supplements with meals.

Nutrient	Suggested Dosage	Formulation
Acidophilus	At least four billion flora daily on an empty stomach, three times daily	
Aged garlic extract	1 teaspoon three times daily	Liquid
Amino acids	4-6 capsules daily	Multiple formula from natural sources
Antioxidants	4 capsules daily*	With selenium and grapeseed extract
Bilberry	100 mg three times daily	
Coenzyme Q10	2 capsules daily	With vitamin E, phospholipids and selenium
Ginkgo biloba	60 mg twice daily	
Multi-mineral	3-4 ounces daily	In liquid solution, with vitamin B12, biotin
Multi-vitamin/mineral	6 caplets daily	Freeze-dried plant sources
Vitamin A	25,000 IU daily*	
Vitamin B6	100 mg daily	
Vitamin C	Individual bowel tolerance**	With bioflavonoids (quercetin, rutin proanthocyanidins)
Vitamin E	2 capsules (800 IU) daily	d-alpha tocopherol

* The FDA recommends pregnant women not exceed 10,000 IU of vitamin A daily.

** To determine individual dosage, on first day take 1,000 mg hourly until diarrhea occurs, then reduce dosage to just below that for individual daily dosage. Vitamin C is not toxic in large doses but must be taken throughout the day to benefit. Divide dosage to three or four times a day.

CHAPTER 42:

Cerebral Palsy

What exactly is cerebral palsy, and what causes it? Rather than an actual disease, it is really a syndrome – a series of symptoms that become progressively worse, characterized by an inability to control the muscles. Because it is believed to be caused by brain damage, it is considered incurable. Here we go again with that word *incurable*.

Strike incurable from your consciousness. There is valid research supporting the fact that, with large amounts of stimulus, brains stunted by neglect or damaged by injury can, to a certain degree, recover and grow. Cerebral palsy cannot be cured, per se, but through therapy its victims can learn to walk and live autonomously. Putting on our detective hat, grasping our magnifying glass, let's first examine how cerebral palsy is originally diagnosed.

Sometimes the first symptoms are "floppy baby syndrome" where the baby's muscles have little tone and the baby flops around when being held. The parents and doctors wait, holding their breath to see if the problem gets better. Two years later, when the symptoms get worse, and the limbs become poorly developed – sometimes rigid due to excessive muscle tone or weak with a tendency to spasm and contract – the diagnosis of cerebral palsy is made. Physical therapy may keep the severe muscle spasms from leading to bone deformities, but basically the child is put into a wheelchair and considered severely handicapped. Very little else can be done, the anguished parents are told.

Cerebral palsy involves nervous system and/or muscular impairment caused by a lack of oxygen to the fetal brain. The cause of this oxygen deprivation is where the controversy starts. In a number of countries concern about cerebral palsy has led to lawsuits against obstetricians who delivered affected children, based on a view that the child's cerebral palsy resulted from something the obstetrician did or did not do. There were even some lawsuits alleging malpractice. In most developed countries, rates of stillbirth and deaths among newborns have declined, but the same reductions have not been seen in cerebral palsy.

In a study of births in Western Australia, researchers found that between 1967 and 1985, rates of stillbirths and deaths among newborn infants dropped dramatically, but there was no change in the rate of cerebral palsy births.[1]

What is more likely, and commonly believed, is that cerebral palsy starts with the brain of the unborn baby. Dr. Alan Leviton, Director of the Neuroepidemiology Unit, Children's Hospital, and Associate Professor of Pediatrics and Neurology at Harvard Medical School, believes that whatever causes cerebral palsy occurs sometime before labor and delivery. He suggests that some children who have cerebral palsy may actually have minor alterations in their brains, and that these problems are likely to have developed months before birth.[2] The bottom line is that there is a communication gap between the brain and the body, which causes an inability to control muscles. How does Dr. Leviton's "minor alteration" end up causing such extreme and debilitating symptoms as those seen in cerebral palsy? Keep reading and you will see!

Inactivity Worsens the Original Problem

Much of the brain's development takes place before birth and these and numerous other subsequent developmental changes are genetically determined. However, brain growth continues throughout adolescence and beyond. The cerebral cortex, that which is involved in muscle control, in particular is capable of considerable growth during early childhood. Both nonhuman and human studies have shown that the brain's structure is affected by activity.[3] What does this mean in terms of cerebral palsy? It means that those two years between the time this brain damage is first evidenced and the time any kind of diagnosis and therapy takes place is critical. Because a child's nervous system is in such a dynamic period of change, much can be accomplished if early diagnosis and intervention takes place. In other words, a great deal of these later and most debilitating symptoms can be prevented.

When a child with damage to motor areas of the brain is restricted in his or her movement or experience, lack of activity may make the problem worse. Dr. Marion Diamond, a neuroanatomist from the University of California at Berkeley, reported in May of 1986 that she could actually measure the amount of brain growth which took place in laboratory animals after only four hours of stimulation.[4] In animal studies, rats raised in an enriched environment that required super motor skills, had huge noticeable growth in the cerebral cortex areas of their brains.[5] Similarly, it has been shown that humans from an intellectually enriched environment had an increase in brain growth in areas of the cortex devoted to verbal understanding when compared with subjects from a less specialized background. Individuals engaged in occupations demanding physical ability had more growth in primary motor areas of the brain.[6]

This has also been proved in studies of severely neglected children, who were forced to live with little or no outside stimulus. It's horrifying to see what being locked up in a dark closet for years can do. A child can literally turn into a vegetable, without even the ability to walk. These sad cases of neglect fortunately have happy endings as therapists can reverse the damage through massive, constant stimulus therapy.

Help in Hungary

A *Washington Post* article reported on Frank Clark and his wife, residents of Manchester, England, who were desperate for help for their son, two-year old Sebastian. He was so handicapped by cerebral palsy that he was unable to stand or even sit up on his own. Receiving no help from doctors and clinics in England, they flew from Manchester to the Peto Institute in Hungary. Clark heard that the institute had developed a uniquely successful treatment for cerebral palsy, Parkinson's disease and other motor disabilities under the name of "conductive education."[7]

The Clarks feel that their gamble – and sacrifice – has paid off. By his third year of intensive treatment, Sebastian was able to go to the toilet, button his shirt buttons, eat and stand on his own. He also learned to speak fluent Hungarian as well as English.

It remains unclear whether the Peto Institute's remarkable reported success with motor disabilities can be duplicated elsewhere. But after more than 40 years of dogged persistence, the institute appears to be on the verge of vindication in its insistence that traditional therapy has long failed to realize the potential for helping the severely handicapped.

At the heart of Peto's conductive education theory is the notion that what motor-handicapped persons need is not targeted therapies but holistic, integrated treatment. "Traditionally, people think handicapped children are ill and need therapy," said Dr. Maria Hari, the institute's director. "That's not true: they have an incurable illness and the key is for them to learn how to live with it."

The Hungarian method abolishes the traditional division of treatment and various specialists, in favor of a unified approach and a single therapist–the "conductor"–who guides the child through complex activities meant to address several problems at once.

According to Clark, the people at the institute "insist that the child must learn to do everything, that he must be self-reliant. It was a terrible shock to Sebastian–and to us–when we first came here. But then he started to do things for himself we never imagined he could do."

The Peto Institute says that 70 percent of the disabled children it treats eventually learn to walk, a remarkably high success rate. It often takes a severely disabled child as long as five years to reach that goal, but once it is achieved it is usually a permanent gain. Dr. Hari estimates that 90 percent of children affected by cerebral palsy can be helped by the technique.

Nutritional Help

With conventional medicine delving so little into nutrition, who's to say cerebral palsy isn't caused by a deficiency that starts with the pregnant mother? At least one nutrient, the enzyme arginase, has been found in studies to be deficient in cerebral palsy victims. Get out your magnifying glass! Symptoms of an arginase deficiency, though rare, are very similar to those associated with cerebral palsy. It causes a progressive inability to control the muscles, failure to grow, seizures, and arm and leg spasms.

Angela Scheuerle, M.D., Institute For Molecular Genetics at Baylor College of Medicine in Houston, studied two cerebral palsy patients who were found to have arginase deficiency. Dr. Scheuerle found that treating with arginase, while it did not reverse all the symptoms, did help with some.[8] Arginase is obtained through the supplement arginine, an amino acid essential for infant growth. All the amino acids must be present in the diet to be of benefit. If one essential amino acid is missing or present in a low amount, the assimilation of protein will be threatened. Amino acid formulations are also available in health food stores. Free form formulations are more easily absorbed and are recommended.

It is interesting that arginine is important to growth because one of the common symptoms of cerebral palsy is growth retardation. However, malnutrition is another likely factor. Because of an inability to control their muscles, children with cerebral palsy can take from two to twelve times as long as other children to chew and swallow even pureed food. Mothers of children with cerebral palsy report spending as long as seven hours per day helping their children eat.

Researchers at the American Dietetic Association believe their common growth retardation is probably a result of this inability to eat well.[9]

This is just one reason why extra nutrition is so important to people with cerebral palsy. Extra nutrition can also benefit the brain and muscles, especially in light of their lack of stimulation and exercise. Nutrients that help muscle tone are: magnesium vitamin B1, vitamin B6 and bioflavonoids. Brain nutrients are the B vitamins; the antioxidant vitamins A, C, E and the mineral selenium; the herbs ginkgo biloba and ginseng, and another amino acid acetyl-L-carnitine. Many animal and human studies have found these nutrients to be of benefit.

Cerebral-Saving Nutrients
For maximum absorption, take supplements with meals.

Nutrient	Suggested Dosage	Formulation
Amino acids	4-6 capsules daily	Multiple formula from natural sources
Antioxidants	4 capsules daily*	With selenium and grapeseed extract
Borage oil	2 capsules daily	
Coenzyme Q10	2 capsules daily	With vitamin E, phospholipids and selenium
Flaxseed oil	1 tablespoon daily	
Ginkgo biloba	60 mg three times daily	
Malic acid	250 mg twice daily	
Multi-mineral	3-4 ounces daily	In liquid solution, with vitamin B12, biotin
Multi-vitamin/mineral	6 caplets daily	Freeze-dried plant sources
Vitamin A	25,000 IU* daily	
Vitamin C	Individual bowel tolerance**	With bioflavonoids (quercetin, rutin proanthocyanidins)

* The FDA recommends pregnant women not exceed 10,000 IU of vitamin A daily.

** To determine individual dosage, on first day take 1,000 mg hourly until diarrhea occurs, then reduce dosage to just below that for individual daily dosage. Vitamin C is not toxic in large doses but must be taken throughout the day to benefit. Divide dosage to three or four times a day.

CHAPTER 43:

Chemical, Heavy Metal Poisoning

A very dear friend of mine had a daughter who was diagnosed as having epilepsy when she was 12 years old. The girl went through years of embarrassing and sometimes dangerous public seizures. Pharmaceuticals helped the symptoms but never addressed the cause. Eleven years later, during an internship with a prominent medical research institute, my friend's daughter discovered something that made her look harder at this original diagnosis, which she and her mother never questioned. After seeking out a research specialist she discovered she didn't have epilepsy at all! All these years her body had been reacting to the presence of aluminum in her body. When she completely stopped eating and drinking out of aluminum cans and cookware, eliminated all foods and medicines containing aluminum, her symptoms stopped. She has not had a seizure for 10 years.

This is the tragedy of our current conventional medicine: the tragedy of misdiagnoses. Many of our chronic diseases: Alzheimer's, arthritis, cancer, chronic fatigue, depression and epilepsy can be caused by chemical poisoning. The good news is that our bodies are capable of throwing off most chemicals alien to our systems and good health. With certain detoxifying tools, which I will describe, we can handle short term toxic exposure. The bad news is that there are more long term sources of toxic chemicals than ever before.

What causes chemical poisoning? Exposure to automobile emissions day after day has been shown to be a leading culprit. Children playing in yards that have been sprayed with pesticides, new carpeting that smells of chemicals long after it has been laid – all are products of our modern, and very toxic environment, wearing down our immune systems and contributing to disease.

Old buildings are not the only dwellings that can cause its occupants to get sick. According to the Environmental Protection Agency (EPA), up to 30 percent of new and remodeled buildings trigger illness in some of their occupants. Affected individuals exhibit any of a range of nonspecific complaints, including headache, respiratory irritation, asthma or flu-like symptoms, chest tightness, and fatigue. Over the past decade, many studies have demonstrated that this "sick building" syndrome contributes to increased absenteeism and reduced work efficiency, not to mention physical discomfort. Experts aren't sure exactly what causes this problem, only that increased ventilation seems to help.[1] What do you think? Could it be...chemicals?!

Food in supermarkets abound with potentially dangerous chemicals. Researchers at the Arizona State University's Biochemical Department have determined that aspartame, an artificial sweetener that goes by the brand name NutraSweet, has been associated with seizures. Aluminum and lead poisoning may also cause seizures.[2]

Not surprisingly, removal of toxic metals and chemicals in the body has been found to reverse symptoms of disease. In a Canadian newspaper there was a case report of two children whose autistic symptoms and hyperactivity disappeared when they were treated for lead poisoning.[3]

Important in any program of self-help health is an awareness of symptoms and ailments that can be traced to chemicals. The number of pharmaceuticals that cause side effects severe enough for hospitalization are so numerous every chapter in this book would double if I included them all.

According to an article in the *Philadelphia Inquirer* entitled "As Prescription Drugs Cure, Some Side Effects Harm (June 24, 1990)," Americans spent nearly $2 billion a year on prescription drugs. Dr. Brian Strom, associate director of medicine and pharmacology at the University of Pennsylvania School of Medicine, estimates that side effects each year put 1.6 million people in hospitals and kill up to 160,000 Americans, at a cost of more than $20 billion.

Suffice it to say you should be aware of the dangers of both prescription and over-the-counter remedies available in your drugstore. The "Just Say No to Drugs" campaign should include those in the nation's medicine cabinets. The *Physician's Desk Reference* is available in libraries and bookstores and lists all the *known* side effects of prescription and over-the-counter medications.

Chemicals Threaten us Daily

The largest study ever conducted on the health effects of airborne particles was described in a March 1995 issue of the *American Journal of Respiratory and Critical Care Medicine*. It found air pollution from high sulfate and fine particle levels raised the risk of premature death from all causes by 15 to 17 percent. The fact is, our health is compromised every day by the air we breathe, the water we drink and the even the food we eat – especially if it comes out of a factory.

The United States uses 2.2 billion pounds of pesticides annually, according to the U.S. Environmental Protection Agency. Of these, says Susan Cooper, staff ecologist for the National Coalition Against the Misuse of Pesticides (NCAMP) in Washington, D.C., all the pesticides are basically toxic to the brain. Yet they are not usually subjected to testing.[4]

What about food additives? Nobody seems to know for sure. According to Michael Jacobson, Ph.D., director of the Center for Science in the Public Interest in Washington, D.C., "Food additives are not normally tested for neurotoxicity or for how they interact with other food agents." In light of this information vacuum and regulatory sieve, add one more item to the list of intelligence-boosting foods – organically grown and additive-free foods are the best bet for your brain.

According to the Food and Drug Administration, approximately 5,000 food additives are permitted in America's food supply. Included among these are antibiotics given to meat-producing animals, anti-foaming agents, foaming agents, bleaches, chemical sterilizing agents, coating materials, colorings, emulsifiers, flavorings, artificial smoke, modifiers, organic solvents, preservatives, sweeteners, synthetic dyes and thickeners.

At an annual meeting of the International Union Against Cancer in Rome, Dr. W.C. Hueper of the National Cancer Institute, stated there are 20 groups of possible cancer-causing additives as well as 17 groups of suspect food contaminants. He concluded by stating many chemicals introduced into foodstuffs "possess carcinogenic properties."

Two products, often found in cosmetics, skin and hair products, were addressed in the *Sarasota/Florida ECO Report*, April 1994. Sodium lauryl sulfate, a detergent that is associated with cancer, skin irritation and eye problems in children is found in approximately 90 percent of commercial shampoos. Propylene glycol, a chemical contained in antifreeze and brake fluid, associated with kidney problems, liver abnormalities and skin problems, is a common ingredient in beauty creams, cleansers and cosmetics.

Why do we need to know all this? We need to be enlightened consumers, aware of chemical hazards so when we shop for food, cosmetics and skin care products we'll know what to buy and what not to buy. As the average consumer becomes more wary and descriminating, cosmetic and skin care companies, for example, are more careful about what they *don't* put in their products. When looking for skin care formulas, look for manufacture-guaranteed, natural, chemical-free ingredients. Look for natural ingredients at the top of the label's list, indicating its highest amount, and don't be afraid to spend a little more money.

If exposure to a certain chemical can be limited or eliminated, and could possibly prevent or stop certain symptoms, doesn't it make sense to try this approach before piling on more chemicals or giving up altogether?

Lead Poisoning – Many Causes, A Definitive Treatment

What is the first source you think of when you hear about lead poisoning? Paint chips? Old lead pipes? Water?

An internal audit by The Inspector General's Office reports that state officials and the Environmental Protection Agency (EPA) are not protecting children against unsafe levels of lead in their school water supply. The EPA estimates that over 250,000 children each year are exposed to lead levels in drinking water high enough to affect intellectual and physical development. Thirteen school districts in the mid Atlantic region found that three of the districts had not adequately tested for lead in the water supply. Lead contamination was found in eight of ten districts that performed the tests. The audit reported that states are not complying with The Safe Drinking Water Act of 1974 or Lead Contamination Control Act of 1988.[5]

Surprising Sources of Lead

While occupational exposure to lead sources account for most adult lead poisoning, other sources can be overlooked. The restoration of old houses that have lead based paint may account for what doctors in Boston are calling "Yuppie Lead Poisoning." They found 20 percent of lead-poisoned patients in the Lead and Toxicology Clinic of Children's Hospital were victimized as their parents renovated their new 'old' house. Certain precautions should be undertaken when renovating old buildings. When rooms are undergoing renovation they should be well-ventilated. Masks should be worn while using heat guns and torches as vaporized lead particles can be absorbed by breathing and go directly into the bloodstream.[6]

Adults are particularly at risk because unless they report occupations that exposes them to known toxins, doctors typically ignore the possibility that their symptoms can be caused by poisoning. Early symptoms of lead poisoning, for example, can easily be dismissed as a viral problem. Symptoms can include seizures, gastrointestinal disorders, weakness and fatigue, irritability, poor appetite, forgetfulness, and flu-like symptoms. Later symptoms include anemia, gout, kidney problems, nervous system damage and high blood pressure. Even moderate exposure may have long term health effects. Lead blocks the body's absorption of iron and copper, which is necessary to produce hemoglobin, the red substance that carries oxygen to our trillions of cells. A lack of hemoglobin causes fatigue and anemia.

Although leaded gasoline is a thing of the past, its memory lingers on – in the soil, vegetation and water. We also get lead from old water pipes, earthenware dishes and mugs whose lead glaze was fixed at too low a temperature, in toothpaste tubes, from food and beverage can sealants and from fruit on trees sprayed with lead and arsenic (lead-arsenate).

Dr. J.H. Graziano, Ph.D. and colleagues at the Department of Medicine, Columbia University College of Physicians and Surgeons in New York, found that the lead content of wine stored in lead crystal decanters rose considerably after four months in the decanters. They concluded that wine stored in lead crystal decanters can increase its lead concentration steadily over time, and that alcohol left in these decanters for long periods of time may actually contain toxic doses of lead.[7]

Pottery and china from certain countries can contain lead in their paint, which could be insidiously poisoning you. Dr. Thomas D. Matte, Lead Poisoning Prevention Branch, Centers For Disease Control and Prevention, reported in *The Lancet* the case of the 7-year-old child of a U.S. Embassy official in Mexico City who was poisoned by fruit punch consumed at a picnic that was contained in a Mexican pottery urn. Dr. Matte believes even brief exposure to the lead contained in Mexican pottery can create a persistent health risk.[8] Recently I was surprised to see a sign above some dishware for sale in a small discount store that read: warning: this dishware may contain lead. Why buy it?, I wondered. Yet, people do.

With certain occupations the risk of lead exposure is known and precautions are taken. Unfortunately, the handyman who uses many of these same products to do his work doesn't have the information to take the same necessary precautions. For example, certain brick mortar contains lead, as does lead solder, batteries, antifreeze, pottery, ceramics and brass. Exposure from gun fire is also a source of lead exposure. Several cases of poisoning have occurred from individuals who frequent indoor firing ranges.

Heavy Metal – Not Music to Your Ears

Chronic exposure to heavy metals, due to lifestyle choices, can cause an accumulation of them in the body, and may compromise health. Any level of toxic metals in the body is not normal, and a large accumulation can be dangerous. When I speak of lifestyle, I have to include the choice to smoke. Read the chapter on Lung Cancer to get a picture of the number of chemicals you ingest if you smoke. Cadmium, a toxic metal, is just one of many. Cadmium is contained in the secondhand smoke of cigarettes and pipe tobacco, and is also found in instant coffee, instant tea, batteries, some soft drinks, refined grains, fungicides, pesticides and some plastics. Cadmium toxicity may be associated with fatigue, irritability, headaches, high blood pressure, prostate enlargement, emphysema, hair loss, learning disorders, painful joints and lowered immune function.[9]

Many pieces of jewelry have nickel plating and wearing them against the skin causes absorption. Some metal cooking utensils, including stainless steel, are coated with nickel. Cooking acidic foods can sometimes cause the nickel to be absorbed into the food. Cigarette smoke and hydrogenated oils contain nickel. Nickel toxicity may be associated with fatigue, respiratory illnesses, heart conditions, skin rashes, psoriasis, fatigue and headaches.

Mercury can be absorbed into the brain and body over time from mercury-based silver amalgam dental fillings. Small amounts of mercury are also found in some inks, some cosmetics, some hemorrhoidal suppositories, fabric softeners, wood preservatives, solvents, drugs, and some plastics. Accumulations of mercury crosses the blood

brain barrier and causes mental symptoms including memory problems, irritability, irrational behavior and confusion. Physical symptoms include fatigue, insomnia, gastrointestinal disorders, numbness,
tingling, muscle weakness, impaired vision and hearing, allergies and
asthma.[10]

Chelation Nutrients – The Treatment of Choice

Chelation therapy, controversial and condemned by convention
for the treatment of heart and circulation problems, is the conventional therapy of choice in the case of lead or heavy metal poisoning.
Chelation (key-lay-shun) comes from the Greek word chele, meaning to claw or bind. It is accomplished by giving the patient EDTA
(ethylenediaminetetraacetic acid) intravenously. Chelation therapy
is performed on an outpatient basis, is painless, and takes approximately 3-1/2 hours. For optimal results, physicians who use chelation therapy recommend 20-30 treatments given at an average rate of
one to three per week.[11]

In 1948 the U.S. Navy began using EDTA to safely and successfully treat lead poisoning. At the same time, EDTA was being used
to remove calcium from pipes and boilers. EDTA is approved by the
FDA for heavy metal toxicity.[12]

For maximum benefit, EDTA therapy should be accompanied by
a carefully tailored program of vitamin and nutritional supplements.

Chelating Heavy Metals with Nutritional Supplements

Dr. Jonathan Wright treats extreme cases of lead poisoning with
a combination of 30-40 grams of vitamin C intravenously, with calcium, at frequent intervals, and less severe cases with oral doses of
vitamin C, calcium, vitamin D and a vitamin B complex formula.
One of his patients, a three-year-old boy who had been exposed to
lead from the air and soil of a crowded trailer park near a busy free-
way, was given five grams of vitamin C initially with 600 mg of

calcium, 400 IU of vitamin D and a B complex formula that contained at least 25 mg of vitamin B6. The boy's symptoms – dark circles under the eyes, poor appetite, lethargy, sallow appearance – subsided in four to six months.[13]

Electric battery factories are notorious for lead-polluted air. Researchers at the Brain Bio Center in Princeton, New Jersey did a study of 22 factory employees with lead poisoning. They were given 2,000 milligrams of vitamin C and 60 mg of zinc each day, and within 24 weeks, their blood levels of lead plummeted by 26 percent.

Dr. Wright believes that because EDTA is toxic in high doses, it should not be used in minor cases of lead or heavy metal poisoning. Especially in children, he recommends they be treated with high amounts of vitamin C (in the form of ascorbic acid) to bowel tolerance. This means up to the point where diarrhea or gas occurs, then the dosage is reduced to just below that. Vitamin C is non-toxic at high levels because the body excretes any it cannot use. Diarrhea is evidence of that process.

Dr. Wright has personally used ascorbic acid to detoxify cadmium, lead and nickel, as well as drug overdoses. Interestingly, long-term drug addicts include high doses of vitamin C with their drugs. Perhaps they know something we are just learning.

Support any detoxification program with a healthy diet high in natural sources of fiber, emphasizing raw fruits and vegetables, lots of pure spring water and little else. Good sources of supplemental fiber are psyllium, oat bran and hyssop.

Detoxifying Nutrients
For maximum absorption, take supplements with meals.

Nutrient	Suggested Dosage	Formulation
Aged garlic extract	1 teaspoon three times daily	Liquid
Fiber	4-8 tablets daily	Psyllium, with herb hyssop
Melatonin	3 mg at bedtime	
Milk thistle	150 mg twice daily	
Multi-mineral	1-4 ounces daily	In liquid solution, with vitamin B12, biotin
Multi-vitamin/mineral	3-6 caplets daily	Freeze-dried plant sources
Vitamin C	Individual bowel tolerance*	With bioflavonoids (quercetin, rutin proanthocyanidins)
Vitamin E	2 capsules (800 IU) daily	d-alpha tocopherol

* To determine individual dosage, on the first day take 1,000 mg hourly until diarrhea occurs, then reduce dosage to just below that for individual daily dosage. Vitamin C is not toxic in large doses but must be taken throughout the day to benefit. Divide dosage to three or four times a day.

CHAPTER 44:

Chickenpox

I will never forget my childrens' bout with chickenpox. My son and daughter came down with this typically childhood disease at the same time. This was before my knowledge of natural remedies. Desperate for them to go back to school I tried everything in the medicine cabinet and the drug store to quickly heal the pox sores. Remember when we put iodine and mercurochrome on everything? My kids thought the bright orange spots were great fun. I even tried a sunlamp, thinking the heat might dry the sores faster. As it turned out, the virus had its own agenda, and nothing I did hurried it up. We didn't have the advantages of access to health food stores and supplements then, or things would have been different.

Meet Varicella Zoster

Varicella zoster is the virus responsible for chickenpox. The first signs of infection are fever and headache. In general, the younger the child, the easier the illness. When a neighbor bragged that her 18-month-old's bout of chickenpox lasted only three days and encompassed a mere handful of sores, her sister, who had suffered with it as an adult, went to her doctor asking for a referral so she could expose her newborn as soon as possible. Those unfortunate enough to get chickenpox as an adult don't wish that kind of misery on their offspring.

Once your child has been exposed to chickenpox, it can take up to three weeks for you to find out whether he or she has caught the infection. By then you could be on your way to Disneyland, and most airlines won't let you fly with a chickenpox-infested child. Many a vacation has been ruined by this benign but bothersome childhood plague. It's when the rash appears that parents know the time is at hand. Sores appear in crops over two to six days. Each crop goes through stages. The first stage is flat red splotches that become pimples. Then the pimples burst, forming crusts that itch as it heals. If the child itches with dirty hands, a bacterial infection can develop. Scars can occur due to itching but will be worse if an infection develops. Commonly, these rashes spread over the body, even in the mouth and on the scalp. Once all the sores have crusted over, the virus is considered non-contagious and a social life may be resumed again. Typically, a bout of chickenpox runs its course in five to seven days.

An Exception to the Rule: Treating the Symptoms

To date, there is no known cure or prevention for chickenpox. To its credit, conventional medicine has admitted that treatments can be worse than the problem and has traditionally assumed a "let nature take its course" position. A new vaccine recently developed and in general use is still in experimental stages. Researchers have found it does no harm, but still don't know if it doesn't just postpone the inevitable. As reported in *The Lancet*, in U.S. studies about five percent of children, including almost a quarter of those with household exposures, contracted chickenpox despite being immunized. The claim is that the chickenpox wasn't as severe as it could have been.[1] This is highly subjective, and I don't know about you, but I'd rather do without conventional help, thank you. Besides, there are many things that can be done to alleviate symptoms and lessen the severity, without dangerous manmade chemicals.

The itching can be maddening but thankfully remedied. Cooked oatmeal, cooled, moistened and wrapped in a cloth that is held on the irritated areas, will help soothe the itching. For all-over relief, a broth made from boiled oats and barley (one-half cup of each, brought to a boil for 20 minutes in two quarts of water) added to bathwater can soak away the itches. When I have itching skin, I use the inside of a banana peel. It's amazing how well it works. Baking soda in the bath is said to be effective as it neutralizes the skin acids that can cause itching. One-half cup of baking soda added to a tub of cool water is the recipe. Sprinkling a mixture of slippery elm and comfrey root powder on the sores before the scabs have formed can also lessen itching. Pastes of baking soda or cornstarch may be dabbed on eruptions. Gargle with baking soda or salt for mouth sores.

Instead of questionable antihistamines, try vitamin C, which has the same effect. Zinc with copper will help heal the wounds and avoid infection. One herbal remedy particularly good for viral and bacterial infections is aged garlic extract. Buy it in concentrated liquid form. It can be added to juice, or given in a teaspoon of maple syrup. It will speed healing of the wounds and counter any infection that might set in. I use it whenever I come down with a virus to keep it from getting worse.

Shortening Stay-At-Home Time with Nutrients

Certain nutrients have been found in studies to actually reduce the amount of time the virus needs to run its course. Sinasi Ozsoylu, M.D., Department of Pediatrics, Hacettepe Children's Hospital in Ankara, Turkey, performed his own double blind study of chickenpox patients. He gave them high doses of vitamin A during the incubation period one to three days before the rash started and found crusting of all lesions occurred earlier in the group given the A versus the group who had received a placebo. And unlike the placebo group, there were no complications in the vitamin A supplemented subjects. Dr. Ozsoylu recommends that vitamin A be given on the first day of eruption to shorten the crusting period and protect against complications.[2]

Vitamin E, an antioxidant, increases the efficacy of vitamin A and helps prevent scarring.

Internal doses of vitamin A, E, beta carotene, the B vitamins, vitamin C, and zinc all promote immune function and tissue healing.

Avoid salves and ointments. They can keep the skin from "breathing" and cause the scabs to come off prematurely. Lotions, including calamine, are fine, as long as they are not applied around the eyes.

Herbs that can be applied topically to relieve skin irritation and promote healing include calendula, chamomile, comfrey, chickweed, yarrow and plantain. Burdock leaves, which have traditionally been used as a poultice to ease the itching and burning of poison oak, may also help.[3]

I use equal parts of zinc oxide in the tube, topical aloe vera and vitamin E mixed together and slathered on overnight. It's messy but effective.

Once the pox have crusted over, says Dr. Ellen Dale, a Golden, Colorado naturopath, you may apply tea tree oil, which by virtue of its disinfectant properties, helps prevent infection and hence scarring. After the scabs have fallen off, you may use vitamin E.[4]

Garlic, in the form of aged liquid extract, is a wonderful body cleanser. It not only boosts the body's immune system, but will help keep the scarring to a minimum.

Varicella Vanquishing Nutrients for Children
For maximum absorption, take supplements with meals.

Nutrient	Suggested Dosage	Formulation
Aged garlic extract	1 teaspoon twice daily	Liquid
Antioxidants	2 capsules daily	With selenium and grapeseed extract
Echinacea	250 mg daily for a maximum of three weeks	
Lysine	500 mg daily	
Multi-mineral	1/2-1 ounce	In liquid solution, with vitamin B12, biotin
Multi-vitamin/mineral	1-2 tablets	Children's chewable
Vitamin C	Individual bowel tolerance*	Chewable with bioflavonoids (quercetin, proanthocyanidins)

* To determine individual dosage, on the first day take 1,000 mg hourly until diarrhea occurs, then reduce dosage to just below that for individual daily dosage. Vitamin C is not toxic in large doses but must be taken throughout the day to benefit. Divide dosage to three or four times a day.

CHAPTER 45:

Cholesterol

Did you know you have an old Western movie going on inside you? The bad guy, with black hat and black horse, rides the range wreaking havoc on your insides. His name is LDL Cholesterol. He thickens the blood and clogs the arteries, raising your blood pressure and increasing your risk of a heart attack and circulation problems. Fortunately, your town has HDL Cholesterol, the sheriff with the white hat and white horse, who comes to the body's rescue, clearing the arteries. Certain foods will make LDL powerful, while other foods support HDL. Which is which will become clear so you can make good choices in your diet.

Understanding Cholesterol

Pick up any newspaper or magazine these days and you'll probably find some reference to cholesterol. Everyone is concerned with lowering cholesterol, and most want to know how. Cholesterol-lowering drugs have serious side effects, so alternatives are widely-sought. Before you panic because your doctor said you have high blood cholesterol, take the time to understand what this means.

The National Cholesterol Education Program has set the "safe" level of cholesterol for the average adult at 200 mg/dl (milligrams per deciliter). This combines both HDL (high-density lipoproteins) and LDL (low density lipoproteins) levels. A reading above 200 indicates a potential for developing heart disease, a level of 200-239 is borderline, and those over 240 are at high risk. When getting a cholesterol test, make sure and find out what your HDL levels are. The normal HDL level for men in the U.S. is 45-50 and 50-60 for women. It is suggested that higher levels such as 70 or 80 will protect against heart disease. An HDL level under 35 is considered risky.[1]

Dr. Alan Gaby, one of the most knowledgeable physicians I know, believes that conventional medicine's idea of high cholesterol is exaggerated. He says cholesterol-lowering drugs may be more dangerous than the cholesterol problem in the first place. During a seminar at the Alternative Medicine Conference in the Bahamas he presented his findings.

Dr. Gaby counters convention by saying a cholesterol level of 300 is high, 270 is OK, and 250 is borderline, contending many people are giving dangerous cholesterol-lowering drugs unnecessarily. Artificially lowering cholesterol is dangerous because we need cholesterol to manufacture sex hormones, vitamin D, DHEA and cell membranes, he says. He believes cholesterol is needed to protect the body against stress, and that lowering cholesterol artificially affects mental acuity and severely disables the ability to cope with physical and mental stress. Studies have shown a three to 13-fold rise in violent deaths among people taking cholesterol lowering drugs.

Ishwarlal Jailal, M.D., University of Texas Southwestern Medical Center at Dallas, won the American Heart Association's "Young Investigator Award" in 1989 when he discovered that supplemental forms of vitamin A, beta carotene and vitamin C block cholesterol buildup in the arteries of animals. His studies revealed that antioxidant vitamins are amazingly effective in reducing the negative, heart-stopping effects of cholesterol. He found that vitamin E was 45 percent effective, beta carotene was 90 percent effective and vitamin C was 95 percent effective in inhibiting the buildup of cholesterol.[2]

Dr. Gaby recommends adding selenium, vitamin A, zinc and copper to any cholesterol-lowering program.

If cholesterol levels are dangrously high, there is a supplement on the market that will lower cholesterol safely, according to Dr. Gaby. It is called pantethine, a biologically active form of the B vitamin pantothenic acid, and has been used in Italy for the past 13 years. He recommends taking 300 mg two or three times a day, saying it lowers cholesterol by 10-15 percent without side effects, raises HDL by 30 percent, and lowers triglyceride levels.

Cholesterol-Lowering Copper

One of the most satisfying benefits to doing my television program, *Maximize Your Life*, is the wonderfully interesting and enlightened physicians I get to interview. Almost every show gives me the opportunity to learn some cutting-edge piece of research that only a privileged few know about. To increase this privileged group, I am only too happy to pass this information on to you.

One of my guests, Richard Kunin, M.D., an orthomolecular psychiatrist and nutrition physician practicing in San Francisco, has been a medical researcher for 27 years. Dr. Kunin has authored many books revealing the information gleaned from both experience in his practice and findings from his research.

Dr. Kunin found copper to be an answer to the question of high cholesterol. He says that supplementing with copper can lower cholesterol an incredible 800 times more than saturated fat has shown to raise it! And, he says, three out of four Americans are deficient in copper, which means you probably are too. Symptoms of a copper deficiency include heart palpitations, fatigue, depression *and* high cholesterol.

Zinc and copper need to be taken together because one does not work without the other.

Fiber Reasons for Low Cholesterol

Studies have shown that increasing fiber intake can reduce cholesterol levels. Certain kinds of fiber, particularly have been shown to help. Australian researchers found that adult rats fed oat bran lowered cholesterol levels better than wheat bran.[3]

Dennis L. Sprecher, M.D., and colleagues at the Lipid Research Center in Bethesda, Maryland, discovered that the addition of psyllium lowered LDL cholesterol by an incredible 39 percent. They concluded that psyllium, when added to a low-fat diet, works so well it can eliminate the need for cholesterol-lowering drugs.[4]

Beans, peas and lentils contain fiber that helps the colon and lowers blood cholesterol. A cup of pinto or navy beans eaten every day was found to lower cholesterol by 19 percent in subjects tested by Dr. James Anderson, a fiber expert at the University of Kentucky. They also favorably effected the ratio of HDL to LDL cholesterol. The fiber in beans is fermented in the colon into short chain fatty acids, which are re-absorbed by the body. These acids may help keep the body from making cholesterol. Carbohydrates in the beans are fermented by anaerobic bacteria in the intestines to form hydrogen, carbon dioxide and methane gases, some of which have to be passed from the system. To remove some of the troublesome carbohydrates, soak dry beans in water for three to five hours and discard this water before cooking. To retain all the nutrients, use this water but be prepared for the side effects.

Yams or sweet potatoes contain much water soluble fiber, as well as beta carotene, a potent antioxidant which prevents the fats in your body from eating away your insides. Consumed four or five times weekly, yams will contribute to a program of cholesterol control. Japanese researchers rated the fiber in sweet potatoes as best of 28 fruit and vegetable fibers for binding with cholesterol and removing it.

Cholesterol-Friendly Food

It isn't coincidence that vegetarians typically have lower blood cholesterol than their meat-eating counterparts. If you don't depend on meat for your entrees, you'll be amazed at the variety of health-giving food from which you can choose. From A to Z, cholesterol-lowering foods are: apples, almonds, avocados, bananas, barley, beans, chili peppers, eggplant, garlic, fruit pectin, oat bran, olive oil, onions, kelp, lentils, peas, green plantains, soybeans, spinach, sweet potatoes, walnuts, yams, and yogurt with active cultures.

Soybeans and the products derived from them, such as soy milk, lecithin and tofu, help break down fatty deposits so they can be flushed from the body more readily. This process also lowers cholesterol. Soybean products seem to work best on patients with extra-high cholesterol – 300 or more. Slightly more than an ounce daily of lecithin– a food substance derived from soybeans – has been shown to reduce blood levels of cholesterol by 18 percent. Researchers at the University of Milan, Italy saw cholesterol levels in their subjects plummet by 15 to 20 percent, simply by having them eat soybeans used in various recipes in place of meat and milk products. Many meat meals can be reproduced by substituting soybean products.

Yogurt is a real winner in lowering cholesterol. Three cups a day have caused cholesterol levels to decline by as much as five to ten percent a week, with the proportion of good guy HDL rising in proportion to LDL. Beware of yogurt substitutes, however. Read the label. Many so-called yogurts are simply milk, corn sweeteners, food starch and gelatin, among other unnatural or unhealthy ingredients. Look for yogurt with active cultures. Plain yogurt is your best bet. Use your blender to make a smoothie with it using fresh fruit.

In one study, three medium-sized raw carrots eaten daily was shown to reduce cholesterol by almost eleven percent. That must be how Bugs Bunny does it.

Chili peppers reduce the blood serum cholesterol level by suppressing the liver's ability to produce cholesterol. When researchers in Bangkok, Thailand, added freshly ground jalapeno pepper to rice flour noodles, subjects who ate the noodles daily experienced lowered cholesterol and an increased ability to dissolve blood clots.

Garlic doesn't work hanging on the wall or around your neck, you have to eat it. A ration of five fresh raw cloves minced into other foods daily for 25 days has been shown to lower blood serum cholesterol by nearly 10 percent. Dr. M. Secur fed this amount of garlic to

200 patients with super high blood serum levels. In almost every patient, cholesterol levels dropped to desired levels, after which Dr. Secur kept it stable with only two cloves of raw garlic daily.

Scientists at Loma Linda University in California fed four capsules of Kyolic® aged garlic extract daily to patients with high cholesterol. Six months later these individuals had achieved an average cholesterol reduction of 44 points.

During the First World Congress on the Health Significance of Garlic and Garlic Constituents in Washington, D.C., August 28-30, 1990, researchers presented many papers that showed Kyolic® aged garlic extract works better than raw garlic as a cholesterol-lowering agent.

Some studies have found that the antioxidants in wine lower cholesterol. Grape juice works just as well. Grape juice contains resveratrol, a naturally-occurring chemical in wine that lowers blood cholesterol, announced Leroy L. Creasy of Cornell University. The bioflavonoid is found in the skin of the purple grape.[5] It doesn't surprise me that yet another bioflavonoid helps to lower cholesterol. Bioflavonoids are the bullet in the gun of vitamin C. They enhance vitamin C's benefit to the body and are themselves potent health boosters. When supplementing with vitamin C, always include bioflavonoids.

Be Fat Smart

An important issue in cholesterol is fat. Too much of the wrong kind of fat can increase cholesterol levels, but did you realize there is good fat that will lower cholesterol?

Before I continue, let me give you a quick fat lesson. The bad fats are saturated, derived from animals. The good fats go by a variety of names and can be confusing. You hear a great deal about PUFAs, or polyunsaturated fatty acids. PUFAs are a generic term for all the essential fatty acids (EFAs). We say "essential" because they cannot be made by the body and must be eaten in the diet. They are required for growth, development and maintenance of cell membranes, including those of the central nervous system. A deficiency of EFAs has been linked to heart disease.

Some of the foods found to lower cholesterol are high in essential fatty acids. These are fish, unroasted nuts and seeds, and the oils from them. Notorious cholesterol lowerers are nuts, olive oil and fish oils. The best supplemental sources of essential fatty acids are cod liver oil and borage oil. Borage oil contains linolenic acid, deemed deficient in most of us.

Researchers at the YMCA Cardiac Rehabilitation Unit in Palo Alto, California, studied 30 men and women who went on a nine-week low-saturated-fat, high essential fatty acid diet, eating almost four ounces a day of almonds, which are high in monounsaturated fat – an EFA. At the end of the nine weeks, the investigators reported that the average total cholesterol level of 235 was reduced by about 20 points.[6] In France, researchers have associated walnut consumption with lower cholesterol levels. Walnuts also contain EFAs.

Health authorities including the American Heart Association and the National Research Council agree that monounsaturated fats, found in highest concentrations in olive oil and canola oil, may offer some benefit, particularly when they replace saturated fat in the diet.

An Australian study found that while both fish and fish oil extracts lower cholesterol, eating fish is more effective. The study, done by the Department of Medicine, University of Western Australia in Perth, found people who ate fish every day for 12 weeks showed a 20 percent reduction in total cholesterol while those who took fish oil supplements showed a 14 percent reduction. The theory is that something is removed during the purification process of the fish oil that reduces cholesterol.[7]

People living in the Mediterranean – Greece, Italy and Israel, for example – have been studied at length due to their low rates of heart disease and high blood pressure. In an Israeli study of men in their early twenties, it was found that enrichment of their diet with almonds, avocados and olive oil reduced their LDL cholesterol by 12 percent.[8] Each of these foods are high in EFAs.

Say No to Margarine

Now that you know what is good for you, pay attention to what is bad for you. Margarine is NOT heart smart. You already know saturated fat is bad for you. Saturated fat, like butter, may increase bad cholesterol, but at least it doesn't touch the good cholesterol. Food processors hydrogenate oils to make them thicker, creamier, and more appetizing to the consumer. Unfortunately, this process also saturates the oils' fatty acids, changing them to trans fatty acids. A study conducted in the Netherlands and published in the *New England Journal of Medicine* compared groups of people with diets high in trans fatty acids, or trans fats, with essential fatty acids and saturated fat. The researchers found that the diet high in essential fatty acids had a beneficial effect on blood cholesterol. The diet high in saturated fat raised the level of bad guy LDL cholesterol. But only the diet high in trans fatty acids both increased bad cholesterol and decreased good-guy HDL cholesterol – a double whammy that has been noted by researchers.

A small amount of trans fats comes from dairy products and beef but the major dietary source is margarine, particularly the hard margarines and shortenings made by hydrogenated plant oils.

Dutch researchers found that eating 33 grams of trans fats every day for three weeks raised serum cholesterol. The U.S. Department of Agriculture did a study for the Institute of Shortening and Edible Oils, and agreed with the Dutch findings.[9] I would love to tell you how much margarine it would take to eat 33 grams of trans fats but, unlike in Canada and other enlightened countries, the U.S. government doesn't require food labels to describe the amount of trans fats contained in its products.

> The Harvard School of Public Health now proclaims that partially hydrogenated vegetable oil, found in margarine and shortening, may be attributed to approximately 30,000 deaths each year.[10]

"These are probably the most toxic fats ever known," said Walter Willett, M.D., professor of epidemiology and nutrition at Harvard School of Public Health. Willett, who has researched the effects of trans fats on the body, disagrees with those who say that the partially hydrogenated fats found in margarine or shortening are less likely to raise cholesterol than the saturated fats found in butter. He proclaimed, "It looks like trans fatty acids are two to three times as bad as saturated fats in terms of what they do to blood lipids."[11]

George V. Mann, Sc.D., M.D., a leading heart researcher, wrote in *The Lancet*: "Trans fatty acids are proposed as the cause of the current epidemic of heart disease. Studies have shown that dietary intake of saturated fats and cholesterol are not the cause of the build-up of fatty deposits within blood vessels. Much suggestive evidence exists that consumption of comparatively large amounts of trans fatty acids causes the problem by impairing fat metabolism. Populations with low consumption of trans-fatty acids have a lower incidence of coronary artery disease even when consuming diets high in animal fat or other oils."[12]

Cholesterol Crunching Nutrients
For maximum absorption, take supplements with meals.

Nutrient	Suggested Dosage	Formulation
Aged garlic extract	1 teaspoon three times daily	Liquid
Antioxidants	4 capsules daily*	With selenium and grapeseed extract
Borage oil	2 capsules daily	
Coenzyme Q10	2 capsules daily	With vitamin E, phospholipids and selenium
Flaxseed oil	1 tablespoon daily	
Gugulipids	250 mg three times daily	
Lecithin	2 tablespoons daily	
Magnesium	200 mg daily	
Multi-mineral	3-4 ounces daily	In liquid solution, with vitamin B12, biotin
Multi-vitamin/mineral	6 caplets daily	Freeze-dried plant sources
Niacin	500 mg four times daily	
Vitamin C	Individual bowel tolerance**	With bioflavonoids (quercetin, proanthocyanidins)

* The FDA recommends pregnant women not exceed 10,000 IU of vitamin A daily.

** To determine individual dosage, on the first day take 1,000 mg hourly until diarrhea occurs, then reduce dosage to just below that for individual daily dosage. Vitamin C is not toxic in large doses but must be taken throughout the day to benefit. Divide dosage to three or four times a day.

CHAPTER 46:

Chronic Fatigue Syndrome

"Disease is the retribution of outraged Nature."
                                        –Hosea Ballou

Chronic fatigue syndrome (CFS) is one of those obscure medical problems upon which researchers and physicians seem unable to agree. Some say it is caused by a virus, others say it is allergy-related or a symptom of depression, and others, not knowing what to think or say, suggest it is all in the head. One thing is for sure, it severely debilitates its victims.

A Rose By Any Other Name

Sometimes, as medical knowledge progresses, the understanding of a series of symptoms changes. Infectious mononucleosis, termed the "kissing disease," was the first illness recognized as causing chronic fatigue. The symptoms were flu-like: low-grade fever, muscular aches and pains, headache and fatigue. The most discouraging part of the illness was that even if the person felt better for a while, the symptoms returned. It was not unusual to have recurring episodes of the illness for two to three years.

In the mid 1980s as the AIDS epidemic spurred extensive research into viruses, more became known about the mononucleosis syndrome. Mononucleosis became Chronic Epstein-Barr Virus (CEBV). A March 1988 report by a Centers for Disease Control

(CDC) working group renamed it Chronic Fatigue Syndrome. The CDC group also outlined strict criteria for its diagnosis. To meet their definition, a patient must have debilitating fatigue for more than six months and must exhibit at least eight of eleven symptoms, including sore throat, mild fever and muscle aches.

Why some experience chronic fatigue and others do not, seems to be related to their immune systems. It has been common experience that chronic fatigue syndrome occurs during times when the immune system is debilitated by other illnesses, whether diagnosed or not.

Immune System Breakdown

The reason nobody can fully explain how people get chronic fatigue syndrome is because so many things cause chronic fatigue. Many, many situations, deficiencies and illnesses wear down and impair the immune system. The symptoms of chronic fatigue syndrome are the signals of a poorly functioning immune system. That is why, if none of the suggestions I make here work, your best bet is to consult a nutritionally-oriented physician or alternative medicine physician for the proper tests to determine what exactly is causing your immune system to break down, and get on a personal program to fill in your nutritional blanks.

Melvyn R. Werbach, M.D., saw a number of CFS sufferers before shifting his practice to psychiatry and research exclusively. He believes one of the underlying causes of CFS is depression. He says the influence of a depressed mind over the body can make people more susceptible to viruses by affecting the immune system, triggering other symptoms.

A report in the *New England Journal of Medicine* quotes Dr. Stephen E. Straus of the National Institute of Allergy and Infectious Diseases in Bethesda, Maryland. Dr. Straus says that chronic fatigue may represent an abnormal response to infection. Scientists think some patients never completely recover from the flu, but instead develop long-standing symptoms of chronic fatigue.

A study of 15 teenagers ages 13 to 17 diagnosed as having CFS, found 11 reported their symptoms as following an acute illness, according to doctors from the University of Washington School of Medicine and Children's Hospital and Medical Center in Seattle, Washington. Seven had positive tests for mononucleosis. A third of the teenagers, all of whom were female, also were found to be clinically depressed.

Infections that lower the immune system, like candidiasis, parasites, bacterial infections and chronic intestinal problems can cause CFS, according to Murray R. Susser, M.D., of Santa Monica, California. By treating these infections and boosting the patient's nutritional intake with a good diet and proper supplementation, Dr. Susser reduces the burden on the immune system.[1]

One of the first documented symptoms of CFS occured following an epidemic of polio in 1934. In that year polio was sweeping through Los Angeles, and in the medical wards of Los Angeles County General Hospital nurses and doctors fell ill with a mysterious ailment no one could explain.

They were so fatigued they couldn't work; some could not even walk three blocks. They were confused and their muscles ached. Some physicians diagnosed them as having an odd strain of the polio virus. Others dismissed their illness as "epidemic hysteria." That strange outbreak 57 years ago is now thought by many researchers to have been chronic fatigue syndrome.

The connection between the decline of the immune system and chronic fatigue has lead to yet another phrase to describe CFS: chronic fatigue immune dysfunction syndrome (CFIDS). Elaine DeFreitas and her co-workers at the Wistar Institute in Philadelphia used three types of tests with 30 people suffering from CFIDS and found that the majority of the volunteers showed some sign of infection by human T-lymphotropic virus type II, a suspect in a rare form of leukemia. A separate group of 20 healthy individuals showed no sign of the virus, the team reported.

Food Allergies

Reknowned food allergists, such as Dr. James C. Breneman, author of *Basics of Food Allergy*, recognize a food allergy disorder called Tension Fatigue Syndrome. Symptoms include irritability, sleeplessness, lack of enthusiasm and pleasure, and pale skin with dark circles under the eyes. Milk and chocolate have been found to be the culprits of this malady, especially among children.[2]

How many times have your heard people say, "It must be Monday," when describing their tiredness following a weekend? This "dumb Monday" concept was first fostered by Walter Alvarez, M.D., when relating to his personal experience with a food allergy. He suffered from chronic fatigue for years as a child, teenager and young adult. It was not until he finished medical school that he began to understand his food allergy to chicken. His reactions would appear as a result of a family chicken dinner every Sunday. Sure enough, he developed a headache and fatigue every Monday.

A clinical test found that 75 percent of a group of 50 patients with tension fatigue syndrome were found to have other allergy symptoms. Over half the patients treated by an elimination diet to remove the offensive food allergens had superior to excellent results, while an additional16 patients had a good response.

For more on this possible source, see the chapter on Allergies. In the meantime, consider the top food allergens identified by specialists: milk, chocolate, sugar, wheat, corn, eggs, tomatoes, nuts, pork, beef, beans, citrus and potatoes.

The body's reaction to a food allergy can be severe and long-term. In a study reported in the *European Journal of Pediatrics*, researchers tested infants from parents with a family history of milk allergy. After one dose of cow's milk, the results were devastating, as shown by "before" and "after" biopsies of their stomach linings.

The important thing to remember about food allergies is that over the course of years, they can cause digestive problems that can lead to malnutrition that lead to deficiencies, that lead to poor immune system function. This domino effect can eventually result in chronic fatigue syndrome that takes extensive nutritional therapy to remedy.

The Malabsorption Connection

When Dr. Jonathan Wright treats his CFS patients, he first gives them shots of vitamin B12. If the patient notices a difference, he considers it a strong indication that there is a lack of hydrochloric or stomach acid. Without adequate stomach acid, proteins are not digested, and essential amino acids, nutrients and minerals such as iron and B12 are not absorbed. Without nutrients, the body literally starves. Chronic fatigue is just the first symptom of severe malnutrition.

A lack of stomach acid is more common than we think and can cause all of the symptoms that appear when the stomach contains too much acid. People should not take antacids too readily as heartburn, gas, bloating after eating and even constipation can all be symptoms of too little stomach acid. The burning sensation common to too much acid is also present when the stomach is overly alkaline, and can be made worse by antacids. Dr. Wright estimates that every third adult he sees in his Kent, Washington clinic secretes too little hydrochloric acid.

Researchers at the Mayo Clinic and Johns Hopkins University pumped the stomachs of over 3,000 individuals and analyzed their contents. It was determined that by the age of 60 years, 60 percent had a significant decline in hydrochloric acid. Supplementing with a hydrochloric acid formula such as Betaine and other digestive enzymes available in vitamin stores will help absorb nutrients, but studies show minerals in solution are considerably more bioavailable to the body than those even present in food. When in solution, they don't need stomach acid to break them down, and aren't influenced by food allergies. Look for a good, easily absorbable, derived-from-nature mineral blend.

Food allergies are not the only things that can attack the stomach lining, leading to diminished gastric acid. Viruses such as measles, mumps and chicken pox – common childhood diseases – can destroy the stomach lining, which may or may not return to normal. Antibiotics are designed to kill bacteria – the good and the bad. Always when taking antibiotics, supplement with a "lactobacillus acidophilus chaser." It won't interfere with the antibiotics and will keep your internal body chemistry at peak performance. Acidophilus can be purchased in pill or powder form in health food stores or in yogurt with active cultures.

Nutritional Support

A condition sometimes found among CFS patients is an adrenal gland insufficiency. The adrenal gland makes hormones. When illness or stress compromises the body, the adrenal gland has to work harder, but if it is compromised, just when it is needed the most, it isn't there. Dr. Jonathan Wright believes for quickest recovery from CFS, supplementing with DHEA (dehydroepiandrosterone) is helpful.[3] DHEA is a natural hormone, and has been found to boost T-helper lymphocytes and their fight against infections. In a study reported by James L. McCoy, Ph.D., of Baton Rouge, Louisiana, researchers tested blood samples from 88 people who met CDC's criteria for chronic fatigue syndrome. Seventy-two percent of them were determined to have an immune system dysfunction. When given a specially determined optimum dose of DHEA, 60 percent showed clinical improvement of their symptoms.[4]

Among those who have been diagnosed as having CFS, researchers also have found abnormally low levels of magnesium in their red blood cells. According to a study reported in *The Lancet*, 32 patients with CFS received 15 magnesium sulphate injections into the muscles each week for six weeks, while the remaining 17 took a placebo (fake pill). Twelve of the 15 people in the treated group said they had improved levels of energy, a better emotional state and less pain, while only three of the 17 said they felt better.[5]

Symptoms of a magnesium deficiency include muscle cramping, severe fatigue and headaches. Sound familiar? More than likely, the magnesium deficiency associated with CFS is a result of the above-described malabsorption since stomach problems can prevent magnesium from being absorbed.

Massive doses of vitamin C is beneficial in the treatment of any immune-debilitating illness like chronic fatigue syndrome. Dr. Robert Cathcart advocates doses as high as the patient will tolerate, up to bowel tolerance. This means to the point where diarrhea or gas occurs, then the dosage is reduced to just below that level. Vitamin C is non-toxic at high levels because the body excretes any it cannot use. It speeds through the body, destroying bad guys until it ends up in the bowel, where it isn't needed. Diarrhea is not an illness, it is the body's way of getting rid of something it cannot use.

Vitamin C is also helpful for all the problems that have been shown to lead to CFS, such as candida, chemical sensitivities, lupus, fibromyalgia, parasites and herpes, just to name a few.

Any nutritional support should be geared toward support of the immune system. This means basic, high-quality multivitamin and multimineral formulations. Always take your mineral formula separate from your vitamin formula. Some minerals block absorption of certain vitamins. Other nutrients specifically recommended for fatigue busting are described below.

Immune-Energizing Nutrients
For maximum absorption, take nutrients with meals.

Nutrient	Suggested Dosage	Formulation
Acidophilus	At least four billion flora daily on an empty stomach, three times daily	
Aged garlic extract	1 teaspoon three times daily	Liquid
Amino acids	4-6 capsules daily	Multiple formula from natural sources
Antioxidants	4 capsules daily*	With selenium and grapeseed extract
Borage oil	2 capsules daily	
Coenzyme Q10	2 capsules daily	With vitamin E, phospholipids and selenium
Flaxseed oil	1 tablespoon daily	
L-Glutamine	500 mg three times daily	
Melatonin (adults only)	3 mg daily at bedtime	With B vitamins
Multi-mineral	3-4 ounces daily	In liquid solution, with vitamin B12, biotin
Multi-vitamin/mineral	6 caplets daily	Freeze-dried plant sources
Vitamin C	Individual bowel tolerance**	With bioflavonoids (quercetin, proanthocyanidins)
Vitamin E	2 capsules (800 IU)	d-alpha tocopherol

* The FDA recommends pregnant women not exceed 10,000 IU of vitamin A daily.

** To determine individual dosage, on the first day take 1,000 mg hourly until diarrhea occurs, then reduce dosage to just below that for individual daily dosage. Vitamin C is not toxic in large doses but must be taken throughout the day to benefit. Divide dosage to three or four times a day.

CHAPTER 47:

Chronic Pain

"Pain adds rest unto pleasure, and teaches the luxury of health."

—Martin F. Tupper

My good friend Marge wins friends with one handshake. Enthusiasm sparkles in her soft brown eyes, and her genuine interest in people is clear in her voice. But under all her spontaneous sincerity, she is hiding a private war.

For the past seven years Marge has had sporadic bouts with a nerve inflammation disorder called peripheral sensory neuropathy. Defined, it is an unexplained burning sensation affecting the outer extremities of the body. In Marge's case, she has random episodes where her hands feel like they are on fire. Since there is no explanation for the flare-ups, there are no clues as to how to treat the condition. And when doctors have no clues, they have no cures.

Marge is one of some 60 million Americans suffering from chronic pain – pain that persists for six months or more, even though the original injury has healed. It is a pain that won't go away. Instead it takes root, waking with you in the morning, turning back the sheets with you at night, lurking like a prowler in your body.

Experts are slowly piecing together the chronic-pain puzzle, but they still aren't sure why certain pain becomes chronic. In the meantime, pain costs about $100 billion a year in lost wages and medical expenses, according to John L. Reeves, president of the American Pain Society.[1]

Fight Pain with Emotion

Chronic pain, whatever the cause, is a problem for a large number of people. The Centre for Epidemiologic Studies indicates that 14.4 percent of the United States population between the ages of 25-74 suffer from definite chronic pain related to the joints and musculoskeletal system, the most common source. Another 7.4 percent endure chronic pain from an unknown source, unsure of how long it will last. That is almost 22 percent of the population wincing in pain every day. Interestingly enough, the Centre found 18 percent of chronic pain sufferers also have depression.[2] Which came first, the pain or the depression, is hard to tell. It is true that stress lowers the immune system, which can bring on problems of chronic pain, but at the same time, I can't think of anything more depressing than coping with this suffering.

Apparently emotions do have an effect on pain. A study reported in the *Journal of Behavioral Medicine* said that out of 142 people suffering chronic pain, the strongest predictor of who hurt the worst was the degree to which they held in their anger.[3] In other words, vent and ye shall be free! The Bible says, "pulling out every root of bitterness." Does this mean that the angry young man at my dry cleaners never feels pain? Not when I pay the bill!

The author of the study, Robert D. Kerns, Ph.D., associate professor of psychiatry, neurology and psychology at Yale University explains it like this: "Unexpressed negative emotions may actually suppress the immune and endocrine systems. These systems are believed to play a role in dimming the experience of pain. Without them functioning at full force, pain tolerance may be reduced." This might explain the depression connection, since when you are depressed, you aren't exactly fighting back.

Learning that it's OK to relax is essential to getting back in touch with the body's innate pain relievers. These misery reducers, called endorphins, are stimulated by deep breathing, fresh air, hormones, certain nutrients, exercise, and positive thinking – things that chronic pain sufferers have long since given up. Perhaps a class in Lamaze? This technique teaches women how to handle the pain of childbirth through natural, innate coping mechanisms like breathing exercises, positive mental imagery and body positioning. I wish I had Lamaze when I was expecting!

When I'm in pain or depressed, I tell myself over and over again to smile, even if I have to clench a pencil between my teeth. I cite a phrase from Psalms over and over again: "Thank you Lord for restoring my soul. Soon the subconscious catches up and says, "Hey, we better catch up, she's not depressed," and Voila! I'm no longer depressed!

Dual Role of B Vitamins

I found the following research very interesting because I know good mental health is dependent on B vitamins. In fact, if you read the chapters on Depression and Stress and follow their recommendations, it will probably help your chronic pain. Anything that causes depression probably contributes to chronic pain, based on what we now know.

In studying the pain of fibromyalgia patients, Dr. Jean-Bernard Eisinger, Chief of Medicine at Hopital G. Clemenceau, La Garde, France, found a study group taking B complex vitamins, including 750 milligrams per day of thiamine hydrochloride in divided doses, experienced less pain following orthopedic surgery. Fibromyalgia patients are found to have trouble absorbing thiamine – vitamin B1. Japanese researchers report therapeutic benefits to so-called neuralgia, a technical term for nerve pain, using thiamine. It is worth noting here that thiamine dependent enzymes also require an adequate supply of magnesium.[4]

I know of a study in which it was proven aspirin didn't work unless accompanied by magnesium.

Thiamine is found in the germ and bran of wheat, the husk of rice, and that portion of all grains which is commercially milled away to give the grain its lighter color and finer texture. A diet rich in brewer's yeast, wheat germ, blackstrap molasses and bran will provide the body with adequate thiamine. Eating sugar will cause a thiamine depletion, as will smoking and drinking alcohol. Thiamine can be destroyed by cooking and by an enzyme present in raw clams, oysters and raw fish.[5]

Magnesium Minimizes Pain

Magnesium is very important to the muscles, a source of pain for many, and a remarkable pain reliever, thanks to its ability to move calcium out of joints and muscles. Dr. Hans Seyle, author of the book *Stress Without Distress*, and a Nobel prize winning biologist, found in rat experiments that in stressful situations, calcium is drawn from the bones and deposited in the tissues, contributing to arthritis and circulation blockages.

It also helps promote absorption of calcium, phosphorous, potassium, the B vitamins, and vitamins C and E, all of which, when deficient, can cause painful circulation, bone and muscle problems. A deficiency of magnesium can cause muscle cramps, depression and blood clots.

Don't miss vitamin B12. Vitamin B12 helps break up calcium deposits in bursitis patients, and alleviate so-called neuralgia, a technical term for nerve pain. I. S. Klemes, M.D., injected study patients with a daily dose of one centimeter of the vitamin for seven to 10 days, followed by the same injection three times weekly for the next two to three weeks, then one or two weekly for two to three weeks, depending upon the patient's progress. Relief came quickly as calcium deposits were absorbed.[6]

Gary Zaloga, M.D., reports that magnesium has been used to inhibit pain from spinal cord injuries[7] and James Braly, M.D., recommends magnesium in a program of nutritional pain supplementation.[8]

Both magnesium and B12 are nutrients that must be taken with other B vitamins and minerals. Because of potential absorption problems, it's best to take minerals in solution.

The following nutritional supplements can be taken daily when in pain: vitamin C to 90 percent of bowel tolerance; evening primrose oil (borage oil is better and cheaper) for essential fatty acids; vitamin E, magnesium; and the amino acid DL-phenylalanine.[9] Bowel tolerance is the point where diarrhea or gas occurs, then the dosage is reduced to just below that. Vitamin C is non-toxic at high levels because the body excretes any it cannot use. It speeds through the body, destroying "bad guys" until it ends up in the bowel, where it isn't needed, and is excreted.

Vitamin C is especially helpful in preventing the pain that occurs after surgery or injury. This is important because of the connection between chronic pain and past injury. I believe that if everyone who had an injury or surgery supplemented with vitamin C after, it would go a long way in preventing the chronic pain that can occur later.

Help from Amino Acids

The amino acid DL-phenylalanine (DLPA) is also helpful for pain relief. It has been proven effective in increasing blood levels of endorphins and reducing inflammation in about 80 percent of patients suffering from chronic pain, according to Dr. Braly. An article in *Advances in Pain Research and Therapeutics* says many chronic pain patients have obtained relief using 1,500-2,500 mg/day of DLPA.[10]

DLPA is a new discovery which strengthens and protects the body's natural pain killers – endorphins. It's a mixture of two forms of the amino acid phenylalanine and is said to be as powerful as morphine, while at the same time is non-addictive and has no side effects. It also seems to help in cases of depression.

Dr. Arnold Fox, former assistant clinical professor of medicine at the University of California, Irvine, and author of the book *DLPA to End Chronic Pain and Depression*, suggests people take 375 to 400 mg of DLPA with each meal. It's available in most health food stores and even some drugstores.

Daniel Asimus, medical director of the Persistent Pain Program at Glendale Adventist Medical Center in California, has treated more than 100 patients with DLPA and has found it to be quite helpful for the treatment of chronic pain.

Needling Pain

Have you ever had the experience of itching one part of the body, and at the same time have another part of the body respond? You might be itching your arm, and at the same time feel it in a spot on your back. What you may be feeling are electromagnetic energy meridians. Just as brain surgeons have mapped the brain and which parts of it affects the body, acupuncturists have mapped the skin and which parts of it affect particular parts of the body.

Successfully used in the Far East for thousands of years, acupuncture is relatively new to Americans. It is used to treat many ailments including chronic back, neck and facial pain, migraine headaches, arthritis and nerve diseases. Small, thin needles are placed in special points of the body, under sterile conditions, to stimulate or relax the body and relieve pain. Techniques vary. Japanese acupuncturists for instance, use smaller, much finer needles. To alleviate the shock of piercing the body, the needle is loaded in a tube that presses against the skin and prepares it for the needle.

The placement and number of needles required to treat a specific condition depends on the nature and location of the pain. According to acupuncturist Michael M. Javedan, M.S., C.A., O.M.D., Carmichael, California, relief may occur immediately or as late as the third or fourth session of treatment. Acupuncture treatments are typically administered over six sessions. If pain is alleviated but later returns, patients are advised to undergo further treatment.

Some studies show an acupuncture needle, when inserted, stimulates the body to produce endorphins, naturally occurring chemicals that act as opiates and pain suppressors. Other studies indicate that the inserted needles also increase blood "microcirculation" to tissues, nerves and muscles.

Acupuncture heals the body by increasing or unblocking circulation, bringing blood and nutrients to even the smallest and thinnest blood vessels in damaged tissue. Acupuncture also relaxes muscles. The mechanism of this relaxation is not precisely understood, but medical scientists are researching acupuncture to further understand the reasons behind those biochemical changes.

The fact that acupuncture works does not surprise me. Researchers have established that the skin, the body's largest organ, has its own immune system. In other words, it has the ability to detect from the outside when healing needs to occur on the inside. It is quite possible that acupuncture is simply utilizing the skin's ability to heal.

Pain Relieving Nutrients
For maximum absorption, take supplements with meals.

Nutrient	Suggested Dosage	Formulation
Amino acids	4-6 capsules daily	Multiple formula from natural sources
Borage oil	2 capsules daily	
DL-phenylalanine (DLPA)	1,500-2,500 mg daily	
Flaxseed oil	1 tablespoon daily	
Glucosamine sulfate	500 mg three times daily	
Magnesium	200 mg daily	
MSM (Methylsulfonylmethane)	500 mg three times daily	
Melatonin (adults only)	3 mg daily at bedtime	With B vitamins
Multi-mineral	3-4 ounces daily	In liquid solution, with vitamin B12, biotin
Multi-vitamin/mineral	6 caplets daily	Freeze-dried plant sources
Vitamin C	Individual bowel tolerance*	With bioflavonoids (quercetin, proanthocyanidins)
Yucca	300 mg three times daily	

* To determine individual dosage, on the first day take 1,000 mg hourly until diarrhea occurs, then reduce dosage to just below that for individual daily dosage. Vitamin C is not toxic in large doses but must be taken throughout the day to benefit. Divide dosage to three or four times a day.

CHAPTER 48:

Circulation Problems

What do intermittent claudication and Raynaud's phenomenon have in common? In each, blood flow in the veins and arteries become restricted, jeopardizing the arms or legs. The late Ella Fitzgerald lost her legs to blocked circulation brought on by her diabetes. In 1993, the year she turned 75, Fitzgerald had both legs amputated. When her legs completely lost their circulation, they became gangrenous and had to be cut off. I believe Ms. Fitzgerald's legs could have been saved if she had taken early steps to not only nutritionally correct her diabetes, but use alternative treatments for the resultant vascular disease. What is very important in the case of any circulation problem is that early warning signs are not ignored. They include muscle cramping, tingling in legs or arms, numbness, and pain when walking. Don't wait until you can't walk 200 feet without stopping in excruciating pain – do something about it now! And I'm here to tell you much can be done!

Magnificent Magnesium

Magnesium is the heart smart mineral because it works so well to not only protect the veins and arteries from becoming blocked, but can be used to "flush" them clean. British physician S.E. Browne writes in the *Journal of Nutritional Medicine* that he has used shots of magnesium sulfate for over 35 years to successfully treat gangrene, leg ulcers, Raynaud's disease and intermittent claudication, adding that it has been used in cases of cardiovascular disease for the last 60 years.[1] This is not new to the medical world, only to you and me. Now I'm letting the secret out.

What's interesting about Raynaud's is how conventional medicine regards it. You hear it referred to as a syndrome: a collection of symptoms, or a phenomenon: just a couple of relatively harmless symptoms, easily dealt with, or a disease. If they call it a disease, you know they are taking it seriously, which they should. People die from Raynaud's, but when the symptoms are described, it's hard to take it seriously. They are described as "cold hands," "color changes occurring bilaterally in the hands evoked by cold and emotions," and "extremities become cold and turn blue." The point I want to make here is that conventional medicine doesn't evaluate what causes these circulation symptoms, choosing to simply treat the symptoms with warmth or drugs. When the restricted arteries don't pop open again and let the blood flow properly, doctors call this secondary Raynaud's. Constricted long enough, the fingers, toes, ears or nose will become gangrenous. Something has to be done long before this happens.

Two Swedish researchers studied the effect of short term intravenous magnesium sulfate in treating Raynaud's. Jerzy Leppert, M.D., Ph.D., Department of Research, IAMU University of Uppsala Central Hospital, in Vasteras, Sweden, reported that magnesium is beneficial for the treatment of primary Raynaud's phenomenon.[2]

Urban Myrdal also of Uppsala Central Hospital, Vasteras, Sweden, conducted his own tests, instead evaluating magnesium's ability to increase circulating levels of calcitonin gene-related peptide. Calcitonin gene-related peptide (CGRP) is a potent vasodilator (opens veins and arteries) that may be involved in regulating the peripheral circulatory system, that which governs the hands and feet and their response to cold. There is evidence that CGRP is deficient in people with Raynaud's phenomenon.[3] Myrdal backed up Leppert's finding by discovering intravenous infusions of magnesium sulfate significantly increased these peptides among women with pronounced primary Raynaud's phenomenon.[4] Researchers reported in *The Lancet* that direct intravenous doses of CGRP has been found to relieve severe cases of Raynaud's.[5]

Sometimes, when looking at research, I look at word connections to help me overcome the barriers of medical jargon. When you do your own investigating and find yourself knee-deep in long-winded medical journals, create your own medical dictionary. For example, when the entertainment articles described Ella Fitzgerald's problem, they attributed it to her diabetes. She had her legs cut off due to diabetes. But when the medical journals describe it they call it diabetic peripheral vascular disease. Now, I'm looking at a piece of research describing Raynaud's as a "severe peripheral vascular insufficiency." The key words here?: peripheral vascular. When you see this, you know they are talking about the capillaries, veins and arteries that circulate blood through the extremities: the legs, hands, ears and nose. Now, I don't know about you, but it sounds like Ella Fitzgerald's problem, no matter what the source, was caused by the same thing as Raynaud's, and, by the way, intermittent claudication.

Intermittent Claudication – Another Peripheral Vascular Disease

Churchill's Medical Dictionary defines intermittent claudication (IC) as "Cramp-like pain and weakness in muscles, most often those of the calf, with consequent lameness. Symptoms develop progressively with walking and disappear with rest. It is due usually to atherosclerotic narrowing of the arteries of supply." This pretty much narrows it down. I can eliminate all the other problems that occur when blood vessels are clogged, like arteriosclerosis and strokes, saving them for other chapters.

This is the definition Dr. Jonathan Wright uses for a chapter in his book *Dr. Wright's Book of Nutritional Therapy*, in which he describes his treatment of a farmer for IC. The man came to the doctor complaining that he couldn't "walk to the barn without sitting," adding, "Fix my legs or I'm moving to a rest home." He had been having early symptoms for an incredible three or four years, and had been putting up with the severe pain for the last two to three months before seeing Dr. Wright, the first physician he consulted. Dr. Wright found blockages in the blood flow to both legs, then tested the farmer for diabetes, high cholesterol and mineral deficiencies. He found the man was borderline diabetic, a little high in cholesterol and had a deficiency of chromium and manganese. Chromium is essential for blood sugar regulation, so that wasn't surprising.[6]

Dr. Wright told the farmer to switch from white bread to whole grain bread, and eat more fruits and vegetables. He then prescribed 2,000 IU of vitamin E, 150 milligrams of chelated zinc, three times a day, 1 mg of chromium, 1,000 mg of vitamin C three times a day, vitamin B15 or pangamic acid, and 100 micrograms (mcg) of selenium. After three months, the farmer reported he could go "to the barn and back," and by nine months was only feeling twinges. Dr. Wright reports that after some experimentation, the farmer kept his problem in check by maintaining a vitamin protocol of eight grams of vitamin C, 800 IU of vitamin E, 100 mg of vitamin B15 and 50 mg of zinc.

This or any other treatment is not foolproof, and may not work for everyone. Dr. Wright did specific tests on the farmer, to determine his nutritional status, before making his recommendations. Sometimes intervention is necessary. Fortunately it doesn't have to be surgical.

Chelation Therapy

While interviewing Dr. Ross Gordon, a world renowned pioneer in the field of chelation therapy practicing medicine in Albany, California, I had the marvelous opportunity to meet a man who had his limbs restored to him by Dr. Gordon through chelation.

Dr. Gordon, his patient Virgil Young and Virgil's wife Arvilla appeared together on my talk show to tell their story. Virgil had intermittent claudication – the arterial blood flow in his lower extremities was being cut off. He couldn't walk without pain, and all the doctors could do was talk of amputating his legs.

"We had no choice, we had to try anything," said Arvilla, sitting in front of me in the television studio, her hands wringing a handkerchief. Virgil continued: "I was very frightened. The big toe on my left leg was dark blue. One doctor callously said to me 'Well, it ain't dead yet!.' Arvilla's chiropractor told us about Dr. Gordon."

By the time they turned to Dr. Gordon, Virgil's big toe was on the verge of gangrene. Dr. Gordon started him at once on chelation therapy.

Chelation therapy, simply stated, consists of intravenously administering a solution commonly referred to as EDTA. This compound has the ability to attract fatty deposits (cholesterol plaque) in the veins or arteries, much as a magnet attracts metal filings. As the EDTA. passes through the veins and arteries, it absorbs this plaque, which is then excreted in the urine.

By the time the couple got to the end of their story, tears were streaming down their cheeks. I couldn't help but join them as the emotions of their ordeal were relived.

"I saw a miracle happen!" said Virgil. "Before, I ate and ate but was never satisfied. I went from 172 pounds to 149 pounds. Now I'm back to my old weight. I'm healthier, and can walk again! Every chance I get, I tell people about Dr. Gordon."

The amount of time it takes for chelation therapy to work depends on the extent of the damage. It is usually administered three times a week for a segment of 21 treatments. It took one man three years to overcome a very bad case of arteriosclerosis. To prevent artery problems, it is important people eat less saturated fat and more plant food – vegetables and fruits.

Vitamin E for Energy

Vitamin E is the heart- and vascular-smart vitamin, touted by most doctors and researchers to be beneficial for the circulatory system. Vitamin E works by not only preventing the oxidation of bad cholesterol, but increasing good cholesterol. It acts like aspirin by thinning the blood so platelets don't stick together. In dosages ranging from 300 to 1,600 IU/day it has been shown in studies to help patients suffering from intermittent claudication without the side effects noted with aspirin and other similar drugs.

At health food conventions in the 1960s and 1970s, Drs. Evan and Wilfrid Shute of the Shute Clinic in Canada presented incredible "before" and "after" color photos illustrating how vitamin E improved the health of patients with heart disease, intermittent claudication and varicose veins.[7] An article in the *American Journal of Clinical Nutrition* reported vitamin E helps produce insulin in diabetics.[8]

Nutrients that Protect

There are a number of reasons circulation becomes diminished. High amounts of cholesterol in the blood coat the arteries with plaque, rough arterial walls collect matter, and diet, drugs and a lack of exercise and oxygen can cause blood to thicken, forming clots. Fortunately, we know of foods and nutrients that work to thin blood and avoid clots.

When researchers in Bangkok, Thailand, added freshly ground jalapeno pepper to rice flour noodles, subjects who ate the noodles daily experienced an increased ability to dissolve blood clots.

At the First World Congress on the "Health Significance of Garlic and Garlic Constituents," held in Washington, D.C., researchers reported that Kyolic® aged garlic extract may prevent the development of blood clots. I take Kyolic® liquid garlic extract because it is many times more absorbable than in pill form.

Other foods that have the power to thin blood are ginger and onions. They contain special phytochemicals as well as flavonoids found to not only get blood flowing but reduce inflammation that can lead to constricted arteries. Quercetin, a flavonoid, has been shown in studies to be particularly helpful in the fight against phlebitis, inflammation of the veins which can lead to blockages.

One of the risks of heart surgery is the blood clotting that can follow it. In a study to discover ways of avoiding this problem, patients were given supplements of calcium and vitamin E before surgery. In comparing those who received these supplements with those who had not, it was found that patients who were not given the supplements before surgery had six times as many blood clots in the lungs, and nine times as many deaths attributable to blockages resulting from the clots.

The path of least resistance is what's important. Efficient and effective blood flow requires not only even pressure, but smooth arterial walls. A deficiency of vitamin C has shown to contribute to roughness of the interior of the arteries. If the inside wall of an artery is rough, it is susceptible to breaks and collection of calcium and blood clots. Vitamin C is shown to be essential in maintaining smooth, flexible arterial walls necessary to proper blood circulation. Dr. Anthony Verlangieri, while at Rutgers University, demonstrated this effect by withholding vitamin C from laboratory rabbits' diets and noting the alteration in their arterial walls. When he restored the vitamin C to their diets, he documented their restoration to a healthy smoothness.

In China, the curative powers of ginkgo biloba have been known for thousands of years. In Europe, medical professionals extensively utilize the extract to aid in poor blood circulation. In France, the pharmaceutical Ginkor contains ginkgo biloba and is prescribed specifically for peripheral vascular disorders. In Spain, France and Switzerland, 100 percent ginkgo biloba is used in pharmaceuticals prescribed for vascular disorders. [9]

Circulation-Boosting Nutrients
For maximum absorption, take nutrients with meals.

Nutrient	Suggested Dosage	Formulation
Amino acids	4-6 capsules daily with exercise	Multiple formula from natural sources
Antioxidants	6 capsules daily*	With selenium and grapeseed extract
Aged garlic extract	1 teaspoon three times daily	Liquid
Borage oil	2 capsules daily	
Coenzyme Q10	4 capsules daily	With vitamin E, phospholipids and selenium
Flaxseed oil	1 tablespoon daily	
Folic acid	5-10 mg daily	
Multi-mineral	3-4 ounces daily	In liquid solution, with vitamin B12, biotin
Niacin	500 mg four times daily	
Magnesium	200 mg daily	
Multi-vitamin/mineral	6 caplets daily	Freeze-dried plant sources
Taurine	500 mg twice daily	
Vitamin B6	100 mg daily	
Vitamin C	Individual bowel tolerance**	With bioflavonoids (quercetin, proanthocyanidins)

* The FDA recommends pregnant women not exceed 10,000 IU of vitamin A daily.

** To determine individual dosage, on the first day take 1,000 mg hourly until diarrhea occurs, then reduce dosage to just below that for individual daily dosage. Vitamin C is not toxic in large doses but must be taken throughout the day to benefit. Divide dosage to three or four times a day.

CHAPTER 49:

Colds and Flu

I get the feeling the flu season is going to be bad this year. I just saw a squirrel hoarding cough lozenges.

In a ten-year study in the United States, colds and flu accounted for 60 percent of all illnesses. According to the study, each person in the U.S. averaged 5.6 colds or flu per year. Very young children averaged 8.3 per year.[1] That's a lot of sick people! Research has overturned our assumption that colds are spread by coughing and sneezing. Instead, the agreement is that they are spread by the hands, from touching the eyes and nose.[2] In experiments, most cold and influenza viruses deposited in the mouths of volunteers and laboratory animals do not result in infection. Apparently, cold and flu germs and viruses do not thrive in the mouth. Instead, they rely on the hands for entry through the nose and eyes.[3]

People are safer kissing than holding hands. Most individuals rub the eyes or pick the nose at least once an hour, almost guaranteeing their chances of passing on a bacterial or viral infection.[4]

Probably the best way to avoid a cold or flu is to wear goggles and gloves at all times. As unrealistic as this is, the next best way to prevent colds is to strengthen your immune system nutritionally. Optimum nutrition is essential for limiting the effect of each of the ten stages of the normal immune response to the common cold.

In a recent study, the United States Department of Agriculture discovered a sad fact: most Americans are not only failing to get optimal nutrition, but are actually deficient in many nutrients needed to strengthen the immune system and prevent and treat colds and the flu. At least one third of us consume less than 70 percent of the Recommended Dietary Allowances for vitamin A, vitamin C, vitamin B1 (thiamine), vitamin B2 (riboflavin), vitamin B3 (niacin), vitamin B12 and the minerals calcium, magnesium, zinc and iron.[5] Considering the fact that the RDA is too low to begin with, this is very telling indeed.

Vitamin C Proven to Help

Of all the vitamins, vitamin C with bioflavonoids is perhaps the best known immune booster. It is well established that vitamin C is vitally important to healthy white blood cells.

If you didn't believe it before, pay attention to this! Since 1971, 21 placebo-controlled studies have been done evaluating vitamin C's effect at a dose of 1 to 4 grams per day on the common cold. In every one of these 21 studies, vitamin C reduced the duration and severity of symptoms of the common cold by an average 23 percent. And wide ranges of other benefits to health were recognized.[6]

How it works is this: vitamin C is an antioxidant. This means it prevents the destruction of healthy cell tissue. Researchers have noted that during a cold or flu, a large number of neutrophils – bad guys – occur in the body. Neutrophils release large amounts of oxidizing materials that can damage cell tissue. What scientists have noted is that during a cold or flu infection, large amounts of vitamin C is used up. As the cold progresses, there is significant decrease in vitamin C concentration. Harri Hemila, a researcher with the University of Helsinki, Finland, did his own studies of this process and believes the body uses vitamin C to fight infection, and when stores are low, the body suffers for it. He believes six grams (6,000 milligrams) a day of vitamin C during a cold or flu can maximize the body's battle, noting that the diet of our ancestors contained 0.4 to 2 grams (400-2,000 mgs) of vitamin C per day.[7]

In his book, *How to Live Longer and Feel Better*, two-time Nobel laureate Linus Pauling, Ph.D., championed the use of vitamin C for preventing and helping to overcome colds.

Pauling cited a controlled study by biochemist G. Ritzel, in which schoolboys taking 1,000 mg/day of vitamin C averaged a 45 percent decrease in the number of days of illness per cold. In addition, Pauling summarized the results of 16 controlled research projects which showed a 31 percent decrease in colds in vitamin C users compared to volunteers who took placebos. Subjects who took more vitamin C averaged a 40 percent decrease in illness.

Robert Cathcart III, M.D., a California physician, has successfully treated over 15,000 patients with massive doses of vitamin C; curing viral pneumonia, mononucleosis, influenza, colds, hepatitis, shingles, and cold sores. He has developed a guideline for practical application of vitamin C which he refers to as "bowel tolerance."

The individual's own body will determine how much vitamin C it requires. The cutoff point is determined by the onset of diarrhea. The tolerance level in each individual differs. Some days you can tolerate more, some days less. A cold can be labeled a 20-to-30-gram cold, or 60-gram flu, according to how much a person can take before he reaches the bowel tolerance level.

The vitamin C will permeate every cell of the body before it reaches the bowel. Massive doses are needed because viruses within the sick cells excrete toxins.

In short, if you have not reached bowel tolerance (diarrhea), you have not taken enough vitamin C.

In an amazing discovery, vitamin C has been found to be helpful in the continuing battle against bacteria that have become immune to antibiotics. For more on this incredible story, see the Infections chapter.

Power-Pack Vitamin C with Bioflavonoids

Now you know that vitamin C, while it can't cure a cold or flu, can keep you from ending up in bed. It turns out there's even more you can do. You can make sure your vitamin C includes bioflavonoids.

Like the B vitamins, which work together in B-complex formulas, vitamin C and bioflavonoids should be considered C-complex.

At the Creighton University School of Medicine, Omaha, Nebraska, a group of nurses was given tablets containing the two substances. The nurses were checked for one year, as was another group which received a placebo. The nurses receiving the vitamin C and bioflavonoids had 55 percent fewer colds than the placebo group, and their infections lasted an average of 3.9 days, compared to 6.7 days for the placebo group.[10]

In the *American Journal of Digestive Diseases* Morton S. Biskind and W.C. Martin reported that 20 of 22 patients with respiratory infections of varying intensity recovered in an 8- to 48-hour period after treatment with bioflavonoids and vitamin C. The patients received 600 mg of each of the two substances every day.

Quercetin, a particularly potent bioflavonoid, acts as an antihistamine, allowing you to clear your medicine chest of all the dangerous over-the-counter remedies you used to take. Quercetin is the most effective nutritional antihistamine.[11]

Some European studies have found that bioflavonoids slow bacterial and viral infections.[12] Quercetin has been shown to be effective against many viruses, including viruses that cause the flu.[13]

Dr. Emanuel Cheraskin has done hundreds of scientific studies that he funded himself in order not to rely on either industrial or government money. In one of his most compelling studies done at Louisiana State University, he gave half the football team vitamin C with bioflavonoids and the other half plain vitamin C. Those who had vitamin C plus bioflavonoids had 87 percent fewer injuries than the group who received vitamin C alone. Think about that for a moment. A baseball player on bioflavonoids and vitamin C is 87 percent safer if he runs into a cement wall when he's trying to catch a ball! According to Dr. Cheraskin, "taking vitamin C without bioflavonoids is like clapping with only one hand."

Benefitting from Botanicals

We've all had our heart strings pulled by the sight of a child with a cold – a pathetic-looking stream of disease-carrying mucus seeping from both eyes and nose, cascading down his face. Whenever I see this, I can't resist passing on what I know: that certain nutrients will keep this infection from occurring. What happens is the mucus that forms from a cold or allergy thickens, perhaps from not enough water in the body, and stays in the nasal cavities long enough for bacteria to develop. It's the proliferation of bacteria, trapped inside the tissue pocket, that creates pain and inflammation. Anything that kills the bacteria will alleviate the infection. The key to this, is that the medicine must be circulated systemically, through the blood, and must kill only the bad bacteria, leaving the good to do its job. That's where aged liquid garlic extract comes in.

Liquid aged garlic extract is a powerful and effective detoxifier and immune system booster. The garlic is aged to reduce the toxic effects of large amounts of fresh garlic. Aged liquid garlic is odorless too, so you don't have to worry that you'll lose your friends and acquaintances. Liquid garlic is recommended for afflictions from AIDS to cancer because of its ability to pull toxic time bombs out of the body. If you choose to eat raw garlic, rather than take the liquid, don't cook it. Heat destroys many of the natural enzymes.

Tea made with elder flowers helps to clear congestion in the respiratory tract. It is also effective for sinus, throat and inner-ear infections. The action of the flowers is enhanced if combined with hyssop and yarrow flowers. For lung congestion or asthma, mix elder flowers with mullein flowers and chamomile flowers. These teas are rather bitter, but adding peppermint leaves improves the taste. Gargling with a cool tea made from elder flowers soothes a sore throat.

Besides its other healing qualities, elder contains vitamin C, vitamin A and bioflavonoids. Four ounces of elderberries contain about 35 milligrams of vitamin C and 600 International Units of vitamin A. Elder flowers contain rutin, a bioflavonoid also found in buckwheat that helps the body assimilate vitamin C.[15]

Forgotten Nutrient Knowledge

Over 50 years ago scientists first discovered vitamin A's value in treating and preventing colds and flu. In 1942, Italian physician Di Salvatore Princi published his study results that showed mice had more resistance to an influenza germ if they were given vitamin A. In 1937, German doctor Torsten Lindquist found that the vitamin A content of the blood was drastically lowered during the first five days of illness. When the patient began to get better, the level of vitamin A rose dramatically, even though no vitamin A was added to the diet. His assumption was that it was used somehow in the healing process.[16]

Dr. Garry Gordon, M.D., of Tempe, Arizona, recommends taking vitamin A and garlic at the same time as vitamin C, at the first sign of cold or flu symptoms, usually for a period of not less than three and not more than five days. Taking vitamin A directly, rather than in the form of beta carotene is most desirable. He recommends taking 500,000 IU when sick, and that high doses are safe as long as the person's weight is over 120 pounds, there is no serious liver condition, and high doses are taken for three days only.[17]

Vitamin A works against colds by strengthening and restoring the mucous membranes of the throat, nose and sinus cavities. The role of mucous is to flush out germs and foreign matter so they can't hurt and take hold in the system. If membranes are weak and thin, their ability to defend the body are compromised. Vitamin A prevents colds and infections by making sure the membranes within are strong enough to push germs and mucous out, and alleviates the symptoms by keeping membranes moist so there is less dryness and pain.[18]

Like vitamin C, zinc also possesses direct antiviral activity against several viruses that can cause the common cold. In a double-blind clinical trial, zinc gluconate lozenges significantly reduced the average duration of common colds by seven days.[19] These lozenges can be purchased at vitamin and health food stores. If you decide to supplement with zinc, do it through a multi-mineral formula that also contains copper, and the below listed minerals. Taking minerals in solution helps your body overcome the limitations presented by illness that may compromise their ability to become absorbed into the body's blood, cells and tissues.

Cold-Crushing Nutrients
For maximum absorption, take supplements with meals.

Nutrient	Suggested Dosage	Formulation
Aged garlic extract	1 teaspoon three times daily	Liquid
Antioxidants	4 capsules daily*	With selenium and grapeseed extract
Echinacea	200 mg daily	
Multi-mineral	3-4 ounces daily	In liquid solution, with vitamin B12, biotin
Multi-vitamin/mineral	6 caplets daily	Freeze-dried plant sources
Vitamin A	25,000 IU daily*	
Zinc gluconate	15 mg three times daily	Lozenges
Vitamin C	Individual bowel tolerance**	With bioflavonoids (quercetin, proanthocyanidins)

* The FDA recommends pregnant women not exceed 10,000 IU of vitamin A daily.

** To determine individual dosage, on the first day take 1,000 mg hourly until diarrhea occurs, then reduce dosage to just below that for individual daily dosage. Vitamin C is not toxic in large doses but must be taken throughout the day to benefit. Divide dosage to three or four times a day.

CHAPTER 50:

Colic

I was in the supermarket when a woman came up to me asking for advice. She looked tired. She told me her one-month-old baby was colicky and constipated and asked me if I thought honey would help. I told her honey is a big no-no for newborns. I asked her if the baby was on formula, which she was. I then asked her if it was a milk-based formula. She didn't know what I meant so I had her show me the brand she was using. It was a cow's milk-based brand she had been given at the hospital, so she thought it would be good for her baby. What she didn't realize was that sometimes a baby's immature digestive system can make digesting cow's milk proteins painful, and that it was probably the formula that was causing her baby's problem. It was too late for her to start breastfeeding, so I recommended she try a goat's milk or soy milk formula and add a little acidophilus powder (one-tenth an adult dose) in the beginning.

Colic Defined

Because babies with colic are generally less than four months old, they cannot tell us where it hurts. Narrowing it down, colic is, by definition, acute stomach or intestinal pain. The main symptom is excessive crying, occurring at the same time every day, notably in the evening, and often lasting for several hours.

The crying is believed to occur in the evening because that is when the baby is most tired. The baby's distress and pain cause concern, while the screaming drives the whole family crazy. The baby's frustration with the pain and the parents' frustration with the scream-ing can easily make the tensions and symptoms worse. It is impor-tant to remember there are choices and options other than just wait-ing out the three or four months, after which babies seem to outgrow colic.

According to conventional medicine literature, a doctor should be consulted if the baby has been crying constantly for over three hours (three hours!!), and if the baby is over four months old, if the cries become high-pitched or agonized, or if other symptoms such as fever, chills, vomiting, strange color or blood in urine or bowel move-ments occur. If it were me, I'd be calling *someone* after one hour! HELP!

What Are You Eating?

Are you breastfeeding? If you are, you may think you're doing everything right. But do you realize the food you eat could be caus-ing the colic?

A breastfed baby may be reacting to cow's milk protein in the mother's diet or to something else that Mom is eating. After exclud-ing the possibility of a medical problem, I usually suggest to a breastfeeding mother that she make some changes in her diet. She should eliminate common culprits such as milk and all dairy prod-ucts, and gas producers such as broccoli, cabbage, and caffeine (in coffee, chocolate, tea, soft drinks).[1]

In attempting to explain why their study showed an equal 20 percent of breastfed infants and 20 percent of formula fed infants had colic, researchers measured the amount of cow's milk antibodies in the milk of breastfeeding mothers who ate dairy products. Incredibly, the breastmilk given to colicky infants was found to have higher levels of cow's milk antibodies than even a cow's milk-based formula. There were no antibodies in the breastmilk of mothers whose babies were not colicky. Normally, the antibodies in cow's milk are destroyed in the human digestive system. In the mothers whose babies got colic, the antibodies stayed in their bodies and entered their breastmilk. If you want to see if this is the reason your baby has colic, plan on staying off dairy products for at least ten days. Cow's milk antibodies can stay in mother's milk for as long as one week after drinking milk.[2]

Baby Heartburn

Another possible reason for colic is the baby is suffering from heartburn. Wouldn't you, if you were throwing up three or four times a day? The acids from the stomach burns and inflames the esophagus, causing pain.

Philip Kazlow, M.D., director of clinical gastroenterology services at Columbia-Presbyterian Medical Center's Babies and Children's Hospital of New York, says that a large number of the colicky babies referred to him have heartburn. The key symptom? The baby cries during feedings, often arching his back and pulling in his arms and legs. "First, the baby cries from hunger," Dr. Kazlow says. "He'll avidly suck on the bottle or breast, taking maybe two ounces, but then he'll pull away and get crazy again." Because of the pain, the baby can't drink enough to feel full, so he can't sleep long before he cries from hunger. But when he's fed, he regurgitates and cries from pain. It's the classic vicious cycle. When the heartburn is mild, it's often enough to burp the baby after every one or two ounces of a feeding, and to keep him upright as much as possible, even tilting his crib. It also helps to thicken his formula with rice cereal, so "it sticks to the ribs," Dr. Kazlow says, and won't come up.[3]

What can you do to help a heartburn colicky baby? There are over-the-counter antacids, but I don't recommend them. Babies need their stomach acid to breakdown the nutrients contained in their milk, especially the minerals. Antacids can cause malabsorption, and eventually malnutrition.

Instead, rely on gentle herbal teas to relax the esophagus and soothe the stomach and intestines. Never use tap water, which could contain copper or lead. Choose filtered or purified water instead.

Diluted lemon balm tea is a good colic remedy. A member of the mint family, lemon balm helps digestion and increases the appetite. Elder is another beneficial botanical. It decreases gas, improves the appetite and generally aids digestion.The flowers, especially combined with chamomile flowers and catnip, make a gentle tea that helps relieve colic. Children usually don't mind the taste, especially when the tea is flavored with peppermint.[4] Chamomile tea is an excellent home remedy for upset stomachs. It relieves heartburn, indigestion and colic, and is completely harmless. In addition, it has mild relaxant and sedative properties. You can give it to infants and young children with good results."[5]

Balanced B complex vitamins, ground up and mixed in spring water, added to a bottle or given in a spoon half an hour before usual colic episodes can help. Calcium-magnesium can be given in a bottle the same way. Check the label for adult dosage and give the baby one-tenth that amount, twice a day.[6]

The B vitamins are essential for proper digestion. A deficiency of magnesium, calcium, potassium or vitamin B6 can cause intestinal cramping or colic. Reducing salt in the diet of a breastfeeding mother may help preserve potassium. When ready, mashed banana can be given for potassium. For the breastfeeding mother, foods that contain the three amigos: potassium, calcium, and magnesium, are items to keep in mind. They are: wheat germ, sunflower seeds, soybeans, almonds, brazil nuts, pistachios and pecans. Each of these foods can be added to salads, cereal and snack foods. Conveniently, they have a pretty decent shelf life as well. Eat your green leafy vegetables and whole grains for B vitamins. See the chapter Breastfeeding to keep you and your baby healthy.

CHAPTER 51:

Colon Problems –
Crohn's Disease, Colitis, IBS

Anyone who tries to tell you that diet can't help or influence colon problems is living in a vacuum (cleaner). Food can both hurt and help the colon. One colonic principle is that "great haste makes poor waste." Food that can be quickly eaten will not be quickly eliminated, and can cause or contribute to colon problems. There are even studies to prove it! Follow along with the researchers and I'll tell you the story of irritable bowel syndrome, colitis and Crohn's disease – why you get them and what you can do about them without going under a surgeon's knife.

Your No Parking Zone

The colon is an area where food should not be allowed to sit. The buck doesn't stop here. Unfortunately, our Western so-called "civilized" diet of processed, pasty foods has meant an epidemic of colon disorders in this country.

Interestingly, it was researchers from Sweden, not America, who found that people who eat at fast food restaurants regularly, and who eat too much sugar, may increase their risk of colon problems. Researchers from the Karolinska Institute in Stockholm interviewed 152 people with Crohn's disease, 145 with ulcerative colitis, and 305 healthy people about their eating habits in the five previous years. Those who ate fast food at least two times a week were 3.4 times more likely to develop Crohn's disease and 3.9 times more likely to develop ulcerative colitis. Fast food consisted of a hamburger or hot dog with mustard and ketchup, french fries or creamed potatoes and a soft drink. It was also noted that those who ate more than 55 grams of sugar per day were 2.6 times more likely to develop Crohn's disease. The Swedish study found that eating whole grain bread or muesli cereal (full of whole grains) prevented people from developing Crohn's disease.[1]

What happens when you eat unraw and processed food is not a pretty picture. The food "paste" you've been ingesting sits in your large intestine, unable to move. The heat and moisture invites bacteria to grow, which then ferments your waste matter, causing acids and byproducts that eat away at your intestinal lining. This condition is called colitis or Crohn's disease. The only difference between them is the extent of the inflammation. In Crohn's disease, the inflammation extends throughout the intestine wall, and can be so bad that blockages develop.

When your intestinal lining develops holes and sores, your doctor proclaims you have ulcerative colitis. Sometimes so many things go wrong that identifying any one cause becomes impossible. That's when they call it irritable bowel syndrome (IBS). Maybe doctors come up with these terms just to make patients feel helpless. If doctors can't make heads or tails of the source of the problem, and they can spin our brains with fancy terminology, we're more likely to hand over control of our lives and afflictions instead of taking charge of our own health with changes in lifestyle and habits.

Fiber for a Healthy Colon

Patrick Donovan, N.D. of Seattle, Washington, agrees fiber is important in the prevention of IBS. However, in the *healing* of IBS, colitis and Crohn's, he recommends easy-on-the-colon soluble fibers. He recommends juices made from cabbage and green leafy vegetables. The chlorophyll in them have healing properties, and cabbage juice has been shown in studies to help heal ulcers. He suggests starting out with broths made from seaweed, adding vegetable juices later, then blended fruit juices. A patient with a history of colitis for ten years and no relief from conventional medicine came to Dr. Donovan. He told the patient to fast for four days then put him on a vegetable juice and lamb bone broth diet. Once the patient's food allergens were identified, he treated his iron-deficiency anemia with iron-containing herbs and foods such as spinach and kale, then raw and steamed vegetables and salads. Within a month the patient was on whole foods and was considerably relieved of his colitis.[2]

Fiber is basically that part of food that cannot be broken down or assimilated, and is necessary to move and eliminate waste. Read the chapters on Constipation and Colon Cancer for more on the importance of fiber. Anything to do with the colon requires a lesson on fiber.

So far as fiber is concerned, seven tablespoons of oat bran daily have been found to keep bowel movements regular and to prevent diseases of Western society: intestinal tract ailments, heart and artery disorders and degenerative diseases such as cancer. Whole grain breads and cereals are key fiber contributors. Other top sources of fiber include psyllium, hyssop, alfalfa, rhubarb and buckthorn. Look for these ingredients among the others listed below in a food-derived fiber supplemental formula for your colon health.

Fiber is activated by water. Whenever fiber intake increases, the need for fluids increases. Anyone who takes a fiber supplement should drink at least six 10-ounce glasses of water a day, in addition to any other beverages.

The Stomach Acid Connection

Dr. Robert Atkins, author of *Dr. Atkins Health Revolution*, believes IBS starts in the upper part of the gastrointestinal tract – the stomach. He found two tests invented and ignored by orthodoxy proved it. One is the Indican test, which looks for the presence of indole in the urine, and shows food has left the stomach properly broken down. The second test is the Heidelberg test, which evaluates the amount of hydrochloric, or stomach acid, available to break down the food. Dr. Atkins found that some patients with IBS were not breaking down their food and had a deficiency of stomach acid. What happens in these cases is that the food enters the large intestine in a whole state and ferments. The large intestine is not designed to break down food, only to absorb its nutrients. Food that is not broken down cannot impart its valuable nutrients to the body, and it becomes a gassy, painful, acidic mess in the intestine until it can be pushed through.[3] The acids that form when food ferments eats away at the intestinal lining.

I wouldn't be surprised if doctors find colon problems are on the rise thanks to the powerful, long-lasting antacids that are now being touted in television commercials for heartburn. Imagine what happens to your meals when your stomach acid is eliminated for eight hours at a time! You'll have a lot more than heartburn if you regularly swallow these bowel busters!

Dr. Atkins found that supplementing with a Betaine, a hydrochloric acid supplement available in health food stores improved approximately 70 percent of IBS cases in which patients were not breaking down food properly. Taking a tablespoon of vinegar with your meals can help also, as can chewing very thoroughly so every bit of food is liquified.

Food Allergies

Food allergies can cause IBS. Since 1982, there have been at least eight different experimental studies published in peer-review journals such as *The Lancet* and the *Annals of Allergy* consistently suggesting that for every three cases of IBS, two will respond dramatically to the elimination of food allergens. The greatest offenders are found to be wheat, corn, dairy products and yeast, in that order. If you're not convinced, read on.

Dr. Steven A. McClave, M.D., Department of Medicine, University of Louisville School of Medicine, Louisville, Kentucky, found that in patients with IBS, eliminating food allergens resulted in a 62 percent remission rate after one year and a cumulative remission rate of 45 percent over five years.[4] There's more!

The allergy/IBS connection was proposed over 50 years ago, with the first controlled trial of an elimination diet in ulcerative colitis conducted in early 1970. While on a milk-restricted diet for over a year, patients with ulcerative colitis showed improvement, as well as a reduced rate of clinical relapse. Dairy products cause intestinal inflammation because their proteins generate certain antibodies.[5]

You've heard of lactose intolerance? This is the protein that can cause so many problems in the colon. When lactose escapes the stomach undigested, it meets intestinal bacteria which feed on it, causing fermentation. Then the small intestine becomes a war zone of cramps, diarrhea, gas and bloating. These are the symptoms of a milk allergy.

The system's reaction to a food allergy can be severe and long-term. In a study reported in the *European Journal of Pediatrics*, researchers tested infants from parents with a family history of milk allergy. After only one dose of cow's milk, "before" and "after" pictures showed their stomach lining was turned to mush. Zinc, a notorious wound-healer, can help restore the stomach and intestinal lining. Look for a supplement that has zinc and copper in solution, which assimilates better in the body.

To make up for an insufficiency of lactase, drink milk or eat yogurt that contains lactobacillus acidophilus, a bacterial culture that makes the necessary lactase. Or you can buy milk that already contains lactase. Lactase enzymes can be purchased at health food stores in the form of a multi-enzyme supplement. Lactase is just one of many digestive enzymes necessary to the proper assimilation of food. I recommend when supplementing with one enzyme, you take all of them.

Fighting Back with Bacteria

One of the chief causes of colon problems is an overgrowth of candida albicans, a yeast. See my chapter Fungus Infections for more on this. I bring it up here to make a point about bacteria. Normally, candida isn't a problem because intestinal bacteria keep it under control. But when bacteria are killed by antibiotics, for example, the bad guys can proliferate while the good guys are still down for the count. Harmful, or disease-causing bacteria have fancy Latin names like pseudomonas-aeruginosa, proteus, staphylococcus, clostridia and veillonellae.

Found in intestinal bacteria supplemental formulas are the body's disease-killing good-guy bacteria, Lactobacilli, Eubacteria and Bifidobacteria. Lactobacilli can inhibit the growth of harmful bacteria, stimulate immune function and aid in digestion, and Eubacteria can inhibit the growth of harmful bacteria. Bifidobacteria can reduce blood ammonia levels, lower cholesterol levels, regulate the immune system, produce vitamins, especially the B vitamin/folic acid group, restore normal intestinal flora during antibiotic therapy, and inhibit the growth of disease-causing germs. Researchers like Marcel B. Roberfroid of the Department of Pharmaceutical Sciences, Catholic University of Louvain, Brussels, Belgium have found these good bacteria are beneficial in any disorder of the bowel, including IBS, colitis and Crohn's disease.[6]

Proper nutrition, fiber and the addition of lactobacillus acidophilus, the supplement that contains the lactobacilli bacteria, can cure the vast majority of cases of IBS. It stands to reason, also, that more serious problems can be prevented by supplementing with these digestive bacteria, especially when under stress, which diminishes stomach acid, and when taking antibiotics.[7] Look for a fiber formula that contains the aforementioned fiber ingredients, adding acidophilus for good measure. Make sure your fiber formula contains lactobacillus acidophilus.

Nutritional Support for the IBS Patient

Because the colon is responsible for absorbing the nutrients essential to good health, anything that compromises the colon's capacity for this job also compromises health. Certain nutrients can only be absorbed in the bowel, and, not coincidentally, are found to be deficient in colon patients.

Dr. McClave found that two thirds to three quarters of patients hospitalized with Crohn's disease are severely malnourished. He found a deficiency of protein to be most common in patients with irritable bowel syndrome. In patients with colitis, he found incredible deficiencies in essential nutrients that can make the difference between health and healing. Over half – 54 to 67 percent – were deficient in folic acid; 48 to 50 percent were deficient in vitamin B12; half were deficient in zinc; and an incredible 75 percent of patients with colitis were deficient in vitamin D. Patients with Crohn's disease had even greater nutritional imbalances. He also found colon patients had trouble absorbing fat, and excreted high amounts of calcium, magnesium and zinc, making them deficient in these minerals.[8]

Dr. Seidman found similar deficiencies when he evaluated children with IBS. In one study, low folic acid deficiencies were seen in 38 percent of patients with Crohn's and 59 percent with ulcerative colitis. Low blood levels of folic acid are associated with lower levels of vitamin B6, B12 and vitamin C. Vitamin B12 deficiency occurs in about one fifth of Crohn's disease patients. In pediatric cases the prevalence may be two times that much. In fact, most of the B vitamins are found to be low in cases of IBS. Dr. Seidman found that two thirds of all Crohn's disease patients are potentially at risk for vitamin D deficiency. Vitamin E levels have also been shown to be lower in Crohn's disease patients, as well as deficiencies in iron, calcium, magnesium and vitamin K.[9]

Normally it is here that I would add foods high in these nutrients. However, due to the high probability of food allergies being at least a contributing cause to your colon problems, and the uncertainty of the severity of the damage to your colon, I will ask that you consult with a physician versed in nutritional medicine before you attempt self-treatment. Nutritional supplementation can do no harm, certain foods can. For a number where you can obtain a list of physicians versed in nutritional therapy, call at 1-800-445-4325.

Treatment with Amino Acids

Not only are certain amino acids essential to a healthy colon, but they can reverse the effect of food allergies, infection and other trauma to the delicate mucosal tissues of the intestinal tract. A deficiency of glutamine will weaken intestinal villi, causing poor absorption of nutrients, so obviously your intestine's health depends on it. An article in *Gastroenterology* stated that a glutamine-enhanced diet helps the colon recover from colitis by increasing good guy bacteria. In animal studies glutamine supplementation has decreased weight loss, improved nitrogen retention, and increased colonic thickness, protein and DNA content, as well as improving survival time and decreasing mortality from Crohn's disease.[10]

Arginine is another amino acid found to help colon problems. It enhances the immune system, especially following trauma, and promotes wound healing and intestinal cell growth. Look for a complete amino acid formula in your neighborhood health food or vitamin store.

Anti-inflammatories for Your Intestine

Several substances have been found to reduce the inflammation associated with colon problems. Quercetin, a bioflavonoid found in citrus rind, onions and in some supplemental formulas has been found to be a potent anti-inflammatory. It is recommended when food allergies are present, and works even better when combined with vitamin C.

Unsaturated fatty acids (also essential fatty acids, or EFAs) are important to restore the mucosal lining of a damaged colon. An article in the *American Journal of Clinical Nutrition* reports on a study that showed flaxseed oil and fish oil are good for ulcerative colitis symptoms.[11]

Certain kinds of EFAs help reduce inflammation and restore the intestinal lining. They are: eicosapentaenoic acid, found in the oils of salmon, trout, mackerel, sardines; and linoleic acid, found in the oils of borage, safflower, sunflower, flaxseed, pumpkin seed, walnut, soybean and sesame seed. The best source of linoleic acid is borage oil, found in supplemental form. It is more concentrated and is less expensive than evening primrose oil, another highly potent supplemental form.[12]

Colon-Restoring Nutrients
For maximum absorption, supplements should be taken with meals.

Nutrient	Suggested Dosage	Formulation
Acidophilus	At least four billion flora daily on an empty stomach, three times daily	
Aged garlic extract	2 teaspoons three times daily	Liquid
Amino acids	4-6 capsules daily	Multiple formula from natural sources
Antioxidants	4 capsules daily*	With selenium and grape seed extract
Borage oil	2 capsules daily	
Coenzyme Q10	2 capsules daily	With vitamin E, phospholipids and selenium
Enzymes	2 capsules twice daily	Multiple formula
Flaxseed oil	1 tablespoon daily	
Fiber	8 tablets daily	Psyllium, with herb hyssop
L-glutamine	500 mg three times daily	
Multi-vitamin/mineral	6 caplets daily	Freeze-dried plant sources
Multi-mineral	2-4 ounces daily	In liquid solution, with vitamin B12, biotin
Vitamin C	Individual bowel tolerance**	With bioflavonoids (quercetin, proanthocyanidins)

* The FDA recommends that pregnant women not exceed 10,000 IU of vitamin A daily.

** To determine individual dosage, on the first day take 1,000 mg hourly until diarrhea occurs, then reduce dosage to just below that for individual daily dosage. Vitamin C is not toxic in large doses but must be taken throughout the day to benefit. Divide dosage to three or four times a day.

CHAPTER 52:

Constipation

*Grain must be ground to make bread, so one does not
go on threshing it forever; though he drives the wheels
of his threshing cart over it, his horses do not grind
it. All this comes from the Lord-Almighty wonderful
in counsel and magnificent in wisdom.*

— Isaiah 28:26-29

Our eating habits have come a long way since Biblical times.
Our food industry threatens to destroy us with its technology. Food
just isn't food anymore, and our constitutions are suffering because
of it.

Despite directions from the Almighty, available to anyone who
cares to read it, civilization went its own way. With its grain mills
and food processing, whole foods became conveniently chopped,
pressed and formed, like some packaged sliced meats, and the fiber
in fruits and vegetables became soft, sweet and denatured in cans.

Our digestive system was not designed to handle the amounts of
refined sugar, bleached white flour, hydrogenated fat and salt that
makes up the average American diet. Even rats cannot survive on
white bread, which is the most commonly eaten food in America.
Pouring all this food paste into our highly complex systems creates
problems never before seen by humankind: constipation, hemorrhoids,
varicose veins and appendicitis – all of which have increased tremendously over the decades.

A friend of mine suffered from constipation for a great many years and took a laxative every single day of his life. When I suggested to him one day that he omit white bread from his diet, he was skeptical, but agreed to try. Within several weeks his constipation disappeared and has never returned. And this was the *only* change he made in his living habits.

Alright, so how does a victim of constipation become regular? By doing the following:

1. Include fiber in the diet
2. Discover and eliminate food allergens
3. Supplement with a lactobacillus acidophilus formula
4. Take at least 60 mg of folic acid daily
5. Make sure your thyroid is functioning properly, and if hypothyroid, read the chapter Low Thyroid.
6. Exercise daily, especially activities the make you bend at the waist.

High Fiber Advice

Daily sources of fiber in the diet are all that separates a person from the ability to resist what is called the "civilized diseases."

Constipation is one example. Chronic constipation can cause colon disorders such as diverticulosis, pouches in the intestine wall where fecal matter can lodge and putrefy, and diverticulitis, swelling and inflammation of these pouches.

The late Dr. Denis Burkitt, an authority on the colon and waste matter, offered a rather commonsensical approach for telling whether or not the diet contains enough fiber and whether or not one is in danger of developing the "civilized disease."[1]

He recommends observing the consistency of your stool for signs of trouble. Floaters are stools with enough fiber to make them float in the toilet bowl. Sinkers are heavy and hard and indicate that a person may be headed for problems. Watch, also, how much fiber floats out when you flush the toilet.

So far as fiber is concerned, food derived sources such as psyllium, hyssop and alfalfa have been found to keep bowel movements regular and to guard against diseases of Western society: intestinal tract ailments, heart and artery disorders and degenerative diseases such as cancer. Whole grain breads and cereals are key fiber contributors. Other sources of fiber include rhubarb and buckthorn. Look for a fiber formula that contains these ingredients.

Fiber in vegetables and fruit is helpful but, aside from that in carrots, is not quite as effective as the bran contained in whole grains. An experimental controlled study revealed that the eating of bran increased the number of bowel movements and reduced intestinal transit time. Corn bran proved superior to wheat bran, according to a report in the *American Journal of Gastroenterology*.

Fiber is activated by water. Whenever fiber intake increases, the need for fluids increases. Anyone who takes a fiber supplement should drink at least six 10-ounce glasses of water a day, in addition to any other beverages. Otherwise, the constipation can get worse.

Other Causes

Constipation is the first warning – a warning to be heeded. If you are constipated, the first thing to do is consider the cause. The most common cause is insufficient dietary fiber, but many other things can contribute too. Some medications may cause constipation: anti-depressants, painkillers and iron supplements for example. Other things to look for are hypothyroidism, too much calcium in the blood (caused by not enough magnesium and potassium), food allergies, pregnancy (pressure on the intestines), obesity, poor muscle tone, sitting for long periods, injury to the bowel nerves, insufficient water intake, and just not defecating when the urge comes.

Low thyroid function slows down all body functions, including bowel contractions necessary to move wastes out efficiently. In first generation hypothyroids, iodine from a highly absorbable mineral in solution formula helps to correct this condition. Hypothyroids of the second generation and beyond may require prescribed thyroid tablets.

An unsuspected cause, believe it or not, is your tap water. Chlorine compounds in tap water kill helpful intestinal bacteria, leading to a possible overgrowth of harmful bacteria, yeasts or even parasites. If you are easily constipated, you may be reacting to the water you drink. People with green thumbs know that chlorine in tap water can seriously affect their plants. So they boil the water to dissipate the chlorine, wait till it cools to room temperature, and then do their watering.

Certain foods encourage the good bacteria and help normalize the bowel tract. Foods to target are acidophilus bacillus in yogurt or in supplemental form, apples, cabbages, figs, papayas, pineapples and prunes.

Lactobacillus acidophilus supplementation has been found in studies to correct constipation. In one study, 305 of 356 patients were relieved. It also has been shown to help in other problems of the colon.[2] For more, see the chapter Colon Problems.

Because chronic constipation can be a symptom of a serious, possibly life-threatening disease, it is important to identify the cause. Any sudden onset of constipation requires examination and evaluation by a physician. Even if the cause is simply a matter of a poor diet, the side effects of constipation are serious.

"Regular" Recommendations

The person whose body is perfectly nourished need have no fear of constipation. Here are some principles of nutrition I adhere to.[3]

1. All food should be organically grown–grown without chemical fertilizers. Plant your own garden, however small. Garden organically and experience for the first time the taste and health thrill of eating lots of vegetables free from chemical fertilizers and insecticides.

2. Eat lots of organic fruit, grown in pesticide-free soil.

3. Eliminate commercially-made sweets and white flour products including cookies, muffins, crackers and biscuits.

If it doesn't contain whole grains, don't eat it.

4. Establish a regular time for bowel action and observe it without fail every day. In addition, make absolutely certain that you relieve your bowels every time you feel the necessity, no matter how much of a rush you are in or how inconvenient it may be.

5. Exercise. A walk, a stretch – take the stairs instead of an elevator. Your bowels don't move when you sleep because you aren't exercising them. Give yourself some time in the morning or at lunch for a little physical activity before rushing out or back to work or school.

6. Watch the amount of food you eat. Moderation is always important. Too much or too little food can contribute to constipation. Instead of a large meal of meat, potatoes, gravy and bread, choose a small meal of crackers or a bowl of processed cereal flakes. It has to be the kinds of foods that will have enough fiber to encourage bowel movement and enough of them to have something to move.

7. Vitamins and minerals must be included in the daily diet for perfect nourishment. Concentrated vitamin and mineral preparations – made from natural sources – should be taken daily, always with foods during the process of digestion. In animal experiments, young rats fed a diet low in minerals had marked constipation while control animals on the same diet plus minerals did not.[4]

For optimum absorption, I take a supplemental mineral in solution formula, and a formula that is derived from dehydrated sprouts and vegetables. Such food supplements overrride many of the civilized digestive dangers we face and put nutrients right where they belong.

The mineral magnesium is one of the most important nutrients for treating constipation. Magnesium is all-important for the muscles.

A deficiency of magnesium can be a cause of muscle cramping, one of the painful symptoms of constipation. Donald Brown, N.D., recommends 800 milligrams of magnesium for adults to get the plumbing working again. He also stresses the importance of water intake and folic acid, especially in women.[5]

In an experiment with three women who were proved to be deficient in folic acid and suffered from chronic constipation – along with other symptoms such as restless legs, depression and fatigue – all recovered when given 60 mg of folic acid daily.[6]

When supplementing with folic acid, always include vitamin B12 and a good, thorough B complex formula. All the B vitamins must be present together for optimum performance.

James Braly, M.D., Medical Director of Immuno Labs, Inc., Ft. Lauderdale, Florida, recommends routine nutritional supplementation for constipated patients. Additionally, he advises using high doses of vitamin C, and essential fatty acids.[7]

For children with constipation, Virender Sodhi, M.D., N.D., Bellevue, Washington, recommends they take almond oil to increase bowel movement.[8] Almond oil is high in essential fatty acids and magnesium.

In most cases, nutrients have to be taken together for best benefit. Potassium, calcium, and magnesium together balance each other out so one cannot overload the system. They are also important to healthy muscles, joints and bones. Too much calcium has been found to cause constipation. Avoid this problem by including magnesium.

For all your mineral needs, target a mineral in solution formula. Because of the high absorption rate of minerals in solution, and deficiency of magnesium in the diet, the ratio of magnesium and calcium in solution should be four to one, respectively.

Constipation-Fighting Nutrients
For maximum absorption, supplements should be taken with meals.

Nutrient	Suggested Dosage	Formulation
Acidophilus	At least four billion flora daily on an empty stomach, three times daily	
Enzymes	2 capsules twice daily	Multiple formula
Exercise	30 minutes daily	Moderate
Fiber	8 tablets daily	Psyllium, with herb hyssop
Magnesium citrate	200 mg once or twice daily	
Multi-vitamin/mineral	6 caplets daily	Freeze-dried plant sources
Multi-mineral	2-4 ounces daily	In liquid solution, with vitamin B12, biotin
Purified water	Two gallons daily	Filtered, chlorine-free
Vitamin C	Individual bowel tolerance*	With bioflavonoids (quercetin, proanthocyanidins)

* To determine individual dosage, on the first day take 1,000 mg hourly until diarrhea occurs, then reduce dosage to just below that for individual daily dosage. Vitamin C is not toxic in large doses but must be taken throughout the day to benefit. Divide dosage to three or four times a day.

CHAPTER 53:

Cramps–Menstrual & Muscle

MENSTRUAL CRAMPS (Dysmenorrhea)

*"Men endure pain as an undeserved punishment;
women accept it as a natural heritage."*

–Anonymous

Only other women can appreciate what Janet went through every month. For three days out of every thirty, Janet spent the time in bed, her lower abdomen covered in a heating pad, getting up only for glasses of water and to use the bathroom. She couldn't eat and she barely slept. Instead she waited out the time writhing in agony as her monthly "curse" wracked her with muscle spasms.

For many of us, the "time of the month" is one we'd rather forgo. Doctors at the Mayo Clinic in Minnesota estimate that more than half of all women regularly suffer from menstrual cramping, technically called dysmenorrhea. If you do your own survey, you'll probably find *all* women, at one time or another in their lives, have been agonized with menstrual cramps.

For years, most medical researchers excluded women from their studies, minimizing the pains and problems associated with hormonal cycles as an inconvenience or dismissing them as an abnormality. Until recently, pharmaceutical companies did not take the menstrual cycle into account in their testing of drugs. Responding to this travesty of inadequacy, in 1993 Congress passed the National

Institutes of Health Revitalization Act, requiring inclusion of women in clinical research. Perhaps it's not surprising, then, that conventional medicine regularly treats many women's health problems ineffectively, even harmfully, over-medicating, misdiagnosing or ignoring women's problems on a regular basis. No wonder we turn to alternative and natural therapies.

Prostaglandins and EFAs

Why does cramping occur? If we didn't cramp at least a little, our muscles wouldn't be able to push menstrual blood out. Prostaglandins are a family of powerful hormones that raise and lower blood pressure, increase or decrease the formation of blood clots and control inflammation. They are also responsible for the uterine contractions needed to expel menstrual blood every month. Too many prostaglandins can cause the uterus to contract so much that the blood supply is cut off temporarily, depriving the uterine muscle of oxygen and causing severe pain.

Conventional treatments, commonly non-steroidal anti-inflammatory drugs (NSAIDs) alleviate this pain because they inhibit prostaglandin release. Oral contraceptives have even been prescribed for cramps because they increase progesterone and decrease estrogen, resulting in less prostaglandins.

It is a fact that essential fatty acids (EFAs) are used by the body to regulate prostaglandins. In today's dietary world, we don't eat like we should, and foods that contain essential fatty acids are often left out. When was the last time you consumed a handful of raw almonds, or used walnut oil in your salad or ate grape or pumpkin seeds? I think it is quite possible that a deficiency of EFAs at least contribute to menstrual cramping since they can lower the amounts of prostaglandins being released during menstruation.

The two families of essential fatty acids are omega-3 found mainly in fish and fish oils (cod liver oil) and omega-6 found in seeds and seed oils. Gamma-linolenic acid (GLA), or linoleic acid, is found in evening primrose oil, black currant oil, borage oil and spirulina.[1]

GLA has been found to be a potent anti-inflammatory among arthritis sufferers. Arthritis inflammation is also associated with increased prostaglandins. Researchers Peter Callejari, M.D. and Robert B. Zurier, M.D., reported on a study in which nine borage seed oil capsules were given daily to arthritic volunteers for 12 weeks. It was noted that the pain and inflammation was reduced, in part because of regulated prostaglandins.[2]

Independent clinical tests show that borage oil contains up to 26 percent GLA. Compare this to evening primrose oil and black currant oil, which contain no more than 18 percent. Not only that, borage oil costs less because the borage seed is three times larger than black currant or evening primrose seeds. Finally, borage is more bioavailable. In other words, the body more readily accepts it.

Nutritional Therapy

"Menstrual cramps that occur every month may indicate low levels of blood calcium," says Rosemary Gladstar, herbalist and author of *Herbal Healing for Women* (Simon & Schuster, 1993). At least ten days before menstruation begins, she recommends increasing high-calcium foods in the diet, such as dark leafy greens, sesame seeds, seaweeds, and watercress. A diet rich in calcium also relaxes the central nervous system. Don't make the mistake, however, of assuming calcium alone will do the trick. Calcium doesn't go where it needs to without magnesium and potassium.

Shari Lieberman, coauthor of *The Real Vitamin Book* (Avery, 1990) says that since calcium and magnesium work together to regulate muscle contractions and the conduction of nerve impulses, a daily supplement containing 1,000 mg of calcium and 500 mg of magnesium helps women with cramps.[3]

"Nothing works better for menstrual cramps than herbs," counters Gladstar. For occasional cramps, she recommends warm ginger tea for its antispasmodic properties. Grate two to three teaspoons of fresh ginger root and simmer in two cups of water for several minutes. Add lemon and honey to taste. Drink as much as desired. For acute cramps, Gladstar suggests combining equal parts of ginger, valerian and cramp bark tinctures, to be taken in half-teaspoon doses every twenty minutes until the symptoms subside.

Susan Lark, M.D., of Los Altos, California, recommends vitamin B3, B6, vitamin C, calcium, magnesium, potassium, zinc and essential fatty acids for treatment of menstrual cramps.[4]

Muscle Cramps

Most women have been through it, especially while pregnant. Deep in slumber, we are startled awake by incredible pain jolting through the calf. Throwing off the covers, still half asleep, we trounce our foot on the floor, easing some of the spasms, desperately massaging the calf until the pain subsides. These kinds of muscle cramps are the most common and are attributed to mineral deficiencies.

A magnesium deficiency can cause muscle cramps. A lack of calcium, too, is attributed to muscle cramps since it is necessary for normal muscle contraction. Eating antacids to get calcium and magnesium are a no-no because they inhibit the stomach acid which is essential to absorbing these minerals. Too little stomach acid can cause calcium to be deposited in joints and blood vessels, where it doesn't belong.

Among athletes, an electrolyte imbalance from a lack of potassium may play a role in muscle cramps. This can be ruled out by eating potassium-rich foods daily, focusing on fruits and vegetables.[5]

Leg cramps can be caused by inadequate oxygen and red blood cell clumping. Vitamin E works to break up clumping and increase oxygen to the cells. Any supplemental source of vitamin E should be in the form of a natural tocopherol, and should be taken alone.

Dr. F. Konikoff, Gastroenterology Division, Brigham and Women's Hospital, Boston, Massachusetts, found that liver patients who had muscle cramps had lower vitamin E levels than those without cramps. Thirteen of the patients with muscle cramps were given tocopherol acetate, a form of vitamin E. Compared with a group which did not get the vitamin E, those who did had less pain, and the pain they did have was less frequent and didn't last as long. They also had no side effects.[6]

Circulation problems can result in muscle cramping. If you experience cramping while walking, it may be a sign of a circulation problem. If it progresses to pain and limits your mobility, it could be a sign of a serious circulation problem. First read my chapter on Circulation Problems, then see a doctor versed in nutrition. Heavy exercise can cause muscle cramping if the muscles haven't been stretched or you have a nutrient deficiency. Other nutrients that can cause muscle pain when deficient are the B vitamins thiamine, pantothenic acid, biotin and vitamin C.[7]

Cramp-Crushing Nutrients

For maximum absorption, supplements should be taken with meals.

Nutrient	Suggested Dosage	Formulation
Amino acids	4-6 capsules daily	Multiple formula from natural sources
Borage oil	2 capsules daily	
Coenzyme Q10	2 capsules daily	With vitamin E, phospholipids and selenium
Flaxseed oil	1 tablespoon daily	
Fiber	8 tablets daily	Psyllium, with herb hyssop
Multi-vitamin/mineral	6 caplets daily	Freeze-dried plant sources
Multi-mineral	2-4 ounces daily	In liquid solution, with vitamin B12, biotin
Natural progesterone cream	1/3 teaspoon daily	With pregnenolone, DHEA
Vitamin B6	200 mg daily	
Vitamin C	Individual bowel tolerance*	With bioflavonoids (quercetin, proanthocyanidins)
Vitamin E	2 capsules (800 IU) daily	d-alpha tocopherol

* To determine individual dosage, on the first day take 1,000 mg hourly until diarrhea occurs, then reduce dosage to just below that for individual daily dosage. Vitamin C is not toxic in large doses but must be taken throughout the day to benefit. Divide dosage to three or four times a day.

CHAPTER 54:

Cystic Fibrosis

"Alex's day would start with an inhalation treatment to loosen the mucus which had settled in her lungs. Then, for a half hour or more, we would give her postural drainage treatment. There were 11 different positions that Alex had to endure, and one of us, Carol or I, would pound away at her, thumping her chest, her back, her side, palms cupped in such a way as to better 'catch' – dislodge – the mucus. After each position, we would press hard on her lungs, kneading them with our fingers in ways that were often more uncomfortable than the pounding had been. Some positions Alex could do sitting up, others lying flat on our laps. But a full four of the eleven she had to endure nearly upside down, the blood rushing to her head, as I banged away on her little chest, pounding her, rattling her, trying somehow to shake loose that vile mucus that was trying to take her life away."

In 1980, writer Frank Deford and his wife Carol lost their 8-year-old daughter Alexandra to cystic fibrosis. Alex was diagnosed with the disease at four months of age. Doctors told them she wouldn't see her second birthday, but she hung on to see her eighth. Deford chronicled her inspiring life, courageous battle and tragic death in his book *Alex: The Life of a Child* (Penguin Books, 1984), excerpted above.

Cystic fibrosis (CF) is a disease primarily of the lungs. It has nothing to do with cysts. A hereditary illness afflicting about 50,000 Americans, CF causes severe lung and digestive problems. Primarily it produces thicker-than-normal mucus, which causes recurring infections and ultimately destroys the lungs. The other major site of damage is the digestive system, where the pancreas may suffer congestion and eventual failure, and the liver may become scarred as years of mucus plugging and bile passage blockage lead to liver failure. Inadequate pancreatic function leads to malabsorption (see the chapter on Malabsorption) which can cause malnutrition, diarrhea, and stomachaches.

Because the initial symptom, thick mucous, causes such severe problems, doctors are unsure which to tackle first, the original problem or the secondary afflictions. The original problem is bad enough, but with the malabsorption comes severe malnutrition, which must be addressed. In order for the body to fight against CF, it must have the strength of good nutrition.

Nutritional Support for the CF Patient

During a 1991 meeting convened by the Cystic Fibrosis Foundation, specialists discussed needs and developed a consensus regarding nutrition and cystic fibrosis. Some of their specific recommendations for nutrients are as follows: basic multivitamin and mineral supplementation with emphasis on vitamins A and E and vitamin D. Children between two and eight years of age need a multiple vitamin containing 400 IU of vitamin D and 5,000 IU of vitamin A. Vitamin E supplementation: Ages 0-6 months 25 IU/daily; 6-12 months 50 IU/daily; 1-4 years 100 IU/daily; 4-10 years, 100-200 IU/daily; and greater than 10 years, 200-400 IU/daily. Vitamin K supplementation may be given at the following dosages: Ages 0-12 months-2.5 mg/week or 2.5 mg twice weekly when on antibiotics; ages greater than one year-5 mg twice a week when on antibiotics or if high blood cholesterol is present.[1]

Researchers have found that cystic fibrosis patients show an inability to move vitamin A from the liver to the blood, resulting in a deficiency of vitamin A.[2] In some cases, this deficiency has resulted in blindness. Doctors have found that this defect can be overcome with supplementation of vitamins A and E.[3]

Drucy Borowitz, M.D., Department of Pediatrics, The Children's Hospital of Buffalo in New York, reported in *Clinical Pediatrics* that CF patients taking multivitamin supplements were better off than those who did not, recommending that specialty physicians who care for children with cystic fibrosis should screen for vitamin A and E deficiency on a yearly basis and should share this information with the patient and the primary care provider. Borowitz concluded by stating that health professionals should encourage the use of multivitamin supplements in patients with cystic fibrosis.[4]

Vitamins A and E are important for another reason. They are antioxidants. One of the most serious effects of cystic fibrosis is the massive lung cell damage. This can be overcome by supplementing with a good antioxidant formula that includes vitamins A, E and C; the minerals selenium, chromium and zinc; herbals such as garlic, ginkgo biloba, echinacea, goldenseal, and grapeseed; and the amino acids cysteine, methionine and glutathione. All have been studied and found to help battle the effects of degenerative diseases.

Ronald G. Crystal, M.D., Pulmonary Branch of the National Institutes of Health in Bethesda, Maryland, studied the use of antioxidants, and glutathione in particular, in limiting tissue cell damage in CF patients. He advocates antioxidants because they both encourage the body's ability to kill infection bacteria, and protect against cell damage caused by them. He found 600 milligrams of glutathione inhaled in an aerosol two times daily for three days significantly reduced oxidation cell damage in cystic fibrosis patients.[5] Antioxidants work for cystic fibrosis the same way they work against colds. They help kill the bacteria that accumulates in thick mucus, causing sinus, ear and throat infections. To further the battle against these infections, take liquid aged garlic extract which works as an antibacterial, and antioxidants to protect the delicate mucus membranes.

For more on battling the problems associated with cystic fibrosis see the chapters on Asthma, Colds, Infections, Liver Problems and Lung Infections.

Protecting the Liver

One of the worst problems that can occur with CF is the break-down of the liver. This can be helped by nutrients that prevent fat from accumulating on it. This fat accumulation usually occurs when digestion is not complete due to a lack of digestive enzymes and which causes an inability to process fats (malabsorption).

Researchers led by Dr. John D. Lloyd-Still at Children's Memorial Hospital in Chicago discovered that infants with cystic fibrosis had too little omega-3 (fish oil) and omega-6 (nut and seed oil) fatty acids, and too much mono- and saturated fat (from meat, dairy products and processed foods). Fatty acids from oils are unsaturated, and are necessary to break up saturated fat and cholesterol, and to keep it from going where it shouldn't, like the liver. Based on his finding, Dr. Lloyd-Still recommends CF patients supplement with these oils.[6] For both omega-6 and omega-3 fats, I recommend the oils of the flaxseed and the borage. They are inexpensive, available, and optimum.

When the body becomes unable to effectively process fat, people with cystic fibrosis lose weight, energy and the immune system falters. The most important thing for the CF patient is a strong immune system. Essential fatty acids not only are vital in the processing of fat, but they boost the immune system and help restore lost weight.

Lesley J. Smith, M.D., Hospital Ste-Justine, Montreal, Canada, found in his studies that the amino acid taurine, combined with vitamin A and oils, help in this fat metabolism.[7]

In the *Journal of Nutritional Medicine*, Bernard Horn, M.D., Benicia, California, stresses the importance of gamma linolenic acid for fat assimilation and to boost the immune system. Most CF patients are supplemented with linoleic acid but few are supplemented with the more important fatty acid, gamma-linolenic acid.[8] The best source of gamma linolenic acid is borage oil, which can be purchased in capsule form in health food and vitamin stores.

Dr. Horn also recommends magnesium. It is very important for the body to absorb the aforementioned essential fatty oils. When there is too much fat in the liver, magnesium cannot be absorbed. So you need the fatty acid oils to prevent fat build-up, and to allow magnesium to be taken in, and you need the magnesium so you can absorb the fatty acid oils. See the nutrient connection? Take it all to benefit all. Magnesium is also helpful for infections and asthma, common among cystic fibrosis patients.

Cystic Fibrosis-Slaying Nutrients for Children
For maximum absorption, supplements should be taken with meals.

Nutrient	Suggested Dosage	Formulation
Aged garlic extract	1 teaspoon three times daily	Liquid
Amino acids	2-4 capsules daily	Multiple formula from natural sources
Antioxidants	2 capsules daily	With selenium and grape seed extract
Borage oil	2 capsules daily	
Coenzyme Q10	1 capsule daily	With vitamin E, phospholipids and selenium
Enzymes	2 capsules twice daily	Multiple formula
Flaxseed oil	1 tablespoon daily	
Magnesium	100 mg daily	
Multi-mineral	1/2-1 ounce	In liquid solution, with vitamin B12, biotin
Multi-vitamin/mineral	1-2 tablets	Children's chewable
Vitamin A	10,000 IU daily	
Vitamin B6	50 mg daily	
Vitamin C	Individual bowel tolerance**	Chewable with bioflavonoids (quercetin, proanthocyanidins)
Vitamin E	1 capsule (400 IU) daily	d-alpha tocopherol

* To determine individual dosage, on the first day take 1,000 mg hourly until diarrhea occurs, then reduce dosage to just below that for individual daily dosage. Vitamin C is not toxic in large doses but must be taken throughout the day to benefit. Divide dosage to three or four times a day.

CHAPTER 55:

Cystitis – Bladder Infection

A dear friend of mine suffered for over ten years with bladder infections. They started just after her honeymoon and averaged three a year, increasing to five the year she was pregnant with her son. She tried everything her doctors threw at her: antibiotics, painkillers for the awful burning, and countless experimental drugs. Nothing helped until she went to see Ross Gordon, M.D., an Albany, California physician licensed in conventional medicine and educated in nutritional and preventive medicine. Dr. Gordon saw what no other wanted to see: the possibility that my friend's chronic cystitis was a result of food allergies. He asked her to fast for five days, eating nothing, including juices, only drinking distilled water and taking supplements. So that her nutrition didn't suffer and to start the healing process, he recommended a minerals in solution formula, liquid aged garlic extract, vitamin C with bioflavonoids, a B complex and a vitamin formula.

"At first my symptoms got worse," she related to me. But after the third day they cleared up. For the first time in my life, I wasn't having to go all the time," she said excitedly. "I didn't need painkillers and my yeast infection cleared up too!"

Dr. Gordon told her the fact that she lost her symptoms when she stopped eating meant food was causing her problem. But now she would have to determine to which foods she was allergic. He told her to come off the fast carefully, one food at a time, with plenty of time between each food, to find out which caused symptoms. She made a list of foods she thought caused symptoms then later a radioallergosorbent – RAST – test confirmed she was allergic to milk, eggs, tomatoes, peppers and bananas. He also told her to take lacto-bacillus acidophilus, three to four capsules twice daily for a least two to three weeks, to restore the bowel flora all those antibiotics had killed. She now reports she has been cystitis free for the past five years, and makes sure anytime she has to take antibiotics, she heads to the health food store instead of the pharmacy.

A note about water. Since flushing is so important to cleansing a bladder of infection, drinking lots of chemical-free water is impor-tant. Ever notice how your urine gets clear when you're drinking a lot of water? This is good! Your urine should only be yellow after taking vitamins, and even then, if you drink a lot of water you can clear it out. If your urine is clear, it doesn't have acids and irritants and will work best in soothing inflamed tissues and washing away bacteria.

Eliminate the Cause

Cystitis is basically an inflammation of the wall and lining of the urinary bladder. It can be caused by bacteria or irritation. It is preva-lent in women during childbearing years, especially during pregnancy. Drugs such as methenamine mandelate, nitrofurantoin, and cyclo-phosphamide can cause cystitis; with the inflammation subsiding when drug use is stopped. Symptoms of cystitis include frequent and painful urination, cloudy and/or bloody urine, and pain and tender-ness over the bladder.[1]

For years, doctors thought women get bladder infections more than men because of the close proximity of the anus to the urinary opening. As a result, we have been told to wipe from front to back–not easy to master. This assumption was refuted by a study in which stool was placed directly into the bladder of brave medical students. By the second voiding, there was no bacteria left.[2] The conclusion? Infection can be a result of improper voiding, not putting out enough urine to effectively clean the bladder and vagina.

Frequent intercourse is believed to increase the chances of getting bladder infections because it can force bacteria from the vagina into the bladder. This is sometimes referred to as "honeymoon cystitis." Make sure the bladder is full before urinating after sex. An overly large diaphragm or contraceptive sponge has also been blamed for cystitis, as it can obstruct the bladder neck and prevent you from completely emptying the bladder. Contraceptive foams, jellies and creams can cause bladder irritation, as can douches and feminine deodorants.

Dr. Christiane Northrup, a holistic physician practicing in Yarmouth, Maine recommends her patients eliminate all sources of caffeine in the form of coffee, chocolate, tea and caffeinated sodas since it's a major bladder irritant. Women who ingest a lot of caffeine often think they have an infection when they don't, since the burning is due to the irritation. It's also important to avoid strong spices, such as curry and hot peppers, which can also irritate the bladder.[3]

Vitamin C for all Infections

Vitamin C is known to prevent infections, treat them, and even prevent the pain that follows any injury to the body. If you work with your hands, and find yourself with frequent cuts, scrapes and skin injuries, try a lotion that contains vitamin C. Vitamin C applied topically will help prevent infection.

Stanford University's Robert Cathcart III, M.D., has successfully treated over 15,000 patients with massive doses of vitamin C; curing viral pneumonia, mononucleosis, influenza, colds, hepatitis, shingles, and cold sores with this method. He has developed a guideline for practical application of vitamin C which he refers to as "bowel tolerance."

He found that the individual's own body will determine how much vitamin C it requires. The cutoff point is determined by the onset of diarrhea.

Vitamin C for cystitis and other genito-urinary disorders was first discovered by the late Dr. Irving Stone during his 40 years of experiments with this vitamin, also known as ascorbic acid. Two grams – 2,000 milligrams – taken by mouth every two hours permits the vitamin C to accumulate in the urine, where it soothes and heals inflammation and detoxifies poisons.

In an amazing discovery, vitamin C has been found to be helpful in the continuing battle against bacteria that have become immune to antibiotics. For more on this incredible story, see the Infections chapter.

When you target vitamin C as a supplement, choose a formulation that includes bioflavonoids from green tea and grape seed extract. Bioflavonoids are potent anti-inflammatories. They reduce swelling while they act on the immune system, and they enhance the healing properties of vitamin C. An article in *The Lancet* (November 13, 1993) reported on a study that showed bioflavonoids to be potent antibacterial and antiviral substances.

Prostatitis and urinary tract infections have been known to respond to vitamins A, B complex, C, E, beta carotene and the bioflavonoids.6

Dr. Garry Gordon, in Tempe, Arizona, recommends a combination of vitamin C to bowel tolerance, garlic, and 500,000 IU of vitamin A for two to three days.

Combining vitamin E with A boosts the benefit so smaller amounts can be taken, and beta carotene, a vitamin A precursor (meaning it converts into vitamin A in the body), can be taken with vitamin A to boost the benefit. Beta carotene can be taken in as high a dose as needed, without side effects.

Botanical Remedies

If you have a bladder infection, don't drink cranberry juice. It's like putting out a fire with gasoline. It's the acid in the urine on inflamed tissues that causes the burning sensation. Cranberry juice can prevent an infection, but will only inflame a current one. Instead, try one-quarter teaspoon of baking soda in water or corn silk tea which contains silica.[7] Despite this logic, I still see just about everybody else recommending cranberries or unsweetened cranberry juice. I think what makes sense here is differentiating between bacteria in the bladder and bladder irritation. Obviously, given time, an infection will cause irritation. However, in cases where the presence of bacteria, and the start of infection, is diagnosed before pain (inflammation) starts, it would seem likely that cranberries and vitamin C, anything that acidifies the urine and kills the bacteria, would help. As long as the acid doesn't cause more inflammation and irritation, it should be safe to use.

Corn silk tea appears to flush poisons from the urethra, bladder and kidneys, bringing about healing. It can be made by boiling a handful of dried, brown corn silk for 15 minutes to assure sterility. After cooling, it is drinkable.[8] You can get corn silk from the field or your supermarket.

Horsetail, another source of silica, is an old folk remedy used for centuries to normalize irritated bladders. Rather than count on irradiated encapsulated horsetail, supplement your silica using a formula of minerals in solution.

I mentioned another folk remedy to a friend with cystitis: garlic. She began chopping and eating four to six cloves of garlic a day, despite the odor. Not long ago she wrote me a note that said, "After a week of eating garlic daily, my cystitis has disappeared. So has my husband."

One way I assure getting my garlic and still keeping my friends is by taking *odorless* garlic extract in liquid form. Six to eight squirts from a squeeze bottle in half glass of water three times daily have cleared up my rare bouts of cystitis within several days. Not only can it reduce inflammation, but is a powerful antimicrobial, helpful to combat any viral or bacterial infection.

Cystitis Smashing Nutrients
For maximum absorption, supplements should be taken with meals.

Nutrient	Suggested Dosage	Formulation
Acidophilus	At least four billion flora daily on an empty stomach, three times daily	
Aged garlic extract	2 teaspoons three times daily	Liquid
Antioxidants	4 capsules daily*	With selenium and grape seed extract
Echinacea	250 mg daily for a maximum of three weeks	
Enzymes	2 capsules twice daily	Multiple formula
Fiber	8 tablets daily	Psyllium, with herb hyssop
Multi-vitamin/mineral	6 caplets daily	Freeze-dried plant sources
Multi-mineral	2-4 ounces daily	In liquid solution, with vitamin B12, biotin
Purified water	2 gallons daily	
Vitamin C	Individual bowel tolerance**	With bioflavonoids (quercetin, proanthocyanidins)

* The FDA recommends that pregnant women not exceed 10,000 IU of vitamin A daily.

** To determine individual dosage, on the first day take 1,000 mg hourly until diarrhea occurs, then reduce dosage to just below that for individual daily dosage. Vitamin C is not toxic in large doses but must be taken throughout the day to benefit. Divide dosage to three or four times a day.

CHAPTER 56:

Dandruff

In 1814, Lord Byron looked across a ballroom and was bedazzled by Lady Wilmot Horton. "She walks in beauty, like the night," his poem began. Thank goodness for art. Suppose Byron had been a dermatologist. Then we'd read: "She walks in a swirling cloud of tiny, dead bits of skin that she is continually shedding."

Sit perfectly still and you shed more than a million flakes of skin every hour; scratch, or dry off with a towel, or undress, and the flurry becomes a downpour. The flakes come off in tiny clusters too small to see – usually. On the scalp, where there is more shedding than elsewhere, flakes can get trapped by hair and oil, eventually falling off in large, conspicuous clumps. That's dandruff.

If you are reading this chapter it is likely you have dandruff and the shampoos on the market aren't helping, or are giving you a scalpache. Some of the ingredients in these shampoos can do more harm than good because first you must identify exactly what is causing your itchy scalp and dry flaky scales.

Dandruff affects approximately 50 million Americans. Last year, consumers spent more than $300 million on products to control the condition. It isn't serious or life-threatening, but for those who suffer from this minor medical malady, it can be annoying and embarrassing.

Dandruff as a Yeast Infection

The precise cause of dandruff is the subject of debate among physicians. It is possible that among some sufferers, their dandruff is caused by a yeast-like fungus, Pityrosporum ovale, which occurs naturally on everyone's scalp. An overabundance causes inflammation; skin cells overproduce, stick together in clumps, and fall off as flakes.

Pityrosporum is a yeast which accounts for about 46 percent of normal scalp flora. In dandruff sufferers, the Pityrosporum accounts for more than 74 percent.[1]

Why does this overabundance occur? Why do yeast infections in general occur? If you suddenly get dandruff following the use of antibiotics, consider this yeast the probable cause. It will cause candida, athlete's foot and our pal dandruff. Antibiotics kill off all bacteria, the good and the bad. Without the good, the bad eventually proliferate, inviting fungus infections. Keep in mind that antibiotics are also found in the food supply because antibiotic supplements are given to animals as treatment for diseases and as food additives.

Yeast needs two more things to grow: moisture and warmth. Dandruff starts when stress or environment or another factor makes the sebaceous glands on the scalp speed up sebum (skin oil) production. The sebum moves out onto the surface of the scalp, and the composition of the scalp changes. Pityrosporum ovale starts to overgrow in the oil and it starts inflammation. Skin cells are overproduced, stick together in clumps and fall off, causing the flaking. The itchiness is caused by the irritation of the scalp. Dandruff is born.

An article in the *Journal of the American Academy of Dermatology* reported that yeast infections of the scalp are most common in temperate and tropical countries, and is exaggerated by heat and sweating. If you have dandruff, don't wear a synthetic fiber hat. The article also reported that 56 percent of patients with Pityrosporum orbiculare, another yeast found on the skin and hair follicles also had acne.[2] Now, what do you do about it?

Simple measures such as regular shampooing will remove most of the excess scales; excessive washing, or the use of harsh detergent soaps can cause irritation and worsen the scaling. How often to wash the hair varies with the degree of "oiliness" or sebum production. A common range tolerated by most people is two to five times weekly.

The key to destroying the fungus is to "acidify" it. I recommend pouring warm apple cider vinegar over the head and wrapping it in a towel. After one hour wash the hair. Vitamin E oil applied to the scalp nightly for three weeks is also suggested. Selenium-based anti-dandruff shampoos act as an antifungal agent. Read the labels.[3]

Dry Skin Dandruff

Since most people with dandruff find their symptoms intensify in the winter, a logical assumption is that the dry air is contributing to the problem. In fact, mild dandruff can be caused by a dry scalp. Unsaturated fatty acids are essential for all cell formation, including skin cells. A deficiency of these nutrients may be responsible for this type of dandruff.

The best sources of unsaturated fatty acids, also coined essential fatty acids or EFAs, are contained in the seed oils flax, pumpkin, soy and walnut. Cod liver oil is also an EFA. Keep in mind that essential fatty acids are destroyed by heat, so if you think you're going to get them from fried food, think again. The best way to eat these essential oils is with vinegar on salads. Try it! You'd be surprised how good walnut oil tastes in a nutty, fruity salad.

Borage oil is an essential fatty acid that has such a reputation for skin care that the French put it in their skin care products. It contains gamma linolenic acid, the best source of EFAs, and can be found in health food stores.

Pantothenic acid, one of the B vitamins, is required for the proper balance of fats and oils in the body, and is essential for proper skin function. Without it, the skin loses the ability to produce the sebum needed to moisten it. Sebum is the oil created by the body to make the skin waterproof and to lubricate it. It's what makes the skin and hair feel greasy.

Foods rich in pantothenic acid include brewer's yeast, legumes, whole grains, egg yolk and salmon. Don't worry that too much of these foods will give you oily skin or hair. God's natural healing gifts work in tune with the body He created. If you want to supplement with this nutrient, be sure and take a B complex formula with it.

Seborrheic Dermatitis

It's funny how commercials can educate. If you are a television junky, you may remember the words seborrhea when describing dandruff. Dandruff is really a symptom. Seborrhea, psoriasis, eczema, dermatitis are all problems that can cause dandruff. Usually, though, they are first noticed on the skin, not the scalp. Since I have chapters on psoriasis and eczema, I'll refer you to them for these problems. Here, I'll cover seborrhea.

Seborrhea starts with scaly bumps that crust into scales or patches of dead skin, and may begin in infancy as cradle cap which never really goes away.

An experimental study revealed that seborrhea sicca occurred when patients were deficient in vitamin B6 (pyroxidine). When researchers applied a vitamin B6 ointment to affected areas, significant improvement was noted.[4]

Vitamin E has been found to be helpful for this type of dandruff also. In an experimental study, 43.5 percent of patients were greatly improved or cured with vitamin E.[5]

Dandruff-Diminishing Nutrients
For maximum absorption, take supplements with meals.

Nutrient	Suggested Dosage	Formulation
Aged garlic extract	1 teaspoon three times daily	Liquid
Borage oil	2 capsules daily	
Flaxseed oil	1 tablespoon daily	
Multi-mineral	3-4 ounces daily	In liquid solution, with vitamin B12, biotin
Multi-vitamin/mineral	6 caplets daily	Freeze-dried plant sources
Vitamin C	Individual bowel tolerance*	With bioflavonoids (quercetin, proanthocyanidins)

* To determine individual dosage, on the first day take 1,000 mg hourly until diarrhea occurs, then reduce dosage to just below that for individual daily dosage. Vitamin C is not toxic in large doses but must be taken throughout the day to benefit. Divide dosage to three or four times a day.

CHAPTER 57:

Depression

"Earth hath no sorrow that heaven cannot heal."
–Thomas Moore

When life is a parade and you keep getting run over by the floats, don't despair. Nothing lasts forever, including depression. Clinical depression is not a jail sentence, nor is it a message to others to tread softly. It is an imbalance of brain chemicals that can be righted. And while depression can be as debilitating and damaging to everyday existence as any life-threatening illness, it can be alleviated.

What To Look For

People with depression have recurring sadness, crying spells, inability to sleep or get out of bed, and a loss of interest, motivation and pleasure in day-to-day activities. They simply give up and let the world go on without them. One important symptom of depression is drug and alcohol addiction as the sufferer looks for something to deaden the pain.

After years of therapy, my friend finally found a cure for his depression: he cries a lot.

Depression can also cause a wide variety of symptoms that resemble those of physical ailments. In a four-year study, doctors at Massachusetts General Hospital, Boston, found fatigue to be the single most frequent symptom of patients diagnosed with depression. Sometimes patients felt so exhausted they could not get through their daily work.

Headaches are another symptom of depression. In studying 423 patients with depression, Seymour Diamond, M.D., director of the Diamond Headache Clinic in Chicago, found that 84 percent complained of headaches. Dr. Diamond also found that 75 percent of depressed patients lost weight – from five to 20 pounds. Other symptoms included breathing difficulty, dizziness, weakness, urinary disturbance, palpitations and nausea.

Mask the Pain or Cure the Cause

Once the late Dr. Carlton Fredericks gave me his candid opinion of mood-elevating drugs as opposed to vitamins and minerals in coping with emotional disorders such as depression.

"Drugs hide the symptoms, and nutrients usually remove the cause," he said.

Anyone who suffers from depression may at first accept the crutch of doctor-prescribed mood-elevating drugs or antidepressants, but he or she is much better served by concentrating on eliminating the cause rather than masking the pain. Fortunately, psychiatrists now realize that all depression is not caused by emotional conflicts and that such over-simplifications are only for the over-simple. In fact, many psychiatrists now add nutrition to their therapy.

And why not? Sigmund Freud, the father of psychoanalysis, predicted that biologic or physiologic therapy would someday prove to be more effective in coping with emotional illness than psychotherapy. Carl Jung agreed.

Amino Acids – Key to the Cure

When it seems like every time you go to smell the roses, someone has fertilized them, look to brain-boosting amino acids.

All antidepressant drugs work by affecting amino acids, which act as chemical signals in the brain. By directly manipulating the levels of some amino acids, it is possible to treat mild and moderate depression without the side effects associated with antidepressant therapy. Eric Braverman, M.D., author of *The Healing Nutrients Within*, says that a high percentage of depressed patients respond to the amino acids phenylalanine, tyrosine or tryptophan. Phenylalanine and tyrosine help create epinephrine and norepinephrine, and tryptophan is used to make serotonin, potent chemical messengers between nerve cells in the brain. Braverman recommends depressed people not take amino acids in pill form without the supervision of a nutrition-oriented physician.[1]

Dr. Braverman and the late Carl C. Pfeiffer, M.D., Ph.D., called tryptophan the "single most-studied nutrient" in today's research-oriented psychiatric community. Drs. Pfeiffer and Braverman believed tryptophan is valuable in treating mental disorders and in controlling pain.

If you are dieting to lose weight and blame your depression on your scale, reconsider. Just remember – to other people, your side looks greener.

Researchers at the Royal Edinburgh Hospital in Scotland and the University of Oxford, England, found that after three weeks on a standard reducing diet, 16 men and women showed a significant drop in blood levels of tryptophan. Low levels of tryptophan and serotonin, the researchers note, have been linked to depression.

Melvyn Werbach, M.D., author of *Healing Through Nutrition* (HarperCollins, 1993), recommends two grams of L-tryptophan three times daily or 25 milligrams of 5-Hydroxytryptophan at mealtime. Then increase as tolerated over 10 to 14 days to 75 mg, three times daily with meals. He says low levels of tryptophan have been found in international studies to be associated with high rates of suicide.

Many thousands of doctors and patients have used tryptophan successfully for panic attacks, and as a natural tranquilizer, pain killer, sedative, brain chemistry normalizer and sleep remedy. British physician Dr. Shelagh Axford uses tryptophan to treat patients with a long history of resistant depression at the "Tryptophan Monitoring Clinic" at St. Andrew's Day Hospital, Thorpe, Norwich. He reported in the *British Journal of Psychiatry* that in all patients except one there was a noticeable improvement in mood, with no reported side effects.[2] Natural tryptophan is currently available in some amino acid formulas.

Tryptophan works most efficiently in the presence of plenty of vitamin B6. Women who take oral contraceptives need a minimum of 20 mg of vitamin B6 daily in order to metabolize tryptophan normally.

A deficiency of certain amino acids that are precursors to neurotransmitters – chemicals that relay signals from one nerve cell to another – can contribute to depression. Examples of these necessary amino acids are: L-phenylalanine and L-tyrosine. These two nutrients at 500 to 1,000 mg a day for a two week period have been shown to lift depression in many patients. However, I should warn you: phenylalanine in large doses can cause the blood pressure to rise, sometimes appreciably, and is best used with the guidance of a nutrition-oriented medical doctor.

DLPA, a combination of two forms of phenylalanine, is safer than many drugs commonly prescribed for pain and depression and is just as effective. Dr. Arnold Fox, former assistant clinical professor of medicine at the University of California, Irvine, and author of the book *DLPA to End Chronic Pain and Depression*, suggests people take 375 to 400 mg of DLPA – DL-phenylalanine – with each meal. It's available in most vitamin stores and some drugstores. He recommends you check with your doctor before taking it.

Dr. Daniel Asimus, medical director of the Persistent Pain Program at Glendale Adventist Medical Center in California, has treated more than 100 patients with DLPA and has found it to be quite helpful for the treatment of chronic pain and depression.

Dr. H.L. Newbold, author of *Mega Nutrients for Your Nerves*, recommends L-glutamine to fight fatigue and depression. Dr. Newbold advises those who just want a potential lift begin with 200 milligrams three times a day, for a week, increasing to 400 milligrams three times a day the second week. L-glutamine is available as a food supplement in health food stores.

Low Blood Sugar Can Mean Low Spirits

I tried dieting once. It was the worst three hours of my life. The hardest part of dieting is not watching what you eat, it's watching what other people eat!

A prominent Jacksonville, Florida physician, Dr. Stephen Gyland, studied 600 hypoglycemic patients and found that 77 percent had symptoms of depression.

In people with low blood sugar, or hypoglycemia, their level of blood sugar (glucose) is too low because the body processes sugars and starches (carbohydrates) in a faulty way. A person eats a meal top heavy in carbohydrates or a junk food snack rich in refined sugar and his or her blood sugar soars, then, a few hours later, plummets.

Hypoglycemia can be caused by many things: a deficiency of certain vitamin B complex fractions – mainly B1, B2 and niacin, essentials for efficient carbohydrate metabolism; deficiencies of protein, pantothenic acid and B2 (making it difficult to impossible for the liver to remove excess insulin), continuous stress, food allergies and low thyroid function (hypothyroidism). Excessive dieting can also be a cause of hypoglycemia. I have a friend who thinks white rice is diet food. We call him Uncle Ben. See my chapter Weight Loss for the healthy way to diet.

British physician Martin L. Budd, N.D., D.O., reports that low blood sugar – he calls it reactive hypoglycemia – almost always is accompanied by a personality disorder, and that patients with symptoms of depression have shown improvement or have been cured with nutritional treatment.[3] For details on what to do about hypoglycemia, see my chapter on Low Blood Sugar.

Smile with Good Nutrition

Certain B vitamins are deficient in patients with severe depression. The B vitamins have a major role in the central nervous system.[4]

Large amounts of B vitamins, including B12, choline and lecithin, when combined with pantothenic acid (B5), serve as precursors to the neurotransmitter acetylcholine, and are essential to good mental health. However, in high potencies this formula is best used with a qualified physician's guidance. If these nutrients are taken by a manic-depressive in the depressed state, for example, it could plunge the person into a long-term profound depression.[5]

A McGill University study of depressed patients found that their levels of folic acid, another B vitamin, were far lower than those of medically ill patients. This was also borne out in research at the Royal Victoria Hospital in Montreal. This indicates that a lack of folic acid could contribute to depression.[6]

Best known for preventing scurvy and protecting against colds and other respiratory ailments, vitamin C can also ward off depression. Depression is actually the early signs of nutritional depletion.

A copper deficiency can cause depression, and three out of four Americans are deficient in it. Copper activates neurotransmitters for pleasure and energy, and 4-5 milligrams at bedtime can increase energy levels. A warning, however – copper must be accompanied by zinc to be effective. It is always best to take minerals in a multi-mineral formula because of the various interactions between them. Choose a formula in solution for maximum absorbability.

Various nutrients help to manage depression: niacinamide (1,000 mg 3x daily) vitamins B6, B12, folic acid – among the B family of vitamins – vitamin C and kelp (as well as thyroid hormone when kelp doesn't work.) Sometimes any one of these nutrients can chase away depression. Sometimes all of them are necessary.

Anti-Depressants

Robert C. Atkins, M.D., a New York cardiologist, uses an anti-depressant formula for his patients which includes 150 milligrams vitamin B6, 100 mg niacinamide, 25 mg niacin, 300 mg vitamin C, 100 mg choline, 15 mg zinc, 5 mg manganese, 400 micrograms of folic acid (another B vitamin), 100 mcg of vitamin B12 and 300 mg of L-tryptophan.[7]

A vitamin B12 (cobalamin) deficiency is a real bogey man – especially in the over-60 crowd. It can produce psychosis, severe memory loss, impaired abstract thinking skills, mental confusion, delusions, hallucinations and even brain and spinal cord degeneration (causing numbness). Low blood levels of the vitamin are found in one-third of hospitalized psychiatric patients suffering from depression and dementia, according to a Denmark study.[8] In addition, a B12 deficiency may inhibit the brain's use of glucose (the gasoline which energizes the brain) and hinder production of acetylcholine, which is vital to brain and memory function.

In an article in the *New England Journal of Medicine*, Dr. John Lindenbaum and colleagues reported on a study of 369 New York City hospital patients with documented cobalamin deficiency. Over a 17-year period, over half developed problems with the nervous system. The symptoms included memory loss, tingling and numbness of the fingers and toes, walking difficulties and dementia. The majority of the cases improved with B12 supplementation.[9]

A lack of B12 in the diet is not the only threat to your health. B12 absorption is compromised by many things, including intestinal ailments. For more on this malabsorption issue, see the chapter Malabsorption.

J. MacDonald Holmes, a British neurologist, examined the case studies of 25 patients with B12 deficiencies and found *all* of them had mental problems such as confusion and memory deficits. Of these, an incredible half suffered from depression.[10]

B12 can even benefit people whose depression is a result of chemical poisoning. The *Journal of Neuropsychiatric and Clinical Neuro-science* reported the case of a silkscreen printer poisoned by a solvent he was using. His symptoms were tension, depression and trouble thinking straight. After six months of monthly B12 injections, his depression and irritability decreased, his temper swings diminished, and he had more energy. After a year, all his symptoms were gone.[11]

Vitamin B6 (pyroxidine) helps produce two chemical transmitters in the brain: dopamine and serotonin, which regulate moods.[12] A lack of vitamin B6 is associated with depression, hyperactivity, autism and schizophrenia.[13] Although people rarely encounter vitamin B6 insufficiency, such a problem may result if a person has a higher-than-average requirement, such as when infection or chronic disease are present. Also, B6 use and absorption may be hindered by interaction with certain chemicals, including hydrazine, the artificial coloring tartrazine (or FD&C yellow no. 5), birth control pills, or PCB's (pesticides).

Plentiful in whole grains, more than 75 percent of the B vitamins are lost in the milling of grain into flour or for cereal. Processing and heating finish the job. Thus, a diet containing large amounts of white bread, milled grains, pasta and pre-cooked rice is practically void of these vitamins.

To assure an adequate amount of vitamin B6, be sure to eat wheat germ, sunflower seeds, chickpeas, nuts, legumes, avocados, bananas, salmon, tuna and beef. And read the label! If it says processed grain, or milled grain, white or bleached flour, or doesn't say *whole* grain, don't buy it and don't eat it.

In studies at Teikyo University, Tokyo, Japan, Naotaka Hashizume, M.D., found that patients with low blood levels of magnesium suffered from depression. He saw improvements when their magnesium levels were raised even a small amount.[14]

Magnesium is so deficient among Americans that the odds are good most of us need it. A magnesium deficiency, too, can contribute to depression, and must be accompanied by vitamin B6 for maximum benefit.

An article in *Biological Psychiatry* reported that of patients hospitalized with major depression or schizophrenia, magnesium was significantly lower in those who had made suicide attempts. The authors believe magnesium has a role in regulating serotonin levels of the brain.[15]

Vitamin A is needed in the manufacture of the anti-stress hormones of the adrenal cortex and is used up under stressful conditions. Signs of vitamin A deficiency include depression, insomnia, fatigue, nerve pain in the extremities, and sore eyes.

Because it is soluble in fat rather than water, vitamin A can be toxic in excessive doses as it can accumulate in the fatty tissues of the body. It is important, therefore, to take vitamin A with other antioxidants such as vitamins E and C and the mineral selenium.

The safest way to take vitamin A is in the form of beta carotene. Foods high in this nutrient include dandelion greens, carrots, yams, kale, parsley, turnip greens, spinach, collard greens and squash. Good plant sources of this vitamin are the green and yellow vegetables. Remember, the depth of the yellow or green color is a rough guide to the amount of vitamin A in the vegetable. Carrot juice has over 2,000 milligrams of vitamin A.

What you don't eat can make a difference in your depression. Larry Christensen, Ph.D., Department of Psychology, Texas A&M University, has done research over the last ten years which shows that elimination of caffeine and processed sugar cures depression in some patients. He recommends that people with depression eliminate caffeine and sugar from their diets for at least two weeks, then carefully add one, then the other to the diet and see if symptoms recur.[16] A nutritious diet does not include either of these non-food substances so I advocate eliminating them altogether.

A word about minerals. They are hard to digest and require adequate stomach acid to be broken down. Unfortunately, one of the symptoms of stress is low stomach acid – just when you need it the most! Don't take antacids to get calcium or magnesium since they lower acid. Instead, target a mineral formula in solution. Liquid formulations provide the maximum absorption ratios.

The Thyroid Connection

Another possible cause of depression is low thyroid function. John J. Haggerty, Jr. and colleagues at the Department of Psychiatry, University of North Carolina, evaluated 16 patients with hypothyroidism and compared them to 15 control subjects with normal thyroid function. He found 56 percent of those with low thyroid function had symptoms of depression compared to 20 percent with normal thyroid function.[17] This means an incredible 76 percent of the people in this study had depression, which says a lot about the enormous need to understand the causes of this most debilitating, and, apparently, common affliction.

After reviewing numerous studies and reports on the role of the thyroid in mood disorders, Dr. Junichi Nomura, Department of Psychiatry, MIE University School of Medicine, in MIE, Japan, believes that physicians dealing with depressed patients, especially the elderly or women with PMS, should definitely have their thyroid functions tested. He also found that large amounts of thyroid hormones may be therapeutic for the treatment of depression.[18]

Watch the type of thyroid hormones you take. If they are prescribed, ask your doctor for natural thyroid instead of synthetic, which can compromise your own thyroid gland and cause nasty side effects.

The late Broda O. Barnes, M.D., Ph.D, a world-renowned thyroid authority, stated that first generation hypothyroids usually can correct their condition by taking a kelp tablet daily. Kelp is rich in iodine, the thyroid's major nutrient. Hypothyroids of the second generation or beyond can overcome depression and many other symptoms of low thyroid function by taking natural, desiccated thyroid prescribed by a physician. Add a mineral supplement that contains thyroid-important iodine.

Iodine is present in large amounts in seafood, including of course, sushi. That black paper that they wrap the rice in, it's called nori. It's nothing but pure iodine. See the chapter on Low Thyroid for more.

Depression Dismissing Nutrients
For maximum absorption, take supplements with meals.

Nutrient	Suggested Dosage	Formulation
Amino acids	4-6 capsules daily	Multiple formula from natural sources
Antioxidants	4 capsules daily*	With selenium and grapeseed extract
Borage oil	2 capsules daily	
Coenzyme Q10	2 capsules daily	With vitamin E, phospholipids and selenium
DHEA	10 mg daily	
Flaxseed oil	1 tablespoon daily	
Ginkgo biloba	60 mg daily	
Magnesium	200 mg daily	
Melatonin (adults only)	3 mg daily at bedtime	With B vitamins
Multi-mineral	3-4 ounces daily	In liquid solution, with vitamin B12, biotin
Multi-vitamin/mineral	6 caplets daily	Freeze-dried plant sources
Pregnenolone	10 mg daily 2 weeks out of the month	
Vitamin B6	100 mg daily	
Vitamin C	Individual bowel tolerance**	With bioflavonoids (quercetin, proanthocyanidins)

* The FDA recommends pregnant women not exceed 10,000 IU of vitamin A daily.

** To determine individual dosage, on the first day take 1,000 mg hourly until diarrhea occurs, then reduce dosage to just below that for individual daily dosage. Vitamin C is not toxic in large doses but must be taken throughout the day to benefit. Divide dosage to three or four times a day.

CHAPTER 58:

Diabetes (Hyperglycemia – High Blood Sugar)

"It's alright, insulin will cure it." I was talking to a close family member about her granddaughter, as she tried to blame genetic heredity on the diabetes they shared. Rather than admitting that her poor diet and habits might have something to do with it, she tried to minimize the problem by claiming insulin shots cure diabetes. Insulin doesn't in any way minimize the damage diabetes does to the body, it only controls blood sugar so you don't faint or go into a coma.

This woman is at least 200 pounds overweight, and has been in and out of hospitals so frequently her doctors use her as a case history. Her poor eating habits started early. As a child she used to keep a box of sugar cubes under her bed to snack on. By the age of 40 she had a complete set of false teeth. She also drinks too much and smokes. This is the legacy she leaves to her granddaughter, not diabetes.

Diabetes is a State of Being, Not a Lifetime Sentence

The problem with depending on insulin instead of nutrition to control diabetes is that it doesn't deal with the resultant metabolic problems that occur. Arteriosclerosis proceeds at five times the rate it does in the non-diabetic, causing a particular kind of heart disease, circulatory problems which can lead to the loss of limbs, blindness, kidney failure and early death. The only way to stop this degradation of the body is through proper supplementation, diet and exercise. It's like turning off the smoke alarm without removing the cigarette left burning in the sofa.

There are two kinds of diabetes: Type 1 and Type 2. Type 1 occurs when the pancreas loses its ability to produce insulin, for whatever reason. It used to be called juvenile diabetes because it is commonly diagnosed in childhood.

Ninety percent of those with diabetes have type 2, and it is estimated that 90 percent of them are obese. Sometimes called "adult onset diabetes," it is typically diagnosed among middle-aged, overweight, inactive people.[1]

Type 2 diabetes occurs when the insulin/glucose manages to get to the body cell wall but can't find the door because something blocks the way. This happens because of a malfunction or weakness in either the insulin or the receptors – the keyholes if you will – that are present in the body cell walls that allow the insulin "keys" to open the door and bring the glucose in. This is called "insulin sensitivity."

In either case, a lack of insulin causes glucose to build up in the bloodstream and spill over into the urine, while the body literally starves to death because the glucose doesn't get to the cells to fuel the body. Type 1 diabetics typically have to inject themselves with insulin because they are unable to produce it on their own. Important to realize is the fact that prescribed insulin does not cure the problem, only alleviates the symptoms. Careful eating and knowledgeable supplementation can help reduce the need for insulin in Type 1s. A change in diet, nutritional supplementation, weight loss and exercise can reverse the diabetic condition among Type 2s.

The Role of Sugar

Refined sugar exhausts the pancreas, which is charged with producing insulin. The definitive essay on the subject is Surgeon-Captain T.L. Cleave's book *The Saccharine Disease* (Keats Publishing Inc., 1975). Cleave shows example after example of societies in which the addition of sugar to the diet was the obvious starting point for the development of diabetes and of atherosclerosis in the epidemic proportions typical of a Western nation. Two striking examples in Cleave's global studies were in Iceland beginning in 1920 and among the nomadic Yemenite Jews. Before sugar was introduced in their cultures, there was absolutely no diabetes or atherosclerosis. Two decades after their diets became similar to ours, because sugar was added, they began to develop nearly as high an incidence of these illnesses as we have.

Another of Cleave's great contributions was the discovery of the Law of Twenty Years. In every culture he studied, it took exactly twenty years after their dietary change for the first cases of diabetes and atherosclerosis to appear. In American terms, this means that the increase in consumption of sugar and highly refined flour between 1895 and 1910 could easily be invoked to explain the beginning of the era of the heart attack and the increase in diabetes prevalence noted between 1910 and 1930. This increase has continued. In the years between 1935 and 1968 the prevalence has increased by 600 percent.

In the United States, inappropriate diet, such as the processed sugar already mentioned, is probably the major factor associated with insulin sensitivity and thus the major cause of diabetes.

The Need to Return to Our Roots

I've already talked of the Western diet relating to colon problems. Now, it comes up again relating to diabetes. Whole civilizations previously exempt from diabetes, once introduced to affluence and its accompanying Western diet high in fat and sugar, have found themselves in an epidemic of diabetes. In the American Southwest, Native American tribes the Pima and the Tohono O'odham ("People of the Desert," formerly known as the Papago), suffer from one of the highest rates of diabetes in the world, with one out of every two adults beyond age 35 afflicted with Type 2 diabetes. Fortunately, enlightenment has also found its way there, as more and more of them are throwing off the diabetes sickness by discarding the fast foods and the convenient, more sedentary ways of the modern world and returning to the seeds, nuts, berries, beans and corns of their ancestral diet. Kwa vul berries, the seeds of the ironwood tree, cholla buds, mesquite beans, acorns, and lima beans are nutritious foods that are once again appearing among Native Americans of the Southwest, restoring them to health and blood sugar fitness.[2]

What is it about our modern-day diet that contributes to obesity and diabetes? Fat, sugar and inactivity. Poor circulation from a lack of exercise causes a lack of oxygen to the cells and allows a poor diet to affect the health. Our modern diet is full of unhealthy transfatty and saturated fats. Fat in the bloodstream blocks the effectiveness of insulin and increases the chances that diabetes will lead to more severe problems. For more on the right and wrong kinds of fat, read the chapter on Arteriosclerosis. Eliminating the habits and problems that lead to arteriosclerosis will go a long way toward eliminating Type 2 diabetes, and will help lower the need for insulin in Type 1 diabetes.

By avoiding the typical high fat, high sugar and low fiber diet, it is possible to prevent and manage diabetes.

A diabetic who married a diabetic, Associate Professor Somasundaram Addanki, a biochemist and nutritionist at Ohio State University College of Medicine, says he and his wife did not develop diabetes until they left their native India and began eating the typical Western diet.

In a United Press International news story, Professor Addanki admitted to six years of diabetes and diabetic impotency before he stopped eating sugar, white flour products and fatty foods, successfully curing his ailment.

Every diabetic regardless of age or type should be in a fitness protection program. Exercise not only loses the fat but lowers blood sugar and improves the health of body cells, making them insulin sensitive. The cells of "exercising" muscles can extract glucose from the blood much more effectively than can resting muscles.

D.M. Klachko and others from the University of Missouri explored the effects of exercise by taking continuous measurement of blood sugar levels in normal and insulin-dependent diabetics during measured activity. The subjects took half-mile "walks" on a treadmill at a relatively brisk but not too strenuous pace.[3]

The little bursts of exercise took only 7-1/2 minutes, but the drop in blood sugar was substantial. The researchers found that moderate exercise had a more profound effect on blood sugar levels among those with diabetes than in normal individuals. In addition, following exercise, the blood sugar levels among those with diabetes did not rise, unlike individuals with normal levels.

A high fiber diet helps both obese and lean diabetics, according to James Anderson, M.D., noted biochemist at the University of Kentucky, who has researched high fiber diets for many years. Both groups reduced blood fats and the need for insulin through a high fiber diet.

Since the average American diet contains between 11 and 21 grams of fiber daily, some diabetics would need to double or triple their fiber intake. I suggest doing this by adding one high-fiber food a week, particularly whole grains and beans, and increasing fluid intake to help the body adjust to increased gas, a common side effect of added fiber.[4]

Outstanding fiber foods are almonds, apples, blackberries, broccoli, corn, fresh peas, kidney beans, plums, potatoes, prunes, raisins, spinach, sweet potatoes, whole wheat bread, figs and zucchini. Outstanding fiber supplements (food-derived in a formula) are psyllium, hyssop, oat bran, alfalfa, rhubarb and buckthorn. For more on fiber see the chapter on Constipation.

Mineral Solutions

Many studies have shown that certain nutrients are essential for normal blood sugar levels and insulin absorption. Among these, chromium gets star billing. Thirty-five years of research on this mega-mineral suggests a deficiency of chromium increases the risk of developing diabetes. *The Nutrition Report* reports that 13 out of 15 studies evaluating chromium supplementation's effect on diabetes show that it works by maintaining blood sugar levels with a minimum of insulin.[5] This means a Type 1 diabetic needs less insulin, and chromium may be all that's necessary to stabilize glucose levels in a Type 2 diabetic. Unfortunately, because there is not a good way to diagnose a chromium deficiency, many scientists and physicians ignore the potential benefits of chromium supplementation.

Dr. Walter Mertz has been documenting the effect of chromium on diabetes since the late '20s and to this day advocates its use. He has shown conclusively that chromium is a crucial part of a substance termed the Glucose Tolerance Factor – or GTF – which is composed of two niacin molecules (vitamin B2), the amino acids cystine, glycine and glutamic acid as well as chromium. When enough chromium is present in the diet, intestinal bacteria can manufacture GTF in the body.[6]

Dr. Richard J. Doisy, professor of biochemistry at the State University of New York, Upstate Medical Center, reported that some diabetics who required insulin shots to maintain their blood sugar at safe levels were able to get by on lower doses after taking chromium. He estimates probably one-fourth to one-half of people in the U.S. are deficient in chromium.

A general deficiency of chromium seems to exist among Americans over age 50. All children seem to be born with a sufficient level of chromium, according to an international study. In those Americans over 50, however, one in four had levels so low they could not be detected. Of the foreigners over age 50 who were checked, almost all had chromium in their tissues.

The reason for this can be found in the American diet. It is estimated that the average American consumes 150 pounds of refined sugar or sucrose annually. When a person consumes refined sugar, and refined flour for that matter, about one-fifth of chromium that is drawn to the bloodstream to aid the insulin is excreted in the urine.

If our diets contained enough chromium to make up for the loss, there would be no problem, but our diets of refined sugar and flour are not sufficient to replenish the amount lost. Refined sugar contains one-twelfth as much chromium as raw sugar, and white flour has about one-seventh as much chromium as whole wheat flour. A continuous diminishing of our bodily store of the mineral is the inevitable result.

Vanadium is a mineral also found to be beneficial for regulating glucose. According to the *Journal of Gerontology*, an Italian study found that vanadium has insulin-like effects on glucose metabolism.[7] In animal studies, insulin-deficient rats showed markedly decreased blood glucose levels when given vanadium.[8] In healthy individuals, from 100 to 300 micrograms a day is recommended. Foods lavish in vanadium are vegetable oils, whole grains, seafood and liver.[9]

The Magnesium Connection

Magnesium is at the center of all energy systems. A deficiency of this ultra-important nutrient is thought to play a role in the development of insulin resistance. A study of 45 diabetic and 12 normal children found those with insulin-dependent diabetes had lower levels of magnesium than normal children.[10]

H.M. Mather of the Department of Medicine, St. George's Hospital, London, measured the blood magnesium level in 582 consecutive diabetic patients visiting the hospital's outpatients clinic. He also measured the magnesium levels of 140 nondiabetic subjects. He found that the diabetics had a significantly lower blood magnesium level. In fact, 25 percent had lower levels than all of the controls except one.

Dr. Takeo Takemura of the Department of Internal Medicine, Osaka City University, Japan, reported to the Japan Diabetic Society that his research studies show low magnesium levels are associated with an increased incidence of diabetic retinopathy – damage to the eyes that leads to blindness, a major complication of diabetes.

Too much of either magnesium or calcium will cancel the other out. There must be equal amounts of each in order to benefit from both. If there is too much calcium in your diet, you risk a magnesium deficiency. Too much magnesium, and you lose your calcium. The same thing can happen with phosphate. Phosphates tend to lower magnesium levels even further. Phosphates are found in abundance in soft drinks and many processed foods.Foods rich in magnesium include whole grains, dark green vegetables, molasses, nuts and bone meal.

The diabetic condition itself may be the cause of mineral deficiencies. Elevated blood sugars stimulate excessive urination, which can wash essential minerals and trace elements out of the body.

Many diabetics are taking hypertensive medication and/or diuretics. Diuretics are notorious eliminators of all minerals, yet potassium is the only mineral routinely replaced.

Vitamin Needs

New research hints that a little-known B vitamin called biotin may nip the need for the injection needle if you have diabetes. An article in the *Annals of the New York Academy of Science* reports on a study in which seven insulin-dependent diabetics were removed from insulin therapy and instead treated with 16 milligrams per day of biotin or a placebo for one week. The diabetics who received nothing saw their diabetes return, while those given the biotin saw their blood glucose level drop.[11]

Japanese researchers divided 43 people with Type 2 diabetes into three groups to test high doses of biotin. One group received the supplement for a month. Another took it for two to four years. The third group added it to their usual regimen with the glucose-lowering drug glibenclamide. All groups received nine milligrams a day – that's about 1,000 times more than you'd get in an average day. All of the participants had slightly lower than average biotin levels at the study's start. The group taking biotin long-term saw the most benefits. Within two months, glucose levels fell to nearly half their original levels while insulin levels didn't budge. The single-month patients also saw glucose dip, without a change in insulin, but it rose again after treatment was stopped. Those on the drug were able to cut their doses by as much as half.[12]

The B vitamin niacin plays an important role in carbohydrate metabolism. Many refined foods consumed by Americans are depleted in niacin. So called "enriched" grains and other foods usually contain added niacinamide, which cannot be converted by the human body into niacin. In addition, most vitamin supplements contain niacinamide, rather than niacin. A small amount of niacin is necessary for blood sugar balance.[13]

Vitamin B6, pyridoxine, is another B vitamin found to be important to glucose metabolism. A vitamin B6 deficiency is known to reduce pancreatic and circulating insulin levels, and degenerative changes have been noted in the B-cells in the islets of the Langerhans of rats fed vitamin B6-deficient diets. Gestational diabetes was eliminated in pregnant women following two weeks of treatment with 100 milligrams per day of B6, and is associated with decreased retinopathy, a common diabetes complication.[14] Taken together, all of the evidence shows a vitamin B6 deficiency could be very important to preventing as well as reversing the diabetic condition.

It has been found that B6 – a fragile and easily destroyed vitamin – is not present in fatty or processed foods. Vital B6 is lost in food transportation, storage, preservation, processing and cooking. Therefore, it is essential to add a B6 vitamin supplement (at least 200 mg daily) to your diet. All the B vitamins work together so it is essential that while supplementing any one B vitamin, you include a good B complex formula to balance it out with the others.

Glucose-Regulating Foods

Before you consider foods for controlling diabetes, consider the possibility they may be *causing* it. Diabetics should be thoroughly tested for food intolerances which may contribute to the disease by causing inflammation and autoimmune destruction of the insulin-producing cells of the pancreas. Foods that often are associated with diabetes-related problems include corn, wheat, chocolate and dairy products.[15]

Once that is done, consider all the foods and plants that have a reputation for helping to prevent or control diabetes.

Broiled stems of the Mexican Opuntia cactus – the genus Opuntia Streptacantha Lemaire – help to control non-insulin dependent diabetes by lowering blood glucose and insulin levels, say Mexican scientists.[16]

Researcher Alberto C. Frati-Munari and associates at the Hospital de Especialidades in Colonia La Raza, compared two groups after a 12 hour fast – one fed broiled stems of the cactus and the other given only water. Blood glucose levels and insulin decreased in the cactus-fed group but not in the group given water.

Although they have no conclusive answer, the researchers feel that the cactus improves the effectiveness of available insulin. This cactus, whose broiled stems serve as a common food in arid parts of Mexico, can also be found in the deserts of the Southwestern United States. Ask for the plant at your health food store. Sometimes a dried version is available.

Through the years in folk medicine, legumes – beans, peas and lentils – have led the pack for controlling blood sugar. Beans are rich in soluble fiber that lower blood cholesterol and blood sugar. Half to one cup of beans per day can significantly reduce blood cholesterol levels and help control blood sugar levels of people who have Type 2 diabetes, according to Susan Kleiner, Ph.D., R.D.[17]

Research by Dr. James Anderson backs up this contention. A cup of cooked navy or pinto beans daily slashed the need for insulin injections by some 38 percent in one group of test patients. Dr. Anderson theorizes this fare works because beans make for such a slow rise in blood sugar that less insulin is needed, and further, contributes to the production of more insulin cell receptors. This gives insulin more doors into the body cells. Dr. Anderson says that in persons who are on less than 30 cc of insulin a day, the addition of legumes in the diet could mean eliminating it altogether.

In a study to determine soybeans' influence on lowering cholesterol, biochemist Andrew P. Goldberg of Washington University found that soybeans also keep insulin levels under control.

People with high blood sugar should eat at least two meals a day of legumes. Good ideas are lentil stew or soup for breakfast and pinto beans for dinner. Lentils are complex carbohydrates, excellent for controlling blood sugar and encouraging an energetic start to the day. And if weight is a problem, lentils can control the appetite as well.

Carbohydrates in the beans are fermented by anaerobic bacteria in the intestines to form hydrogen, carbon dioxide and methane gases, some of which have to be passed from the system. To remove some of the troublesome carbohydrates, soak dry beans in water for three to five hours and discard this water before cooking. To retain all the nutrients, use this water and eat alone.

A diet high in complex carbohydrates is highly recommended for people with high blood sugar. Ideally, food sources should be raw, organic and unaltered. Foods in this category are all whole grains, beans, fruits, vegetables, nuts and seeds. Look for bread and cereal with whole grains and no additives. Better still, make your own. Trail mix, if everything in it is raw and unchemicalized, is an excellent source of nuts and seeds. Watch out for the yogurt raisins, though – if you believe it's yogurt I have got some beachfront property in Arizona to sell you. Raw almonds are good, refined almond paste is not. Don't buy the quick oat hot cereal. Purchase whole oats at the health food store and cook them yourself.

Aloe vera juice, a traditional diabetic remedy in Arabia, has been found to lower blood sugar in patients with diabetes. Researchers at Fujita Health University in Japan found when aloe was given to diabetic patients, their fasting blood glucose level went down.[18]

The most important thing to remember about diabetes is that you are not helpless. You are not a slave to your hypodermic needle or to your doctor. You can take control of your life and make a difference in it.

Glucose-Lowering Nutrients
For maximum absorption, take supplements with meals.

Nutrient	Suggested Dosage	Formulation
Antioxidants	4 capsules daily*	With selenium and grapeseed extract
Borage oil	2 capsules daily	
Coenzyme Q10	2 capsules daily	With vitamin E, phospholipids and selenium
Flaxseed oil	1 tablespoon daily	
Ginkgo biloba	60 mg daily	
Lecithin	One tablespoon with meals	
Magnesium	200 mg daily	
Melatonin (adults only)	3 mg daily at bedtime	With B vitamins
Multi-mineral	3-4 ounces daily	In liquid solution, with vitamin B12, biotin
Multi-vitamin/mineral	6 caplets daily	Freeze-dried plant sources
Vitamin C	Individual bowel tolerance**	With bioflavonoids (quercetin, proanthocyanidins)

* The FDA recommends pregnant women not exceed 10,000 IU of vitamin A daily.

** To determine individual dosage, on the first day take 1,000 mg hourly until diarrhea occurs, then reduce dosage to just below that for individual daily dosage. Vitamin C is not toxic in large doses but must be taken throughout the day to benefit. Divide dosage to three or four times a day.

CHAPTER 59:

Diabetic Retinopathy

"An eye can threaten like a loaded and levelled gun, or it can insult like hissing or kicking; or, in its altered mood, by beams of kindness, it can make the heart dance for joy."

–Ralph Waldo Emerson

Eyesight: oh, what a shame it would be to unnecessarily lose this most powerful of influences.

According to the American Diabetes Association, diabetic retinopathy is a general term for all disorders of the retina caused by diabetes. What it means to the diabetic is that he or she has been unsuccessful in controlling blood sugar levels, and the disease has started to break down the body.

In the early stages of retinopathy, capillaries balloon to form pouches. Although vision loss does not occur at this stage, the capillary walls may lose their ability to control the passage of substances between the blood and the retina. As a result, the retina becomes swollen and fatty deposits form within it. If this swelling affects the center of the retina, the problem is called macular edema. This can cause some vision loss.

In later stages, the blood vessels are so damaged that they close off. In response, new blood vessels start growing in the retina. These new vessels are weak and can leak blood, blocking vision, a condition called vitreous hemorrhage. The damage can also cause scar tissue to grow. When the scar tissue shrinks, it can distort the retina or pull it out of place (retinal detachment). The worst part is, the retina can be damaged before a person notices any symptoms or changes in vision.[1]

The best thing you can do to prevent getting retinopathy is to control your blood sugar. People who keep their blood glucose levels closer to normal are less likely to have retinopathy and to have milder forms if they do. See my chapter Diabetes for help in this endeavor.

The longer you have diabetes, the more likely you are to have retinopathy. It is estimated that after 60 years, 98 percent of diabetics will have some form of retinopathy, 42 percent will have macular edema and 28 percent will experience severe vision loss.[2]

The good news is that even severe cases of retinopathy can regress and vision can improve through diet and supplements alone!

Antioxidants for the Diabetic Eye

Unless this is the first chapter in this book you've read, you should be familiar with the term free radical by now. Barring a lengthy explanation, all you really need to know is that it occurs over time, is worsened by oxygen and chemicals, and effectively destroys your body tissues, including the delicate eye tissues. Cholesterol, or fat, can increase free radical damage. When you think about it, it becomes obvious. Fat, whether clogging your drain pipes, your heart arteries, or you eye capillaries, not only obstructs circulation, but invites bacteria, which feed on it and produce vile acids. These acids encourage free radical damage. Not surprisingly, studies have found that high blood levels of cholesterol can cause diabetic retinopathy. Japanese researchers conducted a study of 104 noninsulin dependent diabetic patients. They found that those with high cholesterol levels were more at risk for retinopathy.[3]

Fat is such an important factor in retinopathy that patients have reversed the disorder just by eating less of it. In one study, cited in

Postgraduate Medicine, 64 percent of 44 retinopathy patients showed improvement after going on a low fat diet. Impressive alone, but eight of the patients eventually saw their retinopathy completely disappear![4]

This would explain the studies that show antioxidants – nutrients that reverse the oxidative, free radical damage of fat and cholesterol – help reverse diabetic retinopathy.

A preliminary trial conducted by researchers at the Department of Human Nutrition and Health, Hoffman-La Roche & Co., Ltd., in Basel, Switzerland found the antioxidants beta carotene, vitamins C and E, and selenium not only helped stop the retinal degeneration of diabetic patients, but in some cases reversed the damage.[5]

In *E: The Essential Vitamin*, Herbert Bailey reported on a Japanese study in which Drs. Kojima, Okaijima and Suzuki gave 90 to 180 milligrams of vitamin E daily to 38 patients with diabetic retinopathy. After 19 to 24 months on this therapy, an incredible 67 percent of all patients reported significant improvement in their condition.[6]

Some eye doctors believe vitamin E helps to treat a detached retina. For retinal nerve hemorrhages, Gershon M. Lesser, M.D., has found vitamins A, C and E, along with zinc and omega-3, useful.[7]

See Better with Vitamin C and Bioflavonoids

Anthocyanosides are a class of bioflavonoids found in fruits and vegetables, most notably blueberries, grapes and bilberries. They are known for their anti-inflammatory, oxygen-quenching, antioxidant and tissue enhancement properties. Aldose reductase is an enzyme believed to be the culprit in the damaging effect of diabetes. Aldose reductase transforms excess blood sugar into an alcohol sugar the body can't burn, and this accumulates in nerve cells and damages them. This is one of the things believed to contribute to diabetic retinopathy. Researchers have found one bioflavonoid that not only reverses free radical damage, reduces inflammation and boosts tissue health, but inhibits the accumulation of aldose reductase. Call it the diabetic friend. Call it quercetin. It is available in health food stores, vitamin formulas and in yellow and red onions.

In some cases, retinopathy occurs when the delicate capillaries of the eyes aren't strong enough to avoid hemorrhaging and leakage, leading some researchers to contend it is not high blood pressure as much as poor capillary strength that causes retinopathy and loss of the retina. Studying what could reverse this, researchers hit on vitamin C and bioflavonoids – rutin from buckwheat most specifically – as compounds that can strengthen capillaries and prevent leaking.

In a case history, a 72-year-old woman with sudden loss of vision in her left eye experienced dramatic restoration of vision with rutin. Drs. Donegan and Thomas noted in the *American Journal of Opthalmology* that 75 percent of cases of capillary leakage can be restored to normal by using 500 milligrams a day of rutin, and that rutin universally improves capillary strength, stops the progression of retinopathy and benefits diabetics in general.[8]

Dr. L.J. Thomas found that with a prescribed dose of 60 mg of rutin four times a day, 22 percent of the cases of diabetic retinopathy improved and 30.6 percent were stabilized over a period of seven to 34 months.[9]

Another bioflavonoid found effective in preventing or reversing retinopathy is catechin, found in green tea leaves. It was shown to reduce capillary fragility three times better than rutin, and quercetin even better than that. Quercetin and catechin are both free radical fighters and when combined with vitamin C, create the best offense and defense teams. In one study, researchers noted that guinea pigs given low levels of vitamin C showed the same blood levels as those not given vitamin C – until they were also given catechin – then the levels shot up.[10]

Because of their ability to fight free radicals, reduce inflammation and strengthen capillaries, bioflavonoids are literally the "finger in the dike" of diabetic retinopathy. They are the blue and red pigments found in plums, berries, apples, grapes, red onions and pomegranates. They are the citrus rind of oranges, grapefruits and lemons. And they are the chlorophyll in dark green vegetables and leaves.

The Good Fats

In recent years, researchers have learned that an omega-3 fatty acid, docosahexaenoic acid (DHA), is the most prominent polyunsaturated fat in the retina, and that a lack of it in the diabetic diet may contribute to retinopathy. Ironically, chronically high blood sugar in diabetics blocks an enzyme that processes omega-3 from food sources into DHA, thus making the effects of any omega-3 deficiency worse.[11]

Interestingly, omega-3 and omega-6 fatty acids also help assimilate cholesterol in the body, so it can't accumulate in tissues and cause damage.

You can find omega-3 in flaxseed oil, cod liver oil; and in cold water fish such as trout, mackerel, sardines, tuna and eel. It is believed eating foods rich in omega-3 may prevent or improve diabetes, cancer tumors and low blood sugar. Omega-3 fatty acids are also found in fresh dark green vegetables like broccoli, kale, collards and Swiss chard.

Also found to benefit is omega-6 fatty acids, most especially borage oil, which contains the highest amount of gamma linolenic acid (GLA). Very large doses of GLA have been shown to reduce by two thirds the risk of eye disease over a period of about six years. David F. Horrobin, of the Efamol Research Institute, Kentville, Nova Scotia, has done extensive research on the benefits of GLA and has found it to reverse a variety of problems diabetics typically experience, especially retina problems.[12]

The amino acid acetyl-L-carnitine, has also been found to help prevent and restore problems with the eye retina. After performing double blind studies, researchers at the Eye Clinic at Catholic University in Rome concluded that carnitine can be helpful in cases of retinal dysfunction.[13]

Magnanimous Minerals

Low blood levels of the mineral magnesium is also associated with diabetic retinopathy. In the medical journal *Diabetes Research and Clinical Practice*, Dr. Abdelaziz Elamin, M.D., reports that diabetic retinopathy patients have the lowest magnesium levels, and that supplementing with magnesium can help diabetic patients reduce the damaging effect of their condition.[14]

In another study, blood magnesium levels were evaluated in 100 Type II diabetics, 40 without retinopathy and 60 with various stages of retinopathy. Magnesium levels were lower in diabetics than controls and those with retinopathy had significantly lower amounts than those without retinopathy.[15]

Once again, we have a connection to cholesterol and heart disease. Doctors use magnesium injections to counter high blood pressure, strokes and heart disease. It works by dilating the capillaries so blood runs faster and smoother and can pull out cholesterol deposits. It's also important for circulation and blockages, *and* sufficient amounts are needed to convert blood sugar into energy.

Magnesium is nature's calcium traffic cop, directing calcium to the parts of the body where it is needed, and making sure it doesn't go where it doesn't belong. Since every tissue in the diabetics' body is shown to have increased levels of calcium,[16] magnesium is essential so that calcium doesn't contribute to blockages. Because of the high absorption rate of minerals in solution, and deficiency of magnesium in the diet, the ratio of magnesium and calcium in solution should be four to one, respectively. If there is too much calcium in your diet, you risk a magnesium deficiency. Too much magnesium, and you lose your calcium. The same thing can happen with phosphate. Phosphates tend to lower magnesium levels even further. Phosphates are found in abundance in soft drinks and many processed foods.

If you decide to supplement with magnesium, choose a multi-mineral formula that has both magnesium and calcium, and zinc and copper. In the body, zinc is at its highest in the male sex organs and the retina. It is an antioxidant, and a notorious wound-healer. Copper is needed to balance out zinc, and in its own right, an excellent cholesterol-lowerer. Choose a formula in solution so absorption isn't compromised by hard pills or too little stomach acid or digestive enzymes.

Eye-Restoring Nutrients
For maximum absorption, take supplements with meals.

Nutrient	Suggested Dosage	Formulation
Antioxidants	4 capsules daily*	With selenium and grapeseed extract
Bilberry	100 mg twice daily	
Borage oil	2 capsules daily	
Coenzyme Q10	2 capsules daily	With vitamin E, phospholipids and selenium
Flaxseed oil	1 tablespoon daily	
Ginkgo biloba	60 mg daily	
Lecithin	One tablespoon with meals	
Magnesium	200 mg daily	
Melatonin (adults only)	3 mg daily at bedtime	With B vitamins
Multi-mineral	3-4 ounces daily	In liquid solution, with vitamin B12, biotin
Multi-vitamin/mineral	6 caplets daily	Freeze-dried plant sources
Vitamin A	25,000 IU daily*	
Vitamin C	Individual bowel tolerance**	With bioflavonoids (quercetin, rutin proanthocyanidins)

* The FDA recommends pregnant women not exceed 10,000 IU of vitamin A daily.

** To determine individual dosage, on the first day take 1,000 mg hourly until diarrhea occurs, then reduce dosage to just below that for individual daily dosage. Vitamin C is not toxic in large doses but must be taken throughout the day to benefit. Divide dosage to three or four times a day.

Chapter 60:

Diarrhea

A surgeon was overheard discussing a case. *"We operated just in time,"* he said. *"One more day and he might have recovered on his own."*

All city and county water districts do one thing once a year. They flush their pipes to release the crud that has built up. Just think of your intestines as your own personal sewage system. Every once in a while your body decides it has had enough and it's time for an overhaul. Diarrhea is your body's way of flushing out your pipes. Because of this reality, diarrhea medications are decidedly not the best way to go.

The most frequent cause of diarrhea is the presence of foreign bacteria in the intestinal tract. The bacteria could be from improperly cooked, improperly refrigerated, rancid food or, in the case of travelers, bacteria familiar to the locals but unfamiliar to tourists. Without the ability to flush the intestine, bacteria can grow and prosper, eventually infecting the rest of the body.

Other causes of diarrhea include sensitivity to the lactose in milk; antibiotics, which can kill off the desirable bacteria necessary for the proper absorption of food; food poisoning, as the body throws off toxic bacteria as fast as it can; stress and anxiety – the body acts to throw off the stress of the mind; food allergies; and celiac disease, which is a sensitivity to gluten. Whether it be a food sensitivity or a bacterial sensitivity, diarrhea is simply the body's way of ridding itself of undesirables.

The problem with diarrhea, aside from painful stomach cramps and embarrassing intestinal rumbling, is the distinct possibility of malnutrition and dehydration. A person with chronic diarrhea does not properly absorb nutrients and can therefore develop nutrient deficiencies. The fact that water is not being absorbed also means the possibility of dehydration, particularly dangerous among infants and children. In some areas of the world, children die of diarrhea-induced dehydration. Disease and parasites cause the diarrhea, but it is the dehydration that leads to death.

Natural Solutions

Rather than turn to conventional medical treatments for diarrhea, why not try the natural way? There are many natural ways to treat or prevent diarrhea; solutions more practical in a foreign country than lugging around boxes or bottles of medicine.

I can testify on behalf of vitamin C with bioflavonoids and garlic to prevent traveler's diarrhea. I lived with the Masai in Africa for 16 weeks, living in a dung hut with dirt floors. I refused the malaria vaccine. I never got sick and ate all the food they did. The only thing I did differently was supplement with liquid garlic and vitamin C with bioflavonoids every day. Sometimes you can't avoid the water, and have to eat what you can. It worked for me!

I stayed healthy in part because garlic, especially in large doses, stimulates the production of the good army of bacteria which destroy the bad bacteria responsible for the diarrhea.

If you don't relish packing fresh garlic or are concerned about the odor, take along odorless aged garlic extract, which has all the medicinal properties of fresh garlic, without the smell and burn.

Certain organisms such as cholera bacteria, Salmonella, and Escheria coli (the cause of traveler's diarrhea) give off toxins that stick to the intestinal lining. Although they don't damage the lining, they do cause the cells to secrete massive amounts of fluid, which results in voluminous watery diarrhea typical of food poisoning.[1] In this case, even fasting won't help. Instead, efforts have to be made to "flush" the bad bacteria and replace it with good bacteria. While you may think you should avoid fiber when you have diarrhea, since fiber causes the stool to become softer, this would be a mistake. The fiber and roughage helps to get rid of the bad bacteria and the addition of digestive enzymes like acidophilus bacillus will replace them with good bacteria.

Important to remember, also, is the fact that without adequate fiber to move the stool through, the bad bacteria that causes the problem in the first place can take hold. Never stop your daily fiber regime, even if you're in the throes of diarrhea.

Bananas may be a golden solution to diarrhea, because they contain pectin, which can tighten up loose bowels. They also provide key minerals often lost with diarrhea: magnesium and potassium. A lack of potassium can cause intestinal cramping, so don't just assume the pain is from the affliction. Carob, rich in pectin, normalizes bowel movements, as demonstrated in numerous well-structured experiments. Pectin is also found in the peel of citrus fruits, apples, carrots, potatoes, sugar beets and tomatoes.

Patrick Donovan, N.D., of Seattle, Washington, treats children with barley water or rice water. In the case of one young patient, he had the mother prepare a large pot of brown rice and barley, boil it in water, and keep adding water. He instructed her to strain the water and give it to the child. The diarrhea cleared within hours.[2] Brown rice and whole barley is high in vitamin B6, magnesium, phosphorous, potassium and selenium, all the nutrients that are sacrificed and depleted with diarrhea.

Since food allergies can be a cause of diarrhea, so they must be first identified and eliminated. (See my Allergies chapter.) To divert diarrhea, the best course of action is to start with lots and lots of fluids. Drink purified water, followed by fruit and vegetable juices. Then eat soups, yogurt and cooked fruit. Avoid fats and fried food.

The diet of a person with diarrhea should be rich in vegetable protein, complex carbohydrates (beans!), oils (nut and seed), vitamins and minerals to compensate for the loss of all nutrients that occurs with this condition. Digestive enzymes such as Betaine HCl, pepsin and acidophilus should be taken with meals to aid in digestion. The diet should be supplemented with water-soluble B-complex vitamins and vitamin C as well as sodium, magnesium and potassium. As much fluids as possible should be ingested to replace the water lost to prevent dehydration.

Replenish Lost Fluids with Water

It is important to realize the dangers present when dehydration occurs. Without adequate amounts of water in the system all vital organs are stressed as they work harder to move everything through. A lack of this vital fluid can mean a total body shutdown as each organ loses the ability to function.

One way to tell if you're getting dehydrated is to pay attention to your mouth. Without adequate fluids, plaque will cling more readily to the teeth. Listen to your tongue: if your teeth don't feel smooth throughout most of the day; if you notice them getting coated with icky plaque, then you're probably not getting enough fluids. Pay attention especially after an illness, and drink the purest water you can. I recommend water that you know has been purified. I have a system in my home that uses reverse osmosis to take out all traces of chemicals and chlorine.

Some people don't like drinking water – they've gotten used to sweet drinks or coffee. For them I say, have you tried cold water with a squeeze of lemon? It tastes a lot better than room temperature water. OK, your teeth are sensitive, so cold doesn't go so well. Try herb tea either without sugar or with a sugar substitute. Take advantage of the tremendous variety of available herb teas. Raspberry tea tastes like hot Koolaid. Or you can make it and keep it refrigerated. It tastes great! Try a couple sprigs of mint in your regular iced tea. You can reduce the amount of caffeine, and it still tastes good. Experiment!! Buy a sample packet of herb teas and try each one – hot and cold.

They're a healthful way to receive your fluids.

Make it a habit to get enough fluids. Have hot herb (mint!) tea or a glass of cold water first thing in the morning – a welcome relief for morning mouth. Instead of coffee, try a coffee substitute like Postum. Some of the herb teas taste very similar to coffee and, of course, are much better for you. Caffeine can actually deplete your body of fluids so if you think you're getting your water from coffee, think again.

Bowel Nutrients Lost

If you look at the chapter on Colon Problems, you'll see the nutritional effect of a poorly operating colon. What happens is many nutrients are absorbed in the intestine, but only if the water in the stool is absorbed. Whether from diarrhea or diseases that prevent absorption, certain nutrients have a high deficiency danger when these problems occur.

Dr. Steven A. McClave, M.D., Department of Medicine, University of Louisville School of Medicine, Louisville, Kentucky, found that of colitis patients he studied, 54 to 67 percent were deficient in folic acid; 48 to 50 percent were deficient in vitamin B12; half were deficient in zinc; and an incredible 75 percent of patients with colitis were deficient in vitamin D. He also found colon patients had trouble absorbing essential fatty acids, and excreted high amounts of calcium, magnesium and zinc, making them deficient in these minerals.[3] Vitamin K, vitamin C and other B vitamins are also at risk during diarrhea episodes and must be replenished once the flushing has ceased.

Magnesium and potassium are closely bonded with water and can be in short supply when dehydrated.[4] When in the throes of diarrhea, always supplement with a mineral formulation in solution. Liquid formulations provide the maximum absorption ratios.

Diarrhea-Defeating Nutrients

For maximum absorption, supplements should be taken with meals.

Nutrient	Suggested Dosage	Formulation
Acidophilus	At least four billion flora daily on an empty stomach, three times daily	
Charcoal	4 tablets daily	In gelatin
Enzymes	2 capsules twice daily	Multiple formula
Exercise	30 minutes daily	Moderate
Fiber	8 tablets daily	Psyllium, with herb hyssop
Mint tea	As desired	
Multi-vitamin/mineral	6 caplets daily	Freeze-dried plant sources
Multi-mineral	2-4 ounces daily	In liquid solution, with vitamin B12, biotin
Purified water	Two gallons daily	Filtered, chlorine-free
Vitamin C	500 mg twice daily	With bioflavonoids (quercetin, proanthocyanidins)

CHAPTER 61:

Diverticulitis

Name the animals with pouches. Go on, humor me! ...the kanga-roo, opossum, seahorse – man! Yes, we sometimes have pouches. Not on the outside to hold babies, like these other animals, but on the inside when we don't eat right. That's what diverticulitis is: pouches in the colon, or large intestine. Diverticulitis occurs when constipation puts enough pressure on the colon to pop open pouches in the lining – called diverticula – at weak spots where blood vessels poke through the wall of the bowel. Diet is probably 99 percent the reason we develop diverticulitis, although heredity, obesity, gallbladder disease and arteriosclerosis can increase the possibility of developing it.[1]

Diverticulosis – which simply means having diverticula – is common in older people. About 60 percent of people over age 60 have some degree of diverticulosis, but with no discomfort as a result.[2]

Diverticulitis – infection of the diverticula – occurs when dry hard stool or food matter becomes caught in these pouches, rotting and inviting bacteria. The symptoms are associated with infection: fever, and pain in the lower left side of the abdomen, where the colon is located. Conventional medicine treats severe diverticulitis with antibiotics to kill the bacteria and fluids to rest the bowel and allow it to heal. Alternative and nutritional medicine works with the body to not only let it rest, but encourage it to heal. Not surprisingly, diverticulosis is seldom seen in vegetarians and is almost unknown in India and parts of Africa where a high fiber diet is standard.[3]

For preventive advice, see the chapter on Constipation. Adopting a high-fiber diet will keep diverticulosis from becoming diverticulitis. Ideally, with a high fiber and largely vegetarian diet, you won't have any diverticulum at all! Do you feel diverted? Well, let's get back on tract – the *digestive* tract that is!

Fighting Back with Bacteria

Harmful or disease-causing bacteria have fancy Latin names like pseudomonas-aeruginosa, proteus, staphylococcus, clostridia and veillonellae. Ugh! Your colon has its own defense system and if you take care of it, it will serve you well. However, if you wear it down with pasty, processed, sugared foods and antibiotics, your arsenal will be emptied. The kind of bacteria that lodges in diverticulum, causing severe infections, can be killed by our good bacteria, if there is enough of it. The trouble with antibiotics is they kill the good as well as the bad bacteria. They are the worst thing you can do, and I recommend they be your last resort. Researchers report our bodies are becoming immune to standard antibiotics so they aren't working any more. What is also possible is that they kill so much of our immune arsenal they cause secondary infections. Fungus infections like candida, for example, can be a direct result of long-term use of antibiotics, and severely debilitate the immune system (see the chapters on Fungus Infections, Chronic Fatigue Syndrome and AIDS).

Found in digestive enzyme supplemental formulas available at health food and vitamin stores are the body's disease-killing good-guy bacteria, Lactobacilli, Eubacteria and Bifidobacteria. Lactobacilli can inhibit the growth of harmful bacteria, stimulate immune function and aid in digestion, and Eubacteria can inhibit the growth of harmful bacteria. Bifidobacteria can reduce blood ammonia levels, lower cholesterol levels, regulate the immune system, produce vitamins, especially the B vitamin/folic acid group, restore normal intestinal flora during antibiotic therapy, and inhibit the growth of disease-causing germs. A lack of this important bacteria can be the reason many of us are deficient in B vitamins. Anybody who takes antibiotics on a regular basis is probably deficient in B vitamins. These are the bacteria we want to fight against diverticulitis. Certain foods, like yogurt with cultures, contain these good bacteria. Any "cultured" food with live enzymes will help in a program of bowel healing. My health food store contacts tell me you can buy cultured cottage cheese, even vegetables with cultures. Look also for a supplemental formula that contains aloe and psyllium, both designed to coat and soothe the colon after the enzymes have done their job of killing the bacteria. In fact, once the infection has subsided, these botanical medicinals coupled with high fiber ingredients such as hyssop, alfalfa and rhubarb, will ensure your diverticulum disappear.

Deflating Your Diverticula

Thinking creatively will help identify diverticulitis-healers. When diverticulum form, they are essentially ulcers. Once infection sets in, they become abscesses (see my chapters on Abscesses and Ulcers for more details). Therefore, targeting nutrients and foods that heal delicate tissues is one path to take. Since inflammation is a symptom, targeting natural anti-inflammatories makes sense also.

Try the sane approach to inflammation – N-SAIN. Instead of gut-busting, cell-wrenching NSAID pharmaceuticals, target safe and effective natural nutrients instead.

Researchers and others have discovered the benefits of pineapple, specifically its healing enzyme bromelain, known for its potent anti-inflammatory effect.

If you've been thinking milk might be the soothing answer for inflamed diverticulum, think again. Studies show fewer peptic ulcers heal on a milk diet than on a diet without milk. Instead of milk, try deglycerizinated licorice, or DGL. It has the same rate of healing as the medications Tagamet, Pepsid or Zantec, but fewer recurrences and no side effects.[4]

Turmeric is also a renowned anti-inflammatory. To be more exact, it is the curcumin, that which gives tumeric its yellow color, that has been found in studies to work better than even ibuprofen, a popular over-the-counter pain medicine. In one study on rats, researchers found 20 mg of curcumin worked as well as 200 mg of ibuprofen.[5]

Another study compared curcumin to the phenylbutazone, a pain reliever. Researchers found that in rats, the active ingredient worked just as well as the drugs. No toxic effects from curcumin have been reported.[6] Curcumin and tumeric are available on your supermarket spice shelves but for more exact dosages, look for anti-inflammatory formulas in your health food store.

Cabbage juice and sophoradin, a bioflavonoid extracted from the root of an ancient Chinese medicinal plant, has shown to be clinically effective in healing gastric ulcers.[7] Bioflavonoids are notorious anti-inflammatories. Curcumin is a bioflavonoid, as is the active ingredient in licorice. Look for supplemental formulas that contain vitamin C to battle infection and bioflavonoids like rutin and quercetin for healing.

Diverticulitis-Defeating Nutrients
For maximum absorption, supplements should be taken with meals.

Nutrient	Suggested Dosage	Formulation
Acidophilus	At least four billion flora daily on an empty stomach, three times daily	
Aged garlic extract	2 teaspoons three times daily	Liquid
Amino acids	4-6 capsules daily	Multiple formula from natural sources
Antioxidants	4 capsules daily*	With selenium and grape seed extract
Borage oil	2 capsules daily	
Coenzyme Q10	2 capsules daily	With vitamin E, phospholipids and selenium
Enzymes	2 capsules twice daily	Multiple formula
Flaxseed oil	1 tablespoon daily	
Fiber	8 tablets daily	Psyllium, with herb hyssop
L-glutamine	500 mg three times daily	
Multi-vitamin/mineral	6 caplets daily	Freeze-dried plant sources
Multi-mineral	2-4 ounces daily	In liquid solution, with vitamin B12, biotin
Vitamin C	Individual bowel tolerance**	With bioflavonoids (quercetin, proanthocyanidins)

* The FDA recommends that pregnant women not exceed 10,000 IU of vitamin A daily.

** To determine individual dosage, on the first day take 1,000 mg hourly until diarrhea occurs, then reduce dosage to just below that for individual daily dosage. Vitamin C is not toxic in large doses but must be taken throughout the day to benefit. Divide dosage to three or four times a day.

CHAPTER 62:

Down's Syndrome

She wasn't a scientist, she wasn't a researcher, she wasn't a doctor. But she was possessed with the dauntless determination of a mother's love – that same determination shown by mothers throughout the centuries that may largely be responsible for the survival of the human race.

Dixie Tafoya was the director of Adoption Options, a Louisiana-based adoption agency specializing in the adoption of physically-challenged children, when she adopted her daughter Madison, then 12 weeks of age. Resolved to the belief that she would raise a physically and mentally challenged little girl who would need special help, she heroically set out to do what little she could.

Then came the moment she realized her presumptions might be wrong. Dixie's routine for changing Madison's diapers always ended with a playful rub of her tummy. One morning, when Madison was eight months old, her mother told her, "Well, honey, I'm too tired. You're going to have to rub your tummy yourself." When Madison responded with a rub of her stomach, Dixie realized that her daughter was not retarded yet, but if she didn't do something she would be.

Discovering the Truth

Dixie began helping Madison by finding out everything she could about why Down's syndrome occurs. She learned that Down's results from genetic abnormalities in chromosome structure. She likens it to a cake recipe. If you mix cake batter with too much of some ingredients, it will bake into something like a cake, but won't be what the recipe intended. With Down's syndrome, there are too many ingredients in the human "recipe."

Normally, a human being has 46 chromosomes, but people with Down's syndrome have 47. The extra chromosome, called trisomy 21, causes a genetic overdose that leads to numerous metabolic imbalances.

She discovered that her ex-husband's nine-year-old nephew Zach with Down's syndrome was not only *not* retarded, but doing so well in school he was consistently on the honor roll, and had none of the typical Down's features. Dixie found out from Zach's mother that from the time he was nine months of age, Zach had been on a special nutritional program originally developed by Dr. Henry Turkel.

Since the 1940s, Dr. Turkel presented over 5,000 cases of children with Down's syndrome, who had shown remarkable improvement, to the NIH and the FDA. The agencies rewarded his success by restricting him to practicing only in Michigan on patients from Michigan.

He discovered early on that Down's syndrome was not a birth defect resulting in a vast array of subsequent physical and mental problems; but rather is a metabolic disease. Taking cues from Linus Pauling, he developed a therapy that included antioxidants, enzymes, a thyroid supplement, a diuretic and a stimulant.

Using Today's Technology

When Dixie first adopted Madison, she had skin rashes, constipation, and a history of frequent respiratory and ear infections. It appeared to her intelligent mother that Dixie's immune system was compromised, and having some knowledge of the benefits of nutritional supplementation, proceeded to discover what she needed.

Realizing today's technology might add to what Dr. Turkel discovered, Dixie turned to geneticists and biochemists to isolate exactly what was missing in Madison. Reading medical journals and consulting with various doctors, including Dr. Turkel, Dixie developed her own formula for Madison using nutrition to compensate for the genetic overdose. She emphasizes that Down's syndrome is a genetic defect alright, but not something than can't be corrected. The original genetic defect causes nutritional deficiencies, that, when corrected, results in a reversal of the symptoms of Down's syndrome. However, *the key to reversing Down's is to start the program before the child reaches 11 months of age.*

Her only regret is that she didn't start sooner. She has noticed that children who are started on metabolic therapy very early in life – while in infancy – show few developmental delays, if any, and even fewer signs of Down's syndrome.

Madison's Progress

Even though Dixie lost valuable time before targeting just the right nutritional therapy for Madison, it still wasn't too late. She started when Madison was two years of age and within two weeks of starting nutritional/metabolic therapy noticed she was getting definite calf muscles. Within three to four weeks Madison no longer felt like a rag doll. At two years she couldn't climb one step. Six weeks after starting nutritional therapy she could climb a flight of stairs, up and down.

The greatest change in her facial features occurred during the first three months on the program. Madison went from a flat face, typical of Down's syndrome, to almost normal. It was such a dramatic change that some people who had not seen her in a while did not recognize her.

Madison's hair grew ten inches in one year. Down's syndrome children typically don't have any hair, or slow-growing straight hair – never curly. Madison's hair is so long she sits on it, and it ends in curls.

Just before her second birthday, Madison was diagnosed with nystagmus (constantly twitching eye movements) and moderate to severe near-sightedness. Specialists said she needed surgery. A year later, just after her third birthday, her eye exam was normal. She had perfect vision – without glasses.

Today, Madison is a bright, talented, normal six-year old. She plays video games, does puzzles, talks normally, walks normally and thinks normally. She will always have Down's syndrome, but she will never again show it.

Nutrients to Consider

The nutrients that Dixie gives to Madison may not be all that your Down's syndrome child needs. Everyone is different, with different needs and different weaknesses. However, to give you an idea of the *kinds* of nutrients needed for Down's syndrome, here are some of the supplements Dixie gives to Madison.

Dixie discovered early that Madison would need amino acids. A French scientist, Dr. LeJeune, showed almost identical amino acid deficiencies in 79 Down's syndrome individuals. One of them, serine, is found to be particularly deficient in Down's patients. Dr. Evan Jones of North Carolina University, an expert in the field of amino acids, has said that a serine deficiency can contribute significantly to many of the problems associated with Down's syndrome, including mental retardation. The first thing Dixie did was give Madison food sources of B vitamins, and supplements of antioxidants and amino acids.

Malabsorption is a big issue with Down's children. Due to their imbalances they are lacking in many enzymes necessary for the proper breakdown and assimilation of food and the life-giving nutrients contained in it. Minerals and protein are especially hard to break down without proper amounts of amino acids, digestive enzymes and stomach acid. Because of this, vegetables and fruit which naturally contain digestive enzymes are important, as are nutritional supplements that contain digestive enzymes. For Down's children *and* adults, I whole-heartedly recommend a formula in solution which delivers vitamins – especially brain boosting B12 – and minerals directly into the cells, bypassing the factors that can result in the malabsorption problems typical of Down's, such as allergies, chemical sensitivities, bowel problems and low stomach acid.

For a concentrated source, and for maximum absorption, look for a supplemental formula that combines freeze dried sprouts and vegetables, and the digestive enzymes that come with them, so as to provide the B complex and all other essential vitamins and minerals needed for proper brain development. A good antioxidant formula combines vitamin C with bioflavonoids, odorless garlic, acidophilus and green tea extract for immune-system boosting.

Dixie added yogurt (determining that at the expiration date it produced less mucus) supplemented with the contents of an acidophilus capsule to coat the intestines and help with digestion, avoided any rice cereals and gave her absolutely no uncultured cow's milk. She gave her vitamin C with bioflavonoids three times a day and a multivitamin supplement.

Conventional physical therapy showed no progress so Dixie decided to forego it and treat her like a normal child, encouraging her to walk. She also added new supplementals. She gave Madison a liquid amino acid formula.

She also found that her daughter needed more than the usual digestive enzymes. As with all Down's syndrome children, her absorption was compromised, so she needed more than the usual amounts of enzymes. Dixie fed her lots of raw vegetables, and avoided raw legumes and nuts because they have enzyme inhibitors. Madison was still too young for most capsules and pills so she concentrated on enzyme-rich raw vegetables instead.

Zinc and vitamin B6 was also emphasized for Madison because zinc helps normalize body growth and blood sugar factors like IGF-1, found deficient in Down's syndrome patients. Vitamin B6 is needed with zinc and helps the mind/body connection. Then she found a formula with coenzyme Q10, a powerful antioxidant needed because of the tremendous amount of free radicals produced by Madison's extra chromosome.

Researchers now emphasize all the antioxidants for this same reason. Recommended antioxidants include selenium, vitamins A, C and E; beta carotene and glutathione. Other nutrients important to brain chemistry and muscle function are highly absorbable minerals in solution, essential fatty acids and the B vitamins, particularly B12.

Help for the Down's Syndrome Parent

Thanks to Dixie, who is sharing her knowledge, you can get specialized, metabolic help for your loved one. Dixie has founded Trisomy 21 Research, dedicated to uncovering therapies that work to reverse the symptoms of Down's syndrome. For information call them at (504) 769-TRIS. Representatives there say you'll get all the information you need to either convince your doctor to try nutritional therapy, or do it on your own.

For continuing coverage of Down's syndrome, and a subscription to *Smart Drug News*, contact CERI – the Cognitive Enhancement Research Institute, who graciously gave me the information contained here. Call them at (415) 321-CERI.

The Cell Therapy Option

I wanted to cover the option of cell therapy because I have personally seen it work with Down's kids. I have been to Germany and seen busloads of improved Down's children receiving cell therapy. I know its value firsthand because I've had it done numerous times. Live cell therapy is not to be used instead of nutritional therapy. Nutritional therapy is the most valuable treatment option available. Live cell therapy is an adjunct to nutrition; and may help get more thorough results.

Live cell therapy is accomplished by injecting live cells from animal embryos into humans. Over the past three decades over two million patients have been treated with live cell therapy to retard aging and restore defective organs and cells. A multitude of controlled laboratory and clinical experiments throughout the world irrefutably prove its efficacy.

You've heard the macrobiotic principle of eating only live food – that is food that when planted can still grow? Live cell therapy uses the same basic principle. By injecting healthy cells into the body, they are able to replace the old and sick cells. In the case of Down's syndrome, defective cells are replaced. The cells are not rejected as foreign because the antigens that cause rejection do not develop until three days after birth.

It is important, however, that cells from fresh embryos be used. Old or dated cells will obviously not work. Compare it to the difference between eating corn straight off the stalk and salted corn nuts. How much energy is left from the corn once it has been plucked, fried, salted and packaged? Not much.

If you are interested in cell therapy, look for clinics with a successful history of using the freshest embryos possible. Don't take anyone's word, investigate for yourself. Unfortunately, they have to practice in Mexico or Europe, away from the arm of the FDA. Two clinics I know of that practice live cell therapy are Contreras Oasis Hospital in Tijuana, Mexico, P.O. Box 439855, San Ysidro, CA 92143, (800) 700-1850) and Claus Marten's Four Seasons Clinic and Health Resort at Fareerweg 3, P.O. Box 244, D 8183 Rottach Egern, W. Germany, phone: 80-222-6780-24041.

Down's Dumping Nutrients

For maximum absorption, supplements should be taken with meals.

Nutrient	Suggested Dosage	Formulation
Acetyl L-Carnitine	500 mg three times daily	
Aged garlic extract	2 teaspoons three times daily	Liquid
Amino acids	4-6 capsules daily	Multiple formula from natural sources
Antioxidants	4 capsules daily*	With selenium and grape seed extract
Borage oil	2 capsules daily	
Coenzyme Q1 (NADH)	2.5 mg daily	
Coenzyme Q10	2 capsules daily	With vitamin E, phospholipids and selenium
Enzymes	2 capsules twice daily	Multiple formula
Flaxseed oil	1 tablespoon daily	
Fiber	8 tablets daily	Psyllium, with herb hyssop
Ginkgo biloba	60 mg three times daily	
Multi-vitamin/mineral	6 caplets daily	Freeze-dried plant sources
Multi-mineral	2-4 ounces daily	In liquid solution, with vitamin B12, biotin
Vitamin C	Individual bowel tolerance**	With bioflavonoids (quercetin, proanthocyanidins)

* The FDA recommends that pregnant women not exceed 10,000 IU of vitamin A daily.

** To determine individual dosage, on the first day take 1,000 mg hourly until diarrhea occurs, then reduce dosage to just below that for individual daily dosage. Vitamin C is not toxic in large doses but must be taken throughout the day to benefit. Divide dosage to three or four times a day.

CHAPTER 63:

Eating Disorders

In Hollywood, where the camera – like a binge itself – adds 10 pounds before you can say "Twinkie," eating disorders are common-place. Jane Fonda was bulimic from age 12 until 35 and admits that at one point she threw up 20 times a day. Sally Field began her three-year bout with bulimia at 20, spurred, she said, by the perception that "everybody then was Twiggy, except me." Ally Sheedy, the *War Games* star who at 11 danced with the American Ballet Theater, later developed bulimia and wrote a searing 1991 poem, *Portrait of a Bulimic*, in which she described "the bloat/the skin/stretched so tightly/over her abdomen she fears/it will rupture."[1]

Lynn Redgrave, who over a period of 20 years would gorge and then purge, remembers sitting beside the late comedian Gilda Radner during a flight to Toronto at the end of the '70s. Over dinner, the women shared eating intimacies, and Radner broke down in tears when she owned up to being bulimic.

Pat Boone's daughter Cherry Boone O'Neill said that in the midst of her seven-year siege with bulimia, she would eat "until I could barely stand up." Consuming a box of doughnuts, a bag of cookies, a pint of macaroni salad and half a gallon of ice cream at a sitting – sometimes four times a day.

Sixties teen idol Sandra Dee has flirted dangerously with anor-exia since age nine. Hers was a desperate attempt to control what she perceived as an unmanageable body and an even more unmanage-able life, including a stepfather who sexually abused her. For more than a year, Dee ate virtually nothing but lettuce. Twice as a young teenager she overdosed after swallowing Epsom salts as a purgative. She said that as a teenager, her weight was "the only thing I could control."

American Ballet Theater prima ballerina Leslie Browne, 34 – who first won public attention at 22 when she replaced the emaciated, 87-pound anorexic-bulimic Gelsey Kirkland in the 1977 movie *The Turning Point* – claims that while she doesn't suffer from a disorder herself, she suspects that 25 percent of dancers do."

Karen Carpenter died of a heart attack years after conquering her anorexia.The disorder created a dangerous magnesium/potassium electrolyte imbalance that weakened her heart. By the time she conquered her illness, it was too late. Doctors estimate that probably 50 percent or more anorexics suffer irreversible physical damage to the vital organs or glands.

Marathon runner Patti Catalano, 38, developed anorexia at 25 and then bulimia, managing to break the U.S. marathon record in 1981 while weighing only 104 lbs.

In the end, most anorexics and bulimics find that battling with their disease is akin to an endless marathon.

At least 80 percent of anorexics are also bulimic. Even though anorexia is defined as self-starvation, most anorexics also binge on food, and follow by purging. This purging, whether through vomiting or laxatives, have horrific and long-term consequences. Therapy must not only halt these actions, but treat the many physical side effects. Often, it is only after these side effects become so pronounced that the victim cannot ignore them, that he/she seeks help. Five years is the average amount of time before a victim of bulimia seeks help. It may take this long for a disorder to produce symptoms of a life-threatening condition.

The Image of Thin

It is estimated that 40 percent of all American women are trying to lose weight. Over the last 30 years there has been a marked trend toward an increasingly unrealistic thin ideal of women's beauty. Subsequently, pressure is put on young women to restrict their food intake, dieting so they may achieve the ultimate thinness. Most attempts at long term weight loss fail. Read my chapter on Weight Loss to see why diets fail and how *healthy* weight loss can be achieved using the body's own metabolic triggers.

You can add anorexia, bulimia, even chronic dieting to the long list of today's modern "civilized" diseases – diet-related diseases that undermine the immune system and result in disability and death. In today's teenage world, dieting is a fad, and fasting a common practice. Obsessed over being thin, ashamed for being overweight, teenagers – male and female – are risking their health by going on dangerous diets which last far too long. They seem unable to stop or see the terrible effects on them. For many, anorexia begins with chronic dieting.

Contained within these pages are answers to the confusion, ignorance, misunderstanding and misconceptions surrounding eating disorders. No longer are we helpless to identify, explain or do something about anorexia and bulimia. No longer do we have to stand by helplessly while our loved ones eat voraciously then use laxatives and/or vomiting to empty their stomachs of valuable, life-giving food, as in bulimia. Or they deny all sustenance and its benefits while slowly and painfully starving to death, as in anorexia.

Zinc Deficiency Possible Cause

It is a given that someone who has been abstaining from food is going to have nutritional deficiencies. What surprised researchers, however, was the finding that zinc deficiencies are low during *early* stages of malnutrition, indicating to them that a zinc deficiency may lead to chronic dieting behavior. They are able to confirm this connection when hospitalized anorexic patients experience an appetite for food after receiving zinc supplementation.

A zinc deficiency can cause confusion and difficulties with taste and smell. If dieting causes a zinc deficiency, it may become easier to abstain from food if taste is impaired.

Researchers at the University of Surrey, U.K., found that when 15 zinc-deficient anorexic females were given 15 milligrams of zinc, all saw an increase in their appetite and taste sensitivity, compared to controls, who were given placebos and saw no such change.[2]

A deficiency of zinc can be a "sustaining" factor for abnormal eating behavior. In other words, while some may unnaturally diet, zinc deficient individuals will take this to extremes, sustaining a diet to starvation. Writing in the *Journal of the American College of Nutrition*, Craig J. McClain, M.D., concluded that people with eating disorders frequently are zinc deficient, which can contribute to their inability to control themselves.[3]

The Lancet reported how a 13-year-old girl who was anorexic was able to overcome her disorder through zinc supplementation. The researchers found that after two weeks of supplementation with zinc (initially 15 milligrams daily, then 50 mg three times daily), her appetite and mood began to improve. After four months of supplementation, she gained 13 kilograms and her depression cleared. What I find most interesting is that ten months after they stopped giving her the zinc, she became anorexic again, which improved once the zinc was reintroduced.[4] This pretty much blasts conventional assumptions that the zinc deficiency occurs after dieting.

This reminds me of a peculiar experience I had a few years ago in Egypt, where feminine beauty is accented by well-padded hips and thighs and full-blown, pendulous breasts. Learning that an "American nutritionist" was a guest at the palace, a captain in the army came to me to discover how they could get their pale, skin-and-bones 14-year-old anorexic daughter to eat.

"Even when I beat her she won't eat," the father informed me. And the squat, huge-busted mother nodded assent. For an instant, I was fascinated by the mother's wretched skin with such huge pores that it was as if I were viewing them with a magnifying glass.

"Don't beat her," I said. "Just give her 30 milligrams of zinc and a 50 mg capsule of vitamin B complex daily."

It is difficult to find vitamin and mineral supplements in Egypt, so I gave the parents part of my personal supply. I later learned that anorexia is common there, and that parents beat young girls because non-eating causes thinness, which makes them bad marriage candidates.

A study reported at a National Health Federation convention illustrated that if a female rat is zinc-deprived, her offspring in the third and fourth generation will be undersized, thin, and with a poor appetite – to the point of starvation. Egypt's notoriously zinc-deficient soils, the girl's anorexia and the mother's poor complexion (zinc and blemishes), seemed related.

Before leaving Egypt, I heard that the young girl was taking her supplements and eating better every day. In three weeks she gained 10 pounds. Several months later, she was back to normal and filling out.

Carl L. Birmingham of the Department of Internal Medicine, St. Paul's Hospital, Vancouver, B.C., Canada, performed a randomized, double-blind, placebo-controlled trial of 35 female anorexia nervosa patients who received either 100 mg of zinc gluconate or a placebo. Incredibly, he found that all the patients taking the zinc were able to increase their weight twice as much as those taking the placebos – a statistically significant finding.[5]

Apparently, zinc can change serotonin levels in the brain. A deficiency of serotonin is associated with fatigue, depression, mood swings and psychosis. Zinc is present in large amounts in areas of the brain involved in food seeking, weight regulation and in the metabolism of serotonin. Zinc, therefore, is essential for good mental health.

Copper is important to balance out your zinc supplements. Be sure and include 2-4 mg. of copper with any zinc.

Because zinc is a mineral, it can be hard to digest, especially if starvation has reduced the amount of hydrochloric acid present in the stomach and bacteria in the intestine. Supplementing with digestive enzymes and Betaine, a hydrochloric acid supplement, can help. But another way is to look for a good, easily absorbable, derived-from-nature mineral blend in solution. Studies show minerals dissolved in water before ingestion are considerably more bioavailable to the body than those even present in food, because they aren't risked by a lack of hydrochloric acid in the stomach or food allergies. Liquid formulations provide the maximum absorption ratios.

When there is a discussion of neuroses, depression or psychotic behavior, the conversation usually gets around to serotonin and its importance to the brain. Serotonin is a chemical which affects sleep, appetite and emotions. Bulimics typically have a problem with this chemical. Also, when the brain is low in tryptophan, a chemical responsible for manufacturing serotonin, irrational cravings can result. A study of bulimics found that when they were given measured doses of tryptophan, their bingeing and purging behaviors decreased. Tryptophan is found in relatively large amounts in milk and bananas and is available in amino acid formulas.

For more answers to the anorexia question, see the chapter Mental Illness.

Anorexia-Healing Nutrients
For maximum absorption, take supplements with meals.

Nutrient	Suggested Dosage	Formulation
Aged garlic extract	1 teaspoon three times daily	Liquid
Amino acids	4-6 capsules daily	Multiple formula from natural sources
Antioxidants	4 capsules daily*	With selenium and grapeseed extract
Borage oil	2 capsules daily	
Coenzyme Q10	2 capsules daily	With vitamin E, phospholipids and selenium
Flaxseed oil	1 tablespoon daily	
Ginger	500 mg twice daily for appetite	
Ginkgo biloba	60 mg daily	
Magnesium	200 mg daily	
Melatonin (adults only)	3 mg daily at bedtime	With B vitamins
Multi-mineral	3-4 ounces daily	In liquid solution, with vitamin B12, biotin
Multi-vitamin/mineral	6 caplets daily	Freeze-dried plant sources
Vitamin B6	100 mg daily	
Vitamin C	Individual bowel tolerance**	With bioflavonoids (quercetin, proanthocyanidins)

* The FDA recommends pregnant women not exceed 10,000 IU of vitamin A daily.

** To determine individual dosage, on the first day take 1,000 mg hourly until diarrhea occurs, then reduce dosage to just below that for individual daily dosage. Vitamin C is not toxic in large doses but must be taken throughout the day to benefit. Divide dosage to three or four times a day.

CHAPTER 64:

Eczema

I remember the first time a doctor told me I had eczema. "Oh, no, doctor, " I exclaimed, horrified at the prospect of living with a skin disease that sounded as bad as eczema. I pictured myself peeling and itching, covered from head to toe with white skin flakes. "I just have sensitive skin!" My doctor laughed. "Maureen, eczema is just another name for atopic dermatitis." Was I supposed to feel better? "It's a symptom, not a disease," he added.

All my life I'd had sensitive skin. It seemed like everything made it itch or hurt. Even a little sun left me red and peeling. The most hypoallergenic cosmetic had to be removed in a few hours or a rash developed. I had hives so often I started attracting honeybees! But I had always assumed nothing could be done about it. I figured it was in my genes or something, and had to be lived with, like the length of my eyelashes or the shape of my nose. That is until I talked to Dr. Ross Gordon, the eminent physician who founded the American College for Advancement in Medicine, which taught a whole generation of doctors about natural healing.

He made me realize my largely genetic problem could be helped. With his advice, and with some furious digging for research on my part, I found that certain nutrients, when applied to skin and taken orally, can actually protect, enhance and fortify skin against the ravages of day to day life. I can honestly say that today, at the age of 60, I have better, younger and more beautiful skin than when I was in my twenties.

Years ago almost any skin disease involving a patch of red, scaling, itching and weeping skin was attributed to eczema. No one really knew what produced the symptoms. Accordingly, at one stage of medical research, more than half of all skin diseases were labeled "eczema." Now we have other names such as hives, rashes and pimples to describe the various ways in which substances affect the skin.

Eczema is described as a common skin inflammation. Its symptoms are redness, itching, small blisters, and a fluid discharge that dries into scales and crusts. It is not a disease unto itself, but a symptom, manifesting itself through the skin, that the body is being irritated by an internal or external source. This is also the definition for an allergic reaction. There are three steps to dealing with it: remove the irritant, remedy a nutritional deficit, and boost the skin's natural immune system. I will address these points in this chapter.

Eczema as an Allergic Symptom

I remember reading about the case of a woman with severe eczema on her hands and forearms, a pattern typical of a chemical reaction. However, this was a woman who did not normally come in contact with strong chemicals, soaps or other irritants. Her lifestyle entailed using her hands for holding cocktails, waving people out of her way and playing Mah-Jongg. After talking to her at length, the doctor discovered that she had inherited a beautiful set of Mah-Jongg tiles, made decades ago in Japan. It turned out that the tiles were covered with a lacquer made from a distant relation of poison ivy! Once she stopped using them, her eczema stopped.

Obviously, the first thing to consider when confronted with eczema is the possibility that it could be caused or made worse by a reaction to food or chemicals.

Do you love strawberries but find they don't love you? If you'd rather see that relief map of the United States on your wall instead of your back, better stay away!

If your child has eczema, the first suspect is an allergy to the lactose in milk. It is so common, doctors recommend it be the first food taken out of the diet when allergies are suspected.

Too often children with food allergies have eczema. Their little bodies aren't fully developed enough to tolerate certain foods. In a study of Japanese children, researchers found an incredible 71 percent had food allergies, mostly to milk and eggs.[1]

The medical journal *Archives of Diseases in Childhood* reported on a study in which 73 percent of children with eczema were improved when food allergens were removed from their diets.[2]

Once an allergen is discovered and eliminated, your task is not completed. You may find the eczema still does not go away. This is due to the underlying problems that caused the reaction in the first place, problems I will now address.

Read the chapter on Allergies for more on tests and symptoms.

The Stomach Acid Link

Also linked to eczema is a deficiency of hydrochloric acid, the stomach acid responsible for breaking down food so the intestines can absorb the nutrients, and eliminate what's left. What happens is this: perfectly good food, chock full of vitamins, minerals and other essentials, instead of being broken down, goes right through the stomach in its whole form. The immune system says, "Hey what's this doing here?" and forms antibodies – our body's immune system warriors – which attack it. This is exactly what happens to cause allergy symptoms like watery eyes. The defending army rallies to rid itself of the enemy and your skin receives the war wounds: eczema. Research has shown this connection.

In one reported study 106 patients with bad cases of eczema had their stomach acid levels tested. It was found that a full 74 percent were eating without adequate stomach acid and of these, 25 percent had no acid at all! Researchers found a direct link between the amount of stomach acid not available for digestion, and the severity of the eczema.[3]

In another study, eight out of 11 patients were found to be low in stomach acid. Of these, seven had other stomach problems that contributed to the severity of the eczema outbreak and the lack of acid.[4] Based on this research, I would suggest having your whole digestive system examined if you have chronic eczema, because there are many factors that can effect your ability to assimilate nutrients. Remember, it's not what you eat, it's what you absorb!

Other signs of low stomach acid include split, peeling nails, hair falling out, and dilated capillaries on cheeks and nose. Dr. Jonathan Wright tells me that he estimates every third adult he sees in his clinic has too little stomach acid.

An easy way to encourage your stomach to acidify is to drink a tablespoon of vinegar before eating. At restaurants I ask the waiter to bring me vinegar and oil – if the waiter asks why, I tell him "Cause I feel like cooking."

Supplementing with a hydrochloric acid formula such as Betaine will help absorb nutrients, but studies show minerals dissolved in water before ingestion are considerably more bioavailable to the body than those even present in food. Look for a good, easily absorbable, derived-from-nature mineral blend in solution. Liquid formulations provide the maximum absorption ratios.

At the risk of sounding like your mother, always chew your food! You'd be amazed at the difference a good chewing can do in preparing your digestive system for assimilation. People who commonly eat quickly and swallow whole pieces of food, can at best cause painful air bubbles, and at worst create food allergies! Those who do not masticate, nature castigates. Twenty to 30 bites is a good "rule of tongue."

EFAs to the Rescue

There is another common denominator to eczema sufferers: a deficiency of essential fatty acids (EFAs). They are called essential because they must come from food. EFAs are the major building blocks of body fat, including that which is contained under your skin. This is not the fat you want to take off, as in weight loss. This is the collagen that keeps pimples, cuts and irritations from leaving scars, pits and craters. EFAs also produce prostaglandins, which work to reduce inflammation. Without prostaglandins, a simple skin irritation becomes an inflamed, itchy, crusty mess.

There is one kind of essential fatty acid that is primary in the production of prostaglandins: linoleic acid or gamma linolenic acid (GLA). Researchers studying various deficiencies among bottle-fed infants found that when they received inadequate GLA, they had drying, flaking skin. Infants with cradle cap, a form of eczema, have been found to be deficient in biotin, a B vitamin, and GLA.

The most common, albeit not the best, source of GLA, commonly used in studies, is evening primrose oil.

The essential fatty acids in evening primrose oil plus fish oil can reduce the severity of eczema. Clinical trials in England using evening primrose oil were deemed so impressive that it has received approval as an eczema therapy by that country's National Health Service.[5]

Researchers S. Wright and J.L. Burton, as reported in the British medical journal *The Lancet*, performed a double-blind, crossover study of 60 adults and 39 children with eczema who were treated with evening primrose oil. The fortunate patients not only experienced less itching, but almost half had a significant reduction in the overall severity of their symptoms.[6]

Despite these impressive studies, I don't recommend evening primrose oil. That is because there is another supplemental source more potent in GLA, and much less expensive – more bang for the buck if you will.

Independent clinical tests show that borage oil contains up to 26 percent GLA. Compare this to evening primrose oil and black currant oil, which contain no more than 18 percent. Not only that, borage oil costs less because the borage seed is three times larger than black currant or evening primrose seeds. Finally, borage is more bioavailable. In other words, the body more readily accepts it.[7]

Other sources of GLA are the oils of sesame seed, safflower, sunflower seed, cottonseed, and soybean. For optimum benefit, the oils should have been extracted without heat (cold-pressed), and eaten raw, like in a healthful salad. Heat and sunlight slowly draws nutrients out of these unsaturated fatty acids, so be sure to buy your oil in non-transparent containers and store them in the refrigerator.

Fish oil, too, can help in this EFA error. Don't try to pronounce it, just know that eicosapentaenoic acid, found in coldwater fish oil (mackerel, herring and salmon), helps incorporate linolenic acid in the skin. Suffice it to say if you have eczema, it helps to eat fish.[8]

Fish oil, or omega-3 oil, also helps the body assimilate arachidonic acid, found in animal products such as milk, eggs and meat. Arachidonic acid is what causes the body to defend itself with allergy symptoms. More on fish oil and skin reactions in the Psoriasis chapter.

Nutritional Skin Care

There are also nutrients, and foods that contain these nutrients, that have been shown to help eczema. Probably what is happening in these studies, is the nutrients are restoring deficiencies that may have caused or contributed to the problem in the first place. In any case, a regimen containing all the nutrients mentioned in this chapter may go a long way toward curing eczema, once the source of irritation is eliminated.

If you understand that it is the lack of prostaglandins that causes your skin to go from a simple red, irritated rash to what would be considered eczema, you know anything that encourages prostaglandin formation or accomplishes the same thing, is desired for eczema treatment. This is where the vitamins C, B3 (niacin), B6 and the minerals zinc and magnesium come in. They are necessary before EFAs can produce prostaglandins. I would add biotin to this list, based on my knowledge of the benefit of biotin to the hair and skin, as well as that study relating a biotin deficiency to cradle cap. Vitamin A and its precursor, beta carotene, are always good nutritional choices, since they are so important to the skin. A deficiency of vitamin A causes thickening of the skin, commonly found in eczema.

Drs. Jonathan Wright and Alan R. Gaby recommend taking 30 mg of zinc 2-3 times a day; 2-3 mg of copper once a day, one tablespoon of flaxseed, sunflower or safflower oil (EFAs) once a day; and 200-400 IU a day of vitamin E to go with the EFA oil. They also suggest taking a zinc supplement to strengthen skin tissue.[9]

In his book, *Dr. Wright's Book of Nutritional Therapy*, he reports that in over 40 cases of eczema he has seen between 1974 and 1979, every case responded to zinc-centered therapy. He says sometimes no improvement is seen for three to six weeks, but often the problem is gone within three or four months. He explains that it takes time for the zinc to become incorporated into the body's healing enzymes.[10]

Incidentally, zinc is also necessary for the enzyme that produces stomach acid. Copper is important to balance out zinc. Be sure and include 2-4 mg. of copper with any zinc.

If allergies prevent you from eating egg yolk, try other biotin-boosters like unpolished rice, brewer's yeast, whole grains, peas, beans and lentils. Keep in mind that antibiotics can affect the amount of biotin available to the body as they interfere with the production of the intestinal bacteria where biotin is produced.

Color it Orange

After Halloween, don't throw that pumpkin away! Get yourself a butcher's cleaver and hack it into cooking-sized pieces. Steamed pumpkin with a little real maple syrup and cinnamon drizzled on top makes a tasty hot dinner. One cup of pumpkin contains 2,651 IU of vitamin A.

Due to the climate, pumpkins grow readily in the Soviet Union. Researchers there were successful in treating eczema patients with beta carotene extracted from pumpkins, given to them as a food supplement and as an ointment rubbed on the affected areas.[11]

In another skin-clearing study, 24 out of 33 patients with eczema were improved or cured with pumpkin extract, and in yet another study, six out of seven individuals with skin scaliness were markedly improved or cured with beta carotene.[12]

Carrots, too, have plenty of vitamin A and beta carotene. I get really dry skin when I have to spend hours on airplanes, so I bring along carrot sticks to munch. One cup of carrots contains an incredible 30,942 IU of vitamin A. Six ounces of carrot juice contains 24,750 IU. There are also some vitamin A lotions on the market, look for them.

Carotene, or beta carotene, as it has become popularly known, converts in the body to vitamin A and is found in yellow and orange fruits and vegetables such as apricots, cantaloupe, persimmons, winter squash and yams. When you measure it for the body, you talk about individual units, hence IU. The studies I've mentioned may have been helped by the fact that pumpkins also contain zinc.

Vitamin C does more than assist EFAs. It is a natural health and skin enhancer. I constantly recommend it for everything from colds to sensitive skin. I use a lotion on my skin that contains vitamin C – not many lotions do – as well as vitamins A, B5 and E, along with various antioxidant herbals including ginkgo biloba and ginseng. It has successfully turned my red, raw sensitive skin, into soft, firm, strong skin able to withstand even high winds on the Austrian Alps ski slopes!

Eczema-Ending Nutrients
For maximum absorption, take supplements with meals.

Nutrient	Suggested Dosage	Formulation
Aged garlic extract	1 teaspoon three times daily	Liquid
Antioxidants	4 capsules daily*	With selenium and grapeseed extract
Borage oil	2 capsules daily	
Flaxseed oil	1 tablespoon daily	
Lecithin	2 tablespoons with meals	
Magnesium	200 mg twice daily	
MSM (Methylsulfonylmethane)	500 mg three times daily	
Multi-mineral	3-4 ounces daily	In liquid solution, with vitamin B12, biotin
Multi-vitamin/mineral	6 caplets daily	Freeze-dried plant sources
Nettle	250 mg three times daily	
Quercetin	400 mg twice daily	With vitamin C
Vitamin B6	100 mg daily	
Vitamin C	Individual bowel tolerance**	With bioflavonoids (quercetin, proanthocyanidins)

Nourish with a moisturizing lotion containing vitamins A, C and E.

* The FDA recommends pregnant women not exceed 10,000 IU of vitamin A daily.

** To determine individual dosage, on the first day take 1,000 mg hourly until diarrhea occurs, then reduce dosage to just below that for individual daily dosage. Vitamin C is not

CHAPTER 65:

Endometrosis

"A woman's guess is much more accurate than a man's certainty."

–Rudyard Kipling

Some five million women suffer from endometriosis, a chronic condition in which endometrial cells – in the form of patches or lesions of endometrial tissue – that normally line the uterus mysteriously appear on its outer surface, or in other parts of the body such as the ovaries, fallopian tubes, and bowels. During menstruation, female hormones stimulate these lesions, causing inflammation, pain, scarring and sometimes bleeding.

Too often, women assume that painful periods are normal and fail to tell their doctors that they're suffering. As a result, the early signs of endometriosis go unnoticed.

Though the disease can progress without symptoms, its typical signs include recurring, unusually intense pelvic pain, especially just before and during menstruation; nausea, vomiting and constipation during menstruation; pelvic pain during intercourse; or heavier than normal menstrual bleeding. Left untreated, endometriosis can damage a woman's reproductive organs and make it difficult or impossible for her to conceive.

Conventional treatment involves outpatient laser surgery, called laparoscopy, in which the damaging tissue is "burned off" using a thin optical tube holding a laser that is inserted in the patient's naval.

While initially successful, this treatment is often temporary and may need to be performed many times, with no guarantee of success. Dr. David Redwine of St. Charles Medical Center, Bend, Oregon, advocates this "near-contact" laparoscopy, claiming 75 percent of his patients experienced complete relief from their symptoms. He says the reason so many women have recurring problems after surgery is because only a portion of the misplaced endometrial tissue has been removed. He claims surgeons who excise only typical black lesions could leave from 50 to 60 percent of the disease behind. It's hard to imagine any responsible surgeon leaving anything behind that could cause further problems, but according to Dr. Redwine, conventional medicine believes only certain kinds of lesions – black powder burn – need to be removed. It also believes endometrial tissue does not "implant" in the peritoneum, which he says is false.[1]

The Estrogen Connection

One thing most doctors agree on: endometriosis is affected by estrogen in the body and by the menstrual cycle. The condition essentially is never seen before puberty and is extremely rare after menopause (when estrogen levels naturally drop), unless a woman is receiving estrogen-replacement therapy. Treatment that reduces estrogen production typically decreases the extent of endometriosis, though women with the disease don't necessarily have higher estrogen levels than women without it.[2]

What can figure into this equation are the thousands of man-made estrogens that can stack the deck against women and increase their estrogen levels by hundreds of times. Pesticides, household chemicals and common plastics are some examples of man-made estrogens.[3] It is quite possible that the same forces increasing our risk for breast cancer increase the chances of getting endometriosis. Before 1950, a lot of pesticides, like DDT, were not so prevalent in the environment. What we've learned is that today's modern environment, filled with plastics, chemicals – including 2.2 billion pounds of pesticides – and electronics, contain innumerable man-made estrogen building blocks. What can we do to protect ourselves? Fortunately, there is much we can do.

The mainstay of any treatment program is to decrease the amount of circulating estrogen to the point where the symptoms of endometriosis subside, but not so far as to cause menopause. To decrease estrogen production, the first step is to eat a low-fat diet, preferably vegetarian, containing no more than 20 to 25 grams of fat a day and eliminating all dairy products. Many women get relief simply by eliminating dairy products. Julian Whitaker, M.D., says that a high-fat, animal protein diet substantially increases a woman's estrogen load.[4] This is due in part to the fact that chemicals toxins are stored in fatty tissue.

Phytoestrogenic Bioflavonoids

Another anti-estrogen plan of action involves the use of natural plant estrogens, called phytoestrogens, which may prevent man-made estrogens from entering cells.This has been particularly true in the case of flavonoids. Sometimes referred to as bioflavonoids, they are substances found in brightly-colored fruits and vegetables. Bioflavonoids are not only phytoestrogenic, but act as potent anti-inflammatories, extremely important in reducing the inflammation associated with the pain of endometriosis.

Legumes – peas, beans and certain roots – are isoflavonoids, which act as a non-steroidal estrogen. Soybeans, particularly, have been found to have this anti-estrogenic property, and have been associated with a lower incidence of breast cancer in some populations. Remember, breast cancer is related to endometriosis because high blood estrogen levels have been found to increase this type of cancer. Soybeans are eaten in great quantities in Japan and China, and is one of the reasons researchers believe these countries have low rates of breast cancer.[5] Tofu, soybean curd, is an excellent food source. It has the unique ability to absorb the flavors it is cooked in. Try it in a casserole.

Rutin, a bioflavonoid from buckwheat, and citrus rind and citrus pulp, contain an assortment of bioflavonoids, including quercetin, a highly potent antiinflammatory, and are excellent sources of estrogen-blocking flavonoids.[6]

When targeting bioflavonoids, always include high amounts of vitamin C. Vitamin C has been shown in studies to reduce inflammation, pain and the risk of infection. Many foods high in vitamin C also contain bioflavonoids. In nature they work together to combat the effects of oxygen free radicals, which kill cells and contribute to aging.

The best way to handle endometriosis is to prevent it from occurring in the first place. Certain nutrients and foods can keep the disorder in check if diagnosed in the early stages, or after ALL misplaced endometrial tissue has been eliminated.

Dietary Regimens for Prevention

The Endometriosis Society believes the key to the disorder lies in early diagnosis and prevention.

A leaflet put out by the society makes a good point. It says, "Many women do not feel or realize that persistently painful periods, painful bowel movements or painful sexual intercourse are very good reasons for visiting their doctors. Women may be embarrassed, worry about wasting a doctor's time or simply disregard their symptoms in the mistaken belief that they are a normal part of being a woman." Pain is our natural heritage, remember?

The Society recommends the following two dietary regimens:

1. Calcium and magnesium supplements during the week before your period for cramps.

2. High doses of vitamin C with added bioflavonoids to compensate for high estrogen levels and to reduce blood flow.

> Supplements of vitamins A, B and E, plus zinc and selenium, and evening primrose oil.

In the early 1980s, the late nutrition educator Carlton Fredericks, Ph.D., reported that a high intake of the B complex vitamins, plus extra boron, choline, inositol, and the amino acid methionine supports the liver and, not coincidentally, also lowers estrogen levels. A series of studies in the '30s and '40s showed that the liver converts the most active form of estrogen, estradiol, to the much less active form, estriol. In experiments, he demonstrated that B vitamins also reduced many symptoms of premenstrual syndrome – themselves caused by excess estrogen.[7]

John R. Lee, M.D., says that using natural progesterone cream can offset this endometriosis-catalyst, and has seen it used successfully with his patients, some after failed surgery. Progesterone stops the proliferation of the endometrial cell tissue. Dr. Lee advises his endometriosis patients to use natural progesterone cream from day six of the cycle (the first day being the first day of menstruation) to day 26 each month, adding that it takes four to six months before the progesterone is completely absorbed into the system and the desired results are obtained.[8]

Dr. Robert C. Atkins, author of *Dr. Atkins' Health Revolution*, uses these supplements in his practice to support the liver and help fight against endometriosis. To these nutrients, Dr. Atkins adds primrose oil, vitamin E, an antioxidant formula that contains vitamin C and bioflavonoids, and any mineral the patient may be deficient in. In his practice, he has seen over half of his patients clearly improved with this regimen.[9]

If you haven't gotten it by now, scores of studies have shown evening primrose oil to be beneficial for reducing inflammation, healing and protecting delicate internal tissues. This is because it contains gamma linolenic acid (GLA) a hormone-like essential fatty acid. However, studies have found that borage oil is a better source of GLA than evening primrose oil. If you look at the health food and vitamin store shelves, you'll find it is less expensive as well. These are the reasons why I advocate borage oil for GLA, instead of evening primrose oil.

DLPA – A Natural Pain Reliever

DLPA – DL-phenylalanine – is a new discovery which strengthens and protects the body's natural pain killers, endorphins. It's a mixture of two forms of the amino acid phenylalanine and is said to be as powerful as morphine, while at the same time is non-addictive and has no side effects. It also seems to help in cases of depression.

Dr. Arnold Fox, former assistant clinical professor of medicine at the University of California, Irvine, and author of the book *DLPA to End Chronic Pain and Depression*, suggests people take 375 to 400 mg of DLPA with each meal.[10] It's available in most health food and vitamin stores. He recommends you check with your doctor before taking it. Remember, only a natural doctor in tune with using natural substances will be able to give you knowledgeable guidance.

Dr. Daniel Asimus, medical director of the Persistent Pain Program at Glendale Adventist Medical Center in California, has treated more than 100 patients with DLPA and has found it to be helpful.

For more on the painful aspects of endometriosis, read my chapters Chronic Pain and Cramps. For more on the causes and solutions see the chapters Circulation Problems, Inflammation, Infertility and Stress.

Pain and Endometriosis Ending Nutrients
For maximum absorption, take supplements with meals.

Nutrient	Suggested Dosage	Formulation
Amino acids	4-6 capsules daily	Multiple formula from natural sources
Borage oil	2 capsules daily	
Flaxseed oil	1 tablespoon daily	
Lecithin	2 tablespoons with meals	
Magnesium	200 mg daily	
MSM (Methylsulfonylmethane)	500 mg three times daily	
Multi-mineral	3-4 ounces daily	In liquid solution, with vitamin B12, biotin
Multi-vitamin/mineral	6 caplets daily	Freeze-dried plant sources
Natural progesterone cream	1/3 teaspoon daily	With pregnenolone, DHEA
Vitamin B6	100 mg daily	
Vitamin C	Individual bowel tolerance*	With bioflavonoids (quercetin, rutin proanthocyanidins)

* To determine individual dosage, on the first day take 1,000 mg hourly until diarrhea occurs, then reduce dosage to just below that for individual daily dosage. Vitamin C is not toxic in large doses but must be taken throughout the day to benefit. Divide dosage to three or four times a day.

CHAPTER 66:

Epilepsy

I will never forget the first time I saw someone have an epileptic seizure. I was in a cafeteria line at school and watched in horror as a girl fell to the ground, spasms wracking her body, a pool of urine forming under her. I was shocked and embarassed for her, especially when I came to understand that it happened to her frequently, and that there was nothing the doctors could do. Wherever she is, I hope she reads this book.

What I witnessed, I came to learn later, was a grand mal seizure. Grand mal seizures involve loss of consciousness, spasms of the muscles, and rapid jerking of various body parts. Petit mal seizures are brief attacks of impaired consciousness – so-called twilight states – with flickering of the eyelids and twitching of the mouth.

I used to think of epilepsy as a disease that some people had and others did not. However, the reality is not that simple. Epilepsy can be caused by severe infections, malnutrition, low blood sugar, stroke, blood vessel spasms, and anything that causes a lack of oxygen or damage to the brain. The horrifying reality is that any of us could spend the rest of our lives dealing with it. Amazingly, many go through life suffering from it, without knowing why.

Researchers at the Arizona State University's Biochemical Department have determined that aspartame, an artificial sweetener that goes by the brand name NutraSweet, has been associated with seizures. Aluminum and lead poisoning may also be the cause.[1] The point is, wouldn't you rather know this before the damage is done? Doctors do not routinely test for metabolic imbalances and chemical poisoning, which are common causes of epilepsy. Prevention is always the best and most efficient way to avoid ill health and disease.

Nutritional Deficiencies Leading Cause

In cases where seizures cannot be pinpointed to trauma or illness, the odds are good that nutritional deficiencies causing metabolic imbalances are the culprit.

Low manganese can trigger epilepsy. Both manganese and the B vitamin choline, when deficient, interefere with nerve cell membranes and can be responsible for setting off epileptic seizures in some people. Researchers Yukio Tanaka, Ph.D., at St. Mary's Hospital in Montreal and Claire DuPont, M.D., Ph.D., of the department of biochemistry at Montreal Children's Hospital in Quebec, Canada, found that a manganese deficiency in animals caused a loss of muscle control, and rats born to manganese-deficient mothers had seizures.[2]

Manganese is important to regulating blood sugar and low blood sugar can also cause seizures. In studies, diabetics have been shown to have only one-half of the manganese of normal individuals.[3] Foods high in choline include lecithin, egg yolk and wheat germ. For optimum usage, include it with the other B vitamin foods, lentils, beans and peas.

For more on treating this common cause of seizures, see the chapters on Diabetes and High and Low Blood Sugar.

The importance of foods containing this manganese cannot be overstressed. A rule of thumb is that edible seeds and fruits and vegetables that have them will be rich in this precious mineral, such as green beans, squash and cucumbers. A calcium plus manganese deficiency results in sex organ problems, male or female. Manganese plays a vital part in so many body functions that I recommend everyone have a few ounces of cranberry juice daily as insurance. Manganese carries the spark of life – never neglect to buy manganese-rich foods.

As I have said before, anything that jeopardizes the health of brain neurons can be a cause of seizures. In 1994, German researchers set out to determine the cause of intractable seizures in two children who developed them within the first year of life. The word intractable is used to describe seizures that cannot be controlled by drugs or any other means and defy explanation. Well, the Germans figured it out. They discovered that when they gave both children selenium supplements they experienced a reduction in the number of their seizures and improvement in their EEG recordings after two weeks. The researchers now believe children with intractable seizures should be screened for a selenium deficiency as soon as possible. They reasoned that the selenium worked because it is a potent antioxidant, and the brains of these children probably had been damaged by free radicals.[4] Selenium rich foods include seafood, whole wheat and brown rice.

Vitamin E is known to multiply selenium's benefit because it, too, is a potent antioxidant. In experiments by researchers at the University of Toronto the same results as the German's selenium trial were uncovered. The Canadian researchers found similar improvements in childhood intractable epilepsy and also believed the seizures were caused by free radical damage of nerve cell membranes.[5] Vitamin E also acts to increase circulating oxygen to the brain and is found in wheat germ, sunflower seeds and seed and nut oils.

Magnesium and calcium are two other minerals important to the brain and body's circulation system. Magnesium acts as a calcium channel blocker, making sure that calcium doesn't enter and block the body's blood vessels and small arteries. Magnesium is considered to be an anti-spasmodic, as it can help alleviate muscle spasms. This mighty mineral has been used to alleviate or prevent high blood pressure related convulsions, prevent or treat heart blockages and a lack of it is implicated in serious mental disorders. It is very important to the health of the circulatory system and I fully endorse it in solution to prevent epileptic seizures. For foods high in both magnesium and calcium, target wheat germ, seeds and nuts.

Always, when supplementing with one mineral, include a formula of minerals in solution. You know you need magnesium, but if you don't also include calcium and the other minerals, there won't be any benefit at all, or you'll become deficient in another. If you take all the minerals together, in the highly absorbable formula of minerals in solution, you'll be ensuring you have a good foundation on which to build.

Factor in Low Blood Sugar

Low blood sugar, or hypoglycemia, is another problem that can factor into the epilepsy equation. Hypoglycemia causes fatigue, and in extreme cases, loss of consciousness. Up to four percent of hypoglycemics experience convulsions, with 23 percent having muscle twitching or cramps.[6]

In a letter to the editor of the *American Journal of Natural Medicine* (December 1995), Dr. Emanual Cheraskin explains that the connection between hypoglycemia and epilepsy has been documented since 1963, with studies showing patients with epilepsy consistently have notably lower blood sugar levels when tested. Additionally, he says, the *Physician's Desk Reference* notes that one of the effects of the anticonvulsant Dilantin is increased blood sugar.

Drugs and B Vitamins

Sometimes the seizures are so severe you are tempted to try anything to stop them, even pharmaceutical drugs. Be warned, however, that this could be at the expense of your health.

Anticonvulsant drugs can cause depression, memory loss, liver problems, addiction and withdrawal, rashes, blood disorders, respiratory failure, depression and heart failure, just to name a few.[7]

Check out your library's *Physician's Desk Reference* if you (or someone you know) are taking or thinking about taking any anticonvulsant.

Some of these physical side effects may be due to one important factor: that many of the commonly-used anticonvulsant drugs cause a deficiency of folic acid, a B vitamin vital to the brain. Physicians are aware of, but try to trivialize, the studies that show more than half of all patients on long-term therapy with the drugs phenytoin (i.e.: Dilantin, Aleviatin, Fenantoin), phenobarbitone (i.e.: Aparoxal, Gardenal, Luminale) and primidone (i.e.: Liskantin, Mylepsin, Mysolin) have unhealthy levels of folic acid.[8]

Simple, right? You just take lots of folic acid to remedy the problem. Wrong. Other studies have shown that when folic acid is added to the diet to remedy the problem, the number of seizures increases again![9]

In the past few years there have been a number of studies implicating folic acid deficiency as a contributing factor in mental illness. Studies have shown that a prolonged deficiency can cause neurological changes and mental deterioration. Because of their close interrelationship, vitamin B12 should accompany any folic acid supplementation. A deficiency of folic acid in pregnancy encourages birth defects including deformities, brain damage, spina bifida and neural tube defects. Other deficiency symptoms are stunted growth, graying hair, gastrointestinal problems and anemia.[10]

Niacin (vitamin B3) can help the epileptic get off anticonvulsant drugs. Abram Hoffer, Ph.D., M.D., author of *Orthomolecular Medicine for Physicians*, says one gram a day will allow the patient to take half the usual dose of medication with the same results. He warns that the niacin must first be taken for several months to get fully metabolized in the system. He explains that niacin works because by itself it has anticonvulsant properties.[11]

About forty years ago, an infant formula inadvertently deficient in vitamin B6 was being sold in the U.S. Many children who consumed this formula developed epileptic seizures which disppeared when they took a vitamin B6 supplement.[12]

Remember, the B vitamins must be taken together, so if you decide to supplement, fortify with a B complex formula. Each B vitamin has its own role in body function, centered on the nervous system.

Since nerves bring messages to all the organs and stimulate glands to secrete their important biochemicals, the whole body communication system can break down with a B vitamin deficiency.

Diet Therapy

Food allergy is an important factor to consider in children with epilepsy. In one study, 63 children with epilepsy followed an elimination diet for four weeks and then added food back to the diet one at a time. Of the 45 children with epilepsy who had food allergies, 80 percent had fewer seizures while on the diet and 56 percent became seizure free. Based on this study, Dr. Alan Gaby estimates that food allergy could be a major cause of seizures in more than half of epileptic children.[13]

The ketogenic diet is a therapy found to help. It involves a diet high in fat (87 percent of total calories) and low in protein and carbohydrates. It's called ketogenic because it promotes the formation of ketones in the body. For reasons not understood, the presence of ketones keep seizures from occurring. The diet has been used since the 1920s and has found success among patients who have tried everything else. However, since it eliminates many nutritious foods, it should be overseen by a qualified nutritionist.

Epilepsy-Easing Nutrients

Nutrient	Suggested Dosage	Formulation
Amino acids	4-6 capsules daily	Multiple formula from natural sources
Antioxidants	4 capsules daily*	With selenium and grapeseed extract
Borage oil	2 capsules daily	
Flaxseed oil	1 tablespoon daily	
Magnesium	200 mg daily	
Melatonin (adults only)	3 mg at bedtime	With B vitamins
Multi-mineral	3-4 ounces daily	In liquid solution, with vitamin B12, biotin
Multi-vitamin/mineral	6 caplets daily	Freeze-dried plant sources
Taurine	3 grams daily	
Vitamin B6	100 mg daily	
Vitamin C	Individual bowel tolerance**	With bioflavonoids (quercetin, rutin proanthocyanidins)

* The FDA recommends pregnant women not exceed 10,000 IU of vitamin A daily.

** To determine individual dosage, on the first day take 1,000 mg hourly until diarrhea occurs, then reduce dosage to just below that for individual daily dosage. Vitamin C is not toxic in large doses but must be taken throughout the day to benefit. Divide dosage to three or four times a day.

CHAPTER 67:

Eye Problems

Men are born with two eyes, but only one tongue, in order that they should see twice as much as they say.
–Charles Caleb Colton

The eyes are the windows of the heart. Quite literally from birth we see, evaluate, judge and learn about life based on what our eyes see around us. The skin protects all our internal organs except the eyes, the only living tissue of our body exposed to the air. As a result, they are constantly at risk, first mechanically, then finally as we age, from the years of exposure to oxygen, ultraviolet light and chemicals.

Approximately 500,000 Americans are legally blind, 14 million have significant visual impairment and about 80 million have eye diseases of varying intensity, according to the American Academy of Ophthalmology.[1] Much of these statistics can be attributed to poor eating habits and nutritional deficiencies. For more detailed information read the chapters Diabetic Retinopathy, Night Blindness, Cataracts, Glaucoma and Macular Degeneration. Here, I will cover the gamut so no matter what eye-related affliction you or your loved ones experience, you'll have the tools to either prevent it from occurring in the first place, keep it from getting worse, or in some cases, alleviate it completely with certain power-packed nutrients.

Vitamin A and Vision

Vitamin A is important to the eyes and visual system in several ways. The ability of the eye to adapt to changes in light is dependent upon a chemical known as retinal purple, or rhodopsin. Retinal purple is comprised mainly of protein and a close relative of vitamin A, and is the army that keeps us seeing even in darkness. But the army has one enemy: light. When light hits the retina – such as when driving and being "blinded" by oncoming headlights – the retinal purple army splits up, temporarily fleeing.[2] The next time you enter a dark room after being outside on a sunny day, see how long it takes for your vision to return. How long it takes depends upon two things: the amount of retinal purple present to begin with and the amount of light. Too much light and not enough vitamin A means the breakdown of night vision.

Conditions such as heart bypass surgery, cystic fibrosis and cirrhosis of the liver make people susceptible to vitamin A deficiency and night blindness. In one case report, a 16-year-old male with cystic fibrosis complaining of night blindness was given 25,000 IU of vitamin A. After seven months his serum vitamin A levels returned to normal and he was able to see in the dark again.[3]

In areas of the world where diet is poor, blindness due to a vitamin A deficiency is tragically common, especially among the children. Vitamin A deficiency exists in many of the 10 million children worldwide under the age of six who have impaired vision. One-tenth of these children usually go blind.[4] Over the decades since this was first discovered by the medical establishment, American physicians have made it their duty to go to these countries armed with vitamin A supplements. Once the children receive the supplements, their sight is often joyfully restored.

Doctors like to scare people away from A by emphasizing that you can take too much. Vitamin A is a so-called fat soluble vitamin, meaning it doesn't dissolve well in water and as a result, our body stores excess A in the liver. As a damaged liver can cause a vitamin

A deficiency, too much can cause liver damage. Combining vitamin E with A boosts the benefit so lower amounts can be taken, and beta carotene, a vitamin A precursor, can be taken with vitamin A to boost the benefit. Beta carotene can be taken in as high a dose as is needed, with no side effects.

A French physician, Dr. C. Carlier, conducted a study in which children with eye problems were given either vitamin A or beta carotene to see which worked better to alleviate the deficiency and restore their eyesight. He gave 256 children 200,000 IU of retinyl palmitate (vitamin A), and 254 children 1.2 million IU of beta carotene for seven weeks, then tested their eyes. Of the children receiving the vitamin A, 51.2 percent were restored to normal. Of the children receiving the beta carotene, 50 percent were restored to normal. The statistics are so close, the doctor concluded that beta carotene works just as well as vitamin A and can be used instead to avoid the toxicity issue.[5]

Vitamin A deficiencies may be more common than we think. Vitamin A can be destroyed in many different ways, including poor liver function; alcohol; eating large amounts of mineral oil or ferrous sulphate, a common preservative; x-rays; and any kind of infection.

The B Vitamins for Stress and Fatigue

How many of us are guilty of reading under dim light? Or continuing to work despite tired, fatigued eyes? The delicate tissues of the eyes are easily stressed, whether through overuse or exposure to smoke and chemicals. The B vitamins, dubbed the anti-stress vitamins, have shown to help. B complex vitamins may in fact be all that is needed to treat bloodshot eyes, eye muscle weakness, eyelid itch and tearing.[6]

Diabetic retinitis, a hemorrhaging of the eye, is a complication of diabetes often brought on by stress, and can be prevented with B vitamins.[7]

Vitamin B2 (riboflavin) aids vitamin A in preventing cataracts as well as skin disorders of the lids and skin around the eyes. It is also important in preventing eye fatigue. Vitamin B6 (pyridoxine) ensures healthy skin and eyelids.

Glare sensitivity may be associated with a B vitamin deficiency, as well as watery eyes, chronic eye fatigue and bloodshot eyes. Signs of B1 (thiamine) deficiency can include involuntary oscillation of the eyes (nystagmus), double vision, and paralysis of the eye muscles.

Each B vitamin has its own role in body function, centered on the nervous system. Since nerves bring messages to all the organs and stimulate glands to secrete their important biochemicals, the whole body communication system can break down with a B vitamin deficiency. To get all your B vitamins, eat lentils, pinto beans, black-eyed peas, black beans, lima beans, rice bran, corn, millet, barley and blackstrap molasses. Sulfa drugs, sleeping pills, insecticides and synthetic estrogen create a condition in the intestinal tract that can destroy B vitamins. All breads are "enriched" with B vitamins because the vitamin is lost when whole grains are milled for flour. Look for supplementation that uses the whole food. One such formula combines all the B vitamins in the form of sprouts and vegetables, as well as adding odorless garlic, acidophilus and green tea extract for immune-system boosting.

Vitamin C Protection

Vitamin C has been found to be instrumental in preventing cataracts and macular degeneration. The facts speak for themselves. It has been noted that ascorbic acid – vitamin C – accumulates in eye tissue at concentrations several times higher than the blood level, and that vitamin C in the eye is much higher in animals who sleep at night and are awake during the day, than animals who roam at night.[8] What does this mean? It means that you need vitamin C to prevent oxidative damage to your eyeballs; the kind of damage that occurs when they are exposed to sunlight. Since your body doesn't make vitamin C, you have to get it from foods and supplements.

Protection against cataract formation is vitamin C's most impor- tant function as far as your eyes are concerned. According to Allen Taylor, Ph.D., director of the Laboratory for Nutrition and Cataract Research at the USDA Human Nutrition Research Center on Aging at Tufts University, "the highest protective effect was seen in people with unusually high blood levels of vitamin C. By correlating data from studies, we have calculated that daily intakes of about 500 mg of vitamin C would be required to achieve such levels."

In his book *Growing Younger*, Gershon M. Lesser, M.D., sug- gests people with ulcers of the cornea take 4,000 to 6,000 milligrams of vitamin C daily.

Zinc and Other Minerals

An essential mineral that affects both general body function and the visual system is zinc. A zinc deficiency can cause very low in- traocular pressure (the opposite of glaucoma). Zinc is also involved in vitamin A metabolism, so that a zinc deficiency can result in symp- toms similar to vitamin A deficiency, such as night blindness.

Preliminary studies have shown that daily zinc supplements can be effective in retarding the severe visual loss due to macular degen- eration (loss of central vision). Jonathan V. Wright, M.D., author of *Healing With Nutrition* (Keats Publishing, Inc., 1990), reports that 40 to 50 percent of his patients with macular degeneration improved following his protocol that included selenium, vitamin E, zinc and taurine orally. Seventy to 80 percent improved when the same four nutrients were given by IV injection.

Another mineral, calcium, is important in the phototransduction process (sending light impulses to the brain from the retina). Sele- nium and copper are also crucial for ocular health, working in con- junction with the antioxidant vitamins.

Selenium works with vitamin E, zinc with copper, and calcium with magnesium. When targeting supplements, it is best to choose formulas that use these combinations to your best advantage. Miner- als are absorbed best when in solution.

Antioxidants

Synthetic antioxidants were first used in the food service industry to prevent color changes in foods high in carbohydrates or to retard rancidity in fatty foods. These undesirable color or flavor changes result from a reaction of food components with oxygen in the air.

The same chemical reactions that make food inedible ravage our immune systems, wrinkle our skin and invite illness and disease.

These chemical reactions may be a fact of life, but the impact on our body need not be.

Enter nature's wonder: antioxidants! They are super-duper nutrients that seek out and destroy the free radicals that damage our skin, joints, tissues and bones – and we're discovering new ones all the time.

Vitamin C, vitamin E and beta carotene are the most well-known antioxidants. Most alternative doctors also recommend coenzyme Q10, selenium, superoxide dismutase (SOD) and the amino acids cysteine, glutathionine, methionine and taurine. Beta carotene is probably the most well known to date. Everywhere you turn, someone's talking about beta carotene. Believe it or not, scientists have found another biologically-occurring nutrient with even more radical punching ability. Lycopene, a carotenoid (a type of bioflavonoid) that is found in the red pigment of the tomato, exhibits the highest physical quenching rate of any of the antioxidants, as revealed in a German study on antioxidants. Foods high in lycopene are tomatoes, dried and canned apricots, grapefruit, guava juice and watermelon.

Vitamin E can help strengthen and restore eye muscles, especially those holding the retina. Protruding eyes are a sign of a vitamin E deficiency, and vitamin E has been shown to be helpful for crossed eyes, blurred vision and a detached retina.[9]

Researchers at the Sidney, Australia Save Sight and Eye Health Institute found that antioxidants, most especially vitamin E, helped restore, protect and strengthen the corneas of laboratory rabbits. In an article in *Current Eye Research*, they emphasized that antioxidants not only prevent oxidative damage, but are important for the integrity of the eye lens, retina and cornea in humans.[10]

Retina Problems

Diabetic retinopathy, a situation where the lining of the eyeball deteriorates, is one of the numerous side-effects associated with diabetes. About half the nation's estimated 14 million people with diabetes may have diabetic retinopathy, including its early stages. Ultimately, all patients with Type 1 or juvenile diabetes develop retinopathy. For those with Type 2 diabetes, up to 21 percent show retinopathy at the time of their initial diagnosis.

The disease can progress, even to a severe stage, and not have noticeable symptoms. To complicate matters even more, many people with diabetes don't know that the disease can affect their eyes. Some patients continue to have good vision in one eye, compensating for the poor vision in the diseased eye. The good news is that nutrition can make all the difference in whether or not the disease progresses.

Japanese researchers gave 90 to 180 milligrams of vitamin E daily to 38 patients with retinopathy. After 19 to 24 months on this therapy, an incredible 67 percent of all patients reported significant improvement in their condition.[11]

In recent years, researchers have learned that an omega-3 fatty acid, docosahexaenoic acid (DHA), is the most prominent polyunsaturated fat in the retina, and that a lack of it in the diet may contribute to retinopathy. Ironically, chronically high blood sugar in diabetics blocks an enzyme that processes omega-3 from food sources into DHA, thus making the effects of any omega-3 deficiency worse.[12]

You can find omega-3 in flaxseed oil, cod liver oil; and in cold water fish such as trout, mackerel, sardines, tuna and eel. It is believed eating foods rich in omega-3 may prevent or improve diabetes, cancer tumors and low blood sugar. Omega-3 fatty acids are also found in fresh dark green vegetables like broccoli, kale, collards and Swiss chard.

Also found to benefit are the essential fatty acids, most especially borage oil, which contains gamma linolenic acid (GLA). Very large doses of GLA have been shown to reduce by two thirds the risk of eye disease over a period of about six years. Extensive research on the benefits of GLA has found it to reverse a variety of problems diabetics typically experience, especially retina problems.[13]

The amino acid acetyl-L-carnitine has also been found to help prevent and restore problems with the eye retina. After performing double blind studies, researchers at the Eye Clinic at Catholic University in Rome concluded that carnitine can be helpful in cases of retinal dysfunction.[14]

For retinal nerve hemorrhages, zinc and omega-3, have been found useful, and retinosa pigmentosa can be helped with vitamin A, vitamin E, lecithin and omega-3 fish oil.[15]

Although there have not yet been reports of taurine-deficient blindness in humans, researchers have found that people suffering from retinitis pigmentosa show abnormal blood levels of taurine. Taurine levels within the eye also have been shown to be decreased in this disease. It is known that taurine can protect the eye and body from various toxins.[16]

In the human body, taurine regulates heartbeat, brain chemistry and vision, and is helpful in digesting fats and ridding the body of cholesterol. Since it is found in body tissues, especially the eyes and heart, it was long thought that we didn't need taurine from food. However, studies at the Oregon Primate Research Center in Portland in 1984 showed that baby monkeys fed milk with no taurine developed eye trouble.

How do we know we're getting enough taurine from the foods we eat? The highest levels of taurine is found in mother's milk and your health food store. But since taurine is an amino acid, look to foods high in essential amino acids like seafood, eggs, beans and peas.

Anthocyanosides – no, they are not a class of insects – are a class of bioflavonoids found in fruits and vegetables, most notably blueberries, grapes and bilberries. They are known for their anti-inflammatory, antioxidant and tissue enhancement properties. Quercetin, available in health food stores, vitamin formulas and in yellow and purple onions, is known to inhibit aldose reductase.

Aldose reductase is an enzyme believed to be the culprit in the damaging effect of diabetes. Aldose reductase transforms excess blood sugar into an alcohol sugar the body can't burn, and this accumulates in nerve cells and damages them. This is one of the things believed to contribute to diabetic retinopathy.

Bilberry Jam, Anyone?

Anthocyanosides are present in the European version of our blueberry, called the bilberry. For hundreds of years, bilberry fruit, a popular source of fresh jam, has been considered a food substance of the purest kind.

One of the most notable discoveries for the use of bilberry fruit was made during World War II. Shortly before their night missions, British RAF pilots would snack on bread covered with bilberry jam. Throughout the war, these pilots seemed to be far more successful at hitting their targets than the enemy. The British pilots swore that eating bilberry jam prior to night missions improved their night vision.

Since then, numerous studies have been published confirming bilberry's effectiveness in helping a variety of visual problems including night blindness, eye fatigue, nearsightedness, cataracts and glaucoma. Studies suggest it may help with color blindness as well.

Animal and laboratory studies have revealed how bilberry works. On a basic level, bilberry helps to strengthen the tiny capillaries that deliver nutrients to eye muscles and nerves. It also decreases the permeability of blood vessels, thereby reducing the damage caused by deterioration of blood vessels. Bilberry also helps the eyes' ability to see at night by increasing retinal purple. Plus, bilberry acts as a photomultiplier on the retina by heightening the perception of normal objects, thus extending the range and sharpness of vision. This multipurpose fruit also contains calcium, magnesium, phosphorous, potassium and lots of the antioxidant vitamin C.

Dry Eye

Nutritional health is nowhere more important than in keeping the tears flowing. Dry eye has been associated with severe malnutrition since many nutrients take part in making sure the lacrimal (tear duct) gland functions properly. Nutrients needed for a good cry are: vitamin B6, vitamin C, folic acid, zinc, potassium, calcium, linolenic acid (borage oil), and of course, water. An article in *Optometry and Vision Science* suggests the following dietary guidelines to keep those tears flowing. These include: 1) Reduce protein, total fat and cholesterol while increasing complex carbohydrates. 2) Increase the intake of red, orange, yellow and dark green vegetables as sources of vitamin A. 3) Increase consumption of grains, legumes and raw vegetables to increase zinc and folic acid uptake. 4) Vitamin B6 and potassium may be increased in the diet by eating nuts, bananas and beans. 5) Consume more foods high in vitamin C. 6) Eliminate alcohol and caffeine. 7) Reduce sugar and salt. 8) Increase water consumption to six to eight glasses per day.[17]

Sight-Restoring Nutrients
For maximum absorption, take supplements with meals.

Nutrient	Suggested Dosage	Formulation
Antioxidants	4 capsules daily*	With selenium and grapeseed extract
Bilberry	100 mg twice daily	
Borage oil	2 capsules daily	
Coenzyme Q10	2 capsules daily	With vitamin E, phospholipids and selenium
Flaxseed oil	1 tablespoon daily	
Ginkgo biloba	60 mg daily	
Magnesium	200 mg daily	
Multi-mineral	3-4 ounces daily	In liquid solution, with vitamin B12, biotin
Multi-vitamin/mineral	6 caplets daily	Freeze-dried plant sources
Vitamin A	25,000 IU daily*	
Vitamin C	Individual bowel tolerance**	With bioflavonoids (quercetin, rutin proanthocyanidins)

* The FDA recommends pregnant women not exceed 10,000 IU of vitamin A daily.

** To determine individual dosage, on the first day take 1,000 mg hourly until diarrhea occurs, then reduce dosage to just below that for individual daily dosage. Vitamin C is not toxic in large doses but must be taken throughout the day to benefit. Divide dosage to three or four times a day.

CHAPTER 68:

Fatigue

"A deficiency of any one vitamin or mineral will result in fatigue."

–Richard Kunin, M.D.

If you are constantly tired, consider the possibility that you are anemic. Anemia is basically a nutritional deficiency which causes a reduction in the number of hemoglobin molecules and/or in the number or size of red blood cells. This condition can result from many factors that have nothing to do with whether the body is taking in or storing enough iron. Anemia can be caused by deficiencies of folic acid, vitamin B6, vitamin B12 and copper, and conditions that pull these nutrients out of your body, of which there are many. See the chapter Anemia for more.

Nutritional Energy Boosters

Magnesium, safe at doses of 300-1,500 mg chelated, is good for fatigue. Magnesium is responsible for 80 percent of all the body's enzymatic reactions and activities. That makes it extremely important! A deficiency of magnesium has also been linked to muscle weakness.

A deficiency of vitamin B12 is associated with pernicious anemia, a common reason for fatigue. Even without anemia, a B12 deficiency can cause memory loss, weakness of the limbs and even paralysis. However, according to a study cited in the *Journal of Nutri-*

tional Medicine, the most common symptom is fatigue.[1]

Among those with many years behind them, thiamine – another B vitamin – has been found to help with fatigue. In a double-blind trial 80 randomly selected, healthy, elderly Irish women between the ages of 65 and 92 years of age were put on a baseline diet for four weeks, followed by a six week double-blind trial with 10 mgs of thiamine daily. Compared to the controls, thiamine supplemented females showed increased appetite, energy intake, body weight, general well being and less fatigue.[2]

Thiamine is found in the germ and bran of wheat, the husk of rice, and that portion of all grains which is commercially milled away to give the grain its lighter color and finer texture. A diet rich in brewer's yeast, wheat germ, blackstrap molasses and bran will provide the body with adequate thiamine. Eating sugar will cause a thiamine depletion, as will smoking and drinking alcohol. Thiamine can be destroyed by an enzyme present in raw clams, oysters and raw fish.[3]

It may well be that carnitine, an amino acid and protein building block, is the key to energy and stamina. A deficiency of carnitine is more common than most people think, since aspirin interferes with the body's use of it. Anyone with unexplained fatigue might find carnitine supplements helpful – at least worth a try.[4]

High amounts of carnitine is found in meat, most especially the red meats, which is why I recommend supplementation.

Eating for Energy

How you eat and when you eat is just as important as what you eat, when it comes to avoiding fatigue. Especially if you are under stress and when you need physical strength.

If you took a survey of teenagers, you'd probably find most of them are dieting. If you asked them about their energy levels, they would answer, "What energy levels?" Unfortunately, it has become a common misconception that skipping meals and starvation is akin to losing weight. If you read my Weight Loss chapter, you'll see this just isn't so. All dieting does is lower the metabolism so fat burns more slowly, and diminish blood sugar and energy levels. Low blood sugar, or hypoglycemia, causes fatigue, and in extreme cases, loss of consciousness.

Eating regular meals (especially breakfast, and lunch) and high complex carbohydrate foods, versus greasy fatty foods, will go farther in reducing fat and increasing energy than any dieting program – liquid or not. To boost your energy, eat power breakfasts and lunches, rather than skipping meals. To fight fatigue during a long workout (mental as well as physical) eat whole grain cereals and breads, fresh-squeezed fruit and vegetable juices, raisins, figs, beans and lentils, and plenty of water. A lentil soup breakfast, while it sounds inappropriate, is most appropriate for an energetic day. Not eating breakfast means that you've already had 12 or more hours without food. Tackling anything after fasting that long is going to leave you with low blood sugar and depressing fatigue, if not exhaustion.

Leave behind the typical on-the-run breakfast of donuts and coffee. You might get a "charge" out of the refined sugar in the donut and the caffeine in the coffee, but it will be a temporary one, as your blood sugar rises then plummets when the energy is quickly absorbed. Carbohydrate snacks containing sugars and starches provide the body with almost instant energy because they cause a sudden rise in the blood sugar level. However, the blood sugar level drops again rapidly, creating a craving for more sweet food and possibly fatigue.[5]

Other Causes of Fatigue

Stress can be caused by many situations and physical conditions. It can be emotional or physical. However, if long-term, it can drain the adrenal glands' hormonal resources, leaving it as useless as a drained battery. Adrenal exhaustion can produce overwhelming fatigue which studies show is correctable with the nutrients pantothenic acid (vitamin B5) and vitamin A.[6]

In one study, prisoner volunteers deprived of pantothenic acid for 25 days became so exhausted and seriously ill that the test had to be called off. Even on a regimen of 4,000 milligrams, the volunteers recovered slowly.[7] For more on alleviating the devastating effects of stress see the chapter Stress.

On several occasions when he spoke at National Health Federation meetings, Broda O. Barnes, M.D., Ph.D., an authority on thyroid function told me, "In my 40-plus years as a medical doctor, four out of five of my thousands of patients with fatigue turned out to be hypothyroid."

In his numerous published papers and at physicians' conventions and meetings, he advised doctors to rule out hypothyroidism – low thyroid function – before considering any other diagnosis for extreme fatigue. He also advised them to request that their patients take the Barnes Basal Temperature Test, the armpit test described in the Low Thyroid chapter.

Candida Albicans, a fungus that causes yeast infections, is known to disable the body system to such a degree that fatigue sets in. This benign yeast found in the colon can overgrow under stress and sickness to literally overwhelm the body. The best army to battle this bombshell is the body's own bacteria, found in cultured food and supplements that contain acidophilus bacillus and other helpful bacteria. See the chapter Fungus Infections for more.

Allergy Route to Low Energy

One of the little-known causes of fatigue is allergy to food and the environment. Have you heard of sick building syndrome? One of the symptoms is fatigue, and it is caused by an allergic reaction to the plethora of chemicals found in building materials – especially new buildings.

A young woman who owned a novelty manufacturing company came to me for a referral to a doctor. Her complaint was fatigue beyond fatigue. She had to lock her office door to take frequent naps, morning, noon and afternoon to get through the day. If she had a business appointment at night, she made it fairly late so she could nap for an hour before going out.

"Maureen, I've got everything I need business-wise, financially and socially, but I can't continue living a fractional life. Do you suppose I have sleeping sickness?"

"Not likely," I replied. "I'll set up an appointment for you with one of the best alternative physicians I know."

We continued talking. Since her fatigue was continual, I reasoned it could be caused by low blood sugar, anemia, a poorly functioning thyroid gland or possibly a yeast infection. However, when I questioned her, she said tests had eliminated these possibilities. I asked her if she ever experienced any other symptoms, no matter how mild. She told me her eyes watered when she came into the office in the morning, but that her fatigue didn't get any worse after that. A thought struck me – something we hadn't considered yet – the possibility that she could be chemically poisoned. I directed her to a special kind of doctor, a clinical ecologist. Sure enough, he discovered that a chemical disinfectant used in her private bathroom was causing her fatigue. Once it was eliminated, after a few weeks and a nutritional regimen to restore her immune system, her former energy level returned.

Fatigue is one of many symptoms attributed to a reaction to the many chemical pollutants assailing us everyday. Pollutants include but are not limited to building and furnishing materials, household products, heavy metals, lead and radon.[8]

According to the Environmental Protection Agency (EPA), up to 30 percent of new and remodeled buildings trigger symptoms such as fatigue in some of their occupants.[9] Self-contained air-circulation systems in large buildings, coupled with the increasing chemical content of building materials contribute to a newly-identified disorder called "sick building syndrome." Sick building syndrome is a collection of complaints, including eye, nose, and throat irritation, headaches, fatigue, dizziness, and skin irritation.

The National Institute for Occupational Safety and Health investigated a number of sick building syndrome complaints and found that fully half were caused by inadequate ventilation.[10]

Undiagnosed food allergies can be another cause of fatigue. Researchers have found that when patients with chronic fatigue had their food allergies identified and eliminated, their symptoms ended or were improved.

When it comes to identifying allergens, scratch the conventional tests. The food elimination diet and Coca Pulse Test are much more reliable. Because allergens can cause the heart rate to soar, taking your pulse in the morning upon rising, and comparing it to your rate after eating certain foods will help you target offending foods.

Narrow your list down to the following foods suspect for most allergy sufferers: beef, sugar, chocolate, eggs, citrus fruits, coffee, corn, malt, milk, pork, potatoes, soybeans, spices, tomatoes, wheat and yeast. Then read the chapter on Allergies.

Fatigue-Fighting Nutrients
For maximum absorption, take nutrients with meals.

Nutrient	Suggested Dosage	Formulation
Acidophilus	At least four billion flora daily on an empty stomach, three times daily	
Aged garlic extract	1 teaspoon three times daily	Liquid
Amino acids	4-6 capsules daily	Multiple formula from natural sources
Antioxidants	4 capsules daily*	With selenium and grapeseed extract
Borage oil	2 capsules daily	
Coenzyme Q10	2 capsules daily	With vitamin E, phospholipids and selenium
Flaxseed oil	1 tablespoon daily	
L-Glutamine	500 mg three times daily	
Melatonin (adults only)	3 mg daily at bedtime	With B vitamins
Multi-mineral	3-4 ounces daily	In liquid solution, with vitamin B12, biotin
Multi-vitamin/mineral	6 caplets daily	Freeze-dried plant sources
Vitamin C	Individual bowel tolerance**	With bioflavonoids (quercetin, rutin proanthocyanidins)
Vitamin E	2 capsules (800 IU)	d-alpha tocopherol

* The FDA recommends pregnant women not exceed 10,000 IU of vitamin A daily.

** To determine individual dosage, on the first day take 1,000 mg hourly until diarrhea occurs, then reduce dosage to just below that for individual daily dosage. Vitamin C is not toxic in large doses but must be taken throughout the day to benefit. Divide dosage to three or four times a day.

CHAPTER 69:

Fever

So, which is it? Starve a cold and feed a fever, or starve a fever and feed a cold? Neither! Perhaps one of the most well-known medical myths is that old saw, "Feed a cold, starve a fever." Trouble is, it simply isn't true.

I can't think of any illness where you'd want to starve a person. You should always try to remain well nourished when you're ill. In fact, you may actually need to eat *more* when you have a fever because the body burns calories faster.

If you don't believe that with age comes wisdom, here's one study to prove you wrong. The Dixie paper products company – no doubt in keeping with their promotion of disposable cups to prevent passing on cold viruses – did a survey of people's belief in the feeding/ starving axiom. They found the belief diminishes with age. Among adults 18 to 34, 40 percent agree with the advice. After age 50, believers drop off to 30 percent.[1] Perhaps nonbelievers prefer orange juice and a box of tissues.

What exactly does it mean to have a fever? A fever is the elevation of normal body temperature. Normal temperature varies from individual to individual, although it is generally considered to be within the range of 97 to 99 degrees Fahrenheit. When the body temperature is raised not more than five degrees, the body can protect itself from the effects. However, when a fever reaches 106 degrees, convulsions can occur. Above 108 degrees and irreversible brain damage can result.

Fever accompanies a wide range of mild to severe illnesses and should be considered a warning that something is wrong in the body. Fever is a symptom, not a problem, so don't automatically reach for the medicine cabinet. In some cases, a fever reducer can cause problems, such as aspirin causing Reye's Syndrome in children with the flu. Feverish skin can be either hot or and dry or wet with perspiration. At high temperatures, the body eventually perspires to cool itself down.

Reye's Syndrome is a rare affliction that can occur among children with viral infections taking aspirin. Most victims are between ages 5 and 12. Symptoms include severe fatigue, vomiting, agitation, delirium, coma – even death.

Something to keep in mind about fevers is that they typically lower blood sugar, creating a temporary case of hypoglycemia, complete with muscle weakness, dizziness and fatigue. To counter this effect, read my chapter on Low Blood Sugar.

Feed a Fever

Because fever increases the body's use of energy, more food and nutrients are needed. Additional protein is necessary to replace and rebuild damaged body tissues and to form antibodies, your body's army against infection. Purified – not bottled – water is essential to replenish lost fluids. When fluid is lost, sodium and potassium are also depleted with it, and need to be replenished.

Because the body uses more energy when it is battling internal bad guys, a deficiency of several nutrients can be expected. Vitamin C and magnesium are two nutrients especially important to heal the body, and not coincidentally are lost during periods of stress. Low potassium levels will deplete the body of magnesium, threatening muscle tissue.

Dried fruit (unsulphered) and fruit juices are good sources of magnesium, potassium and sodium. One cup of apple juice contains 296 milligrams of potassium, and ten dried figs contain 1,332 milligrams. One cup of prune juice contains 706 mg of potassium and one cup of raisins contains 1,362 milligrams.[2]

The old folks knew it best: one tablespoon of blackstrap molasses contains 52 mg of magnesium, 585 mg of potassium and 19 mg of sodium. Stir it into water or juice for easy assimilation. Better yet, look for a good, easily absorbable, derived-from-nature mineral blend in solution. Liquid formulations provide the maximum absorption ratios.

Fevers have been shown in studies to increase the need for vitamin A and the B vitamins. If you are taking antibiotics, be sure to supplement with an acidophilus formula because it will replenish the intestinal bacteria that are responsible for the synthesis of the B vitamins.[3]

Dr. C.B. Stephensen and colleagues at the Department of International Health at the University of Alabama, Birmingham, conducted a study of 58 subjects with pneumonia and infections and found that 34 of those with fevers lost what amounted to half the RDA of vitamin A. Dr. Stephensen believes this loss of vitamin A may compromise an already sick patient and create a better chance of further infection and complications.[4]

Fever-Fighting Nutrients
For maximum absorption, take supplements with meals.
Lower the dosage by half for children.

Nutrient	Suggested Dosage	Formulation
Aged garlic extract	1 teaspoon three times daily	Liquid
Antioxidants	4 capsules daily*	With selenium, grape seed extract
Magnesium	200 mg daily	
Multi-mineral	3-4 ounces daily	In liquid solution, with vitamin B12, biotin
Multi-vitamin/mineral	6 caplets daily	Freeze-dried plant sources
Vitamin A	10,000-25,000 IU daily*	
Vitamin B6	100 mg daily	
Vitamin C	Individual bowel tolerance**	With bioflavonoids (quercetin, proanthocyanidins)

* The FDA recommends pregnant women not exceed 10,000 IU of vitamin A daily.

** To determine individual dosage, on the first day take 1,000 mg hourly until diarrhea occurs, then reduce dosage to just below that for individual daily dosage. Vitamin C is not toxic in large doses but must be taken throughout the day to benefit. Divide dosage to three or four times a day.

CHAPTER 70:

Fibrocystic Breast Syndrome

Why call it a disease when it's not? "Breast disease" is a phrase that makes most women apprehensive. After examining a woman's breasts or reading a mammogram, a doctor may announce that the patient has "fibrocystic disease" or "benign breast disease." If it's benign, why call it a disease?

Disease is a terrible word to use for something that is relatively harmless. Sometimes a doctor uses it to describe chronically lumpy breasts that may be painful and tender before menstruation. More often, "fibrocystic disease" simply refers to the natural overall lumpiness that can occur in breast tissue as a woman ages.

This kind of thing is all too common among conventional medicine: make the problem seem daunting enough to be accepted as incurable. These changes are natural and are no more a disease than gray hair or age lines.

In 1985, the Cancer Committee of the College of American Pathologists called "fibrocystic disease" unacceptable terminology and expressed concern that women might be denied medical insurance on this basis.[1]

If your insurance reimburses you for breast exams and mammograms, notice what diagnosis your doctor or radiologist writes on the forms. If he or she writes "fibrocystic disease," request that he or she instead refer to it as "cystic mastitis" or "mammary dysplasia," which are other, less alarming terms used to denote this problem.

The reason women seek medical intervention for fibrocystic breasts is because as they get older the number of benign cysts increase and the surrounding tissue, inflamed and engorged with fluid, causes acute pain. It's the pain of this natural inflammation that drives women to doctors' examining tables.

Iodine and Magnesium ala Dr. Wright

Drs. Jonathan Wright and Alan Gaby have chronicled little-known, yet successful therapies for common ailments, enlightening a choice-less consumer public desperate for options. Dr. Wright explained how he treated a 36-year old patient with very painful fibrocystic breasts. The problem started when she was 17, and got progressively worse until the monthly pain in her breasts became intolerable. She had suffered with the condition for almost 20 years when she found herself on Dr. Wright's examining table.[2]

Dr. Wright found dozens of lumps in each breast, varying in diameter from one-quarter inch to an inch. There was swelling in the tissue between and around the lumps, and of course both breasts were extremely tender.

The first thing he did was to get her to stop consuming caffeine in all forms, including the caffeine contained in pain relievers, which she didn't know about. Caffeine is also contained in some teas, chocolate drinks and chocolate candy, coffee, and of course in many sodas.

Then he told her about a treatment first discovered by Dr. John Meyers, a pioneer in the clinical use of minerals during the 1930s and '40s. Dr. Meyers discovered that when fibrocystic breast patients' ovaries were treated with iodine, followed by an intravenous injection of magnesium, their pain and inflammation could be eliminated. In less severe cases, oral doses of iodine and magnesium were enough. Dr. Wright's modern protocol adds vitamin B6, vitamin E, gamma linolenic acid and selenium.

And how did Dr. Wright's fair patient fare?

Almost immediately after a vaginal swab of iodine
and a magnesium injection, she noted less pain.

Seven months later, after maintaining an oral prescription of iodine
drops, magnesium and the other supporting nutrients, being careful
to stay away from caffeine, she happily reported that all her pain was
gone, and her cysts were considerably smaller.

The Estrogen Connection

One thing upon which most doctors agree: fibrocystic breasts are
affected by estrogen in the body and by the menstrual cycle. The
condition essentially is never seen before puberty and goes away
after menopause (when estrogen levels naturally drop), unless a
woman is receiving estrogen-replacement therapy. Treatment that
reduces estrogen production typically decreases the extent of the problem.

What can figure into this equation are the thousands of man-made
estrogens that can stack the deck against women and increase their
estrogen levels by hundreds of times. Devra Lee Davis, Ph.D. a senior advisor to the U.S. Department of Health and Human Services,
pinpoints pesticides, household chemicals and common plastics as
some of these man-made estrogens.[3] It is quite possible that the same
forces increasing our risk for breast cancer increase the chances of
having fibrocystic breasts.

Before 1950, a lot of pesticides, like DDT, were not so prevalent
in the environment. What we've learned is that today's modern environment – filled with plastics, chemicals and electronics – contain
innumerable man-made estrogen building blocks. Another factor in
this hazard is the hormones fed to animals to increase their meat
marketability. I have given up meat almost entirely after discovering
the garbage that is being fed to animals and the amounts of pesticide
residues that are stored in meat fat. Nobody has been able to assure

the meat-eating consumer public that these hormones don't end up in our bodies in harmful amounts. What can we do to protect ourselves? Fortunately, there is much we can do.

Christiane Northrup, M.D., co-founder of Woman to Woman Health Care Center in Yarmouth, Maine, found answers outside the realm of drugs and surgery. She now regularly incorporates alternative therapies in her treatment of fibrocystic breasts.

The mainstay of Northrup's treatment program is to decrease the amount of circulating estrogen. To decrease estrogen production, her first step is to prescribe a low-fat diet, preferably vegetarian, containing no more than 20 to 25 grams of fat a day and eliminating all dairy products. This diet usually reduces estrogen levels sufficiently but not to the point where menstruation stops. A high-fat, animal protein diet substantially increases a woman's estrogen load.[4] Many women find relief by simply eliminating dairy products.[5] Don't forget the hormones fed to milk cows! Synthetic vitamin D is just that: a hormone!

Another anti-estrogen plan of action involves the use of natural plant estrogens, called phytoestrogens, which may prevent man-made estrogens from entering cells.This has been particularly true in the case of bioflavonoids. They are substances found in brightly-colored fruits and vegetables. Bioflavonoids are not only phytoestrogenic, but act as potent anti-inflammatories, extremely important in reducing the inflammation associated with the pain.

Foods bountiful in bioflavonoids are citrus rind, cherries, grapes, plums, black currants, apricots, buckwheat, blackberries and rose hips. Phytoestrogenic foods include apples, carrots, yams, green beans, peas, potatoes, red beans, brown rice, whole wheat, rye, flaxseeds and sesame seeds.

Legumes – peas, beans and certain roots – are a form of bioflavonoid called isoflavonoids, which act as a non-steroidal estrogen. Soybeans, particularly, have been found to have this anti-estrogenic property, and have been associated with a lower incidence of breast cancer in some populations. Breast cancer is related because high blood estrogen levels have been found to increase this type of can-cer. Soybeans are eaten in great quantities in Japan and China, and is one of the reasons researchers believe these countries have low rates of breast cancer.[6] Tofu, soybean curd, is an excellent food source. It has the unique ability to absorb the flavors it is cooked in. Similar in texture to custard, it can be cubed and added to soups and casseroles as a substitute for meat.

In the early 1980s, nutrition educator Carlton Fredericks, Ph.D., reported that a high intake of the B complex vitamins, plus extra choline and inositol, helped the liver break down estrogen into es-triol, a non-carcinogenic form of the hormone. In experiments, he demonstrated that B vitamins also reduced many symptoms of pre-menstrual syndrome – also caused by excess estrogen.[7]

Dr. Northrup agrees. She says 100 milligrams of vitamin B6 helps eliminate the fluid retained in postmenopausal breasts, and when it is accompanied by at least 50 milligrams of the other B vitamins, estro-gen is better metabolized by the liver.[8]

John R. Lee, M.D. has successfully used natural progesterone in cream form, applied topically, for his menopausal and osteoporotic patients, and he reports a strong benefit for fibrocystic breasts. He maintains that when natural progesterone is used during the two weeks before menstruation, fibrocystic breasts return to normal within 2-3 months. [9]

Breast-Healthy Nutrients

Certain nutrients are important to cellular tissue, including that which makes up the breast. Some even have a direct impact on breast tissue specifically. Gamma linolenic acid (GLA), is an essential fatty acid that not only strengthens body tissue, but allows the body to absorb the kind of fat that forms the bumps and lumps characteristic of fibrocystic breasts. What this means is that when you don't have enough GLA in your body, the tendency of your body tissue to store fat and accumulate cysts is increased. This nutrient is so important to your health, a deficiency of it may contribute to heart disease, weight gain, high cholesterol, poor circulation, cancer, and a plethora of other problems.

GLA also relates to estrogen. This is due to the connection I've mentioned between fat and estrogen. Hydrogenated fat, such as in margarine and foods containing hydrogenated oil (read the labels!), tend to reduce the body's ability to convert essential fatty acids from the diet into GLA. Red meat, caffeine, large amounts of dietary fat and even epinephrine (produced by the adrenal glands during stress), undermine the smooth conversion of essential fatty acids into GLA. It is easy to see why many women living in high-stress industrialized countries and eating a diet rich in fat and processed foods are suffering from fibrocystic breast disease.

The best source of GLA is borage oil. Independent clinical tests show that borage oil contains up to 26 percent GLA. Compare this to evening primrose oil and black currant oil, which contain no more than 18 percent. Not only that, borage oil costs less because the borage seed is three times larger than black currant or evening primrose seeds. Finally, borage is more bioavailable. In other words, the body more readily accepts it.[10]

Other nutrients reduce inflammation and regulate the body fat so it also helps control the accumulation into cysts. These nutrients are vitamin C, calcium and the B vitamins. All regulate prostaglandins, hormones that regulate the growth of breast tissue.[11]

For some women, vitamin E is all it takes to reverse symptoms. In a double-blind study reported in the *Journal of the American College of Nutrition*, 75 women with PMS and fibrocystic breast disease were given vitamin E. Following two months of varying therapeutic doses, 300 IU was determined to substantially relieve breast tenderness and other common premenstrual symptoms.[12]

Dr. Wright recommends 800 IU daily. But for some women, vitamin E is more effective when taken with 200 micrograms of selenium daily.[13]

Fibrocystic-Stopping Nutrients
For maximum absorption, supplements should be taken with meals.

Nutrient	Suggested Dosage	Formulation
Aged garlic extract	2 teaspoons three times daily	Liquid
Antioxidants	4 capsules daily*	With selenium and grape seed extract
Borage oil	2 capsules daily	
Enzymes	2 capsules twice daily	Multiple formula
Flaxseed oil	1 tablespoon daily	
Fiber	8 tablets daily	Psyllium, with herb hyssop
Lecithin	2 tablespoons with meals	
Magnesium	200 mg daily	
Multi-vitamin/mineral	6 caplets daily	Freeze-dried plant sources
Multi-mineral	2-4 ounces daily	In liquid solution, with vitamin B12, biotin
Natural progesterone cream	1/3 teaspoon daily	With pregnenolone, DHEA
Vitamin B6	200 mg daily	
Vitamin C	Individual bowel tolerance**	With bioflavonoids (quercetin, rutin proanthocyanidins)
Vitamin E	2 capsules (800 IU)	d-alpha tocopherol

* The FDA recommends that pregnant women not exceed 10,000 IU of vitamin A daily.

** To determine individual dosage, on the first day take 1,000 mg hourly until diarrhea occurs, then reduce dosage to just below that for individual daily dosage. Vitamin C is not toxic in large doses but must be taken throughout the day to benefit. Divide dosage to three or four times a day.

CHAPTER 71:

Fibromyalgia

Patty Dopp was a healthy 34-year-old ski instructor – an athletic, adventuresome person, always the first to suggest a bike ride, a ski trip, or a bumpy Jeep trek to a jungle archeological site. Further, she had been health-conscious years before it was fashionable, cutting out saturated fat and red meat, making sure to stretch properly before and after exercise.

Her body was more than her friend. Its strength, grace, and health was a central component of her identity. She had taken her health for granted since she was a young girl, serving as the captain of the soccer team and the belle of the senior prom.

And then it happened: pain. Pain that cut through her back and legs like a molten spear. Pain that turned her into a different person – someone who was fearful, no longer the natural optimist in control of her world.

The pain cut beyond her muscles, tendons and nerves. It attacked her soul. She felt betrayed. She had spent all her life in service to her body; had nurtured it, challenged it, developed it. She had protected it from pollutants, shielded it from injury. Now it had turned on her, breaking its half of the commitment.

Like many with this confounding affliction, it began during a time of stress. Patty's father was recovering from heart surgery when she began to experience numbness down the back of her left thigh after the daily half hour drive to and from the hospital.

Following pronouncement by an internist, neurologist and doctor of physical rehabilitative medicine that it was a bulging spinal disc, the numbness turned to pains which coursed down both legs to her toes. It took seven months of hits and misses before she was given a diagnosis that she was certain was correct: fibromyalgia, sometimes known as fibrositis.

Fibromyalgia is a rheumatic condition that causes pain and spasms in tendons, ligaments and muscles, sometimes creating enough irritation to inflame nerves. The condition is usually accompanied by insomnia that robs the body of rest, thereby blocking it from healing itself. In fact, recent research indicates that the sleep disorder might actually cause the tissue irritation. Five million Americans, 80 percent of them women between 25 and 50, have fibromyalgia. Although doctors have chronicled the symptoms of fibromyalgia since 1904, and it was the most common cause of non-combat disability for soldiers during WWI, it wasn't until the 1980s that it became widely recognized in the medical community.[1]

The Magnesium/Calcium Connection

Stress is one of the common denominators of fibromyalgia. We know what stress does to the body: adrenaline increases heart rate and blood pressure, causing veins to dilate and blood sugar to rise. Circulation through lungs, liver and skeletal muscles increases by as much as one hundred percent.[2] High amounts of adrenaline inhibit digestion and reproduction, and while we aren't necessarily conscious of all the changes that take place, what we might notice are sore, weak muscles, constipation and fatigue. It is interesting that fibromyalgia patients have exhibited most of these stress-related symptoms.

Dr. Hans Seyle, author of the book *Stress Without Distress*, and a Nobel prize winning biologist, found in rat experiments that in stressful situations, calcium is drawn from the bones and deposited in the tissues. When this happens, the calcium can crystalize, causing blockages and pain.

A lack of certain nutrients also triggers accumulations of calcium in the soft tissues of the body, which causes or contributes to pain.

Thomas J. Romano, M.D., a faculty member of the American Academy of Pain Management in Wheeling, West Virginia, studied 100 fibromyalgia patients and found that many were deficient in magnesium.[3]

Magnesium and calcium work in balance throughout our bodies. Without magnesium, calcium accumulates in places it shouldn't. The consequences of taking calcium without magnesium is that calcium moves from where it belongs: hard tissue (the bones), to where it doesn't: soft tissues (muscles, arteries and the skin).

Magnesium Minimizes Pain

One study showed that aspirin didn't work properly unless accompanied by magnesium. Magnesium is very important to the muscles, a source of pain for many. It counters the stimulating effect of calcium, as well as helps promote absorption of calcium, phosphorus, potassium, the B vitamins, and vitamins C and E. A deficiency of magnesium can cause muscle cramps, depression and blood clots.

Magnesium has been used to inhibit pain from spinal cord injuries,[4] and James Braly, M.D., Medical Director of Immuno Labs, Inc., Ft. Lauderdale, Florida, recommends magnesium glycinate in a program of nutritional pain supplementation.[5]

Dr. Guy Abraham studied the effects of combining malic acid with magnesium in 15 fibromyalgia patients, 32 to 60 years old. A placebo group received nothing, while the supplement group was placed on 1,200 to 2,400 mg of malic acid and 300 to 600 mg of magnesium daily. Incredibly, after only 48 hours, the group taking the supplements had a significant decrease in tender points, and after eight weeks the pain among the supplement group decreased substantially. In the placebo group, the pain increased after just two weeks.[6]

B Vitamins Alleviate Stress and Pain

I. S. Klemes, M.D., found that vitamin B12 helps break up calcium deposits in bursitis patients, and alleviate so-called neuralgia, a technical term for nerve pain. Klemes injected a daily dose of one centimeter of vitamin B12 for seven to 10 days, followed by the same injection three times weekly for the next two to three weeks, then one or two weekly for two to three weeks, depending upon the patient's progress. Relief came quickly as calcium deposits were absorbed.[7]

In studying the pain of fibromyalgia patients, Dr. Jean-Bernard Eisinger, Chief of Medicine at Hopital G. Clemenceau, La Garde, France, found a study group taking B complex vitamins, including 750 milligrams per day of thiamine hydrochloride in divided doses, experienced less pain following orthopedic surgery. Fibromyalgia patients are found to have trouble absorbing thiamine – vitamin B1. Japanese researchers report therapeutic benefits to neuralgia using thiamine. It is worth noting here that thiamine requires an adequate supply of magnesium.[8]

Seeking Serotonin

Another theory is that people with fibromyalgia are deficient in a neurotransmitter called serotonin, which filters out unnecessary sensations and allows the brain to relax enough to sleep.[9] Without serotonin, everything feels extreme, both pain and pleasure. Even noises sound too loud, and it is difficult to sleep more than a few hours in a row.

Tryptophan, an amino acid found naturally in the body, is important to mental health, pain regulation and sleep. Stress depletes it, and is found to be deficient in people with depression and fibromyalgia. Not enough tryptophan, and serotonin levels are low. European physicians prescribe tryptophan for insomnia, pain, stress and depression.[10]

Synthetic tryptophan has been banned in this country, but naturally-derived sources are slowly finding themselves in amino acid formulas on vitamin store shelves.

Tryptophan works most efficiently in the presence of plenty of vitamin B6. Women who take oral contraceptives need a minimum of 20 mg of vitamin B6 daily in order to metabolize tryptophan normally.

Vitamin C is also important to the metabolism of serotonin, and is recommended for inflammation-induced pain. If you choose to supplement, vitamin C with bioflavonoids is a must for optimum effect.

Muscle weakness associated with fibromyalgia may be treated with the amino acid methionine, magnesium and phosphorus. The amino acid arginine may be used for general pain and fatigue; and thiamine and B6 may be used for muscle pain.[11] All the nutrients mentioned here can be purchased through either your local health food or vitamin store, by mail order, or your local drug store by special order.

In a study reported in *Current Therapeutic Research*, Italian researchers evaluated 47 patients with fibromyalgia who received 200 mg of methionine (S-adenosylmethionine) intramuscularly, plus 400 mg orally twice daily for six weeks, and found it significantly reduced their stress and pain.[12] This result was duplicated in another study of 30 patients. Of these, a full third saw the severity of the pain and the number of tender points reduced.[13] Methionine is high in potatoes and legumes (beans and peas). Like tryptophan, it also needs vitamin B6 to work.

Whenever I recommend one B vitamin, I recommend all of them. They are so important to each other, a deficiency of one creates an imbalance of the others. The B complex vitamins have been coined "the stress vitamins," they are so important. Since stress seems to be a precursor to fibromyalgia, taking a good B vitamin supplement formula is an excellent idea.

Dr. Alan Gaby has had success treating fibromyalgia patients with what he calls the "Myers cocktail." It is a combination of intravenous calcium, magnesium, B vitamins and vitamin C.

A colleague at the American Academy of Pain Management in San Antonio, Texas, Billie J. Sahley, Ph.D., has helped patients by correcting their nutrient deficiencies of malic acid (found in apples), magnesium and manganese, adding melatonin for sleep difficulties.[14]

Remember my friend Patty? She is doing much better. She found that a consistent exercise program combined with a diet centered around raw vegetables, beans and whole grains, and good nutritional supplements allows her to have a normal lifestyle mostly free from pain.

Fibromyalgia-Fleeing Nutrients

For maximum absorption, supplements should be taken with meals.

Nutrient	Suggested Dosage	Formulation
Aged garlic extract	2 teaspoons three times daily	Liquid
Amino acids	4-6 capsules daily	Multiple formula from natural sources
Antioxidants	4 capsules daily*	With selenium and grape seed extract
Borage oil	2 capsules daily	
Enzymes	2 capsules twice daily	Multiple formula
Flaxseed oil	1 tablespoon daily	
Fiber	8 tablets daily	Psyllium, with herb hyssop
Magnesium	200 mg daily	
Malic acid	250 mg three times daily	
MSM (methylsulfonylmethane)	500 mg three times daily	
Multi-vitamin/mineral	6 caplets daily	Freeze-dried plant sources
Multi-mineral	2-4 ounces daily	In liquid solution, with vitamin B12, biotin
Natural progesterone cream	1/3 teaspoon daily	With pregnenolone, DHEA
Niacinamide	1,000 mg twice daily	
Quercetin	400 mg twice daily	With vitamin C
Vitamin B6	200 mg daily	
Vitamin C	Individual bowel tolerance**	With bioflavonoids (quercetin, rutin proanthocyanidins)

* The FDA recommends that pregnant women not exceed 10,000 IU of vitamin A daily.

** To determine individual dosage, on the first day take 1,000 mg hourly until diarrhea occurs, then reduce dosage to just below that for individual daily dosage. Vitamin C is not toxic in large doses but must be taken throughout the day to benefit. Divide dosage to three or four times a day.

CHAPTER 72:

Food Poisoning

Most of us have had at least one bout of food poisoning. The mushrooms don't taste as good as they smelled, but you eat a few anyway. Later you're glad you listened to your taste buds as your stomach is wracked with painful spasms and you make it to the bathroom just in time. Only after you've regurgitated every possible speck of food in your stomach do you finally feel relief. "Must have been something I ate," you think to yourself. These are the obvious symptoms. Not so obvious are flu symptoms that lead you to believe you've picked up a stomach virus. What you picked up might not be so unavoidable.

The Distastful Facts

Once again, earnings win out over safety as the federal government sacrifices public health so an industry can maintain its profit margin. I'm talking about the USDA's standards for inspection of poultry cleanliness.

An estimated 6.5 to 33 million people in the United States become ill and 6,000 to 9,000 die each year from food-borne illnesses. Statistics suggest that poultry is directly related to food poisoning, and it costs the American citizenry nearly one billion dollars a year in medical and health care costs, and loss of income and productivity. The primary source of poultry contamination is fecal matter in the intestines of birds which are processed in poultry plants at speeds of at least 70 and often 90 birds per minute. At these speeds the intestines are ruptured, contaminating the birds and their immediate surroundings with fecal matter which is washed away. Studies have shown that even after 40 washings, once poultry is contaminated with fecal matter, harmful organisms are still present.[1]

The Department of Agriculture acknowledges that feces are a highly dangerous source of harmful organisms which can cause food poisoning, but argues that condemning poultry carcasses contaminated with fecal matter during processing would result in economic hardship on the poultry industry. Despite a law that requires "the federal government to condemn poultry products that bear or contain any poisonous or deleterious substances that may render them injurious to health," the USDA allows contaminated birds to be processed and sold for the American dinner table.[2] If you look at the next package of chicken you see in the market, you'll see a warning label mandated by law. It warns that the chicken is probably contaminated and that you should take certain precautions so you don't get sick. You'll find this new warning sticker on every package of meat sold.

Forewarned is Forearmed

You get food poisoning two ways: by eating food that actually contains poison, produced by the bacteria growing in it (botulism and staphylococcal food poisoning are this type); or by picking up a bug from food contaminated with organisms (such as salmonella bacteria) that multiply in the body.

Botulism is rare but deadly, killing a third of the 10 to 15 people who get it each year in the U.S. About 75 percent of the cases of botulism are traced to improperly home-canned foods.[3]

To avoid botulism: when in doubt, toss it out. Scientists estimate that one cupful of the pure botulism toxin could kill all the people on earth. So don't even taste food from a swollen can or from a jar with a swollen lid. Ditto for food that is foamy, moldy or has a bad odor. Dispose of the food in such a way that there is no chance it will be eaten by the homeless or animals.

Unlike botulism, salmonella infection is common. It forces more than four million Americans a year to their knees in front of the toilet. Stomach pain, diarrhea and fever are other lowlights of salmonellosis.

To avoid salmonella keep your bird cool. Store raw poultry in the refrigerator down low, where it can't drip onto other foods. Rinse it thoroughly before cooking, and dispose of juices from the package. Frozen poultry should be thawed overnight in the refrigerator or in a plastic bag under cold water, not just left out. Remember, the juices may be poisonous. Don't lick your fingers after touching a raw bird, and don't re-use anything that has come into contact with raw poultry – cutting board, knife, plate – without washing it in hot water and soap first. When you barbecue, don't put cooked meat on the same plate from which you took the raw meat. If you cook meat on a regular basis, keep a spray bottle containing bleach and water nearby (a tablespoon of bleach in a quart of water is sufficient). Bleach kills the nastiest bacteria, and is the best way to ensure your safety.

Considering that a study at Iowa State University found salmonella in 41 percent of packaged cut-up chickens, you'd better cook that bird until the inside is white.

Don't egg yourself into trouble. Skip the Caesar salads and soft-boiled or over-easy eggs.

Salmonella enteritidis outbreaks, associated with the consumption of raw eggs, is the most frequently reported salmonella type infection in the United States. There were 66 outbreaks of the disease in 1991 alone. In one case 15 patrons and 23 employees developed symptoms within a nine day period after eating Caesar salad at a restaurant.[4]

Eggs need to be cooked at least three minutes at 140 degrees to be safe. Use only uncracked eggs and keep them stored no longer than five weeks.

Fight Fire with Fire

Scientists are discovering the benefit to introducing body-friendly bacteria in the prevention and treatment of food poisoning. Your body contains good and bad bacteria. When all bacteria are killed by antibiotics, for example, the bad guys can proliferate while the good guys are still down for the count. Harmful, or disease-causing bacteria have fancy Latin names like pseudomonas-aeruginosa, proteus, staphylococcus, clostridia and veillonellae.

Found in digestive enzyme supplemental formulas are the body's disease-killing good-guy bacteria, Lactobacilli, Eubacteria and Bifidobacteria. Lactobacilli can inhibit the growth of harmful bacteria, stimulate immune function and aid in digestion, and Eubacteria can inhibit the growth of harmful bacteria. Bifidobacteria can reduce blood ammonia levels, lower cholesterol levels, regulate the immune system, produce vitamins, especially the B vitamin/folic acid group, restore normal intestinal flora during antibiotic therapy, and inhibit the growth of disease-causing germs.[5]

Without enough good bacteria, you get gas, diarrhea, constipation, stomachaches, cramping, bloating, and all the other symptoms of stomach distress, with or without food poisoning. Now, let's say you have the right amounts of bacteria, and everything is working smoothly. Along comes a stomach bug, which may or may not have come from food, and suddenly you know it!

In recent years, there has been a growing awareness of the medicial use of beneficial bacteria, termed "probiotics" (from the Greek, "for life"). The medicinal use of beneficial bacteria is not new, but long employed with dairy foods. In ancient times, the Roman historian, Pliny, recommended fermented milks to treat gastrointestinal infections. Early in this century, the Russian scientist Metchnikoff, reported that consumption of large amounts of yogurt replaced toxin-producing intestinal bacteria, and would result in better health and extended longevity. All of these uses of dairy food bacteria depend on the action of live microorganisms, especially lactic acid bacteria.[6]

Beneficial bacteria help prevent some food-borne illnesses. Both bifidobacteria and lactobacilli – available in supplement form in vitamin stores – stop or slow down common disease- and illness-causing bacteria.

In test tube experiments, lactobaccilli acidophilus, found in yogurt with active cultures and in supplemental form, inhibited the growth of 27 different types of bacteria. Ten of the bacteria were common disease-causers.[7]

Yogurt with active cultures have proven in studies to render many kinds of disease-causing bacteria ineffective or kill them outright. The beneficial bacteria contained in yogurt and other cultured foods can help you avoid or recover from diarrhea from whatever source. Acidophilus has also been shown in studies to help when there is too much or too little hydrochloric acid in the stomach. Too little stomach acid results in the same symptoms as too much: gas, bloating and pain. This is because there isn't enough acid to fully break down your food, especially if you've eaten meat, and it ferments in the stomach and intestines.

Beneficial bacteria can help keep the numbers of bacteria that grow on this fermented food to a minimum.

Support Your Internals with Nutrients

The symptoms of food poisoning are bad enough, but the effects can be far-reaching: Stomach muscles are left sore and bruised, the esophagus is burned from vomited stomach acid, the intestinal tract is damaged and delicate stomach tissues are wounded. These are the effects after the bad bacteria have been destroyed. The food-borne pathogens themselves wreak nutritional havoc on your body. Salmonella and Escherichia coli, for example, not only poison food, but destroy ascorbic acid, or vitamin C.[8] Since this occurs, it is very important that once the bad bacteria have been eliminated, vitamin C in high dosages be taken. If diarrhea is a symptom, the absorption of vitamin A, vitamin C and beta carotene is impaired, since it is in the intestine that they are absorbed.

Following a bout of food poisoning, Dr. Garry Gordon recommends a combination of garlic, 500,000 individual units (IU) of vitamin A and vitamin C to bowel tolerance, for two to three days. What is meant by bowel tolerance is up to the point where diarrhea occurs. Large amounts of vitamin C are not toxic to the body, but are required to battle infection. When the body cannot use vitamin C it throws it off in the form of diarrhea. This is how you know you've taken enough to make a difference. Start at 1,000 milligrams every hour and continue until you experience diarrhea or gas, then lower the dosage to just below that.

A pre-existing nutrient deficiency can increase your chances of being colonized by bad bacteria. The Center for Food Safety and Applied Nutrition reported in the *Journal of the American Dietetic Association* that deficiencies of iron and zinc "provide a situation" for candida and salmonella infection. Candida is a yeast infection that can be encouraged by a high sugar diet and not enough beneficial bacteria.[9]

Research abounds with evidence that zinc is a major player for the health and healing of cellular tissue. When you are deficient in zinc, infections and ulcers do not heal as well and your chances of getting them is increased. A zinc deficiency also affects the immune system by causing a reduction in natural killer cells, and the size of the thymus gland, an extremely important immune system organ.

Alleviating Symptoms

Naturopathic physician Cathy Rogers, N.D. recommends a remedy that she learned from John Bastyr, founder of the John Bastyr College of Naturopathy. I tried this remedy in a desperate attempt to get relief from a stomach bug, and although I was impatient for it to take effect, it worked amazingly well. Slowly sip two to three tablespoons of sauerkraut juice (get the juice from sauerkraut packed in a glass jar) until vomiting and diarrhea are relieved. It should work within an hour or two – it worked for me in about 45 minutes. You can also use fresh cabbage juice, but most people don't feel up to preparing vegetable juice when they have severe stomach upset.

Food poisoning can result in painful inflammation of the intestinal tract. Fortunately, certain substances have been found to help. Quercetin, a bioflavonoid found in citrus rind and in some supplemental formulas, is a potent anti-inflammatory. It works even better when combined with vitamin C. Vitamin C is not only an anti-inflammatory, but aids in the absorption of iron.

An article in the highly-respected British medical journal *The Lancet* (November 13, 1993) reported on a study that showed bioflavonoids are also potent antibacterial and antiviral substances.

Unsaturated fatty acids (also essential fatty acids, or EFAs) are important to restore the mucosal lining of a damaged colon, which can occur after a severe bout with diarrhea. An article in the *American Journal of Clinical Nutrition* reports on a study that showed flaxseed oil and fish oil to be beneficial for ulcerative colitis symptoms.[10]

Dr. E. Seidman, Division of Gastroenterology, STE-Justine Hopital, Montreal, Quebec, Canada, reports that certain kinds of EFAs help reduce inflammation and restore the intestinal lining.[11] They are: eicosapentaenoic acid, found in the oils of salmon, trout, mackerel, sardines; and linoleic acid, found in the oils of safflower, sunflower, flaxseed, pumpkin seed, walnut, soybean and sesame seed. The best source of linoleic acid is borage oil, found in supplemental form. It's more concentrated and is less expensive than evening primrose oil, another highly potent supplemental form.

Include a fiber formula that combines bacteria-battling goldenseal, colon cleansing hyssop and psyllium, with friendly acidophilus bacteria and soothing aloe for your intestinal healing.

Certain amino acids can reverse the effect of food allergies, infection and other trauma to the delicate mucosal tissues of the intestinal tract. A deficiency of glutamine will weaken intestinal villi, causing poor absorption of nutrients, so obviously your intestine's health depends on it. An article in *Gastroenterology* stated that a glutamine-enhanced diet helps increase good guy bacteria.[12]

Arginine is another amino acid found to help heal the colon. It enhances the immune system, especially following trauma, and promotes wound healing and intestinal cell growth. For more on nutrients to help restore a traumatized intestinal tract, read my Diarrhea chapter.

Liquid aged garlic extract is my totem when traveling. I travel all over the world, 365 days a year, and find myself eating things I'd never touch at home. I often have little choice in what I eat, but I do have choices in what I take. For any infection, I recommend aged garlic extract. Not only can it reduce inflammation, but is a powerful antimicrobial, helpful to combat any viral or bacterial infection.

Research backs up the benefits of garlic. At the 1990 First World Congress on the "Health Significance of Garlic and Garlic Constituents" in Washington, D.C., researchers presented studies which emphasized the antimicrobial action of garlic and its effectiveness in killing the bacteria salmonella, the candida yeast and even the amoeba parasite that causes amoebic dysentery.[13]

Bad Bacteria-Beating Nutrients
For maximum absorption, take supplements with meals.

Nutrient	Suggested Dosage	Formulation
Acidophilus	At least four billion flora daily on an empty stomach, three times daily	
Aged garlic extract	1 teaspoon three times daily	Liquid
Amino acids	4-6 capsules daily	Multiple formula from natural sources
Antioxidants	4 capsules daily*	With selenium and grapeseed extract
Echinacea	250 mg daily for 14 days	
Enzymes	2 capsules twice daily	Multiple formula
Fiber	4-8 tablets	Psyllium, with herb hyssop
Multi-mineral	3-4 ounces daily	In liquid solution, with vitamin B12, biotin
Multi-vitamin/mineral	6 caplets daily	Freeze-dried plant sources
Water	2 gallons daily	Purified
Vitamin C	Individual bowel tolerance**	With bioflavonoids (quercetin, rutin proanthocyanidins)

* The FDA recommends pregnant women not exceed 10,000 IU of vitamin A daily.

** To determine individual dosage, on the first day take 1,000 mg hourly until diarrhea occurs, then reduce dosage to just below that for individual daily dosage. Vitamin C is not toxic in large doses but must be taken throughout the day to benefit. Divide dosage to three or four times a day.

CHAPTER 73:

Fractures

Even if you don't skateboard or climb trees, your risk of bone fractures may one day be just as great.

At least 26 percent of all women over the age of 60 get spontaneous fractures because they have "brittle bones." Of the million fractures treated by the medical profession, it is estimated that 700,000 are a result of postmenopausal osteoporosis.

While older women seem to be most prone to fractures, it is not a necessary result of the aging process. I repeat: brittle bones do not naturally occur with age; they are a result of many factors, and **age is not one of them.**

Bones are not inanimate objects in your body that serve to hold you up. They are living tissue constantly taking up and releasing nutrients. Bone is continually being formed (osteoblastic) and reabsorbed (osteoclastic) throughout your life. In fact – and this may surprise you – the human skeleton is completely replaced every 10 to 12 years. This means a 70-year-old woman has had seven skeletons in her lifetime! We have more skeletons in our closets than we thought!

Calcium and the Importance of Magnesium

Some of the factors that can cause weak bones are those that create deficiencies of calcium and other minerals that are essential to the *absorption* of calcium. I emphasize absorption because there are a multitude of reasons calcium cannot be taken up by the bones, or is lost in urine. Other factors will cause calcium to actually be drawn out of the bones.

You've seen billboards pronouncing "Everybody needs milk"? Well, how about changing it to read: Everybody needs... sesame seeds, kelp, spinach, chard, brewer's yeast, sardines, carob, caviar, soybeans, almonds, torula yeast, parsley, Brazil nuts, watercress, salmon, chickpeas, egg yolk and beans? These are the many variety of foods that are high in calcium – and low in fat!

Only 25 percent of women taking calcium are in fact preventing fractures. While calcium supplements were found to increase bone mass in these women, it had no effect on the other 75 percent. This is because there are many factors that can prevent calcium from being taken up by the bone.

As much as 50 percent of all magnesium in the body is found in the bones.[1] Magnesium, a neglected nutrient in the diet of Americans – especially women – contributes to the making of solid, enduring bones by activating vitamin D and allowing calcium to enter the bones. The concentration of magnesium in body cells and bones was found in one study to be subnormal in 16 out of 19 women with osteoporosis, and calcium crystal formation in the 16 was defective. This appears to make patients more likely to sustain fractures. Calcium crystals formed in the three women with adequate levels of magnesium were found to be normal.[2]

In a recent study, 31 post-menopausal women took 250-750 mg/day of magnesium for two years. As a result, the researchers found, 75 percent of the womens' bone density *increased* by as much as eight percent![3] This is remarkable because a woman's bone density typically *decreases* by three to eight percent every year during menopause.

Magnesium and calcium work in balance throughout our bodies. Without magnesium, calcium accumulates in places it shouldn't, and is pulled out of places it should be, like the bones.

Dr. Hans Seyle, author of the book *Stress Without Distress*, and a Nobel prize winning biologist, found in rat experiments that in stressful situations, calcium is drawn from the bones and deposited in the tissues.[4]

Calcinosis occurs because of a very common deficiency of magnesium. Several studies show the prevalence of this deficiency, starting as early as the teen years. A magnesium deficiency is very serious, and, based on the research, is probably the number one cause of osteoporosis. It even plays a role in cancer!

A large study by the U.S. Department of Agriculture found that only 25 percent of 37,785 individuals had magnesium intakes at or greater than the recommended daily allowance, which is notoriously low. A 1995 review of 15 studies found that a typical American diet contains only a fraction of the RDA.[5]

Because of the high absorption rate of minerals in solution, and deficiency of magnesium in the diet, the ratio of magnesium and calcium in solution should be four to one, respectively.

Calcium and Vitamin D

One reason for being fracture prone may be a shortage of natural vitamin D, which is necessary for calcium to be absorbed in the body and used in your trillions of cells.

What's important to remember, when it comes to vitamin D, is that there are two kinds: synthetic and natural. The vitamin D found in dairy products, such as milk, is a synthetic hormone deviously labeled as vitamin D. Because it is synthetic, it reduces the absorption of magnesium, important in the fractures story.

Milk is a bad source of calcium for another reason. It is high in phosphorus and protein, which actually depletes calcium. Plus, it is estimated that 27 to 47 percent of osteoporotics cannot tolerate milk.

A deficiency of natural vitamin D is also responsible for something called osteomalacia, or bone softening. It is similar to rickets in children, as it causes bones weakness.

Among elderly patients with hip fractures, 10 to 20 percent have impaired bone mineralization because of vitamin D deficiency.[6]

A major source of vitamin D is sunlight on the skin. However, with the risks and warnings associated with ultraviolet rays, many people avoid or sharply reduce their exposure to the sun. And they don't make it up by eating vitamin D-rich foods. It is estimated that we can safely tolerate 15 minutes a day of sunlight for adequate vitamin D.

Calcium and Phosphorus

Too much phosphorus will also cause you to lose calcium. Yet, not enough will do the same. The ratio of calcium to phosphorus must be one to one for optimal absorption.

Most American diets contain a one to four ratio of calcium to phosphorus. This is because commonly-eaten foods such as meat and potatoes are high in phosphorus.

To demonstrate this phosphorus to calcium *imbalance* in foods, here are some I've talked about.

Half a chicken breast contains 16 mg of calcium and 252 mg of phosphorus. One large baked potato, including the skin, has 14 mg of calcium and 101 mg of phosphorus.

So-called soft drinks could be hard on your bones. A Harvard University study of nearly 5,400 female college grads, ages 21 to 80, revealed that for ex-varsity women over 40 – a time when estrogen levels and bone mass decline – drinking non-alcoholic carbonated beverages more than doubled the risk of bone fractures. It also took the fizz out of exercise's bone-strengthening benefits. The high amount of phosphorus in soft drinks depletes calcium, as the body tries to balance out the ratio of phosphorus to calcium.

Instead, concentrate on the foods that have close to a one to one ratio. They are: ten radishes, one apple, one pear; and one cup of the following: boysenberries, cranberries, loganberries, pineapple, watermelon, Swiss chard, eggplant, summer squash, green beans and iceberg lettuce.

Another way to handle this problem is to eat high-calcium, low phosphorus foods such as kale, sesame seeds, maple syrup and seaweed to ensure adequate calcium. One tablespoon of kelp has 156 mg of calcium and 34 mg of phosphorus.

Other Factors Blocking Absorption of Calcium

An excess of saturated, or transfatty, fats in the diet (found in margarines, and most processed foods) also blocks absorption of calcium. The calcium combines with the saturated fatty acids to form an insoluble calcium soap, a process called saponification. Unsaturated fats, found in oils, do not have this effect.

Stomach acid is a necessity in the absorption of calcium. Since the amount of hydrochloric acid in the stomach typically lowers over time, this may be why some people associate aging with calcium/bone loss.

In studies of postmenopausal women, it has been shown that about 40 percent are severely deficient in stomach acid, a condition known as hypochlorhydria. It has also been shown that patients with insufficient stomach acid output can only absorb about four percent of an oral dose of calcium.

Since a lack of hydrochloric acid in the stomach prevents absorption of minerals, even super-supplementations with minerals will not help. Instead, Doctor Jonathan Wright and his associate, Dr. Alan Gaby, recommend intramuscular injections of vitamin B12, small then larger oral doses of the digestive enzyme supplements pepsin, Betaine Hydrochloride with or without pepsin, acquired at health food stores, or Glutamic Acid HCl with or without pepsin.[7]

Another way to be sure you get the nutrients you need is to target a mineral supplement in solution. Studies show minerals dissolved in water before ingestion are considerably more bioavailable to the body than those even present in food, because they aren't risked by a lack of hydrochloric acid in the stomach or food allergies. Liquid formulations provide the maximum absorption ratios.

Other Nutrients on the Bone-Healthy Team

Although calcium and magnesium are the most spectacular nutrients on the team, the players who get most of the ink, these minerals need the rest of the players to do the job right. Vitamins and minerals you might never suspect also have a role: vitamins A, B6, folic acid, C, D, K and the minerals manganese, boron, copper, silica and zinc.

One of the little-known functions of vitamin A is to help control the process of tearing down old bone cells and forming new ones. When the diet is short-changed on vitamin A, new bone cells are formed faster than the old. Dead cells can be eliminated, causing abnormal bone formations which can bring on pain and bone problems.

The RDA for vitamin A is recommended at 5,000 IU. Doctors like to scare people away from A by emphasizing that you can take too much. It is a so-called fat soluble vitamin, meaning it doesn't dissolve well in water, can't be excreted in urine, and as a result our body stores excess A in the liver. Toxic levels are considered to be above 100,000 IU, for healthy people not already deficient, and damaging only when taken for long periods of time. Beta carotene, a vitamin A precursor, can be taken with vitamin A to boost the benefit, and can be taken in as high a dose as is needed, with no side effects.

Likewise, vitamin B6 provides a strong boost toward making good bones happen. A diet low in this vitamin caused rats to develop weak bones. In one study, more than half of supposedly healthy women volunteers were found deficient in vitamin B6.

Just how does this nutrient influence bones for better or worse? When well supplied, vitamin B6 adds strength to connective tissue, the supporting structure of bones. It also breaks down and neutralizes homocysteine, a harmful acid which builds up and breaks down collagen in the joints.

I recommend taking vitamin B6 in B complex formulas or tablets in potencies of 50 to 100 mg. All the B vitamins need to be taken together to avoid a deficiency of any of them. A good B complex formula has at least ten times the RDA. It is nontoxic in large doses because any excess is excreted in the urine.

To make cells stick together – in both soft tissue and bones – the body must produce collagen, the most plentiful body protein. A liberal supply of vitamin C is necessary for collagen production.[8]

Without enough of this adhesive, our soft tissue, bone tissue cells and we, ourselves, tend to become unglued!

Vitamin C also works as a biochemical escort system, making certain calcium is delivered where needed.

The too-low-for-optimum-health RDA for vitamin C is 50 to 80 mg for adults. Many biochemists feel that the proper amount could range anywhere from 1,000 mg to 20,000 mg. At high potencies, this vitamin is non-toxic, but has a laxative effect until the system has time to adjust. At the point that it causes diarrhea – coined bowel tolerance – it is a maximum amount tolerable and dosage should be reduced, then gradually increased again.

One of the best kept secrets in biochemistry is the fact that vitamin K, well-known for its contribution to blood-clotting, is a star performer in assuring strong, solid, healthy bones. Without it, bones could not be formed, repaired or rebuilt. Vitamin K makes possible the synthesizing of osteocalcin, a protein matrix on which calcium attaches itself to build new bone cells.[9] Osteocalcin is like the chicken wire nailed to the sides of a house so the plaster or stucco can grip the surface. Beyond this function, osteocalcin acts like a magnet to attract ions of calcium.

Because vitamin K is plentiful in vegetables and because friendly bacteria synthesize it, many conventional nutrition authorities assume that everybody's blood levels of vitamin K are adequate.

Not so, as revealed by new and accurate blood testing instrumentation and techniques. Many people become deficient in vitamin K because they don't eat enough vegetables or take antibiotics which annihilate the friendly bacteria along with the enemies.

In one study, 16 osteoporosis patients were found to have only 35 percent as much blood serum vitamin K as age-matched controls without osteoporosis.

Both negative and positive animal and human studies show the towering importance of vitamin K. Rats put on a vitamin K-deficient regime lost increased amounts of calcium in their urine.[10]

The healing of rabbits with bone fractures was speeded up when a vitamin K supplement was given, although these animals were already on a diet with a high enough level of this vitamin.[11]

Among human subjects, researchers found that when they broke a bone, blood levels of vitamin K fell by as much as 71 percent, and that the levels remained low as long as fracture healing took place.[12] This suggests vitamin K is used by the body in the healing of fractures. Obviously, a deficiency could keep healing from taking place.

Another unsung hero is manganese – a must for synthesizing connective tissue, structural material in both cartilage and bone, and for assuring that needed minerals will stay put in bones.

When rats were fed a manganese-deficient diet, their bones were smaller, less mineral-dense and more subject to fracture than those of animals fed enough of this trace mineral.[13]

Boron, Copper and More

Until recent years, even leading biochemists had no idea that the trace mineral boron could be useful anywhere in human nutrition, let alone in bone health and integrity.

Researchers at the Department of Human Nutrition at Winthrop University, Rock Hill South Carolina, found that boron supplementation helped optimize bone mineralization during peak bone growth periods. Susan L. Meacham, a researcher there, emphasizes in the *American Journal of Clinical Nutrition* that all the minerals known or suspected to affect bone density, such as calcium, phosphorous, magnesium, and boron should be emphasized.[14]

Just as boron helps bone integrity, it appears to contribute to turning vitamin D into its most useful form. In a study of baby chickens, it was found that a boron deficiency worsened a vitamin D deficiency and made for abnormally formed bones.[15]

A daily intake of only three milligrams of boron appears to bring about dramatic changes in bone formation and strength, according to U.S. Department of Agriculture studies.[16]

As with boron, only traces of copper are necessary to promote and maintain solid bone structure. A mere two milligrams daily is generally recommended. Surveys indicate that the diet of most people include about half that much.

Even nutritional authorities don't know exactly how copper works on body bones, but they are aware of several rat studies which demonstrate that a copper deficiency permits the escape of bone minerals and, therefore, the weakening of bones.[17]

One experiment revealed that copper supplementation blocks the escape of minerals from bones, keeping them solid and strong.[18]

Noted for its contributions to wound-healing, smooth skin and thymus gland function – the key to the immune system – zinc gets little recognition for its part in assuring bone health.

Vitamin D and copper don't work without zinc, and a deficiency of this mineral could well be one of the major causes of unexplained fractures, inasmuch as several studies show that people get too little zinc in their diets. One study disclosed that 68 percent of adults ingest less than the recommended daily allowance of zinc, which is 15 to 25 mg. Further, many authorities feel this RDA is too low.[19]

Michael Lesser, M.D., in addressing the Senate Select Committee on Nutrition and Human Needs, stated that the soil of 32 states is zinc-deficient and that commercial fertilizers return no zinc to the earth.

Several U.S. Department of Agriculture surveys confirm this fact. It is impossible for even a magician to pull a rabbit out of a hat if it wasn't put there first. Another study revealed that the blood and bones of elderly osteoporosis patients were deficient in zinc.

Added to that, all forms of zinc are not created equal. Some are hard to absorb. Look for zinc in your mineral in solution supplement.

Here's a real-life example of how these minerals can not only cause fractures but help heal them.

For three years one of the greatest centers ever to play professional basketball, Bill Walton, was sidelined in the National Basketball Association (NBA) by an unusual foot fracture that just wouldn't heal. X-rays indicated he had osteoporosis, a condition rarely seen in athletic young men.[20, 21]

To determine how this could happen, he had his blood analyzed at the University of California, San Diego, and the results of the blood sample was sent to Dr. Paul Saltman, a professor of biology there. The analysis showed a high quantity of calcium, but low amounts of copper and zinc, and no manganese whatsoever.

Dr. Saltman offered Walton supplements equivalent to one regular dietary allowance each of calcium, zinc, copper and manganese. Following three months of the regimen, Walton's blood showed normal amounts of these essential nutrients and with continued supplementation, his bones finally healed. During his successful NBA career, he did not display any of his old tendencies toward bone fracture.

Saltman knew of the possibility of a mineral deficiency because of research he did with rats. Saltman and colleagues Linda Strause, Robert Cone and Donald Resnick were able to produce changes in bone suggestive of osteoporosis by maintaining rats on diets deficient in manganese and copper.

What About Silica?

Silica is another less-known mineral, found where calcium is deposited in sites of growing bone. It appears to strengthen the connective tissue matrix by crosslinking collagen strands. Chicks fed a silica-deficient diet developed gross abnormalities of the skull and had unusually thin leg bones.[22]

An important study conducted at the school of Public Health at the University of California, Los Angeles, shows that silica-supplemented bones have a 100 percent increase in collagen.[23]

Dr. Louis C. Kervran, member of the New York Academy of Sciences writes that silica brings about "spectacular results in repairing broken bones." Then he adds the sensational fact that "fractures are repaired and healed faster with organic silica extracts than with the administration of calcium."[24]

The riddle intrigued Kervran all his life. Because no one could give him the answer, he decided to dedicate himself to solving this great perplexing mystery. In so doing, he became an eminent medical scientist and Nobel Prize nominee.

In 1959 Kervran tackled the problem of explaining the biological transformation of silica into calcium. He found that in the human body, both magnesium and silica are principal sources of calcium, necessary to its absorption. Other researchers also found that silica is important in phosphorus absorption; another critical piece in the bone loss puzzle.

Kervran and other researchers discovered something vitally important to this skeletal solution: inorganic silica supplements move calcium from the bones to other tissues, while organic silica derived from vegetation puts calcium right where it's needed: the bones.

It is therefore imperative that your silica sources be derived from natural plants or health food products. Look for a liquid mineral formula derived from natural sources that contains silica, potassium, phosphorus and magnesium, as well as calcium.

All of the known micronutrients added to calcium supplements boosts the bones better than calcium alone. Anthony Albanese, Ph.D., director of nutritional research at the Osborn Memorial Home, in White Plains, New York, gave 12 healthy women 600 mg of calcium plus all the known micronutrients at the RDA level. Eleven comparable women on the same diet took 700 to 800 mg of calcium only. After nine to eleven months, x-ray measurements showed that the women taking all the micronutrients had two to three times greater bone density than those on calcium alone.

Boning-up on this information will give you a strong skeleton, capable of handling all of life's hefty problems.

Natural Progesterone Boosts Bone
Formation, Reduces Fractures

In 1978, after attending a lecture by Dr. Ray Peat on the subject of natural progesterone derived from wild yam root, John R. Lee, M.D., began offering a progesterone skin moisturizer to his menopausal osteoporotic patients who were unable to use estrogen. The doctor found that among his patients using the progesterone cream, serial lumbar DPA tests showed an *increase* in bone density, rather than mere delayed loss, which would have been expected. He notes one patient had a pathological arm fracture at 72 and now at 84, her bone density has increased 40 percent and she has no fractures. Dr. Lee found that natural progesterone typically increases bone mass by 15 percent in two to three years.[25]

Bone-Boosting Nutrients
For maximum absorption, take supplements with meals.

Nutrient	Suggested Dosage	Formulation
Acidophilus	At least four billion flora on an empty stomach three times daily	
Borage oil	2 capsules daily	
Fiber	4-8 tablets daily	Psyllium, with herb hyssop
Flaxseed oil	1 tablespoon daily	
Glucosamine sulfate	500 mg three times daily	
Magnesium	200 mg daily	
MSM (Methylsulfonylmethane)	500 mg three times daily	
Multi-mineral	1-4 ounces daily	In liquid solution, with vitamin B12, biotin
Multi-vitamin/mineral	3-6 caplets daily	Freeze-dried plant sources
Natural progesterone cream	1/3 teaspoon daily	With pregnenolone and DHEA
Niacinamide	1,000 mg twice daily	
Vitamin C	Individual bowel tolerance*	With bioflavonoids (quercetin, rutin proanthocyanidins)
Vitamin D	15 minutes of sunshine daily	
Vitamin E	2 capsules (800 IU) daily	d-alpha tocopherol
Weight bearing exercise	30 minutes daily	

* To determine individual dosage, on the the first day take 1,000 mg hourly until diarrhea occurs, then reduce dosage to just below that for individual daily dosage. Vitamin C is not toxic in large doses but must be taken throughout the day to benefit. Divide dosage to three or four times a day.

CHAPTER 74:

Frostbite

Fifteen years ago the owner of a television station on which I frequently appeared got frostbite when he fell asleep while nursing broken ribs with an ice pack. I told him to cover the skin with a banana peel. His wife did what I instructed and the skin under the peel became pink and healthy. A frostbitten area missed by the peel was oozing and broken. I've used this banana peel remedy for skin injuries from frostbite to sunburns. It works every time!

Frost Burn

Frostbite sounds innocuous, compared to the reality. The reality is that when you get it, it's like getting burned. Have you ever had a wart removed with liquid nitrogen? It works by literally freezing the skin until it forms a blood blister, then scabs and drops off. Frostbite is freezer burn.

The end result of frostbite, so far as tissue damage is concerned, is very similar to that of a burn. The treatment, too, resembles burn therapy, except that conventional doctors are more likely to hack off parts of your fingers and toes.[1]

The injury may be superficial if you are otherwise healthy and have mild pain or tingling followed by numbness, and you find that the tissues beneath the area are soft and pliable. A person with circulation problems may get frostbite quicker, and have more serious problems as a result. For more on this consideration, see the Circulation Problems chapter.

Think Zinc

Research abounds with evidence that zinc is a major player for the health and healing of the skin. Zinc was used topically as calamine lotion as far back as 1500 B.C. by the Egyptians. When you are deficient in zinc, cuts and ulcers do not heal as well and chances of their becoming infected is increased. A zinc deficiency also affects the immune system by causing a reduction in natural killer cells, and the size of the thymus gland, an extremely important immune system organ. A lowered immune system decreases resistance to infection.

Mary Y. Mazzotta, Ph.D., of the California College of Podiatric Medicine in San Francisco, CA., has found that a topical administration of zinc chloride as a spray or ointment reduces the size of wounds, shortens healing time, and produces less splitting of the skin as it heals. She also states that zinc oxide is effective in enhancing wound healing. Zinc oxide is available as an over-the-counter ointment for skin rashes and sunburn. Remember seeing all those white noses at the pool and on the beach? That's zinc oxide. Every first aid kit should have some.[2]

Zinc is well-known in medical circles and well-used in pharmaceutical circles for wound and burn healing. Zinc oxide is incorporated into fillings to stave off infection and in *Martindale, The Extra Pharmacopoeia* I counted over 100 skin pharmaceuticals worldwide that contain zinc oxide.[3]

More importantly, researchers have noted that burn patients have strongly depressed blood levels of zinc and copper. Burn and frostbite patients typically lose zinc and copper as they lose fluids.[4]

Copper and zinc work in synch in the body. Without one, the other is incapacitated. Be sure and include 2-4 mg. of copper with any zinc.

Nutritional Support to Increase Circulation

Anything that helps increase circulation will help restore blood and cellular tissue in body parts afflicted with frostbite. Of the many circulation-boosters, magnesium is probably most magnanimous, found by researchers to increase circulation where blockages and damage has occurred.

Magnesium has the ability to increase circulating levels of calcitonin gene-related peptide (CGRP), which helps govern the hand's and feet's response to cold. A deficiency of this body chemical may make your skin more susceptible to frostbite.[5]

Studies show minerals dissolved in water before ingestion are considerably more bioavailable to the body than those even present in food, because they aren't risked by a lack of hydrochloric acid in the stomach or food allergies. Look for a good, easily absorbable, derived-from-nature mineral blend in solution. Liquid formulations provide the maximum absorption ratios.

Vitamin E is the heart- and vascular-smart vitamin, touted by most doctors and researchers to be beneficial for the circulatory system.

At health food conventions in the 1960s and '70s, Drs. Evan and Wilfrid Shute of the Shute Clinic in Canada presented incredible "before" and "after" color photos illustrating how vitamin E had successfully treated patients with gangrene and severe burns.[6]

Vitamin E acts by reducing the inflammation of damaged tissues, thus reducing harm to them. This antioxidant also helps stabilize skin membranes so healing can occur. In one study, injured tendons healed in the presence of vitamin E were stronger than those healed without it. It was also noted that with the vitamin E, there were smaller and fewer scars. Vitamin E is notorious for boosting the immune system, essential in any injury.[7] For optimal benefit, apply vitamin E to the skin as well as taking it internally.

Vital Vitamins

When it comes to wound healing, if zinc is number one, vitamin A has to be number two. Retinoids, vitamin A derivatives, are used in a myriad of skin care products for skin problems from acne to wrinkles. Vitamin A can increase skin collagen, reduce inflammation, increase postoperative immune suppression, foster healing and improve the appearance of scars. Vitamin A is sometimes applied directly to wounds with sponge implants.[8]

Vitamin C is needed to build strong collagen, the underlying support of skin. Poor wound healing is one of the symptoms of scurvy, caused by a deficiency of vitamin C. A deficiency of vitamin C can actually cause a breakdown of already-healed wounds. Blood vitamin C levels decrease during times of physical and emotional stress. Vitamin C in combination with the B vitamin pantothenic acid has been shown to increase skin strength and decrease scar tissue. A deficiency of both causes wounds to take longer to heal.[9]

Many studies show vitamin C helps prevent frostbite. How can this work? It seems, according to many reputable journals, that high amounts of vitamin C – at least 500 milligrams a day – can stimulate the body to generate greater body heat to make us more cold-resistant.[10]

B vitamins in the body are reduced during times of stress, and I can't think of anything more stressful than being out in the cold long enough to get frostbite. Therefore, burn patients should also supplement with a vitamin B complex in addition to pantothenic acid.

Aloe Vera

Researchers around the world are hard at work analyzing the many medicinal properties of the approximately 600 varieties of aloe plants, which are being used successfully to treat burns, x-ray and radiation dermatitis, gastric ulcers, sunburn, frostbite, gastrointestinal disorders, constipation, sports injuries, diabetes, etc., as well as a therapeutic ingredient in cosmetics.

The medicinal effects of aloe have been documented since the 4th Century B.C. Aloe vera is mentioned in the Ebers Papyrus and in the writings of Hippocrates and Alexander the Great.[11] It remains a renowned skin wound remedy in use today.

Aloe vera is used in trauma centers in California, Illinois, New York, Texas and other states for a variety of uses of benefit to the skin. One reason aloe has a range of beneficial effects, is its ability to very quickly penetrate the skin. Aloe quickly penetrates injured tissue, relieves pain, reduces inflammation, and dilates capillaries, thereby increasing blood supply to the injured area so healing can occur.

Research conducted by Ivan E. Danhof, Ph.D., M.D., retired professor of clinical pharmacology and physiology at the University of Texas, shows aloe vera penetrates human skin almost four times faster than water.[12]

Aloe vera is an effective oral and topical agent for healing any skin wound. In a remarkable experiment involving wounded mice, Robert H. Davis, Ph.D., found that when the mice drank aloe vera in their drinking water, the size of their wounds were reduced by 62.5 percent than those not given the aloe. When a topical 25 percent aloe vera preparation was applied to their wounds, they were reduced by 50 percent.[13]

In 1993, John P. Heggers, Ph.D., and colleagues at the University of Texas Medical Branch at Galveston, conducted various animal and human studies on the medicinal benefits of aloe. The research team found in both human and animal studies that, aloe vera is a substance of "enormous therapeutic potential." In the human studies, the researchers found that frostbite wounds treated with aloe extracts had far less tissue damage than those treated with conventional methods.[14]

Skin-Healing Nutrients
For maximum absorption, take supplements with meals.

Nutrient	Suggested Dosage	Formulation
Acetyl L-Carnitine	500 mg three times daily	
Aged garlic extract	1 teaspoon three times daily	Liquid
Antioxidants	4 capsules daily	With selenium and grape seed extract
Borage oil	2 capsules daily	
Flaxseed oil	1 tablespoon daily	
Multi-mineral	3-4 ounces daily	In liquid solution, with vitamin B12, biotin
Multi-vitamin/mineral	6 caplets daily	Freeze-dried plant sources
Vitamin A	25,000 IU daily*	
Vitamin C	Individual bowel tolerance**	With bioflavonoids (quercetin, rutin proanthocyanidins)

Once healing has begun, nourish skin with a therapeutic moisturizer that contains aloe vera gel, chamomile, vitamins A and C, and avocado oil.

* The FDA recommends pregnant women not exceed 10,000 IU of vitamin A daily.

** To determine individual dosage, on the first day take 1,000 mg hourly until diarrhea occurs, then reduce dosage to just below that for individual daily dosage. Vitamin C is not toxic in large doses but must be taken throughout the day to benefit. Divide dosage to three or four times a day.

CHAPTER 75:

Fungus Infections

Tina went to her doctor because she kept getting itchy cold sores on the edges of her tongue. She figured she had some kind of cold virus that wouldn't go away. Her less-than-enlightened doctor prescribed antibiotics, diagnosing it as a throat infection. Not only did the cold sores not go away, but her privates itched too. Her doctor prescribed an anti-fungal agent to get rid of the candidiasis, and she went to see a nose and throat specialist for the sores.

"I was absolutely appalled when I learned the truth," Tina told me. "Not only did my doctor misdiagnosis my original problem, but by giving me the antibiotics, he made it worse! I never trusted him again, and chose another primary care physician."

Tina's original cold sore problem, called thrush, was caused by an overgrowth of the candida albicans fungus in her mouth. Candida is caused by two things: a diet high in refined carbohydrates, and a lowered immune system, which can be caused by illness or stress. An overabundance of fungus can further diminish the immune system, and has been linked with chronic fatigue.

Conventional medicine admits that the people most often infected are those with natural defenses depressed by excessive use of antibiotics and steroids or by certain diseases or operative procedures. Even spermicides have been credited with upsetting the delicate bacterial balance that invite too much candida. Nonoxynol-9 is the most commonly used over-the-counter spermicide. One medical journal reported that candida albicans were found to not only survive in up to a 25 percent concentration of this product, but grow and adhere better to cells when exposed to it.[1]

The conventional medicine *Home Health Handbook* states that: "Broad-spectrum antibiotics taken for other causes can disrupt the natural bacterial balance of the vagina, and promote (candida) vaginitis from an overgrowth of yeast."[2]

In Tina's case, the antibiotics made the situation worse by destroying her army of beneficial bacteria, allowing candida albicans to go where it doesn't belong and proliferating.

Normally, candida isn't a problem because intestinal bacteria keep it under control. But when bacteria are killed by antibiotics, for example, the bad guys can proliferate while the good guys are still down for the count. Keep in mind that antibiotics are in the food supply because antibiotic supplements are given to animals as treatment for diseases and as food additives.

Killed with Garlic

Candida is an opportunistic organism that overgrows only when the body is beset by allergies, nutritional deficiencies or environmental pollution – anything that lowers the body's natural defenses, including today's modern lifestyle and eating habits.

John Parks Trowbridge, M.D., emphasizes the need to eliminate allergens and irritants, which undermine the immune system, following up with nutritional and bacterial boosters to restore the natural and effective defense system. He especially recommends liquid aged garlic extract as a particularly effective fungus fighter, stating that it worked better than the prescription drug nystatin in several studies,[3] adding that a good squirt of the liquid form sloshed as long as you can in the mouth several times a day can effectively cure thrush.[4]

Numerous studies have been conducted on the antibacterial, antiviral and antifungal properties of garlic, and researchers have found it even works on candida. The *Journal of General Microbiology* reported on a Kuwaiti study of liquid garlic extract and its effect on candida albicans. No matter how the researchers diluted it, the garlic was able to reduce the overgrowth.[5]

Nutritional Solutions

Magdy S. Mikhail, M.D., and colleagues at the Department of Obstetrics and Gynecology, Albert Einstein College of Medicine, Bronx, N.Y., compared 22 women with vaginal candidiasis to 20 normal women without it. They found that the women with candidiasis had significantly lower levels of beta carotene. Dr. Mikhail hypothesized that antioxidants, such as beta carotene, may be beneficial in altered vaginal flora and overgrowth of candida albicans and the subsequent development of vaginal candidiasis.[6]

A nutritional protocol that includes beta carotene or vitamin A, vitamin E, the B vitamins, vitamin C, magnesium and zinc as daily supplements will boost the immune system. Biotin, one of the B vitamins, can help prevent the conversion of the yeast form of candida to the fungus form. Antibiotics, particularly sulfa drugs, can reduce the amount of biotin absorbed in the intestine, causing a deficiency that can add to the problem.[7]

I would add copper because it is needed with the zinc, and calcium because it is needed with the magnesium. Because of the likelihood of digestive problems, it is best to target easily-assimilated forms of these nutrients. You can get your minerals in solution, which means you need a minimum of digestive enzymes to break them down and absorb them. Look for a vitamin formula that includes acidophilus for that intestinal benefit, of which I will describe in a moment.

Free-form amino acids such as taurine, lysine, arginine, methionine and glutamine, are recommended in the event protein is not completely broken down due to allergies, a lack of stomach acid or digestive problems. Yeasts are especially fond of undigested protein and proliferate in its presence.[8] Along these lines, try gamma linolenic acid, an esssential fatty acid present in borage oil, which helps assimilate fats and break down protein.

Fighting Back with Bacteria

Stubborn resistance and a strong offensive are the best answers to defeating the persistent candida fungus. This means putting back the beneficial bacteria that was missing in the first place.

In a study involving 30 women at the University of California, Davis, Edwin B. Collins, Ph.D., and colleagues reported in the *Journal of Dairy Science* that lactobacillus acidophilus produces metabolites that inhibit candida albicans. An article in *The Lancet* reported 20 women with candida were cured with preparations containing lactobacillus acidophilus.[9]

Douching with yogurt and vinegar can help restore beneficial bacteria once the offending fungus has been eliminated. The reason infections become chronic is that normal bacteria is not replaced, especially when antibiotics have destroyed it. The normal vaginal bacteria is called Doderlein's bacillus. The closest thing obtainable is lactobacillus acidophilus, commonly available in health and vitamin stores.[10] Always check the date on the container, package or bottle for freshness.

Here is my formula for restoring vaginal bacteria: buy half a cup of fresh plain yogurt. It doesn't have to be pasteurized, just plain. You don't even have to be concerned about its bacteria content, since you'll be adding your own. Purchase a lactobacillus acidophilus supplement in either powder; tablets that can be crushed to powder; or in capsules that can be opened to release the powder. Avoid liquid suspension because it doesn't mix well.

To the yogurt, add about two tablespoons of the acidophilus powder. Approximately two teaspoons of the yogurt mixture can be placed into the vagina using a suitable, clean device. Some possibilities include a spermicide applicator, tampon applicator or a medicine syringe with the top cut off. Keep the rest of the yogurt in the refrigerator and apply it five nights in a row, beginning the first night of the day you finish using anti-fungal medication. The following mornings douche with purified water and approximately two tablespoons of vinegar. This regimen should be done anytime hormone medication or antibiotics are taken.

The reason supplemental acidophilus is added to yogurt instead of just using yogurt with acidophilus is that a number of prominent national brands do not contain the bacteria, and active yogurt cultures found in some brands may not be L. acidophilus. Certain brands may have the bacteria in some varieties but not in others. If you want to use yogurt with cultures, look to be sure the label says "live cultures" and that it contains lactobacillus acidophilus.

Fungus-Fighting Nutrients
For maximum absorption, take supplements with meals.

Nutrient	Suggested Dosage	Formulation
Acidophilus	At least four billion flora daily on an empty stomach, three times daily	
Aged garlic extract	1 teaspoon three times daily	Liquid
Borage oil	2 capsules daily	
Caprylic acid	100 mg three times daily	
Fiber	4-8 tablets daily	Psyllium, with herb hyssop
Flaxseed oil	1 tablespoon daily	
Grapefruit seed extract	100 mg three times daily	
Multi-mineral	1-4 ounces daily	In liquid solution, with vitamin B12, biotin
Multi-vitamin/mineral	3-6 caplets daily	Freeze-dried plant sources
Vitamin C	Individual bowel tolerance*	With bioflavonoids (quercetin, rutin proanthocyanidins)

* To determine individual dosage, on the first day take 1,000 mg hourly until diarrhea occurs, then reduce dosage to just below that for individual daily dosage. Vitamin C is not toxic in large doses but must be taken throughout the day to benefit. Divide dosage to three or four times a day.

CHAPTER 76:

Gallbladder Problems

My friend June has been determined all her life to keep her body parts. When she was 13 and they wanted to take out her tonsils she stood her ground. In her 40s, after diabetes severely impaired her circulation, doctors wanted to remove her legs. She got chelation treatments instead. When the doctors told her she needed to have her gallbladder removed, she knew there were alternatives and came to me for advice. She was fortunate enough to live near the office of Dr. Ross Gordon, who practices in Albany, California, a pioneer in our field and one of its pre-eminent healers. What he told her is what you'll learn as you read this. Today, she retains her gallbladder and her health!

Probably the least understood and even less acknowledged organ of our body is the gallbladder. It is a small pear-shaped sack that hangs between the lobes of the liver. Gall is another word for bile, and as the bladder stores urine, the gallbladder stores excess bile, which is produced by the liver. What is bile? It is an enzyme necessary for the digestion of fats. As fat-containing foods enter the small intestine, the gallbladder empties its bile, and, simultaneously, the liver begins to produce more.

Gallstones develop when cholesterol combines with bile. While most bile is stored in the gallbladder, some of it travels directly from the liver to the small intestine. Gallstones may form in the passages between liver and gallbladder, between liver and intestine, or in the gallbladder itself. They are more frequently found in diabetics, obese persons, the elderly, and women, especially those who have had children.

Most people who have gallstones experience no symptoms. However, when a stone obstructs any of the bile passages, these symptoms may occur a few hours after the intake of fried or fatty foods: nausea, vomiting, and severe right upper stomach pain that radiates to the right shoulder and back. If the stone completely obstructs one of the passages, jaundice may also occur. Doctors often recommend that patients with gallbladder problems have their gallbladder removed. What they don't consider are the sources of the problems, and the many ways they can be prevented. For more on lowering gallstone-generating cholesterol, see the Cholesterol chapter in this book.

The Royal Gallbladder Flush

When it comes to gallstones I have the solution. I like to call it the Royal Gallbladder Flush, because it gets rid of cholesterol stones and makes me feel like a queen. I've had so many people tell me it works for them that I want to pass it on to you!

It works on a seven day schedule. From Monday to Saturday, I drink all the apple juice I can, along with my regular diet.

On Saturday, three hours after my usual lunch, I dissolve two teaspoonsful of di-sodium phosphate, or Epsom salts into a small amount of hot water. After drinking this concoction, which tastes bad, I wash it away with a cleansing glass of grapefruit juice. I repeat this procedure in two hours.

For dinner, I eat half a grapefruit and drink another glass of grapefruit juice.

Just before going to bed, I blend a half cup of warm, unrefined olive oil with half a cup of grapefruit juice and drink it. I follow that with half a cup of unrefined olive oil blended with half a cup of freshly squeezed lemon juice.

Then I go to bed, lying on my right side with my right knee pulled as closely to my chest as I can for half an hour.

On Sunday morning, I take two more teaspoonsful of Epsom salts in a small amount of hot water at least an hour before I eat.

That morning's bowel movement contains small, green, irregularly-shaped cholesterol stones the size of kiwi fruit or grape seeds and a few just smaller than cherries. I do the Royal Flush every three to six months.

Dr. Ross Gordon's nurse asked him if the flush worked, and he suggested she try it. She came in Monday with 68 little green stones. They sent it to the lab and confirmed they were gallstones.

The Food Allergy Connection

Many imminent physicians and researchers have discovered how diet affects the gallbladder. In some cases, what is eaten can be the source of problems. James Breneman, M.D., author of *Basics of Food Allergy* (Charles C. Thomas, 1984), and former chairman of the Food Allergy Committee of the American College of Allergists, believes an allergy to certain foods can bring on gallbladder problems. He looked at 69 gallbladder patients – those with gallstones or those whose gallbladder removal did not alleviate their symptoms – and found all of them lost their symptoms when certain food allergens were removed. The foods in order of their guilt are as follows: egg, pork, onion, fowl, milk, coffee, orange, corn, beans and nuts. Dr. Breneman believes it is the egg white that causes the reaction, due to its resistance to digestion. He believes every gallbladder patient should identify and eliminate any food allergens before further steps are taken.[1]

A study reported in *The Lancet* showed that of 80 patients with gallbladder disease, all had symptoms of acute colitis as well. The colitis was found to have been caused by food allergy. When the allergies were identified and the food source removed, 100 percent of these patients were relieved of their gallbladder problems. When they again ate their food allergens, the symptoms came back.

Even gallstones can be caused by food allergens, Dr. Breneman believes. He says allergens cause swelling of the bile ducts, which impairs the release of bile. Infection can set in, predisposing the area to cholesterol accumulation, leading to stone development. This brings me to the association between cholesterol and gallstones.

Fat, Sugar, Cholesterol and Gallstones

The same issues covered in the chapters Appendicitis and Cholesterol are at play here in gallstones. Once again, our Western diet high in fat, sugar and cholesterol is giving us digestive problems. Many scientific studies are showing how.

Essential fatty acids, like fish oil and oils from nuts and seeds, have been shown to lower cholesterol and help circulation and heart problems. Lawrence L. Rudel, Ph.D., and colleagues at the Department of Comparative Medicine, Bowman Gray School of Medicine in Winston-Salem, North Carolina, did a study of adult male African green monkeys divided into two groups. One group's high-fat diet was derived mostly from lard, while the other's came from fish oil.

After two to three years necropsies were performed and it was found that 67 percent of the animals fed the lard diet had cholesterol gallstones, while only 22 percent of the animals fed the fish oil did.[2]

Some of the foods found to lower cholesterol are high in essential fatty acids. These are fish, unroasted nuts and seeds, and the oils from them. Notorious cholesterol lowerers are nuts, olive oil and fish oils. The best supplemental sources of essential fatty acids are flaxseed oil and borage oil. Flaxseed contains omega 3 and borage oil contains omega 6 or gamma linolenic acid, deemed deficient in most of the population.

A high intake of refined sugar has also been shown to increase the chances of gallstones. A four-year study conducted by public health researchers in the Netherlands concluded that sugar can cause problems with the gallbladder's bile ducts, resulting in cholesterol accumulation and gallstones.[3] A 25-year follow-up study found the same correlation between sugar, but also found gallstones may be retarded by adequate calcium and magnesium.[4]

It is best to supplement with a minerals in solution formula that contains both magnesium and calcium, along with all the other minerals essential to each other. Because of the high absorption rate of this type of formula, and deficiency of magnesium in the diet, the ratio of magnesium and calcium in solution should be four to one, respectively.

Vitamins C and E for Gallstones

One theory about gallstone formation holds that dead cells from the gallbladder's inner membrane act as the nucleus around which stones form. But this doesn't happen when vitamin E is plentiful. Vitamin A protects the integrity of skin and tissue, which is why a diet without it will result in blindness. However, without enough vitamin E to guard it, vitamin A is attacked by oxidation, permitting membrane cells to die and drop into the bile.

In a study to determine if vitamin E deters gallstone development, a group of hamsters was purposely fed a diet deficient in vitamin E. A second group received an ample amount of this vitamin. The first group developed gallstones, the second did not.

This is believed to occur due to vitamin E's incredible cholesterol-lowering effect. In one study, rabbits were given a high cholesterol diet, then fed 2,100 IU of vitamin E a week. By the eighth week, their cholesterol levels lowered by 50 percent. The researchers also took note of how this affected the gallbladder. They found the vitamin E increased bile salts and improved the gallbladder's ability to avoid cholesterol accumulation.[5]

Low vitamin C levels may be a contributory factor in human gallbladder disease because vitamin C increases an enzyme activity that keeps cholesterol from accumulating. Dr. J. A. Simon, an internist at San Francisco VA Medical Center, found that vitamin C deficient guinea pigs often have cholesterol gallstones, and when he looked at people with risk factors for cholesterol gallstones, such as obesity,

estrogen treatment, pregnancy and diabetes, they too had low vitamin C levels.[6]

Digestive Problems Mistaken for Gallbladder Problems

Dr. Jonathan Wright treated a patient diagnosed with gallbladder
problems simply by eliminating her food allergens, then treating her
stomach problems. She complained of chronic indigestion – pain when
she ate; bloating; gas and heartburn. The first doctor she consulted
told her it was her gallbladder and, incredibly, recommended she
have it removed! Dr. Wright saw it was a common problem, uncom-
monly identified by conventional medicine – she didn't have enough
stomach acid to properly break down her food![7] Normal stomachs
make large amounts of hydrochloric acid and pepsin to digest the
food we eat. Without the stomach acid and digestive enzymes, the
food sits, isn't properly broken down, and causes all sorts of painful
symptoms.

This is Dr. Wright's prescription for gallbladder health: vitamin
C, lecithin, borage oil capsules, vitamin E, and multiple vitamin and
multiple mineral supplemental formulas.

To reiterate, add vitamins A, B complex, C and E.

A diet high in cholesterol and deficient in vitamin C has been
shown to cause gallstones. Vitamin C is necessary for the conversion
of cholesterol into bile acids. Lecithin reduces cholesterol levels; B
vitamins increase the body's production of lecithin and also stimulate the emptying of the gallbladder. In studies, bran added to the diet
has lowered the cholesterol concentration of the bile.

Only two food sources contain liberal amounts of lecithin: soybeans and eggs. Therefore, some people prefer to take a lecithin
supplement. B vitamins are preferred to stimulate emptying of the
gallbladder. For a complete gallbladder supplement, look for one that
uses the whole food. One such formula uses freeze dried sprouts and
vegetables, combined in such a way as to provide B complex and all

essential vitamins and minerals, as well as adding odorless garlic, acidophilus and green tea extract for immune-system boosting.

Gallbladder-Healthy Nutrients
For maximum absorption, take supplements with meals.

Nutrient	Suggested Dosage	Formulation
Acidophilus	At least four billion flora daily on an empty stomach, three times daily	
Aged garlic extract	1 teaspoon three times daily	Liquid
Amino acids	4-6 capsules daily	Multiple formula from natural sources
Antioxidants	4 capsules daily*	With selenium and grapeseed extract
Borage oil	2 capsules daily	
Coenzyme Q10	2 capsules daily	With vitamin E, phospholipids and selenium
Enzymes	2 capsules twice daily	Multiple formula
Fiber	4-8 tablets	Psyllium, with herb hyssop
Flaxseed oil	1 tablespoon daily	
Gugulipids	250 mg three times daily	
Magnesium	200 mg daily	
Multi-mineral	3-4 ounces daily	In liquid solution, with vitamin B12, biotin
Multi-vitamin/mineral	6 caplets daily	Freeze-dried plant sources
Niacin	500 mg four times daily	
Ox bile extract	100 mg daily	
Tumeric	100 mg three times daily	
Vitamin C	Individual bowel tolerance**	With bioflavonoids (quercetin, rutin proanthocyanidins)

* The FDA recommends pregnant women not exceed 10,000 IU of vitamin A daily.

** To determine individual dosage, on the first day take 1,000 mg hourly until diarrhea occurs, then reduce dosage to just below that for individual daily dosage. Vitamin C is not toxic in large doses but must be taken throughout the day to benefit. Divide dosage to three or four times a day.

CHAPTER 77:

Gas, Intestinal

The old comedic line "I have enough gas to get to Poughkeepsie" is not necessarily referring to petrol for the car trip.

Those who do not mastigate, nature castigates. The digestive system is a superb orchestra of reactions, begun the moment you put food into your mouth. At the same time as saliva is produced to help you chew, your stomach is producing hydrochloric acid to break down the food, and your liver and pancreas are producing bile and digestive enzymes so the intestines can draw water and nutrients from it, delivering them to your tissues, blood and cells.

If you do not chew your food thoroughly prior to swallowing, this essential process of digestion becomes incomplete, compromising the whole system. At the very least, when you chew too quickly, you tend to gulp and swallow air. It's amazing how painful a little air in the intestine can be. Ouch! At worst, undigested food putrifies in the stomach and intestine, giving off foul smelling gas and painful acid. It's not antacids you need, it's music!

One way to slow down your eating and step up your digestion is to play soft, slow music as you eat. There's an added bonus: you'll lose weight. Mona Simonson, Ph.D., director of the Health, Weight and Stress Clinic at Johns Hopkins University, carried out an experiment showing that musical munching actually works. Not only does slow, soothing music slacken your eating pace, but it makes you less likely to desire seconds. Simonson found that when a soothing, slow, calming flute instrument played while eating, the study volunteers slowed their chewing to 3.2 bites per minute – much smaller bites too – and lingered over the meal for almost an hour. None of the diners requested seconds.

Eating too much food overwhelms the digestive system, leaving it incapable of breaking down and digesting the amounts before the heat and moisture draw bacteria to feed on it. This bacteria that naturally feeds on undigested food creates toxins and acids, as well as a host of other problems.

Some years ago, *Reader's Digest* published a classic article, "Mealtime Madness," showing that the family dining table is not only a place for eating, but also for carrying on family arguments and rehashing the day's frustrations – negative factors which make individuals eat under stress – too nervously and too fast. The result? Indigestion and intestinal gas. Bloating and odor tell a person immediately that his or her digestion needs a tune up.

I recommend you chew each mouthful of food at least 20 times and meat, at least 30 times, almost liquefying it before swallowing. Meat, especially, needs a lot of chewing to ensure it is completely broken down before it hits the stomach.

A Stomach Acid Deficiency

A lack of hydrochloric or gastric acid is called hypo-acidity or hypochlorhydria. Without adequate gastric acid in the stomach, proteins are not digested, and essential amino acids, nutrients and minerals such as magnesium and B12 are not absorbed. Without diagnosis and treatment, malnutrition and death can result.

This lack of acid is more common than we think and can cause all of the symptoms that appear when the stomach contains too much gastric acid. Doctors warn that people should not take antacids too readily as heartburn, gas, bloating after eating and even constipation can all be symptoms of hypoacidity. The burning sensation common to too much acid is also present when the stomach is too alkaline, and can be made worse by antacids. Other physical signs of low secretion of hydrochloric acid include split peeling nails, hair falling out, and dilated capillaries on cheeks and nose. Dr. Jonathan Wright estimates that every third adult he sees in his Kent, Washington clinic secretes too little hydrochloric acid.

Researchers at the Mayo Clinic and Johns Hopkins University pumped the stomachs of over 3,000 individuals and analyzed their contents. It was determined that by the age of 60 years, an incredible 60 percent had a significant decline in hydrochloric acid.

Dr. Robert Atkins, author of *Dr. Atkins Health Revolution*, believes intestinal problems start in the stomach. He found two tests invented and ignored by orthodoxy proved it. One is the Indican test, which looks for the presence of indole in the urine, and shows food has left the stomach properly broken down. The second test is the Heidelberg test, which evaluates the amount of hydrochloric, or stomach acid, available to break down the food. Dr. Atkins found that some patients with bowel problems were not breaking down their food and had a deficiency of stomach acid. What happens in these cases is that the food enters the large intestine in a whole state and ferments. The large intestine is not designed to break down food, only to absorb its nutrients. Food that is not broken down cannot impart its valuable nutrients to the body, and the acids emitted causes sores and ulcers.[1]

If you suspect a lack of stomach acid is causing your problems, supplement with Betaine HCl, with or without pepsin. Include a digestive enzyme formula to help break down food. Bromelain is a digestive enzyme helpful for increasing absorption and assimilation of nutrients and food. Both bromelain and papain are digestive enzymes, called proteolytic enzymes, which break down protein. For an appetizer, try slices of pineapple and papaya. Papaya contains papain and pineapple contains bromelain.

A product which proves helpful to millions of people in conquering gas comes right out of folk medicine: charcoal. Studies reveal activated charcoal, a health food store item, cuts the production of gas by 75 percent. Herbs such as garlic, anise, fennel and caraway stimulate digestion by increasing gastric juices, decreasing the amount of putrefactive bacteria and stimulating intestinal motility. Exercise invigorates intestinal peristalsis and helps break down large gas bubbles.

Fennel is especially plentiful in the Mediterranean and Eastern Europe, and its licorice-like taste has made it a popular flavoring in breads and candy, as well as in commercially produced herbal teas. It has long been used by many cultures as a digestive aid and is often recommended by herbalists and holistic physicians (following the lead of the "father of medicine," Hippocrates) as a gentle stomach and colic remedy for infants. Colic is believed to be caused by intestinal gas. Fennel works by relaxing the lining of the digestive tract so gas can be expelled.

Gassy Foods

Certain problem foods may be the culprits. Call it food sensitivity. One food notorious for producing intestinal gas is beans. To make beans less bean-like, after soaking them, use fresh water to cook them. Sulfur-containing foods like broccoli, Brussels sprouts, cabbage, cauliflower, eggs and dried fruit (due to its sugar concentration) can produce that rotten egg odor (hydrogen sulfide) so familiar to chemistry students. Fiber from grains is indigestible to us, but certain intestinal microorganisms don't find it so. Individuals who increase their fiber intake too fast run the risk of producing intestinal gas.

Milk can produce gas in lactose-intolerant persons. Many adults lose the ability to produce lactase, so the lactose escapes the stomach undigested, meets intestinal bacteria which feed on it, causes fermentation, and the small intestine becomes a war zone of cramps, diarrhea, gas and bloating. To make up for an insufficiency of lactase, drink milk or eat yogurt that contains lactobacillus acidophilus, a bacterial culture that makes the necessary lactase. Or you can buy milk that already contains lactase. Lactase enzymes can also be purchased at health food stores and taken as a supplement. A zinc and copper supplement can help restore the stomach lining after an allergen has reduced the stomach lining to mush.

Another option is to supplement with digestive enzymes, which will "eat" gas producing foods before they have a chance to ferment. Some over-the-counter products that are sold to prevent gas and heartburn are nothing more than digestive enzymes: natural chemicals produced in the body to digest proteins, fats, carbohydrates, fiber, etc.

Nutritional Solutions

Pantothenic acid has been shown to relieve intestinal gas and distension. This B5 vitamin also aids in bowel mobility and efficient digestion. Without pantothenic acid, acetylcholine cannot be produced. This chemical transmits messages to nerves that control the motor and secretory activities of the intestine. A study showed gas pains were relieved in postoperative patients and prevented in others when they were given 250 mg. of pantothenic acid daily. All the B vitamins are important because they help regulate the body's response to stress, and the digestive process.

Eat garlic in your food and take aged garlic extract to eliminate the pesky bacteria that proliferate and create gas. Magnesium is important to muscular contractions and can help your intestine move out excess gas. If low stomach acid or digestive enzymes is a possible cause of your maldigestion, target liquid garlic extract – a squirt or two a day – and supplement with a minerals in solution formula that contains magnesium.

Psyllium, a natural fiber source, has been found in studies to relieve intestinal gas caused by poor fat metabolism. Researchers at George Washington University Medical Center in Washington, D.C. found that among otherwise healthy men with high cholesterol, indigestion and gas problems, the introduction of psyllium into their diets resulted in significantly lowered cholesterol levels and less gas.[2] Look for a fiber-rich formula that contains acidophilus, pyllium and hyssop, another high fiber botanical. The kind of problems that can cause high cholesterol levels may also result in malabsorption and subsequent gas and indigestion. Therefore, I highly recommend you also read my Cholesterol chapter in this book as well.

For more on gas-causing problems, read my chapters Colon Problems and Malabsorption.

Flatulence-Fighting Nutrients
For maximum absorption, take supplements with meals.

Nutrient	Suggested Dosage	Formulation
Acidophilus	At least four billion flora daily on an empty stomach, three times daily	
Aged garlic extract	1 teaspoon three times daily	Liquid
Caraway	1/2 teaspoon daily	Seeds chewed, or crushed then steeped in boiling water
Coenzyme Q10	2 capsules daily	With vitamin E, phospholipids and selenium
Deglycyrrhizinated licorice	1-2 tablets before meals	Chewable
Enzymes	2 capsules twice daily	Multiple formula
Fennel	1/2 teaspoon daily	Seeds chewed, or crushed then steeped in boiling water
Fiber	4-8 tablets daily	Psyllium, with herb hyssop
Ginger	500 mg after meals daily	
Multi-mineral	3-4 ounces daily	In liquid solution, with vitamin B12, biotin
Multi-vitamin/mineral	6 caplets daily	Freeze-dried plant sources
Vitamin C	Individual bowel tolerance*	With bioflavonoids (quercetin, rutin proanthocyanidins)

* To determine individual dosage, on the first day take 1,000 mg hourly until diarrhea occurs, then reduce dosage to just below that for individual daily dosage. Vitamin C is not toxic in large doses but must be taken throughout the day to benefit. Divide dosage to three or four times a day.

CHAPTER 78:

Gastritis

The biggest mistake people can make when having symptoms of gastritis is to assume it is caused by too much stomach acid, and take antacids. The hydrochloric acid in your stomach serves a dual purpose: to break down foods so their nutrients can be absorbed; and to kill bacteria so it doesn't wreak havoc further down.

Gastritis is defined as an inflammation of the stomach lining. It causes a stomachache. When the inflammation is chronic and it reduces the surface area of the stomach, it is called atrophic. Studies have shown this stage precedes ulcers and stomach cancer. See my chapter Cancer of the stomach for more.

Follow along while I summarize the vicious circle that precedes gastritis. Certain drugs and stress can diminish stomach acid, as well as irritate and inflame the stomach lining. Can you say "Non-Steroidal Anti-Inflammatory Drugs?" They include steroids, aspirin, ibuprofen (Motrin) and other over-the-counter and prescription drugs commonly recommended for muscle and joint pain.

Bacteria That Doesn't Belong

Here's what happens: When you eat certain foods that require a lot of stomach acid to break them down, like meat, or foods high in sugar; instead of being broken down they literally rot, causing bacteria to proliferate in the stomach – bacteria that shouldn't be there and would normally not exist in the presence of adequate hydrochloric/ stomach acid. So the lack of stomach acid not only doesn't kill the bacteria, but contributes to its formation! Conventional medicine has the misguided belief that too much stomach acid causes gastritis and ulcers, when it is actually a lack of acid!

Atrophic gastritis is directly caused by an inability to excrete sufficient stomach acid to kill bacteria.

It is estimated that approximately 20 percent of people between 60 and 69 years of age, and 40 percent over 80 suffer from atrophic gastritis. All of these people have an increased risk of getting stomach cancer, as well as mental problems associated with a lack of vitamin B12, which is diminished with stomach acid loss.[1,2] Other nutrients that can be deficient are folic acid, iron and calcium.[3]

Gastritis can also diminish your zinc stores, and antacids and other stomach remedies can contribute to this risk.[4] This is a problem, because zinc is your body's best wound healer, and can soothe and heal inflamed tissues.

Copper is important to balance out your zinc supplements. Be sure and include 2-4 mg. of copper with any zinc.

Remember, you're not what you put into your mouth, you're what you absorb and digest and deliver to the cells. That's why it is so important when you take your minerals that you take them in solution. A mineral tablet is only one to five percent absorbable. Remember that the process of digestion is a process of breaking down solids into liquids. Your body has to take a hard rock tablet and turn it into solution. When you take your minerals, make sure you're getting them in solution.

Dr. Jonathan Wright concludes, after over two decades of clinical experience that gastritis can also be caused by food allergies – most commonly cow's milk. The allergic reaction includes a loss of stomach acid, which will obviously make the problem worse.[5]

Milk is a very common allergen. You've heard of lactose

intolerance? Many children who are asthmatic are allergic to the lactose in milk. They don't have enough of the enzyme lactase to break it down.

The system's reaction to a food allergy can be severe and long-term. In a study reported in the *European Journal of Pediatrics*, researchers tested infants from parents with a family history of milk allergy. After only one dose of cow's milk, "before" and "after" pictures showed stomach lining was turned to mush.

Narrow your list down to the following foods suspect for most allergy sufferers: beef, chocolate, eggs, citrus fruits, coffee, corn, malt, milk, pork, potatoes, soybeans, spices, tomatoes, wheat, sugar, chocolate and yeast. See my Allergy chapter for more.

Reducing the Risk with Nutrients

The biggest enemy to your stomach is Helicobacter pylori, an organism that causes the stomach flu, which most of us, unfortunately, have experienced. Scientists have isolated this "bug" as being the primary initiator of not only gastritis but stomach cancer.[6] We know that gastritis can contribute to a B12 deficiency. However, researchers at the University of Southern California School of Medicine, Los Angeles found that a deficiency of B12 may predispose patients to Helicobacter pylori. Their study evaluated 98 subjects with low blood levels of B12, comparing them to 17 controls with normal B12 levels. Amazingly, the researchers found that 42 percent of B12-deficient subjects who did not have low stomach acid still had evidence of Helicobacter pylori.[7] Since B12 is crucial to a healthy digestive system, it stands to reason that a lack of this vitamin would compromise it.

Antioxidants, specifically beta carotene, vitamin C and vitamin E may reverse or reduce the risk of atrophic gastritis and/or gastric cancer.[8] This is probably due to the protective effect of antioxidants. Vitamin C, especially, has more than just protective benefits. It also increases circulation, and strengthens and protects cellular tissue. Not surprisingly, a study that found persons with Helicobacter pylori not only had low levels of stomach acid, but also had low concentrations of vitamin C available in the stomach.[9]

Super Stomach-Saving Nutrients
For maximum absorption, take supplements with meals.

Nutrient	Suggested Dosage	Formulation
Acidophilus	At least four billion flora daily on an empty stomach, three times daily	
Aged garlic extract	1 teaspoon three times daily	Liquid
Antioxidants	4 capsules daily*	With selenium and grapeseed extract
Borage oil	2 capsules daily	
Caraway	1/2 teaspoon seeds	Chewed, or crushed then steeped in boiling water
Coenzyme Q10	2 capsules daily	With vitamin E, phospholipids and selenium
Deglycyrrhizinated licorice	1-2 tablets before meals	Chewable
Enzymes	2 capsules twice daily	Multiple formula
Fennel	1/2 teaspoon seeds	Chewed, or crushed then steeped in boiling water
Fiber	4-8 tablets daily	Psyllium, with herb hyssop
Flaxseed oil	1 tablespoon daily	
L-glutamine	500 mg three times daily	
Peppermint tea	As desired	Organically-grown, chemical-free leaves
Multi-mineral	3-4 ounces daily	In liquid solution, with vitamin B12, biotin
Multi-vitamin/mineral	6 caplets daily	Freeze-dried plant sources
Vitamin B6	100 mg daily	
Vitamin C	Individual bowel tolerance**	With bioflavonoids (quercetin, rutin proanthocyanidins)
Vitamin E	2 capsules (800 IU) daily	d-alpha tocopherol

* The FDA recommends pregnant women not exceed 10,000 IU of vitamin A daily.

** To determine individual dosage, on the first day take 1,000 mg hourly until diarrhea occurs, then reduce dosage to just below that for individual daily dosage. Vitamin C is not toxic in large doses but must be taken throughout the day to benefit. Divide dosage to three or four times a day.

CHAPTER 79:

Glaucoma

Glaucoma is a dangerous disease. That's because there are no early symptoms. You could have it right now and not know it. Glaucoma is caused by a defect in the eye's normal draining mechanism, causing a build-up of intraocular pressure. This increased pressure damages the optic nerve and interferes with the transmission of visual images to the brain. Only in one form of glaucoma (angle-closure glaucoma) does the condition cause pain. But this type accounts for less than 10 percent of cases. An estimated three million Americans have glaucoma, but incredibly, half don't know it.

The big news about glaucoma is literally eye-opening. Doctors now know that perhaps millions of cases of vision loss could be prevented through adequate nutrition and early detection. Early diagnosis can make all the difference in a nutritional treatment plan.

Vitamin C Leads the Charge Against Glaucoma

After having regular eye exams, the next best thing to do is be sure you get enough vitamin C.

In glaucoma, the eyeball hardens because of increased pressure on it created by fluids behind it. Several studies, however, have found that vitamin C reduces this pressure.

In his 1980 dissertation at New York University, Ben C. Lane, Ph.D., then a doctoral student in ophthalmology, found in a study of 60 people that increasing their average vitamin C intake from 75 milligrams to 1,200 mg reduced intraocular pressure by an amazing one-third.

At the Provincial People's Hospital in Harbin, China, two ophthalmologists, Tsun-Mou Shen, M.D., and Ming-Ching Yu, M.D., found that a sodium ascorbate solution containing vitamin C reduced intraocular pressure in glaucoma patients by between 21 and 84 percent.[1]

Researchers in Copenhagen did a study where 25 subjects, average age 63 years, with moderate pressure, received 500 milligrams of ascorbic acid – the most common form of vitamin C – orally four times a day. After only six days their pressure was reduced significantly. Vitamin C eye drops have also proven to be beneficial.[2]

When you supplement, make sure you take the bioflavonoid rutin with your vitamin C. This common plant constituent makes vitamin C more available to the body and is also shown in studies to reduce eyeball pressure.

In a pilot study, the administration of rutin for four or more weeks reduced pressure by at least 15 percent in the majority of glaucoma patients tested.[3]

Deficiencies of chromium and vitamin C have been implicated in increased eye pressure. Ophthalmologists have found that low levels of vitamin C and chromium can increase eye pressure among people who use their eyes to do close, detailed work.[4] Chromium is an essential mineral that regulates blood sugar, fat and cholesterol. The best sources of chromium are whole wheat, beets and mushrooms.[5]

A study reported in *Annals of Ophthalmology* found that glaucoma patients have lower blood levels of the B vitamin thiamine.

Where is thiamine found? It's in the germ and bran of wheat, the husk of rice, and that portion of all grains which is commercially milled away to give the grain its lighter color and finer texture. A diet rich in wheat germ, blackstrap molasses and bran will provide the body with thiamine. Eating sugar will cause a thiamine depletion, as will smoking and drinking alcohol. Thiamine can also be destroyed by an enzyme present in raw clams, oysters and raw fish.[6]

Cod liver oil has been shown in studies to also help lower intraocular pressure. Dr. Prasad S. Kulkarni, Ph.D. at the University of Louisville at Kentucky, after observing that Eskimos have a low incidence of glaucoma decided to see for himself. He gave laboratory rabbits food soaked in cod liver oil then observed that their eye pressure lowered, then rose again when the cod liver oil was removed from their diets. Control animals given liquid lard or safflower oil did not have their intraocular pressure affected.[7] Cod liver oil is high in omega-6 fatty acids, shown to be important to healthy cellular tissue. It is also high in vitamin A, the eyesight vitamin, and vitamin D. Flaxseed oil also contains omega-6 fatty acids, and you don't risk the chance of eating cod liver oil that's loaded with dangerous chemicals.

As therapy for glaucoma, James F. Balch, M.D., suggests 3 to 7 grams (3,000-7,000 milligrams) of vitamin C plus bioflavonoids three times daily. He also recommends choline (1 to 2 grams daily); pantothenic acid (100 mg three times daily); rutin, (50 mg three times daily); vitamin B complex (50 mg three times daily with meals); and vitamin E (400 IU daily); as well as inositol and a multivitamin and mineral complex containing vitamin A and beta-carotene, which has shown to be useful in relieving pressure behind the eyeball.

Vitamin A is essential for eye-tissue health, and is recommended for any program of eye strengthening. Beta carotene is a more body-available form of vitamin A and can safely be taken in large doses.

Can the Coffee

Stop drinking caffeinated-products too. That includes your morning cup of coffee, tea and cola soft drinks. There are a lot of reasons not to drink soft drinks, but here's one:

Caffeine may encourage glaucoma in normal people and make it worse in those who have it already, according to Mary G. Lynch, M.D., assistant professor of ophthalmology at Emory University, Atlanta. She found glaucoma patients should be very careful not to drink large amounts of coffee or caffeinated beverages, because they risk raising their eye pressure to damaging levels.[8]

She is especially concerned about the person who drinks at least 32 ounces – the equivalent of four cups – of coffee or highly caffeinated beverages over a short period of time.

Glaucoma Suppressing Nutrients
For maximum absorption, take supplements with meals.

Nutrient	Suggested Dosage	Formulation
Antioxidants	4 capsules daily*	With selenium and grapeseed extract
Bilberry	100 mg twice daily	
Borage oil	2 capsules daily	
Coenzyme Q10	2 capsules daily	With vitamin E, phospholipids and selenium
Flaxseed oil	1 tablespoon daily	
Ginkgo biloba	60 mg daily	
Lecithin	2 tablespoons with meals	
Magnesium	200 mg daily	
Melatonin (adults only)	3 mg daily at bedtime	With B vitamins
Multi-mineral	3-4 ounces daily	In liquid solution, with vitamin B12, biotin
Multi-vitamin/mineral	6 caplets daily	Freeze-dried plant sources
Vitamin C	Individual bowel tolerance**	With bioflavonoids (quercetin, rutin proanthocyanidins)
Vitamin E	2 capsules (800 IU) daily	d-alpha tocopherol

* The FDA recommends pregnant women not exceed 10,000 IU of vitamin A daily.

** To determine individual dosage, on the first day take 1,000 mg hourly until diarrhea occurs, then reduce dosage to just below that for individual daily dosage. Vitamin C is not toxic in large doses but must be taken throughout the day to benefit. Divide dosage to three or four times a day.

CHAPTER 80:

Gout

My friend Joe had pains in his foot so severe he thought he had broken a toe. But an x-ray found no broken bones or bunion problems. Joe couldn't understand it. The pain was so bad, he couldn't put on his shoe, and had to wear his slippers. If he managed to get to sleep, he awoke in the middle of the night, the pain hounding him like a relentless dog.

As he described it to me, "I felt like I was in the middle of an Edgar Allan Poe story." He said it felt like his toe had been dislocated, and cold water poured over it. Then he got chills, shivers and a little fever. The pain which was at first moderate, would become more intense. As it increased, so would the chills and fever. First it was a gnawing pain, then a pressure and tightening. So acute was the pain that the affected part could not bear the weight of bedsheets nor the jar of a person walking into the room. He said he passed many nights in sleepless torture; as turning his foot or changing his posture was akin to red hot pincers being applied.

Finally in desperation, Joe asked me for advice.

Although commonly referred to in history books, gout still occurs today, mostly among middle aged men. It is a hereditary condition in which uric acid builds up in the blood and crystals are deposited in a joint, forming a bump or growth that irritates the joint – particularly the base of the big toe – causing it to become inflamed and painful. It can also occur in the heel, knee, hand, ear or any joint in the body.

Cherry Berry Flavonoids

Over 40 years ago, Texan Ludwig W. Blau, Ph.D., made a discovery that to this day ripples through many nutritional journals and books about gout. Crippled, confined to a wheelchair and suffering from gout, Blau one day wheeled himself to the cupboard. Seeing nothing appetizing, he turned to refrigerator, spied a bowlful of plump, red cherries, sampled them, and, hooked, ate the bowlful.

The next morning, wonder of wonders, the pain and inflammation in his foot were almost gone. Instead of pooh-poohing the cherry story, Blau's family physician tried the therapy on 12 patients. Every one of them saw improvement. Dr. Blau reported in *Texas Reports on Biology and Medicine*[1] that, following a non-restricted diet of one-half pound of fresh or canned cherries per day, all 12 gout sufferers saw their blood uric acid levels return to normal, with no further attacks of gout. Dr. Blau recommended either canned cherries, sour, black and Royal Anne or fresh Bing varieties. In one of his test cases, only juice was drunk, and this proved to be equally effective.[2]

Now, the science behind the cherries. The cherry treatment seems to work because the nutrients in cherries keep uric acid from crystallizing and becoming deposited in joints. They have an excellent calcium-phosphorous ratio, and they contain about 191 mgs of potassium to every 100 grams of sodium.

They are also high in bioflavonoids – which not only strengthen the tendons and cartilage found in joints, preventing their destruction by uric acid, but also act as natural anti-inflammatories, avoiding the swelling of the surrounding soft tissues that causes so much of the pain.[3] How soon can someone expect relief? In 10 days or less. However, one patient just under 60 years of age ate cherries six to eight months before her pain diminished.

Other red and blue berries high in flavonoids, like blueberries, hawthorn berries and strawberries have also been credited with helping gout. Famous Swedish botanist Linnaeus supposedly cured his gout by eating large amounts of strawberries every morning and evening.

Bioflavonoids work best with plenty of vitamin C. Not coincidentally, berries are high in vitamin C. If you take a vitamin C supplement – and everyone should – get one that includes bioflavonoids.

I've seen for myself that vitamin C with bioflavonoids works as well as cherries for gout. On a tour I joined in Israel, a man in our group was unable to walk because of his gout. Unable to find any cherries, I gave him my own emergency supply of vitamin C with bioflavonoids, instructing him to take two of the 500 milligram tablets every hour until he got diarrhea (called bowel intolerance), then cut down and keep taking them until the bottle was gone. In three days he was walking the hills, stairs and steep roads like a teenager.

Caused by Alcohol and Certain Foods

Uric acid is a waste product derived from the breakdown of an amino acid called purine. Normally, uric acid is dissolved in the blood and eliminated from the body by the kidneys. But for some reason, among overweight men (the large proportion who have gout), uric acid builds up in the joints. Researchers have found that avoiding purine-rich foods can help alleviate gout. One study found that healthy men could cut their blood levels of uric acid in half by eliminated all purine-high foods.[4] Foods with the most purine are meats, especially organ meats, and yeast-laden baked goods. Also avoid gravies and broths, sardines, mussels, herring, mushrooms, dried beans, fish, lentils, peas, oatmeal and spinach.[5]

One of the first things I did for my friend Joe was give him this list of purine no-nos. Then I told him to eat only raw fruits and vegetables for two weeks, after which he should concentrate on eating grains, seeds and nuts, and drink only purified water. I also warned him to stop drinking his daily six-pack of beer, and instead drink a quart of unsweetened cherry juice every day, and take a vitamin C supplement with bioflavonoids.

Studies have shown that men who drink alcohol, most especially beer, have a much higher chance of developing gout than those who do not. In a study reported in *Annals of Rheumatic Diseases*, researchers found 41 percent of a group of gout sufferers drank more than seven 12-ounce cans of beer daily, compared to 17 percent from the healthy control group.[6] The explanation? Beer contains not only alcohol, which raises uric acid, but fermented yeast – a double whammy that can make all the difference. Some researchers say eliminating alcohol is all it takes to reverse and prevent gout in some individuals.[7]

As for Joe, once he quit drinking beer and eating glazed, raised donuts for breakfast, he lost weight, and the juice and vitamin C helped dissolve the nasty crystals in his toe joint. He's healthier, happier, and sleeps a lot better.

Gout-Be-Gone Nutrients
For maximum absorption, take supplements with meals.

Nutrient	Suggested Dosage	Formulation
Antioxidants	4 capsules daily*	With selenium and grapeseed extract
Bilberry	100 mg three times daily	
Borage oil	2 capsules daily	
Bromelain	250 mg three times a day between meals	
Coenzyme Q10	2 capsules daily	With vitamin E, phospholipids and selenium
Enzymes	2 capsules twice daily	Multiple formula
Fiber	4-8 tablets	Psyllium, with herb hyssop
Folic acid	10 mg daily	
Quercetin	400 mg twice daily	
Flaxseed oil	1 tablespoon daily	
Melatonin (adults only)	3 mg daily at bedtime	With B vitamins
Multi-mineral	3-4 ounces daily	In liquid solution, with vitamin B12, biotin
Multi-vitamin/mineral	6 caplets daily	Freeze-dried plant sources
Purified water	Two gallons daily	
Tumeric	100 mg three times daily	
Quercetin	400 mg twice daily	With vitamin C
Vitamin B6	100 mg daily	
Vitamin C	Individual bowel tolerance**	With bioflavonoids (quercetin, rutin proanthocyanidins)
Vitamin E	2 capsules (800 IU) daily	d-alpha tocopherol

* The FDA recommends pregnant women not exceed 10,000 IU of vitamin A daily.

** To determine individual dosage, on the first day take 1,000 mg hourly until diarrhea occurs, then reduce dosage to just below that for individual daily dosage. Vitamin C is not toxic in large doses but must be taken throughout the day to benefit. Divide dosage to three or four times a day.

CHAPTER 81:

Gray Hair

*"Darling, I am growing old
Silver threads among the gold..."*

So goes the song. But is gray hair a necessary misfortune of growing old? If so, what about the increasing number of young people who have a smattering of gray hair, or, worse, a mane as white as snow?

In my research, I came across many studies showing vitamin and mineral deficiencies to be responsible for gray hair. The amount of scientific evidence is surprising. Animal experiments consistently show that hair pigment can be lost and re-gained through dietary manipulation. The simple addition of certain vitamins and minerals makes this possible!

Gray Hair in Undernourished Children

Reports are common of graying hair, which scientists call "acromotrichia," in young children in tropical areas where malnutrition is prevalent and conditions are such that a good diet is impossible. Dr. W. Hughes of the Colonial Medical Service found white-maned, malnourished children in Lagos, Africa. The diet of these children consisted chiefly of cassava, the root from which tapioca is made. The children were anemic, some of them had abnormal swelling, and they were docile and apathetic. Their hair, which would normally have been completely black, had turned light yellow or gray. Their eyelashes were yellow or reddish-brown.

At his hospital, Dr. Hughes put the children on a diet of milk, liver and yeast. Within three weeks the first change of hair color was noted. The scalp hair came in "strong, black and curly." Gradually the children's anemia disappeared, they put on weight and became healthy. Dr. Hughes concluded that the gray hair may have been due to a deficiency of B vitamins – probably pantothenic acid.[1]

Lucius Nicholls, M.D. found a number of tragic cases of badly nourished children in refugee camps, ranging in age from seven to 12 years, whose hair, eyelashes and eyebrows had lost their pigment. In many cases it was snow white. The children had other signs of bad nutrition such as emaciation and bad teeth. On a good diet, which included eggs, vegetables and fruit, their hair color began to return within three weeks. Dr. Nicholls also found that a pantothenic acid deficiency in black rats resulted in their fur turning white.[2]

Restore Hair Color with Copper, B Vitamins and Vitamin C

Extreme stress, and/or drug use and poor nutrition can cause hair to gray prematurely. However, the condition can be reversed.

Working with laboratory rats, Dr. J. M. Hundley of the National Institutes of Health, found that liver and brewer's yeast both *prevented* graying fur and *restored* it. When investigating further, he found that in some cases, it was the copper content of these foods that made the difference. Feeding animals a diet low in copper, he produced grayness in ten days. Then he added five percent copper in dried liver or brewer's yeast, and normal color returned. Hundley says that dark hair contains more copper than gray hair, and he found that more copper was required in the diet to prevent gray hair than to prevent anemia. Copper is necessary to assimilate iron.[3] Include zinc with any copper supplement.

New York physicians J.J. Eller, M.D., and Luis A. Diaz, M.D., were interested in the possibility that the B vitamin para-amino-benzoic acid (PABA) could effect a change from gray to normal hair color. They got varying results, but one 48-year-old man, who had been gray since he was 26 years old, went from completely white to "iron-gray" in five months.[4]

Miami physician Lydia Allen DeVilbiss, M.D., tried PABA on her test subjects. Careful photographs were taken of those in the study before the test began, so that the degree of hair color change could be permanently recorded. In one case, a 59-year-old woman physician whose hair had been gray since she was 30 got a significant amount of color back after seven months on PABA. Another subject got so much original color back, within a month his friends accused him of dying his hair.[5]

Like all of the B vitamins, PABA needs others of its kind to function. Folic acid is important for PABA synthesis, which is why whenever I recommend one B vitamin, I recommend all of them.

Vitamin C may also play an important role in the maintenance of hair pigment. E. Geiringer, M.D., directed 24 volunteers who agreed to take doses of vitamin C to see what effect it would have on their gray hair. Of 12 who continued taking the vitamin C long enough to see results, all had some degree of repigmentation. In three cases the hair was restored to almost its former color.[6]

If you are gray and especially if you are prematurely gray, consider this a warning that something is missing in your diet. Somewhere along the complicated line of metabolic processes; somewhere in the mysterious workings of vitamins, hormones, enzymes and minerals, your body is not getting enough of one thing or another.

For all the hair-healthy nutrients, look for a supplement that uses the whole food. Target a formula that uses freeze dried sprouts and vegetables, combined in such a way as to provide the B complex and all other essential vitamins and minerals, as well as adding bioflavonoids, odorless garlic, acidophilus and green tea extract for immune-system boosting.

Hair Color Nutrients
For maximum absorption, take supplements with meals.

Nutrient	Suggested Dosage	Formulation
Enzymes	2 capsules twice daily	Multiple formula
Fiber	4-8 tablets daily	Psyllium, with herb hyssop
Multi-mineral	1-4 ounces daily	In liquid solution, with vitamin B12, biotin
Multi-vitamin/mineral	3-6 caplets daily	Freeze-dried plant sources
Vitamin C	Individual bowel tolerance*	With bioflavonoids (quercetin, proanthocyanidins)
Vitamin E	2 capsules (800 IU) daily	d-alpha tocopherol

* To determine individual dosage, on the first day take 1,000 mg hourly until diarrhea occurs, then reduce dosage to just below that for individual daily dosage. Vitamin C is not toxic in large doses but must be taken throughout the day to benefit. Divide dosage to three or four times a day.

CHAPTER 82:

Hair Loss

Was Yule Brenner less than masculine because he was bald? And has less hair than his James Bond days kept Sean Connery from beating out younger men for romantic movie roles?

The point I want to make here is that hair loss doesn't have to be a tragedy. The only thing lost is hair – not virility, not attractiveness, and not youth. It is *not* a necessary stage of life or a symptom of aging. There can be reversible reasons for losing hair. When you stop worrying about body in your hair and start worrying about the hair on your body, it's time to consider the cause.

The most common cause is male pattern baldness. Why this happens is largely due to genetics, and not a whole lot – unfortunately – can be done about it. It does help if what hair there is, is healthy.

However, rather than assume the worst, consider the possibility of a nutrient deficiency, especially if the pattern of hair loss is not typical of male pattern baldness. That is, the hair is not lost in an evenly retreating hairline or a circle of shining scalp at the crown of the head.

Healthy Hair Nutrients

Researchers have found that certain essential amino acids in the diets of laboratory animals controlled the thinning and thickening of their hair. Magnesium-deficient rats lost hair in bunches.[1] On diets low in biotin or inositol (B vitamins), they became hairless.[2]

A diet rich in B vitamins have resulted in restoration of hair.

Heavy doses have revved up hair growth in some cases.[3] Men deficient in vitamin B6 often lose their hair.[4] And men shorted on folic acid sometimes become totally bald. However, a normal intake of this vitamin restored their hair in most instances.[5]

One nutrition-oriented medical doctor sometimes encourages hair growth with a diet accenting protein – calves liver, brewer's yeast, wheat germ, and two tablespoons of granulated lecithin. This makes sense since hair is comprised mostly of protein, and these foods are high in B vitamins.

Soy protein has been found in European studies to reinforce hair and stimulate regrowth. One study found it increased hair growth by 15 percent, resulting in regrowth for 33 percent of the hair.[6] One good source of soy protein is tofu, soybean curd. It can be made into delicious baked dishes or added to soups and stews. Other good sources of protein are: lowfat cheese, eggs, fish, beans, brewer's yeast and yogurt.

Hair Loss When Nutrients Are Lost

Hair loss occurs when the diet is inadequate in the B vitamins – especially B6, biotin, inositol and folic acid; and the minerals magnesium, sulfur and zinc.[7]

Studies in the former Soviet Union have revealed a slowing of hair loss through silica therapy, and that organic silica added to shampoos will help prevent baldness, stimulate healthier hair growth and assure beautiful shine, luster and strength. Biochemist Klaus Kaufman, Ph.D., has personally added silica to his shampoo on a regular basis and says he has effectively stopped further hair loss. He is also applying it externally to regrow already lost hair.[8]

Silica is found in mineral supplements and in the outer coverings of potatoes, green and red peppers and cucumbers. Bean sprouts are also high in silica. Eating whole foods is the best and eating sprouts even better, since the young shoots concentrate more of the older plants' nutrients. When targeting food supplements, look for a formula that uses freeze dried sprouts and vegetables, combined in such a way as to provide all the essential vitamins and minerals.

Drugs and Stress

Persons losing large amounts of hair rarely realize that certain drugs or medicines could be victimizing them: blood thinners like dicumarol, heparin and heparinoid; carbimazol – used to temper hyperthyroidism, and certain antibiotics such as penicillin, sulfonomides and mycin drugs.[9]

Once these drugs are discontinued, the hair usually grows back. Severe illness or stress can bring on temporary hair loss – even baldness. Stress can contribute to permanent hair loss because often it is never-ending, inasmuch as the person never learns to manage his or her daily stress.

In *Let's Get Well*, (Harcourt, Brace & World, p. 165), the late Adelle Davis confesses that stressful work on her book with many sleepless nights led to an alarming condition – her hair falling out and receding at the temples.

Immediately, she slept more and went on her anti-stress formula: 500 mg of vitamin C, 100 mg of pantothenic acid, and two mg each of vitamins B2 and B6 with each meal, between meals and every three hours during the night when awake.

Additionally, Adelle took half a teaspoon of inositol, five mg of folic acid, 50 mcg of biotin and 300 mg of PABA. New hair came in thick and vigorously and even returned to its original color.

Women lose hair or go bald for more reasons than men do. With greater career opportunities in business and industry, men no longer have the stress market cornered. Further, birth control pills not only create havoc with hormones, they cause a deficiency in vitamin B6, a critical nutrient for healthy hair growth.

Rigid dieting can also cause severe hair loss. Dr. Frank A. Evans brought back hair growth in dieting women with a supplement of para-aminobenzoic acid (PABA).

Hair Restoring Nutrients
For maximum absorption, take supplements with meals.

Nutrient	Suggested Dosage	Formulation
Amino acids	4-6 capsules daily	Multiple formula from natural sources
Borage oil	2 capsules daily	
Enzymes	2 capsules twice daily	Multiple formula
Fiber	4-8 tablets	Psyllium, with herb hyssop
Flaxseed oil	1 tablespoon daily	
Multi-mineral	3-4 ounces daily	In liquid solution, with vitamin B12, biotin
Multi-vitamin/mineral	6 caplets daily	Freeze-dried plant sources
Nettle	250 mg three times daily	
Silica (horsetail)	300 mg daily	
Vitamin B6	100 mg daily	
Vitamin C	Individual bowel tolerance*	With bioflavonoids (quercetin, proanthocyanidins)
Vitamin E	2 capsules (800 IU) daily	d-alpha tocopherol

*To determine individual dosage, on the first day take 1,000 mg hourly until diarrhea occurs, then reduce dosage to just below that for individual daily dosage. Vitamin C is not toxic in large doses but must be taken throughout the day to benefit. Divide dosage to three or four times a day.

CHAPTER 83:

Hangover

The Proverbs say, "The drunkard will come to poverty." Since I've never had a drink I should be wealthy. My wealth is in my loved ones and friends. I have a sister who grudgingly listens to my cheerful advice about her morning "mean attacks," plotting my demise as she pretends to hear, a seismic disruption grinding its jagged plates in her noggin, and a drumbeat of "WHY?" banging in her brain.

Rather than considering the cause, my sister looks for instant relief from the symptoms, which mankind has sought with grail-like fervor since discovering fermentation. Zealous drinkers have plowed through a plethora of folk remedies, trying to kick-start their mornings with oysters, chili peppers, milkshakes, pizza, bizarre potions laden with raw eggs and spices, cabbage juice, exercise, watermelon, carbohydrates and, of course, coffee.

Given enough time, a hangover will go away on its own. Waiting out your hangover is relatively easy, if not painless. After all, what are couches and televisions for? You need rest because alcohol disrupts the patterns of your REM sleep. REM – rapid eye movement – is the sleep stage at which you dream. Chronic disrupted REM sleep has been associated with suicidal tendencies, memory loss and mental illness.

Once alcohol is absorbed by your body, you have its effects to contend with, and later that of its byproduct acetaldehyde (ADH). As the alcohol disappears you sober up, but as the acetaldehyde forms you begin to experience its effects as a hangover. Sobering up is possible in theory by boosting the amount of ADH.[1] Achieving this is another matter, but you cannot sober up by any of the popular remedies of sweating in a sauna, vigorous exercise, drinking black coffee, or putting your head under cold water.

The morning after overindulgence of alcohol is the slow process of waiting for the acetaldehyde to disappear, but there are a few tips for coping with hangovers. No successful hangover cure has yet been marketed, and we know why this is unlikely to work for chemical reasons, unless it can speed up the removal of the excess acetaldehyde from the body.

The Hangover Prevention Plan

If you do drink, or have a loved one who does, advise them to sober up before falling asleep. Going to bed with alcohol in you, even one glass of wine, greatly increases the chances of waking up miserable and in pain. Alcohol is also called ethyl alcohol or ethanol, which is the correct chemical name for this molecule. Now doesn't this sound appetizing?: "Let's toast with a glass of ethanol."

Alcohol is dangerous because it easily overloads the liver and dehydrates the body. The liver can deal with large amounts of alcohol, but it needs time to do so. If a person takes in too much alcohol at one time he may even die, and a lethal dose can be as little as 400 milliliters – the amount of alcohol in a liter bottle of spirits. A normal liver can process a glass of wine, half a pint of beer or one shot of booze every hour. Drink more than this, and you invite a hangover, or worse.

Not coincidentally, many of the symptoms of dehydration are experienced during a hangover.

This is because alcohol severely depletes the body of life-giving water. If you drink two glasses of wine you will lose twice that much in water. Normally, our kidneys reabsorb and reuse all liquids we drink. But if the liquid includes alcohol, that recycling process stops, and you get dehydrated.

This may be what causes hangover headaches. If brain cells or other nerve cells near the brain get dehydrated, they stop working properly.[2]

To avoid a dehydration headache, drink a large glass of water every hour that you are drinking. Then, before bed, have some more water – as much as you can. If you have to get up in the middle of the night to void, make a point of drinking more water while you're in the bathroom. As soon as you get up in the morning, have another glass.

B vitamins have been shown in studies to help your body dilute the alcohol and remove its toxic by-products.[3] It also helps the body relax so you can get some sleep. Many alternative doctors recommend vitamin B12 for relaxation, and at least 50 milligrams of vitamin B complex. The catch? You have to take it *before* you go to bed. The idea is to prevent the ill-effects, so you don't wake up with more than guilt nagging you.

Magnesium and vitamin C are vasodilators, recommended to avoid the morning after headache. Headaches are caused by the constriction of the tiny blood vessels of the head. Vasodilators open up constricted blood vessels, relieving you of your headache before it starts. Doctors recommend 1,000 milligrams of vitamin C and an easy-to-absorb form of magnesium. This is because any damage to the stomach will make it difficult to absorb minerals, and alcohol is notorious for causing stomach damage. Look for a mineral in solution formula that contains magnesium.

Still Feel Rotten in the Morning?

If you forgot your prevention program, start by drinking a minerals in solution formula that contains vitamin B12 and magnesium. The B12 will work on the morning-after stress, and the magnesium will help battle your head and muscle aches. Follow up with fruit juice, lots of water and 1,000 milligrams of vitamin C. For the dizziness and nausea, drink some ginger tea, and eat dry whole-grain toast. Vitamin C is depleted in the body by alcohol and stress; and a deficiency of magnesium is associated with certain kinds of headaches.[4]

These nutrients are most commonly deficient among people who drink alcohol: vitamins A and D, the B vitamins folic acid, B6, thiamine (B1), zinc, potassium, calcium and magnesium.[5]

Not enough vitamin A can result in insomnia, fatigue and depression. If you want an incredibly rich source of vitamin A, try carrot juice. One cup contains a whopping 24,750 Individual Units![6]

Natural vitamin D (not the hormone in milk) is a fat-soluble vitamin, and it can be acquired either by ingestion or exposure to sunlight. It is known as the "sunshine" vitamin because the action of the sun's ultraviolet rays activates a form of cholesterol present in the skin, converting it to vitamin D. However, air pollution, clouds and glass inhibit the sun's action on the skin.

Zinc is needed for all tissue repair, including a damaged liver. Since zinc is necessary for wound healing, drinkers recover slower from everything from a cut finger to major surgery. Zinc supplementation is paramount. If you are with a friend or loved one at a gathering where liquor is being served, encourage him or her to eat the liver pate, which is high in zinc and copper, instead of the dip. Zinc is also essential in a number of major biochemical processes that affect brain function. An imbalance of copper and zinc can cause nervous system disorders.[7]

Copper is important to balance out your zinc supplements. Be sure and include 2-4 mg. of copper with any zinc.

Calcium is essential for the normal functioning of neurons, the "electrical wires" of the nervous system. A deficiency of calcium and vitamin D can cause mental symptoms.

Alcohol, coffee and sugar causes the body to lose potassium and magnesium. What happens then? Have you ever noticed how alcoholics look bloated and puffy? This is because when they lose potassium, but not sodium, their body retains water. Potassium and sodium must be on equal footing in your body to balance moisture loss and gain. A potassium deficiency also causes poor reflexes, soft, sagging and weak muscles, and compulsive disorders. Ugh!

For your program of clean living, emphasize edibles that provide all of the above nutrients. On your party menu choose among these foods that contain both potassium and calcium, as well as magnesium: wheat germ, sunflower seeds, soybeans, almonds, Brazil nuts, pistachios and pecans. They make handy party snacks, and have a decent shelf life as well.

Hangover-Helpful Nutrients
For maximum absorption, take nutrients with meals

Nutrient	Suggested Dosage	Formulation
Aged garlic extract	1 teaspoon three times daily	Liquid
Antioxidants	4 capsules	With selenium and grapeseed extract
Borage oil	2 capsules	
Coenzyme Q10	2 capsules	With vitamin E, phospholipids and selenium
Enzymes	2 capsules twice daily	Multiple formula
Fiber	4-8 tablets	Psyllium, with herb hyssop
Flaxseed oil	1 tablespoon	
L-glutamine	500 mg three times daily	
Magnesium	200 mg	
Melatonin	3 mg at bedtime	With B vitamins
Multi-mineral	1-4 ounces	In liquid solution, with vitamin B12, biotin
Multi-vitamin/mineral	3-6 caplets	Freeze-dried plant sources
Milk thistle	150 mg twice daily	
Purified water:	Two gallons	
Tumeric	100 mg	
Vitamin C	Individual bowel tolerance*	With bioflavonoids (quercetin, proanthocyanidins)
Vitamin E	2 capsules (800 IU)	d-alpha tocopherol

* To determine individual dosage, on the first day take 1,000 mg hourly until diarrhea occurs, then reduce dosage to just below that for individual daily dosage. Vitamin C is not toxic in large doses but must be taken throughout the day to benefit. Divide dosage to three or four times a day.

CHAPTER 84:

Head Lice

A letter from a viewer prompted me to include this topic. The letter read:

"Dear Maureen. I need advice on how to deal with that great plague of elementary school – head lice. The other moms and I are desperate. It doesn't matter what we do or how thorough we are – the wretched bugs just keep getting passed around our neighborhood school. Toxic over-the-counter shampoos don't work, and their plastic combs are useless. We spend hours vacuuming beds and carpets; washing sheets, towels and clothes; and bagging every stuffed animal, doll and otherwise fun and interesting toy in the house. What does it take?!"

Six to 12 million Americans get treated for head lice every year, and three-fourths of them are under 12 years of age. This makes pediculosis capitis (the species of head lice) one of our most communicable diseases. All parents should know that outbreaks of head lice have nothing to do with a family's income or social status or poor hygiene. Head lice like a clean scalp better than a dirty one.

What You Can Do To Prevent Outbreaks

Head lice outbreaks have a great deal to do with the way children share hats (play hats included), scarves, helmets, headbands, headphones, brushes and combs, and the way they hang their coats and sweaters on the same hook at school. Lice are big travelers, but they can't fly. They can only walk or drop from one place to another.

Typically, these tiny creatures – no bigger than a sesame seed – fall out of one head, drop to a coat, walk to the next coat, and up to a new scalp, where they will deposit three to five eggs a day for 30 days. They can only make the trip, however, if the coats are touching each other.

Persistent scratching of the scalp is the first indication of an infestation. Upon closer inspection, parents may find tiny, gray-colored bugs crawling among the hairs. These are the adults. The eggs are called nits, and are white and stick to the individual hairs about one-quarter of an inch from the scalp. The eggs take 7 to 14 days to hatch.

Prevention, especially in schools, includes banning play hats and clothes which are shared by many children, and making sure children have separate cubbies or lockers for their clothes. Teach children what to look for so they can help identify an outbreak before it spreads to everyone else.

Standard Treatments Are Poison

The standard conventional treatment for head lice – prescription or over-the-counter shampoos – has come under fire for several reasons. The first is that many contain lindane, a known toxin, as an active ingredient. Lindane, which is manufactured with the raw materials of benzene and chlorine, has been associated with aplastic anemia, leukemia and other blood disorders, according to the National Pediculosis Association (NPA), a Boston-based health-education agency established to build awareness about head-lice prevention.[1] Dr. Samuel Epstein, speaking to members of the American College for Advancement in Medicine (ACAM) at their 1994 Fall Conference in San Diego, California, said that lindane is a highly potent carcinogen that can cause brain cancer in children.

Since 1994, when it launched a national reporting registry, the NPA has received reports of more than 330 adverse reactions – most commonly caused by lindane – to various lice and scabies treatments, including seizures, behavioral changes, neuromuscular complaints, attention-deficit disorder, chronic skin eruptions and even death. The U.S. Food and Drug Administration has also received reports (albeit not as many), but continues to call lindane "safe and effective when used as directed." The other active ingredients commonly found in lice shampoos are pyrethrin and permetherin, which although not as toxic as lindane, are still poisons. After all, they are there to kill bugs.

Recommended Alternative: Elbow Grease and Tea Tree Oil

If you are lucky enough to find lice in the early stages, it may be possible to manually remove them. They are big enough to be seen – a magnifying glass helps – and can be combed out with a fine-tooth steel comb. Have two people check for lice at the same time, because lice move to one side of the head when you're working on the other. The adults are easily crushed between your fingers. As for the eggs, take each individual hair and snip eggs out one at a time using safety scissors. Do whatever it takes to get rid of the critters. If a girl has long hair, cut it. If it's a boy, get him a buzz cut.

It is essential to stop the spread of lice by washing brushes, combs, hair accessories, clothing, towels and bed linens in hot – not warm – water. Without a scalp to feed on, lice die in 48 hours. Anything that can harbor lice and is not easily washed, like stuffed animals, dolls and porous toys should be encased in air-tight plastic bags for a minimum of three days. Vacuum rugs and furniture thoroughly, then dispose of the vacuum bag outside.

I called Peggy, of Peggy's Health Food Store in Los Altos, California, and she says her customers find tea tree oil to be the best alternative to toxic pesticides. She says it can be used on the scalp to kill lice, and put into the washing machine to kill lice on bedding. She said it's a powerful disinfectant and germicide, and somehow manages to kill lice as well.

Tea tree oil is a natural essential oil distilled from a tree native to New South Wales, Australia, and parts of New Zealand. It is a member of the myrtle family (Melaleuca alternifolia) and is extremely disease resistant.[2]

The leaves of the tree have been used medicinally for centuries by New South Wales aborigines. The name "tea tree" is said to come from a visit to the region by Captain Cook, whose crew made a tea from the tree's leaves.

It is recommended that after washing your child's hair thoroughly and rinsing with hot water, apply tea tree oil and comb the hair with a very fine-toothed comb (or a pet's flea comb) in order to remove insects and eggs. Then tie a cotton scarf around your child's head and leave it on overnight. Watch for redness around the scarf's edge – the neck and forehead area – and wash the oil out immediately if the child complains of burning. Follow by washing with a tea tree oil-based shampoo. Your local health and vitamin store is a valuable source of information. Consult the owner or manager for the most highly-recommended tea tree oil product sold.

More Home Remedies

Some have found success suffocating the little buggers with mineral oil. Pour mineral oil over the entire scalp and leave it on for 10 minutes. You can warm the oil in a double boiler for comfort. After 10 minutes, shampoo out the mineral oil, then use a fine-toothed comb to gather the dead lice and eggs. Repeat this procedure every two days for ten days. At the end of ten days the eggs and lice should be gone.[3]

Another option is to mix one-half teaspoon of eucalyptus oil and one-half teaspoon of pennyroyal oil with two tablespoons of pure olive oil, then follow the same steps.[4]

Eric Jones, N.D., the Dean of Academic Affairs at Bastyr College in Seattle, suggests one part essential oil of lavender mixed with three parts olive oil. After scrubbing the scalp with the mixture, a vinegar rinse can help loosen eggs from the hair shaft.[5]

CHAPTER 85:

Hearing Loss

When I told him I was working on this chapter, Dr. Richard Kunin, a long time associate, told me about his patient, a musician named Duke who played bass guitar for a rock band. He came to Dr. Kunin because, following a lengthy tour of concerts, he discovered he was hearing more than the echo of applause.

"My ears were ringing for days afterward," Duke explained. "Then I noticed I was having trouble hearing people and the sound at movies." Unable to turn back the tragic hands of time, Dr. Kunin could only prescribe hearing aids and lip reading.

"There was nothing I could do by that time," he said. "A test showed he was 55 percent deaf. If he had come to me years earlier, I would have recommended nutrients, but he waited too long to seek a professional."

Duke is just one of 23.3 million Americans who have hearing loss, according to a 1990 survey by the National Center for Health Statistics. About 1.3 million of them are 18 or younger. Although statistics are lacking, anecdotal evidence suggests more young people are losing their hearing today than ever before.[1]

In the 1950s, audiologist Samuel Rosen tested the hearing of the Maaban, an African tribe tucked away in quiet isolation on the Sudanese-Ethiopian border, untouched by the roar of traffic or amplified music. Men well into their seventies, he found, could routinely hear sounds as faint as a murmur across a distance the length of a football field.

Few of us will be so lucky. By age 65, one in three Americans suffers hearing loss serious enough to interfere with communication. In one recent study, researchers found that some symptoms commonly blamed on Alzheimer's disease: unresponsiveness and confusion, for example, can actually be the effects of hearing loss. Among those fortunate enough to reach their nineties, nine out of ten will have impaired hearing.[2]

Just ask older rock stars Rod Stewart, Pete Townshend and Ted Nugent. It wasn't age that made them lose their hearing. Years of screeching feedback, howling riffs and exploding smoke bombs have left them with permanent hearing damage.

Studies of young people after they've left rock concerts show many leave hearing impaired. James Donaldson, M.D., of the University of Washington School of Medicine, says if the hearing doesn't get better within 12 or 16 hours after a show, the loss is usually permanent."[3]

However, you don't have to be a rock musician or fan to be affected. One-third of all hearing loss cases stem at least in part from the loud noises of modern life: power lawn mowers, jet engines, city traffic, loud appliances, music and stereo headsets.[4]

Loud noises destroy the tiny hair cells in the inner ear that signal the auditory nerve to send sound messages to the brain. Once those cells die, they never grow back.

The result is a kind of deafness called "sensorineural hearing loss." This affects both volume and clarity, first at high pitches, then later at lower pitches where speech is heard.

Noise may also cause tinnitus," a ringing in the ears. Besides being a constant annoyance, tinnitus often signals impending hearing loss.

How do you know if you're in danger? Here are some clues:[5]
- if your ears are ringing
- if things sound muffled, as if you're in a barrel
- if sounds are distorted, as if they're coming through a poor-quality speaker.

Protection with Magnesium

Ear plugs at a rock concert? Kind of defeats the purpose, doesn't it? Well, there's good news for worried parents of teenagers. Give them a dose of magnesium before they head out the door. Researchers looking for a nutritional solution to noise-induced hearing loss evaluated 300 young healthy and normal hearing recruits who underwent two months of basic military training. They were given either a placebo or 167 mg of magnesium aspartate in a drink daily. What they found turned them on their ears! They discovered that the recruits taking magnesium had less potential for permanent hearing damage, and wrote in the *American Journal of Otolaryngology* that magnesium may be useful where the use of earplugs is limited or not possible.[6]

Other researchers found that a magnesium deficiency results in susceptibility to noise-induced hearing loss. K.B. Franz, at the Department of Food Science and Nutrition, Brigham Young University, Provo, UT, fed one group of rats a magnesium deficient diet, and another group of rats adequate amounts of magnesium, then subjected them both to high levels of noise. He found the rats eating a diet that included magnesium were better protected from hearing loss. Significant hearing loss occurred on the magnesium-deficient diet, with one rat going completely deaf. But none of the group eating adequate magnesium went deaf and all had a higher threshold before hearing loss occurred.[7]

Magnesium and calcium work in balance throughout our bodies. Without magnesium, calcium accumulates in places it shouldn't. Always when supplementing with magnesium, include calcium one to one.

Nutrient Deficiencies: Most Tragic Sources of Hearing Loss

Hearing can be affected by indoor chemical air pollution[8], solvents, gasses and heavy metals,[9] damage to the inner ear, and even use of the antibiotic erythromycin, which has been associated with hearing loss.[10] But the most tragic are those preventible cases where a deficiency of nutrients was the probable cause.

Traveling in Israel recently, I had the opportunity to talk to a medical university doctor researching the effect of nutrients on hearing. He didn't want his name used, but he did give me a fascinating case history. He said a little girl had been brought into the hospital with almost total deafness. She had come from a small village, and knowing this, the hospital gave her a particularly nutrient-rich diet. The doctors were surprised to note that following a day's menu, her hearing started to improve. The good doctor decided to try intravenous vitamin supplementation and started with vitamin A, which is known to cause blindness in deficient populations. He added oral doses of vitamin E for good measure.

Sure enough, the girl's hearing loss improved, and after several months of supplementation, her hearing was restored. These results have been documented in several studies.[11,12]

A deficiency of vitamin D is also credited with hearing loss because it reduces the concentration of calcium in the fluid of the inner ear.[13] Without adequate calcium, the small, numerous bones of the inner ear become spongy and interfere with sound transmission. Doctors call this condition otosclerosis. People with this malady are notoriously deficient in vitamin D. In one study, 21 percent of people with otosclerosis were found to be vitamin D deficient.[14]

Vitamin D is a fat-soluble vitamin, and it can be acquired either by ingestion or exposure to sunlight. It is known as the "sunshine" vitamin because the action of the sun's ultraviolet rays activates a form of cholesterol present in the skin, converting it to vitamin D. However, air pollution, clouds and window glass inhibits the sun's action on the skin. Foods containing high amounts of vitamin D are: cod liver oil, salmon, sardines, herring, egg yolk, organ meats and bone meal.

A zinc deficiency is also credited with hearing loss. Those with chronic tinnitus, rather than intermittent, have shown to be deficient in zinc.[15] It may be that temporary injury to the aforementioned inner ear hair cells is dependent upon zinc for healing. Without zinc, cellular wounds cannot repair themselves, including those in the inner ear.

Copper is important to balance out your zinc supplements. Be sure and include 2-4 mg. of copper with any zinc.

Hearing Helper Nutrients
For maximum absorption, take supplements with meals.

Nutrient	Suggested Dosage	Formulation
Antioxidants	4 capsules daily*	With selenium and grapeseed extract
Borage oil	2 capsules daily	
Coenzyme Q10	2 capsules daily	With vitamin E, phospholipids and selenium
Flaxseed oil	1 tablespoon daily	
Ginkgo biloba	60 mg daily	
Magnesium	200 mg daily	
Multi-mineral	3-4 ounces daily	In liquid solution, with vitamin B12, biotin
Multi-vitamin/mineral	6 caplets daily	Freeze-dried plant sources
Vitamin A	25,000 IU daily*	
Vitamin C	Individual bowel tolerance**	With bioflavonoids (quercetin, proanthocyanidins)

* The FDA recommends pregnant women not exceed 10,000 IU of vitamin A daily.

** To determine individual dosage, on the first day take 1,000 mg hourly until diarrhea occurs, then reduce dosage to just below that for individual daily dosage. Vitamin C is not toxic in large doses but must be taken throughout the day to benefit. Divide dosage to three or four times a day.

CHAPTER 86:

Heartburn and Hiatal Hernia

My friend Bob has suffered for years with hiatal hernia. Of all his real and imagined ailments, from cancer to colds to the fevers of spring, none is so predictable and preventable as the panicky pain of what he calls the "Pig-Out's Punishment." He hates when it happens – mostly because he knows it's his own fault.

Well, not entirely. The "hiatus" in question is an opening in the diaphragm, the tough muscle that separates the chest from the abdomen. Pregnancy, obesity, strains and certain exertions can weaken the diaphragm muscle and allow the stomach to push up through the hiatus. Bob thinks his hernia was caused by two years of vomiting following chemotherapy sessions – given to him for a bout of testicular cancer. What probably happened is the vomiting weakened his hiatus, leaving him more susceptible to attacks.

Bob's first attack happened after a particularly sumptuous Thanksgiving dinner that included a midnight raid for his favorite dessert – dark turkey meat clawed off the bone and stuffed into his mouth by the light of the open refrigerator. Call it his payment-plan suicide that started early. That first attack woke him out of his Thanksgiving night's sleep. At about two a.m., he felt a choking sensation in the hollow of his throat (at the top of the esophagus) and a burning sensation all the way down to what felt like a clenched fist under his breastbone (where the stomach was pushing up).

The sensation was so extreme, he wondered if he was having a heart attack. If there had been other symptoms – sweating, dizziness, radiating arm or neck pain, a crushing or vise-like pressure on his chest – he would have called for an ambulance. But since he wasn't absolutely sure, he got out of bed, put on clean underwear and clothes for the hospital, unlocked the safe that contained his will and tore certain key pages out of his journal, flushing them down the toilet.

He kissed his sleeping family and went into the living room to read a book and listen to music, awaiting what he thought might just be the end of his life. He didn't die. Within an hour, the pain melted into discomfort and then completely drained away.

After attacks following Christmas dinner and a birthday feast, he went to Dr. Ross Gordon, a god of gastroenterology, who bid him welcome to the Hiatal Hernia Club.

Perhaps half the population over 40 have a hiatal hernia, although most of us don't realize it. Even more have intermittent heartburn, sometimes the result of a hiatal hernia. The symptoms Bob described results when hydrochloric acid, which is used in the stomach to break down food, backs up into the esophagus. Food allergies can cause heartburn, as can a hiatal hernia.

Stomach acid is very caustic stuff. Too much too often can lead to esophageal scarring, anemia, even lung damage. These dire effects can be avoided with certain precautions. Dr. Gordon ordered Bob to lose 10 pounds, wear loose clothing and avoid bending over for a while. He also said he should make a special effort not to eat too much, not to eat within two hours of bedtime, and never lie down right after a meal. He also warned him to avoid "flag" foods that give him heartburn and stomach discomfort.

On special occasions, Bob still cheats. And he pays for it. But at least he can recognize the problem for what it is, take precautions to avoid it, or eat too much and keep making payments on his layaway plan to death's door.

That Burning Sensation

This is a term used most frequently when referring to heartburn, especially in antacid commercials. What causes "that burning sensation" is stomach acids that "reflux" or move upwards into the esophagus (called gastrointestinal reflux). Heartburn can be caused by a hiatal hernia, or the malfunction of a small one-way valve, called the lower esophageal sphincter – LES – located between the esophagus and the stomach. When functioning properly, this valve allows food and water to pass into the stomach, but prevents backward flow. If the valve is loose or weak, ferocious stomach acids back up into the esophagus.

Certain foods are known to weaken or relax the valve, making reflux more likely. Fatty foods and drinks containing caffeine are so-called "flag foods," known to produce heartburn in some individuals. High-fat foods remain in the stomach longer and also tend to relax this critical valve. Chronic heartburn results from a long-term weakened valve.

Finding Relief

Since heartburn can be a result of mechanical difficulties, how you eat and your activities after eating can make a difference in avoiding the problem. Leave a good deal of time between the time you eat and the time you lie down. It's as logical as the force of gravity – lying down spreads out your stomach, letting its contents flow backward into your esophagus. If you feel compelled to lie down after eating, keep the upper part of your body higher than the lower part – stack some pillows under your back or put bricks under the top part of your bed. Avoid wearing tight clothing, especially after eating. Better yet, lose the weight so your clothes won't be tight. And don't eat too much. The Masai in Africa eat only the amount of food they can cup in two hands – they say this is the size of your stomach. When I lived with them I ate like them. For the first three days my stomach was in knots and I wanted to stand in the food line with baseball mitts.

The Masai also eat a lot of fiber. The late Dr. Denis Burkitt believed that heartburn and hiatus hernia are caused by increased stomach pressure due to the straining of constipation. He also said it is a direct result of the typical Western low-fiber, high sugar diet.[1] For better digestion and to help avoid heartburn and a hiatal hernia, eat more whole grains, vegetables and fruits. Some of the highest fiber foods include: raspberries, pears, melon, strawberries, cabbage, asparagus, cucumber, cauliflower, radishes, apples, carrots, green peas and spinach.

Dr. Robert Downs, who heads the Southwest Center of Healing Arts in Albuquerque, New Mexico, recommends a special concoction to relieve the heartburn of a hiatal hernia: one part aloe vera juice and four parts papaya juice blended fifty-fifty with sugar-free ginger ale or club soda, sipped often during the day. Cabbage juice may also help, he says.[2] Cabbage and aloe vera juice also help stomach acid-induced ulcers, which often accompany chronic heartburn.

Raw potato juice is said to help with heartburn. Do not peel the potato, just scrub the skin clean and put it in the juicer. Mix it half and half with water and drink immediately.[3]

Have you ever noticed heartburn after belching? This is interesting. What happens is you eat too fast, swallowing air. When it warms to body temperature it expands, and the force required to burp it can push stomach acid into the esophagus.[4] I've had this happen, and you probably have too. When you eat, always take small bites and chew thoroughly, even if you're the last one at the table.

Antacids are no help to the heartburn sufferer. They neutralize the acid in the stomach, not the esophagus, where the pain is, and they interfere with digestion, risking much more than acid burn. Besides, the body just secretes more, and a vicious cycle begins. Some medications can *cause* heartburn. Instead, try magnesium in solution. Because magnesium is very alkaline, it acts as an antacid and can be used in place of over-the-counter antacid compounds.

Heartburn Healing Nutrients
For maximum absorption, take supplements with meals.

Nutrient	Suggested Dosage	Formulation
Aged garlic extract	1 teaspoon three times daily	Liquid
Deglycyrrhizinated licorice	1-2 tablets before meals	Chewable
Enzymes	2 capsules twice daily	Multiple formula
Fiber	4-8 tablets daily	Psyllium, with herb hyssop
Ginger	500 mg after meals daily	
Magnesium	200 mg daily	
Multi-mineral	3-4 ounces daily	In liquid solution, with vitamin B12, biotin
Multi-vitamin/mineral	6 caplets daily	Freeze-dried plant sources
Vitamin C	Individual bowel tolerance*	With bioflavonoids (quercetin, rutin proanthocyanidins)

* To determine individual dosage, on the first day take 1,000 mg hourly until diarrhea occurs, then reduce dosage to just below that for individual daily dosage. Vitamin C is not toxic in large doses but must be taken throughout the day to benefit. Divide dosage to three or four times a day.

CHAPTER 87:

Heart Problems

What I'm telling you comes right from the heart.
You can either take it or bypass it.

No matter what genetic deck your mom and dad dealt you, disability and early death from heart disease *can* be prevented. And with a little tender loving care a poorly functioning heart and clogged arteries can be reversed without surgery to give you years of devoted service.

No other topic in this book has attracted so much nutritional research and new vitamin and mineral discoveries than this one. In 1995 alone, over a dozen studies were published in various medical journals showing the irrefutable benefits of vitamins and minerals to the heart. If I put all the research I have on the heart and nutritional supplementation, it would likely fill any library.

The fact that researchers are determined to find answers to our epidemic of heart problems is not surprising. Coronary artery disease is the number one killer of men and women in the United States even though there has been a two percent per year reduction over the last two decades. It is the leading cause of death among women after the age of 60 and in men after 40. Not to be outdone, women are joining men in this horrendous epidemic. Heart disease is now responsible for one of every three deaths in women, as well as men.[1]

To bring this issue closer to you, consider this: six out of ten of your high school classmates, or personal family members, will die of this disease – including you!

I should give you a little heart background. A number of factors cause heart problems: poor circulation, clogged arteries (arteriosclerosis), arrhythmias and high blood pressure, just to name a few. To get the most out of this issue, I suggest you also read my chapters on the topics I've just mentioned.

Researchers use specific terms when describing heart problems. For our purposes here, you need to know that a myocardial infarction simply means an acute heart attack. Heart attacks occur when an obstruction blocks the blood from entering the heart, or when oxygen cannot reach the heart, causing the heart muscle (myocardium) to essentially die. Certain nutrients, as you will discover, can help protect the heart muscle when circulation stops, so when it is restored, there isn't permanent damage.

Arrhythmias are changes in the heartbeat. Arrhythmias can come after a heart attack or precede it. Most commonly the heart beats too fast. This is called tachycardia, and is defined as any heart rate over about 80 beats per minute while resting. Sometimes the arrhythmias become so fast the heart stops beating altogether and quivers. This is called fibrillation. Doctors, in an effort to stop this, use "defibrillation" or "defib," techniques.[2]

Since I'm mentioning conventional techniques, I am compelled to point out that some heart medications have been proven to cause death. One fatal pharmaceutical is Tambocor, an antiarrhythmic drug created in the research laboratories of the 3M Company. The horrific story of Tambocor, and other heart medications, is described in a book entitled *Deadly Medicine,* by Thomas J. Moore (Simon & Schuster 1995).

Moore states: "Over just a few years, an estimated 50,000 people died from taking drugs intended to prevent cardiac arrest. After hundreds of thousands of patients routinely took these drugs, a definitive medical experiment proved they did not prevent cardiac arrest as doctors had believed. Instead the drugs *caused* cardiac arrest."

Fortunately, you *can* say no to drugs, because there are safe, effective ways to prevent heart attacks.

Heart Marvelous Magnesium

I have never seen such a rush to evaluate any nutrient for heart problems as I have seen regarding magnesium over the past few decades. First doctors and researchers saw the evidence. It was so compelling they couldn't ignore it. Then they tentatively, cautiously and reluctantly at first conducted more trials. Finally, a large scale study was conducted over several years to demonstrate, once and for all, its efficacy. Magnesium has survived these trials and has made it through the gate with flying colors.

For the past 50 years, doctors have successfully used magnesium in the treatment of cardiac arrhythmias. This was in response to numerous uncontrolled studies, and to the knowledge that it doesn't cause side effects.

At the Royal Hobart Hospital in Southern Australia, researchers added one single nutrient, magnesium, to the nutritional intake of patients with any kind of heart problem, including angina, arrhythmia, and heart attack. That year the death rate among heart patients admitted to the hospital went from 30 percent to one percent.

In 1986 two randomized trials showed patients treated with intravenous magnesium following a heart attack were less likely to die, and that it reduced the frequency of arrhythmias. In 1991, editors of the medical journal *The Lancet* stated that "the reduction in arrhythmias and deaths in magnesium-treated patients is a real and substantial finding."[3]

One study *The Lancet* editors eagerly anticipated was a placebo-controlled evaluation called the Leicester Intravenous Magnesium Intervention Trial in which over 2,500 people were treated with magnesium and evaluated following their treatment. The outcome? The study's authors, writing in *The Lancet*, concluded that using an intravenous magnesium sulfate solution would save the same number of lives as aspirin or thrombolytic drugs.[4] This study was concluded in 1992. Since then, many other studies have emphasized the importance of magnesium for life-threatening heart problems, noting that magnesium has no side effects.

This, in contrast with the issue of taking blood thinnners like aspirin and non-steroidal anti-inflammatories to prevent the blood clots associated with strokes and heart attacks; and pharmaceuticals like pravachol, which block the production of cholesterol. What has to be realized is the danger of depending on these drugs. They don't eliminate the problem, and have side effects not to be taken lightly. Regular aspirin use triples the likelihood of internal bleeding. Cholesterol lowering drugs are a bad idea as well. In a study of male heart patients taking cholesterol-lowering drugs, it was found that their non-cardiac mortality rate was 20-25 percent higher than that of the placebo-takers. What factors in here is the physiological effects of stress, and the fact that our body needs cholesterol to protect its nervous system. Thinning the blood doesn't remove the plaque that causes blood clots, and neither does eliminating the body's ability to produce cholesterol. Drugs bandaid the symptoms, don't address or attempt to resolve the cause, and worse, produce life-threatening side effects.

The question remains: Why take dangerous drugs when you can use nutrients that both deal with the cause and help alleviate the symptoms? Magnesium is a natural calcium channel blocker and it strengthens the heart muscles and blood vessels. Other nutrients, like antioxidants and bioflavonoids, work on cholesterol and arterial plaque.

In 1994, Michael Orlov, M.D. of the University of California, Irvine, Division of Cardiology, cited the many benefits of magnesium to the heart in *The Journal of The American College of Nutrition*: "Magnesium deficiency is associated with multiple cardiovascular problems. Large doses of magnesium may be effective in treating many different types of cardiovascular disorders. Magnesium has antiarrhythmic (keeps heart rhythms regular), antivasospastic (blood vessels aren't affected by pulling or stretching) and other beneficial cardiovascular effects. Several trials evaluating the efficacy of early magnesium therapy and decreasing mortality from myocardial infarction (heart attack) also showed improved survival. Complications from magnesium therapy are low."[5]

The research continues. In 1995, Swedish researchers performed a double-blind, random study on 252 patients who suffered an acute heart attack, treating part of the group with infusions of magnesium sulfate. Patients taking the magnesium showed an astounding 48 percent reduction in mortality risk compared to the placebo treated patients. Writing in the *International Journal of Cardiology*, the authors stated that magnesium protects the heart from injury during a heart attack[6] – injury that could mean the difference between life and death.

The Path of Prevention

We know that magnesium helps, but can it prevent problems? Dr. Mildred S. Seelig, American College of Nutrition, believes that a deficiency of magnesium can cause heart problems, recommending the antioxidant vitamin E to protect against "magnesium deficiency cardiomyopathy."[7] She maintains that when people with cardiovascular problems and low magnesium intake try to improve their health with strenuous exercise, such as jogging, they could be endangering their health. Magnesium requirements are markedly increased during physical stress, and the heart is much more susceptible to arrhythmias during physical exertion if the body's magnesium level is low.[8] During my television show *Maximize Your Life,* Michael Schachter, M.D., agreed, stating that many cases of sudden heart attacks during stressful exercise can be directly attributed to a magnesium deficiency.

Magnesium deficiency is more common than you might expect. A large study by the U.S. Department of Agriculture found that only 25 percent of 37,785 individuals had magnesium intakes at or greater than the recommended daily allowance, which is notoriously low. A 1995 review of 15 studies found that a typical diet contains only a fraction of the RDA.[9]

With processing, 75 percent of the magnesium in food is lost, suggesting that the American diet provides only 40 percent of the recommended daily allowance for the mineral, reported Sherry Rogers, M.D., in *International Medicine World Report* in 1992. Rogers estimates that 80 percent of the population is deficient in magnesium.[10]

The average mixed American diet supplies about 120 mg of magnesium per 1,000 calories. Green leafy vegetables are particularly good sources of the mineral, as are dry beans and peas, soybeans, nuts and whole grains. High losses of magnesium occur in the refinement of foods, and some losses result when cooking water is discarded.

Important to remember is that magnesium must be balanced with calcium and potassium for the proper regulation of heart muscle contraction.

Researchers at a heart institute in Israel found that potassium levels were severely low among patients with heart arrhythmias, as compared to those who did not have arrhythmias, concluding in the *International Journal of Cardiology* that potassium is an important factor in the development of arrhythmias.[11]

The Calcium/Magnesium Connection

Not enough calcium, and magnesium will be depleted.

Not enough magnesium results in calcium being deposited in soft tissue and arteries. Calcium blockages are one reason heart attacks occur. The most fascinating thing about magnesium is the fact that it moves calcium out of the tissues, and into the bones, where it is needed, or into urine where it is excreted if the body has too much. It is even suggested that it is this calcium-blocking effect that makes magnesium so protective of the heart.[12]

Dr. R.M. Touyz, of South Africa, believes the addition of magnesium in a treatment program for high blood pressure would decrease the need for calcium channel blockers and their subsequent side effects.[13]

The body's ratio of calcium to magnesium is extremely important. Because of the high absorption rate of minerals in solution, and deficiency of magnesium in the diet, the ratio of magnesium and calcium in solution should be four to one, respectively. Experts estimate the typical American diet, low in greens and high in dairy products, brings the calcium/magnesium ratio to five calcium to every one magnesium, above the four to one ratio of Finland, which has the highest incidence of heart disease in young to middle aged men.[14]

Finnish researchers, obviously desperate for answers to their epidemic of heart problems, have also hit on the magnesium/calcium answer.

Veterinarian and medical doctor Dr. H. Korpela, at the Department of Human Health, University of Kuopio, Finland examined 18 pigs who died of sudden heart failure and found low concentrations of magnesium and high levels of calcium in their heart muscles and livers, as compared to healthy pigs and those who died of other diseases.

Antioxidants such as selenium and vitamin E may work with magnesium and calcium to prevent the oxidation of fats that is believed to contribute to the destruction of the heart.[15]

Heart Smart Prevention Program with Antioxidants

Obviously, the person who claimed "the best things in life are free," didn't know about free radicals. They're free all right. However, they're anything but the best things in life. Just in case the only free radical you ever heard of was Abby Hoffman, let me explain how they work.

Free radicals are molecules that lack one of their customary electrons. Since the natural order here is pairs, the molecule, now called a free radical, will steal an electron from another compound, rendering that compound unstable and setting up a chain reaction that damages vital cell structures. By one estimate, each cell sustains more than 10,000 of these hits a day, and not all the damage is repaired.

This electron-stripping is referred to as oxidation. Oxidation is what rusts metal, makes oils rancid and turns a sliced apple brown – so imagine what it does to your body! Free radicals also cause the heart muscle to deteriorate over time, making it more susceptible to damage in the event of arrhythmias and blockages.

Enter nature's wonder: antioxidants. While our individual cells are capable of fighting destructive free radicals, they need certain raw materials to form protective enzymes. Large amounts of antioxidants are required: vitamins A, C, E, beta carotene, selenium, zinc, copper, coenzyme Q10 and aged garlic extract are the ones I'll be talking about.

Each has a special cell protective or regenerating function. For example, vitamins A, C and E team up to protect blood vessels and other body tissues from free radical damage. Jeffrey Bland, Ph.D., exposed red blood cells to destructive ultraviolet light, some with vitamin E added. Those without vitamin E aged faster than those with this essential antioxidant. Further, the unprotected red blood cells bulged like an over-inflated bicycle tire, while those with vitamin E resisted the reaction far longer, demonstrating that vitamin E's antioxidant action actually extends cell life and therefore, human life.

Recent studies have shown the benefit of vitamin E in preventing heart disease. A study at the University of Southern California School of Medicine found that heart patients who took 100 IU of vitamin E plus niacin had fewer heart problems over two years than those who did not take the vitamins. In The Physicians Health Study

of more than 20,000 male doctors, preliminary data on 333 participants showed vitamin E protected their patients against heart disease. In a Canadian survey of over 2,200 men it was found that those
who had been taking vitamins of any kind reduced the risk of death
from heart disease by an incredible 78 percent, cutting their risk of a
heart attack by 58 percent and reducing their risk of angina (spasm of
the coronary artery) by 15 percent.[16]

A March 23, 1996 issue of *The Lancet* published the results of a
randomized, double-blind, placebo-controlled study of 2,000 patients
with coronary heart disease. Half the patients received 400 to 800 IU
of vitamin E daily, and all were followed for an average of 510 days.
Those in the vitamin E group had a 75 percent reduction in heart
attacks.[17]

Antioxidants work in virtually all aspects of heart disease. They
help blood circulation, inhibit blood platelets from sticking together
and reduce plaque in the arteries. Most study findings support the
hypothesis that antioxidant vitamins may reduce the risk of coronary
artery disease and subsequent heart problems.

The Nurses Health Study, which began in 1976 with a group of
90,000 participants without heart disease, showed that 16 years later
those with the highest risk of heart disease were those with the lowest intake of beta carotene, and vitamins E and C. In the highest beta
carotene group there was a 22 percent reduction in the risk of heart
problems compared to the lowest group. There was a 34 percent reduction in risk of heart problems among women taking the most vitamin E. If the total intake of these vitamins is put into an antioxidant
score, the people taking the most antioxidants had a 50 percent reduction in the likelihood of ending up in the hospital with a heart
attack.[18]

Two large epidemiologic studies show a strong association between a high intake of vitamin E, particularly from supplements, and
a reduced risk for heart attack or heart disease death. Among 87,245
women participating in the Nurses Health Study, those who took
vitamin E supplements for more than two years were 40 percent less

likely to develop major heart disease than those with the lowest intake of this antioxidant vitamin. The same researchers found a similar preventive effect when they scrutinized vitamin E use among 39,910 men enrolled in the Health Professionals Follow-up Study. The investigations are based at Harvard Medical School, Brigham and Women's Hospital, and Harvard School of Public Health. The results appeared in the May 20, 1993, issue of the *New England Journal of Medicine*.

In the Scottish Heart Health Study, over 10,000 middle-aged men were evaluated for their intakes of vitamins C, E and beta carotene. It was found that these antioxidants had a highly protective effect on their hearts. Critically evaluating the study data was Susan Todd of the Department of Applied Statistics. She concluded in the *Journal of Clinical Epidemiology* that the study was valid, and that, indeed, it appears antioxidant vitamin intake protects against coronary heart disease in men.[19]

One kind of heart problem has been directly linked to a deficiency of the mineral selenium, a particularly potent antioxidant. Keshan's disease was first discovered in Keshan County in the Heilongjiang Province of China, where it was rampant in 1935. Once it was discovered that selenium deficiency was the underlying cause of the disease and selenium supplementation could prevent it, it stopped being a major public health problem.[20]

Ever wonder why so many people have heart attacks in hospitals? Here's one possible explanation. An article in *Clinical Chemistry* states that patients who are fed intravenously in the hospital may have dangerously low levels of selenium, enough to increase their risk of a heart attack.[21]

Copper and zinc are two minerals noted for their antioxidant and healing properties. They work together, and a deficiency of one will create a deficiency in the other. Denis M. Medeiros, Ph.D., R.D., of the Department of Human Nutrition, College of Human Ecology, Ohio State University, Columbus, found animals fed low-copper diets may develop cardiac abnormalities. High blood cholesterol is also associated with copper deficient diets. In rat experiments, copper deficient diets have resulted in heart problems.[22]

Studies at the Cincinnati Medical Center and Institute of Environmental Health in Ohio have concluded that the body's intake and ability to absorb zinc and copper appear to be significant factors in preventing both cardiomyopathy, a degenerative disease of the heart muscle that can cause heart failure, and angiopathy, a degeneration of small arteries that can impede blood flow. An article in *Science News* reports that the diets of many in the United States are deficient in one or both of these essential trace metals.[23]

Antioxidant-Rich Foods

Vitamin C's antioxidant properties are aided by bioflavonoids. In a five-year study of 805 Dutch men between the ages of 65 and 84, it was found that those who consumed the most bioflavonoids – compounds in apples, and other fruit, berries, garlic, onions and green tea leaves – suffered half as many fatal heart attacks as men who consumed the lowest amounts. Men who had a higher intake of bioflavonoids had a lower risk of death from coronary heart disease and of having a first heart attack, reported Dr. Michael Hertog, an epidemiologist at the Netherlands National Institute of Public Health in an article in *The Lancet*. Hertog credited eating one large apple a day with a high intake of flavonoids. I guess an apple a day *will* keep the doctor away![24]

Garlic itself has proven to have many heart-smart properties, no doubt in part due to its bioflavonoids. People who enjoy the zestful cuisine of southern Europe have fewer fatal heart attacks than do those in the north, where the food is blander. Among the benefits of the hearty Mediterranean diet is the consumption of large amounts of garlic. Now this culinary tradition is being hailed by scientists as one of the reasons Americans should look to their European cousins for mealtime tips.

In eight different studies, people given daily garlic or garlic extract lowered their cholesterol levels by an average of nine percent. Some investigators have also found a rise in protective HDL – cholesterol. In addition, something in garlic keeps platelets from being sticky, so they are less able to clump together to form a clot when a blood vessel is injured. And garlic has been discovered to step up the ordinarily low level of clot-dissolving (fibrinolytic) activity present in blood, an action that would favor the breakdown of any clot that did develop.[25]

Researchers at Loma Linda University School of Medicine, Department of Microbiology, studied Kyolic® aged garlic extract and found that its major component, S-allyl cysteine, is a potent free radical scavenger, helping to protect heart cells from oxidative injury.[26] For more on the benefits of garlic, see the chapter Arteriosclerosis.

Another antioxidant proven to help the heart is coenzyme Q10, a nutrient found in studies to help fight congestive heart failure (CHF), a common condition where the heart becomes too weak to pump enough blood to the tissues of the body. Because of this pumping action failure, blood returning to the heart backs up, leading to a build up of fluid in the lungs. This "waterlogging" of the lungs causes weakness and shortness of breath.[27] The key to fighting this often fatal condition is nutrients that strengthen the heart. Alternative treatment pioneer Dr. Ross Gordon has treated his patients with magnesium injections, but also recommends coenzyme Q10, which speeds oxygen to the heart muscles.

In a 1976 study from Japan, 17 patients with mild CHF were given 30 mg/day of coenzyme Q10. Every patient improved within four weeks and 53 percent became completely symptom-free.[28] Coenzyme Q10 has also been found to help people with severe CHF. In a double-blind study, 641 such patients were given either coenzyme Q10 or a placebo for one year. The number of patients requiring hospitalization for worsening heart failure was 38 percent less in the coenzyme Q10 group than in the control group.[29] In another study, the survival rate nearly tripled when patients with severe CHF were given the nutrient.

Researchers Link B Vitamin Deficiencies to Heart Problems

Probably the most recent nutritional find is the connection between the B vitamins, particularly folic acid, and the risk of heart problems. The connection began as researchers discovered that high levels of homocysteine increases the risk of heart disease.

Teams from Tufts University in Boston and the 43-year Framingham (Mass.) Heart Study examined more than 1,000 participants between the ages of 67 and 95 over a three-year period. They found that among the study participants with the most severe cases of constricted arteries, 43 percent of the men and 34 percent of the women had high homocysteine levels in their blood, and twice the risk of heart disease.

Vitamins B12, B6 and folic acid help regulate levels of homocysteine, a naturally occurring amino acid in the blood, says Dr. Jacob Selhub, professor of nutrition and director of the Vitamin Bioavailability Laboratory at the Jean Mayer USDA Human Nutrition Research Center on Aging at Tufts. Homocysteine plays an important role in the body's metabolism and is harmless when kept at normal levels in the body. At high levels, however, it turns toxic, and those who fail to eat the recommended daily allowance of these three vitamins are missing out on an important way to keep homocysteine levels in check. Ultimately, say the researchers, neglecting to consume B vitamins could lead to health risks such as clogged arteries. These risks tend to occur among men more frequently than women. Dr. Selhub recommends a minimum daily intake of 1.9 milligrams (mg) of vitamin B6, two micrograms (mcg) of B12 and 400 mcg of folic acid, which has the strongest influence on homocysteine metabolism.[30]

It has been found that B6 – a fragile and easily destroyed vitamin – is not present in fatty or processed foods. Vital B6 is lost in food transportation, storage, preservation, processing and cooking. There-fore, it is essential to add a B6 vitamin supplement (at least 200 mg daily) to your diet. When supplementing, always take the B vitamins together. They work together, and without one, others can become deficient. Look for a good complex formula at least ten times the RDA.

> Dr. Meir Stampfer, a researcher at Brigham and Women's Hospital at the Harvard School of Public Health in Boston, says that the Tufts study makes "an important contribution" to the present understanding that the lack of folic acid intake is the main reason why homocysteine is related to the thickening of ca-rotid arteries.[31]

Dr. Irwin H. Rosenberg, professor of physiology, medicine, and nutrition at Tufts who helped guide the research team, adds,

> "There is growing recognition that the relationship between diet and heart disease needs to be broadened to include not only dietary fat and cholesterol, but also dietary sources of vitamins, which may protect against heart disease and stroke."[32]

My sentiments exactly. Thank you, Dr. Rosenberg.

The Dangers of Iron Overload

A provocative study by Finnish researchers, published in the American Heart Association's scientific journal *Circulation*, con-cluded that the amount of stored iron in the body ranks second only to smoking as the strongest risk factor for heart disease and heart attacks.

Experts acknowledge that the study, though involving only 1,900 men from eastern Finland, was carefully done. A team of epidemiologists led by Jukka Salonen of the University of Kuopio tested healthy Finns ages 42 to 60 for serum levels of ferritin, an iron-storing protein. Salonen's team then followed the patients for five years. By that time, 51 had suffered heart attacks. Analysis showed that men with more than 200 micrograms of ferritin per liter of blood – a level generally considered normal – were more than twice as likely to have heart attacks compared with men with levels below 200. The risk of heart attack more than quadrupled in men with high levels of both iron and LDL fat.[33]

According to the *Tufts University Diet & Nutrition Letter*, iron-deficiency anemia has been over-diagnosed in the U.S. In fact, a 1988 survey of people with iron overload revealed that one in three had met with more than 11 doctors before getting a correct diagnosis![34]

How can you tell if you have too much stored iron? Only certain blood tests, such as the serum ferritin test and transferrin saturation test, provide the answer. If you find you have iron overload, donate blood and don't take supplements with iron, and cut back on meat consumption.

Margarine is Not Heart Smart

Now that you know what is good for you, pay attention to what is bad for you. Margarine is NOT heart smart. You already know saturated fat is bad for you. Saturated fat, like butter, may increase bad cholesterol, but at least it doesn't touch the good cholesterol. Food processors hydrogenate oils to make them thicker, creamier, and more appetizing to the consumer. Unfortunately, this process also saturates the oils' fatty acids, changing them to trans fatty acids.

A small amount of trans fats comes from dairy products and beef but the major dietary source is margarine, particularly hard margarine and shortening made from hydrogenated plant oils.

A Nurses' Health Study of 85,000 nurses found that margarine increased the risk of a heart attack. Two hundred thirty-nine men and women admitted to a hospital for their first heart attack were compared to 282 controls.

Women who consumed more than 2.5 pats of margarine per day had more than triple a greater risk of having a heart attack compared to those who consumed less than one pat per day. Butter, which contains no trans-fatty acid, did not significantly increase a persons risk in this study. People who consume the highest level of trans-fatty acids had a 2.44 times risk of having a heart attack compared to those who consumed the lowest levels.[35]

The Harvard School of Public Health now proclaims that partially hydrogenated vegetable oil, found in margarine and shortening, may be attributed to approximately 30,000 deaths each year.[36]

"These are probably the most toxic fats ever known," said Walter Willett, M.D., professor of epidemiology and nutrition at Harvard School of Public Health. Willett, who has researched the effects of trans fats on the body, disagrees with those who say that the partially hydrogenated fats found in margarine or shortening are less likely to raise cholesterol than the saturated fats found in butter. He proclaimed, "It looks like trans fatty acids are two to three times as bad as saturated fats in terms of what they do to blood lipids."[37]

George V. Mann, Sc.D., M.D., a leading heart researcher, wrote in *The Lancet*: "Trans fatty acids are proposed as the cause of the current epidemic of heart disease. Studies have shown that dietary intake of saturated fats and cholesterol are not the cause of the buildup of fatty deposits within blood vessels. Much suggestive evidence exists that consumption of comparatively large amounts of trans fatty acids causes the problem by impairing fat metabolism. Populations with low consumption of trans-fatty acids have a lower incidence of coronary artery disease even when consuming diets high in animal fat or other oils."[38]

Heart-Smart Nutrients
For maximum absorption, take supplements with meals.

Nutrient	Suggested Dosage	Formulation
Aged garlic extract	1 teaspoon three times daily	Liquid
Amino acids	4-6 capsules daily	Multiple formula from natural sources
Antioxidants	4 capsules daily*	With selenium and grapeseed extract
Borage oil	2 capsules daily	
Coenzyme Q10	2 capsules daily	With vitamin E, phospholipids and selenium
Enzymes	2 capsules twice daily	Multiple formula
Fiber	4-8 tablets daily	Psyllium, with herb hyssop
Flaxseed oil	1 tablespoon daily	
Folic acid	5-10 mg daily	
Magnesium	200 mg daily	
Melatonin (adults only)	3 mg daily at bedtime	With B vitamins
Multi-mineral	3-4 ounces daily	In liquid solution, with vitamin B12, biotin
Multi-vitamin/mineral	6 caplets daily	Freeze-dried plant sources
Niacin	500 mg four times daily	
Taurine	500 mg twice daily	
Vitamin B6	100 mg daily	
Vitamin C	Individual bowel tolerance**	With bioflavonoids (quercetin, proanthocyanidins)
Vitamin E	2 capsules (800 IU) daily	d-alpha tocopherol

* The FDA recommends pregnant women not exceed 10,000 IU of vitamin A daily.

** To determine individual dosage, on the first day take 1,000 mg hourly until diarrhea occurs, then reduce dosage to just below that for individual daily dosage. Vitamin C is not toxic in large doses but must be taken throughout the day to benefit. Divide dosage to three or four times a day.

CHAPTER 88:

Hemorrhoids

After capturing the Ark of the Covenant from the Israelites, the ancient Philistines were plagued by piles, or hemorrhoids. As atonement, they returned the ark and made an offering of gold. Modern day sufferers are still willing to sacrifice a fortune in hopes of finding relief.

One of the most misunderstood physical disorders is hemorrhoids. The general belief is that they are varicose veins of the anus, an opinion held for many years. W.H.F. Thompson, a British physician, blasted this notion when, in the anal area of 100 babies who had died soon after birth, he discovered three small cushions of mucous-like material containing blood vessels.[1] It is believed by physiologists that these cushions help guide waste matter out the anal canal and, when ruptured due to excessive straining, turn into hemorrhoids.

Constant straining or pressure on the abdominal muscles from constipation, heavy or improper lifting, pregnancy and labor or being overweight can cause super-swelling of these cushions with blood and fluid, making them larger and more sensitive to rupturing. When they become dislodged they push toward and even out the rectum, causing painful itching, swelling and bleeding.

The Benefits of Bioflavonoids

Conventional medical doctors usually recommend surgery for hemorrhoids. When you get a nosebleed do you have your nose cut off? Now a new treatment can spare you this amputation, thanks to

Bernard A.L. Wissmer, M.D., of the Medical Policlinic of the University of Geneva, Switzerland. To 250 patients with internal and external hemorrhoids, Wissmer administered four to six 100 mg capsules of bioflavonoid compounds daily for a week, then two to three daily for three or four more weeks. Relief from hemorrhaging and pain came in two to five days. Anascopic and rectoscopic exams showed a dramatic change to normal.[2]

Wissmer has reported thousands of patients cured with this bioflavonoid compound which includes rutin, a byproduct of milling buckwheat, and citrus peel bioflavonoid (hesperidin). Ninety-seven out of 148 patients with chronic internal hemorrhoids experienced complete healing. Significant improvement was shown in 32 of the cases, although there remained occasional slight bleeding. Sixteen patients showed some improvement: less pain and less bleeding.

With this same regime, Dr. Wissmer scored phenomenally with the most resistant form of hemorrhoids: external. Twenty-eight out of 32 patients were completely cured. Keep in mind, these were very severe cases of hemorrhoids. For those of you who suffer hemorrhoids only occasionally, bioflavonoids can help decrease the number of times you are tempted to reach for the medicine cabinet.

Vitamin C enhances the therapeutic effects of bioflavonoids. In nature, all vitamin C foods contain bioflavonoids.

Vitamin C can help prevent one of the most common causes of hemorrhoids: constipation. Large amounts of vitamin C will keep stools soft, liquid, and easily moved.[3] While choosing supplements, look for a vitamin C formula with rutin and citrus bioflavonoids, and for gentle movements to avoid further irritating existing hemorrhoids, look for a fiber formula that contains hyssop, psyllium, oat bran, alfalfa, rhubarb, buckthorn, goldenseal and gentian. Hyssop is the king of cleansers, but the other herbals are known to strengthen, tone and condition the colon's cells. "Purge me with hyssop and I shall be clean..." – Psalms 51:7.

Vitamins for Bleeding Hemorrhoids

In one study, individuals deprived of vitamin B6 developed bleeding hemorrhoids and were cured of them when their diet was supplemented with 10 mg of this vitamin after each meal.[4] Preventive medicine practitioners have found pregnant women to be severely deficient in vitamin B6 and, therefore, prone to developing hemorrhoids.

It has been found that B6 – a fragile and easily destroyed vitamin – is not present in fatty or processed foods. Vital B6 is lost in food transportation, storage, preservation, processing and cooking. Therefore, it is essential to add a B6 vitamin supplement (at least 200 mg daily) to your diet. Include a naturally-derived B complex formula with your B6 to include the whole family of beneficial Bs. They need to be united together for each one to work.

Don't forget zinc and copper. Zinc is a notorious wound healer, and is used in hospitals to treat burns. Two nutrients must be considered along with zinc: vitamin B6 and copper. Too much copper will deplete zinc stores; they must be equal for optimum usage. Include 2-4 mg of copper with any zinc supplement.

Vitamin K is also suggested for bleeding hemorrhoids, since it is essential to strong blood vessels. Food sources are alfalfa, kale and all dark green leafy vegetables. Salad anyone?

Soothing Suggestions

For those sure of what they've got but not so certain about what to do about it, there are other ways to prevent or treat hemorrhoids.

The best way to avoid any digestive disorder, including hemorrhoids, is to eat plenty of fiber and drink lots of fluids. So far as fiber is concerned, psyllium has been proven to be a terrific source. Dr. Marvin M. Schuster from the Johns Hopkins School of Medicine extolled the virtues of psyllium for digestive problems at the Annual Meeting of The American College of Gastroenterology in New Orleans. He said psyllium can reduce constipation and add more water bulk to the stool.[5]

You won't find this in any medical book, but the folk remedy of applying the inside of a banana peel topically to the hemorrhoid brings instant relief. I have a friend who tried it and she says her hemorrhoids never returned.

Long, warm healing baths with baking soda will both cleanse and de-acidify the area. I recommend 10 to 20 minutes in the bath three or four times daily. Sitz baths are recommended for women who have just given birth and are sore. Apply an ointment containing vitamins A, D or E after drying the area thoroughly. Vitamin E used as a suppository can lubricate and relieve pain. Taken as a supplement, it can prevent and dissolve blood clots.[6]

Americans spend some $200-million a year on over-the-counter hemorrhoid remedies alone. Nearly half of that money goes for Preparation H, whose makers have long claimed the stuff "actually helps shrink swelling of inflamed hemorrhoidal tissues." The folks at *Consumer Reports* evaluated the popular hemorrhoidal remedy, and found the only therapeutic ingredient it contains is shark liver oil, which is rich in vitamin A. An FDA panel concluded that shark liver oil is an effective skin protectant that relieves mild irritation.[7]

Witch hazel and poplar ointments are said by herbalists to help treat irritation and swelling. Cold chamomile tea is suggested as a soothing rectal wash. Look for natural lotions that include oak bark. Oak bark contains large amounts of tannin, which has astringent properties. Tannin is well tolerated by the skin, with no risk of causing irritation. In fact, It is an ingredient in many skin medications for treatment of hemorrhoids, mouth ulcers and burn scars.

For more tips on helping at least one cause of hemorrhoids, read the chapter on Constipation.

Hemorrhoid-Helping Nutrients
For maximum absorption, take supplements with meals.

Nutrient	Suggested Dosage	Formulation
Acidophilus	At least four billion flora daily on an empty stomach, three times daily	
Aged garlic extract	1 teaspoon three times daily	Liquid
Borage oil	2 capsules daily	
Enzymes	2 capsules twice daily	Multiple formula
Fiber	4-8 tablets daily	Psyllium, with herb hyssop
Flaxseed oil	1 tablespoon daily	
Ginkgo biloba	60 mg daily	
Multi-mineral	3-4 ounces daily	In liquid solution, with vitamin B12, biotin
Multi-vitamin/mineral	6 caplets daily	Freeze-dried plant sources
Quercetin	400 mg twice daily	With vitamin C
Vitamin C	Individual bowel tolerance*	With bioflavonoids (quercetin, rutin proanthocyanidins)
Vitamin E	2 capsules (800 IU) daily	d-alpha tocopherol
Water	2 gallons daily	Purified

* To determine individual dosage, on the first day take 1,000 mg hourly until diarrhea occurs, then reduce dosage to just below that for individual daily dosage. Vitamin C is not toxic in large doses but must be taken throughout the day to benefit. Divide dosage to three or four times a day.

CHAPTER 89:

Herpes Simplex (Cold Sores or Genital Herpes)

Would you believe herpes gladiotorum? No, it's not another form of herpes. It's the same herpes simplex that may give you a cold sore or worse, plague you with painful genital herpes. Apparently herpes is so common among wrestlers, they have their own name for it. This is because of the unclothed, close proximity of wrestlers during matches and the ease by which the virus is transmitted. The virus from one wrestler's cold sore may enter a cut or mat burn on another player's body.

Herpes simplex causes both genital sores and mouth sores (commonly referred to as fever blisters or cold sores). What is important to realize is that they are interchangeable. Open sores of the mouth can be transmitted to the genitals. Therefore, genital herpes is not always sexually transmitted, and to call it a venereal disease would be incorrect.

The fact is, during a primary, or the very first attack of herpes simplex, it is possible for infected persons to spread the disease to other parts of their own body – from their mouth, for example, to their eyes, fingertips or genitals.[1] An interesting statistic exemplifies this. According to the 1988 book *Scientific American Medicine*, genital herpes was found in three percent of nuns.[2]

Kissing is the most obvious means of transmitting cold sores, but not the only one. And the mouth is not the only area that can be infected. Doctors and dentists can acquire herpes whitlow (herpes simplex infections of the fingers) from contact with the infected saliva of their patients.

When doctors talk about herpes simplex 1 versus herpes simplex 2, they are not differentiating between two different viruses, they are identifying on which part of the body it manifests itself. Herpes simplex 1 is the cold sore, and herpes simplex 2 is genital herpes.

The bad news is that once you are infected with herpes simplex, it is incorporated into your DNA, and cannot be cured. You don't know when, for how long, and how bad an outbreak will occur. The key is in preventing the outbreaks. The good news is that researchers have identified nutrients that can inhibit the virus and prevent it from causing infectious sores.

Nutrients that Minimize Outbreaks

Vitamin A, the skin and eye vitamin, has been shown in studies to slow the growth of herpes simplex. In one study, retinoic acid – a derivative of vitamin A – after 48 hours dramatically slowed the growth rate among virus cells compared with the cells that had not been exposed to it.[3] It is important to slow the growth of the virus to allow the immune system a chance to overcome it and reduce the severity of the infection.

Zinc has also been shown to be helpful. In a study reported in the *Medical Journal of Australia*, out of 158 patients with cold sores, 70 percent were relieved in 13 days with supplementation of zinc monoglycerolate, a particularly absorbable version.[4] It is quite possible that a zinc deficiency contributes to herpes outbreaks, since a deficiency can cause lesions and sores. Topically, zinc sulfate has also been shown in studies to be useful.[5]

Zinc must be balanced with a number of other minerals, especially copper, to be effective. Look for a good, easily absorbable, derived-from-nature mineral blend in solution. Formulations in solution provide the maximum absorption ratios.

Vitamin C and bioflavonoids can help reduce the inflammatory nature of herpes sores. An incredible 30 out of 38 patients went without genital herpes outbreaks four years after starting to take one to two grams of vitamin C daily,[6] and when bioflavonoids were added, 28 out of 38 patients avoided getting sores even after the telltale burning of their herpes symptoms started.[7] James Braly, M.D., recommends eight to 12 grams a day of vitamin C, depending on the severity of the outbreak.[8]

Dr. Robert Cathcart, a California physician, has successfully treated over 15,000 patients with massive doses of vitamin C; curing viral pneumonia, mononucleosis, influenza, colds, hepatitis, shingles, and cold sores with this method. He has developed a guideline for practical application of vitamin C which he refers to as "bowel tolerance."

The individual's own body will determine how much vitamin C it requires. The cutoff point is determined by the onset of diarrhea. The tolerance level in each individual differs. Some days you can tolerate more, some days less, according to how much a person can take before he reaches the bowel tolerance level.

In short, if you have not reached bowel tolerance (diarrhea), you have not taken enough vitamin C.

Vitamin C combined with zinc works even better, and has been shown to greatly inhibit herpes outbreaks so they aren't as severe.[9]

Topical applications of vitamin E have also been shown to help alleviate herpes simplex symptoms. In one study, dental patients with cold sores were relieved of pain in 15 minutes, with complete recovery after 10 days following topical treatment of vitamin E.[10]

Another alternative is the amino acid lysine. Lysine, a true antiviral "heavy hitter," works against a broad range of infections. It suppresses the amino acid arginine, which promotes viral growth and reproduction. If you have a tendency toward herpes eruptions, it helps to minimize your intake of arginine-rich foods such as nuts, chocolate, carob, seeds and grains and supplement with L-lysine, and a multiple amino acid formula.

Doctors at the Indiana School of Medicine gave 800 to 1,000 mg of lysine daily to 45 patients with active herpes infections. Most of the patients noted that the pain stopped overnight, and all but three had a complete disappearance of symptoms within a few days. Not everyone will respond this dramatically during active infections, but the researchers found that daily maintenance doses of 300 mg to 500 mg of lysine resulted in fewer herpes outbreaks.[11]

Preventive Protocol

Herpes sufferers can control outbreaks through natural means:

1. Improve the diet and take a therapeutic dosage vitamin supplement.

2. With a cotton swab, dab flare-up blisters for five to ten minutes with the sodium ascorbate form of vitamin C and water, followed by dabbing a vitamin E capsule cut in two.

3. Take vitamin A in slowly increasing dosages to 30,000 IU, and 100 mg of zinc three times daily for a week.

4. Take a lysine supplement.

Herpes-Hating Nutrients
For maximum absorption, take supplements with meals.

Nutrient	Suggested Dosage	Formulation
Acidophilus	At least four billion flora daily on an empty stomach, three times daily	
Aged garlic extract	1 teaspoon three times daily	Liquid
Antioxidants	4 capsules daily*	
Echinacea	100 mg daily	
Fiber	4-8 tablets daily	Psyllium, with herb hyssop
Lysine	500 mg twice daily during inactive stage, increasing to 1,000 mg three times daily during active stage	
Multi-mineral	1-4 ounces daily	In liquid solution, with vitamin B12, biotin
Multi-vitamin/mineral	3-6 caplets daily	Freeze-dried plant sources
Vitamin A	25,000 IU daily*	
Vitamin C	Individual bowel tolerance**	With bioflavonoids (quercetin, rutin proanthocyanidins)
Vitamin E	2 capsules (800 IU) daily	d-alpha tocopherol

* The FDA recommends pregnant women not exceed 10,000 IU of vitamin A daily.

** To determine individual dosage, on the first day take 1,000 mg hourly until diarrhea occurs, then reduce dosage to just below that for individual daily dosage. Vitamin C is not toxic in large doses but must be taken throughout the day to benefit. Divide dosage to three or four times a day.

CHAPTER 90:

Hiccups

Can you imagine having the hiccups for 60 years? Retired farmer Charles Osborne did. For most of us, the hiccups are a passing annoyance, halted by personal folk remedies. But for some, hiccups are a chronic problem that defy the usual remedies.

What causes hiccups? We're not sure, although drinking or eating too fast does seem to bring them on. What actually happens is the muscles of the diaphragm spasm, causing contractions that are followed by closing of the glottis – folds of cartilage in the throat that allow you to speak. It is this "slamming" of the glottis that causes the sounds made while hiccuping. You may notice that if you try to clear your throat when you have them, it will bring one on. What works to stop them seems to depend on who you are. There are many different cures. If you haven't found one that works for you, keep reading.

Folk Remedies That Work

In my many years of fascination with folk remedies, I've collected so many hiccup remedies, I haven't enough hiccups to try them all. A friend says drinking gulps of water – as many as she can – while holding her breath works for her. Then there's the old paper bag trick, where you breathe in and out while holding a paper bag over your mouth. Doctors say these two tricks work because they increase carbon dioxide in the blood, and that seems to reduce the hiccups. Drinking water – cold or warm – with plugs in your ears is also supposed be effective. Another variation is sipping honey with a little lukewarm water. No fingers in the ears this time.

I hate to even tell you about the next one, because the solution is less than healthy, but it has worked for me and many in my TV audience. It's a teaspoon of dry, granulated sugar. A respected physician, Edgar E. Engleman, M.D., a faculty member of the University of California School of Medicine in San Francisco, and associates tried the sugar solution and scored with a complete and immediate end to the hiccups in 19 out of 20 patients. This was no small achievement, because many of the patients had hiccupped their way through a number of days – one for six weeks![1]

A venturesome physician who was induced by a friend to eat a slice of lemon soaked in agostura bitters, lost his hiccups and recommended the cure in the letters section of a medical journal. Many people believe lemon juice is the best cure for severe, obstinate hiccups. No laughing matter for those afflicted for years with hiccups, the answer may just be a mineral long overlooked and commonly underestimated.

Magnesium for Chronic Hiccups

One of the implications that has come out of research studies is that calcinosis is a factor in long-term, chronic hiccuping. Calcinosis occurs when calcium is deposited into the soft tissues of the body. It causes heart problems, circulation problems, fibromyalgia, hypertension, scleroderma, skin wrinkling and aging. In the case of hiccups, it is believed that calcium deposits irritate nerve fibers that govern what has been called the hiccup reflex. This involves sensory fibers which carry signals from the breathing muscles to the medulla of the brain, and then motor fibers which return from the medulla to control the diaphragm. Chronic hiccups can result when the sensory nerves travelling to the medulla are irritated in some way, for example by surgery or this deposition of calcium. In a study of patients with, in some cases, years of chronic hiccups, a calcium-blocking drug successfully alleviated five out of seven cases.[2]

Calcium acts as a trigger for muscle contraction, and it is likely that local calcium concentrations, without the magnesium to control it, increase the force of muscle contractions, prolonging what should be a temporary case of hiccups.[3]

Calcium-channel blockers work against chronic hiccups because they attach to the surface membrane of sensory fibers and prevent calcium from entering. Without calcium, nerves and muscles relax and arteries dilate. Without magnesium, calcium accumulates in nerves and muscles, possibly keeping a case of hiccups from going away, because magnesium is the traffic cop that tells calcium where to go – and not to go.

Probably the most beneficial nutritional discovery of our time is the finding that magnesium is a calcium channel blocker, and therefore may be the missing link for people with long-term, chronic hiccups. For more on this story, read the chapter Hypertension.

Since calcium and magnesium are both taken up in the same place in the body, it is essential that magnesium be supplemented in the most efficient way possible. Researchers have established the best way is intravenously. Next to that, magnesium in solution is the most absorbable form and is recommended for any case of calcium overload. Because of its high absorption rate, and deficiency of magnesium in the diet, the ratio of magnesium and calcium in solution should be four to one, respectively.

Hiccups-Helping Nutrients
For maximum absorption, take supplements with meals.

Nutrient	Suggested Dosage	Formulation
Fiber	4-8 tablets	Psyllium, with herb hyssop
L-Carnitine	500 mg twice daily	
Magnesium	200 mg	
Multi-mineral	1-4 ounces	In liquid solution, with vitamin B12, biotin
Multi-vitamin/mineral	3-6 caplets	Freeze-dried plant sources
Vitamin C	Individual bowel tolerance*	With bioflavonoids (quercetin, rutin proanthocyanidins)
Vitamin E	2 capsules (800 IU)	d-alpha tocopherol

* To determine individual dosage, on the first day take 1,000 mg hourly until diarrhea occurs, then reduce dosage to just below that for individual daily dosage. Vitamin C is not toxic in large doses but must be taken throughout the day to benefit. Divide dosage to three or four times a day.

CHAPTER 91:

High Thyroid

A dear friend – I'll call her Anne – came to me terribly frightened because her teenage daughter was in danger of "going over the edge." She had been losing weight, seemed anxious all the time, could not sleep, and as a result had talked about suicide. Doctors said it was teenage hormones and the stage would pass. But Anne was not satisfied. The symptoms seemed too "physical" not to have an organic cause. I asked her if her daughter had been tested for an overactive thyroid gland.

"Overactive? What is the thyroid gland, anyway?" she asked.

The thyroid gland sits at the base of the neck. If you wore a tie, it would be where the knot lies – two lobes on either side of the trachea. Considered a master gland, because of its importance to the body's metabolism, the thyroid's main functions are to create thyroid hormone that form protein RNA and oxygenate cells. Too much thyroid hormone speeds up most chemical reactions in the body, causing mental as well as physical changes, and depleting the body of valuable nutrients.[1]

Nutrition and Hyperthyroidism

An overactive thyroid gland quickly uses up certain vitamins, causing them to become dangerously deficient. The B vitamins are responsible for our mental health, and it is possible some of the mental symptoms of hyperthyroidism are due to B vitamin deficiencies, especially vitamin B1 (thiamine). Therefore, a high intake of this vitamin is necessary. Likewise, demand for vitamin B6 (pyridoxine) is high in hyperthyroidism and also when protein intake is generous. Depletion of this vitamin in hyperthyroidism is sometimes so great that only a daily injection can prevent muscle weakness – a common symptom. Other vitamins, too, are drawn upon heavily in hyperthyroidism, particularly vitamin C and E, which are literally drained from the tissues.[2]

If you have any family or personal history of thyroid problems, make sure you take supplemental vitamins C and E. Too little of these antioxidant vitamins can not only mimic the symptoms of an overactive thyroid, but a shortage of these can worsen a thyroid problem. In some cases, hyperthyroidism can be alleviated by adequate amounts of these vitamins.

Bone loss is one of the long term effects of hyperthyroidism. This is because an overactive thyroid causes an extreme depletion of calcium. Some experimenters have found that natural vitamin D (not the hormone found in milk) counteracts the usual rapid excretion of calcium, so blood levels of calcium can return to normal.[3]

Vitamin D is a fat-soluble vitamin, and it can be acquired either by ingestion or exposure to sunlight. It is known as the "sunshine" vitamin because the action of the sun's ultraviolet rays activates a form of cholesterol present in the skin, converting it to vitamin D. However, air pollution, clouds and window glass inhibits the sun's action on the skin. Foods containing high amounts of *natural* vitamin D are: cod liver oil, salmon, sardines, herring, egg yolk, organ meats and bone meal.

Too much thyroid hormone uses up essential fatty acids (EFA), which the thyroid gland needs to function normally. In one study, rats deprived of EFA became hyperactive with excessive thyroid hormone production.[4] The two families of essential fatty acids are omega-6 (linoleic acid), found in seeds and seed oils and omega-3 (alpha-linolenic acid) found mainly in fish, fish oils (cod liver oil) and green leafy vegetables. Gamma-linolenic acid (GLA), or linoleic acid, is found in evening primrose oil, black currant oil, borage oil and spirulina.[5] The most effective source of GLA is borage oil.

Independent clinical tests show that borage oil contains up to 26 percent GLA. Compare this to evening primrose oil and black currant oil, which contain no more than 18 percent. Not only that, borage oil costs less because the borage seed is three times larger than black currant or evening primrose seeds. Finally, borage is more bioavailable. In other words, the body more readily accepts it.[6]

Researchers accept the fact that hyperthyroidism results in a severe magnesium deficiency,[7-10] creating its own set of risks. A lack of magnesium is linked to heart attacks, atherosclerosis, hypertension, arrhythmias, fibromyalgia, diabetes, alcoholism, premenstrual syndrome, aging and chronic fatigue syndrome, just to name a few.[11]

A large study by the U.S. Department of Agriculture found that only 25 percent of 37,785 individuals had magnesium intakes at or greater than the recommended daily allowance, which is notoriously low. In a review of 15 studies it was found that a typical diet contains only a fraction of the RDA.[12]

Trading One Problem for Another

There are three conventional overkill therapies recommended for hyperthyroidism: medication, radiation and surgery. If you opt for these measures, you should know that the odds are high the treatments will so damage your thyroid, you may find yourself having too little thyroid hormone instead of too much. An article in *Patient Care* cites the alarming statistics.

Radiation therapy, usually with iodine and called radioiodine therapy, has the highest chance of causing patients to become permanently hypothyroid. Following this treatment, an incredible 33 percent of all patients develop hypothyroidism within the first year, and an additional three percent each year thereafter lose thyroid function. With antithyroid medication, five to ten percent of patients develop hypothyroidism. Radioiodine therapy and surgery respectively "burn" and cut out the overly active thyroid, removing all or part of the gland.[13] This is sure to cause permanent hypothyroidism, not to mention a severe detriment to your immune system.

Other risks of surgery include damage to the larynx nerve resulting in permanent hoarseness, or the risk of damage to the parathyroid glands. Hypoparathyroidism due to injury to the parathyroid glands can cause cramps, twitching, kidney problems and cataracts.[14]

As for my friend Anne, her daughter did not undergo surgery or radiation and she thankfully took my advice and avoided medications. Instead, she started taking the supplements I recommended, including a magnesium in solution formula, and in a couple of months was her old self again.

Thyroid-Thankful Nutrients
For maximum absorption, take supplements with meals.

Nutrient	Suggested Dosage	Formulation
Amino acids	4-6 capsules daily	Multiple formula from natural sources
Borage oil	2 capsules daily	
Coenzyme Q10	2 capsules daily	With vitamin E, phospholipids and selenium
Flaxseed oil	1 tablespoon daily	
Magnesium	200 mg daily	
Melatonin (adults only)	3 mg daily at bedtime	With B vitamins
Multi-mineral	3-4 ounces daily	In liquid solution, with vitamin B12, biotin
Multi-vitamin/mineral	6 caplets daily	Freeze-dried plant sources
Vitamin C	Individual bowel tolerance*	With bioflavonoids (quercetin, proanthocyanidins)
Vitamin E	2 capsules (800 IU) daily	d-alpha tocopherol

* To determine individual dosage, on the first day take 1,000 mg hourly until diarrhea occurs, then reduce dosage to just below that for individual daily dosage. Vitamin C is not toxic in large doses but must be taken throughout the day to benefit. Divide dosage to three or four times a day.

CHAPTER 92:

Hypertension

"He who is stretched like a rubber band will soon find himself shooting for the moon."

–Barbara Klein Moss

Hypertension is often called the "quiet killer" for the good reason that it doesn't always show signs of the undercover damage it may be doing: 1) weakening blood vessel walls; 2) aneurysms – abnormal expanding or hazardous ballooning of the artery wall which, when ruptured, can cause strokes, heart attacks or instant death; and 3) congestive heart failure and kidney damage.

The National Institutes of Health define hypertension as a blood pressure greater than 140/90.[1] Higher levels of either systolic or diastolic blood pressure are associated with an increased death rate, and these rates begin to rise at blood pressure levels as low as 120/80. An estimated 50 to 70 percent of elderly Americans have hypertension, and the risk of hypertension, at least in Americans, increases with age.[2]

The first hint that hypertension is dietary-related comes when you examine the data from other countries. Not all populations experience this age-assumed increase in blood pressure. Population studies from nonindustrialized societies suggest that average blood pressure does not, in fact, rise with age.[3] In the United States, diastolic hypertension levels off at about age 55, but systolic hypertension continues to rise, even after age 80.[4]

What could make the difference? Could it be...diet? It has been well established that the U.S. diet is deficient in a number of essential nutrients. The most important nutrients to hypertension are the minerals.

The Mineral Alliance

There is a catch to treating high blood pressure with minerals. They must be taken together, and they must be in the correct proportions. Consider calcium and magnesium. The average U.S. citizen's ratio of calcium to magnesium is out of balance. Because of the high absorption rate of minerals in solution, the ratio should be one calcium to every four magnesium. Experts estimate the typical American diet, low in greens and high in dairy products, brings the calcium/magnesium ratio to five calcium to every one magnesium, above the four to one ratio of Finland, which has the highest incidence of heart disease in young to middle aged men.[5]

Finnish researchers, understandably desperate for answers to their epidemic of heart problems, hit on the magnesium/calcium explanation. Veterinarian and medical doctor Dr. H. Korpela, at the Department of Human Health, University of Kuopio, Finland examined 18 pigs who died of sudden heart failure and found low concentrations of magnesium and high levels of calcium in their heart muscles and livers, as compared to healthy pigs and those who died of other diseases.[6] American researchers have since found that a decreased concentration of magnesium is found in the heart and blood of human heart attack victims.[7]

The Link to the Heart

What does heart disease have to do with hypertension? Plenty!

Hypertension has a definite link to heart disease, cardiovascular disease and strokes. One massive European study showed that having hypertension can increase the chances of dying of cardiovascular disease by an incredible 52 percent, and of congestive heart failure by 63 percent![8]

Coronary artery disease is the number one killer of men and women in the United States even though there has been a two percent per year reduction over the last two decades. It is the leading cause of death among women after the age of 60 and in men after 40. Not to be outdone, women are joining men in this horrendous epidemic. Heart disease is now responsible for one of every three deaths in women, as well as men.[9]

One of the most common conventional treatments for hypertension are calcium-channel blockers. These drugs are supposed to attach to the surface membrane of the muscles in the artery walls and prevent calcium from entering. Without calcium interfering, magnesium makes muscles relax and arteries dilate, relieving pressure. Commonly prescribed blockers are: amlodipine (Norvasc), diltiazem (Cardizem, Dilacor), felodipine (Plendil), isradipine (DynaCirc), nicardipine (Cardene), nifedipine (Procardia, Adalat), and verapamil (Calan, Isoptin, Verelan). The drugs are also prescribed for the treatment of coronary artery disease or heart-rhythm abnormalities.

What doctors don't tell you is that magnesium does what all these drugs do, but better.

Probably the most beneficial nutritional discovery of our time is the finding that magnesium is a calcium channel blocker.

The addition of magnesium in a treatment program for high blood pressure would decrease the need for calcium channel blockers and their subsequent side effects.[10]

What side effects? In a 1995 study, researchers from the University of Washington searched through the medical records of a health maintenance organization and identified 1,531 men and women who had been treated for high blood pressure between 1986 and 1993. A total of 291 of the patients had suffered a heart attack during that period; the remaining 1,240 had not.[11]

When the research team reviewed computerized pharmacy records to find out what drugs the patients took, they discovered that the people who had suffered heart attacks were more likely to have taken calcium-channel blockers than other drugs commonly used for treatment of hypertension. Through a statistical analysis, the researchers calculated that the people who took calcium-channel blockers for their high blood pressure had an incredible 60 percent higher risk of having heart attacks than did the people who took other kinds of drugs.

In a study of hypertensive rats, researcher E.P. Gordon at the Department of Pharmacology, Medical College of Hampton Roads, Norfolk, VA, found that in the blood cells of laboratory rats, a lack of magnesium resulted in higher amounts of calcium, and he noted that when there were high amounts of calcium in the cells, they became inactive and unable to perform needed tasks. Dr. Gordon concluded in an article in the *Journal of the American College of Nutrition* that dietary magnesium makes veins and arteries stronger.[12]

So, how bad is it? Very bad! In a 1982 to 1989 study of a variety of nutritional elements, compared to the recommendations of the National Academy of Sciences (the people who come up with the RDAs--recommended daily allowances), it was found that magnesium was low among teenage girls and boys, adult women, and older men and women.[13] A large study by the U.S. Department of Agriculture found that only 25 percent of 37,785 individuals had magnesium intakes at or greater than the recommended daily allowance, which is notoriously low. In a review of 15 studies it was found that a typical diet contains only a fraction of the RDA.[14] Certainly those plagued with hypertension should consider upping their intake of magnesium, and perhaps cutting back on dairy products.

Potassium and Sodium

The controversy continues regarding the role of sodium in high blood pressure. Some say it has no effect, others say too much can severely increase blood pressure. However, if you look at the studies, you'll see a definite pattern: tests that show no effect, do not also evaluate potassium levels. Studies that consider potassium realize that a low potassium, high sodium ratio is what causes dangerous hypertension.

Researchers at the University of Pennsylvania, Philadelphia, con-ducted a double-blind, randomized, crossover trial of 12 hyperten-sive patients who were placed on a 10 day diet providing either low or high amounts of potassium, with sodium and other minerals kept constant. On the 11th day patients received an infusion of saline, severely increasing their blood sodium levels. Patients who had a low potassium intake not only saw their systolic and diastolic pres-sure increased, but lost even more potassium. It appeared that the increased sodium intake was actually drawing potassium out of their blood! With their depleted potassium stores, their bodies were un-able to eliminate the excess sodium, and also depleted their stores of calcium and phosphorus, thereby further increasing blood pressure.[15]

Sodium and potassium, in the correct ratio, regulate the body's fluid balance, as well as influence the heart's strength. Current re-search shows the common American diet does not contain the bal-ance optimal for maintaining normal blood pressure. Heikki Karppanen, M.D., Department of Pharmacology and Toxicology, University of Helsinki, Finland, believes that it only takes a moder-ate restriction of sodium together with a marked increase in potas-sium to have very powerful antihypertensive effects in some patients. Karppanen states in *Annals of Medicine* that "sodium restriction in conjunction with potassium and magnesium supplementation may help reduce the dosage and frequency of antihypertensive medicines and thereby reduce the side effects from these medications."[16]

Other research studies have shown that potassium alone, without considering the sodium issue, work to reduce blood pressure.

In one crossover, double-blind, randomized trial, 24 hyperten-sive patients were given potassium chloride or a placebo during two four-week periods. At the end of the fourth week potassium supple-mentation resulted in a decrease in systolic, diastolic and mean blood pressure in all the subjects.[17]

In another placebo-controlled study, 586 individuals received potassium for an average of 28 days. Of these, 412 had hypertension and 240 received a placebo. British researchers found all the hypertensive patients taking potassium had a reduction in blood pressure. The higher the baseline blood pressure and the longer the patients took the mineral, the better the results.[18]

Just to clarify: eating too much salt will not cause high blood pressure. But if you don't get enough potassium in your diet and eat too much salt, you'll be risking it. It is no longer acceptable to recommend lowering salt (sodium chloride) alone. First calcium, potassium and magnesium deficits should be corrected. The evidence suggests salt would not be a factor if these minerals were present in sufficient quantities. Also, low magnesium appears to cause or have a connection with low potassium.[19]

If you are already hypertensive, definitely cut down on the salt and eat foods high in potassium. Watch out for soft drinks. They rob your body of potassium.

As evidence suggests, a therapeutic diet high in potassium, magnesium and calcium should lower blood pressure. Researchers in India decided to find out. They evaluated 199 patients with essential hypertension who were given either a diet high in potassium, magnesium and calcium, or the usual diet with drug therapy. After eight weeks they found significantly lower mean systolic and diastolic pressures in the mineral-rich diet group versus the conventional diet/drug group, with an approximately 10 point difference in both diastolic and systolic measures between the two groups.[20] What I find so fascinating is that even antihypertensive drugs couldn't compete with the three mineral allies.

Remember, you're not what you put into your mouth, you're what you absorb and digest and deliver to cells. A tablet is only one to five percent absorbable. Since the process of digestion is a process of liquefaction, your body has to take a hard rock tablet and turn it into solution. This may not be possible due to a number of factors, such as inadequate stomach acid, food allergies and intestinal problems. This is why it is so important that when you decide to supplement, you target minerals in solution – all the minerals in solution.

Sugar and Hypertension

There is no doubt in my mind that the eating habits of the typical American is killing us. Consider these statistics: 46 percent of every food dollar is spent on meals and snacks away from home. Convenience stores have increased by 50 percent over the last decade. The typical American consumes 48 pounds of high fructose corn syrup annually – mostly in soft drinks – and in 1990, consumed their body weight in sweeteners and salt.[21] No wonder America is experiencing an epidemic of degenerative diseases! With habits like these, who needs auto accidents?

Dr. P. Al-Karadaghi and associates at the Department of Medicine at Georgetown University Medical Center in Washington, D.C., set out to determine the effect of a diet high in sugar on blood pressure. In his studies of hypertensive rats, he found it took only two weeks on a high sugar diet for the rats to see a marked increase in their blood pressure, and discovered he could turn this effect off and on just with the addition of sugar in their diets.[22]

Richard A. Ahrens, Ph.D., of the University of Maryland's College of Human Ecology, found the same results in humans, concluding that sugar contributes to sodium retention.[23]

Blood Pressure-Healthy Nutrients
For maximum absorption, take supplements with meals.

Nutrient	Suggested Dosage	Formulation
Aged garlic extract	1 teaspoon three times daily	Liquid
Amino acids	4-6 capsules daily	Multiple formula from natural sources
Antioxidants	4 capsules daily*	With selenium and grapeseed extract
Borage oil	2 capsules daily	
Coenzyme Q10	2 capsules daily	With vitamin E, phospholipids and selenium
Enzymes	2 capsules twice daily	Multiple formula
Fiber	4-8 tablets daily	Psyllium, with herb hyssop
Flaxseed oil	1 tablespoon daily	
Hawthorne	250 mg twice daily	
Magnesium	200 mg daily	
Melatonin (adults only)	3 mg daily at bedtime	With B vitamins
Multi-mineral	3-4 ounces daily	In liquid solution, with vitamin B12, biotin
Multi-vitamin/mineral	6 caplets daily	Freeze-dried plant sources
Rutin	100 mg twice daily	With vitamin C
Taurine	500 mg twice daily	
Vitamin B6	100 mg daily	
Vitamin C	Individual bowel tolerance**	With bioflavonoids (quercetin, rutin, proanthocyanidins)
Vitamin E	2 capsules (800 IU) daily	d-alpha tocopherol

* The FDA recommends pregnant women not exceed 10,000 IU of vitamin A daily.

** To determine individual dosage, on the first day take 1,000 mg hourly until diarrhea occurs, then reduce dosage to just below that for individual daily dosage. Vitamin C is not toxic in large doses but must be taken throughout the day to benefit. Divide dosage to three or four times a day.

CHAPTER 93:

Impotence

From *The American Heritage Dictionary* comes the definition of impotence, of which I ask you to disregard: "Lacking physical strength or vigor; helpless."

A man's strength, unlike Samson's hair, is not dependent on sexual performance. Remember, no single influence can undermine a man's ability to perform the sex act; and this encumbrance is in no way reflective of a man's power, strength or masculinity. Most women would agree.

Dr. Beverly Palmer, a psychology professor at California State University, Dominguez Hills, who teaches a course in human sexuality and serves as a clinical psychologist to a medical doctor specializing in male sexual dysfunction, says it's a mistake for a man to think of his condition as impotency. "It is better to call this disorder 'erectile dysfunction'," she says. "That sticks to the specific part of the body having the problem, rather than to a man's conception of himself."[1] This makes perfect sense since it is simply a matter of the male organ not being able to become either partially or fully erect. Men with erection problems can still have an orgasm and ejaculate.

I'm telling this to the millions of you who suffer from erectile dysfunction: you are not alone! The ongoing Massachusetts Male Aging Study revealed that 51 percent of healthy men between the ages of 40 and 70 reported occasional-to-frequent problems with erections. On a national basis, that comes out to 18 million men. While emotional factors can play a role in many cases, most doctors (and even many psychotherapists) now think that the overwhelming majority of impotence cases – about 80 percent – are caused by personal plumbing problems.[2]

The Importance of Good Circulation

Anything that reduces blood circulation can result in an inability to achieve erectile efficiency. Because of the incredibly small blood vessels of the male genitalia, it can be the first to react to a decrease in blood or narrowing of the vessels. Ever heard of a tension headache? Many migraines are caused by a narrowing of the arteries in the head, causing pressure to build up. The same things that cause headaches: anxiety, anger, fatigue, stress, and, of course, tension, will also cause impotency. For more, see my chapter on Stress.

Perhaps the major physical cause of erectile dysfunction is impairment of blood circulation to the male organ due to cholesterol, calcium and other substances that narrow the arteries. If you have high cholesterol, see my chapter on Cholesterol for natural, effective ways to lower it, and protect against erectile difficulties. See my chapter on Circulation Problems for solutions to this possible cause.

Chelation Therapy for Blocked Arteries

Practitioners of alternative medicine tell me many of their patients have been returned to full sexuality after a series of chelation treatments, which dissolve blockages in the tiny capillaries of the male organ. Chelation therapy usually involves a total of 21 painless treatments in which a natural amino acid compound known as EDTA is injected into the arteries. EDTA acts as a magnet collecting plaque and calcium from the arteries and flushing them out through the kidneys.

Recently, I had Dr. Ross Gordon, the eminent pioneer in the field of chelation therapy on my television program, *Maximize Your Life*. With him was one of his grateful patients who had gone to him to reverse the plaque build up in his arteries. We expected his patient to simply testify that the chelation worked for him. However, he surprised everyone by spontaneously blurting out that one of the side effects he was delighted to experience was his restored sexual function. Obviously still ecstatic at the results, he explained to the television viewers that he hadn't meant to tell this part, as his wife (in the studio) beamed her approval.

Dr. Ross Gordon and his brother, Dr. Garry Gordon, are cofounders of the American College of Advancement in Medicine (ACAM). ACAM has members in all parts of the world who practice chelation. A letter or phone call to my office can help you locate an ACAM member near you. Call 1-800-445-HEAL.

Are there any foods that naturally chelate? Certain tropical fruits such as bananas, kiwi, mangoes and papaya have a high concentration of chelating minerals and an enzyme called bromelain, which creates a chelation-like effect. Bromelain "acts like a pipe cleaner" for blood vessels.[3] Be warned, however, that a heavy intake of bromelain can delay the healing of a stomach ulcer.

Foods That Fuel

If you believe in locker room talk, ginseng is supposed to be an aphrodisiac that fires up the libido and boosts erectile efficiency. Not so. Ginseng will boost your energy and endurance levels, as Russian experiments show, and energy and endurance are important to sexual competency, but ginseng is no aphrodisiac.

And while I'm at it, stay away from dubious sex potions found in those little ads in popular tabloids. Not only is there no true magic potion, but some of those concoctions could be dangerous, especially since you don't know what's really in them. Stick to God-given foods and the nutrients derived from them – like garlic.

In China, the Ammites are said to credit garlic for their sexual vigor and health. In India, men rub a garlic and fat ointment on the genitalia and lower back to promote and maintain erection.

Garlic is used in the East as an aphrodisiac, and is said to create a long-lasting effect. Japanese researchers point to garlic's power to stimulate and invigorate hormonal and gastric secretions. This results in a general revitalization of the entire body.

Although the smell of garlic turns most people off, the power of garlic to turn people on has throughout history turned certain sects of celibate clergy off. Thus, we often see garlic as a forbidden food in the bylaws of various religions. In support of this claim of arousal, herbalists point to the warmth that develops throughout the body, particularly in the stomach area, after eating garlic.

A Low Fat Diet Can Help

It is estimated that half of all men with diabetes have erectile dysfunction.

According to Bruce and Eileen MacKenzie, founders of Impotents Anonymous – yes, there *is* such a group! – approximately 80 percent of the estimated 13 million diabetic men in the U.S. suffer from premature hardening of the arteries, especially in the small blood vessels of the male organ. The restricted blood supply not only hampers the engorgement process, but can lead to permanent nerve damage and impotence.[4]

While the odds may seem bleak, the future is bright – as it can be reversed!

By avoiding the typical high fat, high sugar and low fiber diet, it is possible to prevent and manage diabetes, writes Associate Professor Somasundaram Addanki, a biochemist and nutritionist at Ohio State University College of Medicine.

In a United Press International news story, Professor Addanki admitted to six years of diabetic impotency before he stopped eating sugar, white flour products and fatty foods, successfully curing his ailment.

Dr. Louis Lipson, chief of the division of geriatric medicine at the University of Southern California, says that probably half of diabetics who have erectile dysfunction can be helped.[5]

He says many are led into thinking the situation is hopeless. In a study of 320 diabetic men, Lipson traced half of their dysfunction to three causes other than the diabetes: 20 percent were from psychological factors, another 20 percent from the medications they were on, and 10 percent from related disorders.

Lipson warns that erectile dysfunction is not a necessary evil with diabetes. Sometimes the expectation creates the reality, he says. Because of the expectation, it becomes a self-fulfilling prophecy.

Smoking and Drinking are Not Macho

Alcohol is a major cause of the inability to achieve an erection. Even social drinking can cause an embarrassing inability to perform, as many wives can attest to. There is nothing funny about a man whose libido goes into overdrive after having a few drinks, then gets home only to find he's incapable.

Drinking can undermine sexual desire because it tends to reduce the body's production of sex hormones. Even persons who consume just a drink or two a day can suffer the sexually repressive effects of alcohol.

The chemicals inhaled while smoking cigarettes are notorious for causing the blood vessels to constrict, and while smoking can't as yet be conclusively found to cause impotence, at least one study links it.

Researchers at Queen's University in Kingston found that among men who had erectile dysfunction, 81 percent smoked, compared to 58 percent of men in the general population who smoked at the time of the study.

Researchers evaluating 4,400 Vietnam veterans found that impotence occurred at a 50 percent higher rate among current smokers than in nonsmokers or past smokers.[6]

Smoking also depletes the body of valuable nutrients, especially zinc, which I will discuss in more detail later. These nutrients, as you will learn to appreciate, can make an enormous difference in the health of your sex life.

Thou Shalt Not Medicate

Other erection enemies are prescription and over-the-counter medications. Medications prescribed for high blood pressure, depression, and cancer are some culprits. As are over-the-counter pain medications and antihistamines.

Beware of any anti-inflammatory drug or medication which acts to constrict blood vessels. Read the literature included with any medication and especially read the precautions and side effects. Look for what it actually does and how it works on the body.

A physician at New York University found that 16 patients had impotence problems directly linked to long-term daily use of over-the-counter nose drops!

The drugs contained in the drops temporarily improve breathing and reduce swelling by constricting the small blood vessels in the nose. Like all drugs, however, they can be absorbed into the bloodstream and go where they aren't needed – like the male organ. Continued use caused blood vessels to constrict, which prevented their erections.

A 1981 review of the 200 most frequently prescribed drugs found that 15 percent were associated with male sexual impairment, including impotence. And considering the speed by which the FDA approves of new medications, this statistic is probably valid today.

For those of you who might be taking prescription drugs, I'll name some that have been identified by Arthur G. Lipman, doctor of pharmacy, as contributing to erectile dysfunction. I warn you, there are many!

The list includes Aldomet, Aldactone, Chlorpromazine, Librium, Valium, Serax, Tranxene, Mellaril, Haldol, Catapres, Dibenzyline, Ismelin, Macrodantin, Furadantin, Priscoline, Regitine and Trecator-SC. Look also for phenothiazines, anticholinergics, antineoplastic and estrogens. Quite a mouthful isn't it? When you're prescribed medications, and choose to use them – you always have a choice you know – make sure you get all the information from the pharmacist.

Doctors may ask pharmacists not to include the manufacturer's warnings because they are afraid if the patient knows about the side effects, he or she will actually create the symptoms! Your rights as an informed consumer include getting all the facts.

The Physicians Desk Reference (PDR) is a large book used by doctors to look up medications and their side effects. Years ago, certain forces attempted to ban the PDR from public viewing. Thanks to efforts by the National Health Federation, it is available for public use at any library or for purchase at most bookstores. It is a must-read treasure house of all the symptoms and side effects of the most commonly used medications.

Glandular Sources

Physicians who, instead of sending their impotent patients to psychotherapists, dig a little deeper, often find that erectile dysfunction can be connected to the sex glands, most especially the pituitary, thyroid and thymus glands. Called the hypothalamic-pituitary-gonadal axis, many disorders can be attributed to a dysfunction in this hormonal highway linking the brain, pituitary and sex organs.

The pituitary serves our body like an inconspicuous general commanding an army. Often called the master gland, it governs the activity of the sex organs. It also has a direct link with the hypothalamus, a brain gland important to the nervous system and growth. Since the entire development of sex glands and sex hormones is governed by this bean-sized little wonder, a malfunction can cause lowered amounts of male hormones, and subsequent loss of body hair and small testicles, not to mention erectile dysfunction.

In one case, a patient of Dr. Richard F. Spark, M.D., department of medicine, Beth Israel Hospital in Boston, had been seeing internists, psychiatrists and psychologists for a span of 12 years to cure impotency left after treatment for a pituitary tumor. The doctor evaluated his hormonal system and found it to be out of wack. After treatment, which included testosterone, his erectile function returned in an incredible 48 hours.

In one ground-breaking study, medical experts measured the serum testosterone levels of 105 consecutive patients with impotence. It was found that 37 of them had previously unsuspected axis disorders.

Since it is the control-tower pituitary that directs the important-to-your-health glands, it behooves us to keep it in tip-top shape.

To keep your hormonal highway healthy, feed it foods rich in the B complex vitamins, especially pantothenic acid (B5) and niacin, vitamins A, C, E, unsaturated fatty acids and zinc. Adrenal exhaustion can result in little strength or desire for sex. An inadequately supplied thyroid gland can also cause a lack of desire or strength for sex. Iodine, the B vitamins and vitamin E are essential for production of its hormone, thyroxine.

Men deficient in vitamin B6 (pyridoxine) have become impotent; and during stress, the sex urge and sperm production diminish.[7]

Think Zinc

When it comes to a man's sexual functioning, zinc is really the last word. Zinc deficiency will likely impair sexual growth and maturation, because this mineral appears to be essential for the manufacture of testosterone. Teenage boys, therefore, should be sure and get enough of this mega-mineral.

Michael Lesser, M.D., testifying before the Senate Select Committee on Nutrition and Human Needs, exploded the blockbuster that the soil of 32 states is zinc-deficient and that fertilizers put no zinc back in the ground.

A four-year study of 11 midwest states in which several thousand grain samples revealed that zinc levels in corn dropped 10 percent during the study.

As fundamental as two and two equaling four is the fact that if soil is short of zinc, so is the plant growing in it, and the animal feeding on the plant! All the more reason to consider zinc supplementation.

Insufficient zinc can also lead to a greatly reduced sperm count, improper development of the male sexual organs in young males, and prostrate problems. Furthermore, scientists report even a small zinc deficiency can wreak havoc on sexual vigor.

In his studies, Dr. Ananda Prasad, M.D., professor of medicine and chief of hematology at Wayne State University School of Medicine in Detroit, Michigan, found the testes to be very sensitive to zinc.

Dr. Prasad and colleagues induced mild zinc deficiencies by restricting zinc-foods from the diets of five healthy men aged 51 to 65. By eating controlled meals, the subjects actually lost about one milligram of zinc a day from their bodies. During the six-month study, sperm counts dropped in four out of five men. Testosterone levels dropped in all five.[8]

In three men, the sperm counts plummeted below the point of technical sterility. And the subjects complained of diminished sexual desire.

After the volunteers resumed standard meals and were fortified with 30 mg of zinc a day, they returned to normal within 16 to 20 weeks.

Dr. Prasad recommends that once the doctor has ruled out most organic and psychological causes of impotency, plasma zinc levels should be checked. If a zinc deficiency does exist, the doctor can begin treating it with 20 to 30 mg of zinc daily for six months to a year.

Watch out if you smoke! Smoking depletes the body's supply of zinc. Toxic heavy metal cadmium, present in cigarette smoke, interferes with zinc metabolism and can accumulate in the testicles.[9]

Calcium and Magnesium

There are even more nutrients essential to erections. Two very important minerals for good health are calcium and magnesium. We usually think of calcium as primarily needed to make strong bones and teeth, but it is also important in sexual functioning. Calcium provides an essential link between the brain, hormonal glands, and the mechanical processes. However, what is important to realize is that without magnesium, the benefits of calcium are lost because without it, calcium deposits in soft tissues and forms blockages that can cause erectile problems.

Doctors have long noticed the detrimental effect certain pharmaceuticals have on sexual function, but have wondered why calcium channel blockers are not among them. They know calcium is important to sexual performance, and therefore, cannot understand why a drug which blocks the entry of calcium would not cause problems.[10] The answer to this puzzle is a diet low in magnesium.

Without calcium interfering, magnesium dilates the arteries, relieving pressure and blockages. Probably the most beneficial nutritional discovery of our time is the finding that magnesium is a calcium channel blocker.

The addition of magnesium in a treatment program for high blood pressure would decrease the need for calcium channel blockers and their subsequent side effects.[11]

Calcium channel blockers do not cause problems because the subjects of their studies are like most of the U.S. population – they are deficient in magnesium, and therefore are not effected by something that blocks excess calcium.

So, how bad is this deficiency? It's dreadful. In a 1982 to 1989 study of a variety of nutritional elements, compared to the recommendations of the National Academy of Sciences (the people who come up with the RDAs – recommended daily allowances), it was found that magnesium was low among teenage girls and boys, adult women, and older men and women.[12] A large study by the U.S. Department of Agriculture found that only 25 percent of 37,785 individuals had magnesium intakes at or greater than the recommended daily allowance, which is notoriously low. In a review of 15 studies it was found that a typical diet contains only a fraction of the RDA.[13] Certainly those of you plagued with sexual problems should consider upping your intake of magnesium, and perhaps cutting back on dairy products.

Plumbing-Promoting Nutrients

For maximum absorption, supplements should be taken with meals.

Nutrient	Suggested Dosage	Formulation
Aged garlic extract	2 teaspoons three times daily	Liquid
Amino acids	4-6 capsules daily	Multiple formula from natural sources
Antioxidants	4 capsules daily	With selenium and grape seed extract
Borage oil	2 capsules daily	
Coenzyme Q10	2 capsules daily	With vitamin E, phospholipids and selenium
Enzymes	2 capsules twice daily	Multiple formula
Flaxseed oil	1 tablespoon daily	
Fiber	8 tablets daily	Psyllium, with herb hyssop
Folic acid	5-10 mg daily	
Ginkgo biloba	60 mg twice daily	
L-Carnitine	500 mg twice daily	
Magnesium	200 mg daily	
Multi-vitamin/mineral	6 caplets daily	Freeze-dried plant sources
Multi-mineral	2-4 ounces daily	In liquid solution, with vitamin B12, biotin
Nettle	250 mg three times daily	
Niacin	500 mg four times daily	
Pygeum	250 mg twice daily	
Saw palmetto	160 mg twice daily	
Vitamin C	Individual bowel tolerance*	With bioflavonoids (quercetin, rutin, proanthocyanidins)
Vitamin B6	100 mg daily	
Vitamin E	2 capsules (800 IU) daily	d-alpha tocopherol

* To determine individual dosage, on the first day take 1,000 mg hourly until diarrhea occurs, then reduce dosage to just below that for individual daily dosage. Vitamin C is not toxic in large doses but must be taken throughout the day to benefit. Divide dosage to three or four times a day.

CHAPTER 94:

Infections

One of my first experiences, over 30 years ago, with the miracle of nutritional healing, involved my husband Frank and a Siamese kitten named Sammy Jr. During an attempted post-bath blow dry, Sammy reacted by severely biting the index finger of Frank's right hand to the bone. He was admitted to the hospital where they performed emergency surgery and put him on IV antibiotics around the clock for six weeks. However, to our horror, the antibiotics didn't work and his hand swelled with a deeply rooted bone infection. It became so severe that after six weeks the doctors could only suggest amputation. They wanted to cut off his right hand! Wheeling him out of the hospital, his hand had swelled to three times its normal size and was so tender he couldn't even place it on the arm rest.

I knew there was another way. I gave him massive doses of vitamin C and took him to a physician knowledgeable in nutrition to boost his intake with IV doses. Our new doctor obliged by giving my husband an IV of massive amounts of vitamin C. Within three days the pain had completely subsided, wounds from the surgery healed and the infection, which had been traveling down his hand with alacrity, eating away the bone, knuckle and joint, was gone.

Because of this, and the death of a dear friend, I became determined to unearth all the other therapies available to medical consumers that are being kept from us. That was 30 years ago, and what I've learned since then literally fills volumes – the volumes I've written for you.

Vitamin C Instead of Antibiotics

You brush and floss your teeth every day to prevent cavities and gum disease. If you don't you should. But what you should also do to protect those pearly whites is take vitamin C – shown in studies to prevent dental infections by lowering the amount of plaque and bacteria in the mouth. The *New York Journal of Dentistry* reported on a study in which plaque accumulation was measured among subjects all brushing well, some supplementing with vitamin C, some not. The study found that those supplementing with vitamin C actually had less tarter and bacteria than those only brushing. The study found that when the subjects took vitamin C the inflammation of their gums from concentrations of bacteria improved 58 percent![1]

A Protective Army

How does vitamin C perform its magic? By increasing the numbers of the antibody warriors that come to our defense when infection sets in. In South Africa, University of Witwatersrand medical students were given one gram a day of ascorbic acid (vitamin C) and monitored for blood immunologic levels. Unlike the control group who did not get the vitamin C, the ones who did experienced a marked increase in their defense antibodies. Vitamin C is renowned for alleviating the symptoms of colds and flu, and studies have shown it to be of benefit for tuberculosis, herpes, tetanus and diphtheria. Any type of infection can be helped with vitamin C.[2]

Vitamin C works to prevent infections, treat them, and even prevent the pain that follows any injury to the body. If you work with your hands, and find yourself with frequent cuts, scrapes and skin injuries, try a lotion that contains vitamin C. Vitamin C applied topically can help prevent infection.

Massive doses of vitamin C has successfully curing viral pneumonia, mononucleosis, influenza, colds, hepatitis, shingles, and cold sores. How much vitamin C you require is determined by the onset of diarrhea. The tolerance level in each individual differs. Some days you can tolerate more, some days less, depending upon how much you need to cleanse the system of toxins. When the system is cleansed, diarrhea results. When that occurs, just cut back the dosage.

In an amazing discovery, vitamin C has been found to be helpful in the continuing battle against bacteria that have become immune to antibiotics. Antibiotics are not the most desirable way to fight infection, but they are used. However, medical science is in a quandary because many of the bacteria we are fighting have become immune to antibiotics. Rather than using stronger antibiotics, perhaps physicians should consider using stronger doses of vitamin C.

A recent Harvard study found vitamin C may reduce bacterial resistance to antibiotic therapy. In their laboratories, researchers exposed strains of staph bacteria to ascorbic acid for six hours. In four out of six of the strains, the bacteria showed less resistance. The researchers found that the doses of antibiotics could be reduced by 50 to 75 percent after resistant strains of bacteria were exposed to the vitamin C. They also found that previously ineffective doses of penicillin and tetracycline showed increased inhibitory effects on resistant bacteria, and even killed 23 to 93 percent of the initial bacteria population with vitamin C.[3,4] This is very exciting stuff. With vitamin C, not only are old antibiotics useful again, but you don't have to take as much of them! Now, if only conventional medicine would wake up and smell the oranges!

When you target vitamin C as a supplement, choose a formulation that includes bioflavonoids. Bioflavonoids are potent anti-inflammatories. Among other therapeutic benefits, they reduce swelling, boost the immune system, and enhance the healing properties of vitamin C. Researchers Joe A. Vinson and Pratima Bose at the University of Scranton carried out several well-designed studies that revealed when vitamin C was combined with citrus bioflavonoids, blood levels of vitamin C were higher and lasted longer than vitamin C alone.[5] Synthetic vitamin C, commonly used in lower-priced supplements, does not contain bioflavonoids.

Vitamin A for All

All kinds of infections respond to vitamin A, especially those which effect the tissues of the body, like pneumonia, skin infections and ear infections.

In areas of the world where vitamin A deficiencies are common, children are chronically ill with a host of infections. In a study done in an urban slum area in Bombay, India, vitamin A was given to 2,000 children under 5 years of age, and 403 under one year of age, and compared to a control group of 2,060 children under 5 and 460 under 1. At six month intervals a detailed history was taken of their illnesses. Common illnesses, in addition to vitamin A deficiency, were fever, respiratory tract infections, diarrhea, gastrointestinal infections, skin infection, ear infections, post measles complications and malnutrition. Thanks to the vitamin A, the children were much healthier. Not only did the vitamin A help reduce the incidence of infections, diarrhea, measles, respiratory infections and parasite infections, but there was also a substantial decrease in the death of children due to these problems.[6]

Over 50 years ago scientists first discovered vitamin A's value in treating and preventing colds and flu. For example, in 1942, Italian physician Di Salvatore Princi published his study results that showed mice had more resistance to an influenza germ if they were given vitamin A. In 1937, German doctor Torsten Lindquist found that the vitamin A content of the blood was drastically lowered during the first five days of illness. When the patient began to get better, the level of vitamin A rose dramatically, even though no vitamin A was added to the diet. His assumption was that it was used somehow in the healing process.[7]

Dr. Garry Gordon, M.D. practicing in Tempe, Arizona, recommends taking vitamin A and garlic at the same time as vitamin C, at the first sign of cold or flu symptoms, usually for a period of not less than three and not more than five days. He says that taking vitamin A directly, rather than in the form of beta carotene is most desirable.

He recommends taking 500,000 IU when sick, and that high doses are safe as long as the person's weight is over 120 pounds, there is no serious liver condition, and high doses aren't taken daily over weeks or months.[8]

Garlic – The Body Detoxifier

If garlic were a pharmaceutical, you would see advertisements in all the magazines, and the lucky company with the patent would earn hundreds of millions of dollars a year. Everyone would learn of garlic's vast power and flock to their doctors for a prescription. Fortunately for those of us in the know, garlic is easily available and inexpensively obtained.

Unfortunately, because it's not patentable, few are aware of the many benefits they can derive from raw garlic and, especially liquid aged garlic extract.

I avidly follow international garlic studies, and am convinced the science of garlic is truly the science of Kyolic® – the brand I use – manufactured by the Wakunaga Company of Japan. More than 100 published studies of Kyolic® cover a vast range of subjects from AIDS to cancer, to cholesterol and allergies – many conducted by the reputable and knowledgeable scientists at Wakunaga. The company has 14 international patents and patents pending on Kyolic®.

Why is *aged* garlic so important? To get the kind of benefit that kills diseases, large amounts of garlic is needed. Unfortunately, according to Dr. Herbert Pierson, excessive amounts of raw garlic can be toxic, but when it is aged he says, it "enters the body's cells and stimulates immune response."

Dr. Tariq Abdullah, of the Akbar Clinic and Research Foundation in Panama City, Florida, conducted studies showing that raw and aged garlic extract enhances T-cell activity, the body's warriors of defense. He says, "No other substance, either natural or synthetic, can match garlic's proven therapeutic versatility and effectiveness."[9]

Garlic is the best example of the philosophy, "Let your medicine be your food, and your food your medicine." What can't hurt in any infection therapy, is supplementing garlic with the active ingredients contained in it. Garlic contains germanium, magnesium, selenium, 17 amino acids, 33 sulfur compounds, vitamins B1, A and C. Organic germanium is a dramatic immunostimulant. Controlled studies found organic germanium restores immune function in immune-depressed animals.[10] Studies of human subjects have shown that it enhances natural killer cell activity. Garlic is one of the richest sources of organic selenium and germanium.[11]

Infection Fighting Nutrients
For maximum absorption, take supplements with meals.

Nutrient	Suggested Dosage	Formulation
Acidophilus	At least four billion flora on an empty stomach, three times daily	
Aged garlic extract	1 teaspoon three times daily	Liquid
Antioxidants	4 capsules daily*	With selenium and grapeseed extract
Echinacea	200 mg daily	
Fiber	4-8 tablets	Psyllium, with herb hyssop
Multi-mineral	3-4 ounces daily	In liquid solution, with vitamin B12, biotin
Multi-vitamin/mineral	6 caplets daily	Freeze-dried plant sources
Vitamin A	25,000 IU daily*	
Vitamin C	Individual bowel tolerance**	With bioflavonoids (quercetin, rutin proanthocyanidins)

* The FDA recommends pregnant women not exceed 10,000 IU of vitamin A daily.

** To determine individual dosage, on the first day take 1,000 mg hourly until diarrhea occurs, then reduce dosage to just below that for individual daily dosage. Vitamin C is not toxic in large doses but must be taken throughout the day to benefit. Divide dosage to three or four times a day.

CHAPTER 95:

Infertility

The federal government is funding an exhaustive multi-million dollar research project on male infertility. But the initial results are very discouraging. So far none of the male subjects have gotten pregnant.

Don't Stress It

It's truly amazing – though not surprising – how many couples trying to conceive give up and adopt, only to find themselves expecting. This is not unexpected when you realize how profound the effect stress has on the human body.

A study of 150 men found that stress due to the death of a family member, separation or divorce slowed their sperm enough to affect their ability to conceive.[1] Anibal Acosta, M.D., clinical director of the Andrology Laboratory at the Jones Institute, Norfolk, Virginia, says that, "Due to advancements in diagnosis, we now know that at least 40 percent of cases are due to male infertility."[2]

Never underestimate the power of stress. Experts believe it plays a major part in fifty percent of all medical problems.[3] Not only is the chance for infections and illnesses increased, due to the body's lowered immune system; but nutrients, important to conception, are depleted. Vitamin C is the first nutrient to be depleted. During stress, vitamin E, pantothenic acid (B6), vitamin A, and all the B vitamins are used up in massive amounts. Calcium, magnesium, phosphorous, and potassium demands are also increased under stress.[4]

Studies reported in the *American Journal of Clinical Nutrition* found that, although volunteers had more than adequate intakes of zinc, iron, copper and selenium, their blood levels of these minerals during stress went down by 33, 44, 12 and 9 percent respectively.

Since it is difficult to know how badly your body reacts to the stresses of everyday life, the first course of action in any program of conception is to target these nutrients in your diet and in supplemental form. Not coincidentally, many of these nutrients have been shown in studies to help couples conceive.

Fertility With Antioxidants

Infertility may be an inherent protective mechanism signalling that the body is not strong enough to give birth. When the human body is weakened and its health potential severely lowered by environmental factors – inadequate nutrition, disease, or severe emotional or physical stress – it will be deprived of its ability to reproduce.[5]

Nicknamed the "antisterility vitamin," vitamin E shows great promise as an aid to fertility. In 1955, researchers studied the effects of the vitamin on fertility at a large horse breeding facility in Oshawa, Canada. They administered vitamin E daily to the entire herd, including old mares who were previously thought to be barren, and older stallions.

According to the Jockey Club, a leading authoritative body in thoroughbred racing, registered foals are produced by pregnant mares approximately 52 percent of the time. After treatment with vitamin E, 71 percent of the pregnancies resulted in births.[6]

R. Bayer, M.D., a West German physician, conducted a study involving the effects of vitamin E on 100 infertile couples with a history of miscarriages. In the group, there were 144 conceptions without a single live birth. After daily administration of 100 units of the vitamin to the males and 200 units to the females, the same couples conceived 79 children, of which only two were miscarried.[7]

When Dr. Bayer conducted the same experiment with a second group in which 63 of 101 pregnancies had resulted in miscarriage,

41 women became pregnant and none of them miscarried.

In the 1920s, Drs. C. Raychaudhuri and I.D. Desai of the University of British Columbia, Vancouver, recognized the chemical similarity between vitamin E and the sex hormones. The researchers began administering large doses of vitamin E to rats. When the rats became more fertile, they reversed the experiment to study the effects of a lack of vitamin E on fertility. One result consistently observed was a failure by male rats to produce sperm. The E-deficient rats had considerable tissue damage in the sex organs – in part the result of low levels of vitamin E.[8]

A deficiency of the mineral selenium has been shown in studies to contribute to infertility. Like vitamin E, selenium is an antioxidant. This means that it protects vital body tissues, like those found in the female uterus, and male testes, from cell damage that could contribute to miscarriages and sperm problems.[9]

In a controlled study using laboratory mice, a deficiency of selenium in their diets produced a very high rate of abnormal sperm – as much as 49 percent, compared to the control group whose highest rate was only 15 percent.[10]

Some nutrients not only have oxidation-quenching abilities, but are central to a healthy sexual system. Zinc is one of those nutrients. A diet low in zinc is associated with prostate problems, and is necessary to healthy sperm. Not surprisingly, a deficiency of zinc has been shown in studies to cause male infertility. Because of its importance to female hormones, it is also associated with female infertility. According to the October 1994 *The Nutrition Report*, a zinc deficiency can cause abnormal ovaries, too little egg-releasing hormones, disruption of the estrous cycle, frequent abortion, prolonged gestation and stillbirths. In men, a zinc deficiency leads to poor sperm, too little testosterone, small testicles and dysfunction of the sex glands.[11]

Vitamin C is another antioxidant beneficial to making babies. Several studies have shown ascorbic acid supplementation helps to turn childless couples into parents-to-be.[12] A sequence of events led researchers to discovering the value of vitamin C to male fertility. In

1941, researchers recognized that the concentration of vitamin C in the testicles was around 20 times higher than in the blood. Six years later researchers noted that a majority of infertile males had low testicular vitamin C levels. Researchers next discovered that sperm stickiness is associated with infertility, then found vitamin C helps unstick sperm, leading to better mobility and higher levels of fertilization. Today nutritionists know that ascorbate – a form of vitamin C – can increase sperm count, volume and motility, as well as improve sperm quality.[13]

A study proved it. Researchers used clearly-diagnosed infertile, but otherwise healthy men for their study. They gave one group 1,000 milligrams (one gram) of ascorbic acid every day for 60 days. They gave the other group (the same number of men) a placebo. At the end of two months, none of the placebo group were able to conceive, while all of the vitamin C-supplemented group reported their wives were pregnant.[14]

Don't Forget Garlic

I recommend garlic for any chemical-quenching need. Not only is it an excellent antioxidant detoxifier, but is full of the nutrients most beneficial to fertility. Garlic includes germanium, magnesium, selenium, amino acids, sulfur compounds, and vitamins A, B1 and C. For optimum benefit and absorption, choose liquid aged garlic extract.

Before I go on to the other beneficial nutrients, let me just say that antioxidants are beneficial not only because the body needs them, but because they are invaluable defenders against the chemical onslaught we face daily from our environment. Many, many studies link pesticides, chemicals, toxins, heavy metals and artificial estrogens in our environment to infertility – both male and female. For example, an article in *The Lancet* says that certain pesticides affect male hormones to such a degree that the reproductive abnormalities, such as low sperm counts, incurred by them can be seen 20 to 40 years later in subsequent generations. Pesticides have such serious estrogen mimicking effects that boy babies are being born with female hormonal levels and girl babies have too much male hormones. Fortunately, we have defenses.

The best defense? A complete and thorough supplemental antioxidant formula containing vitamins A, C and E; the minerals zinc, selenium and chromium; the herbs echinacea, ginkgo biloba and grape seed extract; and the amino acids cysteine, glutathione and methionine.

Other Beneficial Nutrients

Australian physician Ian Brighthope, M.B., B.S., (don't you love the name!) has observed that vitamin B6 (pantothenic acid), vitamin C, zinc and the amino acid L-arginine have assisted in achieving successful pregnancies in infertile women.[15]

L-arginine has also been shown in studies to help sperm problems.[16]

Another amino acid, L-carnitine, has been shown to increase sperm output. Italian researchers evaluated 100 patients with sperm motility problems, who received three grams a day of oral L-carnitine for 4 months. They found that the amino acid not only increased sperm output, but improved the amount and quality of the sperm.[17]

A case study reported in the *Journal of Assisted Reproduction and Genetics* described a couple who suffered with infertility for four years. Found to be anemic, the husband was treated with vitamin C and B vitamins until the anemia was corrected. Following this treatment, the couple were able to conceive. The authors attributed this happy outcome to his supplementation of vitamins C, B12 and folic acid, thus restoring his sperm's fertilizing capacity.[18]

Melvyn R. Werbach, M.D., reports that pernicious anemia, most often due to a deficiency of vitamin B12, leads to male infertility and can be reversed with B12 injections.[19]

In one double-blind study of 375 infertile men, 57 percent of the men whose sperm count was very low, responded to daily injections of B12.[20]

Infertile women can also benefit from vitamin B12 and folic acid.[21]

Fertility-Favorable Nutrients
For maximum absorption, take supplements with meals.

Nutrient	Suggested Dosage	Formulation
Acidophilus	At least four billion flora on an empty stomach, three times daily	
Aged garlic extract	1 teaspoon three times daily	Liquid
Amino acids	4-6 capsules daily	Multiple formula from natural sources
Antioxidants	4 capsules daily*	With selenium and grapeseed extract
Borage oil	2 capsules daily	
Coenzyme Q10	2 capsules daily	With vitamin E, phospholipids and selenium
Enzymes	2 capsules twice daily	Multiple formula
Fiber	4-8 tablets daily	Psyllium, with herb hyssop
Flaxseed oil	1 tablespoon daily	
Ginkgo biloba	60 mg daily	
Melatonin (adults only)	3 mg daily at bedtime	With B vitamins
Multi-mineral	3-4 ounces daily	In liquid solution, with vitamin B12, biotin
Multi-vitamin/mineral	6 caplets daily	Freeze-dried plant sources
Saw palmetto	160 mg twice daily for men and women	
Selenium	300 mcg daily	
Vitamin B6	100 mg daily	
Vitamin C	Individual bowel tolerance**	With bioflavonoids (quercetin, rutin proanthocyanidins)

* The FDA recommends pregnant women not exceed 10,000 IU of vitamin A daily.

** To determine individual dosage, on the first day take 1,000 mg hourly until diarrhea occurs, then reduce dosage to just below that for individual daily dosage. Vitamin C is not toxic in large doses but must be taken throughout the day to benefit. Divide dosage to three or four times a day.

CHAPTER 96:

Inflammation

Your arm is sore after playing tennis. You have cramps because it is that time of the month. You came home from that camping trip with poison oak. You woke up with a sore throat. Your son bumped his head and now he has a knot the size of Lake Erie. What do you do? First let me tell you what you *don't* do. You don't reach for the aspirin!

Inflammation is defined as redness, swelling, pain and heat, in localized areas of the body, due to tissue injury secondary to disease process, or trauma from physical, infections or chemical insult.[1] In other words, it hurts and it is swollen.

NSAIDs, or Non-Steroidal Anti-Inflammatory Drugs, are prescription and over-the-counter pain killers recommended by doctors and promoted extensively for all kinds of inflammation, from arthritis to bruises. Some are considered anti-inflammatory, some only take away the pain. Unfortunately NSAIDs do a lot more. Some examples are aspirin, ibuprofen (Motrin) and acetominophen (Tylenol).

One study showed NSAIDs increased the relative risk of peptic ulcer disease by four times compared to a control group. And if you think it happens only with long-term use, the study found the risk was greatest during the first month of use.[2]

Stanford University researchers found that arthritis patients taking NSAIDs were six times more likely to be hospitalized than those who were not. The researchers agreed that NSAIDs present the most common serious side effects of all conventional medicines.[3]

It's become so bad, researchers are looking at nutrients that protect against the effect of NSAIDs. In one study, zinc was shown to protect the stomach and intestinal lining against the incredibly corrosive effect of NSAIDs. Doctors in Spain found that supplementing with zinc increased protective mucous and strengthened cells.[4] Isn't it ironic? Instead of looking at nutrients to replace NSAIDs, they suggest we use nutrients to protect against them.

Zinc is also helpful in the fight against inflammation. During stress or inflammation there is a reduction in zinc concentrations of certain tissues and a redistribution of zinc internally. An article in the *Journal of the American College of Nutrition* states that in one study, head injury patients who received zinc supplementation had better healing, compared to those who received a placebo.[5]

Copper is important to balance out your zinc supplements. Be sure and include 2-4 mg. of copper with any zinc.

For all your mineral needs, target a minerals in solution formula. Minerals in solution are complete and more absorbable than hard tablets.

Non-steroidal Anti-Inflammatory Nutrients (NSAINs)

Try the sane approach to inflammation – N-SAIN. Instead of gut-busting, cell-wrenching NSAID pharmaceuticals, target safe and effective natural nutrients instead.

Several antioxidants have exhibited anti-inflammatory properties, and in some cases have proven to be as good or better than NSAIDs.

Selenium is a mineral valued for its ability to strengthen tissues and prevent further damage after injury. Its health benefits extend to preventing inflammation because it boosts the immune system, lessening the response to injury. In studies, selenium has been shown to be particularly effective for rheumatoid arthritis, as it increases oxygenation in synovial tissues in joint spaces, where inflammation occurs. In one particular four month trial, selenium helped approximately 40 percent of a small group of rheumatoid arthritic patients.[6]

Selenium-rich foods include tuna, herring, brewer's yeast, wheat germ and bran, whole grains and sesame seeds.

I know first hand the benefit of vitamin C with bioflavonoids on infection-caused inflammation. My husband's hand was saved from amputation by megadoses of C. Vitamin C is especially helpful in the case of allergy-caused inflammation, like puffy, itchy eyes and throat swelling. The symptoms of hay fever and other allergies, including inflammation, itchiness, runny nose, and constricted breathing, are caused by the body's misguided production of histamine, which the immune cells release as part of their normal immune response. The same stress that triggers the release of histamine also increases the need for vitamin C, the body's natural defense against excessive histamine. Thus, vitamin C helps reduce inflammation.

In a recent study at Arizona State University, Carol Johnston, Ph.D., gave nine people vitamin C supplements for six weeks, beginning with 500 mg daily and gradually increasing the amount to 2,000 mg per day.

By the time their daily intake of vitamin C had peaked, histamine levels had dropped an average of 40 percent![7] Bioflavonoids, compounds present in berries, most fruits and some vegetables, are potent anti-inflammatories. An article in the medical journal *The Lancet* (11/13/93), found that bioflavonoids effectively reduce the histamine reaction common in allergy reactions.

Bioflavonoids are often found in foods high in vitamin C and one in particular, quercetin, has been shown in studies to act as an antihistamine and anti-inflammatory.[8] Quercetin is so powerful, it is compared to cromolyn, a prescription antihistamine. Prescription antihistamines act by blocking the binding of histamine to cellular receptors, while quercetin actually inhibits the release of histamine and other inflammatory chemicals, and thus is even more effective in controlling inflammation.[9] Quercetin is found in yellow and red onions. Interestingly, applying a cut onion to an insect bite is a folk remedy.

Bioflavonoids like quercetin are also potent anti-inflammatories, useful in all problems that incur inflammation, like burns, arthritis, and, of course, insect bites. Leukotrienes are immune system chemicals believed to contribute to the swelling of insect bites. Quercetin, combined with bromelain extracted from pineapple for increased absorption, has been shown in studies to effectively inhibit the formation of leukotrienes.[10]

I recommend that anyone with allergies to seasonal pollen or insect bites supplement with vitamin C and bioflavonoids on a regular basis.

Target vitamin A to reduce skin inflammation, especially the swelling that occurs with cuts and burns. Vitamin A can increase skin collagen, reduce inflammation, increase postoperative immune suppression, improve healing and improve the appearance of scars. It is so good, it is sometimes applied directly to wounds with sponge implants.[11]

Another NSAID-substitute is vitamin E. It not only boosts the immune system, but it reduces the damage to tissues that results in inflammation, especially those of the skin. Vitamin E helps internally, as well as externally. This antioxidant also helps stabilize skin membranes so healing can occur. In one study, injured tendons healed in the presence of vitamin E were stronger than those healed without it. It was also noted that with the vitamin E, there were smaller and less scars.[12]

An Oily Solution

Many research studies point to essential fatty acids to reduce all kinds of inflammation. It can become very confusing when talking about the different kinds of fatty acids, which are the kinds of fats we need for energy and health – *not* saturated fat from meat and dairy products and certainly *not* transfatty acids from hydrogenated margarine and foods. Suffice it to say that omega-6 fatty acids are found in seeds and seed oils and that the best source is gamma-linolenic acid (GLA) from borage oil. GLA is a notoriously excellent anti-inflammatory.

I've already talked about two kinds of chemicals which create inflammation: histamine and leukotrienes. Another inflammation source is prostaglandin. NSAIDs work by reducing prostaglandins. Borage oil has been shown in studies to reduce all these chemicals. In one study, when nine borage seed oil capsules were given daily to arthritic volunteers for 12 weeks, there was a substantial reduction in prostaglandins and leukotrienes, thereby alleviating their painful arthritic symptoms.[13]

Controlled trials with GLA have shown sufficient benefit to warrant the approval of treatment by the National Health Service.[14]

A recent German study highlighted the anti-inflammatory benefits of omega-3 fatty acids. These oils quickly reduced inflammation in 20 patients suffering from psoriasis. Ten percent of patients with psoriasis also develop another inflammatory disease – arthritis.[15]

Independent clinical tests show that borage oil contains up to 26 percent GLA. Compare this to evening primrose oil and black currant oil, which contain no more than 18 percent. Not only that, borage oil costs less because the borage seed is three times larger than black currant or evening primrose seeds. Finally, borage is more bioavailable. In other words, the body more readily accepts it.[16] Take borage oil, while reducing NSAID dosage, and continue afterwards.

Beneficial Botanicals

"The beneficial effects attributed to aloe in the process of wound healing are so miraculous as to seem more like myth than fact," stated John P. Heggers, Ph.D., and colleagues of the University of Texas Medical Branch at Galveston.[17]

In both animal and human studies, the University of Texas research team found that, based on available data and their studies, aloe vera is a substance of "enormous therapeutic potential." It penetrates injured tissue, relieves pain, is anti-inflammatory and dilates capillaries, thereby increasing the blood supply to the injured area.

In the human studies, the researchers treated burns, frostbite and sores caused by intravenous drug use. They found that partial thickness burn wounds treated with aloe extracts healed faster and had less tissue loss than patients treated with standard techniques. Similarly, frostbite wounds treated with aloe extracts healed better.[17]

Turmeric has been used in both the Indian and Chinese systems of medicine for the treatment of many forms of inflammation. Its anti-inflammatory properties are likened to the pharmaceutical effects of hydrocortisone and phenylbutazone, only much safer.[18] To be more exact, it is the bioflavonoids in curcumin, that which gives tumeric its yellow color, that has been found in studies to work better than even ibuprofen, a popular over-the-counter pain medicine. In one study on rats, researchers found 20 mg of curcumin worked as well as 200 mg of ibuprofen. No toxic effects from curcumin have been reported.[19,20] Curcumin is a bioflavonoid, and also contains a large amount of vitamin C.

Bromelain, the active phytochemical in pineapple is also recommended when joints, muscles or ligaments are swollen and inflamed. Since you would have to eat two whole pineapples a day to achieve this anti-inflammatory effect, it's good we have health stores that carry bromelain extract.[21] Bromelain is recommended as a supplement with all the other anti-inflammatories since it acts as a digestive enzyme, helping to break down and assimilate other nutrients.

Licorice, specifically, glycyrrhiza, has valuable bursitis-busting properties. Licorice contains a remarkable chemical called glycyrrhetinic acid or GA, which is effective for treating inflammation.

Ginger has been noted in studies to be useful in inflammation and rheumatism. Danish researchers evaluated 28 patients with rheumatoid arthritis, 18 with osteoarthritis, and 10 with muscular discomfort using powdered ginger. In the arthritic patients, over 75 percent had varying degrees of relief from pain and swelling. All the patients with muscular discomfort, had pain relief. There were no reported side effects when ginger was eaten regularly from three months to 2.5 years.[22]

For more information on natural and safe anti-inflammatories, see the chapters on Arthritis, Burns, Bursitis, Carpal Tunnel Syndrome, Hemorrhoids, Infections, Migraines, Muscle Soreness, Skin Irritations and Sprains.

Anti-inflammatory Nutrients

For maximum absorption, take supplements with meals.

Nutrient	Suggested Dosage	Formulation
Aged garlic extract	1 teaspoon three times daily	Liquid
Antioxidants	4 capsules daily*	With selenium and grapeseed extract
Borage oil	2 capsules daily	
Bromelain	200 mg twice daily	
Flaxseed oil	1 tablespoon daily	
Ginger	500 mg after meals daily	
Magnesium	200 mg daily	
Melatonin (adults only)	3 mg daily at bedtime	With B vitamins
MSM (methylsulfonylmethane)	500 mg three times daily	
Multi-mineral	3-4 ounces daily	In liquid solution, with vitamin B12, biotin
Multi-vitamin/mineral	6 caplets daily	Freeze-dried plant sources
Niacinamide	1,000 mg twice daily	
Quercetin	400 mg twice daily	With vitamin C and bioflavonoids
Taurine	3 grams daily	
Vitamin B6	200 mg daily	
Vitamin C	Individual bowel tolerance**	With bioflavonoids (quercetin, rutin proanthocyanidins)

* The FDA recommends pregnant women not exceed 10,000 IU of vitamin A daily.

** To determine individual dosage, on the first day take 1,000 mg hourly until diarrhea occurs, then reduce dosage to just below that for individual daily dosage. Vitamin C is not toxic in large doses but must be taken throughout the day to benefit. Divide dosage to three or four times a day.

CHAPTER 97:

Insect Bites

"Sometimes men come by the name of genius in the same way that certain insects come by the name of centipede – not because they have a hundred feet, but because most people can't count above fourteen."
–G. C. Lichtenberg

Mary likes to garden, but is bothered by mosquito bites. She lives in a hot climate so she has to do most of her work in the early evening hours. Unfortunately, when the air cools, the mosquitos come out to feed – on her. Preferring not to coat herself with sticky, smelly chemical repellents, nor tolerate the lack of sleep and excessive itching she endured following a couple of hours outdoors, Mary sought help. What she learned, and more, is contained in the following paragraphs.

The first thing you need to realize is that it isn't the mosquito bite that causes the lump, redness and itching, it's the body's immune response to the anticoagulant the mosquito injects into the skin to keep the blood flowing.

Venom is a term that is loosely used when it comes to insect and snake bites. It can be a substance that, itself, is poisonous to the body, such as snake venom, or it can also mean anything that causes a harmful reaction in the body. For the most part, it is the body's immune-system reaction to a bite that causes the irritation and sometimes dangerous reaction. A reaction to an insect sting can be immediate or delayed. In most cases, the sooner the reaction starts the more severe it will be. The initial response usually begins in 10 to 20 minutes. Delayed reactions can occur several hours to several days later, producing painful joints, fever, hives, and swollen lymph glands. Both immediate and delayed reactions can occur in the same person following a single sting. If a reaction to an insect bite or sting increases, see a physician immediately.

One percent of the population is thought to be allergic to bees, wasps, and hornets. Approximately 60 deaths a year are attributed to insect stings in the United States, although some researchers say the true number is considerably higher because many such deaths are incorrectly labeled heart attacks.[1]

Natural Antihistamines

Histamine in the body is what causes the swelling, redness, itching, weals and even the life-threatening anaphylactic shock of insect bites and stings. Fortunately for us, we have access to natural antihistamines that work without the side effects of pharmaceuticals.

One of them is vitamin C. In a double-blind, placebo-controlled study at Arizona State University in Tempe, Carol Johnston, Ph.D., R.D., and colleagues gave nine people vitamin C supplements for six weeks, beginning with 500 mg daily and gradually increasing the amount to 2,000 mg per day. By the time their daily intake of vitamin C had peaked to bowel tolerance, histamine levels had dropped an average of 40 percent!

What is interesting to note is that the researchers did not see histamine levels drop until vitamin C intakes were at 1,000 milligrams.[2]

A nasty newcomer to the list of troublesome insects is the fire ant. Introduced accidentally many years ago in Alabama, it has spread to at least a dozen southern states and seems impossible to contain. If you've had the unpleasant experience of walking into a fire ant nest, you know you've been had when dozens of the tiny but painful pests are all over you, biting and repeatedly stinging like mad pitbulls. Experts say fire ants bite first, hanging on by their mandibles, then sting from their abdomen as many as 20 times. The sting causes swelling, bruising and blistering, and the pain lasts for 4-6 hours. The potent venom is a very real hazard to those allergic to it, capable of causing severe systemic (throughout the body) reactions.[3]

A friend of mine took her 3-year-old daughter, Sara, to Florida. While there, her daughter wandered into a hill of fire ants. Her mother recalls how Sara came running to her, screaming and crying. Lifting up her dress, her mother was horrified to see her back and legs literally covered in writhing black ants. After the ants had all been knocked off, they left angry welts. My friend had brought her daughter's chewable vitamin C tablets, and gave her three, 500 milligram tablets. With the exception of the slowly healing marks on her skin, Sara had no further reactions or discomfort.

Other antioxidants, specifically vitamin E and selenium have also demonstrated significant anti-allergy effects in experimental and clinical studies. Antioxidants prevent cell damage, which can contribute to symptoms.[4]

Bioflavonoids are often found in foods high in vitamin C and one in particular, quercetin, has been shown in studies to act as an antihistamine and anti-inflammatory. Robert Atkins, M.D., says that quercetin is "the most effective nutritional antihistamine I have seen yet." It also acts to protect vitamin C from becoming broken down in the body.[5]

Quercetin is so powerful, it is compared to cromolyn, a prescription antihistamine. Prescription antihistamines act by blocking the binding of histamine to cellular receptors, while quercetin actually inhibits the release of histamine and other inflammatory chemicals, and thus is even more effective in inhibiting the allergic response.[6]

Quercetin is found in yellow and red onions. Interestingly, applying a cut onion to an insect bite is a folk remedy.

Bioflavonoids like quercetin are also potent anti-inflammatories, useful in all problems that incur inflammation, like burns, arthritis, and, of course, insect bites. Leukotrienes are immune system chemicals believed to contribute to the swelling of insect bites. Quercetin, combined with bromelain extracted from pineapple for increased absorption, has been shown in studies to effectively inhibit the formation of leukotrienes.[7]

Bromelain is a digestive enzyme helpful for increasing absorption and assimilation of nutrients and food. Both bromelain and papain are digestive enzymes, called proteolytic enzymes, which break down protein. You've heard that you should use meat tenderizer on bee stings? Bromelain from pineapple and papain from papaya are proteolytic enzymes, meaning they break down protein, and are essentially meat tenderizers. The reason they work on bee stings is because bees inject a protein to break down blood. If applied soon enough, they will neutralize the protein before the body has a chance to recognize it as a foreign substance. Papaya is also high in vitamin C, so you can't go wrong there!

Bug Bite Prevention

Your best way to prevent insect stings and bites is to avoid contact with insects. Here are some tips so you won't look so inviting to the pesky critters.

- When you are outdoors, avoid wearing bright colors and strong, flowery odors (such as in perfume or scented cosmetics), which attract flying insects like bees, wasps and yellowjackets
- Avoid wearing loose-fitting clothes that may accidentally "trap" insects.
- Wear closed-toed shoes when you walk in grass (where many insects love to lurk).

- Whenever you work or play outdoors, check for bee hives and other insect nests in the vicinity first and then avoid these areas.

Some doctors believe that taking 50 mg of the B vitamin thiamine (B1), twice a day, may also provide your body with protection against insect bites.[8] Vitamin B1 has a noxious aroma. Large amounts are excreted in the sweat and may be effective in repelling mosquitoes.

When I was a child my naturopathic mother wore a string of garlic around her neck toward off the mosquitoes so that she could work outside in the evening. It worked – the mosquitoes stayed away. The peasants of Italy have long been aware of this pungent principle. Rural Italians eat tremendous amounts of garlic as part of their regular diet. In addition, they rub garlic juice on exposed parts of their bodies to ward off the blood suckers. Mosquitos avoid the garlic, not only because of its strong smell, but because garlic is fatal to them.

Many herbs and plants that contain volatile (smelly, that evaporate quickly) oils naturally repel insects. Lavender is one. During my European travels, I've noted that many people use lavender oil as an insect repellant. The oil is anti-bacterial so they use it also to soothe and heal bites. Europeans also grow basil, tansy, fennel or bay in their window boxes to keep insects away. Other volatile oils include eucalyptis, clove, menthol, camphor and tea tree oil. They can be used to prevent and treat bug bites. In this country, the oil of the citronella plant is being marketed as an insect repellant. You can get it in candles, in bottles, or you can buy the plant and hang it around your pool or patio.

Natural Remedies

To treat minor bites and stings, first wash the affected area thoroughly with an antibacterial soap. Look for a liquid soap that incorporates herbs that soothe and heal. I use a formula that includes anti-inflammatory and skin healing botanicals such as aloe vera, witch hazel, hawthorn, comfrey and honey. Comfrey and hawthorn berries are used in some skin ulcer medications.

To neutralize acidic bee stings, apply a paste of cornstarch or baking soda. For alkaline wasp stings, use vinegar or lemon juice.[9] For stings of all sorts, you can rub on any nonpoisonous green plant; the chlorophyll in the leaves will help relieve pain.[10]

Call a doctor if your child has a bite or sting inside the mouth or throat, or shows signs of a bad allergic reaction such as localized swelling, hives, nausea, vomiting, or stomach cramps; swelling of lips, face, eyes, or tongue; or difficulty swallowing or breathing.

Fresh banana or plantain skin applied to a bite or sting will draw infection out and provide soothing relief. When I was in Africa I hesitated to use a banana peel because I didn't want to attract the enormous numbers of flies and insects there. After rubbing the peel onto my rash I was astonished to realize not only did it provide instant relief from the itching, but repelled the flies as well!

These days, consumers are seeking out skin formulations that use botanicals, at the same time researchers are isolating the active ingredients in them that make them so wonderful. For soothing my overworked hands, I use a therapeutic lotion formula that contains an incredible array of soothing, healing and nutritional botanicals such aloe vera, avocado oil, lecithin, Kola, chamomile, lime tree, birch tree, oak bark, geranium, sage, ginseng, rosemary, sandalwood, clove, vitamin A and vitamin C. Some of these ingredients are antibacterials, some are flavonoids, some are wound healers and some are skin fortifiers. They all work together to soothe and heal damaged skin, and are your best defense against a six-legged offense.

Anti-Inflammatory Nutrients
For maximum absorption, take supplements with meals.

Nutrient	Suggested Dosage	Formulation
Aged garlic extract	1 teaspoon three times daily	Liquid
Antioxidants	4 capsules daily*	With selenium and grapeseed extract
Borage oil	2 capsules daily	
Enzymes	2 capsules twice daily	Multiple formula
Fiber	4-8 tablets daily	Psyllium, with herb hyssop
Flaxseed oil	1 tablespoon daily	
Magnesium	200 mg daily	
Melatonin (adults only)	3 mg daily at bedtime	With B vitamins
MSM (methylsulfonylmethane)	500 mg three times daily	
Multi-mineral	3-4 ounces daily	In liquid solution, with vitamin B12, biotin
Multi-vitamin/mineral	6 caplets daily	Freeze-dried plant sources
Niacinamide	1,000 mg twice daily	
Quercetin	400 mg twice daily	With vitamin C and bioflavonoids
Taurine	3 grams daily	
Vitamin B6	200 mg daily	
Vitamin C	Individual bowel tolerance**	With bioflavonoids (quercetin, rutin proanthocyanidins)

* The FDA recommends pregnant women not exceed 10,000 IU of vitamin A daily.

** To determine individual dosage, on the first day take 1,000 mg hourly until diarrhea occurs, then reduce dosage to just below that for individual daily dosage. Vitamin C is not toxic in large doses but must be taken throughout the day to benefit. Divide dosage to three or four times a day.

CHAPTER 98:

Kidney Stones

"I got one, I got one!"

I was visiting a friend in the hospital some years ago when I heard the ringing voice of a young Candy Striper as she quickly ran down the hall. It was a small hospital and she had been put in charge of straining the urine of kidney stone patients in the hopes of "catching" a passed stone. The odds were slim, she had been told, that she would be "lucky" enough to find a stone. She was a determined teen, however, and was diligent in her duty. So when she noted a small irregularly-shaped white "stone" at the bottom of the strainer, she immediately ran it to her supervisor, excited that she would be responsible for the discharge of her patient, who could go home now that his stone had passed without incident.

It is estimated that one in every thousand adults per year is hospitalized with kidney stones. About 60 percent of them will have another stone episode within seven years.[1]

Out of every 10,000 hospital admissions 7 to 21 are admitted for kidney stone problems. Almost 80 percent of kidney stones are composed mainly of calcium oxalate.[2] They occur when oxalic acid binds with calcium in the urine to form stones instead of being excreted.

Because of this oxalic acid connection, doctors may mistakenly (more about this later) recommend patients with chronic kidney stones avoid eating foods high in oxalic acid. One food, however, is said to counter this effect. Asparagus contains a substance that can break up oxalate crystals.[3]

Symptoms include pain originating in the middle back, which radiates around the stomach toward the genitalia, increased urine which may contain blood or pus, nausea and vomiting. Urinary tract infections may be caused by lodged stones that accumulate bacteria.

It appears that our diets have much to do with the prevalence of this often painful affliction. Cases of kidney stones have increased in Europe and the United States since the latter part of the 19th century and have been increasing steadily in Japan since the latter half of this century.

Researchers suspect that the dietary changes occurring with industrialization – the advent of processed food and more meat in the diet – play a significant role.

In one study, the daily dietary habits of 241 male kidney stone patients were evaluated over a seven year period. It was found that among the kidney stone patients, protein and carbohydrate intake was higher, as was calcium. The most telling fact?

Those who formed kidney stones had low amounts of magnesium, and they ate large meals consisting of animal protein at dinnertime and late evening.[4]

Along with these factors, too little potassium, common in refined-food diets; too much salt; and not enough fruits and vegetables make the urine too alkaline, eventually causing minerals to precipitate into stones.[5]

Another "civilized" habit can contribute to stones. Research shows that soft drinks can encourage the recurrence of kidney stones in some persons. This is because most sodas contain phosphoric acid, a component of some stones.[6]

The Magnesium and B6 Connection

Stones in your garden, maybe. Rolling Stones for your music – ugh! But no stones in your body! Once again we see the calcium channel-blocking effect of magnesium as studies show calcium oxalate stones in the kidney and other parts of the urinary tract are reduced by plenty of magnesium.

In Japan, researchers noted that the geological features of certain areas influenced the magnesium to calcium ratio of the tap water and the incidence of kidney stones among its populace. They found that in the basalt-rich areas of the country, the magnesium to calcium ratio was highest, with the people living there having the lowest incidence of stones. In the limestone area, with the lowest ratio of magnesium to calcium, residents had the highest incidence of kidney stones.[7]

Take your minerals in solution. Because of its high absorption rate, and deficiency of magnesium in the diet, the ratio of magnesium and calcium in solution should be four to one, respectively.

Three studies found 500 mg of magnesium decreased the kidney stone recurrence rate by 90 percent.

Dr. Jonathan Wright treats kidney stones with magnesium and vitamin B6. Magnesium makes calcium oxalate more soluble in urine, so it has less tendency to precipitate and form stones.[8]

A large study by the U.S. Department of Agriculture found that only 25 percent of 37,785 individuals had magnesium intakes at or greater than the recommended daily allowance, which is notoriously low. In a review of 15 studies it was found that a typical diet contains only a fraction of the RDA.[9]

Australian physician Dr. Ian Brighthope, M.B., B.S., concurs with Dr. Wright on behalf of magnesium and vitamin B6 in reducing the production of oxalate kidney stones.[10]

Because a very small percentage of the body's oxalic acid actually comes from oxalic acid-containing foods, these foods need not necessarily be restricted. That is good, because many magnesium rich foods contain oxalic acid. A deficiency of vitamin B6 is more to blame. This is because vitamin B6 is essential to the amino acid glycine.[11] Without B6, glycine creates oxalic acid inside the body, contributing more toward the formation of kidney stones than a can a day of almonds.

It has been found that B6 – a fragile and easily destroyed vitamin – is not present in fatty or processed foods. Vital B6 is lost in food transportation, storage, preservation, processing and cooking. Therefore, it is essential to add a B6 vitamin supplement (at least 200 mg daily) to your diet.

The B vitamins are like a military army. None individually are as strong as they are as a group. Always when supplementing one B vitamin, include a derived-from-nature, whole foods source of all the other B vitamins.

Decreasing Calcium Excretion with Rice Bran

Kidney stones can form when there is too much calcium in the urine, and instead of being excreted, solidifies into stones. Defatted rice bran contains phytin, which binds to calcium in the intestine, keeping it from becoming solid. Studies show this effect may be of benefit in preventing the recurrence of stones in people with too much calcium (doctors call this syndrome hypercalciuric or calcinosis).

In a clinical trial conducted at Wakayama Medical College in Japan, a total of 182 hypercalciuric patients with calcium-containing urinary stones received 10 grams of rice bran twice daily after meals for one to 94 months. Within the first month of treatment, there was a significant reduction in urinary calcium. In the 49 patients who received rice bran for more than three years, there was an obvious decline in the stone formation rate, as compared with the three years immediately preceding treatment. In 30 patients (61.2 percent), no new stones formed during rice bran treatment.[12]

The Importance of Water

Whether you are trying to lose weight or avoid stones, nothing is better than water.

Studies show too little water can encourage the precipitation of calcium into stones.

This is logical when you think about it. The next time you go potty look at your urine in the bowl. Is it light yellow and clear? Or is it dark yellow and milky? A clear urine will thoroughly flush your urinary tract clean, while dark urine will leave deposits along the way.

Researchers at a urinary and kidney stone clinic evaluated 819 patients for adequate water intake. They found that 19 percent of them had chronic dehydration. Once they drank more water, they excreted less concentrates.

Following up the patients for the next five years, the researchers concluded that chronic dehydration is a common cause of kidney stones and that it can be treated simply by increasing water intake.[13]

Especially in the summer, when the weather is warm, and when exercising, drink plenty of purified water. You don't have to avoid the mineral water, just make sure you drink at least two quarts of water a day. Add lemon juice, which cuts down on uric acid, which can also contribute to stones.

Stone Splitting Nutrients
For maximum absorption, take supplements with meals.

Nutrient	Suggested Dosage	Formulation
Amino acids	4-6 capsules daily	Multiple formula from natural sources
Antioxidants	4 capsules daily*	With selenium and grapeseed extract
Borage oil	2 capsules daily	
Enzymes	2 capsules twice daily	Multiple formula
Fiber	4-8 tablets daily	Psyllium, with herb hyssop
Flaxseed oil	1 tablespoon daily	
Glycosaminoglycans	50 mg three times daily	
Magnesium	200 mg twice daily	
Melatonin (adults only)	3 mg daily at bedtime	With B vitamins
Multi-mineral	3-4 ounces daily	In liquid solution, with vitamin B12, biotin
Multi-vitamin/mineral	6 caplets daily	Freeze-dried plant sources
Silica (horsetail)	300 mg daily	
Uva Ursi	50 mg three times daily	
Vitamin B6	100 mg daily	
Vitamin C	Individual bowel tolerance**	With bioflavonoids (quercetin, rutin proanthocyanidins)

* The FDA recommends pregnant women not exceed 10,000 IU of vitamin A daily.

** To determine individual dosage, on the first day take 1,000 mg hourly until diarrhea occurs, then reduce dosage to just below that for individual daily dosage. Vitamin C is not toxic in large doses but must be taken throughout the day to benefit. Divide dosage to three or four times a day.

CHAPTER 99:

Lactose Intolerance

Got milk?

Dairy industry ads are getting increasingly glamorous and enticing. Celebrities appear in magazines sporting milk moustaches, and television commercials feature chocolate and peanut butter gluttons desperate for a drink of milk. The commercials are funny, what milk does to some is not.

Have you ever experienced frequent cramps, bloating, gas, or diarrhea 15 minutes to three hours after consuming milk or milk products? Has your tolerance for milk products decreased over the years? Research has shown that as many as 28 percent of individuals do not realize they cannot digest milk sugar.[1]

Lactase, an enzyme produced in the small intestine, is responsible for breaking down milk sugar, lactose, into simpler forms to be absorbed into the bloodstream. Production of lactase may start to drop off after the age of two years. For some people, production may stop much later in life. The severity of the symptoms experienced is dose dependent and varies with each individual.

Studies have shown that many people suffering from lactose intolerance do not make the connection between their indigestion and their diet. At one research center, 66 percent of 242 patients referred for evaluation of various abdominal complaints were found to be lactose intolerant. Seventy percent of these patients had not related their symptoms to milk drinking. Forty-two percent of these test subjects, in fact, didn't relate their symptoms to intake of any particular food.[2]

You may be one of the estimated 30-50 million Americans who suffer from lactose intolerance. Certain ethnic and racial populations seem to be affected more than others. Studies have shown as many as 75 percent of all African-Americans and Native Americans and 90 percent of Asian-Americans show signs of lactose intolerance.[3] In Northern European populations, only about five percent of people cannot digest lactose.[4] I am among that unlucky five percent.

It's important not to confuse lactose intolerance with milk allergy. There are people allergic to milk because of a protein called *casein* contained in milk. A milk allergy gives a rash to people who are allergic and normally doesn't give them diarrhea. Talk to your doctor if you're uncertain.

What Causes Lactose Intolerance?

Anything that destroys intestinal bacteria can cause a temporary case of lactose intolerance. This includes aspirin, non-steroidal anti-inflammatory drugs and antibiotics. Gastroenteritis and small intestine disorders, such as viruses, surgery or parasites may also cause a relative lactase deficiency.

A definite link has been found between lactose intolerance and irritable bowel syndrome (IBS). At the University of Louisville School of Medicine, researchers discovered that up to 34 percent of their patients with IBS also had lactose intolerance.[5] In one study, out of 242 IBS patients, 67 percent could not digest milk sugar. What I find most interesting, and which suggests IBS may have been caused by whatever caused the intolerance, is that a lactose-restricted diet led to a complete remission of symptoms in 43 percent of these patients, partial remission in 41 percent, and that only 15 percent did not see some improvement, compared to controls.[6]

Check food labels for lactose-rich ingredients like whey, whey protein concentrate and milk solids. They're commonly used in many types of processed foods, including some you might consider lactose-free, such as chewing gum and frozen dinners.

Be aware that some over-the-counter and prescription pharmaceutical products contain lactose as well. Among them: Centrum Silver vitamin supplements, Contact cold medication, Maalox caplets and Premarin prescribed for estrogen replacement therapy.[7]

If lactose intolerance keeps you from drinking pasteurized milk, you're better off. Pasteurized milk is good for corporate profits, but bad for consumer health. Pasteurized milk can sit on your grocer's shelf without spoiling because it has had the life force removed from it. The heating of milk during pasteurization destroys much of its vitamins B2 and B12, vitamin C, calcium, phosphorus and iodine. It denatures protein, and destroys 90 percent of the enzymes that help us utilize lactose, protein, fats, starches, phosphorus and calcium.

Supplement with Lactase and
Change Your Milk-Drinking Habits

One option for this problem is to avoid milk and other lactose-laden dairy products. But if milk appeals to your palate, the other is to supplement with the enzyme you're missing. The FDA poo-poos the sale of enzyme supplements in 99 percent of the cases, even when a plethora of studies show them to be of benefit. But when corporate backers like those within the dairy industry are involved, enzyme supplementation becomes highly accepted and recommended.

Available just about anywhere these days, the supplement is a non-prescription lactase enzyme, called B-galactosidase. The pill form may be chewed or swallowed, and the liquid form can be added to milk. Don't pay more for less. Consumers should choose lactase enzymes measured in FCC measurements. This is a measure of the enzyme activity and efficacy.[8]

If you really like milk, choose raw *certified* milk available more and more on your grocery store shelves, and if not, at your local health food store. I'm lactose intolerant and drink nothing but Stueve's. I've been to the Stueve's Alta Dena dairy and seen first-hand the great pains they take to keep their product clean. White towels are used to wipe cows' udders until they are clean of mud and fecal matter, and cows are tested daily. No antibiotics or hormones are used on the cows. They don't need antibiotics because they are healthy.

Milk pasteurization was instituted to kill the germs caused by poor sanitation, such as dead flies lying in open pails, on early dairy farms. Natural certified raw milk is tested daily. Certification means adhering to very high standards of cleanliness, so pasteurization, or boiling, is not needed. In its fresh, natural state, milk has a better taste and contains the properties important to good nutrition that are altered when milk is pasteurized and homogenized. Certified raw milk is also recommended for its digestibility. Because it is not heated, the enzymes that help us digest it are not killed.

Target Lactose-Free Dairy Foods

You like yogurt? Good! Because studies show yogurt doesn't bother lactose-intolerant people. Research by Joseph Kolars and colleagues at the University of Minnesota and the Veterans Administration reported in the *New England Journal of Medicine* that eight out of 10 lactose intolerant individuals were free of distressing symptoms when they ate yogurt. That's because the bacterial culture in yogurt, called lactobacillus acidophilus, produces lactase.[9]

The live cultures in yogurt digest the lactose. But it must be real, unpasteurized yogurt. Someone who's lactose intolerant and eats yogurt could have a cup of yogurt at a time if it contains live cultures. (Unfortunately, frozen yogurts don't pass that test.) Avoid yogurts labeled "heat-treated after culturing," and which do not contain active cultures. I go out of my way to get Alta Dena yogurt. It has all natural flavorings.

Aged cheeses are low in lactose. Choose Cheddar, blue cheese, Brie, Parmesan, colby, Camembert and Limburger. (Of course, seek out low-fat versions of these for your health.)

If you are concerned about losing calcium because you lose the dairy products, have no fear. There are many dairy-free sources of calcium such as green leafy vegetables, watercress, spinach, dandelion greens, peas, parsley, mint, chickpeas, molasses, sesame seeds, cheese, brewer's yeast, sardines, caviar, salmon, torula yeast, soybeans, brazil nuts, egg yolk, sunflower seeds, and walnuts.

Because of the risk of colon problems among the lactose intolerant, the following list is designed to promote a healthy intestinal system.

Colon-Restoring Nutrients
For maximum absorption, supplements should be taken with meals.

Nutrient	Suggested Dosage	Formulation
Acidophilus	At least four billion flora daily on an empty stomach, three times daily	
Aged garlic extract	2 teaspoons three times daily	Liquid
Amino acids	4-6 capsules daily	Multiple formula from natural sources
Borage oil	2 capsules daily	
Coenzyme Q10	2 capsules daily	With vitamin E, phospholipids and selenium
Enzymes	2 capsules twice daily	Multiple formula
Flaxseed oil	1 tablespoon daily	
Fiber	8 tablets daily	Psyllium, with herb hyssop
Multi-vitamin/mineral	6 caplets daily	Freeze-dried plant sources
Multi-mineral	2-4 ounces daily	In liquid solution, with vitamin B12, biotin
Vitamin C	Individual bowel tolerance*	With bioflavonoids (quercetin, rutin proanthocyanidins)

* To determine individual dosage, on the first day take 1,000 mg hourly until diarrhea occurs, then reduce dosage to just below that for individual daily dosage. Vitamin C is not toxic in large doses but must be taken throughout the day to benefit. Divide dosage to three or four times a day.

CHAPTER 100:

Laryngitis

In a recent study, the United States Department of Agriculture discovered a sad fact: most Americans are not only failing to get optimal nutrition, but are actually deficient in many nutrients needed to strengthen the immune system and prevent and treat the viruses that can cause laryngitis. At least one third of us consume less than 70 percent of the Recommended Dietary Allowances for vitamin A, vitamin C, vitamin B1 (thiamine), vitamin B2 (riboflavin), vitamin B3 (niacin), vitamin B12 and the minerals calcium, magnesium and zinc.[1] Considering the fact that the RDA is too low to begin with, this is very telling indeed.

Acute laryngitis is usually caused by a virus but can result from a bacterial infection. Chronic laryngitis can be caused by heavy smoking, overuse of the voice by speaking or singing loudly, coughing violently, or exposure to chemical irritants. Many a singer, including Barbara Streisand, has had to cancel concert tours when their voices simply gave out.

Symptoms include low, raspy voice and hoarseness, dry cough (no mucus), wheezing, dry throat, little or no pain, and weakening voice as the day progresses. The symptoms are not caused so much by the initial cause, but by the inflammation that occurs as the body fends off the infection. The telltale signs of laryngitis: hoarseness and embarrassing inability to talk without squeaking or losing the ability altogether, is caused by swelling of the lining of the larynx, making the vocal cords incapable of working properly. The best course of action? Treat the problem by boosting the body's ability to defend and heal itself through good nutrition, and treat the symptoms through inflammation-reducing nutrients. Happily, many of the nutrients that boost the immune system also reduce inflammation. This is because inflammation is the immune system's response to injury, and by helping the immune system, these nutrients limit the need for the inflammatory response.

Vitamin C Proven to Help

Vitamin C is a good example of an immune-boosting anti-inflammatory. Coupled with bioflavonoids, it reduces swelling and inflammation, which not only helps laryngitis symptoms, but avoids long-term damage to delicate tissues.

As an antioxidant, it minimizes cell damage from injury or illness. This means it prevents the destruction of body cells. Researchers have noted that during a flu infection, a large number of neutrophils – bad guys – occur in the body. Neutrophils release large amounts of oxidizing materials that can damage cell tissue. What scientists have noted is that during a flu infection, large amounts of vitamin C are used up. As an infection progresses, there is significant decrease in vitamin C concentration. Harri Hemila, a researcher with the University of Helsinki, Finland, did his own studies of this process and believes the body uses vitamin C to fight infection, and when stores are low, the body suffers for it. He believes six grams (6,000 milligrams) a day of vitamin C during a flu can maximize the body's battle. He notes that the diet of our ancestors contained 0.4 to 2 grams (400-2,000 mgs) of vitamin C

In a controlled study by biochemist G. Ritzel, schoolboys taking 1,000 mg/day of vitamin C averaged a 45 percent decrease in the number of days it took for them to recover from a viral infection. In addition, the results of 16 controlled research projects indicated a 31 percent decrease in infections in vitamin C users than in volunteers who took placebos. Subjects who used more vitamin C averaged a 40 percent decrease.

In an amazing discovery, vitamin C has been found to be helpful in the continuing battle against bacteria that have become immune to antibiotics. For more on this incredible story, see the Infections chapter.

Power-Pack Vitamin C with Bioflavonoids

Now you know that vitamin C, while it can't cure laryngitis, can keep you from getting it. As it turns out, there's even more you can do. You can make sure your vitamin C includes bioflavonoids.

At the Creighton University School of Medicine, Omaha, Nebraska, a group of nurses was given tablets containing the two substances. The nurses were checked for one year, as was another group which received a placebo.

The nurses receiving the vitamin C and bioflavonoids had 55 percent fewer flu infections than the placebo group, and they lasted an average of 3.9 days, compared to 6.7 days for the placebo group.[5] Imagine a flu that lasts only three days! If this news gets around, employers will be paying a lot less in sick time.

Kathryn Grayson, veteran of screen and stage, is the only one of her vintage generation still singing. She filled The Paladium in London and still tours, sharing her four range-voice with thousands of fans. Her secret is vitamin C with bioflavonoids. Vocal cords are made of collagen, which flap together to produce sound. Vitamin C plumps out collagen while bioflavonoids protects against damage from overuse.

In one study, 20 of 22 patients with respiratory infections of varying intensity recovered in an 8- to 48-hour period after treatment with bioflavonoids and vitamin C. The patients received 600 mg of each of the two substances every day. Now, imagine laryngitis only lasting two days!

Quercetin, a particularly potent bioflavonoid, acts as a natural anti-inflammatory, allowing you to clear your medicine chest of all the dangerous over-the-counter remedies you used to take.

Some European studies have found that bioflavonoids slow bacterial and viral infections.[6] Quercetin has been shown to be effective against many viruses, including viruses that cause laryngitis, according to the *Journal of Medical Virology*.[7] Quercetin is found in citrus fruit rind.

Other Anti-Inflammatory Antioxidants

Selenium is a mineral valued for its ability to strengthen tissues and prevent further damage after injury. Its health benefits extend to preventing inflammation because it boosts the immune system, lessening the response to injury. In studies, selenium has been shown to increase oxygenation in synovial tissues in joint spaces, where inflammation occurs.[8]

Vitamin E not only boosts the immune system, but it reduces the damage to tissues that results in inflammation, especially those of the skin.

Vitamin E helps internally, as well as externally. This antioxidant also helps stabilize skin membranes so healing can occur. In one study, injured tendons healed in the presence of vitamin E were stronger than those healed without it. It was also noted that with the vitamin E, there were smaller and less scars.[9]

Oil for Inflammation

Many research studies point to essential fatty acids to reduce all kinds of inflammation. It can become very confusing when talking about the different kinds of fatty acids, which are the kinds of fats we need for energy and health – *not* saturated fat from meat and dairy products and certainly *not* transfatty acids from hydrogenated margarine and foods. Suffice it to say that omega-6 fatty acids are found in seeds and seed oils and that the best source is gamma-linolenic acid (GLA) from borage oil. GLA is a notoriously excellent anti-inflammatory.

Independent clinical tests show that borage oil contains up to 26 percent GLA. Compare this to evening primrose oil and black currant oil, which contain no more than 18 percent. Not only that, borage oil costs less because the borage seed is three times larger than black currant or evening primrose seeds. Finally, borage is more bioavailable. In other words, the body more readily accepts it.[10] Take borage oil, obtained in health food stores or through mail order, instead of Tylenol or aspirin.

Over 50 years ago scientists first discovered vitamin A's value in treating and preventing viral infections. For example, in 1942, Italian physician Di Salvatore Princi published his study results that showed mice had more resistance to an influenza germ if they were given vitamin A. In 1937, German doctor Torsten Lindquist found that the vitamin A content of the blood was drastically lowered during the first five days of illness. When the patient began to get better, the level of vitamin A rose dramatically, even though no vitamin A was added to the diet. His assumption was that it was used somehow in the healing process.[11]

Dr. Garry Gordon, M.D., residing in Tempe, Arizona while engaged in full time research, recommends taking vitamin A and garlic together, with vitamin C, at the first sign of viral symptoms, usually for a period of not less than three and not more than five days. He says that taking vitamin A directly, rather than in the form of beta carotene is most desirable. He recommends taking 500,000 IU when sick, and that high doses are safe as long as the person's weight is over 120 pounds, there is no serious liver condition, and high doses aren't taken daily over weeks or months.[12]

Vitamin A is believed to work against laryngitis by strengthening and restoring the mucous membranes of the throat. The role of mucous is to flush out germs and foreign matter so they can't take hold and damage the system. If membranes are weak and thin, their ability to defend the body are compromised. Vitamin A prevents infections by making sure the membranes within are strong enough to push germs and mucous out, and alleviates the symptoms by keeping membranes moist so there is less dryness and pain.[13]

Learn Sign Language

Along with nutrients, you can support your larynx by taking the advice of Dr. Robert Ossoff, an ear-nose-and-throat specialist and medical director of the Vanderbilt University Voice Center. Dr. Ossoff has become a leading consultant to country singers whose vocal cords are frayed, whose voices are reduced to a whisper, whose throats ache like Billy Ray Cyrus's heart – or who just want to know how to keep their "instrument" in good singing order. He ministers to some of America's twangiest vocal cords, with such notable clients as Naomi and Wynonna Judd, Larry Gatlin, Kathy Mattea, Crystal Gayle, Randy Travis, Ricky Van Shelton, Reba McEntire, Johnny Cash and K. T. Oslin.[14]

He advises his patients to avoid caffeine and chocolate [they dry up the larynx] and dairy products [they thicken the larynx mucus, necessitating excessive throat-clearing] and he tells them to drink a lot of water. Ossoff also recommended the use of a steam inhaler before speeches or singing engagements to "loosen things up."

Patients looking for a quick fix may want a different doctor. Before he even looks at a larynx, Ossoff probes into some unexpected corners of his patients' lives: Do they eat junk food? Do they sleep on a full stomach? Do they sleep on their right side? (All of these factors can expose the larynx to burning stomach acid.) Ossoff advises singers to allow at least five minutes of warmup exercises, for example, scales and arpeggios, and 15 minutes of cool down – no talking – for every show. And he suggests they install humidifiers on their tour buses.

Did you think whispering was OK? Whispering puts as much tension on the vocal cords as does shouting.[15] If you can't speak normally while suffering from laryngitis, don't speak at all.

Gargling doesn't help because the fluid cannot get far enough down to reach the larynx. Instead, drink plenty of tepid water to keep the throat moist. Don't drink cold water or eat ice, which constricts the vocal cords. Don't drink milk, which creates mucus, don't clear the throat, which irritates, and don't take menthol or mint throat lozenges, which have a drying effect. To soothe stressed vocal cords use a steam vaporizer to moisten the larynx and sip warm water with a small amount of honey. Avoid mint tea, choosing instead bioflavonoid-bountiful berry and citrus teas.

Larynx-Loving Nutrients
For maximum absorption, take supplements with meals.

Nutrient	Suggested Dosage	Formulation
Aged garlic extract	1 teaspoon three times daily	Liquid
Amino acids	4-6 capsules daily	Multiple formula from natural sources
Antioxidants	4 capsules daily*	With selenium and grapeseed extract
Borage oil	2 capsules daily	
Coenzyme Q10	2 capsules daily	With vitamin E, phospholipids and selenium
Echinacea	200 mg daily	
Enzymes	2 capsules twice daily	Multiple formula
Fiber	4-8 tablets daily	Psyllium, with herb hyssop
Flaxseed oil	1 tablespoon daily	
Multi-mineral	3-4 ounces daily, gargled, then swallowed	In liquid solution, with vitamin B12, biotin
Multi-vitamin/mineral	6 caplets daily	Freeze-dried plant sources
Vitamin A	25,000 IU daily*	
Vitamin B6	100 mg daily	
Vitamin C	Individual bowel tolerance**	With bioflavonoids (quercetin, rutin proanthocyanidins)
Vitamin E	2 capsules (800 IU) daily	d-alpha tocopherol
Zinc lozenges	15 mg three times daily	

* The FDA recommends pregnant women not exceed 10,000 IU of vitamin A daily.

** To determine individual dosage, on the first day take 1,000 mg hourly until diarrhea occurs, then reduce dosage to just below that for individual daily dosage. Vitamin C is not toxic in large doses but must be taken throughout the day to benefit. Divide dosage to three or four times a day.

CHAPTER 101:

Leukemia

Leukemia – the word strikes fear into the hearts of any parent faced with the diagnosis. According to the National Cancer Institute (NCI) and the Leukemia Society of America, about 28,000 Americans were diagnosed with leukemia in 1992. Fewer than 35 percent of them are likely to be alive today. What you probably didn't know was that leukemia is most common – and most likely to be fatal – in the elderly.[1] This is because leukemia attacks the immune system, and older people typically have lowered immune systems, leaving them little to fight with.

Leukemia is not a single disease, but a group of malignancies in which the bone marrow and other blood-forming organs produce excessive numbers of immature or abnormal white blood cells. The extra cells suppress the production of normal white blood cells, the function of which is to protect the body against infection.

Malignant cells "take over" the bone marrow and prevent it from producing red blood cells, which transport oxygen around the body, and platelets, which help blood clot. They also invade other organs, such as the liver, spleen, lymph nodes, genitals, and brain.

What we are dealing with here are basically cells that have mutated or have "birth defects" if you will. Why they mutate relates most strongly to environmental factors. Situations from prenatal exposure to electric blankets, to workplace toxins, to the close and long-term presence of power lines have been associated with an increased risk of leukemia.[2] People living around toxic waste dumps have been shown to have a high incidence of leukemia. It's obvious that anything, including the chemicals we eat in our food, that alters cell DNA is going to create a risk, however small, of getting leukemia.

A headline in the *Los Angeles Times*, June 3, 1994 proclaimed "Hot Dogs Linked to Cancer." John Peters, a University of Southern California epidemiologist reported in the scientific journal *Cancer Causes and Control*, that children who eat more than 12 hot dogs a month have nine times the normal risk of developing childhood leukemia. Two other reports in the journal suggest children born to mothers who eat at least one hot dog a week during pregnancy have double the normal risk of developing brain tumors, as do children whose fathers ate hot dogs before conception. Researchers point to reports like these as explaining why the cases of childhood leukemia and brain tumors have increased over the last two decades. The symptoms of leukemia, not coincidentally, may be the same as when the immune system breaks down. A patient with leukemia may go to the doctor feeling extremely sick, complaining of recurrent infections, bleeding, bruising, bone tenderness, fever, chills, sweats, weakness, fatigue, headaches, or swelling in the neck, armpits or groin.

On the other hand, the patient may have no symptoms at all and the disease may be discovered by chance from a routine blood test. It depends on how many cells have been affected.

A normal blood smear contains many red cells and platelets and a few white cells. In leukemia, the blood usually contains many abnormal white cells and not enough red cells and platelets. Such an abnormal blood count is the physician's first clue that the patient may have leukemia. This initial signal is also a symptom of a nutritional deficiency that can be misdiagnosed as leukemia, if nutritional testing is not done.

Nutritional Deficiency Mimics Leukemia

Imagine being told you or a loved one has leukemia, steeling yourself for the prospect of a long-term illness, only to discover it was a nutritional deficiency instead. It has happened, and as a result, doctors are cautioning their colleagues not to make this mistake.

> French researchers found that two out of three patients diagnosed as having leukemia actually had a severe deficiency of folic acid and vitamin B12 – pernicious anemia. With 30 to 45 days of vitamin therapy, there was complete normalization of their blood counts.[3]

An article in the *British Medical Journal* described the case of a 43-year-old woman who suffered for three months with fatigue, no appetite, shortness of breath and nosebleeds. Her blood count indicated leukemia and doctors prepared to start her on chemotherapy. Fortunately, realizing the great detriment chemotherapy has on the immune system, doctors did a series of preparatory tests to determine her nutritional status. When she was found to be malnourished and nutrient deficient, she was given 1,000 micrograms of B12 and five milligrams of folic acid. After two weeks doctors found her blood count much improved. They ordered more tests and finally determined she had pernicious anemia, not leukemia. In two to three months, her blood count was normal and her symptoms subsided.[4]

For more on pernicious anemia, see the chapter Anemia in this book.

There is no way of knowing how many people have been or are being misdiagnosed. The scary part is, conventional cancer therapies are documented as causing leukemia, and leukemia is known to recur following conventional therapies. As I will describe later, it is quite possible that in attempting to cure the cause, conventional medicine may be creating the problem.

Newest Hope is Vitamin A

Would you believe the FDA is allowing vitamin A to be used for leukemia?[5] Well, not quite. Remember, if it can't be pharmaceuticalized, it can't be patented, and profits can't be made.

It all started when researchers at the University of California, Irvine, Clinical Care Center uncovered it as a treatment for a type of "middle-aged" leukemia. In a 15-year national trial, clinical Director Frank L. Meyskens Jr., M.D., and fellow researchers discovered that a combination of vitamin A and Busulfan, a chemotherapeutic agent, postponed the acute phase of chronic myelogenous leukemia (CML) for eight or nine months. Symptoms of CML include mild fatigue, weakness and anemia, and typically occurs among people in their 40s and 50s, unlike other forms of leukemia.

In a presentation of his findings to more than 500 cancer specialists on March 12, 1993, at the Seventh International Conference on the Adjuvant Therapy of Cancer held in Tucson, Arizona, Meyskens concluded that relatively low doses of vitamin A helps increase the survival rate of patients with CML because "vitamin A has chemopreventive, immunologic and anti-tumor properties."[6]

Since vitamin A is considered a food, not a drug, pharmaceutical companies had to come up with another form. About the closest thing is retinoic acid, a relative of vitamin A and the active ingredient of the skin treatment Retin-A. Other researchers discovered the same benefits. At least that's the news from laboratories in China, France and the U.S., including the prestigious (and oh, *so* conventional) Memorial Sloan-Kettering.

It was there that Raymond Warrell, M.D., treated 79 patients with acute promyelocytic leukemia with retinoic acid. In his trials, 86 percent of patients achieved a complete remission. Unlike chemotherapy, which blasts all rapidly dividing cells – thereby inflicting miserable side effects – retinoic acid induces cancer cells to mature and follow an abbreviated life cycle. Says Warrell, "They just grow up and die."[7]

Factors interfering with absorption of vitamin A and beta carotene include strenuous physical activity within four hours of consumption, intake of mineral oil, excessive consumption of alcohol and iron, and the use of cortisone and other drugs.

The Rimland Experience

Bernard Rimland, Ph.D., of San Diego, is known worldwide for his nutritional therapies for psychological and emotional disorders. He started studying cancer intensively some 17 years ago when his teenage daughter was found to have what was then considered to be a terminal type of cancer: Hodgkins disease, stage 4B.

Tests revealed her liver and kidneys were deeply affected – doctors had never seen anyone with kidneys so impaired. They gave her six to eight months to live. Dr. Rimland's in-depth reading of medical literature showed him there was a tremendous amount of knowledge about the disease that wasn't being utilized.

He immediately started her on 40 grams of vitamin C a day, orally, as well as a gram of niacinamide, 50 mg of the other B vitamins, 800 IU of vitamin E and 75,000 IU of vitamin A, as well as calcium, magnesium and other minerals in normal amounts.

He told me:

"Although the oncologists were giving her chemotherapy – those horrible chemicals – and she lost all of her hair, they assured me their efforts wouldn't help a case this far gone. (Despite their contentions), she began to improve at a spectacular rate."

Seeing her great improvement – as the oncologists did, too – Dr. Rimland kept photocopying pages of medical literature about the efficacy of vitamin C to take to the oncologists. They paid no attention to them. He would return to the doctor's office two or three weeks later, and the reports would still be on their desks, not even unfolded.

"Meanwhile," he said, "the (other) kids, most of them with leukemia, were dying like flies. I remembered Irwin Stone's writing which noted that the symptoms of leukemia are identical to those of scurvy."

Dr. Rimland continued: "Stone used to say, 'If you run a vitamin C blood test, someone with leukemia would have almost zero vitamin C. If you gave that person a lot of vitamin C, the blood level would still measure zero. So you have to give them massive amounts to get the blood level anywhere near normal. And, if you did, the symptoms of leukemia would go away. Stone published case histories of people who recovered and did very well."

I am happy to report that Dr. Rimland saved the life of his daughter, and she's completely recovered today. The super-nutritional program worked and probably could have saved the lives of many of the little kids in her ward. Tragically, the doctors ignored the research. It had to be their way or no way. Unfortunately for those little children, it was often no way.

Antioxidants Prevent Cell Damage

Antioxidants are truly nature's wonder. They are beneficial not only because the body needs them, but because they are invaluable defenders against the chemical onslaught we face daily from our environment. The best defense? A complete and thorough supplemental antioxidant formula containing vitamins, minerals and botanical antioxidant sources.

You've already read testimony in favor of vitamin C. Vitamin C-rich foods high in bioflavonoids – antioxidants themselves, which have their own anti-inflammatory and cell protectant properties. One particularly potent flavonoid is quercetin.

The most recent study on quercetin was conducted by the National Toxicology Program. Researchers found that among male rats quercetin protected against cancer. Quercetin is enhanced by vitamin C, and is reported as being beneficial in the treatment of acute leukemia. It works with rutin, a related flavonoid. Both flavonoids have been used for a variety of medical problems throughout the world, and is sometimes referred to as vitamin P. Studies indicate quercetin, rutin and vitamin C together may contribute toward a reduction of leukemia cells.[8]

Did you know zinc is an antioxidant? This underestimated mineral is found to be deficient among people suffering from most degenerative diseases, especially those affecting cell DNA. A deficiency of zinc shows itself in the thymus gland, the master immune system regulator by reducing the amount of hormone it produces.

Researchers at the Immunology Center, National Research Centers on Aging, Ancona, Italy, found that "in 91 young patients affected by acute lymphoblastic leukemia...it was discovered that the plasma zinc level was reduced at the onset and (during) relapse, whereas in complete remission and in off-therapy it was in the normal range." The researchers also found low levels of thymulin, a hormone necessary for a functioning immune system, when there were low levels of zinc.[9]

What is interesting to me is the connection between the male sex glands and zinc. Among populations exposed to radioactive fallout, studies show those with enough zinc in their systems were protected against their offspring bearing the mutagenic brunt of the impact.

This was the finding of British researchers who discovered a high incidence of leukemia in children whose fathers have been exposed to external radiation before conception at the Sellafield Nuclear facility in the United Kingdom. Zinc is found in high concentrations in the semen and is crucially important for proper functioning of DNA. Described in an article in the *British Medical Journal*, the researchers believe adequate zinc keeps metals out of the sex glands which attracts cell- and DNA-destroying radiation. Sperm mutated by radiation produce offspring with cell mutations that translate into leukemia.[10]

According to Utah researchers as many as seven of 17 leukemia deaths in a Utah county nearest a Nevada nuclear test site, and 50 of 1,177 leukemia deaths statewide may be related to the fallout from open air nuclear testing which occurred in the 1950s.[11]

Australian researchers have discovered that zinc inhibits a process known as apoptosis, which basically destroys the immune system and alters cell DNA. In a study of this effect, researchers at The Queen Elizabeth Hospital in Woodville, South Australia, exposed chronic lymphatic leukemia cells to zinc. They discovered that this apoptosis process was completely inhibited in the presence of zinc concentrations.[12]

Copper is important to balance out your zinc supplements. Be sure and include 2-4 mg of copper in a full spectrum mineral in solution formula, with any zinc.

Leukemia Following Conventional Cancer Therapies

You know that chemicals cause leukemia. You also know that radiation causes leukemia. Therefore, is it any surprise that conventional chemical and radiation therapies cause leukemia?

Hundreds of cancer survivors each year develop leukemia as a result of previous therapy. Bad enough that it happens at all, but these malignancies tend to be chemotherapy resistant or difficult to treat. Conventional medicine calls them secondary leukemias, and they are being identified with increasing frequency.[13]

Radiotherapy and many forms of chemotherapy inevitably produce DNA damage, according to Stephen Forman, M.D., of the City of Hope National Medical Center in Duarte, California. He states that patients undergoing bone marrow transplants are often treated with the very things that cause leukemias.[14]

One study looked at 114 cases of leukemia following conventional ovarian cancer treatment. It was found that the chemotherapy alone increased the patients' risk of leukemia by as much as 12 times compared to surgery. Radiotherapy increased the risk ten times. The risk of leukemia was greatest four or five years after chemotherapy began and lasted for at least eight years. Cyclophosphamide, Chlorambucil, Melphalan, Thiotepa and Treosulfan were independently associated with increased risk of leukemia. Chlorambucil and Melphalan were found to be the most leukemogenic drugs.[15]

The good news? Folic acid can protect against this effect.

Dr. Richard Albertini, Ph.D., of the University of Vermont College of Medicine in Burlington, studied white blood cells of women who had been treated for breast cancer. He found a high frequency of mutant cells following chemotherapy but – get this – only in those with low or marginal blood levels of folic acid.[16] It's amazing what doctors can learn when they consider the nutritional factor.

Leukemia-Fighting Nutrients
For maximum absorption, take supplements with meals.

Nutrient	Suggested Dosage	Formulation
Acidophilus	At least four billion flora on an empty stomach, three times daily	
Aged garlic extract	1 teaspoon three times daily	Liquid
Amino acids	4-6 capsules daily	Multiple formula from natural sources
Antioxidants	4 capsules daily*	With selenium and grapeseed extract
Borage oil	2 capsules daily	
Coenzyme Q10	2 capsules daily	With vitamin E, phospholipids and selenium
Echinacea	100 mg daily	
Enzymes	3 capsules twice daily	Multiple formula
Fiber	4-8 tablets daily	Psyllium, with herb hyssop
Flaxseed oil	1 tablespoon daily	
Folic acid	10 mg daily	
Melatonin (adults only)	3 mg daily at bedtime	With B vitamins
Multi-mineral	3-4 ounces daily	In liquid solution, with vitamin B12, biotin
Multi-vitamin/mineral	6 caplets daily	Freeze-dried plant sources
Vitamin A	25,000 IU daily*	
Vitamin C	Individual bowel tolerance**	With bioflavonoids (quercetin, rutin proanthocyanidins)
Vitamin E	2 capsules (800 IU) daily	d-alpha tocopherol

* The FDA recommends pregnant women not exceed 10,000 IU of vitamin A daily.

** To determine individual dosage, on the first day take 1,000 mg hourly until diarrhea occurs, then reduce dosage to just below that for individual daily dosage. Vitamin C is not toxic in large doses but must be taken throughout the day to benefit. Divide dosage to three or four times a day.

CHAPTER 102:

Liver Problems

Dr. Cass Ingram, in his book *Eat Right or Die Young*, coins a phrase, "The Toxic American Liver Syndrome" to describe the extreme amounts of toxins to which American livers are being exposed daily.[1]

Cirrhosis of the liver is the fourth leading cause of death among city dwellers between the ages of 25 and 65, no doubt in part thanks to the amounts of toxic chemicals present in the city environment.[2]

According to the FDA's national market basket survey, at least 38 percent of the food supply contains pesticide residues. This figure is probably an underestimation because routine laboratory tests can detect fewer than one-half of the pesticides applied to food.[3]

In 30 years, conventional pesticide use in the U.S. has doubled from 500 million to more than two billion pounds annually, representing one-third of the world market. Total pesticide use in 1991 (including wood preservatives and disinfectants) exceeded 2.2 billion pounds.[4]

Located under the diaphragm just above the stomach, the liver detoxifies harmful substances such as pesticides, food additives and environmental pollutants. Liver damage can result from chronic alcoholism, social drinking, being overweight, drug or chemical ingestion or an improper diet. It is the largest internal organ of the body. Countless chemical reactions take place in the liver every day, including the synthesis of amino acids, protein breakdown, sugar conversion and storage, and the storage of some vitamins and minerals, including cell-saving antioxidants. It also produces lecithin, cholesterol, enzymes and bile.

Slight liver injury may go largely unnoticed, producing minor symptoms such as digestion problems and fatigue. Long before actual damage is detected, the liver may lose cells; accumulate fat and scar tissue, and produce far less enzymes and bile, resulting in poor food absorption. When the liver isn't working properly, some scary symptoms may appear: water retention, hypoglycemia, hyperthyroidism, and excessive male or female hormones in the opposite sex.

The Copper Connection

Crystal was a bright, vivacious 17-month-old. She and her parents lived in the country, in an old farmhouse on three acres they shared with chickens, cows, two dogs, three cats and a family of goats. Crystal's mother looked forward to feeding her fresh-grown produce from their garden, and water from their spring-fed well. She knew their lifestyle was a healthy one, and so was surprised when Crystal's "little flu" didn't get better.

After noticing Crystal's liver was very firm and enlarged, her doctor admitted her into the hospital for tests. She was diagnosed as having cirrhosis of the liver. Horrified, Crystal's mother consulted a nutritionally-oriented physician for advice. After nutritional testing, the doctor concluded that Crystal had dangerously high amounts of copper in her body, and recommended zinc supplementation to force the copper out. Once supplementation was started, her liver began to repair itself.

How did Crystal get such high copper levels in her body? You may have guessed by now. Once Crystal's physician learned that she had been bottle-fed as an infant, he had their water and plumbing system checked. It was revealed that the well water was high in copper and very acidic, and that the acid water was leaching copper out of old copper water lines. Chlorine, by the way, can do the same thing. In the summer when sources of drinking water are dirtier than usual, water treatment facilities often increase the amount of chlorine. Chlorine will leach copper out of the pipes into the water, leaving a green-blue stain. Crystal's family supplemented with zinc and other health-important nutrients, replaced the plumbing and installed a water softener.

Cirrhosis of the liver involves the loss and hardening of liver cells, resulting in formation of scar tissue. Depending on how much is formed, scar tissue can impair or destroy the liver. Cirrhosis is caused by excessive alcohol, malnutrition, viral hepatitis, or chronic inflammation or obstruction of certain liver ducts.

Early signs are fever, indigestion, diarrhea or constipation and jaundice. Later symptoms include swelling, anemia and internal bleeding, characterized by spider-shaped bruises. Because the liver is a storehouse of these nutrients, a deficiency of vitamins B complex, A, C and K also may occur.

The Lancet reported on a study in which it was found that 22 children with childhood cirrhosis of the liver had been bottle fed with formulas prepared with water from home wells. The authors of the report concluded that too much copper can be a cause of infant cirrhosis.[5]

Copper is a trace mineral found in all body tissues. It assists in the formation of hemoglobin and red blood cells, and is important to iron absorption. Researchers have found that a combination of zinc and manganese will increase excretion of copper in the urine when there is too much copper in the body.[6] Too much copper can be a problem, but not enough zinc will create abnormally high levels of copper also. Always, when supplementing with zinc, include copper. Better yet, target a multi-mineral formula in solution.

Alcohol is dangerous because it easily overloads the liver and dehydrates the body. The liver can deal with large amounts of alcohol, but it needs time to do so. If a person takes in too much alcohol at one time he may even die, and a lethal dose can be as little as 400 milliliters – the amount of alcohol in a liter bottle of spirits. A normal liver can process a glass of wine, half a pint of beer or one shot of booze every hour. Drink more than this, and you invite liver problems.

One of the first things that happens when alcohol overloads the liver is that it loses zinc and copper stores. In one study, 20 alcoholics underwent a liver biopsy and were compared to three nonalcoholic subjects. It was found liver copper and zinc levels were lower in those who drank, but increased significantly when they stopped. The directors of the study concluded that increasing levels of zinc and copper in the liver helps heal it after it has been damaged by alcohol.[7]

Wound-Healing Zinc for Cirrhosis

Research abounds with evidence that zinc is a major player for the health and healing of body tissues. Zinc was used topically as calamine lotion as far back as 1500 B.C. by the Egyptians. When you are deficient in zinc, cuts and ulcers do not heal as well and your chances of them getting infected is increased. A zinc deficiency also affects the immune system by causing a reduction in natural killer cells, and the size of the thymus gland, an extremely important immune system organ.

Doctors at the Hacetteppe Children's Hospital in Ankara, Turkey noted that in patients with cirrhosis of the liver, urinary excretion of zinc is high, encouraging a zinc deficiency. They believe zinc supplementation is warranted in all cases of liver cirrhosis.[8]

In one study, 73 adults with liver cirrhosis were compared to 39 controls for serum zinc levels, zinc urinary excretion and retention of zinc after intravenous zinc therapy. Not only did they find lower levels of zinc and higher rates of excretion among cirrhosis patients, but after giving them eight milligrams of zinc intravenously, blood levels of zinc fell more rapidly in cirrhosis patients than in controls. The researchers concluded that since zinc depletion accompanies cirrhosis, it should be treated with zinc supplementation.[9]

Researchers in the Netherlands cite a case study in the medical journal *Gastroenterology* in which a 54 year old woman with congenital liver fibrosis had her symptoms turned off and on by zinc supplementation. After trying all the conventional recommendations for her condition, following physical exertion she developed tremors around the mouth, nausea, vomiting and excessive sleep for several days. She could not eat or drink, speak or walk, and had some incontinence and nausea. Hospital tests revealed a severe deficiency of zinc. She was on zinc supplementation for three weeks and her symptoms went away. One week after stopping the supplementation, she developed symptoms again. Her doctors finally had to conclude that her liver problems were caused by a zinc deficiency.[10]

Liver Lifeguards

The liver is an incredibly resilient organ. It has to be, considering all it is required to do. The liver filters over a liter of blood a minute, effectively removing bacteria and toxins. It manufactures bile, which also helps remove dangerous chemicals, and is necessary for the absorption and storage of fats, vitamins and minerals. When the liver breaks down, the body follows. But it doesn't break down easily, and it has the capability of regenerating itself, when given the proper nutrients and a little time.

Fortunately for us, health food stores offer us a cornucopia of nutrients to enliven our liver. Liver protecting substances have been identified as the amino acid methionine, trimethylglycine (TMG), form of vitamin B15, and the B vitamins choline, folic acid and B12.[11]

Researchers at the University of North Carolina, Chapel Hill, found in animal experiments that a choline and lecithin deficiency may cause enough of a liver dysfunction to eventually result in liver cancer.[12]

Studies at the Bronx Veterans Affairs Medical Center and Mt. Sinai School of Medicine in New York show promise utilizing soybean lecithin as a liver protector. Baboons were fed three tablespoons of soy lecithin daily over a ten year period. Six of the baboons ate standard baboon diets, while the other six ate diets comparable to alcoholics, as well as consuming alcohol up to 50 percent of their calories, equivalent to eight cans of beer per day. Seven of the nine unsupplemented baboons developed severe liver scarring, two developed full blown cirrhosis. In those baboons consuming alcohol and lecithin there was little scarring and none developed cirrhosis after eight years on the diet.[13]

Basically, all you have to know is that choline is a constituent of lecithin and if you take lecithin, you'll be getting your choline. Scientists separate them because the body does. Lecithin is available as a dietary supplement with food sources of choline identified as egg yolk, liver, brewer's yeast and wheat germ. Choline is manufactured in the body by the combination of – guess what? – folic acid, B12 and the amino acid methionine. All these nutrients must be taken as a group and are absolutely essential to the health and well-being of your liver.

Methionine is available in amino acid supplemental formulas and in poultry, nuts and seeds, and fruits and vegetables. The following liver lifeguards are vitally important in defending against the poisons of our polluted planet.

Linolenic acid found in borage oil actually stops damage to liver cells exposed to toxic substances. It is the treatment of choice for certain types of mushroom poisoning – disorders that would otherwise be fatal.

Biotin is a B vitamin whose primary role is to modulate fat metabolism. Whenever liver damage occurs, the cells swell and become infiltrated with fat. This fat, when present, keeps the cells from healing. Biotin works well to remove fatty deposits resulting from toxins.[14]

Many studies show that liquid garlic extract, selenium and vitamin E offer dramatic protection to the liver and improve its ability to remove poisons from the system.[15]

In one study, blood levels of vitamin E, beta carotene and selenium were assessed in a group of alcoholics. Compared to the control group, the alcoholics showed lower blood levels of beta-carotene and selenium. Blood beta carotene levels declined as alcohol-induced liver damage increased, while vitamin E levels were depleted only in patients with cirrhosis. Deficiencies of antioxidants like these have been shown to influence the amount of damage a liver sustains when over-worked.[16]

What Garlic Can Do

Three studies by Japanese researchers shows how garlic protects against liver cell damage.

In one detoxifying study, researchers headed by Dr. Tohru Fuwa at the Central Research Laboratories of Wakunaga Pharmaceutical Company in Japan (the makers of Kyolic® aged garlic products) reported in the *Hiroshima Journal of Medical Sciences* that four of the six sulfur-containing compounds isolated from garlic protected liver cells from damage caused by a toxic chemical, carbon tetrachloride. This finding was confirmed by Dr. Hiroshi Hikino and associates at the Pharmaceutical Institute of Tohoku University.

In a third study by Dr. Kyoichi Kagawa, published in the *Japanese Journal of Pharmacology*, mice ate garlic six hours after they consumed a dose of carbon tetrachloride. Carbon tetrachloride damages liver cells by producing fats in the liver. The study showed the garlic significantly reduced the amount of fat induced by this toxic chemical.

For the best detoxifying program, choose Kyolic® liquid aged garlic extract. I take it every day.

Beets and beet tops contain special substances, some yet to be identified, that protect liver cells from damage, help heal injured liver cells, and stimulate the flow of bile, reducing liver congestion. Hepatitis, whether caused by viruses or chemicals, often responds to beet juice, if you drink a quart or more a day.[17]

Chlorophyll, found in all green plants, lessens the toxic load on the liver by aggressively binding to various harmful substances, including cadmium, lead, mercury, pesticides and chlorinated hydrocarbons. Perhaps because of its chlorophyll content, it actually pulls poisons out of the liver.[18]

In numerous experiments, silymarin, the active principle in milk thistle fruit, has been found effective in preventing and reversing the damaging effects of hepatitis and cirrhosis of the liver. Apparently silymarin acts directly on cell membranes and can, therefore, both prevent and cure liver damage. In experiments with rats poisoned with chemicals, researchers found that silymarin protected their livers against damage, and it has no side effects, even in large doses.[19]

Hepatitis-Helpful Nutrients

Hepatitis occurs when infection or toxins cause the liver to inflame. Symptoms first resemble the flu: fever, swollen lymph glands, weakness, drowsiness, stomach discomfort and headache, often followed by extreme fatigue and loss of appetite. Soon the liver is unable to eliminate poisons, allowing them to build up and no longer store and process certain nutrients vital to the body.

There are two types of viral hepatitis. The least serious is infectious, or hepatitis A, caused by eating contaminated shellfish (prevented by cooking for at least six minutes), drinking contaminated water, or inhaling airborne germs from infected persons or body secretions. Serum hepatitis, or hepatitis B, is more serious--sometimes fatal. It is contracted from contaminated blood transfusions, the ingestion of contaminated body fluids or dirty needles. Hepatitis C is diagnosed through blood tests that identify the antibody.

To recover from hepatitis, one must rest, abstain from alcohol, and follow a diet rich in essential nutrients: high in vegetable protein and complex carbohydrates, unsaturated fatty acids, including coldwater fish, liberal amounts of fluids, and vitamins B complex, C and E. This regimen should be continued long after recovery, since sensitivity to toxins may persist.[20] Along with whole foods and nutritional supplementation, consume plenty of filtered water. Drinking fresh lemon juice in water every morning and evening followed by a vegetable juice is believed to be beneficial. Do this consistently for two to four weeks and then several mornings a week for several months and whenever liver symptoms occur.[21]

Because hepatitis results from toxic substances in the body, vitamin C therapy is particularly important. Large intravenous doses of vitamin C (sodium ascorbate) along with B complex and calcium supplements can help reduce the severity of the infectious hepatitis symptoms and speed up the healing process.

This treatment originated with Dr. Frederick Klenner, M.D., of North Carolina in the 1940s and has been used successfully elsewhere, most recently by Dr. Akira Murata of Saga University in Japan.

Without vitamin C, all humans would die of scurvy. Our bodies don't create it, so it must be provided in food and supplements. Only humans, primates and a few other animals don't create it internally.[22]

Jaundice – Waste Not, Want Not

Jaundice is basically an excretory system problem. In newborns it is not desirable, but is common and treatable. Jaundice in adults, however, is a bad sign. It usually means something is blocking digestive bile from being excreted normally through the intestinal tract. In jaundice, the skin, whites of the eyes and urine become abnormally yellow because pigments from worn-out red blood cells are not excreted in bile and instead accumulate in the bloodstream and tissues. When the liver stops or reduces its production of bile, or the biliary tract is blocked, these cells cannot be excreted. Jaundice is not a problem, but a symptom of a problem, and should not be ignored.

Aside from a dysfunctional liver, jaundice can be caused by anemia, surgical trauma, swelling or spasms of the bile duct, or obstruction of the duct by a stone, cyst or cancer – anything that blocks bile from entering the intestine or being excreted through the intestinal tract.

Obviously, to cure jaundice the initial problem has to be corrected. In the meantime, certain foods and nutrients can help. The diet should be high in nutrients that build up the red blood cells, especially the B vitamins, C, E and magnesium. Tissue relaxants such as vitamins B6, magnesium and calcium can alleviate muscular spasms of the bile duct which may contribute toward an inability to excrete bile.[23]

Cut out the foods that create waste – avoid all hydrogenated and processed fats and fried foods. Instead emphasize those that make haste – a hasty departure: a whole, raw foods diet with lots of fruits and vegetables. Try drinking a warm glass of water with the juice of half a lemon in it, upon arising in the morning. Eat raw apples and pears or grate together with yogurt and raw seeds or seed and nut butters (no peanut butter), so long as the nut butters do not contain hydrogenated oils. Consume plenty of raw green vegetables and sprouts to help cleanse the blood. Drink barley water (one cup of barley in three quarts of water, simmer for three hours) throughout the day.[24]

Choose a supplemental formula that contains freeze-dried sprouts and vegetables, combined in such a way as to provide all the essential vitamins and minerals, as well as adding odorless garlic, acidophilus and green tea extract for deep-cleansing your excretory system. The less toxins in your liver and blood, the better it will work for you.

Liver-Loving Nutrients

For maximum absorption, supplements should be taken with meals.

Nutrient	Suggested Dosage	Formulation
Acidophilus	At least four billion flora on an empty stomach, three times daily	
Aged garlic extract	2 teaspoons three times daily	Liquid
Amino acids	4-6 capsules daily	Multiple formula from natural sources
Antioxidants	4 capsules daily*	With selenium and grape seed extract
Borage oil	2 capsules daily	
Coenzyme Q10	2 capsules daily	With vitamin E, phospholipids and selenium
Enzymes	2 capsules twice daily	Multiple formula
Flaxseed oil	1 tablespoon daily	
Fiber	8 tablets daily	Psyllium, with herb hyssop
Milk thistle	150 mg twice daily	
Multi-vitamin/mineral	6 caplets daily	Freeze-dried plant sources
Multi-mineral	2-4 ounces daily	In liquid solution, with vitamin B12, biotin
Tumeric	100 mg three times daily with food	
Vitamin C	Individual bowel tolerance**	With bioflavonoids (quercetin, rutin proanthocyanidins)

* The FDA recommends that pregnant women not exceed 10,000 IU of vitamin A daily.

** To determine individual dosage, on the first day take 1,000 mg hourly until diarrhea occurs, then reduce dosage to just below that for individual daily dosage. Vitamin C is not toxic in large doses but must be taken throughout the day to benefit. Divide dosage to three or four times a day.

CHAPTER 103:

Lou Gehrig's Disease (Amyotrophic Lateral Sclerosis)

Few had heard of amyotrophic lateral sclerosis (ALS) until baseball Hall of Famer Lou Gehrig came down with the debilitating nerve disease in 1939. An adoring public was stunned. "This is the only time a disease has been named for a patient, not a doctor," said a spokesperson for the ALS Association in an article in *People* magazine. More than 50 years after Gehrig's death in 1941, fund-raising events still bear his name.

When the debonair David Niven succumbed to ALS in 1983, there was a new surge of public awareness of the disease. While Niven was still alive, public service ads proclaimed, "It's not just Lou Gehrig's disease, it's David Niven's disease." After Niven's death, actor Douglas Fairbanks, Jr., did a series of TV spots about his friend to reinforce the ALS-awareness message.

From his diagnosis of ALS in 1980 until his death in 1986, Senator Jacob Javits of New York campaigned tirelessly for a cure. He served on the board of directors of the National ALS Foundation, and helped secure passage in 1983 of a bill to fund ongoing neurological research – even appearing on the floor of Congress in a wheelchair and hooked up to a respirator.[1]

Other notables who have been struck by the disease include composer Dimitry Shostakovich, physicist Stephen Hawking, and former San Francisco 49ers Matt Hazeltine, Gary Lewis and Bob Waters. As this list suggests, more men than women are affected by the disease, which strikes about 5,000 individuals in the United States each year.[2]

It's a devastating illness that causes the slow destruction of motor neurons – nerve cells in the brainstem and spinal cord that control muscle contractions – to the point that all movement, including breathing, stops, resulting in complete paralysis. People who have ALS typically experience weakness in the hands and legs, muscle cramps and stiffness and twitching muscles. If motor neurons in the brainstem are involved, talking and swallowing become difficult. Although most people die within three to five years, some survive for a decade or longer. Stephen Hawking lived with the disease for more than 20 years.[3]

In the case of Lou Gehrig's Disease, promising therapies exist, and there are nutritional supplements available that at least one doctor has found can alleviate the devastating symptoms of the disease. You will find it only here!

Calcium/Magnesium Balance Important, Aluminum Implicated

Japanese researchers, particularly have been interested in the cause and cure of ALS. On the Kii Peninsula of Japan there is a high incidence of ALS, believed to be correlated to the low magnesium content in the soil and drinking water. The researchers theorized that since the central nervous system is very sensitive to magnesium deficiency states, there might be a connection. This is because without it, calcium accumulates in the brain and brain stem, causing the loss of myelin, the nerve's covering that protects it from short-circuiting. M.Yasui, M.D., of the Division of Neurologic Disease, Yakayama Medical College, Yakaama, Japan, took five brain samples from people who died with ALS, and compared them to five samples from people who died with a normal central nervous system. He found the average calcium content in specific areas of the ALS brains were higher than the controls, and that magnesium concentrations in 26 central nervous system regions were markedly reduced in the ALS cases. He also found high amounts of aluminum in the 26 pinpointed regions. His explanation of all this? He and his colleagues concluded that the high incidence of ALS in the Kii Peninsula may be due to a deficiency of dietary magnesium resulting in accumulations of calcium and aluminum in the brain.[4]

I realize we are not in Japan, but if you or someone you know has ALS, don't discount the chance that too little magnesium is a factor. A large study by the U.S. Department of Agriculture found that only 25 percent of 37,785 individuals had magnesium intakes at or greater than the recommended daily allowance, which is notoriously low. A 1995 review of 15 studies found that a typical diet contains only a fraction of the RDA.[5]

Magnesium and calcium work in balance throughout our bodies. Without magnesium, calcium accumulates in places it shouldn't. Always when supplementing with calcium, include magnesium one to one.

Be cautious about the kinds of magnesium-rich foods you pick. Nuts contain magnesium, but it's no nuts if you're eating the ones that have been processed. The processing techniques leave the nuts both nutrient deficient and often harmful. Once nuts are shelled, rancidity sets in fast, not always detectable by taste, and often masked by flavorings such as salt. Methods used for blanching can include hot lye and bleach, and other chemicals. Additives may be used to extend shelf life.

And what about those cooked beans? Sixty-five percent of the magnesium has been lost; and 36 percent of frozen spinach's magnesium has been lost in the blanching process used for freezing. Best to choose raw, whole food sources of magnesium like whole wheat, pumpkin seeds, almonds, Brazil nuts and hazel nuts, dark-green vegetables and molasses. One cup of pumpkin seeds has a whopping 738 mgs of magnesium.[6]

Lou Gehrig's Disease Caused by Free Radicals

At an international conference at George Washington University Medical Center it was announced that ALS is probably caused by free radicals. Researchers found a link between an inherited form of ALS and a defect in the gene that codes superoxide dismutase, a naturally-occurring body enzyme which breaks down toxic superoxide free radicals.[7]

New concepts are often slow in converting the scientific community to their validity and value. So it was when the free radical theory of aging was proposed by Denham Harman, M.D., some 34 years ago. At that time, he announced free radicals are the saboteurs causing cellular damage leading to degenerative diseases and premature death.

Few biochemists went along with Dr. Harman because no one had the tools to identify free radicals and prove they really exist in living organisms. However, in 1968, Dr. Irwin Fridovitch and his colleagues discovered that the body also has its natural defenses against the actions of free radicals. Among the most common proteins in human cells is superoxide dismutase, an enzyme that converts the superoxide radical to hydrogen peroxide, which is in turn metabolized by another enzyme, catalase, to harmless water and oxygen. This discovery proved Harman right because there is no way for SOD to form hydrogen peroxide without combining with superoxide, which is another name for a free radical.

Today doctors and researchers agree, after countless studies confirming these two early findings, that one of the natural orders of life is the gradual breaking down, thanks to free radicals, of the human body, but that antioxidants and naturally-occurring SOD help limit this breakdown. People with ALS have been found to be dangerously low in SOD, meaning their free radicals have free reign. Superoxide dismutase in ALS patients is less than half that found in normal individuals, allowing the superoxide free radicals to selectively damage motor neurons in ALS patients.[8]

The Antioxidant Answer

Now that we know free radicals are the reason ALS patients lose their motor neurons, we only have to look at those substances which destroy free radicals: antioxidants. My first reaction when looking for studies that pitted antioxidants against ALS was, why aren't there more? I could not find one study using supplemental superoxide dismutase to battle Lou Gehrig's. Why not? If something is missing, doesn't it make sense to replace it? ALS patients are also deficient in the amino acid glutamate,[9,10] yet researchers are hesitant to consider it. Why? Now, I'm sure it's not as simple as that – medicine is very complicated. But simple solutions have been discovered, and in the case of something as incredibly devastating as Lou Gehrig's I should think every avenue would be explored. Yet, here we are. This is why it is so important for us, as unwitting consumers, to question medical authority. Find the research and present it to your physician. If he or she won't look at it, find someone who will. I do not advocate self-treatment. A physician versed in nutritional medicine can do the proper tests and monitor results safely. But do investigate and communicate. If you have Lou Gehrig's you have very little to lose and everything to gain.

In any case, I did find a doctor who says he has developed a protocol that can successfully treat ALS – and he has done it for himself!

A Canadian physician using intravenous vitamin C for the treatment of degenerative diseases inspired C.A. Douglas Ringrose, M.D., formerly of The Linus Pauling Institute of Science and Medicine in Palo Alto, California, and now practicing out of Edmonton, Alberta, Canada, to develop his protocol. I talked to him personally and he says he has successfully fought his own battle with Lou Gehrig's disease, which he has had now for 14 years. He told me his right hand and forearm were paralyzed and now they are "stronger than before." He recommends starting by eliminating anything that alters or suppresses brain activity including tobacco, alcohol, caffeine and antidepressant or antianxiety drugs. Read the label! Many over-the-counter pain relievers contain caffeine, as do seemingly benign diet pills. He says you absolutely don't want to suppress brain activity.

He calls his protocol "fortified ascorbic chelation therapy," and says it consists of an intravenous dosage of 25 to 50 grams of vitamin C in a 500 milliliter IV of five percent dextrose and water once a week, fortified with two to three grams of oral antioxidants, including 400-800 IU of vitamin E. He also adds 2,000 micrograms of vitamin B12 every two to four weeks. He has used this protocol successfully for Parkinson's and Parkinsonism, Alzheimer's and Multiple Sclerosis. He says it works for any disorder of the nervous system. If your physician is open-minded enough, have him or her call Dr. Ringrose, who has given me his permission to include his phone number here. It is (403) 484-8401. He also emphasizes a whole-foods – raw as much as possible – chemical-free diet, and lots of exercise to keep the circulation moving through the brain arteries. Exercise encourages the circulation of the vital nutrients you need to get well, and maximizes the body's healing capacity.[11]

Eating whole foods is the best, eating sprouts even better, since the young shoots concentrate more of the older plants' nutrients. When targeting food supplements, look for a formula that uses freeze dried sprouts and vegetables, combined in such a way as to provide all the essential vitamins and minerals.

Brain-Saving Nutrients
For maximum absorption, take supplements with meals.

Nutrient	Suggested Dosage	Formulation
Aged garlic extract	1 teaspoon three times daily	Liquid
Amino acids	4-6 capsules daily	Multiple formula from natural sources
Antioxidants	4 capsules daily*	With selenium and grapeseed extract
Borage oil	2 capsules daily	
Coenzyme Q10	2 capsules daily	With vitamin E, phospholipids and selenium
Coenzyme Q1 (NADH)	2.5 to 5 mg daily	
Enzymes	2 capsules twice daily	Multiple formula
Fiber	4-8 tablets daily	Psyllium, with herb hyssop
Flaxseed oil	1 tablespoon daily	
Malic acid	250 mg twice daily	
Melatonin (adults only)	3 mg daily at bedtime	With B vitamins
Multi-mineral	3-4 ounces daily	In liquid solution, with vitamin B12, biotin
Multi-vitamin/mineral	6 caplets daily	Freeze-dried plant sources
Vitamin A	25,000 IU daily*	
Vitamin B6	100 mg daily	
Vitamin C	Individual bowel tolerance**	With bioflavonoids (quercetin, rutin proanthocyanidins)
Vitamin E	2 capsules (800 IU) daily	d-alpha tocopherol

* The FDA recommends pregnant women not exceed 10,000 IU of vitamin A daily.

** To determine individual dosage, on the first day take 1,000 mg hourly until diarrhea occurs, then reduce dosage to just below that for individual daily dosage. Vitamin C is not toxic in large doses but must be taken throughout the day to benefit. Divide dosage to three or four times a day.

CHAPTER 104:

Low Blood Pressure – Hypotension

Is low blood pressure a disease or a symptom? If you listen to your doctor, he'll give you the impression it is a disease, treatable with drugs. If you listen to the researchers, you hear a very different story.

The most common kind of low blood pressure is orthostatic hypotension. Have you ever gotten up suddenly, then became dizzy or light-headed? For some, this happens all the time, and for the elderly, it may even cause them to faint (if you see it written on your grandmother's medical chart it will read "postural syncope"). Circulation problems can cause this kind of hypotension, as poor circulation means blood isn't pumping as strong as it should be.

Fatigue is often associated with low blood pressure, generally defined as a blood pressure below 100/60 in an adult, although some healthy younger adults may have normally low blood pressure. Sometimes low blood pressure occurs with anti-hypertensive drugs or drugs to treat heart problems. In attempting to lower pressure on the heart or arteries, the pressure becomes too low and causes problems. A severe allergic reaction to food has also been found to cause low blood pressure, as the body releases massive amounts of histamine to counter the allergen.[1]

For people who are otherwise healthy and suffer from hypotension, nutrition may be the answer. Interestingly, hypotension is one of the symptoms of pernicious anemia, believed to be caused by nutritional deficiencies of vitamin B12. Is it possible that pernicious anemia is the underlying cause of hypotension? The research is very convincing.

Vitamin B12 and The Anemia Connection

Doctors report that the most common symptoms of low blood pressure are fainting, dizziness and fatigue,[2] all symptoms associated with anemia.

In a case report, a 70-year-old male was admitted to the Hadassah University Hospital in Jerusalem because for the past six months he'd been having fainting spells. They only thing doctors could find wrong, medically, was that when he stood up his blood pressure dropped from 160/80 to 110/70. Nutritionally, they found he was deficient in vitamin B12. The patient was given B12 at first daily for the first week, then weekly for a month and then monthly thereafter. After two months his hypotension was resolved. In the next year he had no episodes of fainting.[3]

A. Lossos, M.D. and Argov, Z., M.D., reported in an issue of the *Journal of the American Geriatric Society*, that they observed a B12 deficiency in four other cases of hypotension, and that in all the cases the patients were around 67 years of age and had pernicious anemia. In all of the patients their low blood pressure improved after a few weeks of vitamin B12 therapy.[4]

Spyridon Koudouris, M.D., treats his older hypotensive patients with vitamin B12 and sublingual folic acid (held under the tongue until dissolved).[5]

In a 17-year study of B12-deficient patients, researchers at Columbia-Presbyterian Medical Center and Harlem Hospital determined that pernicious anemia was the most common symptom of the deficiency. Other associated symptoms included muscle weakness, poor reflexes, mood swings and low blood pressure.[6]

When stomach and intestinal problems are present, the tablet form of B12 is not absorbed. Some doctors give B12 shots to their geriatric patients. Another option would be to choose a supplement that contains B12 in solution.

Always when supplementing any B vitamin, include a good B complex supplemental formula. All the B vitamins work together, and too much of one can create a deficiency of another.

Hypotension-Hating Nutrients
For maximum absorption, take supplements with meals.

Nutrient	Suggested Dosage	Formulation
Fiber	4-8 tablets daily	Psyllium, with herb hyssop
Multi-mineral	1-4 ounces daily	In liquid solution, with vitamin B12, biotin
Multi-vitamin/mineral	3-6 caplets daily	Freeze-dried plant sources
Vitamin C	Individual bowel tolerance*	With bioflavonoids (quercetin, rutin proanthocyanidins)
Vitamin E	2 capsules (800 IU)	d-alpha tocopherol

* To determine individual dosage, on the first day take 1,000 mg hourly until diarrhea occurs, then reduce dosage to just below that for individual daily dosage. Vitamin C is not toxic in large doses but must be taken throughout the day to benefit. Divide dosage to three or four times a day.

CHAPTER 105:

Low Blood Sugar

Low blood sugar, or hypoglycemia, causes fatigue, and in extreme cases, loss of consciousness.

I'll never forget the day I learned that lesson. Fortunately, it wasn't from personal experience. I was in a hotel, walking down the hallway, when I chanced upon a young chambermaid washing the windows. I saw her falter, her eyes roll back, then she slumped down, fainting at my feet. She quickly recovered, but her face was as white as a sheet, her lips pale. I asked her if I could help, and she replied that it was her first day on the job and she had eaten nothing since a hotdog the day before at lunch. It was apparent that the relatively taxing job of washing the windows required more energy reserves than she had left. I explained the situation to her supervisor then escorted her to the cafeteria for an early lunch of bean soup and whole grain sprout bread, warning her never to work on an empty tank.

It's Not Sugar That You Need

A friend of mine incorrectly assumed that since she had low blood sugar, she needed more sugar. She couldn't have been more wrong! Another way to describe hypoglycemia is hyperinsulinism, or too much insulin. Your body creates too much insulin in response to too much simple carbohydrates, like sugar and white flour.

To summarize, simple sugars such as white sugar, honey, syrups and milk sugar are absorbed into the system quickly through the mouth or stomach. The complex carbohydrates found in grains, root vegetables, legumes, and fruits are slowly broken down into absorbable sugar (glucose) which is absorbed slowly through the wall of the small intestine. You want the foods that are absorbed slowly so your body isn't fooled into believing it needs insulin.

Glucose, or blood sugar, is carried to the liver where it is converted into glycogen and stored. When the body needs sugar for muscle, brain, or nerve function, the stored glycogen is reconverted to glucose and transported by the blood to where it's needed. The pancreas must secrete the hormone insulin and the adrenal glands secrete adrenaline to permit the metabolism and utilization of glucose. Other endocrine glands are also involved.

When you eat too much simple sugars/carbohydrates, the pancreas reacts by producing too much insulin which causes the blood-sugar level to drop too low – hence, hypoglycemia. This sudden drop in blood-sugar will reduce blood oxygen, which wreaks havoc with the liver and brain. The first symptom may only be sudden fatigue; but in time the symptoms may become very severe with mood swings, quick temper, heart rhythm problems, allergies, insomnia, etc. Unless hypoglycemia is controlled, the overworked pancreas may lose its ability to produce insulin; then the diagnosis will be diabetes.

Other symptoms of low blood sugar include heart palpitations, headaches or migraines, confusion and sweating occurring before breakfast, after exertion, or two to four hours after eating. Low blood sugar is serious enough to be blamed for temporary cases of senility[1], clumsiness[2] and even low intelligence.[3]

The Hypoglycemic Diet

Eating regular meals (including breakfast and lunch) and high complex carbohydrate foods, versus greasy fatty foods, will go further in reducing fat and increasing energy than any dieting program--liquid or not. To boost your energy, eat power breakfasts and lunches, rather than skipping meals. To fight fatigue during a long workout (mental as well as physical) eat whole grain cereals and breads, fresh-squeezed fruit and vegetable juices, raisins, figs, beans and lentils, and lots of water. A lentil soup breakfast, while it sounds inappropriate, is most appropriate for an energetic day. Not eating breakfast means that you've already had 12 or more hours without food. Tackling anything after fasting that long is going to leave you with low blood sugar and depressing fatigue, if not exhaustion.

Leave behind the typical on-the-run breakfast of donuts and coffee. You might get a "charge" out of the refined sugar in the donut and the caffeine in the coffee, but it will be a temporary one, as your blood sugar rises then plummets when the energy is quickly absorbed. Carbohydrate snacks containing sugars and starches provide the body with almost instant energy because they cause a sudden rise in the blood sugar level. However, the blood sugar level drops again rapidly, creating a craving for more sweet food and possibly fatigue.

The hypoglycemic should remove from the diet sugar, refined and processed foods such as instant rice and potatoes, white flour, soft drinks, alcohol and salt. Avoid sweet fruits and juices such as grape and prune juice. Avoid pasta, gravies, hominy, white rice, yams and corn. The diet should include vegetables, legumes, brown rice, avocadoes, seeds, grains, nuts, and yogurt.

The hypoglycemic should not go without food. Instead, eat six to eight small meals throughout the day. Food allergy testing should also be conducted. A high-fiber diet will help stabilize blood sugar swings. Combine fiber with protein sources such as bran crackers with sesame or almond butter.

Chromium – A Star Performer

Many studies have shown that certain nutrients are essential for normal blood sugar levels and insulin absorption. Among these, chromium gets star billing. Thirty-five years of research on this megamineral suggests chromium plays a considerable role in the progression of glucose intolerance and the increased risk of developing diabetes. *The Nutrition Report* says that 13 out of 15 studies evaluating chromium supplementation's effect on glucose levels show that it works by maintaining blood sugar levels with a minimum of insulin.[4] This means that chromium may be all that's necessary to stabilize glucose levels. Unfortunately, because there is not a good way to diagnose a chromium deficiency, many scientists and physicians ignore the potential benefits of chromium supplementation.

Dr. Walter Mertz has been documenting the effect of chromium on diabetes since the late '20s and to this day advocates its use. Chromium is a crucial part of a substance termed the Glucose Tolerance Factor – or GTF – which is composed of two niacin molecules (vitamin B2), the amino acids cystine, glycine and glutamic acid as well as chromium. When enough chromium is present in the diet, intestinal bacteria can manufacture GTF in the body.[5]

Dr. Richard J. Doisy, professor of biochemistry at the State University of New York, Upstate Medical Center, reported that some diabetics who required insulin shots to maintain their blood sugar at safe levels were able to get by on lower doses after taking brewer's yeast, a source of dietary chromium.[6]

Later, he and his colleagues gave a GTF supplement made from brewer's yeast extract to a group of elderly people with faulty glucose tolerance, and he reported that within just two months, half of them had regained normal glucose tolerance levels.

Brewer's yeast is said to be the hypoglycemic's best friend because it is rich in all the B vitamins and has the necessary minerals (chromium, selenium and zinc) that are involved in carbohydrate metabolism.

In another study, Dr. Doisy decided to test the effect of GTF on healthy, young adults. He found they didn't have to produce as much insulin to keep their blood sugar levels within healthy levels. He estimates probably one-fourth to one-half of people in the U.S. are deficient in chromium.

A general deficiency of chromium appears to exist among Americans over age 50. Yet, all children seem to be born with a sufficient level of chromium, according to an international study. In Americans over 50, however, one in four had levels so low they could not be detected. Of the *foreigners* over age 50 who were checked, almost all had chromium in their tissues.

The reason for this can be found in the American diet. It is estimated that the average American consumes 150 pounds of refined sugar or sucrose annually. When a person consumes refined sugar, and refined flour for that matter, about one-fifth of chromium that is drawn to the bloodstream to aid the insulin is excreted in the urine.

If our diets contained enough chromium to make up for the loss, there would be no problem, but our diets of refined sugar and flour are not sufficient to replenish the amount lost. Refined sugar contains one-twelfth as much chromium as raw sugar, and white flour has about one-seventh as much chromium as whole wheat flour. A continuous diminishing of our bodily store of the mineral is the inevitable result.

Magnanimous Magnesium

Magnesium is at the center of all energy systems. A deficiency of this ultra-important nutrient is thought to play a role in the development of insulin resistance. A study of 45 diabetic and 12 normal children found children with insulin-dependent diabetes had lower levels of magnesium than normal children.[7]

Adequate magnesium stores are necessary for proper insulin effect. In a study of magnesium deficient patients it was found that their low levels of magnesium directly affected their glucose levels.[8]

H.M. Mather of the Department of Medicine, St. George's Hospital, London, measured the blood magnesium level in 582 consecutive diabetic patients visiting the hospital's outpatients clinic. He also measured the magnesium levels of 140 nondiabetic subjects. Dr. Mather found that the diabetics had a significantly lower blood magnesium level. In fact, 25 percent had lower levels than all of the controls except one.

Dr. Takeo Takemura of the Department of Internal Medicine, Osaka City University, Japan, reported to the Japan Diabetic Society that his research studies show low magnesium levels are associated with an increased incidence of diabetic retinopathy – damage to the eyes that leads to blindness, a major complication of diabetes.

The diabetic condition itself may be the cause of mineral deficiencies. Elevated blood sugars stimulate excessive urination, which can wash essential minerals and trace elements out of the body.

Many diabetics are taking hypertensive medication and/or diuretics. Diuretics are notorious wasters of all minerals, yet potassium is the only mineral routinely replaced.

Carbohydrate-Kind B Vitamins

As a component of the glucose tolerance factor, the B vitamin niacin plays an important role in carbohydrate metabolism. Many refined foods consumed by Americans are depleted in niacin. So called "enriched" grains and other foods usually contain added niacinamide, which cannot be converted by the human body into niacin. In addition, most vitamin supplements contain niacinamide, rather than niacin. A small amount of niacin is necessary for synthesis of GTF.[9]

Vitamin B6, pyridoxine, is another B vitamin found to be important to glucose metabolism. A vitamin B6 deficiency is known to reduce pancreatic and circulating insulin levels, and degenerative changes have been noted in the cells of rats fed vitamin B6-deficient diets. Gestational diabetes was eliminated in pregnant women following two weeks of treatment with 100 milligrams per day of B6, and is associated with decreased retinopathy, a common diabetes complication.[10] Taken together, all of the evidence shows a vitamin B6 deficiency could be very important to preventing as well as reversing hypoglycemia.

Glucose-Stabilizing Nutrients

For maximum absorption, take supplements with meals.

Nutrient	Suggested Dosage	Formulation
Fiber	4-8 tablets daily	Psyllium, with herb hyssop
L-glutamine	500 mg twice daily	
Magnesium	200 mg daily	
Multi-mineral	1-4 ounces daily	In liquid solution, with vitamin B12, biotin
Multi-vitamin/mineral	3-6 caplets daily	Freeze-dried plant sources
Vitamin C	Individual bowel tolerance*	With bioflavonoids (quercetin, rutin proanthocyanidins)

* To determine individual dosage, on the first day take 1,000 mg hourly until diarrhea occurs, then reduce dosage to just below that for individual daily dosage. Vitamin C is not toxic in large doses but must be taken throughout the day to benefit. Divide dosage to three or four times a day.

CHAPTER 106:

Low Thyroid – Hypothyroidism

"Here is the test to find whether your mission on earth is finished: If you're alive, it isn't."

–Richard Bach

One of my goals in writing this book is to arm the public with the information they need to help prevent one of life's greatest tragedies: the medical misdiagnosis. As you read through these chapters, something might stick in your mind: a plan, an option, an idea, that when followed through with your physician could make all the difference to your life.

Alas, some of the beneficial information has come from the tragic lessons of those for whom the information came too late. Such was the case of Sally, a potential Olympic contender who had her running career cut short because her doctor thought he knew best.

Sally was doing very well in her trials. Her times were good and her energy and stamina were optimal. She was moving further along in her goals to try out for the U.S. Olympic team. Suddenly her times were down, and fatigue set in. She was helpless, and approached her doctor for help. He told her she was overtraining, that her body could not handle the amount of work she was subjecting it to. He told her she would have to quit. All her life Sally had trusted her doctor. He had gotten her this far, and she would have to trust his judgement. She stopped training, and let the trials go on without her. Months went by and she didn't get any better. During a relaxation trip to Europe, she had a breakdown and ended up in a hospital in Germany.

Doctors there told her that when her tests showed she had abnormally high serum cholesterol levels – odd in an athlete – their suspicions proved true: she had primary hypothyroidism, and that this is what was causing her fatigue and depression.

Since that time, physicians who specialize in sports medicine are being cautioned about this possibility. In *The Physician and Sports Medicine*, Dr. Robert S. Lathan cites a study in which six female runners between 24 and 48 years of age with a history of persistent fatigue and deteriorating running performances were evaluated. Researchers found that four of these individuals had abnormally high serum cholesterol levels, and all of them were diagnosed as having primary hypothyroidism.

Dr. Lathan cautions that problems with the thyroid gland develop gradually over a period of months to years, and that when a runner complains of fatigue, testing for hypothyroidism should be done.[1]

What is the Thyroid?

The thyroid gland sits at the base of the neck. If you wore a tie, it would be where the knot lies – two lobes on either side of the trachea. Considered a master gland, because of its importance to the body's metabolism, the thyroid's main functions are to create thyroid hormone that forms protein RNA and oxygenates cells.[2]

The gland regulates growth and metabolism, and it releases hormones that affect numerous bodily functions such as heartbeat, temperature, digestion, calorie burning and hair growth. Thyroid hormones are made from iodine and the amino acid tyrosine. A thyroid hormone deficiency results from a lack of stimulation by the pituitary gland, the master gland located in the brain that secretes the thyroid stimulating hormone (TSH).[3]

Symptoms run the gamut. They include weight gain, depression, fatigue, cold hands and feet, mental disorders, infertility, miscarriage, poor sex drive, heavy or irregular menstruation, high cholesterol, hair loss, dry skin, pale skin, brittle hair, thin and grooved fingernails, muscle weakness, stiff joints, heart problems, constipation, goiters and kidney problems. Since metabolism breaks down with a thyroid problem, having many different ailments can signal a dysfunction.[4]

An article in the *British Medical Journal* addressed a study in which "six percent of children with Down's Syndrome have thyroid disorders, a rate roughly 28 times that of the general population."[5]

Researchers at the Department of Medicine, National University Hospital, Singapore backed this up in 1993 when they found a significant link between Down's Syndrome and autoimmune thyroid disease, usually hypothyroidism.[6]

Even sleep apnea, a situation where breathing stops during sleep, is shown in studies to be caused by hypothyroidism. When the hypothyroidism is treated, not only is sleep apnea alleviated, but overall sleep is improved. Bashir A.Chaudhary, M.D., of the Sleep Disorder Center, Medical College of Georgia in Augusta, suggests it is reasonable to evaluate thyroid function in all sleep apnea patients.[7]

It's Not All in Your Head

It's impossible to know many people with chronic psychiatric symptoms are suffering from a completely organic, treatable thyroid problem. Doctors tell them to go home and get some rest, when what they need is to be diagnosed and treated!

The late Broda O. Barnes, an internationally recognized thyroid authority, said that approximately 30 percent of patients treated for low thyroid function suffer slight to deep depression, fatigue, anxiety, irritability, mental sluggishness and poor memory.[8]

John J. Haggerty, Jr. and colleagues at the Department of Psychiatry, University of North Carolina, evaluated 16 patients with hypothyroidism and compared them to 15 control subjects with normal thyroid function. He found 56 percent of those with low thyroid function had symptoms of depression compared to 20 percent with normal thyroid function.[9]

After reviewing numerous studies and reports on the role of the thyroid in mood disorders, Dr. Junichi Nomura, Department of Psychiatry, MIE University School of Medicine, in Japan, believes that physicians dealing with depressed patients, especially the elderly or women with PMS, should definitely have their thyroid functions tested. He also found that large amounts of thyroid hormones may be therapeutic for the treatment of depression.[10]

In 1886 it was noted by a 28-year-old London surgeon that "the symptoms of mere senility may be accounted for by the loss of functions of the thyroid." In the late 1890s and for a period of about 40 years desiccated thyroid was given to delay or prevent age-related changes.[11]

Subclinical hypothyroidism is common in older individuals and more so in women than men. Community surveys of persons older than 60 in the United Kingdom and the United States showed that 48 percent have subclinical hypothyroidism. In areas where the soil is low in iodine, the prevalence is even higher.[12]

The good news is that not all thyroid failure is permanent. In a small number of older patients thyroid dysfunction can spontaneously return to normal over a year's time. If thyroid failure is due to medication it is usually reversed if the medication can be stopped.[13]

Iodine: Thyroid Essential Nutrient

Make sure your thyroid gland has enough iodine so it can function properly. A deficiency of iodine results in the development of a goiter, an enlarged thyroid gland.

A survey by Dr. J.G.C. Spencer, of Frenahay Hospital in Bristol, England, revealed goiter belts in 15 nations on four continents. Goiter belts are geographical areas where the soil has only about one-seventh the amount of iodine needed to assure efficient thyroid function, easily identified by the high incidence of goiter among its populace.[14]

The United States' goiter belt is in the northern area of the nation from the mountains of New England to Washington and includes the provinces of Canada following this path along the border. These states are: Maine, New Hampshire, Vermont, New York, Pennsylvania, Ohio, Michigan, Indiana, Illinois, Wisconsin, Minnesota, North Dakota, Montana, Idaho and Washington.

Goiter is estimated to affect over 200 million people the world over. In all but four percent of these cases the goiter is caused by an iodine deficiency. Iodine deficiency is now rare in the United States, due to the addition of iodine to table salt. Adding iodine to table salt began in Michigan, where in 1924 the goiter rate was an incredible 47 percent.[15]

The late Broda O. Barnes, M.D., Ph.D, a world-renowned thyroid authority, stated that first generation hypothyroids usually can correct their condition by taking a kelp tablet daily. Kelp is rich in iodine, the thyroid's major nutrient. Hypothyroids of the second generation or beyond can overcome depression and many other symptoms of low thyroid function by taking natural, desiccated thyroid prescribed by a physician.

Iodine is present in large amounts in seafood, including of course, sushi. That black paper they wrap the rice in, it's called nori. It's nothing but pure iodine.

Just as important as getting enough iodine is getting too much. Either extreme can be deadly. Doctors recommend dietary sources and supplementation not exceed one milligram a day. Like all essential minerals, iodine should be combined with other minerals for proper nutritional balance. Look for an easily absorbable, derived-from-nature liquid mineral blend. A formula in solution provides the optimal absorption ratios.

A Do-It-Yourself Test

Dr. Barnes' best contribution toward public awareness of thyroid problems was probably the Barnes Basal Temperature Test, a simple test that can be done by anyone in the privacy of their own home. Since your body temperature reflects your metabolic rate, which is largely determined by hormones secreted by the thyroid gland, the state of the gland can be determined by taking your temperature. All that is needed is a thermometer.

- Shake down the thermometer to below 95 degrees Fahrenheit and place it by your bed before going to bed at night.

- Upon awakening, before getting out of bed, place the thermometer in your armpit for a full ten minutes, making as little movement as possible.

- After ten minutes, read and record the temperature and the date.

- Record the temperature for at least three mornings, preferably at the same time each day. Menstruating women should perform the test on the second, third and fourth days of menstruation.

Your basal body temperature should be between 97.6 degrees F and 98.2 degrees F. Anything lower can indicate hypothyroidism, anything higher can indicated hyperthyroidism.[16]

Natural Alternatives to Synthetic Hormones

The treatment for hypothyroidism, in all but its mildest forms, involves the use of thyroid hormone. Naturopathic physicians prefer the use of desiccated natural thyroid complete with all the thyroid hormones.[17] In my experience, a good, natural thyroid hormone is Armor Thyroid.

For the mild cases, changes in diet and an exercise program can stimulate thyroid hormone production and lessen – or eliminate – a need for hormones.

Joel Fuhrman, M.D., a Belle Mead, N.J. physician, specializing in nutritional medicine, advises a vegetarian diet, low in protein and fat, and high in the antioxidant nutrients – vitamins C, E and beta carotene, among others – that are found in fresh vegetables and fruits.

"This is a diet important for the body to be resistant to any disease," he says. "The typical American diet – high protein, high fat – makes the body require more of the thyroid hormone. A vegetarian diet won't help produce more of the hormone, but because the cells are not being taxed, the body won't need as much."[18]

Certain nutrients are necessary for a healthy thyroid. Zinc, vitamin A and vitamin E function together to manufacture thyroid hormone. A deficiency of any of these result in lower levels of active thyroid being produced. There may be a correlation between the low zinc levels common in the elderly and the high incidence of hypothyroidism. The B vitamins riboflavin (B2), niacin (B3) and pyridoxine (B6), and vitamin C are also necessary for normal thyroid hormone manufacture.[19]

Thyroid-Thankful Nutrients
For maximum absorption, take supplements with meals.

Nutrient	Suggested Dosage	Formulation
Fiber	4-8 tablets daily	Psyllium, with herb hyssop
Multi-mineral	1-4 ounces daily	In liquid solution, with vitamin B12, biotin
Multi-vitamin/mineral	3-6 caplets daily	Freeze-dried plant sources
Vitamin C	Individual bowel tolerance*	With bioflavonoids (quercetin, rutin proanthocyanidins)

* To determine individual dosage, on the first day take 1,000 mg hourly until diarrhea occurs, then reduce dosage to just below that for individual daily dosage. Vitamin C is not toxic in large doses but must be taken throughout the day to benefit. Divide dosage to three or four times a day.

CHAPTER 107:

Lupus

A former neighbor's teenage daughter approached me one day with a question: "Mrs. Salaman, she said with tears in her eyes, "I need help desperately!" I can't eat, I can't sleep, my grades are falling and I'm afraid I am dying!"

She explained to me that after a month of face rashes and flu symptoms, her doctor finally pronounced her suffering from systemic lupus erythematosus (SLE) and prescribed steroids. After getting severe reactions from the drugs and "we don't know" answers from her doctor, she and her mother decided to approach me.

The practice of medicine is not a finite field. Exploration and experimentation is necessary for answers to be found, especially when the root cause of a problem is considered unknown. Sometimes doctors forget this, or else today's climate of liability and FDA lawsuits discourage considering alternatives. In either case, when doctors reach the end of their knowledge and experience they may conclude nothing else can be done, preferring not to consider alternatives. I told my neighbor to see Dr. Ross Gordon, a practicing M.D. in Albany, California, who has years of experience in nutritional and alternative therapies, and has gotten remarkable results in almost every patient to whom I've ever sent.

What is Lupus?

Determining what works in the fight to reverse a disorder as puzzling and elusive as lupus is a mystery indeed. First you have to define the problem. *Churchill's Medical Dictionary* defines lupus as "a multisystem disease of unknown etiology."[1] The *American Journal of Medicine* calls it "a chronic inflammatory disease of the connective tissue resulting from unknown causes."[2] – Oh, *there's* a help: "unknown causes."

A little more information comes from the *Academic American Encyclopedia*, which states that lupus is an autoimmune disease in which the body produces abnormal antibodies that attack normal body tissue as though it were a foreign invader. Now we're getting somewhere! I will get back to this issue in a moment.

For those of you uncertain, confused, or dismissed by conventional medicine, here are the symptoms. Discoid lupus is a skin disorder characterized by a rash over the nose and cheeks in a butterfly pattern. Another form occurs as a result of certain prescription drugs. The most common – SLE – causes joint pain and inflammation, fever and fatigue. A little less than half of people with lupus get facial rashes. No single test diagnoses the disease, but in the majority of cases (50-90 percent), patients test positive for lupus erythematosus cells, white blood cells that destroy other white cells. Of the approximately 500,000 lupus patients in the United States, most are women. About 1 in 700 women aged 15 to 64 is afflicted. If not alleviated, SLE can cause permanent damage to the kidneys, heart, lungs, liver, nervous system, joints and skin.[3]

Anti-Phospholipid Antibodies and Essential Fatty Acids

What are these abnormal antibodies that attack normal body tissue? Researchers are beginning to think they are what's called antiphospholipid antibodies. Phospholipids are charged with fighting invasions of fat molecules in cell membranes. When phospholipids are destroyed or minimized by a high saturated fat-processed food diet, the organs of the body become bloated with fat, and cannot function properly. When the body produces antibodies that kill phospholipids, researchers call them antiphospholipid antibodies.

Researchers believe lupus may well be a form of anti-phospholipid-antibody syndrome. The symptoms certainly fit. According to an article in the *Annals of the Rheumatic Diseases*, high levels of antiphospholipid antibodies have been noted in patients suffering from lupus, who also exhibit the same symptoms as 'primary anti-phospholipid syndrome.'[4] The bottom line? Whatever works to reverse the effects of these antibodies will most likely help lupus as well. This is where our sleuthing pays off. It just so happens that what researchers have noted works for this antibody syndrome, also has been shown in studies to alleviate the damaging effects of lupus: fish oils and other essential fatty acids.

In a double-blind, crossover study, 27 patients with SLE attending the Bloomsbury Rheumatology Clinic in London were placed on a low-fat diet and given 20 grams/day of fish oil capsules or a placebo for 12 weeks each. Fourteen of 17 patients who completed the study showed improvement in their overall condition while on fish oil. Thirteen of the 17 worsened or showed no change while on the placebo. The researchers concluded that although the study was small, "its implications are significant."[5]

A number of animal studies have shown that fish oil added to the diet may slow the progression of kidney disease associated with lupus. The theory holds that fish oils contain a type of fatty acid that may alter the production of prostaglandins, important hormones that help control the inflammatory process in rheumatic diseases like arthritis and lupus.[6]

Researchers from the Arthritis and Metabolic Bone Disease Research Unit in Pellenberg, Belgium, studied 90 patients with rheumatoid arthritis who were treated with three supplements: 2.6 grams of omega-3 fatty acids, 1.3 grams of omega-3 fatty acids plus three grams of olive oil or six grams of olive oil. There was significant improvement only in those taking 2.6 grams of omega-3 fatty acids per day. Patients taking this dosage improved markedly, and were able to reduce their medications. This improvement was apparent after three months of supplementation and tended to increase throughout the 12-month study.[7]

It can become very confusing when talking about the different kinds of fatty acids, which are the kinds of fats we need for energy and health – *not* saturated fat from meat and dairy products and certainly *not* transfatty acids from hydrogenated margarine and oils. Suffice it to say that omega-3 fatty acids are found in fish oil and omega-6 fatty acids are also in vegetable and seed oils. The best source of omega-6 is borage oil.

Both families of essential fatty acids have shown to help lupus sufferers, especially when it comes to the pain of inflammation. In studies at the Department of Metabolic Disease Research at Hoffman-LaRoche in Nutley, New Jersey, researchers there discovered that both omega-6 and omega-3 fatty acids inhibit inflammation.[8]

Researchers have repeatedly demonstrated that a shortage or excess of prostaglandins can be a source of many common diseases, lupus for one. Borage oil is a good source of prostaglandins and early tests have shown it to be not only a valuable treatment for lupus, but a substitute for commonly-used non-steroidal anti-inflammatory drugs (NSAIDs). NSAIDs have dangerous side effects. Frequent use causes stomach ulcers and liver and kidney disease. Deaths have even been associated with NSAID use.

Gamma linolenic acid, or GLA, present in borage oil, evening primrose oil or black currant seed oil, is one of the natural components of the prostaglandin chain disturbed by NSAIDs. Take borage oil while reducing NSAID dosage, and continue afterwards.

Dr. Jonathan Wright recommends flax oil as a source of omega-3, along with the GLA, adding that vitamin E is an important addition, as well as vitamin B6 because most lupus medications inhibit the enzymes that depend on vitamin B6. For his lupus patients, Dr. Wright makes sure he does allergy testing, because he has found many lupus patients are allergic to gluten, a protein found in all grains except corn and rice.[9]

New Research Points to DHEA

From me to you: cutting edge research found nowhere else that could mean a breakthrough for lupus sufferers!

Researchers at the Stanford University Medical Center, Stanford, California, recently designed a study seeking to determine the therapeutic benefits of dehydroepiandrosterone (DHEA) in ten female patients with mild to moderate SLE. DHEA is a naturally-occurring adrenal hormone. The women were given 200 mg of DHEA orally for three to six months, with the patients improving enough to reduce their need for prescribed corticosteroids. The researchers concluded that DHEA "holds promise as a new therapeutic agent for the treatment of mild to moderate systemic lupus erythematosus."[10]

Dr. Wright has found that in women with lupus, 80 percent were low in the hormone testosterone, and recommends that doctors with lupus patients perform a hormone panel.

When it comes to DHEA, it is best to use it with a responsible doctor's supervision as too much of it can cause male pattern baldness – especially in women.

The makers of DHEA are currently battling the FDA system in order to get this natural substance to health food store shelves.

Skin-Healing Nutrients for Lupus-Associated Rashes

Two vitamins have been found in studies to help alleviate the red "mask" of lupus. One, reported in *Clinical Medicine*, found that when 12 patients with SLE were treated with intramuscular shots of vitamin E, eight had "excellent results."[11] In another study, four lupus patients receiving 900-1600 IU of daily vitamin E had a complete or almost complete clearing of their rashes. Two patients who received a lower dosage of 300 IU daily had no benefit.[12]

When vitamin E doesn't work, researchers have found that vitamin B12 can help. In the above mentioned *Clinical Medicine* study, three of the 12 patients who did not respond with vitamin E were given B12 shots. After six weeks, they all had complete clearing of their lesions.[13]

Supplementation of B12 may not be the key factor in lupus skin rashes, but it could reduce their frequency. Israeli M.D. Yair Molad and colleagues found in studies that 18.5 percent of 43 females with SLE had significantly lower levels of B12 than controls.[14]

For more on what you can do for skin rashes, see the chapters Allergies and Insect Bites. In the meantime, target a good antioxidant formula that contains vitamin E to boost your immune system. It appears that with lupus, a poor immune system contributes toward a worsening of the disease. In that vein, consider two possibilities: food allergies and low stomach acid.

Lupus-Fighting Nutrients
For maximum absorption, take supplements with meals.

Nutrient	Suggested Dosage	Formulation
Acidophilus	At least four billion flora on an empty stomach, three times daily	
Aged garlic extract	1 teaspoon three times daily	Liquid
Amino acids	4-6 capsules daily	Multiple formula from natural sources
Antioxidants	4 capsules daily*	With selenium and grapeseed extract
Borage oil	2 capsules daily	
Coenzyme Q10	2 capsules daily	With vitamin E, phospholipids and selenium
Enzymes	2 capsules twice daily	Multiple formula
Fiber	4-8 tablets daily	Psyllium, with herb hyssop
Flaxseed oil	1 tablespoon daily	
Lecithin	2 tablespoons daily	
Magnesium	200 mg daily	
Melatonin (adults only)	3 mg daily at bedtime	With B vitamins
Multi-mineral	3-4 ounces daily	In liquid solution, with vitamin B12, biotin
Multi-vitamin/mineral	6 caplets daily	Freeze-dried plant sources
Niacin	500 mg four times daily	
Vitamin B6	100 mg daily	
Vitamin C	Individual bowel tolerance**	With bioflavonoids (quercetin, rutin proanthocyanidins)
Vitamin E	2 capsules (800 IU) daily	d-alpha tocopherol

* The FDA recommends pregnant women not exceed 10,000 IU of vitamin A daily.

** To determine individual dosage, on the first day take 1,000 mg hourly until diarrhea occurs, then reduce dosage to just below that for individual daily dosage. Vitamin C is not toxic in large doses but must be taken throughout the day to benefit. Divide dosage to three or four times a day.

CHAPTER 108:

Macular Degeneration

"One of the most wonderful things in nature is a glance of the eye – it transcends speech; it is the bodily symbol of identity."
                                        – Ralph Waldo Emerson

Although cataracts and glaucoma get all the press, macular degeneration is really big news. It occurs in approximately 30 percent of Americans over the age of 75, is the leading cause of blindness among the elderly,[1] and affects over 10 million people over the age of 50.[2] Macular degeneration gets its name from the word macula. That's the part of your retina responsible for sharp, central sight – like reading fine print, driving, or working on puzzles. Picture this: your eyes are like a camera. The retina is the light-sensitive film behind the eye. In the dead center of the film sits the macula. When the macula is damaged, you get a blur or blind spot right in the middle of your vision.

Age-related Macular Degeneration Caused by Free Radicals

Macular degeneration is described as one of the "wear and tear" diseases attributed to oxidation, or free radical damage. This is because the macula is in an oxygen-rich environment where the metabolic rate is high, and which generates a significant amount of free radicals.[3]

The important thing to understand at this point is the role that oxygen plays in eye disease. The eyes are the only part of the outer body that is actually *living tissue* which is directly exposed to the damaging effects of oxygen and the environment. No wonder they are so easily damaged.

Although we cannot live without oxygen, being exposed to it causes degenerative problems. In addition to using oxygen to generate greater amounts of energy, exposure produces unstable oxygen compounds known as oxygen free radicals that damage DNA, proteins, carbohydrates and fats.

We can see this process in everyday life in the form of rusting metal, browning fruit and rancid oils.

Highly charged with energy, free radicals are unstable and unpredictable as a madman who runs amuck in a crowd. They are scavenger molecules with unpaired electrons which steal single electrons from other pairs and in the process rust our lawn furniture and shorten our lifespans.

How do free radicals originate? In many ways. First, from the air that we breathe. Secondly, we encourage the production of free radicals in our bodies when we expose ourselves to toxic poisons. For example, when we spray insecticide on our gardens, eat rancid oil, inhale tobacco smoke, use strong cleaners without gloves and ventilation, and ingest drugs. Even stress can cause free radicals to form.

There are two ways our bodies compensate for this problem: by replicating new cells and by creating antioxidant enzymes that snuff out the free radicals, changing them into harmless waste that's thrown off.

The eye, and in particular the macula, contains a number of key antioxidants including vitamins C and E, beta-carotene, and the minerals zinc, selenium and copper. Macular degeneration can be exacerbated by several factors. Older individuals are more susceptible to macular degeneration and tend to eat a diet that is less rich in antioxidants.[4] Other important factors are reduced stomach acid and intestinal absorption, making it harder to absorb minerals.[5] Older people should always target minerals in solution for their supplemental needs in order to overcome these adversities.

Think Zinc

Several studies show higher blood concentrations of antioxidants such as beta carotene, vitamin C and E are associated with lower levels of macular degeneration.[6]

Zinc is an essential mineral that affects both general body function and the visual system. A zinc deficiency can affect intraocular pressure, causing very low eye pressure (the opposite of glaucoma). Zinc is also involved in vitamin A metabolism, so that a zinc deficiency can result in symptoms similar to vitamin A deficiency, such as night blindness.

In one study, 151 older, healthy volunteers were divided into two groups. One group received 100 to 200 mg of zinc daily for 18 to 24 months. The other received no zinc supplementation. It was found that the zinc-supplemented subjects had significantly less macular loss than those who did not take the supplement.[7]

In a year-long study at the University of Florida in Gainesville, David Whitley, M.D., and colleagues reported that pigs receiving a diet low in zinc were found to have changes in the eye similar to those occurring in the early stages of age-related macular degeneration in humans.[8]

Long-term use of Captopril, an ACE inhibitor prescribed for hypertensive patients, often results in a depletion of zinc stores, according to researchers. Zinc loss was also reported in patients taking Enalapril, another ACE inhibitor.[9]

Stress also reduces the amount of zinc stored in the body. One study of volunteers found although they had more than adequate intakes of zinc, iron, copper and selenium, their plasma levels of the minerals during stress went down by 33, 44, 12 and 9 percent respectively.

Only about 10 to 20 percent of the zinc that we ingest from foods is properly absorbed. Large amounts of calcium, phytic acid (from grains, nuts and legumes), copper and cadmium (from pollution and cigarette smoke) can deplete zinc stores in blood and tissues.

Zinc is needed for normal skin, bones and hair. It is a component of several different enzyme systems involved in digestion and respiration. Zinc is required for the transfer of carbon dioxide in red blood cells; for proper calcification of bones; for the synthesis and metabolism of proteins and nucleic acids; for the development and functioning of reproductive organs; for wound and burn healing; for the functioning of insulin; and for normal taste acuity. The bottom line? Make sure you think zinc!

Your children may not be getting enough zinc. Nutrition surveys conducted by the U.S. Department of Agriculture reveal that many children in the United States are not meeting the minimum requirement for the mineral. Average intakes of zinc in children two to seven years old are about 4.65 to 6.7 mg daily, well below the RDA of 10 mg for this age group.[10]

Always take a multi-mineral formula that contains copper before taking zinc alone. It is important, when taking large amounts of zinc, to also ingest 2-4 mg per day of copper as large, prolonged dosages of zinc can cause a copper deficiency and immune system impairment. Too much copper, too, can deplete zinc. They must be in balance or they cancel out the other. A good zinc/copper formula will have 30 mg of zinc to 2 mg of copper.

Antioxidants to the Rescue

Jonathan Wright, M.D., reports that 40 to 50 percent of his patients with macular degeneration improved following his protocol that included the antioxidants selenium, vitamin E, zinc and the amino acid taurine orally. Seventy to 80 percent improved when the same four nutrients were given by IV injection.

Dr. Wright recounts a fascinating case of a woman whose macular degeneration was dramatically improved with intravenous selenium and zinc. In 1986 a 61-year-old female came to the physician with rapidly progressing macular degeneration. She wanted an alternative to her proposed laser treatment. Since she was found to be deficient in stomach acid and therefore had trouble absorbing nutrients, she was given an IV of zinc and selenium. During the first selenium/zinc IV infusion she shouted for the nurse, noting that she could read the print on a poster across the room which she saw blurry before the IV had started. Initially she needed a zinc and selenium IV every two or three days or her vision would deteriorate again. Four years later she was getting an IV every few weeks. Dr. Wright included vitamin E to boost the selenium.[11]

Beta carotene and vitamin C may be useful in treating patients with macular degeneration. Drs. Jack Goldberg and O.M. Tso of the University of Illinois in Chicago discovered that those with this problem are apt to eat fewer carotene-rich fruits and vegetables, such as carrots, apricots, cantaloupe, spinach and peaches. Dr. Tso recommends 50 mg of beta carotene daily.[12]

All aspects of macular degeneration are being addressed at The Eye Research Institute in Boston, including special glasses, laser treatments and other approaches. D. Max Snodderly, Ph.D., and Alice Adler, Ph.D., are feeding monkeys a carotene-rich diet to better understand the biochemistry of the retina. Dr. Adler and her colleagues are also studying the role of fats in the development of macular degeneration.[13]

Allen Taylor, Ph.D., of the USDA Human Nutrition Research Center on Aging at Tufts University in Boston, has found in his studies that vitamins C and E, and beta carotene work to protect the macula from light and free radical damage.[14]

John Weiter, M.D., of The Eye Research Institute in Boston, believes vitamins C and E, selenium, and zinc may help absorb the abnormal chemicals that can damage eyes.[15]

Macula-Mighty Nutrients
For maximum absorption, take supplements with meals.

Nutrient	Suggested Dosage	Formulation
Antioxidants	4 capsules daily*	With selenium and grapeseed extract
Bilberry	100 mg twice daily	
Borage oil	2 capsules daily	
Coenzyme Q10	2 capsules daily	With vitamin E, phospholipids and selenium
Flaxseed oil	1 tablespoon daily	
Ginkgo biloba	60 mg daily	
Multi-mineral	3-4 ounces daily	In liquid solution, with vitamin B12, biotin
Multi-vitamin/mineral	6 caplets daily	Freeze-dried plant sources
Taurine	500 mg twice daily	
Vitamin A	25,000 IU daily*	
Vitamin C	Individual bowel tolerance**	With bioflavonoids (quercetin, rutin proanthocyanidins)

* The FDA recommends pregnant women not exceed 10,000 IU of vitamin A daily.

** To determine individual dosage, on the first day take 1,000 mg hourly until diarrhea occurs, then reduce dosage to just below that for individual daily dosage. Vitamin C is not toxic in large doses but must be taken throughout the day to benefit. Divide dosage to three or four times a day.

CHAPTER 109:

Malabsorption

"The mind is like the stomach. It is not how much you put into it that counts, but how much it digests."
—Albert Jay Nock

Phoebe Pator was a spunky lady I met while visiting a friend in the hospital. From the moment I met her I liked her. Despite her acute illness, the 73-year-old wasn't apathetic. She complained constantly, never let anybody ignore her needs, and maintained a determined demeanor. Phoebe was admitted to the hospital suffering from starvation. When I met her, her stomach was bloated like the pictures of starving children in Africa. She still had her sense of humor though, and bragged that when she got home she would gain 50 pounds. Her doctors put her on a parenteral IV (nutrients given intravenously), then liquid diets, and sent her home.

A month later she was back again. They diagnosed her as having sprue, or celiac disease, which in her case was caused by an allergy to gluten, a protein found in all grains except rice and corn. Gluten irritates the intestinal lining, interfering with the absorption of nutrients and water, and is found in just about every processed food.

Even though they discovered the problem, it was too late for Phoebe. The years of allergic reactions in her intestines had taken their toll. Part of her bowel had to be removed, and the cilia, which absorbs nutrients and water, in what was left, was non-existent. In order to continue living, Phoebe would have to have had nutrients continually given to her through her veins. After going back and forth several times from home to hospital, she gave up, ate the foods she enjoyed, and the next time she went back to the hospital, never went home again. Could Phoebe had been saved? Yes, if she had learned early enough that her chronic diarrhea and intestinal problems was the result of an allergy to gluten. It wasn't the destroyed intestinal lining that killed her, it was the resultant malabsorption that kept her from getting the nutrients she needed to stay alive.

What Causes Malabsorption?

The story of malabsorption is the story of nutritional deficiencies. When the body is unable to absorb nutrients every symptom can be traced to nutritional deficiencies. There are two reasons malabsorption occurs: too little stomach acid to break down foods so their nutrients can be absorbed, and intestinal problems that make it impossible for nutrients and even life-giving water to be absorbed. Malabsorption can be caused by gastrointestinal ailments, allergies, diarrhea, parasites which destroy the intestinal lining, antibiotics which cause an overgrowth of bad bacteria; and even a deficiency of zinc, which can result in intestinal problems. The symptoms of malabsorption, or nutritional deficiencies, include fatigue, anemia, asthma, stunted growth, hair loss, bloating and the eating of clay or dirt (termed pica).

Certain health problems can be traced to specific nutrient deficiencies because of the role the organ has in assimilating the nutrient. For example, chronic constipation impairs the absorption of vitamin A and beta carotene. The bacteria that causes food poisoning, such as Salmonella and Escherichia coli, not only result in a trip to the doctor, but also destroy vitamin C in the small intestine, where it is absorbed. Anything that disrupts the workings of the small intestine, including antibiotics and other pharmaceuticals, can decrease absorption of vitamin C. A lack of hydrochloric acid in the stomach will also impair absorption of vitamin C. The B vitamins, particularly riboflavin, are absorbed in the intestine and require hydrochloric acid for their absorption. Kidney problems reduce the amount of bile salts needed to absorb vitamin K.[1] Alcoholics often have malabsorption of nutrients, especially vitamin A and thiamine, due to an impaired liver.[2] The list of nutrients that can be easily and dangerously lost from the body due to malabsorption is long, and include the minerals zinc, selenium and magnesium; and the vitamins A, C, B12 and beta carotene.

Food allergies can be a major factor in the onset of malabsorption. Not only can an allergy to gluten create the problem, but common in children is an allergy to cow's milk, specifically the milk sugar lactose or the protein casein. Cow's milk may initiate severe allergic gastritis which then results in a lack of hydrochloric acid and pepsin, a digestive enzyme. This has been a factor in many cases of asthma in children. This malabsorption results in a deficiency of vitamin B12, which further aggravates asthma symptoms.[3]

When Ross Gordon, M.D. treats his patients with chronic fatigue, he first gives them shots of vitamin B12. If the patients notice a difference, he considers it a strong indication that they have too little hydrochloric acid or stomach acid. Without adequate stomach acid, proteins are not digested, and essential amino acids, nutrients and minerals such as iron and B12 are not absorbed. When supplementing with any B vitamin always take a B-complex formula. All the B vitamins are dependent upon each other. Without one, the others become deficient.

Sometimes I come across case histories so unnecessarily tragic, they beg uncovering. Such is the case of a 3-1/2 year old child who had been chemically treated for leukemia. Six months after receiving chemotherapy she developed vomiting and diarrhea. Hospitalized, she was put on parenteral nutrition. She had eye disturbances after four weeks and died three days later.[4] The autopsy revealed Wernicke's encephalopathy, which is a fancy name for beriberi, or a thiamine (B1) deficiency. Encephalopathy literally means brain damage.

Inadequate amounts of thiamine reduces blood flow to the brain, and if it continues it can cause death. The *Clinical Neuropathology* article that reported this case didn't attempt to explain how someone receiving nutritional supplementation in a hospital managed to become thiamine deficient to the point of death, but I have one hypothesis. Many vitamin supplements do not contain proper amounts of thiamine. The RDAs (recommended daily allowances) are notoriously low, since they are designed to maintain health, not to improve it. Pharmaceutical companies often use RDA amounts to formulate their supplementals – the same supplementals used in hospitals for very sick people.

It is quite likely that in this case the chemotherapy effectively jeopardized the child's intestinal system to such a degree that the low doses of thiamine present in the hospital's supplementation wasn't enough to fully nourish her body. It wasn't until she was postmortem that they discovered what caused her death – a death that could have been prevented. Even more telling, the author of the article suggests that "thiamine supplementation should be considered in all patients who have persistent malnutrition and malabsorption," insinuating that in the case of this little girl, she was not given thiamine at all!

The Dangers of Digestive Problems

Nutritionists are just beginning to realize the extent by which conventional medicine ignores the nutritional equation in illness. Intestinal problems can be caused by so many ailments – for example anorexia, chronic dieting, disease, surgery, diarrhea, ulcers or pharmaceutical side effects – that most hospitalized patients are probably nutritionally deficient as a rule rather than an exception. This would not be very helpful in a program designed to heal.

An article in *Family Practice News* suggests most physicians believe the need for nutritional supplements is rare or "esoteric" and doesn't need to be addressed in the clinical care of most patients. Despite this prevalent attitude, the data suggests deficiencies are far from uncommon. Among Crohn's disease patients, low vitamin B12 levels can be found in as many as 60 percent, and among those with inflamed bowels from whatever the source, as many as 64 percent are deficient in folic acid, with 65 percent deficient in vitamin D. Vitamin D works with calcium to build strong bones, and deficiencies of folic acid and B12 have been clinically associated with mental problems.[5]

Only one nutrient has been directly associated with malabsorption: zinc. Studies show zinc can either be a result of malabsorption, or it is a contributing factor. This is because zinc is a wound healer, with the intestine requiring zinc to heal its delicate tissues. Without adequate amounts the likelihood of developing gastrointestinal problems increases. Akira Okada, M.D., of Osaka University Medical School in Japan, even goes so far as to state that gastrointestinal diseases are either caused from or frequently a result of a zinc deficiency. Just when it's needed the most, the stress of surgery is found to reduce zinc stores in the body, contributing to hospitalized deficiency. A lack of zinc also lowers the immune system, making recovery harder.[6]

Hypochlorhydria: More Common Than You Think

A lack of stomach acid – hypochlorhydria – is more common than we think and can cause all of the symptoms that appear when the stomach contains too much acid. Doctors warn that people should not take antacids too readily as heartburn, gas, bloating after eating and even constipation can all be symptoms of too little stomach, or gastric, acid. The burning sensation common to too much acid is also present when the stomach is too alkaline, and can be made worse by antacids. Dr. Gordon estimates that every third adult he sees in his Clinic in Albany, California, secretes too little hydrochloric acid.

The Heidelberg test can be performed to determine the amount of gastric acid present in the stomach. Ed Persaud, a student of naturopathy at Dr. Ron Hoffman's Center of Holistic Medicine uses the Heidelberg test to measure stomach acid levels. He told me that in his 14-year experience, testing approximately 10,000 individuals, he estimates 90 percent were found to have low amounts of stomach acid.

Researchers at the Mayo Clinic and Johns Hopkins University pumped the stomachs of over 3,000 individuals and analyzed their contents. It was determined that by the age of 60 years, 60 percent had a significant decline in hydrochloric acid. Supplementing with a hydrochloric acid formula such as Betaine, available in health food stores, will help absorb nutrients.

Food allergies are not the only things that can attack the stomach lining, leading to diminished gastric acid. Viruses such as measles, mumps and chicken pox – common childhood diseases – can destroy the stomach lining, which may or may not return to normal.

The Solution is in Solution

If you have any of the symptoms I've mentioned already and suspect a malabsorption problem, many studies and case histories have shown the importance of taking nutrients in solution.

In 1988, Dr. Ralph F. Shangraw, chairman of the Department of Pharmaceutics at the School of Pharmacy, University of Maryland, reported results of experiments he had conducted with calcium supplements. He found that many calcium tablets on the market could not be absorbed by the average healthy person.[7]

Calcium supplements cannot be absorbed unless they disintegrate and dissolve. According to standards established by the U.S. Pharmacopeia, 75 percent of a drug tablet must disintegrate within a half hour. However, calcium tablets are regarded as nutritional supplements, not drugs and there is currently no disintegration requirement.

A simple test you can do at home will tell you roughly how effectively a supplement is apt to disintegrate and dissolve in the presence of hydrochloric acid in the normally functioning stomach. Place a tablet in vinegar and stir occasionally. After a half hour, at least three-fourths of the tablet should be dissolved. If this has not occurred, the supplement may not be adequately absorbed.

Inorganic minerals also may not be well absorbed. To improve absorption, manufacturers may chelate mineral supplements. This technique binds the mineral to an organic chelating substance that causes a slight increase in absorption. Look on the labels for these examples of inorganic, and therefore difficult to absorb, forms of minerals: carbonate, chloride, hydroxide, iodide, oxide, phosphate, selenate, selenite and sulfate. Examples of organic chelated forms of minerals are ascorbate, aspartate, citrate, gluconate, glycinate, lactate, orotate and any substances that end with the word "chelate."[8]

Studies show minerals dissolved in water before ingestion are considerably more bioavailable to the body than those even present in food or inorganic supplements. Minerals in solution don't need stomach acid to break them down, and aren't influenced by food allergies. Look for a good, easily absorbable, derived-from-nature mineral blend in solution. Formulations in solution provide the maximum absorption ratios.

Health-Restorative Nutrients
For maximum absorption, take supplements with meals.

Nutrient	Suggested Dosage	Formulation
Acidophilus	At least four billion flora on an empty stomach, three times daily	
Aged garlic extract	1 teaspoon three times daily	Liquid
Amino acids	4-6 capsules daily	Multiple formula from natural sources
Antioxidants	4 capsules daily*	With selenium and grapeseed extract
Borage oil	2 capsules daily	
Coenzyme Q10	2 capsules daily	With vitamin E, phospholipids and selenium
Enzymes	2 capsules twice daily	Multiple formula
Fiber	4-8 tablets daily	Psyllium, with herb hyssop
Flaxseed oil	1 tablespoon daily	
L-glutamine	500 mg twice daily	
Multi-mineral	3-4 ounces daily	In liquid solution, with vitamin B12, biotin
Multi-vitamin/mineral	6 caplets daily	Freeze-dried plant sources
Vitamin C	Individual bowel tolerance**	Chewable, with bioflavonoids (quercetin proanthocyanidins)

* The FDA recommends pregnant women not exceed 10,000 IU of vitamin A daily.

** To determine individual dosage, on the first day take 1,000 mg hourly until diarrhea occurs, then reduce dosage to just below that for individual daily dosage. Vitamin C is not toxic in large doses but must be taken throughout the day to benefit. Divide dosage to three or four times a day.

CHAPTER 110:

Measles

Some years ago while visiting Central America, I found myself in a small "campo," or village. The people lived in mud houses with no running water or sewage facilities. They bathed and drank from the same pool of water their livestock did, and the children rarely if ever had shoes on their feet. The people lived primarily by picking coffee for rich landowners, and barely existed on the meager amounts of corn and beans they grew. I'll never forget the sight of a girl around six or seven years of age lying on a cotton cloth on the dirt floor covered in a measles rash, obviously deathly ill. I thought, "How could measles do this?" Why, in America few even get the illness, much less be ravaged by it. I told my driver to translate and asked the child's parents if they would let me take the girl into the city for treatment. I told them I would pay for the hospitalization and bring her back when she was better. I didn't expect them to agree. After all, I was a stranger. But something made them trust me. Desperation perhaps. I took the little girl, her name was Juanita, to the hospital. During the two weeks she was there, she was treated with medicines and healthy food. Her doctors were open to giving her all the foods and vitamins I suggested.

In developing countries such as the one I was in, measles causes more than a million deaths per year. Poor nutrition and unsanitary conditions compromise the immune system to such a degree that complications and secondary infections prolong the illness or lead to death. Ear and chest infections, including pneumonia, are common, as are chronic diarrhea, vomiting and stomachaches. In about one in

1,000 cases measles leads to encephalitis, or inflammation of the brain. Many more tragedies occur when women who managed to avoid the disease as children contract it when they are pregnant and give birth to children with birth defects.

I had measles as a child. I enjoyed staying home from school until I found out I had to be quarantined in my house. My mother wisely put up a big sign on the window to keep my friends away, robbing me of the reward of staying home but I'm sure hastening my recovery.

Measles, or rubella, is a highly contagious viral infection characterized by a fever, cough, spots on the gums, and a red rash that usually begins at the head and neck and slowly moves down to cover the entire body. The measles virus Morbillivirus is passed on through airborne droplets. One person sneezes, and another inhales the droplets. The virus is active from seven to 14 days. Like the chickenpox, another childhood viral disease, treatment usually includes bed rest, drinking plenty of fluids, and lotions to relieve the itching. There was little anyone could do to help – until now.

The Answer is A

Several lines of evidence indicate that measles increases the body's use of vitamin A. In Indonesia and other parts of Asia, measles is an important factor in the development of clinical vitamin A deficiency and blindness, and in northern Nigeria, vitamin A blood levels of well-nourished children with measles were lower than in nutritionally-starved children without measles.[1]

Vitamin A was first recommended as a protective agent against measles 50 years ago.[2] Sadly, the compelling evidence was ignored. Finally, researchers around the world are admitting to the benefit of vitamin A in minimizing the effects of the measles virus.

In controlled trials in South Africa and Tanzania, high-dose vitamin A supplementation reduced the number of deaths in children with severe measles. In a South African study, children receiving the vitamin recovered more rapidly from pneumonia and diarrhea, had a lower incidence of croup, and spent fewer days in the hospital than those taking a placebo.[3]

A randomized double-blind trial of 189 South African children with measles found that when they were given vitamin A, their risk of contracting and succumbing to complications was decreased by half. Of the 12 children in the study that died, ten had been given a placebo.[4]

Researchers chose an urban slum area in Bombay, India, to conduct another study on the health-giving benefits of vitamin A. The vitamin was given to 2,000 children under five years of age, and 403 under one year of age, and compared to a control group of 2,060 children under five and 460 under one.

At six month intervals a detailed history was taken of their illnesses. Common illnesses for these children, in addition to vitamin A deficiency, were fever, respiratory tract infections, diarrhea, gastrointestinal infections, skin infections, ear infections, measles and malnutrition. Thanks to the vitamin A, the children were much healthier. Not only did the vitamin A help reduce the incidence of measles, but their parents were relieved to note they had less cases of these "common" childhood illnesses.[5]

In this country a deficiency of vitamin A is deemed rare, even among poor children. In New York City, where clinical vitamin A deficiency is almost unknown, researchers were shocked to find it in epidemic proportions among children with measles.

Vitamin A levels were measured in 89 measles patients under the age of two years and in a reference group of 60 healthy children. Doctors found over half with measles had either severely low blood levels of vitamin A or were borderline. In contrast, none of the children in the reference group had low levels. For every age, gender, and ethnic subgroup, vitamin A levels were lower in the measles patients.[6]

Not only that, the children with low vitamin A levels were more likely to have high or prolonged fevers, and lower measles-specific antibody levels, meaning less antibodies available to fight off the infection. Children with low or borderline vitamin A levels were more likely to be hospitalized than those with normal levels.

Reporting on this study in the *American Journal of Diseases of Children*, Thomas R. Frieden, M.D., of the New York City Department of Health, proclaimed that since measles seems to decrease levels of vitamin A, and that a deficiency of vitamin A makes the disease worse, "U.S. clinicians may wish to consider vitamin A therapy for children younger than two years with severe measles." Vitamin A therapy is currently recommended for children with measles only in third-world, developing countries.[7]

What You Need to Know About Vitamin A

Doctors like to scare people away from vitamin A by emphasizing that you can take too much. Vitamin A is a so-called fat soluble vitamin, meaning it doesn't dissolve well in water and as a result, our body stores excess A in the liver. Too much can cause liver and bone damage. However, high amounts are damaging only when taken for long periods of time, and when combined with normal levels of vitamin A. The good news is that including vitamin E and beta carotene with A helps the effect so lower amounts can be taken. Early warning signs of vitamin A toxicity are a small pounding headache at the front of the head, cracked lips or peeling palms.

In an editorial in the *British Medical Journal*, Michael Chan of the Liverpool School of Tropical Medicine recommends that all children in developing countries who are diagnosed with measles should receive a supplement of 400,000 IU of vitamin A as a routine part of primary care.[8] For Americans, the advice of a physician versed in nutritional medicine is certainly recommended.

Zinc is needed for the absorption of vitamin A, and is considered a wound healer. A supplement that contains zinc and copper may help in not only boosting vitamin A, but in getting the skin back to pre-measles shape. Vitamin C is always a good idea because it is essential to the formation of the skin's collagen and is severely depleted during fevers. It also helps prevent any problems that might occur with high doses of vitamin A.

Factors interfering with absorption of vitamin A and its precursor beta carotene include strenuous physical activity within four hours of consumption, drinking mineral oil (often recommended by conventional pediatricians to fight constipation), excessive consumption of alcohol and iron, and the use of cortisone and other drugs.[9]

For more on dealing with the symptoms of measles, see the chapters Fever and Insect Bites.

Measles Reducing Nutrients – Childrens' Dosage
For maximum absorption, take supplements with meals.

Nutrient	Suggested Dosage	Formulation
Aged garlic extract	1 teaspoon twice daily	Liquid
Antioxidants	2 capsules daily	With selenium and grapeseed extract
Echinacea	250 mg daily for a maximum of three weeks	
Lysine	500 mg daily	
Multi-mineral	1/2-1 ounce	In liquid solution, with vitamin B12, biotin
Multi-vitamin/mineral	1-2 tablets	Children's chewable
Vitamin A	15,000 IU daily	
Vitamin C	Individual bowel tolerance*	Chewable with bioflavonoids (quercetin, proanthocyanidins)

* To determine individual dosage, on the first day take 1,000 mg hourly until diarrhea occurs, then reduce dosage to just below that for individual daily dosage. Vitamin C is not toxic in large doses but must be taken throughout the day to benefit. Divide dosage to three or four times a day.

CHAPTER 111:

Memory Loss

"Memory is the cabinet of imagination, the treasury of reason, the registry of conscience, and the council chamber of thought."
— Saint Basil

"A retentive memory is a good thing, but the ability to forget is the true token of greatness."
— Elbert Hubbard

Nobody is perfect, and nobody remembers everything. Memory loss can occur with as little reason as the effort to try. If you find yourself staring in disbelief because you got where you were going but forgot why you went there, don't be alarmed. That's why we have shopping lists! Sometimes memory is as elusive as the flattering drivers license photo, and has nothing at all to do with your increasing age.

A certain amount of brain cell loss is accepted by conventional medicine to be a normal process of aging, but studies show with certain nutrients and exercises, brain function can not only be restored, but improved! Follow along while I show you how.

The Brainy B Vitamins

All the B vitamins, found in liver, brewer's yeast and whole grains, are vital for the normal functioning of the nervous system, and may be the single most important factor for the health of the nerves. Because the B vitamins are water-soluble, those not used immediately by the body are excreted, not stored. On the good side, this means you cannot take too much. On the bad side, they must be continually replaced. Sulfa drugs, sleeping pills, insecticides and estrogen create a condition in the digestive tract which can destroy B vitamins. The most important thing to remember is that all the B vitamins must be taken together. Too much of one can cause a deficiency of another. Always take a B complex supplement when targeting a specific B vitamin.[1]

Vernon Mark, M.D., Harvard neurosurgeon and director of the Center for Memory Impairment and Neurobehavioral Disorders in Brookline, Massachusetts, considers the government's recommended daily allowances (RDAs) inadequate, and says solely meeting them is comparable to getting Ds on your report card.

Memory nutrients are the minerals calcium, magnesium, potassium, copper, zinc and iron; and the vitamins B3 (niacin), B6 (pyridoxine), folic acid, B12, and C. Dr. Mark suggests adding three grams of choline daily. Choline, found naturally in oatmeal, rice, soy products, peanuts and pecans, is the precursor of acetylcholine, a key brain messenger for memory.

Minimizing your intake of fat and cholesterol is one of the smartest moves you can make to ensure your brain's health. An ideal, brain-sustaining diet is low in calories, salt, processed foods and alcohol, and loaded with whole grains, beans and peas (legumes), and lots of fresh produce.[2]

Folic acid and vitamin B12 can cause memory loss commonly associated with dementia, and a thiamine deficiency can cause severe chronic memory problems.[3]

A vitamin B12 deficiency is a real bogey man – especially in the over-60 crowd. It can produce psychosis, severe memory loss, impaired abstract thinking skills, mental confusion, delusions, hallucinations and even brain and spinal cord degeneration (causing numbness). Low blood levels of the vitamin are found in one-third of hospitalized psychiatric patients suffering from depression and dementia, according to a Denmark study.[4] In addition, a B12 deficiency may inhibit the brain's use of glucose (the gasoline which energizes the brain) and hinder production of our friend acetylcholine.

A deficiency of B12 can be caused by exposure to toxic chemicals and ingestion of mercury, heavy metals (cadmium, lead) and certain solvents, which prevent transfer of the vitamin from the blood to the brain. Prescription drugs can also keep B12 from getting to the brain. Some offenders are aldomet, neomycin and para-aminosalicylic acid.

Folic acid, a B vitamin found in leafy greens, prevents irritability and forgetfulness; plus, it partners with B12 in the brain's synthesis of our all important ally acetylcholine. In one case, 67 percent of patients admitted to a psychogeriatric ward were deficient in folate. Such a deficiency may arise from poor nutrition, an inability to absorb the nutrient or impaired absorption caused by drugs such as aldomet, bactrim, isoniazid, neomycin, dilantin, methotrexate, dyazide and premarin.

Boron Bests the Rest

Iron, copper, magnesium, iodine and zinc are generally recognized as brain-critical minerals. But boron turns out to be the brain's all-star performer. James Penland, Ph.D., a research psychologist with the U.S. Department of Agriculture's Human Nutrition Research Center in Grand Forks, North Dakota has studied boron in relation to memory and has found that people receiving three milligrams (mg) of boron daily demonstrated alertness, brain activity and learning superior to those receiving only one mg. Penland figures that Americans generally get less than one mg of boron per day – the amount contained in a medium-size apple.[5]

The brain's memory center, the hippocampus, has a special affinity for magnesium. If your memory is like a sieve, you may be lacking this mineral, as various experiments demonstrate.[6]

From the pages of *Medical Science Research* comes the case history of a 76-year-old male patient with Alzheimer's who, after becoming unaware of his surroundings, was placed in a nursing home. At some point doctors started giving him 500 milligrams of magnesium two times daily. Two to three weeks after the magnesium therapy the doctors were surprised to note his improved awareness. His wife and son visiting him were elated when, for the first time in months, he could turn to his wife when she called his name. He continued to improve with enhanced memory and more clarity of thought, and after nine months he was able to go home again.[7]

There is a lesson in this: beware of assumptions. Never assume you know where symptoms come from. It was easy to assume this man's memory problems were a result of his Alzheimer's. What was more likely was a magnesium deficiency was causing poor blood circulation to his brain, causing the cognitive problems. Happily, there was a good ending.

Nurture Your Memory Garden with Plenty of Water

Because a number of nutrients crucial to brain health – including calcium, magnesium, sodium, potassium and chloride exist in the body in solution, too much or too little water can unbalance their concentrations and disturb brain function. Keeping yourself well irrigated allows the kidneys to remove potential brain-poisons from the blood. You'd be hard pressed to drink too much liquid, but drinking too little water is not so uncommon.

I recommend everyone drink water throughout the day, continually. What's important is that the body tissues retain water. If the body doesn't need that glass of water you just drank, it will excrete it. If you drink it a little at a time, over the course of the day, it mimics the amounts your body gets in food and is better retained.

One way to be sure your minerals get absorbed is to make sure they start out in solution. Studies show minerals dissolved in water before ingestion are considerably more bioavailable to the body than those even present in food, because they aren't risked by a lack of hydrochloric acid in the stomach or food allergies. Look for a good, easily absorbable, derived-from-nature mineral blend in solution.

Alternative Memory Enhancers

Anything that enhances circulation and acts as an antioxidant is going to encourage a good memory. In China, the curative powers of ginkgo biloba have been known for thousands of years. According to records dating back to 2,800 B.C., the Chinese were the first people to explore ginkgo's extraordinary medicinal properties, using dried green leaves of the Maidenhair tree to treat poor circulation, memory loss and mental deterioration.

More recently, a six month double-blind, placebo-controlled trial of 31 patients 50 years of age with mild to moderate memory loss found after 12 to 24 weeks there was significant improvement in memory and learning ability.[8]

Ginkgo works by increasing blood flow to the brain, benefitting stroke, dementia and other victims of cerebral insufficiency. In one enlightening study, 40 patients, aged 60 to 80 years were split into two groups and monitored for three months. One group received ginkgo extract, while the other received a placebo. All the patients had been diagnosed as having some kind of dementia. At the end of the test, all the seniors on ginkgo showed "significant improvement" both on mental tests and their emotional outlook.[9]

Researchers determined to identify substances that help turn back the clock have found DHEA (dehydroepiandrosterone) powerful in its ability to increase circulation and enhance memory. An article in *The Lancet* cites experiments that found it reduces the effects of stress and trauma on the brain, and stimulates the immune system as well.[10]

If wish to consider DHEA, have a nutritionally-oriented doctor do a hormone panel. Too much can cause male pattern baldness – in women as well.

Mind Your Brain

Some scientists believe the natural course of aging includes the decay and loss of brain cells. This is just not so! What happens is we stop challenging our brain. We work hard all our young lives so we don't have to as we get older. There are less challenges, and less need for deep and concentrated thought.

Eric Kandel, M.D., a neurobiologist at the Howard Hughes Medical Institute at Columbia University in New York found that when brain neurons are stimulated, they actually grow, doubling the number of brain connections, and increasing memory capability.[11] As you make demands on your body through exercise, it builds muscle and uses up fat. As you make demands on your brain, it builds cells and sprouts synapsis, or cell branches. The technical term for this cell regeneration is "reactive synaptogenesis."[12]

That this phenomenon applies to you and me is becoming increasingly clear. What Kandel has observed, others have seen in mammals, including rats. University of Illinois neuroscientist William Greenough, Ph.D., found that the brains of rats reared in complex environments, and trained in a maze every day, had more extensive dendrites than did unchallenged animals. Their dendrites also sprouted more synapses.[13]

"Stimulation in general is very important to the development of the brain," reports neurobiologist Carla Shatz, Ph.D., of the University of California at Berkeley. Researchers believe that, from birth to adolescence, we are laying down the basic circuitry of the brain. As we grow up, the world subsequently makes its mark physically. Exposure to new tasks and challenges generates the development of new circuits and synapses for handling all of them. From then on, continued stimulation throughout life further strengthens these pathways and enhances their interconnections.[14]

Something to keep in mind: stress is not the same as challenges. Studies show stress, and its subsequent dumping of adrenaline in the system, can cause memory problems. It's when stress is continual and chronic, that it starts to affect the nervous system. To combat stress and alleviate its effects, see the chapter in this book.

Scientists cannot yet quantify exactly how much an enriched environment helps the brains of young children to grow. But "we do know that deprivation and isolation can result in failure of the brain to form its rich set of connections," says Shatz.

Your brain is a muscle and to keep it in peak performance you need to give it exercise. Here's a neat exercise that proves my point. Ever wonder how actors can memorize so many lines so quickly? Soap opera actors often have to memorize a whole script in one day. It's because their memory muscle is so strong. Give yourself ten words a day to memorize. Ten *new* words a day. Ideally in a foreign language. You'll find after a week or two you'll cut the time needed to memorize them in half. You are exercising your mental muscle. This ability to memorize will help in so many everyday ways you'll be glad you made the effort.

Memory Boosting Nutrients
For maximum absorption, take supplements with meals.

Nutrient	Suggested Dosage	Formulation
Acetyl L-Carnitine	500 mg three times daily	
Aged garlic extract	1 teaspoon three times daily	Liquid
Antioxidants	4 capsules daily*	With selenium and grapeseed extract
Borage oil	2 capsules daily	
Coenzyme Q1 (NADH)	2.5 mg daily	
Coenzyme Q10	2 capsules daily	With vitamin E, phospholipids and selenium
Enzymes	2 capsules twice daily	Multiple formula
Fiber	4-8 tablets daily	Psyllium, with herb hyssop
Flaxseed oil	1 tablespoon daily	
Ginkgo biloba	60 mg three times daily	
Multi-mineral	3-4 ounces daily	In liquid solution, with vitamin B12, biotin
Multi-vitamin/mineral	6 caplets daily	Freeze-dried plant sources
Vitamin C	Individual bowel tolerance**	With bioflavonoids (quercetin, proanthocyanidins)
Vitamin E	2 capsules (800 IU) daily	d-alpha tocopherol

* The FDA recommends pregnant women not exceed 10,000 IU of vitamin A daily.

** To determine individual dosage, on the first day take 1,000 mg hourly until diarrhea occurs, then reduce dosage to just below that for individual daily dosage. Vitamin C is not toxic in large doses but must be taken throughout the day to benefit. Divide dosage to three or four times a day.

CHAPTER 112:

Meniere's Syndrome

A few years ago a doctor suggested that Vincent Van Gogh had cut off his ear because he suffered from Meniere's Syndrome. The doctor believed that the vertigo or dizziness, nausea, hearing loss, pressure and loud ringing in his ears are what led him to cut off his ear and present it to a prostitute. It was an interesting theory but has largely been discounted. Van Gogh did not specifically complain of ringing in his ears, nor did he have hearing problems. He did, however, have a long history of mental disturbances leading to a more realistic theory that his depression, mania and hallucinations were a result of severe, chronic malnutrition and poisoning by the heavy metals contained in the paints and environment of the day.

First described by French ear specialist Prosper Meniere in 1861, Meniere's Syndrome is characterized by three main symptoms: attacks of vertigo or dizziness, fluctuating hearing loss (usually in one ear), and tinnitus – ringing, buzzing, or roaring sounds. This triad is often accompanied by a feeling of fullness or pressure in the affected ear. There is no way to clinically test for the ailment so doctors use the symptoms for a diagnosis. Since it is named by its symptoms, to call it a disease would be incorrect. It is a syndrome.

An estimated 5-7 million people in the United States have Meniere's syndrome, and 100,000 new cases are diagnosed each year. It can strike adults of any age but is rare in children. Although the illness is not fatal, it is completely unpredictable in its course and severity.[1] A typical Meniere's attack begins with sensations of ear pressure and loud tinnitus. Within hours, a sudden onset of severe, whirling vertigo occurs and there is generally a loss of hearing in the affected ear. The dizziness can last for minutes or even hours and may be accompanied by nausea and vomiting. One journal contends that if the sufferer can get to sleep, the symptoms will stop and he or she wakes up refreshed and symptom-free.

Doctors believe the symptoms are triggered when the inner ear canal becomes overfilled with a fluid called endolymph. Like a balloon filled with too much water, the fluid creates pressure that causes the inner ear to malfunction. The inner ear controls both hearing and balance by sending signals to the brain to regulate these functions. A dysfunction affects both.

A person's attacks may vary in duration and severity – and one individual's experiences with the syndrome may be quite different from another's. Sometimes symptoms are frequent and highly distressing for weeks or months, only to disappear almost entirely for months or years.

Niacin Needed

Dr. Miles Atkinson, an otologist formerly with New York University, found the same factors that cause migraines – spasms of the blood vessels – contribute to Meniere's. It is commonly held that migraines occur when head arteries contract and expand, causing pain and pressure. When the blood vessels of the inner ear spasm, they increase blood flow and accumulation of fluid in the chambers of the inner ear, causing the distressing symptoms – most especially vertigo. Dr. Atkins found that nicotinic acid, one form of vitamin B3 or niacin, helps control these spasms, and is chronically deficient in Meniere's patients.[2] Niacin has also been found helpful in treating high blood pressure as it improves circulation and reduces cholesterol. A deficiency can cause nausea, vomiting, tension, irritability and headaches. Important to note here is that there are three forms of *synthetic* niacin: nicotinic acid, niacinamide and nicotinamide.

Jeffery Wiersum, M.D., of Syracuse, New York, reports in an

issue of *Cortlandt Forum* that he has found success treating Meniere's with a high complex carbohydrate diet, omega-3 fatty acids (fish or flaxseed oil), 1000 mg of nicotinamide (niacin), 100 mg of vitamin B complex, 400 mg of vitamin B6, three grams of vitamin C with rose hips and nicotinic acid (niacin) in divided doses tapering up to 1000 milligrams per day.[3]

The B vitamins must be taken together, so do the B complex shuffle. The whole B complex family includes B1 (thiamine), B2 (riboflavin), B3 (niacin), B5 (pantothenic acid), B6 (pyridoxine), B12 (cobalamin), B15 (pangamic acid), biotin, choline, folic acid, inositol and PABA (para-aminobenzoic acid). Each B vitamin has its own role in body function, centered on the nervous system. Since nerves bring messages to all the organs and stimulate glands to secrete their important biochemicals, the whole body communication system can break down with a B vitamin deficiency.

For help with the specific symptoms of Meniere's see the chapters Migraines, Nausea, Hearing Loss, Water Retention and Vertigo.

Meniere's Eliminating Nutrients
For maximum absorption, take supplements with meals.

Nutrient	Suggested Dosage	Formulation
Aged garlic extract	1 teaspoon three times daily	Liquid
Antioxidants	4 capsules daily*	With selenium and grapeseed extract
Borage oil	2 capsules daily	
Coenzyme Q10	2 capsules daily	With vitamin E, phospholipids and selenium
Flaxseed oil	1 tablespoon daily	
Ginkgo biloba	60 mg daily	
Hawthorne	250 mg twice daily	
Magnesium	200 mg daily	
Melatonin (adults only)	3 mg daily at bedtime	With B vitamins
Multi-mineral	3-4 ounces daily	In liquid solution, with vitamin B12, biotin
Multi-vitamin/mineral	6 caplets daily	Freeze-dried plant sources
Niacin	200 mg three times daily	
Rutin	100 mg twice daily	
Taurine	500 mg twice daily	
Vitamin B6	100 mg daily	
Vitamin C	Individual bowel tolerance**	With bioflavonoids (quercetin, rutin proanthocyanidins)

* The FDA recommends pregnant women not exceed 10,000 IU of vitamin A daily.

** To determine individual dosage, on the first day take 1,000 mg hourly until diarrhea occurs, then reduce dosage to just below that for individual daily dosage. Vitamin C is not toxic in large doses but must be taken throughout the day to benefit. Divide dosage to three or four times a day.

CHAPTER 113:

Menopause

If there's one issue heavy with misinformation and hysteria regarding middle age, it's menopause. Menopause is not exactly terra incognita. Edith Bunker dithered through a few hot flashes on the classic TV show *All in the Family*. Kathy Bates' mood-swinging character in the movie *Fried Green Tomatoes* tore down walls and built them back up again while Jessica Tandy exhorted her to "take those hormones!" and get on with her life. The fact is, the symptoms of menopause: hot flashes, night sweats, insomnia and irritability, among others, can be prevented! How else can you explain why some women go through the change unscathed, while others cry desperately for help? The answer is the adrenals.

The adrenal glands form the baby-making hormones estrogen and progesterone. As the child-bearing years are left behind, the adrenals make less of these hormones, and fluctuations occur. The condition of the adrenal glands seems to determine how short-lived these symptoms are or whether they occur at all.

Here's what can happen. Long term nutriential deficiencies leave the body unprepared for the stress of menopause. A chronically poor diet, lack of exercise and emotional stress can so exhaust the adrenals that the metabolic response of the body is to produce more hormones. Have you ever experienced a hot flash of embarrassment or a "rush" of adrenaline when on a roller coaster? You know how when you're very angry or frightened your blood rushes to your head and you feel almost dizzy? These are your adrenals' responses to stress. It is these stress responses that cause menopausal symptoms.

As the adrenals' stop making estrogen, the body responds to the stress. What tipped me off to the connection between stress and menopause was a letter I received from a viewer in Lomita, California:

"I watched your program today and one of the subjects was about estrogen. I'm in the menopausal time of my life. My doctor told me that I'd have to take Premarin and progesterone the rest of my life. No Way!! I found a mineral in solution product which has highly absorbable boron that has been great. I went off Premarin three months ago. I didn't have any withdrawal problems. I have never felt better. Minerals with boron have made all the difference." – A.L.

At first I was perplexed. Boron has been shown in studies to help prevent osteoporosis because it puts calcium in the bones, but minerals with boron for hot flashes? Then it hit me. Calcium is helpful in preventing the effects of stress on the body, and boron is helpful in getting calcium to where it is needed when the body is under stress!

I'm compelled to add a tidbit of very important information regarding calcium. You hear about the significance of calcium in preventing post-menopausal osteoporosis, but what you don't hear is the importance of magnesium in this equation. If you supplement with calcium but not with magnesium, the calcium will not go where it should: your bones. Instead it will accumulate where it shouldn't: in skin and other soft tissues, arteries and nerves. Because of the high absorption rate of minerals in solution, and deficiency of magnesium in the diet, the ratio of magnesium and calcium in solution should be four to one, respectively.

Stress and Menopause

Follow along while I put the pieces of the puzzle together. Nutritional needs of the body skyrocket during stress. Resistance falls in direct proportion to the depletion of certain vitamins and minerals. Vitamin C is the first to be lost. During stress, vitamin E, pantothenic acid, vitamin A, and all the B-vitamins are used up in massive amounts. The body withdraws minerals from its bones, teeth, hair, organs, and other tissues to meet the demands of defense, and breaks down protein from itself to create more hormones and antibodies. Calcium, magnesium, phosphorus and potassium demands are also increased under stress.

As the body becomes deficient in essential nutrients, its ability to resist the stressors diminishes. If stress is prolonged for weeks, months or years, the body is unable to convert cholesterol into needed hormones. Menopausal symptoms could be, in part, the body's way of reacting to stress and its subsequent nutritional deficiencies. Continued stress results in complete exhaustion and total collapse. "Nervous breakdowns," heart attacks, cancers, strokes, liver damage, and even kidney damage can be caused by constant stress. Menopausal symptoms are, therefore, the body's reaction to the stress of diminished hormones, worsened by nutritional deficiencies which further deplete needed hormones. It's a vicious cycle. The stress of diminished hormones, coupled with the knowledge that a woman can no longer bear children and the anticipation of the much-touted symptoms, which further depletes hormones, brings on massive negative reactions – all preventable!

What I have learned from my investigations made all the difference in my personal life. When I went through the "change," I wasn't afraid. I used what I learned to not only avoid menopausal symptoms, but that turning point gave me more energy, vitality and enthusiasm for life than I have ever had. I'm 60 years old and I have never felt better in my life – I mean it!

One more important thing. Exercise is essential for any program of stress or menopause relief. The reason the adrenals spit out more hormones when we are under stress is so we may be physically ready to fight or run. Every once in a while I read where somebody under stress performs some incredible feat of strength – lifting a car to save someone, for example. If that person had not taken action when his body told him to, he would have suffered. Stress and menopause both require a physical outlet to "work off" excess hormones so they don't turn inward and damage the body. An extreme example of this is the marathon runner who no longer menstruates. Talk about burning off hormones – she no longer has any!

Another issue with exercise is the fact that it takes effort. This positive effort can make a difference. Karen Matthews, professor of psychiatry, epidemiology, and psychology at the University of Pittsburgh School of Medicine, has identified the characteristics of those who experience few problems in menopause and those who experience many. "The women who do well respond to menopause with action," she says. "That may not be their direct intention, but they end up coping with the stressor by making positive changes. Those who, say, step up their *exercise* regimen don't even show the biological changes, such as the adverse shifts in lipids implicated in coronary disease, that others do."[1]

Phytoestrogens and Other Natural Solutions

Hot flashes. Every menopausal woman gets them, right? Wrong! If they are such an inevitable symptom of menopause, why then do some cultures not have them? Although Americans consider hot flashes nearly universal symptoms of menopause, investigation does not bear this out. Cross-cultural studies have found that Mayan women say they don't have hot flashes; Greek women have hot flashes but shrug them off as trivial; and while a small proportion of Japanese women report hot flashes, they are far more likely to complain of headaches and stiff shoulders. The Japanese language doesn't even have a word for hot flashes. What makes the difference is diet. The cultures that don't have hot flashes typically eat foods high in phytoestrogens: foods that naturally contain estrogen, that can help normalize hormone levels.

An article in the *British Medical Journal* reported on a study in which 25 postmenopausal women were given foods high in estrogen and evaluated for changes. All the women were in good health and were not taking any drugs known to influence estrogen levels. Their ages ranged from 51 to 70 years. The subjects recorded their normal diet for a period of two weeks, and then for six weeks three different food supplements derived from plants were given, each eaten for two weeks. The high-flavonoid supplements were soya flour (45 grams per day), red clover sprouts (10 grams dry seeds per day), and linseed (25 grams per day). Because the cell lining of the vagina is very sensitive to estrogen, the researchers took both blood samples and scrapings from the vagina of these women every two weeks. The researchers noted definite changes in their estrogen levels and cautiously concluded that a diet high in these plants "may modulate the severity of menopause symptoms in some individuals who habitually eat isoflavonoids, foods which contain plant estrogens."[2]

Legumes – peas, beans, and certain roots – are isoflavonoids, which act as a non-steroidal estrogen. Soybeans, a fabulous cancer fighter, is eaten in great quantities in Japan and China, and is one of the reasons researchers believe these countries have low rates of breast cancer.[3] Tofu, soybean curd, is not as bad tasting as it sounds. It has the unique ability to absorb the flavors it is cooked in.

Other oestrogenic food include apples, carrots, yams, green beans, peas, potatoes, red beans, brown rice, whole wheat, rye, and sesame seeds.

There is another reason why these foods stabilize estrogen needs. They are high in dietary fiber. Fiber is capable of altering the way various estrogen hormones are metabolized. David P. Rose, M.D., from the American Health Foundation in New York, found women showed significant reductions in a form of estrogen (estrone) after two months on a high fiber diet. Estrone is associated with hormonal problems. Dr. Rose also found that fiber helps the liver metabolize estrogens so levels can be normalized and balanced according to need.[4]

Certain vitamins can also help. Especially vitamin E. In 1945 Dr. C.J. Christy reported in the *American Journal of Gynecology* that an "entire" group of menopausal women responded to vitamin E treatment and showed either complete relief or marked improvement. In some cases the vitamin worked better than hormone therapy (such as it was at that time). In 1948, Dr. H. Ferguson reported in the *Vir-*

ginia Medical Monthly that "Sixty of 66 patients with severe menopausal symptoms were completely relieved with 15 to 30 IU of vitamin E daily."[5]

Susan M. Lark, M.D., of Los Altos, California, recommends the supplements vitamin B6 and a B vitamin complex, vitamin E, vitamin C and bioflavonoids, magnesium, evening primrose oil and borage oil.[6] Vitamin C and bioflavonoids should be taken together. Rutin, a bioflavonoid found in buckwheat, has been found to enhance the use and absorption of vitamin C by the body.

Michael Sporn, a researcher in Bethesda, Maryland, reported in April 1994 at an international conference on breast cancer therapies, that three kinds of flavonoids: deltanoids, retinoids and terpenoids have the same properties as Tamoxifen, a pharmaceutical drug (with major side effects) that keeps breast cells from absorbing estrogen.[7] Terpenoids are found in abundance in rosemary and citrus oil (the oil you squeeze out of the pores of citrus fruits); retinoids are precursors of vitamin A and are found in orange fruits and vegetables; and deltanoids are found in egg yolks.

A report in *Chicago Medicine* stated that the bioflavonoid hesperidin, found in citrus fruit rind, was more effective than sub-therapeutic doses of estrogen for menopausal symptoms.[8]

Making Your Hormones Work for You

Two natural hormones, melatonin and DHEA (dehydro-epiandrosterone) have connections to the adrenals that may prove to be advantageous to menopausal women. A study reported in the *American Journal of Obstetrical Gynecology* (December 1993) concluded that DHEA could be beneficial to postmenopausal women who exhibit a deficiency of androgens, male hormones produced by the adrenals. It just so happens DHEA and progesterone are androgens. The researchers noted a strong T-cell activity in DHEA, suggesting any problem that involves a dysfunction of the adrenals could be remedied by DHEA, including uterine and breast cancer risked by hormone therapy.[9] A warning, however, too much DHEA can cause hair loss. Have a nutrition-oriented doctor do a hormonal panel first.

Melatonin's effect on estrogen could also reduce the risk of breast cancer experienced by postmenopausal women. Scientists at Tulane University School of Medicine in New Orleans grew human breast cancer cells in the laboratory then added melatonin to some of the cultures. They found that when estrogen was involved in the growth of breast cancer cells, the melatonin effectively retarded its growth, suggesting to Dr. Michael Cohen that combining melatonin with low-dose estrogen could effectively block its tendency to cause breast cancer cell growth. Additional studies showed that melatonin boosts the ability of Tamoxifen to inhibit the growth of human cancer cells in the laboratory.[10] Since Tamoxifen has been shown in studies to promote the growth of uterine and endometrial cancer, perhaps DHEA would be a more likely candidate to prevent breast cancer than a toxic agent that creates its own hazards.

Natural Progesterone to Balance Hormones and Alleviate Symptoms

John R. Lee, M.D. a family physician from Sebastapol, California, has been treating women for over 15 years with natural progesterone cream. In a book he published himself, entitled *Natural Progesterone, the Multiple Roles of a Remarkable Hormone*, he relates the story of a Canadian woman who was seeing six doctors for her menopausal symptoms. She sent Dr. Lee her 10-pound medical record file for his advice. He found one telling page, and related it in his book. It seems the woman had been prescribed increasingly high doses of Provera by her physician, in response to lab tests that showed zero blood progesterone levels. The poor woman was experiencing serious debilitating symptoms by the time the lab technician wrote a note to the doctor. It said,"Doctor, you are giving this lady Provera. You are ordering tests for serum progesterone. Provera is *not* progesterone!" Dr. Lee circled the comment in red and sent a copy to the woman, including information on natural progesterone cream. Several months later he got a very nice note from the lady telling him how much better she felt using natural progesterone and had fired all but one of her doctors.

Dr. Lee believes most, if not all, of the symptoms related to menopause are a direct result of a lack of progesterone. He has all his patients use progesterone cream. Why cream? Oral progesterone is diluted when it reaches the liver, so high doses are needed. Progesterone in the form of cream is less expensive, easy to apply, and works as well as pills or injections.

Menopause-Munching Nutrients
For maximum absorption, take supplements with meals.

Nutrient	Suggested Dosage	Formulation
Fiber	4-8 tablets daily	Psyllium, with herb hyssop
Borage oil	2 capsules daily	
Flaxseed oil	1 tablespoon daily	
Magnesium	200 mg daily	
Melatonin	3 mg daily at bedtime	With B vitamins
Multi-mineral	1-4 ounces daily	In liquid solution, with vitamin B12, biotin
Multi-vitamin/mineral	3-6 caplets daily	Freeze-dried plant sources
Natural progesterone cream	1/3 teaspoon daily	With pregnenolone and DHEA
Vitamin C	Individual bowel tolerance*	With citrus (quercetin, proanthocyanidins)
Vitamin E	2 capsules (800 IU) daily	d-alpha tocopherol

* To determine individual dosage, on the first day take 1,000 mg hourly until diarrhea occurs, then reduce dosage to just below that for individual daily dosage. Vitamin C is not toxic in large doses but must be taken throughout the day to benefit. Divide dosage to three or four times a day.

CHAPTER 114:

Mental Illness

During one of my many excursions throughout the country, a university neurology professor told me a tragic story which exemplifies the need for recognizing the connection between nutrition and mental illness. Jack Turner worked very hard, and as a result suffered from intestinal ulcers. He was a corporate CEO, in charge of many and responsible for much. His daily grind did not afford him the luxury of eating well, and the stress of his work exacerbated his ulcers. When he finally suffered a mental breakdown, nobody was surprised. His doctors, his co-workers and even his wife attributed his collapse to his stressful workaholic lifestyle and his perfectionist point of view.

Jack was admitted to a state hospital, diagnosed with psychosis. He was there several years before a new doctor decided to evaluate his nutritional status. He was found to be deficient in the B vitamins and was given shots of B12.

Miraculously, Jack began to recover. After a few months of an aggressive campaign of nutritional therapy, Jack Turner was discharged, his psychosis ended. Tragically, because of irreversible neurological damage, he was confined to a wheelchair. Not complaining, Jack left the corporate world to become a schoolteacher. His ulcers healed and he retained excellent mental health well into his 80s.

How many Jack Turners are out there, misdiagnosed and misrepresented, denied the help that could make them better?

Bowel Reasons for B Vitamin Deficiencies

There are no other nutrients more important to mental health than the B vitamins. The B-complex vitamins provide the body with energy, metabolizing fats and protein, and are necessary for the normal functioning of the nervous system. They are the single most important factor for the health of the nerves. Symptoms of deficiencies include dizziness, hallucinations, irritability, depression, insomnia and even suicidal tendencies.

Mental illness as a physical disease can result from low brain concentrations of vitamins B1 (thiamine), B6 (pyridoxine), B12 (cobalamin), niacin, pantothenic acid and folic acid.[1] Please, always supplement with a good B-complex formula when adding any one B vitamin to your diet. One without the other can cause more harm than good since they are dependent upon each other to work in your body.

Remember, vitamins aren't properly utilized without minerals and minerals are nearly impossible to absorb in tablet form. That's why I take a mineral in solution formula along with a vitamin/mineral tablet that consists of freeze dried sprouts and vegetables.

A vitamin B12 deficiency is a real bogey man – especially in the over-60 crowd. It can produce psychosis, severe memory loss, impaired abstract thinking skills, mental confusion, delusions, hallucinations and even brain and spinal cord degeneration (causing numbness). Low blood levels of the vitamin are found in one-third of hospitalized psychiatric patients suffering from depression and dementia, according to a Denmark study. In addition, a B12 deficiency may inhibit the brain's use of glucose (the gasoline which energizes the brain) and hinder production of acetylcholine, which is vital to brain and memory function.

Folic acid, a B vitamin found in leafy greens, prevents irritability and forgetfulness; plus, it partners with B12 in the brain's synthesis of acetylcholine. In one case, cited in "Nutrition and the Brain," 67 percent of patients admitted to a psychogeriatric ward were deficient in folate. Such a deficiency may arise from poor nutrition, an inability to absorb the nutrient or impaired absorption caused by pharmaceuticals.

There are two places in the body where nutrients are absorbed: the stomach and the intestine. If the stomach has too little acid, whether from illness, stress or age, absorption is compromised. If there is something wrong with the intestines, nutrients, especially the B vitamins, cannot be absorbed properly.

Studies have shown that among those with intestinal problems, their blood levels of B vitamins are low. Irritable bowel syndrome (IBS) is a fancy term to describe a temporarily dysfunctional large intestine, caused by food allergies, stress or too much fat in the diet.

In one study, 20 patients with IBS were compared to a control group of 20 without IBS. Remarkably, but not surprisingly, it was found that 18 out of 20 of the IBS patients had a history of mental illness during their lifetimes compared to only nine out 20 in the control group. Half of the patients with IBS had regular panic attacks, and another half had social phobias. IBS patients commonly have problems with depression, sleeping problems and substance abuse. The connection sticks. When questioned, most of the IBS patients said their intestinal problems occurred before their mental illness.[2]

What makes this connection between the bowel and mental disorders? B vitamins. An unhealthy intestine cannot absorb B vitamins. And without the B vitamins, mental disorders result.

Churchill's Medical Dictionary defines pernicious anemia (PA) as "anemia resulting from impaired intestinal absorption of vitamin B12." It is called pernicious because it is fatal if left untreated. It has been estimated that the majority of elderly people with symptoms of senility are actually suffering from pernicious anemia. The symptoms range from early signs of paleness, fatigue, diarrhea, heart palpitations and numbness in fingers and toes, to delusions, senility and schizophrenia in later stages.

A lack of B12 has been found to cause a type of brain damage resembling schizophrenia. Symptoms of this disorder include sore mouth, numbness or stiffness, shooting pains, needles-and-pins or hot-and-cold sensations. Editors at the *British Medical Journal* stated that a vitamin B12 deficiency may cause severe psychotic symptoms which may vary in severity from mild mood swings to severe psychotic episodes. If a deficiency is not detected in its early stages, it may result in permanent mental deterioration.[3]

A number of studies have shown a deficiency of folic acid as a contributing factor in mental illness. Studies have shown that a prolonged deficiency can cause neurological changes and mental deterioration. Because of their close interrelationship, vitamin B12 should accompany any folic acid supplementation. A deficiency of folic acid in pregnancy encourages birth defects including deformities, brain damage, spina bifida and neural tube defects. Other deficiency symptoms are stunted growth, graying hair, gastrointestinal problems and anemia.[4]

Psychosis from a Thiamine Deficiency

Imagine your loved one has been hospitalized with schizophrenia, or is tranquilized with strong drugs. Now imagine there is a possibility that just one missing nutrient could be the cause, but it is being ignored.

Time and time again the signs of nutritional deficiencies are ignored because symptoms are conveniently categorized; programmed into conventional medicine so that doctors do not have to discover the cause, just treat the symptoms. Options are ignored because conventional physicians are not taught to look at the whole picture, instead they evaluate a collection of symptoms with the purpose of signifying one problem.

Such is the case of mental illness. Doctors look at the symptoms, evaluate the problems, then rather than discover the cause, treat the symptoms with pharmaceuticals. B vitamin deficiencies cause such a host of mental symptoms that to ignore this possibility constitutes medical malpractice in my book. Take thiamine, or B1, for example.

The symptoms of a thiamine deficiency are listed as anorexia, confusion, depression, irritability and memory loss.[5]

In an experimental study reported in the *American Journal of Clinical Nutrition*, five of nine normal volunteers placed on a thiamine-deficient diet developed depression and irritability.[6]

Vitamin B1, or thiamine, is involved in the conversion of blood sugar to caloric energy in the body. During stressful periods it can give a boost to your energy level. Thiamine deficiency, or beriberi, is known to produce psychiatric and neurological symptoms.

Attacks on the Brain

Today's modern day beriberi is Wernicke's syndrome. It is also called Wernicke's reaction, Wernicke symptom, Wernicke's encephalopathy, Wernicke's disease, and in its advanced stages, Wernicke-Korsakoff psychosis. What happens is a chronic deficiency of thiamine causes brain lesions, swelling and eventually destruction of the brain itself. This condition is most commonly found in chronic alcoholics but has been diagnosed in nonalcoholics as well. The symptoms are similar to those of senile dementia, with memory problems being the first to appear. Classic signs include global (total) confusion, ophthalmoplegia (paralysis of the muscles that move the eyes) or nystagmus (involuntary eye movements), and ataxia (disturbance of gait).[7]

A short note here. You may wonder why I bother with the technical terms. This is for your benefit in dealing with conventional medicine. Let's say your uncle is in a mental hospital and his doctors won't tell you anything, so you insist on seeing his medical records. But the medical records don't help because physicians use such specific jargon you can't understand a word of it! You may recognize some of the terms here. If you don't, write all the words down you don't understand, then consult a medical dictionary. Don't stop until you fully understand what doctors *think* is your uncle's problem.

Similar to Wernicke's is something called Korsakoff's psychosis. In keeping with conventional medicine's habit of categorizing, the industry is now lumping the two into a single diagnosis of "alcohol amnesic syndrome."[8] Even though alcoholism is not the only cause of a thiamine deficiency, and its subsequent mental symptoms, thanks to this new definition, doctors may now discount the possibility of a thiamine deficiency unless alcoholism is present.

Thiamine is needed to produce and use acetylcholine and to avoid emotional excesses. People who indulge in refined sugar and flour (processed) foods, who drink alcohol regularly, or are addicted to coffee, literally drain vitamin B1 from their system. We should remember that sugar and fats, which make up a high percentage of processed foods and supply over 35 percent of our calories, give us no thiamine or other B vitamins. Also, excessive use of tea, alcohol and the eating of raw fish has been linked to thiamine deficiency.

In one experiment, rats trained to get through a maze were divided into two groups, one given a nutritionally complete diet and the other a diet totally lacking in B1. When the rats were tested 20 days later, the group on the good diet sped through in an average of 22 seconds, while the B1-deprived rats took 55 seconds, almost three times as long. However, putting the deprived rats on a diet rich in B1 induced a remarkable memory recovery and ability to run through the maze.

Anything that causes malnutrition, from poor eating habits to alcoholism, can cause a thiamine deficiency. I find it interesting that anorexia is a symptom of a thiamine deficiency. If a lack of thiamine causes depression and nervous system disorders, it stands to reason that a young person who diets consistently could first become thiamine deficient, causing the kind of obsessive behavior that leads to anorexia.

Even subclinical (moderate) thiamine deficiency can cause anxiety or neuroses. In one study, subjects deprived of thiamine complained of poor mental alertness, fatigue and nervousness.[9] Since psychiatrists are the least likely to inquire about diet, I have to wonder how many of their anxiety patients are being treated with drugs when they are simply thiamine-deficient.

A diet high in empty calories and junk foods has been linked to neurotic behavior. One study found 20 patients with a thiamine deficiency reported mental symptoms including aggressiveness and hostility. Twelve reported a diet high in carbonated and other sweet beverages, candy, and typical snack foods. Blood tests indicated that all 20 had low thiamine levels. After the patients were given thiamine supplements, all 20 had marked improvement or lost their symptoms completely.[10]

Patients in modern hospitals are probably at risk of a thiamine deficiency because they are sometimes fed intravenously. This is called total parenteral nutrition, or TPN. This is done whenever the patient cannot eat or digest food the usual way. The problem is, this "liquid food" can be deficient in nutrients, most especially the B vitamins.

In 1988, three patients receiving intravenous feedings in a hospital died because the intravenous solution was deficient in thiamine, according to *The New York Times*. A B1 deficiency can develop within a week with these deficient feedings, which are 70 percent glucose, since the vitamin is necessary for metabolizing glucose.[11]

The Food and Drug Administration reported these patients died of refractory lactic acidosis. Autopsies performed on two of the patients revealed brain abnormalities.[12]

If you are anxious, depressed or suffer from neuroses, consider the possibility that you are thiamine deficient and see a physician versed in nutrition.

Minerals for Mental Health

Some essential elements can act as brain boosters, working as preventive medicine against mental illness.

Of the minerals that can help to protect the nervous system, the most important are zinc and magnesium. Zinc is essential to the synthesis of RNA, DNA and protein, and to the maintenance of vitamin

A levels in the blood. A zinc deficiency can cause confusion and difficulties with taste and smell. When older people are not eating properly, zinc deficiency may be at fault since food is less appetizing when the senses of smell and taste are reduced.

In the 1950s, the late Carl Pfeiffer, Ph.D., M.D., former director of the Brain Bio Center in Princeton, New Jersey, found that trace metal imbalances, for example copper and zinc, can contribute to mental disorders. William Walsh, Ph.D., a former research scientist at Argonne National Laboratories and a colleague of Dr. Pfeiffer estimates that 95 percent of violent individuals suffer from mineral imbalances that predispose them to bad behavior.[13]

Dr. Walsh discovered that violent individuals often had an imbalance of copper to zinc and low levels of sodium, potassium and manganese. He found people who were delinquent, impulsive and irritable were low in all the trace minerals including calcium and magnesium.

An article in *Biological Psychiatry* reported that of patients hospitalized with major depression or schizophrenia, magnesium was significantly lower in those who made suicide attempts. The authors believe magnesium has a role in regulating serotonin levels of the brain.[14]

Remember, you're not what you put into your mouth, you're what you absorb and digest and deliver to cells. A vitamin or mineral tablet is only one to five percent absorbable. Since the process of digestion is a process of liquefaction, your body has to take a hard rock tablet and turn it into solution. This may not be possible due to a number of factors, such as inadequate stomach acid, food allergies and intestinal problems. This is why it is so important that when you decide to supplement, you target minerals in solution. Look for a good, easily absorbable, derived-from-nature mineral blend in solution. Formulations in solution help provide the maximum absorption ratios.

Mentally-Mighty Nutrients
For maximum absorption, take supplements with meals.

Nutrient	Suggested Dosage	Formulation
Aged garlic extract	1 teaspoon three times daily	Liquid
Amino acids	4-6 capsules daily	Multiple formula from natural sources
Antioxidants	4 capsules daily*	With selenium and grapeseed extract
Borage oil	2 capsules daily	
Coenzyme Q10	2 capsules daily	With vitamin E, phospholipids and selenium
Flaxseed oil	1 tablespoon daily	
Multi-mineral	3-4 ounces daily	In liquid solution, with vitamin B12, biotin
Multi-vitamin/mineral	6 caplets daily	Freeze-dried plant sources
Niacin	200 mg three times daily	
Vitamin B6	100 mg daily	
Vitamin C	Individual bowel tolerance**	With bioflavonoids (quercetin, proanthocyanidins)

* The FDA recommends pregnant women not exceed 10,000 IU of vitamin A daily.

** To determine individual dosage, on the first day take 1,000 mg hourly until diarrhea occurs, then reduce dosage to just below that for individual daily dosage. Vitamin C is not toxic in large doses but must be taken throughout the day to benefit. Divide dosage to three or four times a day.

CHAPTER 115:

Migraines & Headaches

*"Pain dies quickly, and lets her weary prisoners go;
the fiercest agonies have shortest reign."*
　　　　　　　　　　　– William Cullen Bryant

A headache by any other name is just as painful. Why the differentiation between migraines and headaches? Confusion abounds as to when the pain is a migraine, a cluster headache or what's termed a 'tension' headache.

Recently, a television news show did a segment on migraines. The commercials, lead-ins and the interview itself showed a young man on the floor repeatedly banging his head against the wall. He hit his head so hard you had to wince watching him. He said the pain was so bad he sought something that would hurt more just to distract him from it. After years of daily torture, he contemplated suicide as an escape. The show's journalists said it was a migraine. Joel Saper, M.D., director of Michigan's Head Pain and Neurological Institute in Ann Arbor, Michigan, would probably consider it a cluster headache. In an article in *World Health News*, Dr. Saper said that men with cluster headaches tend to pace and cry out and often bang their heads and hands against walls, and throw things. Whereas people with migraines seek dark, quiet, cool rooms and reduce stimulation, whether it be from sound or light or smell.[1]

A migraine is a headache that usually lasts hours to days, whereas a cluster headache usually lasts a half-hour to two hours. Migraines generally occur in women more than men, whereas cluster headaches generally affect more men. Cluster headaches are almost always around an eye with a runny nose, tears, and sometimes eyelid drooping. If a headache is severe, if it is associated with severe nausea or vomiting, and is unilateral and throbbing, then it's more likely to be migraine. Because of the symptom similarities: presence of throbbing and pain on one side of the head, some researchers believe that the tension-type headache is a milder version of a migraine. Both can be associated with nausea, both can occur on one of both sides of the head, have moderate pain and be non-throbbing. So at times it's difficult to differentiate between them.

All sorts of alarms go off when a migraine is imminent. Hands get cold to icy; lights flash, like zig zags of lightening; blind spots; tingling, numbness, or weakness on one side of the face or body; changes in emotion, mood and appetite that occur a day or two before the pain and for some, the "aura." Ten to 20 percent of people with migraines experience the mysterious "aura," which are eye-widening symptoms that occur just before the pain starts.[2] Some researchers have come to believe that the aura occurs as a result of a deficiency of magnesium in the cortex of the brain.[3] This is not a surprising revelation when you realize the importance of magnesium to blood circulation, and further, that these aura symptoms are similar to those which occur just before a stroke. More on magnesium later.

Migraines Often Caused by Chemicalized Food

There is a lot of evidence that migraine pain is caused by certain foods and chemicals. A double-blind study reported in *The Lancet* found that 94 percent of a group of 88 children with severe, frequent migraines were relieved of their pain after eliminating foods to which they were allergic.[4]

Seymour Solomon, M.D., director of the Headache Unit at Montefiore Medical Center and professor of neurology, Albert Einstein College of Medicine in Bronx, N.Y., believes that about 20 percent of people with migraines are sensitive to chemicals in certain foods, such as monosodium glutamate (MSG) and nitrites in hot dogs and sausages.[5]

Tartrazine (FD&C Yellow No. 5), a common food coloring (read the labels!) has a history of provoking allergic headaches.[6]

It is estimated that 90 percent of all migraine headaches are directly linked to food allergies or to reactions caused by additives, particularly certain preservatives and colorings, caffeine and chocolate.[7]

All processed foods, whether bottled, bagged, canned or packaged have hidden dangers. MSG is only one of the identified dangers hidden in the plethora of chemicals contained in processed food. A very good friend of mine has migraines for days after ingesting MSG. Unfortunately, he eats out often, and forgets to ask the waitress to "hold the MSG."

According to the FDA, approximately five thousand food additives are used in food products in the United States.[8] As the chemicals in our supermarkets grow, so do reported cases of migraines.

The Centers for Disease Control and the National Center for Health Statistics conducted personal interviews over a 10 year period with between 60,000 to 125,000 people. They found that between 1980 and 1989 the prevalence of chronic migraine headache sufferers increased nearly 60 percent from almost 26 to 41 individuals per 1,000 people. Tragically, 71 percent of the increase occurred among individuals less than 45 years of age. Interestingly, and indicative of the possibility of it being a mineral-deficiency, migraine frequency was geographic. In 1989, the highest number of migraine sufferers was in the Western United States (45 per 1,000 persons), while in the South and Midwest the rate of migraine headaches was 41 and 40.4 per 1,000 persons respectively. The lowest rate was in the northeast at almost 37 per 1,000.[9]

One of the reasons MSG gets such a headstrong reaction is that it contains a chemical known as tyramine. Tyramine dilates blood vessels in the head, causing the pressure credited with the pain of migraines. If you suspect a food reaction is causing your migraines, consider the possibility that one of these tyramine-foods could be the culprit: cheese, bananas, chocolate, yogurt, bean curry, pickled fish, citrus fruit, red wine, beer, fermented sausage, brewer's yeast, fava beans, soy sauce, MSG, Chinese broad bean pods, coffee, licorice, snails and yogurt.

Magnesium for Migraines

Numerous studies have shown the connection between low blood levels of magnesium and migraines. Researchers at the prestigious Interuniversity Center For the Study of Headache and Neurotransmitter Disorders in Perugia, Italy, examined 90 adult migraine and tension headache patients comparing them with a control group. They found migraine sufferers, with and without aura and tension-type headaches, had significantly lower levels of magnesium between attacks, and even less during a migraine. The authors also note that it is probably more than coincidence that subjects with epilepsy or mitral valve prolapse have a higher incidence of headaches and also have low serum magnesium levels.[10]

Magnesium is a mineral essential for brain function, and also regulates serotonin, a mood regulating brain chemical. One study found a deficiency of magnesium in about 40 percent of migraine patients. Robert S. Kunkel, M.D., director of the Headache Clinic, Cleveland, Ohio, knows of physicians who manage acute migraine headaches with intravenous magnesium sulfate.[11]

In another study, 35 out of 40 people suffering from frequent migraines given one gram of intravenous magnesium at the start of their headaches experienced a complete reduction in head pain within 15 minutes. Almost none suffered any more pain recurrence over the next 24 hours.[12] The reason intravenous magnesium is used is because of the difficulty our systems have in absorbing any mineral in tablet form.

Remember, you're not what you put into your mouth, you're what you absorb and digest and deliver to cells. A tablet is only one to five percent absorbable. Since the process of digestion is a process of liquefaction, your body has to take a hard rock tablet and turn it into solution. This may not be possible due to a number of factors, such as inadequate stomach acid, food allergies and intestinal problems. This is why it is so important that when you decide to supplement, you target minerals in solution. Look for a good, easily absorbable, derived-from-nature mineral blend in solution. Liquid formulations provide the maximum absorption ratios.

Magnesium and calcium work in balance throughout our bodies. Without magnesium, calcium accumulates in places it shouldn't. Because of the high absorption rate of minerals in solution, and deficiency of magnesium in the diet, the ratio of magnesium and calcium in solution should be four to one, respectively.

Magnesium deficiency is more common than you might expect. A large study by the U.S. Department of Agriculture found that only 25 percent of 37,785 individuals had magnesium intakes at or greater than the recommended daily allowance, which is notoriously low. A 1995 review of 15 studies found that a typical diet contains only a fraction of the RDA.[13]

Beat It with B Vitamins

The B vitamins are notorious brain boosters. Anything that affects the brain depletes B vitamins. If you don't believe me, read the chapter Mental Illness. In any case, it's not surprising that two B vitamins: riboflavin and niacin help alleviate the pain of migraines.

A doctor in New York, Jeffrey A. Hall, D.O., reports that he has successfully treated his own migraine headaches for the last 15 years with oral doses of niacin. At the onset of his aura he takes 300 to 500 milligrams of niacin and allows the pills to slowly dissolve in his mouth after chewing them slightly. This works best on an empty stomach though it can have benefit when taken after meals.[14] Niacin is also used to reduce blood pressure as it dilates and opens constricted blood vessels, with the only side effect being menopausal-like hot flashes from too much niacin at one time.

Belgium researchers split 49 migraine sufferers into two groups: 26 took 400 mg of riboflavin (vitamin B2) daily before breakfast for three months and the rest took the B2 and 75 mg of aspirin. All of the study participants were relieved to find that the severity of their head pain was reduced by nearly 70 percent. In all probability, the aspirin made no difference, except to the one participant who dropped out because of stomach problems.[15] Dr. Seymour Solomon recommends migraine patients take 100 milligrams of B2 four times a day.

Migraine Relieving Nutrients
For maximum absorption, take supplements with meals.

Nutrient	Suggested Dosage	Formulation
Borage oil	2 capsules daily	
Fiber	4-8 tablets daily	Psyllium, with herb hyssop
Flaxseed oil	1 tablespoon daily	
Ginkgo biloba	60 mg three times daily	
Magnesium	200 mg twice daily	
Melatonin (adults only)	3 mg daily at bedtime	With B vitamins
Multi-mineral	3-4 ounces daily	In liquid solution, with vitamin B12, biotin
Multi-vitamin/mineral	6 caplets daily	Freeze-dried plant sources
Niacin	500 mg four times daily	
Vitamin B6	100 mg daily	
Vitamin C	Individual bowel tolerance*	With bioflavonoids (quercetin, proanthocyanidins)
Vitamin E	2 capsules (800 IU) daily	d-alpha tocopherol

* To determine individual dosage, on the first day take 1,000 mg hourly until diarrhea occurs, then reduce dosage to just below that for individual daily dosage. Vitamin C is not toxic in large doses but must be taken throughout the day to benefit. Divide dosage to three or four times a day.

CHAPTER 116:

Miscarriage

"If nature had arranged that husbands and wives should have children alternatively, there would never be more than three in a family."

– Laurence Housman

Actress JoBeth Williams and her husband, director John Pasquin, struggled for eight years to have a baby. In 1988, after surgery and a series of artificial-insemination attempts, she became pregnant, only to learn in a 12th-week sonogram that the fetus had died. "Over the next few months," she said in a faint voice in an interview, "I wondered if I might lose my mind."

At 34, singer/comedienne Bette Midler kidded with an interviewer that she'd like to have children someday, "before my uterus falls out." Two years after marrying Martin von Haselberg, the 40-year-old Midler gave birth to daughter Sophie, insisting then that it would take "at least two more babies to make my life worth living." A miscarriage the following year left her grieving. "Sometimes it's a brutal world," she said at the time. Referring to the solace of her marriage she added, "It's good to have a haven."[1]

There is nothing more tragic than losing a child, as any who have suffered miscarriage can attest. Every year, more than one in ten women miscarry.[2] Not only is a child lost, but also lost is faith that delivery can be achieved. If you ask your friends, you'll be amazed to discover just how common miscarriage is. Probably some of your own relatives and associates have miscarried between pregnancies.

Many other women miscarry and never know they were pregnant. In these cases, the menstrual flow might be more painful, with more clots than normal, but little more to indicate conception has taken place.

I'm here to help with the information you need to increase the odds that when conception takes place, a full term delivery will follow.

Vitamin C and Bioflavonoids

Vitamin C is a notorious antioxidant and is helpful for a variety of afflictions including bacterial infections, hemorrhaging and poor red blood cell formation, all vitally important to forming a strong placenta. A primary function of vitamin C is maintaining collagen, important for skin and tissue strength.

All these reasons and more are why vitamin C is effective for women with a history of miscarriage. Two prominent researchers, Dr. Carl Javert of Cornell University, and R. Robert Greenblatt of the Medical College of Georgia, independently discovered that vitamin C and bioflavonoids can prevent miscarriage.

Javert tested 1,334 women with a history of miscarriage and found 45 percent deficient in vitamin C. Over and above a diet which already supplied them with 350 mg of vitamin C daily, he gave 100 pregnant women from this larger group vitamin C with bioflavonoids and was happy to report a 91 percent success rate!

Dr. Greenblatt tried this with 13 women, and out of these, 11 gave birth to live infants.[3]

Take vitamin C and bioflavonoids together to keep the blood vessels in the uterus strong and healthy. In order to support a growing baby over nine months, the blood vessel-lined uterus must remain strong and resilient. If too many vessels break, the lining's integrity is ruined, the placenta sloughs off and the pregnancy is terminated. Enter vitamin C and bioflavonoids, a great team for increasing the strength of these unique tiny blood vessels.

Bioflavonoids are important with vitamin C because they amplify the benefit and are necessary for vitamin C absorption. However, one bioflavonoid, quercetin, has been shown in studies to particularly boost vitamin C's powers. Intensive studies of quercetin in a wide variety of disciplines have found quercetin alone helps prevent blood clotting and inflammation, fights viral infections, strengthens blood capillaries and vessels, and has even been shown in studies to inhibit the growth of abnormal, cancerous cells.[4] When supplementing with a vitamin C formula, choose one that contains green tea and quercetin. Quercetin is found in the white inner rind of citrus fruits and in onions.

B6 for "Luteal Phase Defect"

Sometimes miscarriage results because of a lack of progesterone in the body. Each month, the egg develops inside the ovary within a little sac called a follicle. At ovulation time the follicle and the wall of the ovary rupture and discharge an egg. The follicle transforms itself into a gland called the corpus luteum ("yellow body" in Latin), which is the major source of the progesterone that is needed for the first four crucial months of pregnancy. When the placenta, which separates the fetal blood system from the mother's, is fully formed, it takes over secretion of progesterone and other hormones needed to keep the pregnancy going.

Some women have what is known as a "luteal phase efect," which means their corpus luteum is not producing enough progesterone to maintain the pregnancy. Conventional physicians take the unnatural way out, by prescribing progesterone supplements. The healthier route is nutrients that naturally increases progesterone levels. High amounts of B6 lowers estrogen levels. As estrogen levels lower, progesterone levels rise. Atlanta obstetrician-gynecologist Richard Taylor, M.D., has observed that women with histories of miscarriages have low levels of B6. Both alcohol and caffeine deplete the body of B6 – alcohol by deactivating the vitamin, and caffeine by increasing the excretion of B6 in the urine. Magnesium is also added to the formula to enhance the effect and to build up red blood cells.[5]

Herbert S. Mansmann, Jr., M.D., Department of Pediatrics at Jefferson Medical College, in Philadelphia, contends that a deficiency of magnesium alone can jeopardize the infant, causing miscarriages, still births and sudden infant death before and after birth, as well as a some birth defects.[6]

Magnesium deficiency is more common than you might expect. A large study by the U.S. Department of Agriculture found that only 25 percent of 37,785 individuals had magnesium intakes at or greater than the recommended daily allowance, which is notoriously low. A 1995 review of 15 studies found that a typical diet contains only a fraction of the RDA.[7]

Vitamin B6, like most of the B vitamins, can cause a deficiency of the others if taken alone. When supplementing with any one B vitamin, always include a good B-complex formula for proper balance. B6 and the other B vitamins are water soluble, which means they cannot be stored in the liver and any excess is excreted in urine.

Vital B6 is lost in food transportation, storage, preservation, processing and cooking. Therefore, it is essential to add a B6 vitamin supplement (at least 200 mg daily) to your diet.

Vital Vitamin E

Paavo Airola, N.D., Ph.D., a leading nutritionist, claims that infertility may be an inherent protective mechanism signalling that the body is not strong enough to give birth. He says that when the human body is weakened and its health potential severely lowered by environmental factors – inadequate nutrition, disease, or severe emotional or physical stress – it will be deprived of its ability to reproduce.

Nicknamed the "anti-sterility vitamin," vitamin E shows great promise as an aid to fertility. In 1955, researchers studied the effects of the vitamin on fertility at a large horse breeding facility in Oshawa, Canada. They administered vitamin E daily to the entire herd, including old mares who were previously thought to be barren, and older stallions.

According to the Jockey Club, a leading authoritative body in thoroughbred racing, registered foals are produced by pregnant mares approximately 52 percent of the time. After treatment with vitamin E, 71 percent of the pregnancies resulted in births.[8]

Not to insinuate that women are akin to mares, but human studies have shown the same results.

R. Bayer, M.D., a West German physician, conducted a study involving the effects of vitamin E on 100 infertile couples with a history of miscarriages. Previously, the group had 144 conceptions without a single live birth. After daily administration of 100 IU of the vitamin to the men and 200 IU to the women, the same couples conceived 79 children, of which only two were miscarried.[9]

When Dr. Bayer conducted the same experiment with a second group in which 63 of 101 pregnancies had resulted in miscarriage, 41 women became pregnant and none of them miscarried.

Vitamin E has been used extensively for miscarriage problems. Dr. Evan Shute of Canada, whose work with vitamin E and heart disease is famous, recounts case histories of 87 women with histories of miscarriages. With vitamin E supplementation, he saw an incredible 86 percent success rate. In addition, very few mothers suffered from toxemia.[10]

How does vitamin E achieve this wonderful track record? The placenta provides the embryo with nutrients of all types, but especially oxygen. Vitamin E works best by delivering oxygen to growing cells, especially those of the placenta and fetus. This alone makes it a valuable vitamin for pregnancy. Vitamin E also helps strengthen blood vessels.

Think Zinc

Pregnancy is a complicated interaction of many different hormones and body systems. One system not often discussed is the immune system – of which zinc is a crucial factor for the proper functioning. Zinc deficiency can cause any number of defects in this intricate and important defense system, including miscarriage, according to Judy Graham and Michael Odent, writing in *The Z Factor* (Thorsons, 1986). Animal studies have also shown that diets low in zinc cause miscarriages, as well as abnormal fetuses.

Do you know any families with a string of girl babies punctuated by miscarriages in between? The mother may possibly be zinc deficient. The late Dr. Carl Pfeiffer suggested that since male babies need more zinc than females, a pregnant woman deficient in this mineral would be more likely to miscarry a male fetus.

Zinc is needed to transform vitamin B6 from its inactive to its active form in the body. Zinc and B6 work well together because B6 helps zinc absorption. A woman preparing her body for the nutritional challenge of pregnancy should take both a B-complex and zinc.

Copper and zinc are a twosome. Without at least 2 mg of copper to every 15 mg of zinc, they both can become deficient. Not coincidentally, copper has also been shown in studies to increase the risk of miscarriage.

H. Ozgunes, M.D., of the Department of Pharmacology and Toxicology, Faculty of Pharmacy, Hacettepe University in Ankara, Turkey, studied healthy pregnant women and compared them to women who were at risk of miscarriage. He found those at risk had significantly low copper levels. He also found low copper in women who had miscarried, concluding that low copper levels can be used to indicate a risk of miscarriage.[11]

Fertility-Favorable Nutrients
For maximum absorption, take supplements with meals.

Nutrient	Suggested Dosage	Formulation
Acidophilus	At least four billion flora on an empty stomach, three times daily	
Aged garlic extract	1 teaspoon three times daily	Liquid
Amino acids	4-6 capsules daily	Multiple formula from natural sources
Antioxidants	4 capsules daily*	With selenium and grapeseed extract
Borage oil	2 capsules daily	
Coenzyme Q10	2 capsules daily	With vitamin E, phospholipids and selenium
Enzymes	2 capsules twice daily	Multiple formula
Fiber	4-8 tablets daily	Psyllium, with herb hyssop
Flaxseed oil	1 tablespoon daily	
Ginkgo biloba	60 mg daily	
Magnesium	200 mg daily	
Melatonin (adults only)	3 mg daily at bedtime	With B vitamins
Multi-mineral	3-4 ounces daily	In liquid solution, with vitamin B12, biotin
Multi-vitamin/mineral	6 caplets daily	Freeze-dried plant sources
Natural progesterone cream	1/3 teaspoon daily	With pregnenolone, DHEA
Saw palmetto	160 mg twice daily for men and women	
Selenium	300 mcg daily	
Vitamin B6	100 mg daily	
Vitamin C	Individual bowel tolerance**	With bioflavonoids (quercetin, rutin proanthocyanidins)

* The FDA recommends pregnant women not exceed 10,000 IU of vitamin A daily.

** To determine individual dosage, on the first day take 1,000 mg hourly until diarrhea occurs, then reduce dosage to just below that for individual daily dosage. Vitamin C is not toxic in large doses but must be taken throughout the day to benefit. Divide dosage to three or four times a day.

CHAPTER 117:

Multiple Sclerosis

I was fielding questions during the airing of my television show *Maximize Your Health*, and a man called in. He blessed the day he first saw the product in his refrigerator or heard my name. He wife had bought it from Son Broadcasting TV 11 in New Mexico.

She was at a meeting at her church praying for his recovery. At that moment, he was at home in a wheelchair, having just decided not to continue his life as a hopeless invalid. As he searched the kitchen for something that would poison him to death, he spied a bottle of minerals in solution and drank the whole thing. When his wife returned from church he greeted her at the door standing on both feet, which had not held his weight for over a year.

Whether it was the minerals in solution with biotin and 1,000 mcg of B12 per ounce that healed him, or not, we don't know. We must never underestimate the power of prayer. The caller, however, continues to take six to eight ounces a day of his mineral drink in solution with B12.

Multiple Sclerosis (MS) is another of the those degenerative diseases wrongly considered incurable by conventional medicine. True, once the myelin sheath covering the nerves is destroyed, it can't be replaced, but this side effect from inflammation of the central nerves can be prevented. What happens is this: lesions and plaque form on nerves in the brain, spinal cord and eyes. The lesions cause inflammation, eventually destroying the nerves' protective covering, the myelin sheath. This process is known as demyelination. The main symptom of MS, loss of motor skills, occurs because these demyelinated nerves are now exposed, and like live electrical wires, touch each other. What happens when you get a short circuit in your electrical wiring? Pfft! No juice. It gets worse and worse, until the patient ends up in a wheelchair, unable to even go to the bathroom unassisted.

From 1953 to 1959, Dr. Hinton D. Jonez successfully treated multiple sclerosis with natural therapies. His success curing a priest and a nun led to him being given an entire wing of St. Joseph's Hospital in Tacoma, Washington, to treat MS. Patients flocked to him from all over the world (no place else offered any hope). In spite of his achievements, only other hospital doctors' complaints filled his file. When he died in 1959, the wing was closed and his practice was terminated.

Fortunately, before he passed on, Dr. Jonez wrote a book entitled *My Fight to Conquer Multiple Sclerosis*, and an article in the *Journal of Postgraduate Medicine*, outlining his protocol (which included 8,000 mcg of vitamin B12, omega-3 and omega-6 essential fatty acids, and intravenous minerals) and documenting his successes. For information on how you can obtain copies of these publications, call 1-800-445-HEAL.

Lorenzo's Oil for MS?

Did you ever see the heart-wrenching movie Lorenzo's Oil? The movie was based on an actual case history of a couple whose son was afflicted with adreno-leuco-dystrophy (ALD), a rare genetic disease believed to be caused by an enzyme defect that allows saturated fats to accumulate in the body. What the couple discovered, heroically on their own, was that certain fatty acids – oils that help the body assimilate saturated fat – could reverse this enzyme defect. They researched and researched, and on their own they concocted Lorenzo's Oil, a formula of omega-6 and omega-3 oils that stopped the progression of their son's disease.

What I found so fascinating in researching this, was the number of studies that compared MS with ALD. Both afflictions have similar symptoms, both have lesions of the nerves, both destroy the myelin sheath, and in one article, autopsies of patients who died of both diseases had similar brain damage. The article says that for demyelinating diseases, "dietary therapy with oils rich in very long chain monenoic acid fatty acids (such as erucic acid) may be beneficial."[1] Long chain fatty acids are found in olive oil, flaxseed oil and borage oil, for example.

For the time being, there is nothing definite on the use of Lorenzo's Oil for multiple sclerosis. But for your information, this is what *Martindale, the Extra Pharmacopoeia*, 3rd edition says about it: "Lorenzo's Oil is a liquid containing glyceryl trierucate (a source of erucic acid) and glyceryl trioleate (a source of oleic acid), in the ratio of one part to four parts respectively. It has been used in conjunction with dietary modification for the treatment of adrenoleucodystrophy, a genetic disorder characterized by *demyelination*, adrenal cortex insufficiency, and accumulation of *saturated* "very-long-chain fatty acids." It adds that Lorenzo's Oil can be obtained from Scientific Hospital Supplies, 38 Queensland St., Liverpool, L73JG, England, 011-44151-228-1992.[2]

Oleic acid is generally contained in fish oils, like cod liver oil, and in olive oil and grapeseed oil. Certain rapeseed oils have high concentrations of erucic acid. However, the Food and Drug Administration has banned the use of oils containing erucic acid from the food supply.[3]

I called the people at Scientific Hospital Supplies myself, and got the usual desperate disclaimers. The representative I talked to said they will not sell to patients, only to doctors. I told the "representative" that people in this country with MS (and probably the U.K. as well) don't have anything to lose, since conventional medicine offers them absolutely nothing to try. Talk to your doctor if they won't help you. You have nothing to lose by trying Lorenzo's Oil. It's not a pharmaceutical so there are no dangerous side effects. Nobody wants you to believe it's a miracle cure, and SHS even worries you might have "false hope." There is no such thing as false hope. Hope is hope with all its spirit-elevating elements. Positive expectations are the rungs on the ladder leading to hope.

EFAs Explained

It can get very confusing when talking about the different kinds of fatty acids-sometimes termed polyunsatured fats, or PUFAs – which are the kinds of fats we need for energy and health – *not* saturated fat from meat and dairy products and certainly *not* transfatty acids from hydrogenated margarine and foods.

The two families of essential fatty acids are omega-6 (linoleic acid), found in seeds and seed oils and omega-3 (alpha-linolenic acid) found mainly in fish, fish oils (cod liver oil), green leafy vegetables and flaxseed oil. Gamma-linolenic acid (GLA), or linoleic acid, is found in evening primrose oil, black currant oil, borage oil and spirulina, and are known primarily for their anti-inflammatory effect.

EFAS and MS

In line with the theory that a deficiency of EFAs can cause multiple sclerosis, studies performed all over the world have shown them to be of benefit in treating it.

In one study, reported in the *British Medical Journal*, patients with MS were treated with evening primrose oil, a commonly-used source of gamma linolenic acid (GLA), for two years. Patients who were treated with 23 grams a day had significantly shorter and less severe relapses than a control group, which was given 16 grams a day of oleic acid from olive oil.[4]

Fortunately for us lay people desperate for answers, researchers, confused over varied results, decided to evaluate all the studies and come up with a definitive recommendation regarding the use of linolenic acid for MS. These esteemed doctors of conventional research concluded that "dietary supplementation with linolenic acid may have some beneficial effect not only on the severity and duration of re-lapses, but also on the progression of disability when patients are treated early in the course of the disease."[5]

Further encouraging was a proclamation made by the International Federation of Multiple Sclerosis Societies (IFMSS) Therapeutics Claims Committee acknowledging that "dietary supplementation with omega-6 PUFAs (GLA) may have some efficacy, since it appears to slow MS progression and reduces the severity and duration of exacerbations without affecting their frequency rate."[6] Remember, this is conventional medicine talking. They essentially have an unwritten code that any mention of nutrition in healing be preceded by "may" and "appears." If it sounds hesitant, that's because it is. It is the politics talking, not the evidence. The evidence is clear.

So, what can we do if our loved ones are pronounced afflicted with multiple sclerosis? The first thing I would do is look up the people who sell Lorenzo's Oil. Its ingredients are healthy sources of nutrients we need anyway. The second thing I would do is stock up on the best source possible of GLA.

The jury is in, and it calls to the stand on behalf of multiple sclerosis sufferers: borage oil. Independent clinical tests show that borage oil contains up to 26 percent GLA. Compare this to evening primrose oil and black currant oil, which contain no more than 18 percent. Not only that, borage oil costs less because the borage seed is three times larger than black currant or evening primrose seeds. Finally, borage is more bioavailable. In other words, the body more readily accepts it.[7]

The Fatty Evidence

If it is true that ALD and MS have the same or similar causes, then it stands to reason that an accumulation of saturated fat would be an important catalyst to the MS disease process. This becomes more and more likely as you examine the evidence. For example, people with MS have been known to improve when their intake of saturated fats is restricted. This would not happen if MS didn't have the same causal factor as ALD.

Roy L. Swank, M.D., Ph.D., Department of Neurology, Oregon Health Sciences University, has conducted a very long follow-up study of a group of 150 multiple sclerosis patients who were asked to stay on an extremely low saturated fat diet (less than 15 grams of fat per day) in the early '50s. When these same people were examined 30 years later, the data showed that both the strict dieters (those who consumed no more than 20 grams/day of saturated fat) and those who were less compliant (consuming more than 20 grams a day but still significantly less than they did before treatment) had a decrease in progression of the disease. The study showed that even eating as little as eight grams a day *more* than recommended resulted in sharp *increases* in deterioration and death as compared to the strict dieters. The researchers concluded by stating that "when all factors are taken into consideration, there is little reasonable doubt that a low saturated fat diet benefits patients with multiple sclerosis."[8]

If that doesn't convince you, just look at the evidence from the standpoint of geographical populations.

Pick up your magnifying glass, put on your detective hat and follow along while I recite the clues in the MS mystery.

More cases of multiple sclerosis are found in the northern, German-speaking part of Switzerland, where large amounts of animal fat are typically eaten.[9] In contrast, researchers found that in the southern part of Switzerland, where the Italian-speaking Swiss typically eat a diet low in saturated fat, *fewer* cases of MS were recorded. Similarly, the incidence of MS in Norway was found to be higher in the inland agricultural, dairy-eating regions than in coastal fishing communities.[10] A low incidence of MS was also observed among Eskimos and Laplanders, who consume large amounts of polyunsaturated fatty acids in the form of blubber and cod liver oil.[11]

You don't have to be Sherlock Holmes to figure this one out.

Dr. Swank did. He concluded, after considering all the evidence, that MS is linked to a diet high in saturated animal fats and deficient in PUFAs. According to Swank, persons afflicted with MS are, with few exceptions, sensitive to or intolerant of saturated fats.[12]

A B12 Boost

Some researchers have found a connection between B12 and multiple sclerosis. Patrick Kingsley, M.D., of Leicestershire, England, has treated over two thousand multiple sclerosis patients and believes vitamin B12 can be helpful in some cases. He believes MS can be caused by food allergies and chemical reactions, especially mercury poisoning. Like Alzheimer's disease sufferers, the mercury causing or making their MS worse can come from silver amalgam teeth fillings, which emit mercury into the brain. Dr. Kingsley makes sure all his patients replace their fillings before treating them with high doses of vitamin B12, niacin, vitamin B6, zinc and magnesium. He has found high doses of vitamin B12 administered intravenously, can completely clear an MS relapse.[13]

What is interesting about this tidbit of information is that all the nutrients Dr. Kingsley prescribes are necessary for the body to absorb and use fatty acids, which I believe is the crown jewel of successfully treating multiple sclerosis.

There are numerous natural healing doctors using Dr. Kingsley's protocol. For a number where you can obtain a list call 1-800-445-HEAL.

MS-Minimizing Nutrients
For maximum absorption, take supplements with meals.

Nutrient	Suggested Dosage	Formulation
Aged garlic extract	1 teaspoon three times daily	Liquid
Amino acids	4-6 capsules daily	Multiple formula from natural sources
Antioxidants	4 capsules daily*	With selenium and grapeseed extract
Borage oil	4 capsules daily	
Coenzyme Q1 (NADH)	2.5 to 5 mg daily	
Coenzyme Q10	2 capsules daily	With vitamin E, phospholipids and selenium
Fiber	4-8 tablets	Psyllium, with herb hyssop
Flaxseed oil	2 tablespoons daily	
Ginkgo biloba	60 mg three times daily	
Lecithin	2 tablespoons with meals	
Malic acid	250 mg twice daily	
Melatonin (adults only)	3 mg daily at bedtime	With B vitamins
Multi-mineral	3-4 ounces daily	In liquid solution, with vitamin B12, biotin
Multi-vitamin/mineral	6 caplets daily	Freeze-dried plant sources
Vitamin B6	100 mg daily	
Vitamin C	Individual bowel tolerance**	With bioflavonoids (quercetin, rutin proanthocyanidins)

* The FDA recommends pregnant women not exceed 10,000 IU of vitamin A daily.

** To determine individual dosage, on the first day take 1,000 mg hourly until diarrhea occurs, then reduce dosage to just below that for individual daily dosage. Vitamin C is not toxic in large doses but must be taken throughout the day to benefit. Divide dosage to three or four times a day.

CHAPTER 118:

Muscle Soreness

The first time I joined a fitness center it was run by macho men who didn't know a thing about the human body. They had me pumping iron and doing repetitions without warm ups and stretches. Every day I felt like an elephant had been doing a tap dance on my arms and legs. For weeks I let the dog get the paper so I didn't have to bend down to pick it up. I left food out just so I wouldn't have to put it back, and an inch of dust covered the furniture by the time I felt strong enough to pick up a dustcloth. I've learned a thing or two since then. First, not to overdo it, and second, what to take when I do.

Exercising Right to Avoid Muscle Soreness

At age 60, I can do two hours of exercise a day, one hour of high level aerobics and another hour of pumping iron. As long as I listen to my personal trainer, I never have sore muscles. She tells me all the time that "Less is more," and I shouldn't get carried away. The most benefit comes from moderate exercise increased very gradually.

The adage "no pain, no gain," has a point, but not to the extent that every movement elicits groans. This kind of torture is definitely not to your benefit. But to gain muscle, a certain amount of stress is necessary. What happens is that as you stress your muscles, a certain amount of tissue destruction occurs – that's the 'burn' you feel. The body then rebuilds the muscle, adding a little more. The more you burn, the more you gain. You can even feel some burn with a good stretch, as minute muscle fibers pull and tear. After-workout soreness is another matter altogether. It means you are doing too much. After a good workout, stretch long and hard.

Injury or overdoing the exercise results in structural damage to muscle proteins. Muscle damage can also occur if you perform unaccustomed types of exercise or suddenly increase their intensity or magnitude. Symptoms such as pain and muscle tenderness indicate muscle damage. Increasing muscle growth must be done gradually. When injury or overuse occurs, the best response is rest so muscles can heal and the injury is not made permanent.[1]

Instead of a pounding exercise routine, take a brisk walk in the morning or afternoon, making sure to stretch the muscles first. Muscle soreness and cramping can be caused by inadequate stretching before exercise. Also try stretching those muscles just before sleep if you have problems with muscle cramping. Nothing vigorous, just some pulls and stretches.

If you think heavy exercise is the only way, you'd be wrong. Studies are showing that moderate exercise is just as beneficial healthwise, and walking is turning out to be a good form. One study compared walking to jogging, and found that walking had the same health advantages as jogging, but with fewer injuries and less muscle soreness.[2]

Antioxidant Pain Relievers

If I get sore muscles, I head to my nutritional-medicine cabinet and come back with vitamin C plus bioflavonoids.

Bioflavonoids, a group of substances related to vitamin C, has been shown in studies to speed the healing of bruised muscles, not surprising considering they are powerful anti-inflammatories. A report in *Medical Times* reported that athletes taking citrus bioflavonoids and vitamin C healed twice as fast as athletes who took either vitamin C alone or no supplements whatsoever. Another study found that injured football players who took 200 to 600 mg daily of citrus bioflavonoids returned to the game in one-fourth the time of those not taking the supplements.[3]

A study by Mark Kaminski, M.S., an associate professor at Western States Chiropractic College in Portland, Oregon, found that one gram of vitamin C taken three times daily dramatically reduces muscle soreness after strenuous or infrequent exercise.[4]

Vitamin E, too, has been found in studies to help alleviate the pain of sore muscles. A study at the Human Nutrition Research Center on Aging at Tufts University, Boston, found vitamin E may reduce some of the muscle damage that occurs during vigorous exercise. Researchers studied 21 sedentary men, half of whom were given 800 IU of vitamin E for seven days prior to running downhill on a treadmill for 45 minutes. The other half were given placebos. After both groups exercised, the group taking the vitamin E had less damage to muscle tissue.[5]

Muscle contraction during resistance exercises causes damage to the muscles and the delayed pain of a "charley horse." But it is this damage that stimulates the increased repair and growth of new muscle. Another double-blind study at Tufts University shows that vitamin E can aid this muscle-building process. The researchers found that vitamin E supplements (727 mg) dramatically improved the rate of repair of skeletal muscle after damage in older people between the ages 55 to 74 and the effects were far more pronounced than in a group of younger subjects between 22 and 19 years.[6]

Beneficial Botanicals

"The beneficial effects attributed to aloe in the process of wound healing are so miraculous as to seem more like myth than fact," stated John P. Heggers, Ph.D., and colleagues of the University of Texas Medical Branch at Galveston.[7]

In both animal and human studies, the University of Texas research team found that, based on available data and their studies, aloe vera is a substance of "enormous therapeutic potential." It penetrates injured tissue, relieves pain, is anti-inflammatory and dilates capillaries, thereby increasing the blood supply to the injured area.

Turmeric has been used in both the Indian and Chinese systems of medicine for the treatment of many forms of inflammation. Its anti-inflammatory properties are likened to the pharmaceutical effects of hydrocortisone and phenylbutazone, only much safer.[8] To be more exact, it is the curcumin, that which gives tumeric its yellow color, that has been found in studies to work better than even ibuprofen, a popular over-the-counter pain medicine. In one study on rats, researchers found 20 mg of curcumin worked as well as 200 mg of ibuprofen. No toxic effects from curcumin have been reported.[9,10] Curcumin is a bioflavonoid, and also contains a large amount of vitamin C.

Bromelain, the active phytochemical in pineapple is also recommended when muscles or ligaments are swollen and inflamed. Since you would have to eat two whole pineapples a day to achieve this anti- inflammatory effect, it's good we have health stores that carry bromelain extract.[11] Bromelain is recommended as a supplement with all the other anti-inflammatories since it acts as a digestive enzyme, helping to break down and assimilate other nutrients.

Ginger has been noted in studies to be useful in inflammation and rheumatism. Danish researchers evaluated 28 patients with rheumatoid arthritis, 18 with osteoarthritis, and 10 with muscular discomfort using powdered ginger. In the arthritic patients, over 75 percent had varying degrees of relief from pain and swelling. All the patients with muscular discomfort had pain relief. There were no reported side effects when ginger was eaten regularly from three months to 2.5 years.[12]

For more on muscle pain relief, see the chapters Chronic Pain and Inflammation.

Sore Muscle Soothing Nutrients
For maximum absorption, take supplements with meals.

Nutrient	Suggested Dosage	Formulation
Aged garlic extract	1 teaspoon three times daily	Liquid
Amino acids	4-6 capsules daily	Multiple formula from natural sources
Borage oil	2 capsules daily	
Bromelain	200 mg twice daily	
Deglycyrrhizinated licorice	1-2 tablets before meals	Chewable
Flaxseed oil	1 tablespoon daily	
Ginger	500 mg after meals daily	
Magnesium	200 mg daily	
MSM (Methylsulfonylmethane)	500 mg three times daily	
Melatonin (adults only)	3 mg daily at bedtime	With B vitamins
Multi-mineral	3-4 ounces daily	In liquid solution, with vitamin B12, biotin
Multi-vitamin/mineral	6 caplets daily	Freeze-dried plant sources
Tumeric	100 mg one to three times daily	
Vitamin C	Individual bowel tolerance*	With citrus bioflavonoids (quercetin, proanthocyanidins)
Yucca	300 mg three times daily	

* To determine individual dosage, on the first day take 1,000 mg hourly until diarrhea occurs, then reduce dosage to just below that for individual daily dosage. Vitamin C is not toxic in large doses but must be taken throughout the day to benefit. Divide dosage to three or four times a day.

CHAPTER 119:

Muscle Weakness

One of my favorite people in the world, Kathryn Grayson (I call her Sister Kathryn because she's so wise), starred recently in *Love Letters*, a play in which she aged from a five-year-old girl to an old, old woman. Another dear friend, Barbara Rush, starred in another production of that same play in San Francisco. Miraculously, with no costume or makeup changes, both actresses were able to portray an entire human lifespan. How did they manage this transformation? They used the muscles in their bodies to loosen their skin and bend their posture to emulate the symptoms of age. Muscles are miraculous things. We can strengthen them, bend them, stretch them and manipulate them – even the heart muscle! – through the sheer force of will. That is why it is so frustrating when, due to weakness, we find them not complying with our wishes.

Muscle weakness can be the sign of many things. Nutrient deficiencies, such as magnesium, will cause the muscles to be weak, as can a lack of activity, causing atrophy. The next time you see the bare legs of someone who is in a wheelchair, notice how loose and thin the muscles are. If a paraplegic suddenly regained the use of his legs after years of being in a wheelchair, it would take months more to regain use of the muscles. Studies of elderly people have found that weight bearing exercises increase muscle strength better than anything, as long as the weakness is due to a sedentary lifestyle.

Certain illnesses can cause muscle weakness – illnesses that may be caused by nutrient deficiencies. Hypothyroidism, helped by iodine, causes muscle weakness; as does hypoglycemia, assisted by chromium; and heart muscle weakness, which can be caused by a lack of magnesium.

Muscles are largely made up of protein and essential fatty acids (EFAs). EFAs are coined 'essential' because they can't be produced by the body and therefore need to be obtained from the diet. The two families of essential fatty acids are omega-6 (linoleic acid), found in seeds and seed oils and omega-3 (alpha-linolenic acid) found mainly in fish, fish oils (cod liver oil), green leafy vegetables and flaxseed oil. Gamma-linolenic acid (GLA), a very good source of fatty acids is found in evening primrose oil, black currant oil, borage oil and spirulina. EFAs are required for growth, development and maintenance of cell membranes, including those of the muscular system. EFAs are important in fat metabolism. Without them, fat cannot be converted into glucose and instead gets stored throughout the body, including the muscles.

However, almost every mineral and vitamin is involved in muscle contraction, relaxation and repair. For example, potassium, which is very low in processed "junk" food diets, is necessary for the contraction of every muscle in the body. Magnesium and calcium are also needed – together not individually. Too little magnesium will cause calcium to accumulate in muscle tissues, jeopardizing the circulation of oxygen and causing muscles to atrophy.[1]

Muscles and Exercise

All across America, nursing homes are filled with elderly people whose muscles are so weak they need help with simple tasks, such as getting up out of a chair.

They're institutionalized not because of any disease or cognitive impairment but because of muscle weakness. Their minds may still be quite nimble and alert, but their bodies are diminished.

Dr. William Evans, director of the Noll Laboratory for Human Performance Research at Penn State University, has given this age-related muscle loss a name, "sarcopenia," from the Greek for "flesh reduction." By identifying this costly and life-threatening condition as a disease, he hopes it will get the widespread public attention that's already been given to other degenerative conditions associated with aging, such as osteoporosis and arthritis.

Until now, sarcopenia has been overlooked because muscle weakness was considered an inevitable part of growing old. But new research is proving that strength does not have to diminish into decrepitude with age. Muscles will get stronger in response to strength training no matter what your age. Much of the muscle loss attributed to age actually comes from inactivity. No other single intervention holds greater promise of keeping people out of nursing homes than resistance training – exercises that work the muscles against weight.

It is estimated that muscle mass naturally decreases by 15-20 percent between the ages of 30 and 80. However, this muscle mass can be recovered. A just-completed three-year project, funded by the National Institute on Aging and the National Center for Nursing Research, has shown that strength and balance exercises can help frail elderly in their 80s and 90s double and triple their strength to the point where many are able to walk and perform other tasks without assistance.[2]

Muscles Degenerate Without Antioxidants and B Vitamins

While I'm not really talking about muscular dystrophy here, the principles can be applied. In MD, the patients' muscles atrophy and degenerate, eventually being replaced with useless fat. It is similar to multiple sclerosis in that plaques form and cause degeneration. In MS it is a degeneration of the nerves, and in MD it is a degeneration of the muscles. Why does this occur? Certain nutrients seem to hold the key, and animal studies have opened the doors.

Researchers have determined that a deficiency of choline, a B vitamin, can result in muscular degeneration. Studies on laboratory rabbits showed a choline deficiency can produce muscular dystrophy, with the symptoms identical to those deficient in vitamin E.

What researchers finally discovered was this deficiency in choline so impaired their livers that it jeopardized their ability to store and assimilate vitamin E. Without adequate vitamin E, no living creature can properly synthesize choline.[3]

Vitamin E is also an antioxidant, shown in studies to protect the muscles against free radical damage. Vitamin E and vitamin C have been proven in research to defuse free radicals, molecules that can harm muscle tissue. Overtraining, pollution, sunlight and aging causes free radicals to accumulate in muscle tissue. Research indicates that 400 IU of vitamin E and 500 mg of vitamin C will protect muscles from free radicals' effects.[4]

Other antioxidant vitamins have been shown in studies to also reverse the degeneration of muscles. If you read the Heart chapter in this book, you will see how they help prevent heart muscle damage following strokes and attacks. Coenzyme Q10, a very effective heart antioxidant, has also been found to help in treating muscular dystrophy.[5]

In a 24-month open trial, researchers from University Hospital in Linkoping, Sweden, found patients with myotonic muscular dystrophy, the most common form of muscular dystrophy in adults, had improvement in both muscular force and function when treated with high doses of vitamin E and selenium.[6] Selenium is a mineral antioxidant, and helps amplify the benefits of vitamin E.

The Amino Acid/Protein Connection

From the pages of sports medicine come the most widely-used supplements to boost muscle strength: amino acids. When amino acids are lost or missing, muscle tissue breaks down. While vitamin E can reverse this process, amino acids can prevent it from happening in the first place. The story starts with protein. Your muscles are made up of protein. Without it, fat cannot convert to muscle. Protein is composed of approximately 22 amino acids. All but eight can be produced in the human body, the rest have to be obtained from food or supplements. If just one amino acid is low or missing, even temporarily, protein synthesis will fall or stop altogether and muscles can become weak or stop functioning.[7]

Because of this delicate balance and its importance to muscle strength, athletes emphasize amino acid formulas in their daily nutritional routine, and especially after injury, to rebuild muscle. Amino acids help prevent the body from breaking down protein in injured muscles. One amino acid, arginine, seems to outshine the others in this regard. In animals with fractures, diets supplemented with arginine and glycine (another amino acid) reduced the loss of protein from the muscles by 40 percent, researchers at Rutgers University found. And researchers at Einstein Medical School in New York City found that, after moderate surgery, people who got an extra 15 grams of arginine a day had a 60 percent reduction in protein loss compared to patients who did not get the supplement.[8]

What do boxer Evander Holyfield, football star Lyle Alzado and Olympic track gold medalist Florence Griffith Joyner have in common? They all have depended on nutritional supplements, including amino acids, for their muscular prowess.[9,10,11]

Foods containing protein may or may not contain all the essential amino acids. Food that has them all is termed a "complete protein." The best sources of protein are vegetable proteins, found in whole grains like brown rice, and in legumes, such as beans. These two combined are every bit as complete as the protein in meat or dairy products.

Muscle-Bound Nutrients
For maximum absorption, take supplements with meals.

Nutrient	Suggested Dosage	Formulation
Amino acids	4-6 capsules daily	Multiple formula from natural sources
Antioxidants	4 capsules daily*	With selenium and grapeseed extract
Coenzyme Q10	2 capsules daily	With vitamin E, phospholipids and selenium
Fiber	4-8 tablets daily	
L-Carnitine	500 mg twice daily	
Magnesium	200 mg daily	
Malic acid	250 mg three times daily	
Multi-mineral	3-4 ounces daily	In liquid solution, with vitamin B12, biotin
Multi-vitamin/mineral	6 caplets daily	Freeze-dried plant sources
Vitamin B6	100 mg daily	
Vitamin C	Individual bowel tolerance**	With bioflavonoids (quercetin, proanthocyanidins)
Vitamin E	2 capsules (800 IU) daily	d-alpha tocopherol

* The FDA recommends pregnant women not exceed 10,000 IU of vitamin A daily.

** To determine individual dosage, on the first day take 1,000 mg hourly until diarrhea occurs, then reduce dosage to just below that for individual daily dosage. Vitamin C is not toxic in large doses but must be taken throughout the day to benefit. Divide dosage to three or four times a day.

CHAPTER 120:

Muscular Dystrophy

If money is all it takes to cure a disease, this one would have been alleviated billions of dollars ago. Muscular dystrophy is another of those tragic diseases associated predominately with children, even though plenty of adults have it too. To raise money for the Muscular Dystrophy Association, every year comedian Jerry Lewis produces a telethon. Featuring children walking with the aid of torturous-looking metal braces or sitting in wheelchairs, Lewis has used hopeless cases and dramatic images to get people to open their wallets and donate billions of dollars toward discovering a cure. I remember watching the telethon once, and tearfully pledging money out of pity for the little ones. After 30 telethons and over a billion dollars raised, families are still told there is no cure.

A Multiple Deficiency?

In MD, the patients' muscles atrophy and degenerate, eventually being replaced with fat. It is similar to multiple sclerosis in that plaques form and cause degeneration. In MS is it a degeneration of the nerves, and in MD it is a degeneration of the muscles. Why does this occur? Certain nutrients seem to hold the key, and animal studies have opened the doors.

Researchers have determined that a deficiency of choline, a B vitamin, can result in muscular degeneration. In a study reported in the *Journal of Nutrition*, Drs. E. L. Hove and D. H. Copeland of the Alabama Polytechnic Institute described an animal experiment that showed a diet low in vitamin E caused muscular dystrophy in rabbits. Looking further, they found that muscle atrophy occurred predominately due to a deficiency of the B vitamin choline. They noted that one of the functions of vitamin E in the body is to bring about the synthesis of a substance called acetylcholine. They concluded that a deficiency in choline should not only cause wasting of muscles, but a vitamin E deficiency. To see if it did, they put laboratory rabbits on a diet deficient in choline, but not vitamin E, and compared them to a group who received a choline-sufficient diet. They found the symptoms of muscular dystrophy were identical in all respects to those of the rabbits deficient in vitamin E, concluding that it was the choline, not the vitamin E that caused the dystrophy.[1]

Researchers have also discovered that muscular dystrophy, at least in part, can be caused by free radical damage, speeded up.[2] If you look at the aging process, you see a certain amount of muscular dystrophy, in part due to inactivity, but also due to the long-term effect of free radicals – molecules that can harm muscle tissue. Overtraining, pollution, sunlight and aging causes free radicals to accumulate in muscle tissue. Anything that can reverse the effects of free radical damage will help fight against muscular dystrophy.

Vitamin E is an antioxidant, and has been shown in studies to protect the muscles against free radical damage, as has vitamin C. Research indicates that 400 IU of vitamin E and 500 mg of C will protect muscles from free radical damage.[3]

Other antioxidant vitamins have been shown in studies to reverse the degeneration of muscles. If you read the Heart chapter in this book, you will see how they help prevent heart muscle damage following strokes and attacks. Coenzyme Q10, a very effective heart antioxidant, has also been found to help in treating muscular dystrophy.[4,5]

In a 24-month open trial, researchers from University Hospital in Linkoping, Sweden, found patients with myotonic muscular dystrophy, the most common form of muscular dystrophy in adults, had improvement in both muscular force and function when treated with high doses of vitamin E and selenium, a mineral antioxidant.[6]

The Amino Acid/Protein Connection

From the pages of sports medicine come the most widely-used supplements to boost muscle strength: amino acids. When amino acids are lost or missing, muscle tissue breaks down. Vitamin E can reverse this process, but obviously adequate amino acids can prevent it from happening in the first place. Your muscles are made up of protein. Without protein, fat cannot convert to muscle. Protein is composed of approximately 22 amino acids. All but eight can be produced in the human body, the rest have to be obtained from food or supplements. If just one amino acid is low or missing, even temporarily, protein synthesis will fall or stop altogether and muscles can become weak or stop functioning.[7]

Because of this delicate balance and its importance to muscle strength, athletes emphasize amino acid formulas in their daily nutritional routine, and especially after injury, to rebuild muscle. Amino acids help prevent the body from breaking down protein in injured muscles. One amino acid, arginine, seems to outshine the others in this regard. In animals with fractures, diets supplemented with arginine and glycine (another amino acid) reduced the loss of protein from the muscles by 40 percent, researchers at Rutgers University found. And researchers at Einstein Medical School in New York City found that, after moderate surgery, people who got an extra 15 grams of arginine a day had a 60 percent reduction in protein loss compared to patients who did not get the supplement.[8]

What do boxer Evander Holyfield, football star Lyle Alzado and Olympic track gold medalist Florence Griffith Joyner have in common? They all depend on nutritional supplements, including amino acids, for their muscular prowess.[9,10,11]

Foods containing protein may or may not contain all the essential amino acids. Food that has them all is termed a "complete protein." The best sources of protein are vegetable proteins, found in whole grains like brown rice, and in legumes, such as beans. These two combined are every bit as complete as the protein in meat or dairy products.

Muscle Essential Nutrients

Muscles are largely made up of protein and essential fatty acids (EFAs). EFAs are coined 'essential' because they can't be produced by the body and therefore need to be obtained from the diet.The two families of essential fatty acids are omega-6 (linoleic acid), found in seeds and seed oils and omega-3 (alpha-linolenic acid) found mainly in fish, fish oils (cod liver oil), green leafy vegetables and flaxseed oil. Gamma-linolenic acid (GLA), a very good source of fatty acids is found in evening primrose oil, black currant oil, borage oil and spirulina. EFAs are required for growth, development and maintenance of cell membranes, including those of the muscular system. EFAs are important in fat metabolism. Without them, fat cannot be converted into glucose and instead gets stored throughout the body, including the muscles.

Almost every mineral and vitamin is involved in muscle contraction, relaxation and repair. For example, potassium, which is very low in processed "junk" food diets, is necessary for the contraction of every muscle in the body. Magnesium and calcium are also needed- -together not individually. Too little magnesium will cause calcium to accumulate in muscle tissues, jeopardizing the circulation of oxygen and causing muscles to atrophy.[12]

For your mineral needs, look for a good, easily absorbable, derived-from-nature mineral blend in solution. Liquid formulations provide the maximum absorption ratios.

Muscle-Mighty Nutrients
For maximum absorption, take supplements with meals.
(Half doses for children.)

Nutrient	Suggested Dosage	Formulation
Amino acids	4-6 capsules daily	Multiple formula from natural sources
Antioxidants	4 capsules daily*	With selenium and grapeseed extract
Borage oil	2 capsules daily	
Coenzyme Q1 (NADH)	2.5 to 5 mg daily	
Coenzyme Q10	2 capsules daily	With vitamin E, phospholipids and selenium
Enzymes	2 capsules twice daily	Multiple formula
Fiber	4-8 tablets daily	
Flaxseed oil	1 tablespoon daily	
Ginkgo biloba	60 mg three times daily	
L-Carnitine	500 mg twice daily	
Magnesium	200 mg daily	
Melatonin (adults only)	3 mg daily at bedtime	With B vitamins
Malic acid	250 mg three times daily	
Multi-mineral	3-4 ounces daily	In liquid solution, with vitamin B12, biotin
Multi-vitamin/mineral	6 caplets daily	Freeze-dried plant sources
Vitamin B6	100 mg daily	
Vitamin C	Individual bowel tolerance**	With bioflavonoids (quercetin, proanthocyanidins)
Vitamin E	2 capsules (800 IU) daily	d-alpha tocopherol

* The FDA recommends pregnant women not exceed 10,000 IU of vitamin A daily.

** To determine individual dosage, on the first day take 1,000 mg hourly until diarrhea occurs, then reduce dosage to just below that for individual daily dosage. Vitamin C is not toxic in large doses but must be taken throughout the day to benefit. Divide dosage to three or four times a day.

CHAPTER 121:

Nail Problems

Strong fingernails come in handy for picking up dimes. But let's be honest. Most of us want great nails because they complete the picture of well-groomed good looks. In fact, after your face, they're the most looked-at part of your body. For many people, however, great nails have been an impossible challenge.

There are multitude of reasons for not-so-perfect nails. Bad habits can break them, poor hygiene can spoil them, the wrong nail care products can dry them, and poor nutrition can sabotage them.

Any physician knows that the condition of the nails is an indicator of the health of the body. If the nails are pale and yellow instead of healthy pink, the doctor might look for diabetes. If the doctor sees that the nails are dry and brittle, calcium or other nutrients might be lacking in the diet.

Nails, skin and hair are first cousins, as each are made of a sturdy protein called keratin. Because the nail is so porous, water and chemical-containing solutions can be readily absorbed. Soaking allows nails to swell; drying causes them to shrink. Too many unprotected dips in water, and the cumulative stress of swell-and-shrink cycles damages the protein bridges between the nail cells and encourages splits and breaks.

The half moon, or lunula, seen at the base of most nails, is the tip of the nail-growth zone. It is the most vulnerable part of the nail plate. Too-vigorous use of manicure tools here can cause growth disturbances like ridges or white spots.[1]

Biotin for Brittle Nails

For years no one's been able to put a finger on an effective treatment for brittle nails. Now finally someone has. It's a little-known B vitamin called biotin. You could say the idea came straight from the horse's hoof.

After seeing how veterinarians used this water-soluble vitamin to work wonders for horses with problem hooves, Swiss researchers decided to try it out on people with brittle fingernails. In a controlled study of 32 men and women, the researchers gave one group with thin, frail and split nails six to nine months of daily treatment (2.5 milligrams, which averages 12.5 times the average daily intake). The subjects' nail thickness was boosted by 25 percent.[2]

Biotin is absorbed into the matrix of the nail, where it can encourage a better, thicker nail to grow. Richard K. Scher, M.D., head of the nail section at Columbia Presbyterian Medical Center, New York City, treats his brittle-nail patients with biotin supplements.[3]

Nutritional Deficiencies Spotted

A deficiency of protein, vitamins and minerals can affect the condition and appearance of your nails.[4]

Ever notice white spots under your nails? They can be caused by two things: injury to the nail and a zinc deficiency. Because zinc is necessary to wound healing, spots can indicate there's not enough zinc for the healing process to occur.

Copper is important to balance out your zinc supplements. Be sure and include 2-4 mg of copper with any zinc.

Silica is also important to healthy nails. If yours are dark, brittle and have an abnormal surface, they deserve a closer look. It could be that a deficiency of silica is robbing the calcium from your body and you haven't noticed – yet.

I take a mineral in solution formula that contains biotin, silica and vitamin B12, and my nails look great!

The lack of protein, folic acid and vitamin C causes hangnails, and dry, brittle nails and white bands indicate a protein deficiency.

A shortage of vitamin A or calcium in the diet can cause dry, brittle nails, and a B vitamin deficiency can cause horizontal and vertical ridges, making the nail prone to breakage.[5]

While calcium supplementation, in and of itself, does not help the nails, silica, as already described, can keep you from losing valuable calcium.

Vitamin A is especially essential to healthy nails because without it, the body can't utilize protein. The best kind of protein is free form amino acids found in vegetables, egg yolk, oatmeal, nuts, seeds, grains and fruits.

B12 is an important nail nutrient. Without it, the nails become very dry, thin, flat, dark, and spoon-shaped with rounded and curved nail ends.[6]

For a healthy system, B vitamins must be taken together. Without one, the others are useless. B12 is the only one that can be taken alone. However, digestive enzymes in the stomach can destroy it, which is why it is usually given in shot form. Since I hate shots, I take my B12 in solution.

Inadequate stomach acid (hydrochloric acid) can cause nail splitting, not to mention a host of other problems. Not enough stomach acid means nutrients are not being extracted from foods and supplements, which can cause all of the above symptoms.

If you suspect you have this problem, supplement with Betaine HcL, available in health food stores, or take your minerals in solution, which makes them easier to assimilate.

Moisturizing Healthy Nails

OK, you're taking the right supplementation and eating right. Now you have healthy nails, right? Wrong! You still have to treat your nails right to keep them smooth, strong and healthy.

Just as you moisturize your skin, you must also moisturize your nails. Brittle, peeling nails can be a sign of dehydration, caused by a dry, cold environment or exposure to harsh chemicals, including nail polish removers that contain acetone, a chemical used to remove enamel paints. Experts agree that using an acetone-based remover only once a week will limit the drying to acceptable limits. But if you plan to take no chances, choose a nail polish remover that contains acetate rather than acetone.

Avoid strong soaps, detergents and excessive washing of the hands, which alternately stretches and shrinks the nail plate. This repeated stretching and shrinking is like taking a piece of metal and bending it back and forth – eventually it breaks. If you feel the need for an antibacterial soap, choose one that includes soothing herbals and healing ingredients.

Before using any moisturizer, you must rehydrate the nails with water. Dry skin and brittle nails are both due to a loss of water, not oil. Soak your hands in water (sans soap) for 15 to 20 minutes before using a moisturizer. You can even soak if you're wearing nail polish. In fact, nail polish can actually help prevent moisture loss. It works, provided you don't take it off and put it on too often."[7] I discovered an ingredient in some moisturizers that is more of a medicinal than a cosmetic. It's called hyaluronic acid, or sodium hyaluronate. It's so gentle it is used by eye surgeons to separate delicate tissues. It moisturizes by binding with the skin, holding 1,000 times its own weight in water.

Hot water and soap can be nail enemies. Like when you're doing the dishes, taking a bath or washing out a few things and your nails get so soft that they split.

Apply a moisturizer to your hands every time you wash them, or any other time they've been in water.[8]

Nails absorb water and expand in volume. Then when you take your hands out of the water, the water evaporates and the nail volume contracts. If you apply a lotion to your hands as soon as you've lightly dried them, while they're still a bit damp, it helps seal the moisture in your skin and nails.[9] Look for a moisturizing lotion that includes hyaluronic acid, the antioxidants vitamins A, C and E; chamomile for healing; and other herbal helpers like marigold, papaya, lemon peel and cucumber. Your hands need all the help they can get, including ingredients that soften, heal and revitalize.

Nail-Loving Nutrients
For maximum absorption, take supplements with meals.

Nutrient	Suggested Dosage	Formulation
Antioxidants	4 capsules daily*	With selenium and grapeseed extract
Fiber	4-8 tablets daily	Psyllium, with herb hyssop
Multi-mineral	1-4 ounces daily	In liquid solution, with vitamin B12, biotin
Multi-vitamin/mineral	3-6 caplets daily	Freeze-dried plant sources
Vitamin C	Individual bowel tolerance**	With bioflavonoids (quercetin, proanthocyanidins)

Nourish nails with a therapeutic moisturizer that contains aloe vera gel, chamomile, vitamins A and C, and avocado oil.

* The FDA recommends pregnant women not exceed 10,000 IU of vitamin A daily.

** To determine individual dosage, on the first day take 1,000 mg hourly until diarrhea occurs, then reduce dosage to just below that for individual daily dosage. Vitamin C is not toxic in large doses but must be taken throughout the day to benefit. Divide dosage to three or four times a day.

CHAPTER 122:

Nausea

The water is blue, the boat is white, and you're green from seasickness. At first you're afraid you're going to die. After a couple of hours, you're afraid you're *not* going to.

You're pregnant, and you've told your boss that you will work until your due date – if only you could get out of the bathroom!

You're home after having surgery. Your doctor said you have to remain in bed to let the stitches heal. You wonder how they're going to heal when you spend most of the day bent over the toilet bowl.

Whatever the cause, there are natural, nutritional solutions to nausea, found in your health food store, garden or neighborhood market, accessible and easy to prepare no matter where you find yourself.

A B Vitamin That Helps

When it comes to nausea that results in vomiting, vitamin B6 is the nutrient to call on. Like all the B vitamins, B6 is responsible for calming the nerves and soothing the spirit. It is essential for the synthesis of tryptophan, an amino acid that helps with insomnia and depression.

In a study directed by Dr. Sahakian of the University of Iowa College of Medicine, 31 pregnant volunteers receiving 25 mgs of vitamin B6 every eight hours for three days were compared to 28 women who took a placebo. After treatment with B6, only eight of the 31 patients in the vitamin B6 group had vomiting, while almost half did – 15 of the 28 patients in the placebo group. Dr. Sahakian and his colleagues concluded that severe nausea and the total number of patients with vomiting was significantly reduced following the vitamin B6 therapy.[1] It is recommended that 25 mg be taken with each meal for nausea, and 250 mg or more daily for vomiting. By the way, vitamin B6 has also been found effective in controlling the fluid retention associated with prenatal toxemia.[2]

A Folk Remedy Triumphs Over Modern Science

Unlike many folk remedies handed down through the generations, the use of ginger for nausea has been given the green light by modern scientists. In a double-blind study conducted by researchers at Brigham Young University, ginger root beat the most popular pharmaceutical, Dramamine, in alleviating motion sickness.[3]

In a study described in the *European Journal of Obstetrics, Gynecology, Reproductive Biology*, 27 pregnant women so incapacitated by nausea that they required hospitalization, were given either ginger root powder or a placebo. After only four days of treatment, an incredible 70 percent had fewer attacks of nausea, and with less severity. There were no side effects reported.[4]

If you think it only works for morning sickness, read on. Ginger has shown in studies to help postoperative nausea, and seasickness.

In a double-blind trial, doctors at St. Bartholomew's Hospital, London studied 60 women between the ages of 16 and 65 who had major gynecologic surgery with accompanying nausea. One group was given one gram of ginger root and a fake injection. The other group was given an oral placebo and an injection of metoclopramide, a drug to help combat nausea and vomiting.

The good news? Ginger root combated nausea better than the pharmaceutical, with a quarter of those receiving it, benefitting by it. A control group getting nothing had a 51 percent incidence of nausea, while those receiving the ginger root had a 28 percent incidence. The group getting the drug had a 30 percent incidence. The doctors concluded that ginger root effectively prevents nausea after major gynecological surgery with minimal to no side effects, and is easy to administer.[5]

If you were in charge of a study on seasickness, what subjects would you choose? Fishermen? Sailing buddies? Danish researchers chose newly-graduated Naval cadets unaccustomed to sailing in heavy seas for their study on ginger root and seasickness.

In a double blind, randomized, placebo-controlled trial, 80 Naval cadets consumed one gram of ginger root or a placebo every hour for four consecutive hours. The researchers and the Navy were delighted to discover that ginger root reduced the tendency toward vomiting and cold sweating significantly better than placebo. The researchers reported remarkably fewer symptoms of nausea and vertigo, with no side effects.[6]

Health food stores sell ginger root capsules, and advise taking one capsule three times daily. Not one who suffers from motion sickness, I have never taken Dramamine or tried ginger root. My friends have played guinea pig with ginger root capsules and have found them effective, whether for a harbor cruise or an ocean voyage. I'm told ginger root works best if taken an hour before meeting with potentially upsetting motion. If you prefer fresh ginger root be warned that it burns. Best to mix it with fruit juice or use the capsules.

Nausea-Negating Nutrients
For maximum absorption, take supplements with meals.

Nutrient	Suggested Dosage	Formulation
Aged garlic extract	1 teaspoon three times daily	Liquid
Enzymes	2 capsules twice daily	Multiple formula
Fiber	4-8 tablets daily	Psyllium, with herb hyssop
Ginger	500 mg after meals as needed	
Multi-mineral	3-4 ounces daily	In liquid solution, with vitamin B12, biotin
Multi-vitamin/mineral	6 caplets daily	Freeze-dried plant sources
Tumeric	100 mg as needed	
Vitamin B6	200 mg as needed	
Vitamin C	Individual bowel tolerance*	With bioflavonoids (quercetin, rutin proanthocyanidins)

* To determine individual dosage, on the first day take 1,000 mg hourly until diarrhea occurs, then reduce dosage to just below that for individual daily dosage. Vitamin C is not toxic in large doses but must be taken throughout the day to benefit. Divide dosage to three or four times a day.

CHAPTER 123:

Night Blindness

"My darkness has been filled with the light of intelligence, and behold, the outer day-lit world was stumbling and groping in social blindness."

–Helen Keller

Imagine not being able to drive in the dark, walk in the dark, see in the dark. Imagine looking out your window to see who is at the door and seeing nothing, not even the street lights. As a teenager, I knew someone who had night blindness. We lived near a community center and would walk there evenings to play basketball. When we went together I had to hold his arm because he couldn't see, even by the street lights! That young man broke my heart, in more ways than one. When I think back on it today I remember his family was poor, and I'm willing to bet his problem was caused by poor eating habits. If only I'd known then what I know now!

Vitamin A and Night Blindness

Vitamin A is important to the eyes and visual system in several ways. The ability of the eye to adapt to changes in light is dependent upon a chemical known as retinal purple, or rhodopsin. Retinal purple is comprised mainly of protein and a close relative of vitamin A, and is the army that keeps us seeing even in darkness. The army has one enemy: light. When light hits the retina – such as when driving and being "blinded" by oncoming headlights – the retinal purple army splits up, temporarily fleeing.[1] The next time you enter a dark room after being outside on a sunny day, see how long it takes for your vision to return. The length of time depends upon two things: the amount of retinal purple present to begin with and the amount of light. Too much light and not enough vitamin A means the breakdown of night vision. Imagine you walk into a dark theater, wait for your vision to come back and it never does! Patrons might forgive you for groping them and banging into their knees, but until the movie starts, you're in the dark.

Conditions such as heart bypass surgery, cystic fibrosis and cirrhosis of the liver make people susceptible to vitamin A deficiency and night blindness. In one case report, a 16-year-old male with cystic fibrosis complaining of night blindness, was given 25,000 IU of vitamin A. After seven months his serum vitamin A levels returned to normal and he was miraculously able to see in the dark again.[2]

In areas of the world where diet is poor, blindness due to a vitamin A deficiency is tragically common, especially among the children. Vitamin A deficiency exists in many of the 10 million children worldwide under the age of six who have impaired vision. One-tenth of these children usually go blind.[3] Over the decades since this was first discovered by the medical establishment, American physicians have made it their duty to go to these countries armed with vitamin A supplements. Once the children receive the supplements, their sight is often joyfully restored.

Some doctors scare people away from A by emphasizing that you can take too much. Vitamin A is a so-called fat soluble vitamin, meaning it doesn't dissolve well in water, can't be excreted in urine, and as a result our body stores excess A in the liver. Too much can cause liver and bone damage. However, toxic levels are considered to be above 100,000 IU, for healthy people not already deficient, and damaging only when taken for long periods of time. Pregnant women should not exceed 10,000 IU a day. Early warning signs of vitamin A toxicity are that you'll get a small pounding headache at the front of the head, your lips will crack or your palms will peel. Combining vitamin E with A boosts the benefit so lower amounts can be taken.

A French physician, Dr. C. Carlier, did a study in which children with eye problems were given either vitamin A or beta carotene to see which worked better to alleviate the deficiency and restore their eyesight. He gave 256 children 200,000 IU of retinyl palmitate (vitamin A), and 254 children 1.2 million IU of beta carotene for seven weeks, then tested their eyes. Of the children receiving the vitamin A, 51.2 percent were restored to normal. Of the children receiving the beta carotene, 50 percent were restored to normal. The statistics are so close, the doctor concluded that beta carotene works just as well as vitamin A and can be used instead to avoid the toxicity issue.[4]

Vitamin A deficiencies may be more common than we think. Vitamin A can be destroyed in many different ways, including poor liver function; alcohol; eating large amounts of mineral oil or ferrous sulphate, a common preservative; x-rays; and any kind of infection.

Bilberry Jam, Anyone?

For hundreds of years bilberry fruit, the European version of our blueberry and a popular source of fresh jam, has been considered a food substance of the purest kind.

One of the most notable discoveries for the use of bilberry fruit was made during World War II. Shortly before their night missions, British RAF pilots would snack on bread covered with bilberry jam. Throughout the war, these pilots seemed to be far more successful at hitting their targets than the enemy. The British pilots swore that eating bilberry jam prior to night missions made their night vision much better.[5]

Since then, numerous studies have been published confirming bilberry's effectiveness in helping a variety of visual problems including night blindness, eye fatigue, nearsightedness, cataracts and glaucoma. The family of bioflavonoids, the anthocyanosides, present in the berry take some of the credit. Bioflavonoids, nature's chemicals that put the color in fruit, are notorious anti-inflammatories and have numerous therapeutic properties.

Animal and laboratory studies have revealed how anthocyanosides work. On a basic level, they help to strengthen the tiny capillaries that deliver nutrients to eye muscles and nerves. They also decrease the permeability of blood vessels, thereby reducing the damage caused by deterioration of blood vessels, and help the eyes' ability to see at night by increasing retinal purple. Plus, they act as a photomultiplier on the retina by heightening the perception of normal objects, thus extending the range and sharpness of vision. Eating your anthocyanosides in billberry also gives you calcium, magnesium, phosphorus, potassium and plenty of the antioxidant vitamin C, and other bioflavonoids.

If you can't get bilberry jam, try mimicking the benefit with these healthy-anyway nutrients. The minerals support and strengthen the circulatory system and tiny capillaries that deliver nutrients to the eyes. Vitamin C and bioflavonoids are potent anti-inflammatories, keeping infections from jeopardizing the eyes. They also boost the immune system so injury and illnesses heal faster, better. Free radicals have been shown in many studies to especially damage delicate eye tissues, and vitamin C and bioflavonoids are potent free radical-scavenging antioxidants.

Other nutrients said to benefit are the B vitamins riboflavin, niacin, thiamine and the mineral zinc.[6] The B vitamins must be taken together, so do the B complex shuffle. Each B vitamin has its own role in body function, centered on the nervous system. Since nerves bring messages to all the organs and stimulate glands to secrete their important biochemicals, the whole body communication system can break down with a B vitamin deficiency.

Night Sight-Restoring Nutrients
For maximum absorption, take supplements with meals.

Nutrient	Suggested Dosage	Formulation
Antioxidants	4 capsules daily*	With selenium and grapeseed extract
Bilberry	100 mg twice daily	
Borage oil	2 capsules daily	
Coenzyme Q10	2 capsules daily	With vitamin E, phospholipids and selenium
Flaxseed oil	1 tablespoon daily	
Ginkgo biloba	60 mg daily	
Magnesium	200 mg daily	
Multi-mineral	3-4 ounces daily	In liquid solution, with vitamin B12, biotin
Multi-vitamin/mineral	6 caplets daily	Freeze-dried plant sources
Taurine	500 mg daily	
Vitamin A	25,000 IU daily*	
Vitamin C	Individual bowel tolerance**	With bioflavonoids (quercetin, rutin proanthocyanidins)

* The FDA recommends pregnant women not exceed 10,000 IU of vitamin A daily.

** To determine individual dosage, on the first day take 1,000 mg hourly until diarrhea occurs, then reduce dosage to just below that for individual daily dosage. Vitamin C is not toxic in large doses but must be taken throughout the day to benefit. Divide dosage to three or four times a day.

CHAPTER 124:

Nosebleeds

"Those who in quarrels interpose,
Must often wipe a bloody nose."

– John Gay

Nothing is more embarrassing than a sudden onslaught of blood from the nose. "Excuse me, but I think you should know that your nose is bleeding." Oh, the horror of it all! Or you feel a little moisture, thinking you have a runny nose, wipe it with a tissue, and discover a bright red smear the size of the Missouri River. When I see it happening to someone, I'm reminded of how vulnerable I am in front of television cameras, and at the slightest runny nose, imagine the worst has happened. Fortunately, I've not had the displeasure and embarassment of a public nosebleed, but having spent endless summers in my youth at the local swimming pool, remember many red-faced kids in the first aid office having cold compresses applied to their nostrils. I think there must be something about chlorinated water that predisposes kids to nosebleeds. Either that, or they were too embarrassed to admit they were diving in the shallow end!

Common Causes and First Aid

In healthy people, nosebleeds are uncommon. They occur if you injure or bump your nose, blow it too hard, pick it too much; or if irritation, dry air and/or congestion causes fragile blood vessels in the nose to inflame and break. When faced with dry air in an overconditioned hotel or during a visit to Arizona or Nevada, try keeping the inside of your nose lubricated. KY jelly is best because it's not made of petroleum by-products like Vaseline, and it is water soluble. Being in water all the time can also jeopardize blood vessels as it washes out naturally-protective nasal goo. A good friend of mine, Junis Olmscheid, is a Hollywood makeup artist. She advocates KY Jelly; applying a light coating to both waterproof makeup, and retain the skin's moisture level. On a more therapeutic level, aloe vera gel, calendula ointment or zinc oxide can both lubricate and strengthen tissues, although nothing is stranger than walking around with glow-white nostrils from zinc oxide ointment. Use zinc oxide for bedtime instead.

Third-generation cephalosporin antibiotics are documented as causing nosebleeds (among other problems). An article in the nursing journal *RN* warns of Moxam, Claforan, Cefobid, Cefizox, Rocephin and Fortaz as causing something called hypoprothrombinemia – a shortage of prothrombin, which is the factor in blood that causes clotting. Without enough of this factor, you could bleed to death. Nosebleeds are just one symptom of the disorder.[1] Vitamin E is a blood thinner, helpful if you have high cholesterol or a history of strokes. Occasionally high amounts can cause blood to seep out of the nostrils. I don't know about you, but I'd trade a little nosebleed for a stroke any day!

If a nosebleed occurs after a traumatic blow to the head, or is accompanied by bleeding in other parts of the body, call 911 immediately. Otherwise, simple first aid should suffice to close off ruptured blood vessels and stop the bleeding. First, do not tip your head back to stop a nosebleed, unless you like the taste of blood and don't mind choking on it. If you do this, the blood will travel down into your throat. Instead, you should sit up, lean forward and first blow all blood and clots out of both nostrils. Open your mouth and breath through it to avoid getting blood clots in air passages. Direct pressure is the best course of action for any bleeding. For nosebleeds, pinch the lower part of your nose for 10-20 minutes, then slowly release the pressure, avoiding any contact or pressure with the nose for a while. Resist the temptation to pick out blood clots. If your nose itches, gently swab with a lubricant such as already described. If bleeding continues after 20 minutes of direct pressure, pack the nose with gauze and apply a cold pack or cloth containing crushed ice against the nose and cheek. Refrain from any motion or activity for several hours.[2]

If you are so inclined, you could try a yarrow snuff. Nicknamed "woundwort," the dried leaves of the yarrow is folk medicine for clotting blood and relieving pain. Herbalists recommend it be pounded into powder and snuffed into the nose to stop a nosebleed.[3] It makes me want to sneeze just thinking about it. I'd be more inclined to put a bit on the end of a Q-Tip and dab it in gently, if the blood isn't too profuse to flush it right out.

Popeye Doesn't Get Nosebleeds

Here's one more reason to eat your green leafy vegetables: they can keep you from getting nosebleeds. I tell nosebleed sufferers to regularly eat green leafy vegetables like spinach, cabbage, turnip greens, broccoli or kale because they are high in vitamin K.[4] Recall my discussion of hypoprothrombinemia – the bleeding disorder caused by a shortage of prothrombin, which is the factor in blood that causes clotting. I've advised many doctors of this simple solution. When they see this disorder, they prescribe vitamin K to combat it.[5] This is because vitamin K makes prothrombin, among other blood clotting factors, and without enough of the vitamin, levels become low, causing bleeding problems. One of the reasons antibiotics lower amounts of vitamin K is because it kills the intestinal bacteria that create it. To help combat this effect, whenever you absolutely have to take antibiotics, supplement with lactobacillus acidophilus bacteria to restore intestinal normalcy.

To prove my theory, Dr. Ross Gordon did his own epidemiological studies of vitamin K for nosebleeds. After finding no obvious cause in one child with particularly bothersome nosebleeds, and having him checked out by an ear, nose and throat specialist, tests revealed the boy lacked prothrombin. His medical history showed he had taken antibiotics on a regular basis and hated green vegetables, so Dr. Gordon gave him an injection of pure vitamin K, nothing else. The nosebleeds stopped. Since then, Dr. Gordon has found if a person with a history of nosebleeds simply includes a daily portion of green leafy vegetables to his diet, it stops them. When this isn't possible, he recommends a natural fat-soluble chlorophyll preparation containing vitamin K.

Nosebleed-Not Nutrients
For maximum absorption, take supplements with meals.

Nutrient	Suggested Dosage	Formulation
Acidophilus	At least four billion flora daily on an empty stomach, three times daily	
Billberry	100 mg twice daily	
Enzymes	2 capsules twice daily	Multiple formula
Fiber	4-8 tablets daily	Psyllium, with herb hyssop
Ginkgo biloba	60 mg daily	
Multi-mineral	3-4 ounces daily	In liquid solution, with vitamin B12, biotin
Multi-vitamin/mineral	6 caplets daily	Freeze-dried plant sources
Quercetin	400 mg twice daily	With vitamin C
Vitamin C	Individual bowel tolerance*	With bioflavonoids (quercetin, rutin proanthocyanidins)

* To determine individual dosage, on the first day take 1,000 mg hourly until diarrhea occurs, then reduce dosage to just below that for individual daily dosage. Vitamin C is not toxic in large doses but must be taken throughout the day to benefit. Divide dosage to three or four times a day.

CHAPTER 125:

Osteoporosis

How can you tell if you have osteoporosis? When you have to use telephone books to reach the dinner table? Or when you *don't* have to bend over to tie your shoes? Nobody wants to wait until things get that bad!

The signs are noticeable long before the diagnosis: weakness, hip and back pain, muscle tenderness and cramping, periodontal disease, decreased height, stooped posture and the beginnings of a "dowager's hump." Then the patient suffers a severe vertebral compression fracture merely by stepping off a curb; or a fractured wrist in a slight fall. Finally, most mysteriously, the patient falls for no apparent reason with a broken hip. The reason: the hip joint deteriorated to such a point that it could no longer support the bones above!

Often, it isn't until one of these bad breaks that osteoporosis is finally diagnosed for what it is – not just dismissed as fatigue, poor posture or a nagging backache. By this time, as much as 50 percent of the bones' spongy mass has been lost.

Make No Bones Without It

Six million people suffer from osteoporosis. Of them, five million are postmenopausal women. At least 26 percent of all women over the age of 60 get spontaneous fractures, like the hip break already described, because they have "brittle bones." Of the million fractures treated by the medical profession, it is estimated that 700,000 are a result of osteoporosis.

While older women seem to be most prone to osteoporosis, it is not a necessary result of the aging process. I repeat: brittle bones do not naturally occur with age; they are a result of a lot of factors, and *age is not one of them.*

Here are some of the factors to explain why women are more vulnerable to bone loss:

1. From their teens through maturity, many women go on extreme and hazardous reducing diets. As early as age 25, some women show a bone mass loss of 10 to 25 percent.

2. The high phosphorus and low magnesium content of many weight-reducing diets hinder the calcium necessary for bone formation.

3. The body stops producing estrogen. This can be a result of long-term fasting, surgical loss of the ovaries, reducing diets, extreme long term physical exercise (such as with athletes) and menopause.

Bones are not inanimate objects in your body that serve to hold you up. They are living tissue constantly taking up and releasing nutrients. Bone is continually being formed (osteoblastic) and reabsorbed (osteoclastic) throughout your life. In fact – and this may surprise you – the human skeleton is completely replaced every 10 to 12 years. This means a 70-year-old woman has had seven skeletons in her lifetime! We have more skeletons in our closets than we thought!

Natural Progesterone Builds New Bones

In 1978, after attending a lecture by Dr. Ray Peat on the subject of natural progesterone derived from wild yam root, John R. Lee,

M.D. began offering a progesterone skin moisturizer to his menopausal osteoporotic patients who were unable to use estrogen. The good doctor found that among his patients using the progesterone cream, serial lumbar DPA tests showed an *increase* in bone density, rather than mere delayed loss, which would have been expected. He notes one patient had a pathological arm fracture at 72 and now at 84, her bone density has increased 40 percent and she has no fractures.[1]

In the U.S. it is common for women's production of progesterone to fall to near zero at least six to eight years before actual menopause. Dr. Lee contends that when estrogen, not progesterone, is given for pre-menopausal symptoms, by the time menopause occurs, osteoporosis is well underway. Dr. Lee has found that natural progesterone typically increases bone mass by 15 percent in two to three years, with or without supplemental estrogen. With estrogen alone, patients may experience a five percent increase in two to three years, but by five years, bone loss of approximately 1.5 percent per year occurs. Estrogen supplementation only prevents bone loss. Progesterone actually increases new bone formation.[2]

Magnesium More Important Than Even Calcium

What women need to understand is that calcium is only as important as the magnesium that goes with it. Calcium cannot get to the bones without magnesium. It is so important, in fact, that studies have shown magnesium alone can prevent osteoporosis.

Magnesium, a neglected nutrient in the diet of Americans – especially women – contributes to the making of solid, enduring bones by changing vitamin D to an active form and by activating an enzyme that helps create new calcium crystals in the bone. Dietary surveys have shown that 80 to 85 percent of American women consume less than the RDA for this mineral.

The concentration of magnesium in body cells and bones was found to be subnormal in 16 out of 19 women with osteoporosis, and calcium crystal formation in the 16 was defective. This appears to make patients more likely to sustain fractures. Calcium crystals formed in the three women with adequate levels of magnesium were found to be normal.[3]

In a recent study, 31 post-menopausal women took 250-750 mg/day of magnesium for two years. As a result, the researchers found, 75 percent of the womens' bone density *increased* by as much as eight percent![4] This is remarkable because a woman's bone density typically *decreases* by three to eight percent every year during menopause.

The reason for this increase is obvious, once you know a little about how magnesium works, especially as it relates to calcium. Calcium is important to bones, but only if it can get to them.

Magnesium and calcium work in balance throughout our bodies. Without magnesium, calcium accumulates in places it shouldn't, and is pulled out of places it should be, like the bones.

Dr. Hans Seyle, author of the book *Stress Without Distress*, and a Nobel prize winning biologist, found in rat experiments that in stressful situations, calcium is drawn from the bones and deposited in the tissues.[5] Too much calcium circulating in the body is termed calcinosis, and is credited with age-related afflictions from arthritis to wrinkles.

Calcinosis occurs because of a very common deficiency of magnesium. Several studies show the prevalence of this deficiency, starting as early as the teen years. A magnesium deficiency is very serious, and, based on the research, is probably the number one cause of osteoporosis. It even plays a role in cancer!

A large study by the U.S. Department of Agriculture found that only 25 percent of 37,785 individuals had magnesium intakes at or greater than the recommended daily allowance, which is notoriously low. A 1995 review of 15 studies found that a typical American diet contains only a fraction of the RDA.[6]

Doctors and health care experts have been telling you for years to get enough calcium. So, you dutifully drink your milk, eat your cheese, and take calcium supplements. But something is wrong because you are still getting osteoporosis, heart disease, hypertension, cancer, arteriosclerosis and wrinkles! You are still getting sick, and you are still dreading middle age. What is missing, and what has been shown in studies to make all the difference is the addition of magnesium. My research shows the degenerative diseases of aging are caused by an imbalance of calcium to magnesium in the body.

Because of the high absorption rate of minerals in solution, and deficiency of magnesium in the diet, the ratio of magnesium and calcium in solution should be four to one, respectively.

A deficiency of magnesium leaches calcium out of the bones, we know that. Other factors do the same thing, according to Dr. Gaby, who wrote an excellent volume entitled *Preventing and Reversing Osteoporosis*, which includes more details than I have room here.

Calcium and the Other Nutrients

Only 25 percent of women taking calcium are in fact preventing osteoporosis. While calcium supplements were found to increase bone mass in these women, it had no effect on the other 75 percent. This is because there are many factors that can prevent calcium from being taken up by the bone, other than a lack of magnesium.

One reason may be a shortage of vitamin D, which is necessary for calcium to be absorbed in the body and used in our trillions of cells.

A deficiency of vitamin D is also responsible for something called osteomalacia, or bone softening. It is similar to rickets in children, as it causes bones weakness.

Among elderly patients with hip fractures, 10 to 20 percent have impaired bone mineralization because of a vitamin D deficiency.[7]

A major source of vitamin D is sunlight on the skin. However, with the risks and warnings associated with ultraviolet rays, many people avoid or sharply reduce their exposure to the sun. And they don't make it up by eating vitamin D-rich foods.

A warning here about milk. An intake of dairy foods fortified with vitamin D, like milk, results in decreased magnesium absorption, important in the osteoporosis story. This is because the so-called vitamin D added to milk is actually a hormone – and a synthetic one at that. The government has been requiring milk producers to put this hormone into their products to prevent rickets. Synthetic vitamin D can actually contribute to aging by depositing calcium in the soft tissue at the surface of the skin. Get your vitamin D from foods and sunlight instead. Milk is also high in phosphorus and protein, which serves to deplete calcium. Plus, since it is estimated that 27 to 47 percent of osteoporotics cannot tolerate milk, it is not an ideal source of calcium.

A great amount of money has been spent encouraging the consumer public to get their calcium from dairy products and their protein from meat. These are two bone-shattering myths.

Calcium and Protein

Osteoporosis is, in fact, a disease caused by a number of things, the most important of which is excess dietary protein. One long-term study found that with as little as 75 grams of daily protein (less than three quarters of what the average meat-eating American consumes) more calcium is lost in the urine than is absorbed by the body, resulting in a negative calcium balance and bone loss. In every study, the same relationship was found: the more protein that is taken in, the more calcium that is lost.

Researchers have found that African Bantu women take in only 350 mg of calcium per day. They bear nine children during their lifetime and breastfeed them for two years. They never have a calcium deficiency, seldom break a bone and rarely loose a tooth. Their children grow up with strong bones and teeth.

Now, how can they do that on 350 mg a day when the National Dairy Council recommends 1,200 mg a day? It's easy. They eat a low protein diet that doesn't kick the calcium out of their bodies.

The balance of nutrient intake is very important in ensuring calcium is absorbed in the body. Too much of one nutrient, or not enough of another could mean the difference between strong bones and broken bones.

The kind of protein found in vegetables is the best way to ensure adequate amounts. Vegetable protein contains many other vital nutrients, including nitrogen and amino acids, necessary to make collagen, the matrix of the bone where the calcium is deposited. It also influences the intestinal flora, allowing the absorption of calcium.

The argument made by the egg and meat people in favor of their products has been that vegetables have incomplete protein – that is, there isn't one kind that contains all the essential amino acids. A U.S. Department of Agriculture survey found that American vegetarians consume, on the average, 150 percent of their actual protein requirements. Who says protein has to come from one source? The fact of the matter is, all foods contain some amount of protein. In order to get *complete* protein in one meal, you simply have to combine them properly.

To get your daily allowance of complete protein combine whole grains with legumes. For example, the Greek dish *felafel* combines whole wheat pita bread with mashed garbanzo beans and spices. It happens to be a healthy, fast finger food, not to mention a delicious meal. Latin Americans get their protein by combining corn tortillas with beans. In India it's rice or wheat chapatis with lentils. Since cooking can destroy many essential amino acids, try to avoid processed foods and eat your veggies raw.

In the United Kingdom, tests have shown that 70-year-old vegetarians have bones equal to or greater in density than the bones of 50-year-old meat eaters. In two other studies, it was found that vegetarians in their 70s and 80s had bone densities greater than that of meat-eating people 20 years younger.

Calcium and Phosphorus

Too much phosphorus will also cause you to lose calcium. Yet, not enough will do the same. The ratio of calcium to phosphorus must be one to one for optimal absorption.

So-called soft drinks could be hard on your bones. A recent Harvard University study of nearly 5,400 female college grads, ages 21 to 80, revealed that for ex-varsity women over 40 – a time when estrogen levels and bone mass decline – drinking non-alcoholic carbonated beverages more than doubled the risk of bone fractures. It also took the fizz out of exercise's bone-strengthening benefits. The high amount of phosphorus in soft drinks depletes calcium, as the body tries to balance out the ratio of phosphorus to calcium.

This is probably due to the high amounts of phosphates added to counteract the acidity of the carbon dioxide. Phosphates are harmful to calcium reserves and drives calcium out through the kidneys. So, if you value your bones, turn down that cola.

Instead, concentrate on the foods that have close to a one to one ratio. They are: ten radishes, 9 mg of calcium to 8 mg of phosphorus; one ounce of Brie cheese, 52:53; one apple, 10:10; one pear, 19:18; and one cup of the following: boysenberries, 36:36; cranberries, 7:8; loganberries, 38:38; pineapple, 11:11; watermelon 13:14; Swiss chard, 18:16; eggplant, 30:26; summer squash, 36:38; green beans 41:42; and iceberg lettuce, 15:17.

Another way to handle this problem is to eat high-calcium, low phosphorus foods such as kale, sesame seeds, maple syrup and seaweed to ensure adequate calcium. One tablespoon of kelp has 156 mg of calcium and 34 mg of phosphorus.

Other foods high in calcium include: agar-agar, a seaweed used as a thickening agent, which has 400 mg of calcium and 8 mg of phosphorus; dulse, a seafood, with 567 mg of calcium versus 3 mg of phosphorus, and hijiki, another seaweed found in Japanese food, which contains a whopping 1,400 mg of calcium and 56 mg of phosphorus. Just so you don't think all seafood is the same, three ounces of swordfish has 4 mg of calcium and 224 mg of phosphorus.

Since calcium is absorbed from the intestines within about three hours, high phosphorus foods should be eaten three to four hours after.

Other Nutrients on the Bone-Healthy Team

Although magnesium and calcium are the most spectacular nutrients on the team, this mineral needs the rest of the players to do the
job right – vitamins and minerals you might never suspect also have
a role: vitamins A, B6, folic acid, C, K and the minerals manganese,
zinc, copper, boron and silica.

One of the little-known functions of vitamin A is to help control
the process of tearing down old bone cells and forming new ones.
When the diet is short-changed on vitamin A, new bone cells are
formed faster than the old, dead cells can be eliminated, causing abnormal bone formations which can bring on pain and periodontal
problems.

Likewise, vitamin B6 provides a strong boost toward making good
bones happen. A diet low in this vitamin caused rats to develop osteoporosis. In one study, more than half of supposedly healthy women
volunteers were found to be deficient in vitamin B6.

Just how does this nutrient influence bones for better or worse?
When well supplied, vitamin B6 adds strength to connective tissue,
the supporting structure of bones. It also breaks down and neutralizes homocysteine, a harmful acid which builds up and breaks down
collagen in the joints.

I recommend taking vitamin B6 in B-complex formulas or tablets in potencies of 50 to 100 mg. All the B vitamins need to be taken
together to avoid a deficiency of any of them. A good B-complex
formula has at least ten times the RDA. It is nontoxic in large doses
because any excess is excreted in the urine. In supplementals, look
for formulas that use natural God-given ingredients. One formula
gets its B vitamins from freeze-dried whole grain sprouts, which have
the highest and most concentrated amounts of B vitamins.

Individuals with a genetic disorder in which large amounts of
homocysteine accumulate are stricken with the worst osteoporosis at
an early age, as demonstrated by studies. Before menopause, the body
chemicals of women are efficient at translating homocysteine into

less harmful substances. After that, they are not. This may account for rapid bone degeneration in postmenopausal women, say some authorities.

Another of the B vitamins, folic acid, was shown to reduce the level of this harmful substance, even though none of the subjects tested showed a deficiency of folic acid.[8]

Researchers concluded that there appears to be a greater need for folic acid after menopause. If this need is not filled, poisonous homocysteine levels seem to rise. Studies disclose that 22 percent of persons 65 years of age are folic acid deficient.[9] Alcohol drinking, smoking and taking of oral contraceptives all contribute to a deficiency of folic acid.

To make cells stick together – in soft tissue and bones as well – the body must produce collagen, the most plentiful body protein. A liberal supply of vitamin C is necessary for collagen production. Without enough of this adhesive, our soft tissue, bone tissue cells and we, ourselves, tend to become unglued.[10]

In one study, vitamin C-deprived guinea pigs showed only two to three percent tissue content of collagen after 14 days. Animals who continued their usual intake of vitamin C were found to have 14 to 16 percent collagen in their tissues.

Vitamin C also works as a biochemical escort system, making certain calcium is delivered where needed.

The RDA for vitamin C is 50 to 80 mg for adults. Many biochemists feel that the proper amount could range anywhere from 1,000 mg to 20,000 mg. At high potencies, this vitamin is non-toxic, but has a laxative effect at maximum dosage. At the point that it causes diarrhea, it is a maximum amount tolerable and dosage should be reduced, then gradually increased again. The dosage will go up during periods of stress and illness, when the body needs more vitamin C.

When targeting vitamin C, look for formulas that contain bioflavonoids. They enhance the healing properties of C and are remarkable in their ability to stabilize bones' collagen structure.

One of the best kept secrets in biochemistry is the fact that vitamin K, well-known for its contribution to blood-clotting, is a star performer in assuring strong, solid, healthy bones. It is also required to synthesize osteocalcin, a protein found uniquely and in large amounts in bone.[11]

Without it, bones could not be formed, repaired or rebuilt. Vitamin K makes possible the synthesis of osteocalcin, a protein matrix on which calcium attaches itself to build new bone cells. Osteocalcin is like the chicken wire nailed to the sides of a house so the plaster or stucco can grip the surface. Beyond this function, osteocalcin acts like a magnet to attract ions of calcium.

Because vitamin K is plentiful in vegetables and because friendly bacteria synthesize it, many nutrition authorities assumed that everybody's blood levels of vitamin K are adequate.

It isn't so, as revealed by new and accurate blood testing instrumentation and techniques. Many people become deficient in vitamin K because they don't eat enough green leafy vegetables or take antibiotics which annihilate the intestinal bacteria that makes vitamin K in the body.

In one study, 16 osteoporosis patients were found to have only 35 percent as much blood serum vitamin K as age-matched controls without osteoporosis.[12]

Both negative and positive animal and human studies show the towering importance of vitamin K. Rats put on a vitamin K-deficient regime lost increased amounts of calcium in their urine.

The healing of rabbits with bone fractures was speeded up when a vitamin K supplement was given, although these animals were already on a diet with a high enough level of this vitamin.

A vitamin K supplement given to human subjects decreased calcium loss in urine by 18 to 50 percent.[13] These research projects reveal that vitamin K may, indeed, be a sleeper nutrient to use as a supplement when dealing with osteoporosis and broken bones.

Another unsung hero is manganese – a must for forming connective tissue, structural material in both cartilage and bone, and for assuring that needed minerals will stay put in bones.[14]

When rats were fed a copper and manganese-deficient diet, their bones were smaller, less mineral-dense and more subject to fracture than animals fed enough of this trace mineral.[15]

It was discovered that osteoporotic women had only one-quarter of the manganese blood levels of women who were osteoporosis-free.

In a two-year double-blind, placebo-controlled trial of over 200 postmenopausal women, researchers found that calcium supplements with added copper, zinc and manganese were more successful than calcium alone in reversing bone loss.[16]

Zinc is important in over 100 enzymes, most of which are related to cell growth and proliferation. The skeleton contains most of the body's zinc. Studies of osteoporotic women show they use large amounts of zinc quickly, making researchers believe there is a correlation between bone loss and zinc loss. A copper deficiency can result in fragile bones, as copper is essential for bone collagen.[17]

Copper is important to balance out your zinc supplements. Be sure and include 2-4 mg of copper with any zinc.

Until recent years, even leading biochemists had no idea that the trace mineral boron could be useful anywhere in human nutrition, let alone in bone health and integrity.

One particular experiment rocked them like an earthquake. When three milligrams of boron was added to a typical daily diet of post-menopausal women, the amount of calcium they excreted in urine dropped by 44 percent.[18]

At the same time, their blood concentration of the most biologically active form of estrogen rose sharply – to the same level as in the women receiving estrogen therapy.

How does boron work this wonder? Biochemists can only offer an educated guess. When boron joins certain organic chemicals, it appears to make possible the synthesis of the most usable form of boron.

It is a well-established fact that estrogen therapy for osteoporosis in postmenopausal women poses certain dangers of cancer. Does this mean that boron presents the same risk? No, say authorities.

Oral estrogen must be taken in relatively high doses to clear the gastrointestinal tract and reach the bloodstream in its most effective form. In sharp contrast, the amount of estrogen produced with the help of boron is only about five percent of the oral dose. Therefore, it produces the desired effect with virtually no risk of cancer.

Just as boron helps bone integrity, it appears to contribute to turning vitamin D into its most useful form. In a study with chicks (baby chickens, that is), it was found that a boron deficiency worsened a vitamin D deficiency and made for abnormally formed bones.

A daily intake of only three milligrams of *boron* appears to increase bone formation and strength, according to U.S. Department of Agriculture studies.[19]

Silica is another less-known mineral, found where calcium is deposited in sites of growing bone. It appears to strengthen the connective tissue matrix by crosslinking collagen strands. Chicks fed a silica-deficient diet developed gross abnormalities of the skull and had unusually thin leg bones.

An important study conducted at the school of Public Health at the University of California, Los Angeles, shows that silica-supplemented bones have a 100 percent increase in collagen.[20]

Dr. Louis C. Kervran, member of the New York Academy of Sciences, writes that silica brings about "spectacular results in repairing broken bones..." Then he adds the sensational fact that "fractures are repaired and healed faster with organic silica extracts than with the administration of calcium."[21] Look for a mineral formula in solution, derived from natural sources, that contains silica.

The Value of Exercise

Several studies indicate that how you exercise is as important to preventing, neutralizing or reversing osteoporosis as how you eat.

So which exercise techniques are the best bets?

Weight-bearing exercise. That is, exercise in which the weight of the body falls or is pressed against the bones. This includes jogging, running, dancing or tennis.

Peter Jacobson and associates at the University of North Carolina in Chapel Hill, who have done much experimentation in this field, says that weight-bearing exercise can often counter bone loss after menopause. He compared postmenopausal women who played tennis three times a week with age-matched, non-exercising women. The tennis players had much more bone mass than the sedentary test subjects, accenting the fact that exercise can slow or prevent bone loss.

A note of warning here. Sometimes the osteoporosis has gone so far that exercise could cause bone collapse, so it's best to have your doctor do a bone density test before okaying an exercise program.

Experience has shown that women with less muscle and fat (the skinny ones we tend to envy) are more prone to osteoporosis. Studies show that there appears to be a direct relationship between body weight and bone mass. The more weight bearing down equals greater bone mass.

Even body fat seems to help since it increases the strain on the bones, which is what appears to work in strengthening it. Studies have shown that osteoporosis is more likely in lighter people than in heavier ones.

Bone-Boosting Nutrients
For maximum absorption, take supplements with meals.

Nutrient	Suggested Dosage	Formulation
Acidophilus	At least four billion flora on an empty stomach three times daily	
Fiber	4-8 tablets daily	Psyllium, with herb hyssop
Borage oil	2 capsules daily	
Flaxseed oil	1 tablespoon daily	
Glucosamine sulfate	500 mg three times daily	
Magnesium	200 mg daily	
MSM (Methylsulfonylmethane)	500 mg three times daily	
Multi-mineral	1-4 ounces daily	In liquid solution, with vitamin B12, biotin
Multi-vitamin/mineral	3-6 caplets daily	Freeze-dried plant sources
Natural progesterone cream	1/3 teaspoon daily	With pregnenolone and DHEA
Niacinamide	1,000 mg twice daily	
Vitamin C	Individual bowel tolerance*	With bioflavonoids (quercetin, rutin proanthocyanidins)
Vitamin D	15 minutes of sunshine daily	
Vitamin E	2 capsules (800 IU) daily	d-alpha tocopherol
Weight bearing exercise	30 minutes daily	

* To determine individual dosage, on the first day take 1,000 mg hourly until diarrhea occurs, then reduce dosage to just below that for individual daily dosage. Vitamin C is not toxic in large doses but must be taken throughout the day to benefit. Divide dosage to three or four times a day.

CHAPTER 126:

Ovarian Cysts

"I firmly believe that if the whole materia medica could be sunk to the bottom of the sea, it would be all the better for mankind, and all the worse for the fishes."

–Oliver Wendell Holmes

If this chapter saves only one woman from an unnecessary hysterectomy or partial hysterectomy it will be worth it. Ovarian cysts are not cancer waiting to happen, nor are they a good reason to remove ovaries. If your doctor has recommended you have one or both ovaries removed because you have cysts, please, get the opinion of an enlightened, nutrition-oriented physician. Many researchers are now saying hysterectomies, even in postmenopausal women, are not necessary in the case of ovarian cysts.

Ovarian cysts are fluid-filled sacs in or on an ovary. They are quite common and are classified into two types: functional and abnormal. It is normal for the ovary to contain cysts and most will go away on their own. The most common type usually produces no symptoms and does not require any treatment. It is called a functional cyst, which frequently occurs in reproductive-age women during ovulation when an egg is released into the fallopian tube. This small cystlike structure should dissolve as it progresses through the normal cycle. If not, it forms a functional cyst. The good news is that functional cysts will usually dissolve within one to three months.[1]

The standard treatment for functional cysts that do not regress after three months is to prescribe oral contraceptives to prevent ovulation. Research has shown, however, that oral contraceptives are not necessary. In one study, 48 women with functional cysts were randomly assigned to receive either no treatment or oral contraceptive therapy. All were followed up at the 6th and 9th week. The researchers found that the cysts in both groups went away on their own (*Fertility and Sterility*, November 1990).

The most common functional cyst is a follicular cyst. This type of cyst forms when the egg-producing follicle of the ovary enlarges and fills with fluid. The other functional cyst is the corpus luteum cyst, which occurs after the egg has been released from the follicle. When pregnancy does not occur, the corpus luteum usually disintegrates. However, occasionally it swells with fluid or blood and remains on the surface of the ovary as a cyst. The most common abnormal cyst is a dermoid cyst. These cysts are similar to skin tissue on the outside and are filled with oily material and sometimes bits of bone, hair and cartilage.

Cysts may cause symptoms or they may not. Symptoms include stomach pain or indigestion, pain during intercourse, menstrual irregularities such as lack of menstruation, heavy or painful periods, a firm, painless swelling in the lower abdomen, a feeling of pressure or fullness in the abdomen or pelvis, irregular bowel or bladder function or an increase in facial and body hair. Sometimes dermoid cysts twist, causing severe abdominal pain, nausea, and vomiting.

Women Castrated by Misguided Physicians

Sally went to her doctor complaining of menstrual cramping. This might not have worried her except that she had gone through menopause early that year. Her doctor consulted a "specialist," who examined her, then scheduled her for a hysterectomy. His reasoning? Because her ovaries could be felt, they should be taken out.

For the last 20 years, the guiding principle in gynecology has been: If the ovaries can be felt in a postmenopausal woman, that in and of itself indicates the necessity of a complete hysterectomy. The risk of ovarian cancer (considered one in 100) among women over the age of 50 was, and still is, considered justification enough for most doctors.

With the introduction of ultrasound, this treatment approach has been called into question because it has uncovered many unnecessary operations. It appears that postmenopausal women commonly develop small, benign (non-cancerous) cysts on their ovaries. As for the significance of enlarged ovaries, this was addressed by C. Paul Morrow, M.D., professor of the Department of Obstetrics and Gynecology, and director of Gynecologic Oncology, University of Southern California School of Medicine: "...we do not know the relationship of normal ovarian size to the number of years passed since the menopause, nor do we know how accurately the combined parameters of age and size can predict malignancy" (*1989 Year Book of Obstetrics and Gynecology*). In other words, doctors have nothing to justify their belief that taking out enlarged ovaries reduces the chances of cancer. One team of investigators found that 10 of 11 postmenopausal women with detectable ovaries had no risk of cancer.[2]

The sheer dimensions of this medical lunacy were identified in one retrospective study by Drs. M.C. Rulin and A.L. Preston of the University of Pittsburgh. They looked at the medical records of 150 women aged 50 years or more scheduled for hysterectomies between 1982 and 1986 with a diagnosis of mass, cyst, tumor, or cancer of the ovary. Only 47, or fewer than one-third, actually had cancer.[3] Incredibly, many conventional physicians believe that a woman's ovaries are essentially useless after menopause, and that women are better off without them! If this were true, the makers of Premarin would go out of business. Women still need their ovaries after menopause, even if they typically get smaller and generate less hormones.

Drs. W.H. Parker and J. S. Berek performed laparoscopies and removed the cysts of 25 postmenopausal women, aged 47 to 81. All 25 masses were accurately predicted to be benign. All would normally have been treated with a complete hysterectomy, but only three required this treatment (for such reasons as an inconclusive test). On the basis of published studies and their own work, Drs. Parker and Berek dismissed as "conjectural" the commonly held fear that the rupture of a cyst that proves to be cancerous results in the spread of cancer cells (*American Journal of Obstetrics/Gynecology*, 1990, 163: 1574-1577). It is possible that all 25 women in this study may one day be viewed as overtreated because each had at least one ovary removed.[4]

The Estrogen Connection

One thing most doctors agree on: ovarian cysts are affected by estrogen in the body and the menstrual cycle. The logic is that when ovulation doesn't occur, neither do ovarian cysts.

Some women are prescribed birth control pills to stop cysts from occurring. I find this wholly ironic considering the commonly-recommended treatment: hysterectomy or removal of one or both ovaries. Either way, if conventional medicine has its way, ovarian cysts result in infertility.

What can figure into this equation are the thousands of man-made estrogens that can stack the deck against women and increase their estrogen levels by hundreds of times. It is quite possible that the same forces increasing our risk for breast cancer increase the chances of having ovarian cysts. Before 1950, many pesticides, like DDT, were not so prevalent in the environment. What we've learned is that today's modern environment, filled with plastics, chemicals – including 2.2 billion pounds of pesticides – and electronics, contain innumerable man-made estrogen building blocks.

Devra Lee Davis, Ph.D., a senior advisor to the U.S. Department of Health and Human Services, pinpoints pesticides, household chemicals and common plastics as some of these man-made estrogens.[5]

Dr. Samuel Epstein, professor of environmental medicine at the University of Illinois, agrees, describing the levels of estrogenic hormones found in meat as "terrifyingly high." He states that there is, to all intents and purposes, no regulation whatsoever of the use of food additives including antibiotics and including hormones in meat. I have long since given up meat after discovering that toxins are stored in fat. Nobody has been able to assure the meat-eating consumer public that these hormones don't end up in our bodies in harmful amounts. What can we do to protect ourselves? Fortunately, there is much we can do.

Since a high-fat, animal protein diet substantially increases a woman's estrogen load, the first step is to maintain a low-fat diet, preferably vegetarian, containing no more than 20 to 25 grams of fat a day and eliminating all dairy products. This diet usually reduces estrogen levels sufficiently but not to the point where menstruation stops. Many women find relief by simply eliminating dairy products.[6] Don't forget the hormones fed to milk cows! Vitamin D is just that: a hormone!

Another anti-estrogen plan of action involves the use of natural plant estrogens, called phytoestrogens, which may prevent man-made estrogens from entering cells. This has been particularly true in the case of bioflavonoids, substances found in brightly-colored fruits and vegetables. Bioflavonoids are not only phytoestrogenic, but act as potent anti-inflammatories, extremely important in reducing the inflammation associated with ovarian cysts.

Legumes – peas, beans and certain roots – are iso-flavonoids, which act as a non-steroidal estrogen. Soybeans, particularly, have been found to have this anti-estrogenic property, and have been associated with a lower incidence of breast cancer in some populations. Breast cancer is related because high blood estrogen levels have been found to increase this type of cancer. Soybeans are eaten in great quantities in Japan and China, and is one of the reasons researchers believe these countries have low rates of breast cancer.[7] Tofu – soybean curd – is an excellent food source. It has the unique ability to absorb the flavors it is cooked in.

In the early 1980s, nutrition educator Carlton Fredericks, Ph.D., reported that a high intake of the B complex vitamins, plus extra choline and inositol, helped the liver break down estrogen into es-triol, a non-carcinogenic form of the hormone. In experiments, he demonstrated that B vitamins also reduced many symptoms of pre-menstrual syndrome – also caused by excess estrogen.[8]

One hundred milligrams of vitamin B6 helps eliminate the fluid retained in postmenopausal breasts, and when it is accompanied by at least 50 milligrams of the other B vitamins, estrogen is better me-tabolized by the liver.[9]

Ovary-Healthy Nutrients

Certain nutrients are important to cellular tissue, including that which makes up the ovaries. Some even have a direct impact on ova-ries specifically. Gamma linolenic acid (GLA), is an essential fatty acid that not only strengthens body tissue, but allows the body to absorb the kind of oils and fat found in ovarian cysts. What this means is that when you don't have enough GLA in your body, the tendency of your body tissue to store fat and accumulate cysts is increased. This nutrient is so important to your health, a deficiency of it may contrib-ute to heart disease, weight gain, high cholesterol, poor circulation, cancer, and a plethora of other problems.

GLA relates to estrogen as well. This is due to the connection I've mentioned between fat and estrogen. Hydrogenated fat, such as is in margarine and foods containing hydrogenated oil (read the la-bels!), tend to reduce the body's ability to convert essential fatty ac-ids from the diet into GLA. Red meat, caffeine, large amounts of dietary fat and even epinephrine (produced by the adrenal glands during stress), subvert the smooth conversion of essential fatty acids into GLA. It is easy to see why many women living in high-stress industrialized countries and eating a diet rich in fat and processed foods are suffering from ovarian cysts.

The best source of GLA is borage oil. Independent clinical tests show that borage oil contains up to 26 percent GLA. Compare this to evening primrose oil and black currant oil, which contain no more than 18 percent. Not only that, borage oil costs less because the borage seed is three times larger than black currant or evening primrose seeds. Finally, borage is more bioavailable. In other words, the body more readily accepts it.[10]

Other nutrients reduce inflammation and regulate the body fat so it also helps control the accumulation into cysts. These nutrients are vitamin C, calcium and the B vitamins. All regulate prostaglandins, hormones that regulate the growth of body tissue.[12]

Cyst-Stopping Nutrients

For maximum absorption, supplements should be taken with meals.

Nutrient	Suggested Dosage	Formulation
Aged garlic extract	2 teaspoons three times daily	Liquid
Antioxidants	4 capsules daily*	With selenium and grape seed extract
Borage oil	2 capsules daily	
Chaste berry	200 mg twice daily	
Enzymes	2 capsules twice daily	Multiple formula
Flaxseed oil	1 tablespoon daily	
Fiber	8 tablets daily	Psyllium, with herb hyssop
Lecithin	2 tablespoons with meals	
Magnesium	200 mg daily	
MSM (Methylsulfonylmethane)	500 mg three times daily	
Multi-vitamin/mineral	6 caplets daily	Freeze-dried plant sources
Multi-mineral	2-4 ounces daily	In liquid solution, with vitamin B12, biotin
Natural progesterone cream	1/3 teaspoon daily	With pregnenolone, DHEA
Vitamin B6	200 mg daily	
Vitamin C	Individual bowel tolerance**	With bioflavonoids (quercetin, proanthocyanidins)
Vitamin E	2 capsules (800 IU)	d-alpha tocopherol

* The FDA recommends that pregnant women not exceed 10,000 IU of vitamin A daily.

** To determine individual dosage, on the first day take 1,000 mg hourly until diarrhea occurs, then reduce dosage to just below that for individual daily dosage. Vitamin C is not toxic in large doses but must be taken throughout the day to benefit. Divide dosage to three or four times a day.

CHAPTER 127:

Pancreatitis

"To eat is human; to digest, divine."

–C.T. Copeland

First, what is the pancreas? Before I became an ostrich on the beaches of medical literature, I used to confuse the organs. What's the difference between the gallbladder, the bladder, the pancreas and the liver? What happens when the pancreas becomes diseased? I won't confuse you by trying to explain how each of the organs work together to keep you healthy, since we *are* talking about the pancreas here. Suffice it to say that each day the pancreas, when functioning at full capacity, secretes about 2-1/2 pints of pancreatic enzymes in the small intestine. This "juice" digests and breaks down carbohydrates, fats and protein.[1]

However, once inflamed, it becomes a liability because it can no longer produce digestive enzymes and insulin. Without adequate pancreatic enzymes, secondary and potentially deadly problems can set in. Among them are food allergies, intestinal infections and cancer. The pancreas also produces insulin. A lack of insulin causes diabetes mellitus, itself causing major problems.

When the pancreas is severely inflamed, gas forms and hemorrhaging begins – not only in the pancreas, but also in the kidneys and eyes. Pancreatic cells that are damaged are replaced by scar tissue that can become calcified. Persons with pancreatitis store abnormally high amounts of iron, a symptom also of a B6 deficiency.

When too much iron is stored in the body, the vital organs break down. The symptoms of too much iron are very similar to an iron deficiency so care must be taken that a correct diagnosis is made. Symptoms include general weakness, fatigue, paleness, brittle nails, loss of appetitive, dizziness and stomach pain. Apparently it is common for people with an excess of iron, possibly due to an undiagnosed organ breakdown, to be considered iron deficient. Then they are given iron supplements, making the situation worse. Some have actually died from this misdiagnosis.

A provocative study by Finnish researchers, published in the American Heart Association's scientific journal *Circulation*, concluded that the amount of stored iron in the body ranks second only to smoking as the strongest risk factor for heart disease and heart attacks.

Experts acknowledge that the study, though involving only 1,900 men from eastern Finland, was carefully done. A team of epidemiologists led by Jukka Salonen of the University of Kuopio tested healthy Finns ages 42 to 60 for serum levels of ferritin, an iron-storing protein. Salonen's team then followed the patients for five years. By that time, 51 of them had suffered heart attacks. Analysis showed that men with more than 200 micrograms of ferritin per liter of blood – a level generally considered normal – were more than twice as likely to have heart attacks compared to men with levels below 200. The risk of heart attack more than quadrupled in men with high levels of both iron and LDL cholesterol.

Healing with Enzymes

Let's say you do all the no-nos. You smoke, are overweight, have high cholesterol, eat a lot of saturated fat and meat, drink too much and don't exercise. Your pancreas is so overloaded your stools are pale and greasy, and the intense pain that goes from your stomach to your back makes you wish you were dead. You have pancreatitis, and you are lucky because if you fix it now, you might not get cancer.

Your pancreas will heal itself if you let it. But you need to quit those bad habits and give it some help. The best way to help it heal itself is by supporting it with its own digestive enzymes so it doesn't have to work so hard. Give it a ticket to Hawaii by adding a supplemental pancreatic enzyme formula to your diet. You know how you reach for antacids when you have indigestion? Try pancreatic enzymes instead. I know from personal experience that they work better and faster than antacids, which don't really deal with the problem – pancreatic overload – in the first place. You can buy these formulas in health food stores or from nutrition-minded physicians like your chiropractor.

Pancreas-Supporting Nutrients

Zinc is a mineral, but it might as well be an enzyme considering how important it is to them. It is a constituent of at least 25 enzymes involved in digestion and metabolism, and is a component of insulin.[2] Studies have shown a deficiency of zinc compromises the ability of pancreatic enzymes to function.

One study of mice highlights the importance of zinc and choline in pancreatitis. Researchers at the mineral transport research department at the Veterans Administration Center in Sepulveda, California, induced pancreatitis in their test subjects by providing them with a choline-deficient diet, then giving them zinc. They found the zinc significantly increased their survival rates.[3]

Copper is important to balance out your zinc supplements. Be sure and include 2-4 mg of copper with any zinc supplement and include a formula of minerals in solution. All of the minerals work together and without one, another can become deficient. Minerals in solution help overcome the many problems that can result in minerals not being absorbed into the body. Foods high in zinc and copper include molasses, seeds and nuts.

In animal studies, magnesium has shown to contribute so greatly to gastrointestinal health that a lack of it can cause pancreatitis. This is because magnesium is important to cellular strength, including the cells of the pancreas. A deficiency of magnesium has been shown to create abnormalities in muscle organs.[4]

In a human study, out of 29 patients hospitalized with acute pancreatitis, 15 were found to be low in calcium. Of these, 14 were found to be low in magnesium as well. The researchers believed that the lack of calcium was a direct result of low magnesium levels.[5] This is because without adequate magnesium, calcium cannot enter the bones, and instead accumulates in soft tissue. It is quite possible, now that we know about this incredibly-important relationship, that the calcification that occurs in acute cases of pancreatitis is actually cell damage from a lack of magnesium.

Magnesium deficiency is more common than you might expect. A large study by the U.S. Department of Agriculture found that only 25 percent of 37,785 individuals had magnesium intakes at or greater than the recommended daily allowance, which is notoriously low. A 1995 review of 15 studies found that a typical diet contains only a fraction of the RDA.[6] Foods high in both calcium and magnesium include wheat germ, sunflowers seeds and nuts.

Because of the detrimental effect a lack of pancreatic enzymes has on the ability to digest and assimilate nutrients, it is best to supplement with minerals and vitamins in solution.

Antioxidants and the Role of Free Radicals

Numerous studies have noted that oxygen free radicals are involved in the development of tissue damage in acute pancreatitis. Rather than go into the story of free radicals, suffice it to say that they are as inevitable as taxes, are the number one cause of degenerative diseases, and can be countered with such antioxidants as zinc, selenium, vitamin E and vitamin C. In the case of pancreatitis, studies have shown that pancreatitis starts with free radical damage which leads to inflammation and tissue damage.[7] Therefore, it is not surprising that studies show antioxidants help. Pursuing the connection is Dr. Bodo Kuklinski, from the Clinic for Internal Medicine in

Rostock, Germany. He examined a 1990 study which showed an extreme deficiency of the antioxidant selenium among the German populace, and an abnormally high rate of pancreatitis among its women.[8] Noting that selenium is enhanced by vitamin E, he reasoned that the two together might offset the deterioration associated with pancreatitis. Noting first the horrible 34 percent fatality rate, he and fellow researchers treated 90 acute pancreatitis patients with selenium and vitamin E. After treatment over a 7-month period, to their delight they discovered that the rate dropped to 1.1 percent! Not only that, but the cost was far lower than if surgery, which is the usual course of action, had been implemented. Incidentally, almost 80 percent of their patients had pancreatitis because of alcoholism.[9]

Vitamin C is another antioxidant that has been shown in studies to help pancreatitis. In a mice study three groups were given two free-radical scavenging treatment options. Researchers compared the survival rates of pancreatitis-plagued mice treated with ascorbic acid (vitamin C), to those treated with superoxide dismutase (SOD), and a control group who got nothing at all. The researchers found the vitamin C worked best in reducing free radical damage and increasing survival rates.[10]

Human studies show pancreatitis patients have diminished blood levels of vitamin C, which may just decrease the pancreas' ability to heal itself. A study published in the *British Journal of Surgery* compared vitamin C levels in 30 healthy fasting volunteers with 29 acute pancreatitis patients. The healthy volunteers had blood levels of 15 micrograms per milliliter while the pancreatitis group had only 2.8 micrograms per mililiter.[11]

Pancreatitis-Pummeling Nutrients
For maximum absorption, take supplements with meals.

Nutrient	Suggested Dosage	Formulation
Acidophilus	At least four billion flora on an empty stomach, three times daily	
Aged garlic extract	1 teaspoon three times daily	Liquid
Amino acids	4-6 capsules daily	Multiple formula from natural sources
Antioxidants	4 capsules daily*	With selenium and grapeseed extract
Borage oil	2 capsules daily	
Coenzyme Q10	2 capsules daily	With vitamin E, phospholipids and selenium
Enzymes	2 capsules with meals	Multiple formula
Fiber	4-8 tablets daily	Psyllium, with herb hyssop
Flaxseed oil	1 tablespoon daily	
Gugulipids	250 mg three times daily	
Magnesium	200 mg daily	
Niacin	500 mg four times daily	
Ox bile extract	100 mg daily	
Multi-mineral	3-4 ounces daily	In liquid solution, with vitamin B12, biotin
Multi-vitamin/mineral	6 caplets daily	Freeze-dried plant sources
Tumeric	100 mg three times daily	
Vitamin C	Individual bowel tolerance**	With bioflavonoids (quercetin, rutin proanthocyanidins)

* The FDA recommends pregnant women not exceed 10,000 IU of vitamin A daily.

** To determine individual dosage, on the first day take 1,000 mg hourly until diarrhea occurs, then reduce dosage to just below that for individual daily dosage. Vitamin C is not toxic in large doses but must be taken throughout the day to benefit. Divide dosage to three or four times a day.

CHAPTER 128:

Panic Attacks

I was having dinner with a professional colleague and his wife when I first became aware of the devastation of panic attacks. While my friend was talking, I noticed his wife's hands began shaking. Presumably in order to pull herself together she began rooting in her purse. Finally she excused herself and almost ran to the ladies' room. Excusing myself, I followed. I found her standing at the sink, pouring through her purse, tears running down her cheeks, muttering to herself, "I can't do it, I can't do it, what's wrong with me, what's wrong with me?!"

Her breath was coming out in deep gasps as items from her purse fell, one after the other, onto the tile floor. Finally she just stood there, staring at herself in the mirror, her hands clenching and unclenching against her chest. Before she had a chance to be embarrassed at my presence, I gently guided her out of the bathroom into the bar lounge and sat her down, soothing her with gentle words and a glass of orange juice.

"I have no control, Maureen!" she lamented as she took sips of juice. "Whenever my husband takes me to a social or business function, I'm so nervous I can't eat, then I become so overwhelmed with anxiety I lose control! I spend most of the time in the bathroom, crying and trying to compose myself! What on earth is wrong with me?"

I had no idea then what to tell this distraught woman, but resolved to find answers to this devastating phenomenon.

Physical Conditions Can Contribute To Mental Duress

Certain afflictions, such as low blood sugar, high blood pressure, heart valve abnormalities, and even bowel disorders have been associated with panic attacks. The reasons are numerous, and include a B vitamin deficiency, scary physical symptoms, a magnesium deficiency, increased adrenalin and energy loss, which itself can be a side effect of many drugs, including synthroid, a synthetic thyroid hormone. If you suffer from panic attacks, don't see a psychiatrist, see a nutritionally-oriented physician who can best evaluate your state of health and identify any nutritional deficiencies. And don't let anyone tell you it's all in your head!

The next time I encountered this issue, I was contacted on the air by a woman – I'll call her Patty – who was being wracked with panic attacks. Patty was a 40-year-old nurse whose symptoms began after she took on a second job with a group of five physicians specializing in critical care internal medicine. She worked five days a week, averaging 10 to 12 hectic hours a day. You might assume her symptoms were a result of stress on the job. If you did, you'd be partly right. Stress can cause many physical symptoms. However, her panic attacks did not arise simply from the stress.

Patty's symptoms started approximately two weeks after beginning work. Along with anxiety, she had weight loss, loss of appetite, neck pain, headaches, heart palpitations, insomnia and heartburn. She sought help from one of the doctors for whom she worked, who prescribed an assortment of pharmaceuticals for her symptoms. She rejected the drugs, so I referred her to Dr. Ross Gordon in Albany, California, who specializes in identifying causes, not just treating symptoms.

By the time Patty saw Dr. Gordon she was also experiencing "vice-grip" attacks of chest pain and panic attacks that resulted in a loss of consciousness for several minutes. What puzzled her the most was that these episodes occurred while at rest rather than at work.

She was diagnosed as having high blood pressure, hyper-adrenalism and possibly low blood sugar. Dr. Gordon believed her adrenal glands were producing too much adrenalin, causing the high blood pressure and chest pain, and her poor diet was causing low blood sugar, resulting in the panic attacks.

I began to work with her diet, urging her off all sources of sugar, caffeine, saturated fats and alcohol. Instead, I got her to eat fruits, vegetables and grains in the form of a snack every two hours or so to maintain a constant blood sugar level; walk or do some form of aerobic exercise at least 30 minutes daily to burn up the excess adrenalin. She began taking an anti-stress nutritional supplementation regimen which included a multi-vitamin supplement, extra vitamin C and a multi-mineral supplement in solution that includes calcium, potassium and magnesium. For her insomnia, I found an amino acid formula that includes naturally occurring tryptophan.

Patty returned to Dr. Gordon's office one month later. After beginning the regimen, her chest pains and panic attacks disappeared completely, she gained back five pounds and her blood pressure stabilized. Her headaches and neck pain were much better and the tryptophan was helping her sleep. She called the office two months later to tell the doctor that she left her job and found a position with an alternative medicine physician. All her symptoms had completely disappeared by that time.

At the 1984 meeting of the Phobia Society of America, Dr. Frederic Neuman, associate director of the White Plains Phobia Clinic, reported a high incidence of mitral valve prolapse (heart valve abnormality) and hypoglycemia (low blood sugar) among those who suffer from anxiety attacks. The point he was making was that the symptoms of these two physical conditions: shortness of breath, dizziness, palpitations, fatigue and panic should not be dismissed as psychological, and that anyone with panic attacks should be evaluated for these physical conditions.[1]

B Vitamins and Panic Attacks

There are no other nutrients more important to mental health than the B vitamins. B-complex vitamins provide the body with energy, metabolize fats and protein, and are necessary for the normal functioning of the nervous system. They are the single most important factor for the health of the nerves. Symptoms of deficiencies include dizziness, hallucinations, irritability, depression, panic attacks, insomnia and even suicidal tendencies.

Mental illness as a physical disease can result from low brain concentrations of vitamins B1 (thiamine), B6 (pyridoxine), B12 (cobalamin), niacin, pantothenic acid and folic acid.[2] Please, always supplement with a good B-complex formula when adding any one B vitamin to your diet. One without the other can cause more harm than good since they are dependent upon each other to work in your body.

A vitamin B12 deficiency is a real bogey man – especially in the over-60 crowd. It can produce psychosis, severe memory loss, impaired abstract thinking skills, mental confusion, delusions, hallucinations and even brain and spinal cord degeneration (causing numbness). Low blood levels of the vitamin are found in one-third of hospitalized psychiatric patients suffering from depression and dementia, according to a Denmark study. In addition, a B12 deficiency may inhibit the brain's use of glucose (the gasoline which energizes the brain) and hinder production of acetylcholine, which is vital to brain and memory function.

Folic acid, a B vitamin found in leafy greens, prevents irritability and forgetfulness; plus, it partners with B12 in the brain's synthesis of acetylcholine. In one case, 67 percent of patients admitted to a psychogeriatric ward were deficient in folic acid. Such a deficiency may arise from poor nutrition, an inability to absorb the nutrient or impaired absorption caused by pharmaceuticals.

There are two places in the body where nutrients are absorbed: the stomach and the intestine. If the stomach has too little acid, whether from illness, stress or age, absorption is compromised. If there is something wrong with the intestines, nutrients – especially the B vitamins – cannot be absorbed properly.

Studies have shown that among those with intestinal problems, their blood levels of B vitamins are low. Irritable bowel syndrome (IBS) is a fancy term to describe a temporarily dysfunctional large intestine, caused by food allergies, stress or too much fat in the diet.

In one study, 20 patients with IBS were compared to a control group of 20 without IBS. Remarkably, but not surprisingly, it was found that 18 out of 20 of the IBS patients had a history of mental illness during their lifetimes compared to only nine out 20 in the control group. Half of the patients with IBS had regular panic attacks, and another half had social phobias. IBS patients commonly have problems with depression, sleeping problems and substance abuse. The connection sticks. When questioned, most of the IBS patients said their intestinal problems occurred before their mental illness.[3]

A deficiency of thiamine, vitamin B1, has also been shown in studies to contribute to panic attacks. Even subclinical (moderate) thiamine deficiency can cause anxiety or neuroses. In one study, subjects deprived of thiamine complained of poor mental alertness, fatigue and nervousness.[4] Since psychiatrists are the least likely to enquire about diet, I have to wonder how many of their anxiety patients are being treated with drugs when they are simply thiamine-deficient.

A diet high in empty calories and junk foods has been linked to neurotic behavior. In one study, 20 patients with a thiamine deficiency reported symptoms including aggressiveness and hostility. Twelve of that group reported a diet high in carbonated and other sweet beverages, candy, and typical snack foods. Blood tests indicated that all 20 had low thiamine levels. After the patients were given thiamine supplements, all 20 had marked improvement or lost their symptoms completely.[5]

Beriberi, an affliction that is caused by a thiamine deficiency has, in the past, been thought to primarily occur in rice-eating populations of Asia. However, as far back as 30 years ago, severe clinical beriberi was widely found in the United States; in areas of New England, Arkansas, Texas and California. This, despite the fact that 50 years ago the enrichment of flour with thiamine was started.[6]

Patients in modern hospitals are probably at risk of beriberi because they are sometimes fed intravenously. This is called total parenteral nutrition, or TPN. This is done whenever the patient cannot eat or digest food the usual way. The problem is, this "liquid food" can be deficient in nutrients, most especially the B vitamins.

In 1988, three patients receiving intravenous feedings in a hospital died because the intravenous solution was deficient in thiamine, according to *The New York Times*. A B1 deficiency can develop within a week with these deficient feedings, which are 70 percent glucose, since the vitamin is necessary for metabolizing glucose.[7]

The Food and Drug Administration reported these patients died of refractory lactic acidosis. Autopsies performed on two of the patients revealed brain abnormalities.[8]

Mood Smoothing Magnesium

My first clue to the connection between panic attacks and mitral valve prolapse came during an interview with Michael Schachter, M.D., a New York psychiatrist, on my television show *Maximize Your Life*. Dr. Schachter told me he had a relative who experienced panic attacks and heart palpitations. When this relation was given 600 milligrams daily of magnesium, in divided doses, he was relieved of both.

Magnesium is responsible for 80 percent of all enzymatic reactions in the body – literally all the body's activities. A deficiency of magnesium is documented as causing unexplained anxiety, panic attacks, palpitations, muscle spasms, cramps, insomnia, mitral valve prolapse and fatigue.

German researchers at the 10th Hohenheim Magnesium Symposium in Darmstadt, Germany, reported the same findings, adding that magnesium is an important therapeutic agent for psychiatric disorders. At the symposium, Dr. K.H. Hofle reported that magnesium helps with sleep disturbances, excitability, panic attacks, hyperkinetic children, anxiety states, psychogenic asthma and heart syndromes. It is an effective muscle relaxant and has influence on nerve excitability. Hofle added that psychotherapy is not as effective among patients with low magnesium levels.[9]

Remember, you're not what you put into your mouth, you're what you absorb and digest and deliver to cells. A tablet is only one to five percent absorbable. Since the process of digestion is a process of liquefaction, your body has to take a hard rock tablet and turn it into solution. This may not be possible due to a number of factors, such as inadequate stomach acid, food allergies and intestinal problems. This is why it is so important that when you decide to supplement, you target minerals in solution. Look for a good, easily absorbable, derived-from-nature mineral blend in solution. Formulations in solution provide the maximum absorption ratios.

Panic-Preventive Nutrients
For maximum absorption, take supplements with meals.

Nutrient	Suggested Dosage	Formulation
Aged garlic extract	1 teaspoon three times daily	Liquid
Amino acids	4-6 capsules daily	Multiple formula from natural sources
Antioxidants	4 capsules daily*	With selenium and grapeseed extract
Borage oil	2 capsules daily	
Coenzyme Q10	2 capsules daily	With vitamin E, phospholipids and selenium
Flaxseed oil	1 tablespoon daily	
Ginkgo biloba	60 mg daily	
Magnesium	200 mg daily	
Melatonin (adults only)	3 mg daily at bedtime	With B vitamins
Multi-mineral	3-4 ounces daily	In liquid solution, with vitamin B12, biotin
Multi-vitamin/mineral	6 caplets daily	Freeze-dried plant sources
Vitamin B6	100 mg daily	
Vitamin C	Individual bowel tolerance**	With bioflavonoids (quercetin, rutin proanthocyanidins)

* The FDA recommends pregnant women not exceed 10,000 IU of vitamin A daily.

** To determine individual dosage, on the first day take 1,000 mg hourly until diarrhea occurs, then reduce dosage to just below that for individual daily dosage. Vitamin C is not toxic in large doses but must be taken throughout the day to benefit. Divide dosage to three or four times a day.

CHAPTER 129:

Parasites

Would you believe you have a one in five chance of having parasites? Parasites are more common than you, and the majority of physicians out there, realize. Studies show it is quite possible that the majority of gastrointestinal complaints are a result of undiagnosed, unrecognized parasitic infections.

In a report to The American College of Gastroenterology, Dr. Leo Galland, M.D., said that among 197 consecutive patients with a variety of gastrointestinal symptoms, over half were found to have Giardia lambia, a microscopic organism introduced to water supplies by animals via mountain streams and by human sewage entering public water supplies. Symptoms included diarrhea, stomach bloating, chronic fatigue, food intolerance, stomach pain and constipation.[1]

Martin Lee, Ph.D., biochemist, microbiologist and director of the Great Smokies Laboratory in North Carolina, conducted a study on the presence of parasites in very sick people. In one group of lower-income immigrants, 70 percent were found to be infected. More surprising, when he examined a group of more well-to-do Americans, he found 20 percent had parasites. The Centers for Disease Control (CDC) in Atlanta got the same results in their tests.[2] What does this mean? In the past we took a certain comfort in the belief that parasites occurred mostly in Third World countries and that in our sterile, government-inspected industrialized society, we were immune. The fact is, we can have parasites and not have symptoms, and we can get them a lot easier than we ever realized.

Do you swim in the summer? Certain parasites are not killed by chlorine and all it takes is an undetected or neglected pool filter to infect many people. In 1990, a *Los Angeles Times* article reported on the case of a child infected with cryptosporidium who infected others through the local swimming pool. The pool managers treated the water with chemicals, not realizing that because one of the three pool filters was not working their efforts were in vain. The parasite infected swimmers for about a month before the broken filter was discovered (*Los Angeles Times*, September 23, 1990).

California recommends that public pools be inspected three times a year. In one report health officials estimated that 44 percent of the pools in Los Angeles County had not been inspected for three or more years.[3]

According to the Environmental Protection Agency, cryptosporidium is the leading cause of waterborne illness in the United States. This microscopic parasite was the cause of a Milwaukee contamination in which 400,000 people were afflicted with severe stomach problems and diarrhea, and one died. *Dateline* NBC reported the presence of cryptosporidium cysts in New York City's municipal water supply. You may be interested – or disgusted – to learn that healthy people can tolerate up to 1,000 of these little buggers before showing signs of illness. Among persons with severely suppressed immune systems, it only takes a few to cause death.[4]

Parasites Cause Nutritional Deficiencies

If you read my chapter on Malabsorption, you realize the extreme problems that can occur when parasites infect the body. Parasitic infection can reduce food intake, impair absorption from the intestine and, as a result, cause massive nutritional deficiencies over time. Different organisms can cause an inability to absorb different nutrients.

The tapeworm Diphyllobothrium latum can cause pernicious anemia because it blocks vitamin B12 from being absorbed in the intestine. Blood loss from hookworm, trichuris and chistosoma infections may cause iron-deficiency anemia. Ascaris lumbricoides infection may reduce fat absorption and interfere with the absorption of vitamin A, compromising eyesight.[5]

Because parasites cause the cilia in the intestine to become flattened and basically ineffective, any nutrients, including the B vitamins and many minerals, cannot be absorbed into the body. This catch-22 causes deficiencies which impair the immune system resulting in secondary health problems that can't be traced to the parasites. For more, see the chapters Anemia, Asthma, Allergies, Arthritis, Colon Problems, Chronic Fatigue Syndrome, Fibromyalgia...even Leukemia.

Stopping Parasites Without Dangerous Drugs

On a speaking tour I met a woman who had volunteered with the Peace Corps in Guatemala. Evelyn – a woman who was hardly sick a day in her life – endured three months of torturous cramps, diarrhea and fevers before being diagnosed with intestinal amoebas. She said she managed to get through the days despite the diarrhea, but the worst was when doctors prescribed Flagyl, a strong pharmaceutical used to kill everything in the intestine and flush out what's left. The Flagyl left her barren of nutrients and strength, and physically unable to return to her duties.

There are diets and strategies that can help kill and flush out parasites without destroying the intestinal lining and the bacteria that keep it healthy.

1. The first step is to cleanse the intestinal tract. Scour the health food stores for supplements that contain good sources of fiber, like psyllium and hyssop, combined with laxative herbs such as cascara sagrada and aloe, and good-for-your-intestine bacteria like acidophilus. In addition, you should consider following a simple, cooked-vegetable-based detoxifying diet for at least several days and up to two or

three weeks. Such a diet will include mostly vegetables with small portions of grain and beans, little or no fruit or other sweet foods, and no refined or processed foods, caffeine, or alcohol. Eliminate all milk and dairy products as well, with the possible exception of raw goat's milk, which contains immune-boosting antibodies, and has been found helpful in the treatment of parasites.[6]

2. Modify the diet. The most important ongoing dietary recommendation is to eliminate sugar. Parasites thrive on sweets and simple carbohydrates, including white rice, white bread, fruit and fruit juices. Cranberries, papaya, and fresh pineapple are exceptions, since these have enzymes that are anti-parasitic.[7] Eat unprocessed, high-fiber foods, which encourage frequent elimination. To overcome the limitations of intestinal parasites that drain the body of nutrients, supplement with an easily absorbable, derived-from-nature mineral blend in solution. Studies show minerals dissolved in water before ingestion are considerably more bioavailable to the body than those even present in food, because they aren't risked by a lack of hydrochloric acid in the stomach or a disabled intestine. Formulas in solution provide the maximum absorption ratios.

3. Take natural substances to prevent and eliminate parasites. Parasite-fighting foods include fresh garlic (several cloves a day) and pumpkin seeds (a couple handfuls per day), which you may take until your condition is corrected. If your situation prevents you from carrying around and eating fresh cloves of garlic, try aged garlic extract, in liquid or capsule form. *Odorless* aged garlic concentrates the active parasite-killing ingredients in a garlic supplement that won't leave your travel agent diving for cover. In cooking, you may use sage, cloves, fennel, and thyme, all of which act against parasites. Citrus seed extract is an old folk medicine used in other countries for treatment of parasitic infections.

4. Restore the digestive tract to its old self. One of the few things doctors did right when my Peace Corps friend was suffering from the effects of her amoeba was send her to a local Guatemalan pharmacy for a digestive enzyme supplement. Of course, eliminating the source of the problem would have been more prudent, but when she had trouble digesting her mashed black bean sandwiches and pepper steak breakfasts (what her Guatemalan hosts were feeding her), they had her try digestive enzymes to create more bile and acids to break down the unfamiliar fare. What would have helped further would have been beneficial bacteria – acidophilus bacillus – to recolonize her wrecked intestinal tract.

5. And finally, restore the immune system with a good B vitamin complex, minerals in solution, and a high-potency multi-vitamin formula. Once the source of malabsorption is eliminated, boosting your body with important nutrients is the last step toward the road to health.

Parasite-Pounding Nutrients
For maximum absorption, take supplements with meals.

Nutrient	Suggested Dosage	Formulation
Acidophilus	At least four billion flora on an empty stomach, three times daily	
Aged garlic extract	1 teaspoon three times daily	Liquid
Enzymes	2 capsules twice daily	Multiple formula
Fiber	4-8 tablets daily	Psyllium, with herb hyssop
Grapefruit seed extract	100 mg three times daily	
Multi-mineral	3-4 ounces daily	In liquid solution, with vitamin B12, biotin
Multi-vitamin/mineral	6 caplets daily	Freeze-dried plant sources
Vitamin C	Individual bowel tolerance*	With citrus bioflavonoids (quercetin, proanthocyanidins)

* To determine individual dosage, on the first day take 1,000 mg hourly until diarrhea occurs, then reduce dosage to just below that for individual daily dosage. Vitamin C is not toxic in large doses but must be taken throughout the day to benefit. Divide dosage to three or four times a day.

CHAPTER 130:

Parkinson's Disease

"He's not only nearsighted physically, his mind is selective of what it sees too."
–Actor Jim Backus, speaking of the cartoon character Mr. Magoo, to whom he lent his voice. Backus suffered from Parkinson's Disease prior to his death in 1989 of pneumonia.

Jim Backus' fight for life and control helped bring Parkinson's Disease into the limelight. Now boxing champ Mohammed Ali is letting the public know he has Parkinson's. An estimated 500,000 to one million Americans have Parkinson's disease, which robs people of control over their movements. There is no test for Parkinson's. Instead, doctors depend upon the process of elimination to make a diagnosis.

While researchers can't isolate exactly what causes the progressive disease, they do know that it is characterized by death of the brain cells in the basal ganglia – the gray matter above the brain stem. This leads to a drop in dopamine, a chemical made by the cells that helps translate thought into muscle action. Although it usually hits people age 50 and older, Parkinson's can strike people of all ages.

In 1980, at the age of 34, Diane Carlin first started noticing tremors in her right arm and hand. She saw an orthopedist, then a neurologist. They prescribed depressants and beta blockers, but still her tremors persisted. Diane became chronically fatigued and depressed.

She got worse. She couldn't move her right arm, and held it in front of her. Her right leg became stiff and she dragged it when she walked. Her posture became stooped. Her neurologist insisted that, because of her age, her symptoms were caused by nerves and anxiety. Finally, another neurologist admitted she might have Parkinsonism. He believed the stress of an auto accident which preceded her symptoms was responsible. Parkinsonism has the same symptoms as Parkinson's, but a cause is found. Causes include too much copper (which can be caused by not enough zinc), head trauma, anti-psychotic drugs and carbon monoxide poisoning. Diane's new neurologist gave her every test in the book, then finally, after all tests were negative, had to diagnose true Parkinson's disease. She went misdiagnosed for so long simply because she was young. Like most conventional physicians who rely on textbooks instead of common sense, Diane's first doctors ignored the signs, trying to make her believe it was all in her head.[1]

Conventional treatments for Parkinson's follow the same premise: treat the symptoms. Physicians typically prescribe pharmaceuticals to help battle the symptoms. The drugs don't stem the tide of degeneration, and eventually any benefit wears off. Earning orthodoxy's reputation of slash, burn and poison medicine, in an operation known as a pallidotomy, doctors have resorted to literally destroying the part of the brain, the globus pallidum, which is thought to cause many of the symptoms of Parkinson's.[2] *There's* a solution for you!

Free Radical Damage Alleviated with Antioxidants

One of the reasons for the severe symptoms of Parkinson's, many researchers have come to believe, is the extreme free radical damage that occurs. Dr. P. Jenner, a researcher at the Neurodegenerative Diseases Research Center at King's College in London, states in an article in *The Lancet* that free radical damage has been noted in the brains of Parkinson's victims and that the loss of dopamine in the brain may accelerate the damage and further increase the number of free radicals. Diseases that affect the brain have been associated with increased free radicals and subsequent brain cell death. Dr. Jenner believes anything that slows or stops the progression of free radical damage could slow or even stop the progressive damage induced by Parkinson's.[3] This is where antioxidants come in.

In an open trial, Stanley Fahn, Ph.D., and colleagues at New York City's Neurological Institute, gave patients with early Parkinson's large doses of the antioxidants vitamin E and vitamin C in four divided doses. Seventy-six patients followed this regimen from June 1979 to December 1986. What they found, other than almost nonexistent side effects to these large doses, was that the progression of the disease slowed considerably, giving the patients more time – 2.5 to three years – before the need to be treated with conventional therapies.[4]

Other researchers are looking at antioxidant therapy in conjunction with drugs like Deprenyl, which acts as an antioxidant, but has side effects. For your individual treatment program, target an antioxidant formula that combines antioxidant herbs, minerals and vitamins with amino acids for the most complete and thorough free radical busting benefit.

Foods high in vitamin E have been shown to help. Dr. Lawrence I. Golbe, M.D., of Robert Wood Johnson Medical School in New Jersey, interviewed 81 patients with Parkinson's and their same-sex siblings who did not have the disease to see which food items they ate the most before the age of 40. The answer turned out to be foods rich in vitamin E. In another study, the use of supplemental vitamin E or cod liver oil lowered the chances of getting Parkinson's disease.[5]

Other antioxidants boost the benefit greatly. Selenium for example, is known for accelerating the benefit of vitamin E.

Amino Acids Boost Dopamine

I've already established it is a lack of dopamine that causes the debilitating symptoms of Parkinson's. One of the conventional strategies for treating Parkinson's is to prescribe something called levodopa, or L-dopa, which is an amino acid (dihydroxyphenyla-lanine) that helps restore dopamine levels. Sometimes it doesn't work because it has to be absorbed from the small intestine and can be compromised by ulcers, stress, liver or gallbladder problems; anything that reduces digestive bacteria and enzymes in the intestine or damages the intestinal wall. Side effects include nausea, vomiting, anorexia, high blood pressure, heart arrhythmias, involuntary movements of the facial muscles, muscle twitching, respiratory problems, even hallucinations and paranoid delusions. It is reported that as many as 75 percent of patients taking levodopa experience dyskinesias – abnormal involuntary movements – with 25 percent experiencing mental disturbances. Long term studies with relatively high doses showed that after two or three years, any benefit was reduced as the disease progressed and late complications ensued.[6]

Evaluating all the evidence, I would say taking levodopa in pharmaceutical form is not beneficial in the long term, and may even create its own problems. If, despite my warnings, you decide to take L-dopa, there are some precautions you must follow. For one, vitamin B6 can be depleted and also interfere with L-dopa. Protein and B vitamin food sources also can interfere. For the best advice, see a nutrition-minded physician who can evaluate your blood levels of amino acids and recommend the best course of therapy for you.

However, there is a way of getting your dihydroxyphenylalanine without the side effects of levodopa, and that is by eating foods high in this and other amino acids. Australian researchers led by P.A. Kempster, M.D., at the Department of Neurosciences and Medicine, Monash Medical Center, in Melbourne, isolated the vicia faba bean as a rich source of dihydroxyphenylalanine. The bean is a natural food which contains this vital amino acid in a form that may be even better than conventional levodopa medication in some cases.

The Aussies found that in five of six Parkinson's patients, simple meals of broad bean pod mixtures that included the vicia faba produced motor improvement. An approximately 100 gram serving of vicia faba pod contains 250 mg of levodopa, which is equivalent to the content of one of the standard pharmaceutical formulations. The researchers also found that the food did not compete with the pharmaceutical form, and recommended that Parkinson's patients substitute this and other broad beans for all dietary sources of protein.[7] The faba and other broad beans are found anywhere health food items are sold, in a variety of forms.

Other amino acids have proven to be beneficial without the dangerous side effects. Dr. S. Croxson, B.M., and colleagues at Northern General Hospital, Sheffield, United Kingdom, conducted a study of six men with Parkinson's disease. The subjects were placed on a normal diet for two weeks, then in a double blind fashion they received a low protein diet followed by either a dietary supplement of large neutral amino acids (phenylalanine, leucine, isoleucine, tryptophan, valine, methionine, histidine, tyrosine) or a placebo in a crossover trial. Five patients improved their Parkinson's disability on the low protein diet compared to the normal (typically high in fat and simple carbohydrates) diet. In the diet supplemented with large neutral amino acids or placebo, three subjects with Parkinson's disease did significantly better than the placebo.[8]

A high carbohydrate diet can make a big difference in alleviating Parkinson's symptoms. Researchers at the Colorado Neurologic Institutes Movement Disorder Center found that Parkinson's patients who consumed a 7-to-1 carbohydrate-to-protein diet were able to walk and move around better than those who ate high protein meals.[9]

Carbohydrates can be manufactured in the body from some amino acids and work to regulate protein and fat metabolism. They are important in Parkinson's because they can offset the effect of too much protein. The best sources are found in whole grains. Avoid simple carbohydrates such as white sugar, white flour and most processed foods.

When looking at protein foods, target those that contain essential amino acids. They are: vegetables, grains, nuts, peas and the aforementioned beans. Grains such as brown rice can be combined with beans to achieve the most complete (with amino acids) and best source of protein.

Physical Exercise Lowers Risk

Many Parkinson's patients feel that movement is their enemy because of their sense of fragility. Actually the exact opposite is true. Movement is their friend, the means by which they keep the body going for the longest possible time. The single most important strategy for maintaining flexibility, mobility, and mental well-being is exercise. Inactivity shortens ligaments, stiffens and even freezes joints, slows circulation and makes bones more brittle. People who are sedentary should take a daily walk but patients who have on-off symptoms, in which mobility is followed by freezing, should not jog or swim alone.[10]

I have long recommended a program of regular physical exercise as a major life-extender and protector against chronic disease. But recently I was surprised to learn that it can also affect whether or not you get Parkinson's disease. A team of doctors from Harvard Medical School and research institutions in Lyon, France, looked at the incidence of Parkinson's among 50,000 men who attended Harvard College or the University of Pennsylvania between 1916 and 1950. They found that having belonged to a varsity team or having done regular physical exercise was associated with a smaller risk of getting Parkinson's, and doing regular moderate activity or sports as an adult brought the risk down even further. At the highest level of activity, however, the protective effect of exercise disappeared. This might explain how Muhammed Ali managed to get Parkinson's. Moderate exercise, say the researchers, leads to higher levels of dopamine but intense activity does not add any further protection.[11]

Cerebral-Saving Nutrients
For maximum absorption, take supplements with meals.

Nutrient	Suggested Dosage	Formulation
Aged garlic extract	1 teaspoon three times daily	Liquid
Amino acids	4-6 capsules daily	Multiple formula from natural sources
Antioxidants	4 capsules daily*	With selenium and grapeseed extract
Borage oil	2 capsules daily	
Coenzyme Q1 (NADH)	2.5 to 5 mg daily	
Coenzyme Q10	2 capsules daily	With vitamin E, phospholipids and selenium
Enzymes	2 capsules twice daily	Multiple formula
Fiber	4-8 tablets daily	Psyllium, with herb hyssop
Flaxseed oil	1 tablespoon daily	
Malic acid	250 mg twice daily	
Melatonin (adults only)	3 mg daily at bedtime	With B vitamins
Multi-mineral	3-4 ounces daily	In liquid solution, with vitamin B12, biotin
Multi-vitamin/mineral	6 caplets daily	Freeze-dried plant sources
Vitamin A	25,000 IU daily*	
Vitamin B6	100 mg daily	
Vitamin C	Individual bowel tolerance**	With bioflavonoids (quercetin, rutin proanthocyanidins)
Vitamin E	2 capsules (800 IU) daily	d-alpha tocopherol

* The FDA recommends pregnant women not exceed 10,000 IU of vitamin A daily.

** To determine individual dosage, on the first day take 1,000 mg hourly until diarrhea occurs, then reduce dosage to just below that for individual daily dosage. Vitamin C is not toxic in large doses but must be taken throughout the day to benefit. Divide dosage to three or four times a day.

CHAPTER 131:

Pellagra – A Deficiency Disease

"Ignorance breeds monsters to fill up the vacancies of the soul that are unoccupied by the verities of knowledge."

–Horace Mann

It is impossible to estimate the enormous number of people who likely have, in the past *and* present, been committed to mental institutions, when their symptoms were the result of B vitamin deficiencies. Countless tragedies could have been prevented.

As soon as a deficiency is named – such as in pellagra – you know that the syndrome at one time was common enough to be identified. As recently as 50 years ago, pellagra was a common disease in the Southern United States. In 1917, for example, there were more than 170,000 cases in the South, and in South Carolina pellagra ranked second as a cause of death.

In the early 1900s researchers searched for a viral cause of pellagra, believing it was an infectious disease. During this time, it was epidemic in the South, primarily among poor, black sharecroppers who subsisted on a diet of fatback, cornmeal, and molasses.[1]

In those days, when double-blind, placebo-controlled studies were not the norm, researchers and physicians depended upon good old-fashioned common sense and observation to educate themselves and provide medical breakthroughs.

Joseph Goldberger, a U.S. Public Health Service doctor, refuted turn-of-the-century mainstream medicine's assumption that pellagra was caused by a virus. He observed that hospital staff members caring for pellagra patients did not become ill, and that exposure to their bodily secretions did not cause illness.

He conducted his own epidemiological experiments which showed that improved diets among orphanage children and mental patients with pellagra prevented new cases and cured the disease. He then induced pellagra among volunteer prisoners by feeding them the sharecropper diet. His findings met with enormous resistance among Southerners, who denied that pellagra was rooted in the economics of cotton growing.

In 1927, Dr. Goldberger determined conclusively that B vitamins were pellagra's cure.

Symptoms and Causes

Doctors and researchers continue to identify and investigate pellagra because, as we become complacent about our diets, it continues to "crop up." It is believed to be caused primarily by a deficiency of vitamin B3 (niacin and niacinamide), but according to Abram Hoffer, M.D., Ph.D., author of *Orthomolecular Medicine for Physicians* (Keats Publishing, 1989), it is more likely caused by a lack of tryptophan, an amino acid that converts to vitamin B3 in the body.

This essential amino acid is also the raw material for the manufacture of serotonin, a neuro-transmitter which produces a calming effect. Certain types of depression are thought to be linked to abnormal serotonin levels. Although the brain and nerve symptoms caused by a B3 deficiency are not completely understood, researchers suggest the serotonin levels, specifically, may be responsible. A third cause is a deficiency of vitamin B6 (pyridoxine). B6 must be present before tryptophan can be converted to B3.

Dr. Hoffer characterizes pellagra by the four Ds: dermatitis, diarrhea, dementia and death. Once the symptoms of pellagra become obvious, death can be the next step. The most common first symptom is a symmetrical, reddish brown, sometimes black, discoloration of the parts of the skin exposed to the sun. It looks like a suntan or sunburn. Diarrhea may alternate with constipation. Because the B vitamins are absorbed in the small intestine, diarrhea makes the deficiency worse, as it prevents B vitamins from being absorbed.

To call the behavioral symptoms mere dementia understates the effect of pellagra. Earlier stages are more typically schizophrenic, with thought disorder, mood changes and psychotic behavior. In the 1920s and 1930s, when pellagra was rampant in the southeastern U.S., mental hospitals were filled with patients suffering from the disease. At one time, over 25 percent of spring admissions to mental hospitals in the South were pellagra.[2] Before the necessary nutrient was isolated, the symptoms of pellagra were well-documented. It gradually became clear that the picture was very similar to schizophrenia. When niacin was used, the results were dramatic. Many patients were instantly cured who had been thought to be hopelessly doomed to mental wards.[3]

Even today, behavioral rather than nutritional testing may overlook many cases of pellagra in the guise of mental illness.

Glen Green, M.D., a Canadian researcher, said that many penitentiary inmates have sub-clinical pellagra.[4] He also noted that today's children with learning and behavioral disorders are very similar to children who were diagnosed with sub-clinical pellagra over 40 years ago.[5] Between 1941 and 1948, El Kholy, M.D., an Egyptian researcher, studied the relationship between crime and pellagra. After examining 1,150 incarcerated felons, Dr. Kholy reported that 206, or 18 percent, had pellagra.[6] Like Dr. Abram, he confirmed that the symptoms of pellagra are often mistaken for a schizophrenic personality. For more on B vitamins' relationship to mental illness, see the chapters Schizophrenia, Depression and Mental Illness.

Nutritional Treatment Provides Miraculous Results

In 1952, Dr. Hoffer and Dr. Humphry Osmond were struck by the similarity between schizophrenia and the delirium experienced in pellagra. They conducted the first double-blind study in the discipline of psychiatry comparing niacin, niacinamide and a placebo on a group of 30 schizophrenic patients. Since most of the early treatment of pellagra had involved large doses of niacin, they hypothesized that schizophrenics may also need larger amounts of the vitamin. Consequently, they began treating patients with doses of nearly 3,000 mg daily. Out of the 30, only three receiving placebos had improvement. The spontaneous or natural recovery rate is considered to be 35 percent. Using niacin and niacinamide, Hoffer and Osmond managed to double this rate, curing 75 percent of the patients.[7]

George Watson and W.D. Currier conducted an experiment with 60 subjects diagnosed as having some form of mental illness. Half were given large daily doses of vitamin B3, along with a supplemental dose of the remainder of the B complex vitamins. The remaining subjects received placebos. Of those receiving placebos, seven improved, six got worse and 17 showed no change. Among those taking vitamins, 22 showed substantial improvement, two became worse and six remained the same. With each successive month of supplementation, the success rate climbed even higher.

Today, a tremendous amount of scientific research is in progress with tryptophan, the least abundant amino acid present in the average diet. A number of studies suggest that tryptophan malnutrition may cause depression. For example, neuroendocrinologist Richard Wurtman, M.D., and a research team at the Massachusetts Institute of Technology have spent almost two decades studying the way in which diet determines neurotransmitter levels in the brain. Their research indicates that the amount of tryptophan that reaches the brain dictates the rate at which nerve cells will manufacture serotonin.

Simply eating foods that contain high levels of tryptophan, however, may not affect the level of serotonin. Initially, when Wurtsman and colleagues fed rats tryptophan, levels of both serotonin and tryptophan actually decreased. The paradox was explained once researchers realized that tryptophan must compete with five other amino acids for transportation into the brain. Since most proteins contain less tryptophan than other amino acids, a high-protein meal can create less opportunity for tryptophan to reach its goal. The foods that are most effective at getting tryptophan into the brain are carbohydrates, even though they provide no tryptophan. A high-carbohydrate meal (whole grains, vegetables and fruit) raises the insulin level which moves most amino acids out of the bloodstream and into muscle tissue. When insulin is high, levels of amino acids fall, except for tryptophan. As a result, tryptophan has little competition for transportation, and more of it moves from the blood to nerve cells in the brain.

Since the discovery of vitamin B3, it has successfully been used to treat alcoholism, depression, learning and behavioral problems in children, diabetes, allergies, lupus, stress, senility, arthritis, circulation problems and high blood pressure.[8]

B Vitamin Foods and Tryptophan

Tryptophan, available in amino acid formulas, works most efficiently in the presence of plenty of vitamin B6. Women who take oral contraceptives need a minimum of 20 mg of vitamin B6 daily in order to metabolize tryptophan normally. Foods that contain tryptophan include soybeans, fish, wheat germ, cottage cheese, granola, oats, eggs, whole milk and cheese.

The B vitamins must be taken together, so do the B complex shuffle. The whole B complex family includes B1 (thiamine), B2 (riboflavin), B3 (niacin), B5 (pantothenic acid), B6 (pyridoxine), B12 (cobalamin), B15 (pangamic acid), biotin, choline, folic acid, inositol and PABA (para-aminobenzoic acid). Each B vitamin has its own role in body function, centered on the nervous system. Since nerves bring messages to all the organs and stimulate glands to secrete their important biochemicals, the whole body communication system can break down with a B vitamin deficiency.

To get all your B vitamins, eat whole grains. Sulfa drugs, sleeping pills, insecticides and synthetic estrogen create a condition in the intestinal tract that can destroy B vitamins. All breads are "enriched" with B vitamins because the vitamin is lost when whole grains are milled for flour. Pellagra is most common among societies that eat primarily corn and little else. Corn does not contain tryptophan and its niacin is 'locked,' so it is unavailable to the body. Certain cultures' habit of preparing it for cooking with lime is probably what saves them from pellagra.

Pellagra-Preventive and Health-Restoring Nutrients
For maximum absorption, take supplements with meals.

Nutrient	Suggested Dosage	Formulation
Amino acids	4-6 capsules daily	Multiple formula from natural sources
Enzymes	2 capsules twice daily	Multiple formula
Fiber	4-8 tablets daily	Psyllium, with herb hyssop
Multi-mineral	3-4 ounces daily	In liquid solution, with vitamin B12, biotin
Multi-vitamin/mineral	6 caplets daily	Freeze-dried plant sources
Niacin	500 mg four times daily	
Niacinamide	1,000 mg twice daily	
Vitamin B6	100 mg daily	
Vitamin C	Individual bowel tolerance*	With bioflavonoids (quercetin, proanthocyanidins)

* To determine individual dosage, on the first day take 1,000 mg hourly until diarrhea occurs, then reduce dosage to just below that for individual daily dosage. Vitamin C is not toxic in large doses but must be taken throughout the day to benefit. Divide dosage to three or four times a day.

CHAPTER 132:

Poison Ivy, Oak

"Berries white, poisonous sight! Leaves of three, let me be!"

–Anonymous

I remember as a child getting poison oak. I recall the itching rash that coated my legs and ached between my shoe-encased toes. My sister's solution was to tear the skin away with her fingernails, itching as much as she wanted, until her legs were shredded and bleeding. I took the more stoic approach: coating my skin with calamine lotion, and agonizing when it didn't help. When it comes to poison ivy or poison oak, forewarned is really forearmed. Learning as much as you can about it will help immensely.

A poison ivy or oak rash is really an allergic contact dermatitis caused by urushiol (you-ROO-shee-ol), a substance found in the sap of poison ivy and poison oak. For our purposes here, and because they are similar in their effect, I will lump the two together, using the term poison ivy to connote both.

Urushiol is a colorless or slightly yellow oil that oozes from any cut or crushed part of the plant, including the stem and leaves. The weeds are most dangerous in the spring and summer, as there is plenty of sap then, the urushiol content is high, and the plants are easily bruised.

Urushiol is one of the most concentrated and toxic skin agents known, and can cause reactions with as little as one-billionth of a gram of oil. It is estimated that a mere five ounces of this oil is enough to have caused allergic reactions in every person who has lived in the last several thousand years!

Not only is the oil highly toxic and concentrated, but its adverse effects are long-lasting as well. Gloves which have crumbled a single leaf can cause reactions 6-12 months later, and even centuries-old specimens of plants containing the oil have caused rashes when handled.[1]

Studies show that approximately 85 percent of the population will develop an allergic reaction if exposed to poison ivy. Although they're not sure why, scientists believe that an individual's sensitivity changes with time and tends to decline with age.

The first bout of poison ivy usually occurs in children between ages 8 and 16, and can be quite severe. If there is no repeat exposure to urushiol, sensitivity will probably decrease by half by the time these individuals are in their 30s.

Only 10-15 percent of the population are not sensitive to poison ivy. Never assume you are among these few, as people who reach adulthood without being infected in childhood have about a 50 percent chance of having an allergy. Reactions in these uninitiated can be severe, with swelling of the face, arms, and genitals, and will require immediate medical attention.[2]

Because the offending substance is oil, it has properties important to keep in mind. First, it can get to your skin through your clothes – even leather! If it doesn't seep through your clothes, it can stick to them. A friend of mine bought some property and spent weeks with her husband clearing the land. There she was, pulling up poison ivy with gloved hands, wiping the sweat off her brow with the same gloves. She thought she was immune because her skin was not actually coming into contact with the plant. She spent weeks in bed, taking antihistamines and drugs so the blisters in her eyes and throat wouldn't kill her. It was a close call. Never underestimate the power of poison ivy.

Urushiol sticks to almost all surfaces and is virtually invisible. Everything that has come in contact with it must be washed. This includes tools, the steering wheel, all clothing, and even the dog can be a secondary carrier. Do not use any soap that has oil or cold cream, as it just spreads the oil around. Lye soap, natural castile or Fels Naptha are recommended. Clean tools with solvents that will break the oil down. As far as whether to use cold or hot water, there are arguments for both. I'm told that cold water is ideal because it closes the pores. However, are the pores even involved? I'd bet on hot water because it more readily dissolves oil. Very hot water, however, is supposed to spread the oil.

You can be infected through your animal. The oil sticks to hair just as surely as clothes. My Great Dane Fred once infected me when, following a romp on the two acres of wooded area surrounding my house, he greeted me covered with poison oak. You couldn't tell because it was the oil left on his hair that I got on my hands and arms in my welcoming embrace. I immediately called a team to come out and rid the area of it.

Never burn poison ivy, as the urushiol can be carried in smoke and not only will your skin be exposed but you will inhale it as well. And the poison ivy will just grow back.

Poison Ivy Myths

As a child, I remember being told over and over that I shouldn't scratch because I would spread the blisters. Envious of my sister who scratched as much as she pleased, but determined to do the right thing, I gritted my teeth and resisted the impulse. If I had only known, I probably would have joined her. It turns out the rash is not spread by itching. It can only be spread if you still have urushiol on your hands or under the fingernails, which I suppose is possible if you don't wash well enough. Scratching is not recommended, in any case, because it can cause nasty infections and ugly scars.

Poison ivy cannot be passed from one person to the other. I used to think the stuff that gave me blisters was contained in the blisters. If I broke a blister, I could spread it to the unaffected parts of my skin or to my best friend. Another myth I wish someone had told me about!

Just because you were allergic as a child, doesn't mean you retain that degree of sensitivity. I hate to think of the number of adults who, recalling their miserable childhoods, refrain from hiking, camping or enjoying nature's bounty because of the fear of contracting poison ivy again. A person's sensitivity changes over time and even from year to year. People who are very sensitive as children may not be sensitive as adults.

Vitamins Can Help

Contact dermatitis caused by urushiol creates its own set of problems. But when swelling occurs as a result, the danger can become deadly. If you're talking about the throat or mouth, it can mean suffocation. If the plant is burning, and is inhaled, it can cause the throat to swell.

The reason for the swelling is the histamine the body produces to combat the foreign substance. The itching, redness and swelling are symptoms of the histamine. Pharmaceutical *anti*-histamines are designed to halt these symptoms, but have side effects and aren't always recommended. Fortunately, there are nutrients that act as natural antihistamines.

The same stress that triggers the release of histamine also increases the need for vitamin C, the body's natural defense against excessive histamine. Thus, vitamin C helps reduce inflammation.

In a study at Arizona State University, Carol Johnston, Ph.D., gave nine people vitamin C supplements for six weeks, beginning with 500 mg daily and gradually increasing the amount to 2,000 mg per day. By the time their daily intake of vitamin C had peaked, histamine levels had dropped an average of 40 percent.[3]

In another remarkable study, researchers gave 126 people, known to be sensitive to poison oak, injections and oral doses of vitamin C before and after exposure to urushiol. Only one developed a rash.[4]

I would recommend anybody with allergies to poison oak or ivy, seasonal pollen or insect bites supplement with vitamin C on a regular basis.

Quercetin, a bioflavonoid found in citrus fruits, is a potent agent against inflammation. Quercetin's effect is very similar to the anti-allergic drug cromolyn, as it has been shown to actually inhibit the release of histamine. But it goes further than that. Quercetin is also able to inhibit inflammatory compounds like leukotrienes, which are a thousand times worse than histamine in creating allergic inflammation.[5]

Target vitamin A to reduce skin inflammation, especially the swelling that occurs with urushiol blisters. Vitamin A can increase skin collagen, reduce inflammation, reduce scarring and improve healing. It is so good, surgeons have been known to apply it directly to wounds.[6]

Another natural anti-inflammatory is vitamin E. Vitamin E not only boosts the immune system, but reduces the damage to tissues that results in inflammation, especially those of the skin. Vitamin E helps internally, as well as externally. This antioxidant also helps stabilize skin membranes so healing can occur. In one study, vitamin E taken five to seven days prior to injection with histamine showed far less swelling around the injection site.

Fight Fire with Fire

The manufacturer of a popular poison ivy remedy told me once that his tonic was made of a blend of acetic acid and isopropanol. Translated from the chemist's jargon, it meant a mixture of vinegar and rubbing alcohol. When the supply was exhausted in our home, I concocted a half vinegar/rubbing alcohol solution, which of course is still effective. Now that you know that a 50-50 mix of vinegar and rubbing alcohol is an effective treatment, what other simple or back-yard remedies are there? Consider the following:

Once you've gotten the sap on you and know you're in trouble, try cutting up a green tomato and squeezing the juice on the affected area.

What if you already have a red rash and it's starting to hurt and itch? Try mixing equal parts of buttermilk, vinegar, and salt, and rub on the area. Another effective treatment is to place a cup of willow leaves in a cup of water and boil. Strain and let cool while the solution becomes dark brown. Use cotton swabs and place on the affected area. The common willow, found in many backyards, is the plant source for aspirin, a pharmaceutical anti-inflammatory.

Still another medicinal plant is the jewelweed, or Touch-Me-Not. These tender, fragile plants have many branches and are light green. They are very juicy, and strangely, the juice is light orange. The leaves vary in size from very tiny to about three inches long and are egg-shaped with a point on the outer end and widespread serrations on the margins.

The name was given to it because rain and dew will stand on the leaves in round drops and shine like little jewels on the unwettable leaf surface. It has pretty yellow flowers that are followed by slipper-shaped seed pods about 3/4" long. If these seed pods are touched when ripe, they suddenly split, the two sides curling back into tight spirals with an audible snap, throwing seeds all over the surrounding area...which is why they are also called Touch-Me-Nots. Conveniently, it most often grows right next to poison ivy, making for an immediate remedy to the potential itch. When you think you have entered a poison ivy patch and had contact, look around for the jewelweed. Break the stem and spread the gel-like residue on the areas you think have come into contact with poison ivy. This will stop the spread of infection.

The late Euell Gibbons, author of books on wild edible plants, claimed that after adding handfuls of jewelweed to his bathwater, he could walk through poison ivy with impunity. Fresh-cut jewelweed is also brewed as a tea, which is applied to the sores and taken internally.

To prepare jewelweed to preserve, boil down a quantity of the plants in a potful of water to about half the original volume, then strain. Pour the juice into ice cube trays and freeze. Then transfer the cubes into a plastic bag for easy storage. Now, even though the jewel-weed may be spent for the year, you'll be ready in case of an unexpected brush with some urushiol.

Skin Anti-Inflammatory Nutrients
For maximum absorption, take supplements with meals.

Nutrient	Suggested Dosage	Formulation
Aged garlic extract	1 teaspoon three times daily	Liquid
Antioxidants	4 capsules daily*	With selenium and grapeseed extract
Borage oil	2 capsules daily	
Enzymes	2 capsules twice daily	Multiple formula
Fiber	4-8 tablets daily	Psyllium, with herb hyssop
Flaxseed oil	1 tablespoon daily	
Melatonin (adults only)	3 mg daily at bedtime	With B vitamins
Multi-mineral	3-4 ounces daily	In liquid solution, with vitamin B12, biotin
Multi-vitamin/mineral	6 caplets daily	Freeze-dried plant sources
Niacinamide	1,000 mg twice daily	
Quercetin	400 mg twice daily	With vitamin C and bioflavonoids
Vitamin B6	200 mg daily	
Vitamin C	Individual bowel tolerance**	With citrus bioflavonoids (quercetin, proanthocyanidins)
Vitamin E	2 capsules (800 IU) daily	d-alpha tocopherol

* The FDA recommends pregnant women not exceed 10,000 IU of vitamin A daily.

** To determine individual dosage, on the first day take 1,000 mg hourly until diarrhea occurs, then reduce dosage to just below that for individual daily dosage. Vitamin C is not toxic in large doses but must be taken throughout the day to benefit. Divide dosage to three or four times a day.

CHAPTER 133:

Preeclampsia (Toxemia in Pregnancy)

I don't watch television as a rule (no time), but sometimes I find myself in front a TV while I work. It was an episode of the television show ER that drew my attention to preeclampsia. On this particular show, one of the doctors was confronted with a pregnant woman having complications. He originally misdiagnosed her and sent her away. She arrived again going into convulsions. The whole one-hour show was about the doctor's battle to save this woman and her baby. My ears perked up when I heard him order the charge nurses to give her an IV of magnesium sulfate. In real life it probably would have lowered her dangerous blood pressure and saved her life. But for the purposes of drama, after hours of heroics, the baby was saved but the mother died. I was transfixed throughout the show, and found myself crying at the end. It moved me to such a degree that when I read the cut-and-dried research on toxemia, eclampsia and preeclampsia, I could appreciate the emotional effect this disorder must have.

When you visit your obstetrician, chances are you will have your weight and blood pressure checked, and be asked to leave a urine sample. You are being checked for toxemia.

The very word is misleading. Toxemia is not an overdose of toxins, or poisoned blood. In fact, it isn't even a disease. It's a syndrome – or collection of abnormalities that involve: 1) hypertension, or high blood pressure; 2) a high amount of protein in the urine, indicating an inability to assimilate protein; and 3) an abnormal amount of edema or swelling. The term stems from an assumption that pregnancy in and of itself can be toxic to the body, producing disorders that threaten it. Morning sickness, for example, is viewed as a side effect of pregnancy, even though it can be controlled by adequate amounts of vitamin B6.

Again, we have fancy terminology I suspect was originated by male traditional doctors to confuse women into believing they were helpless to effect change in their conditions. Eclampsia and preeclampsia are fancy names for the stages of these three original abnormalities.

Preeclampsia is basically the same as toxemia. Eclampsia is brought in when these original malfunctions become life-threatening. What is considered normal blood pressure in pregnancy varies somewhat over the course of nine months. A baseline pressure – what is normal for the individual – is obtained at the first prenatal visit. Generally, the pressure drops a little over the next several months. But as delivery nears, somewhere about the seventh month, it usually begins to rise a bit.

During the first or second trimester, if the pressure rises 30 systolic (the upper number) or 15 diastolic (the lower number) over the baseline reading (or by more than that in the third trimester) and stays up for at least two readings taken at least six hours apart, the pregnant woman's condition warrants close observation, and possibly intervention. The traditional doctor might then proclaim to the mystified patient that she has preeclampsia. This is one of the reasons prenatal care is important: in the event these symptoms occur they can be controlled to prevent more serious complications.

If increased blood pressure is accompanied by sudden weight gain (more than three pounds a week in the second trimester or more than two pounds a week in the third); severe edema (swelling due to water retention), particularly in hands and face as well as ankles; and/or protein in the urine, the problem may be proclaimed eclampsia. If blood pressure continues to rise and these symptoms continue, it can result in convulsions and coma.

When preeclampsia proceeds to eclampsia, it is considered to be the result of very complex disturbances and an unbalanced dietary intake. Since there is no association between caloric intake and preeclampsia, the conclusion reached is that it is the *kind* of food eaten, rather than the amount. This inference is reinforced by the fact that well-nourished women typically don't have these problems. This is also backed up geographically. Populations which are typically undernourished have a higher rate of preeclampsia and eclampsia.

In Europe and other developed countries eclampsia occurs in one in 2000 deliveries while in developing countries it varies more widely from one in 100 to one in 1700. Over half a million females die each year of pregnancy related causes and 99 percent of these causes occur in the developing world. Eclampsia probably accounts for 50,000 deaths from pregnancy a year worldwide.[1]

During the German occupation of Belgium and Holland, the incidence of preeclampsia and eclampsia decreased. However, after liberation from German occupation, when food became more plentiful, the frequency increased. Again, it is the quality of the food that is important. Once the Germans gained access to sugar and other accessory foods, they ate less fresh plant foods high in preeclampsia-preventive nutrients I will tell you about.[2]

Magnesium: The Treatment of Choice in America

For over half a century magnesium has been used in preeclampsia and eclampsia yet its use remains controversial. In the United States magnesium is the anticonvulsant of choice for women with eclampsia while in the United Kingdom it is used by only two percent of obstetricians.[3] This is puzzling considering the compelling evidence in favor of magnesium.

In one study, 1,089 women were given the pharmaceutical Dilantin for eclamptic convulsions compared to 1,049 women who received magnesium sulfate. Ten of the women in the Dilantin group still experienced convulsions compared to none in the magnesium sulfate treated group. The author of the study, Michael J. Lucas, M.D., and fellow researchers of the Department of Obstetrics and Gynecology, University of Texas Southwestern Medical Center in Dallas, concluded in an article in *The New England Journal of Medicine* that magnesium sulfate is superior to Dilantin for the prevention of eclampsia in hypertensive pregnant women.[4]

Martin Rudnicki, M.D., a Danish physician practicing at the Department of Obstetrics and Gynecology, University of Copenhagen, has studied the benefits of magnesium. He found that magnesium reduces blood pressure, boosts the heart and decreases vascular resistance. In a double-blind study, researchers found that magnesium reduced blood pressure in pregnant women not only when given intravenously, but also orally before delivery. Researchers also found it perfectly safe to the unborn infant, nor were there any reported problems of low calcium levels. A deficiency of calcium can occur when high amounts of magnesium are taken without like amounts of calcium. However, in the cases of preeclampsia, this was not an observed problem. As if this wasn't enough to convince, babies born to women taking magnesium were shown in studies to have higher birth weights.[5]

Despite this irrefutable evidence, many doctors continue to use magnesium as crisis, rather than preventive medicine. The conventional mindset is so ingrained against therapeutic nutrition that physicians don't use magnesium until a woman comes into the emergency room wracked with convulsions.

Fortunately, there are doctors out there educated and knowledgeable about nutritional medicine, and for the lucky few who can afford and find them, help is available. Jonathan Wright, M.D. is one of the brave who continues to heal patients, despite harassment from the FDA. He has found in his practice that adding vitamin B6 to magnesium works even better than magnesium alone.[6] The body's need for vitamin B6 increases during pregnancy, and a deficiency has shown in studies to contribute to water retention, a symptom of preeclampsia.[7]

The Right Kind of Protein

There is one more factor involved in preventing preeclampsia: adequate amounts of dietary protein. We're not talking about eating meat at every sitting – targeting certain kinds of food is just as important as certain kinds of supplements. As far back as 1935, a lack of sufficient protein in the diet was linked to an increased incidence of toxemia by Dr. Maurice Strauss of Harvard University.[8] This observation has been repeated over and over since then.

Women with toxemia of any degree sometimes have lower serum albumin levels, and this type of protein in the bloodstream is necessary to keep fluid from leaking into the tissues, where it causes extreme swelling.[9]

Good food sources of protein include eggs, legumes – peas, beans and lentils – and grains. The vegetarian can get complete proteins by combining legumes and grains. Rice and beans, for example. I also recommend cheese, nuts and seeds.

Antioxidants

Another observation was made while examining the differences between healthy pregnant women and pregnant women with preeclampsia. In a normal pregnancy, blood tests show high amounts of antioxidants, while in preeclamptic women, there are fewer antioxidant vitamins in the blood, and more evidence of free radical damage. Certain chemical reactions take place as a result of this condition, and researchers are finding it in preeclampsia.[10]

Magdy S. Mikhail, M.D., and fellow researchers at Albert Einstein College of Medicine, Bronx, New York., took this observation into the laboratory and did a study comparing 30 women with preeclampsia to 44 women with uncomplicated pregnancies between 15 and 35 years of age and at 28 to 42 weeks for blood levels of vitamin C, E and beta carotene.[11]

They found vitamin C levels were significantly decreased in

patients with mild and severe eclampsia, and that vitamin E and beta carotene levels were significantly decreased only in severe preeclamptic patients. What is interesting is that some of both groups were taking prenatal vitamins at RDA dosages. Yet, there was no difference in antioxidant nutrient concentrations between those who did or did not use prenatal vitamins. The researchers believe that the small RDA dosages may not be enough to overcome the preeclamptic condition.

Essential Fatty Acids

While many nutrients are likely to be helpful in combating preeclampsia, it is beginning to look as though the essential fatty acids may be the crucial factors. Essential fatty acids are important partly because they make up a major part of the membranes surrounding all cells and partly because they give rise to substances known as prostaglandins.

The two main problems in preeclampsia are a rise in blood pressure and fluid retention. Kidney problems then compound the problem. Prostaglandins are important in lowering blood pressure and helping the kidneys function properly.

Two groups of medical researchers (in Texas and Nottingham, England) have been working on the idea that preeclampsia is due to a lack of prostaglandins. Both groups have now collected a substantial evidence that this is indeed true. Animal experiments have shown that in pregnancy a disease very similar to preeclampsia develops when animals are deprived of essential fatty acids in the diet, or are given drugs to block the conversion of the fatty acids to prostaglandins in the body.[12]

Many researchers are therefore now convinced that a lack of prostaglandins plays a key role in the development of preeclampsia. This might occur because of a lack in the diet of the most common essential fatty acid, cis-linoleic acid, and then to the prostaglandins. Some people take too little cis-linoleic acid, but the more common problem is in gamma-linolenic formation. Borage oil is the best solution for this problem, because it contains gamma linolenic acid.[13]

Researchers at the Division of Perinatal Medicine, Swedish Medical Center in Seattle, conducted a study of 22 preeclamptic women and 40 normal women for fatty acid status. After adjusting for variables, women with the lowest level of omega-3 fatty acids were 7.6 times more likely to develop preeclampsia as compared to those women with the highest level of omega-3 fatty acids.

A 15 percent increase in the ratio of omega-3 and omega-6 fatty acids was associated with an incredible 46 percent reduction in the risk of preeclampsia.[14]

It can get very confusing when talking about the different kinds of fatty acids, which are the kinds of fats we need for energy and health – *not* saturated fat from meat and dairy products and certainly *not* transfatty acids from hydrogenated margarine and foods. Suffice it to say that omega-3 fatty acids are found in fish oil and omega-6 fatty acids are found in vegetable and seed oils. The best source of omega-6 is borage oil. Take borage oil, obtained in health food stores or through mail order, for omega-6 fatty acids.

To increase your omega-3 fatty acids, target flaxseed oil. It is an excellent source of this type of fatty acid. In one study, women with preeclamptic high blood pressure responded well to the use of omega-3. It has also proven to be an excellent substitute for aspirin – which is sometimes prescribed as treatment for preeclampsia – since it is just as effective and has no negative side effects.

Preeclampsia-Preventive Nutrients
For maximum absorption, take supplements with meals.

Nutrient	Suggested Dosage	Formulation
Aged garlic extract	1 teaspoon three times daily	Liquid
Amino acids	4-6 capsules daily	Multiple formula from natural sources
Antioxidants	4 capsules daily*	With selenium and grapeseed extract
Borage oil	2 capsules daily	
Coenzyme Q10	2 capsules daily	With vitamin E, phospholipids and selenium
Enzymes	2 capsules twice daily	Multiple formula
Fiber	4-8 tablets daily	Psyllium, with herb hyssop
Flaxseed oil	1 tablespoon daily	
Hawthorne	250 mg twice daily	
Magnesium	200 mg daily	
Melatonin (adults only)	3 mg daily at bedtime	With B vitamins
Multi-mineral	3-4 ounces daily	In liquid solution, with vitamin B12, biotin
Multi-vitamin/mineral	6 caplets daily	Freeze-dried plant sources
Rutin	100 mg twice daily	With vitamin C
Taurine	500 mg twice daily	
Vitamin B6	100 mg daily	
Vitamin C	Individual bowel tolerance**	With bioflavonoids (quercetin, rutin, proanthocyanidins)
Vitamin E	2 capsules (800 IU) daily	d-alpha tocopherol

* The FDA recommends pregnant women not exceed 10,000 IU of vitamin A daily.

** To determine individual dosage, on the first day take 1,000 mg hourly until diarrhea occurs, then reduce dosage to just below that for individual daily dosage. Vitamin C is not toxic in large doses but must be taken throughout the day to benefit. Divide dosage to three or four times a day.

CHAPTER 134:

Premenstrual Syndrome

Her company wanted to make her an associate, but no one would associate with her! She doesn't play hard to get, she plays hard to tolerate! She can enter a crowded room and within ten minutes have it all to herself!

Jokes abound about premenstrual syndrome, or PMS. But for those close to someone with the disorder, it's no laughing matter. It's hard to be sympathetic with someone who is biting your head off. The lack of control over one's emotions, just one of many symptoms, have sufferers screaming in frustration and growling for help.

Today, PMS is one of the most talked about maladies in the world. It's about time. For hundreds of years this debilitating condition affecting millions of women went unrecognized, not to mention undiagnosed and untreated. Even more, women suffering from it were made to feel like it was their fault. Since men do not experience PMS, without doubt it has contributed toward a belief that women are "the weaker sex."

Meanwhile women – ever since Eve – have suffered an incredible array of patience-taxing physical and emotional symptoms. They include anxiety, anti-social behavior, bloating, breast swelling and sensitivity, confusion, cramps, cravings for certain foods, crying spells, depression, dizziness, exhaustion, fluid retention – especially in the legs – headaches, irritability, sleeplessness, and, among others, wide mood swings.

It is estimated that between one-third and one-half of all American women between the ages of 20 and 50 – as many as 14 million women – have premenstrual symptoms of varying degrees. That's a lot of unhappy women!

One of the problems medical science has concerning PMS is that it is not an illness, per se. It's not something you "get" or "catch," then start medication to treat. This is because the causes can be varied, uncertain and sometimes impossible to pinpoint.

The good news – when it comes to nutritional information, there is always good news – is that PMS can be helped, easily and conveniently.

Before I go on, however, it's important to understand what premenstrual syndrome is, and how it can happen.

Caused by Hormonal Fluctuations

Premenstrual syndrome is actually a number of symptoms, varying in severity, that occur a week to ten days prior to the start of the menstrual period. Because of this tell-tale timing, we know it somehow relates to the hormonal changes our bodies go through during this time.

History books describe PMS as "the vapors." When I hear the term I picture the way movie-makers typically depict the turn of the century woman: waving a lace handkerchief in front of her nose, eyes rolled upward as she falls in a dead faint. Ever notice how whenever a woman faints in soap operas it turns out she's pregnant?

It seems incredible that in this generation of women in the workplace and legislature there could still be physicians who would label premenstrual syndrome "psychosomatic." Makes you wonder how many other valid and "obvious" diseases are being overlooked.

What seems likely is that hormonal fluctuations contribute, if not cause, most symptoms of PMS.

Studies show that five to 10 days before menstruation, women with PMS have higher blood levels of estrogen and lower levels of progesterone than non-PMS sufferers. Estrogen and progesterone are needed to stimulate and prepare the lining of the uterus for pregnancy.[1]

In attempting to understand the effect of sexual hormones on behavior, reproductive endocrinologist Ken Muse of the University of Kentucky, evaluated a group of volunteers' progesterone levels in the first few hours after lunch. Healthy women typically showed normal levels of blood progesterone after eating a midday meal, but the volunteers with PMS showed a steep drop, possibly contributing to the eating binges reported by some women with PMS.[2]

One way to counter this low progesterone level is to supplement with natural progesterone cream. John R. Lee, M.D., has been using progesterone cream in his practice for over 15 years, and advocates its use for everything from osteoporosis to fatty tumors to PMS. He reports that in his practice the majority of his patients reported remarkable improvement in their PMS symptoms, and experienced less swelling and water weight gain.[3]

Dr. Joel T. Hargrove of Vanderbilt University Medical Center has published results indicating a 90 percent success rate in treating PMS with natural progesterone.[4]

Controlling Hormones with Nutrition

When evaluating blood factors, one need only go a little further to make the zinc connection. Realizing that trace amounts of zinc regulate the secretion of certain hormones, including progesterone, C. James Chuong, Ph.D., and his co-workers at the Baylor College of Medicine in Houston decided to look for zinc abnormalities in the blood of women with PMS.

They recruited 10 women with PMS and 10 controls who reported no sign of the monthly disorder. They collected blood samples from the volunteers every two to three days during three menstrual cycles and measured zinc concentrations in the blood. During the premenstrual phase, the researchers discovered significantly lower zinc levels in blood from women with PMS than in the control samples.[5] Zinc is also a factor in controlling the pituitary hormones which stimulate the thyroid. Low levels of thyroid hormones can cause PMS.

The work of Drs. Nora and David Brayshaw at the Biopsychiatry Center of Watchung, New Jersey, raised a red flag showing that PMS may be caused by a disorder of the thyroid and pituitary glands – and subsequently can be treated effectively.

The doctors initially noticed the striking similarity between the symptoms of hypothyroidism and PMS – weight gain, lethargy, moodiness, irritability, anxiety – but that the similarity had not yet gained the attention of researchers. So they set out to examine women with PMS to see if, indeed, there was a connection.

The Brayshaws studied 66 women, 54 of whom suffered from classic PMS symptoms to determine the presence or absence of either a thyroid or pituitary disorder. The pituitary controls thyroid function by secreting TSH – a hormone that stimulates the thyroid. They found a distinct elevation of pituitary TSH in the blood of PMS patients – an indication that the pituitary is working overtime to drive the thyroid into action.

Other tests confirmed the connection. The doctors found that 94 percent of the PMS patients had some measure of thyroid dysfunction, either pituitary-linked or otherwise – while none of the 12 patients without PMS symptoms had any thyroid problems. For solutions to thyroid problems, consult my chapter Low Thyroid.

A Nutritional Protocol

PMS sufferers must do several things before starting on a program of supplementation. They must stop drinking caffeinated beverages, eliminate all refined sugar and white flour from the diet, and be tested for food and hormone allergies to make sure the thyroid, which makes certain hormones, is in good working order.[6] Only then are the following nutrients targeted.

Vitamin B6 may help relieve some of the symptoms of PMS including depression, anxiety, irritability, mood swings and anger.[7] Magnesium works with B6 and helps calm nerves. Calcium works with magnesium to relieve fatigue. A deficiency of essential fatty acids, found in borage and flaxseed oils, contributes to PMS, and vitamin E helps with PMS symptoms.

Vitamin B6 and the other B vitamins are important to the nervous system. A deficiency of B vitamins has been connected to many mental illnesses, including schizophrenia. A deficiency of B12 causes pernicious anemia and has been linked to senile dementia as well. Therefore, it's not surprising that studies show B6 helps with PMS.

The Blood Sugar Connection

Vicki Georges Hufnagel, M.D., an obstetrician-gynecologist, told the 14th Annual California Dairy Council Nutrition Conference that two of the major causes of PMS are strict dieting and eating poorly.[8]

Over-dieters jeopardize their energy reserves, lowering blood sugar to such a degree that PMS symptoms result. Low blood sugar is a major contributor to PMS, and while hormone fluctuations can contribute, a poor diet is more to blame. The truth is that the PMS patient, typically suffering from a ravenous appetite and a strong craving for the no-nos: salt, sugar and chocolate, must raise her progesterone level and stabilize her blood sugar before PMS symptoms can be eradicated.

Patients should eat a mid-morning snack to satisfy hunger and increase fiber and calcium. PMS sufferers should keep their blood sugar level up by eating six small meals a day, instead of three large ones, refrain from adding salt to foods and eat more potassium-rich fruits, vegetables, nuts, seeds, beans and peas. Beans are the best source of protein, and are essential in any blood-sugar raising diet. Try lentils for breakfast for an excellent energy boost.

For more on battling hypoglycemia, see my chapter Low Blood Sugar.

GLA for PMS

Probably the most beneficial nutrient for PMS, and with the most studies to back it up, is gamma-linolenic acid (GLA), an essential fatty acid found in black currant oil, evening primrose oil and borage oil. Most of the studies involve evening primrose oil. However, I always recommend borage oil. Evening primrose oil is very expensive, and borage oil contains more GLA. Independent clinical tests show that borage oil contains up to 26 percent GLA. Compare this to evening primrose oil and black currant oil, which contain no more than 18 percent. Not only that, borage oil costs less because the borage seed is three times larger than black currant or evening primrose seeds. Finally, borage is more bioavailable. In other words, the body more readily absorbs it.[9]

In two British experiments, evening primrose oil was given to 70 women who failed to get relief from one or two other attempted treatments. Taking it two to three times daily, 67 percent were completely relieved of PMS symptoms and 22 percent gained partial relief. In this study, an amazing total of 89 percent of treatment-resistant women got partial to complete relief of their PMS with GLA.[10]

Researchers investigating the effects of GLA on PMS believe they know why women suffer the symptoms they do and why evening primrose oil relieves the problem in 60 to 80 percent of those tested.[11]

David Horrobin, Ph.D., director of the Efamol Research Institute in Nova Scotia says it was the team of doctors who won the 1982 Nobel Prize in Medicine for their research into prostaglandins who discovered a link between premenstrual tension and low levels of prostaglandin E1 (PGE1).

A deficiency of GLA can cause a shortage of PGE1s in the body. It is believed the hormonal changes and stress associated with a woman's oncoming period can cause a GLA deficiency. GLA is one of the building blocks from which the body creates prostaglandins such as PGE1s." Regular GLA supplementation increases prostaglandins and reduces PMS symptoms.[12]

A 60 to 80 percent success rate treating hundreds of PMS sufferers with evening primrose oil is proclaimed by Donald Lombard, M.D., and Ann Nazzaro, Ph.D., in Northampton, Massachusetts. By sticking to a nutritional regimen that involves taking primrose oil capsules an average of twice a day for just two or three months, women whose lives, jobs and families were disrupted each month by PMS have returned to a normal existence. They suffer no drug-related side- or after-effects, and in most cases they are totally symptom free."[13]

Premenstrual Mood Managing Nutrients
For maximum absorption, supplements should be taken with meals.

Nutrient	Suggested Dosage	Formulation
Aged garlic extract	2 teaspoons three times daily	Liquid
Antioxidants	4 capsules daily*	With selenium and grape seed extract
Borage oil	2 capsules daily	
Enzymes	2 capsules twice daily	Multiple formula
Flaxseed oil	1 tablespoon daily	
Fiber	8 tablets daily	Psyllium, with herb hyssop
Lecithin	2 tablespoons with meals	
Magnesium	200 mg daily	
Melatonin	3 mg daily at bedtime	With B vitamins
Multi-vitamin/mineral	6 caplets daily	Freeze-dried plant sources
Multi-mineral	2-4 ounces daily	In liquid solution, with vitamin B12, biotin
Natural progesterone cream	1/3 teaspoon daily	With pregnenolone, DHEA
Vitamin B6	200 mg daily	
Vitamin C	Individual bowel tolerance**	With bioflavonoids (quercetin, proanthocyanidins)
Vitamin E	2 capsules (800 IU)	d-alpha tocopherol

* The FDA recommends that pregnant women not exceed 10,000 IU of vitamin A daily.

** To determine individual dosage, on the first day take 1,000 mg hourly until diarrhea occurs, then reduce dosage to just below that for individual daily dosage. Vitamin C is not toxic in large doses but must be taken throughout the day to benefit. Divide dosage to three or four times a day.

CHAPTER 135:

Prenatal

*The cost of prenatal care and funerals is skyrocket-
ing – they've got you coming and going!*

Emotionally, having a baby can be the most wonderful thing in the world. It's God's gift to you, and your gift to Him.

The first thing a woman should do when she becomes pregnant is have her overall health evaluated, including her blood levels of all vital nutrients. The conventional obstetrician evaluates the ongoing growth and health of the fetus, important in case problems occur. However, convention typically doesn't evaluate the health of the mother. It is absolutely essential that for the baby to grow and prosper, the mother must be nutritionally healthy. Prenatal care is more than just monitoring a baby's heartbeat, it must involve monitoring the mother's nutritional status as well. The best thing to do is educate yourself as you are doing now. You are the senior partner in your care. Your junior partner is your nutritionally-oriented physician.

First, it's not how much you eat, it's *how* you eat and what you are able to absorb. Taking the "eating for two" adage to heart, many consume all the foods they enjoy, not considering the quality of them. Eating for two doesn't mean two cupcakes or two hotdogs. It means two servings of lentils or two carrots. It's true that calorie intake should be increased, but this means complete calories from complete foods.

The fetus takes the nutrients it needs to survive and grow. If there aren't any, growth is restricted. If there's only enough for the baby, the mother's growth is restricted. Eating for two means twice as much of all the nutrients essential for optimum growth. Weight gain will not be excessive if the food ingested is nutritious.

Preventing Defects with Nutrition

A parents' biggest fear during pregnancy is that the child will not be healthy. Technology doesn't really help, with ultrasound and the risky amniocentesis, since generally it isn't until birth that fears are realized or alleviated. A healthy baby starts with a healthy mother. Eating right is important, but in these days of environmental chemicals, nutritionally-deficient soils and produce, and hormone-supplemented meat and milk, diet just isn't enough. For optimum nutritional support of your baby, supplement a healthy diet with life-giving nutrients.

An article in the *British Medical Journal* reported on a study which found that when taken by women around the time of conception, a daily dose of multivitamin tablets including folic acid could almost halve the rate of major congenital abnormalities in babies.

Dr. Andrew Czeizel of the National Institute of Hygiene in Budapest, who conducted the controlled trial in Hungary, called it a "major finding because it will be helpful in preventing neural tube defects and congenital abnormalities."[1]

Czeizel analyzed 4,156 pregnant women who had been given multivitamins including folic acid, a B vitamin, or who had taken placebos which have no physiological effect. Incredibly, he discovered the rate of major congenital abnormalities was nearly double in the group that received placebos compared with the group receiving multivitamins.

The abnormalities included cleft palate, no kidneys and Down's syndrome. According to the study, neural tube defects such as the absence of the skull and brain, and spina bifida, in which part of the spinal cord is exposed through a gap in the backbone, could also be appreciably reduced by the use of multivitamin supplements.

You can't rely on food to have the proper amounts of nutrients. Despite the abundance of fruits and vegetables in our supermarkets, many studies show Americans are deficient. We get along OK until we try to procreate, then the deficiencies rear their ugly heads. An article in the medical journal *Neuropsychopharmacology*, states that prenatal nutritional deficiencies alter brain activity to such a degree that they could be responsible for mental illness and even schizophrenia.[2] When you examine the backgrounds of career criminals, you find poverty. Poverty of home includes poverty of nutrition. To realize the connection between criminal behavior and nutrition, read the chapters Schizophrenia and Mental Illness.

The Importance of Folic Acid

If there is one nutrient most vitally important to fetal growth and development, it is the B vitamin folic acid.

Robert L. Goldenberg, M.D., and colleagues at the Department of Obstetrics and Gynecology, The University of Alabama at Birmingham, studied 289 pregnant women, half of whom were given folic acid, the other half a placebo. The researchers found that the women who had higher blood levels of the vitamin had fewer low birth weight infants, and concluded that folic acid lowered their risk of poor fetal growth and/or mental retardation.[3]

The World Health Organization reports that one-third to one-half of pregnant women are folate-deficient in the last trimester of pregnancy.[4]

In 1991 the MRC Vitamin Study Research Group demonstrated that folic acid supplementation during conception prevents neural tube defects and spina bifida. The MRC study was built on almost 20 years of work on the possible role of folic acid and minerals in fetal malformations. Following this revelation, an editorial in *The Lancet* suggests that all women visiting prenatal clinics be given folic acid and that women who have had a previously affected fetus should be given folic acid supplements if they intend to have another pregnancy. In response to the research and results, the FDA has recommended that folic acid be added to all bread (bread devoid of *whole* grains and which has had the B vitamins processed out of it) and bread products.[5] Unfortunately, the amounts the FDA has mandated is wholly inadequate.

There is some evidence that excess pigmentation – dark spots on the skin – may be related to a deficiency of folic acid. Eat salads for the best food sources of folic acid. The B vitamin is found in green lettuce, as well as avocados, brown rice, wheat bran, soybeans, bean sprouts, artichokes, beets, cauliflower and corn. Cooking (or baking) can destroy folic acid so eat your veggies fresh and raw.

Eating whole foods is best, eating sprouts even better, since the young shoots concentrate more of the older plants' nutrients. When targeting food supplements, look for a formula that uses freeze dried sprouts and vegetables, combined in such a way as to provide all the essential vitamins and minerals.

When targeting one B vitamin, add a B-complex supplement for the rest. The B vitamins depend upon each other for optimum performance. Without one, the other cannot be used in the body. For example, without vitamin B12, folic acid cannot be absorbed. Other B vitamins are necessary for the absorption of B12. More important than what you ingest is what you absorb. Almost any interference with the metabolism of folic acid in the mother encourages fetal deformities such as cleft palate, brain damage or impaired learning ability in the child. Reasons for poor metabolism of folic acid include sulfa antibiotics, intestinal disorders, diarrhea or vomiting. Folic acid and the other B vitamins are absorbed in the small intestine and anything that alters the natural bacteria or health of the tract can impair absorption.[6]

Other essential vitamins can protect various developing fetal body parts. A daily intake of 5,000 to 10,000 international units (IU) daily of beta carotene, noted for promoting healthy mucous membranes, has been shown to offer protection for the respiratory tract, vitally important if there is a risk of premature delivery or multiple births.

Vitamin A is produced in the body from beta carotene. Because vitamin A is stored in the liver, it is safer if you get your source from beta carotene. A vitamin A deficiency has also been associated with cleft lip and cleft palate.

Attempt to eat foods that are raw and unchanged. When food products containing vitamin A are cooked or canned, there may be as much as a 40 percent depletion of the nutrient.

Vitamin E cooperates with vitamin A, protecting it from destructive oxidation in the lungs and other mucous membranes. Additionally, vitamin E on its own has been shown by researchers at four major universities to protect lung tissue from nitrogen oxide and ozone in smoggy areas.

Fortuitous Fats

The World Health Organization issued a report which recommended all pregnant women increase their intake of essential fatty acids.[7] The reasoning is that essential fatty acids are vital for all growing cells, but particularly for the brain cells of the growing infant. Without enough essential fatty acids, brain development may be retarded.

It can get very confusing when talking about the different kinds of fatty acids, which are the kinds of fats we need for energy and health – *not* saturated fat from meat and dairy products and certainly *not* transfatty acids from hydrogenated margarine and foods. Suffice it to say that omega-3 fatty acids are found in fish oil and omega-6 fatty acids are found in vegetable and seed oils. The best source of omega-6 is borage oil. Take borage oil, obtained in health food stores or through mail order.

Minerals That Matter

Zinc and copper are two minerals that, not coincidentally, are shown in studies to influence fetal health. Diabetes – even temporary cases due to pregnancy – can be complicated by a deficiency of zinc. While blood sugar problems increase the chances of abnormalities, a zinc deficiency can further increase the chances. In addition, diabetes alters the levels of zinc and copper in both the mother and fetus.[8]

Pregnant women often have a zinc deficiency, according to a February 1992 article in *The Nutrition Report*. The mineral deficiency shows up in the second and third trimester of the pregnancy or during subsequent complications. According to the report, this can result in retarded growth and maturation of the child, impaired fetal development and reduced infant survival.[9]

In studies of sheep, researchers noted that bone abnormalities developed in lambs born of severely copper-deficient ewes. This is worth noting here because both zinc and copper need each other in order to be properly absorbed. Zinc without copper can result in a zinc deficiency. Since not enough of these minerals are absorbed.[10]

Magnesium is an essential nutrient, and is at the center of all energy functions. A deficiency of magnesium early in pregnancy can cause the fetus to abort. Later, a deficiency can cause abnormalities. Women with low magnesium tend to give birth to low birth weight babies, and have placental abnormalities. Pregnancy aggravates magnesium deficiency.

Too much of either magnesium or calcium will cancel the other out. If there is too much calcium in your diet, you risk a magnesium deficiency. Too much magnesium, and you lose your calcium. The same thing can happen with phosphate. Phosphates tend to lower magnesium levels even further. Phosphates are found in abundance in soft drinks and many processed foods.

What *Not* To Do

I want to include smoking here because of how important it is to not only the baby, but to the mother as well. Sometimes the difference between a positive pregnancy and a negative experience is the presence or absence of cigarettes. Important to note is that when you smoke you inhale more than just tobacco smoke. Many dangerous chemical preservatives are added to cigarette tobacco. Read the chapter on Lung Cancer for more on this factor.

Smoking not only directly contributes to ill-health in the mother and development in the child, but affects the body's ability to absorb nutrients, contributing to malnutrition that will also affect the fetus.

One study found women who smoked during conception were two and a half times as likely to have an ectopic or tubal pregnancy, where the egg is fertilized outside the womb, often in the fallopian tubes. Complications from this, if not diagnosed in time, can be severe. The developing embryo can rupture the tubes resulting in infertility and, if not diagnosed in time, death to the mother.

It's well documented that smoking during pregnancy – particularly beyond the fourth month – can cause a wide variety of complications; everything from miscarriage and bleeding in the first trimester to premature separation of the placenta and membranes in the last trimester.

There is also strong evidence that smoking affects the baby's development. The most common side effect to prenatal smoking is low birth weight. But the problems don't stop there. Low birth weight is a bad start to what should be a healthy life. On average, children of smokers have long-term physical and intellectual defects. By age 14, one study showed, children of smokers tended to be more prone to respiratory disease, to be shorter than children of non-smokers, and less successful in school.

Recent research shows that the children of mothers who smoke during pregnancy may have an increased risk of mental retardation. Researchers interviewed 221 mothers whose 10-year-old children have mental retardation with no known cause, and 400 mothers whose 10-year-old children appear normal (controls). Smoking during pregnancy was associated with more than a 50 percent increase in the risk of mental retardation. If the mother smoked one or more packs a day during pregnancy, there was more than a 75 percent increase in the risk of mental retardation.[11]

The cause seems to be carbon monoxide and cyanide poisoning, and a reduction of oxygen to the fetus through the placenta. In effect, when people smoke, their babies are living in a smoke-filled womb. Their heartbeat speeds, they cough and sputter, and worst of all they can't grow and thrive as they should.

Don't Drink

"Behold, thou shalt conceive, and bear a son; now beware, drink no wine or strong drink," an angel tells Samson's mother in the Book of Judges. Good advice. She was able to start eating right when her son was just a gleam in his father's eye.

Traditional medicine warns against chronic use of alcohol during pregnancy. Consistent, daily drinking can increase the risk of miscarriage, prematurity, complications during labor and delivery, and developmental lags in later infancy and childhood.

Heavy drinking by a pregnant woman, the kind typical of an alcoholic, can result in death or deformities in the child. Unfortunately, babies born with severe defects due to alcohol occur often enough for health professionals to give it a name: Fetal Alcohol Syndrome.

Traditional medicine excuses occasional alcohol use in pregnancy, even though the safe daily alcohol dose is not known. There are two problems with this: one, each fetus, like each mother, has a different genetic makeup and responds differently to drugs and alcohol; and two, alcohol is heavy with chemicals, processed sugar and empty calories. Why would anyone subject themselves, much less risk the health of their unborn baby, to something that could do such harm?

No, the best advice is to abstain from drinking at any time, especially when pregnant. If celebrating is in order, try carbonated apple juice or if you crave a cocktail, try a "virgin" daiquiri. Insist on fresh fruit and hold the whipped cream.

Prenatal Nutrients
For maximum absorption, take supplements with meals.

Nutrient	Suggested Dosage	Formulation
Acidophilus	At least four billion flora daily on an empty stomach, three times daily	
Aged garlic extract	1 teaspoon three times daily	Liquid
Amino acids	4-6 capsules daily	Multiple formula from natural sources
Antioxidants	2 capsules daily	With selenium and grapeseed extract
Borage oil	2 capsules daily	
Coenzyme Q10	2 capsules daily	With vitamin E, phospholipids and selenium
Fiber	4-8 tablets daily	Psyllium, with herb hyssop
Flaxseed oil	1 tablespoon daily	
Folic acid	5-10 mg daily	
Ginkgo biloba	50 mg three times daily	
L-glutamine	500 mg twice daily	
Multi-mineral	1-4 ounces daily	In liquid solution, with vitamin B12, biotin
Multi-vitamin/mineral	3-6 caplets daily	Freeze-dried plant sources
Vitamin C	Individual bowel tolerance*	With bioflavonoids (quercetin, rutin proanthocyanidins)
Vitamin E	2 capsules (800 IU) daily	d-alpha tocopherol

* To determine individual dosage, on the first day take 1,000 mg hourly until diarrhea occurs, then reduce dosage to just below that for individual daily dosage. Vitamin C is not toxic in large doses but must be taken throughout the day to benefit. Divide dosage to three or four times a day.

CHAPTER 136:

Prostate Problems

"I do not believe in a fate that falls on men however they act; but I do believe in a fate that falls on them unless they act."

–Gilbert K. Chesterton

In 1993 an estimated 35,000 men died in America from prostate cancer, according to *The American Cancer Society*. It is the second leading cause of cancer deaths in men, behind lung cancer. The news doesn't get any better. Nearly 60 percent of men between the ages of 40 and 59 years of age have an enlarged prostate gland. Because of the often subtle symptoms, many don't even know it. Researchers at John Hopkins University and at Roswell Park Memorial Institute found men with an enlarged prostate were four times more likely to develop cancer than those with normal prostates.[1] For early identification, watch for the following symptoms:

- Weak or interrupted urinary stream;

- The feeling you cannot empty your bladder completely;

- A feeling of delay or hesitation when urinating;

- A need to urinate often, especially at night;

- Dribbling.

Any or all of these symptoms can indicate an enlarged prostate (benign prostatic hypertrophy or BPH), or chronic inflammation (prostatitis).

If a cancerous tumor develops, it usually grows on the outer portion of the prostate and may not exhibit symptoms. By the time a tumor causes symptoms, it has grown so large it forces pressure on the urethra. An early-stage tumor can be detected during a regularly-scheduled rectal exam, a PSA blood test or by the use of ultrasound or x-ray.

The prostate, whose function is to secrete a milky white fluid to carry sperm cells out of the penis, surrounds part of the urethra, the tube that carries urine from the bladder.

With advancing age, the prostate enlarges or inflames, a condition called prostatitis.

Because enlargement is common to any prostate problem, difficulty urinating is the first symptom. As the prostate enlarges, it squeezes the urethra, causing urine to back up into the bladder, making it feel full most of the time; and partially blocking the urethra, making it difficult to urinate. As the urethra narrows, you have to push harder to urinate. This can cause the bladder walls to thicken and stretch out of shape, becoming less efficient (when not overdistended, the bladder's capacity is one pint). If urine stays in the bladder, infections and even bladder cancer (from carcinogens in the urine) can develop. The kidneys may fail if they can't drain into the bladder because it's full.

Surgery is the usual course of action for prostate problems. *The New York Times* (June 23, 1992) reported that each year 400,000 American men spend at least $3 billion on prostate surgery. Unfortunately, many men have to repeat the procedure within five years.

Possible complications include infection, blood clots, excessive bleeding, loss of bladder control, impotence and sterility. During surgery, a muscle that is involved in ejaculation may be cut. If this happens, semen may move backward into the bladder, instead of traveling out of the body (pamphlet, Krames Communications, 1991).

Proscar, a well-advertised, best-seller pharmaceutical, was dubbed "not impressive" by an editorial in the October 22, 1992 *New England Journal of Medicine*. Furthermore, as many as five percent of patients taking Proscar become impotent. Dr. Alan Gaby did his own investigation of Proscar and reported that the FDA approved the drug even though it showed little, if any, improvement on the few patients it was tested on.

Conventional therapy inadequacies make prevention the most solid bet. Pre-cancerous prostate problems, fortunately, can be managed with diet.

Think Zinc

Nutrition-minded physicians often prescribe zinc for prostate disorders since the prostate gland is a major storehouse of the mineral. It just so happens one of the major symptoms of a zinc deficiency is an enlarged prostate. Andrew Weil, M.D., recommends 60 mg of zinc daily. When symptoms subside, reduce that amount in half and continue taking it.[2] A super high level of zinc is found in the prostate gland and semen of men with no prostate problems.

Sometimes, due to a number of factors – many associated with age – minerals are poorly absorbed. Only about 10 to 20 percent of the zinc we get from food is properly assimilated. Imagine the tragedy of being mineral deficient, taking supplements, and remaining deficient. Zinc works wonders when it is absorbed quickly and efficiently. Studies have concluded that minerals are best assimilated when they are in solution. Formulations in solution, not just liquid, provide the maximum absorption ratios. This way they are not impaired by a lack of stomach acid, other minerals, too few pancreatic enzymes, a poorly functioning intestinal system, etc., etc. Look for a derived-from-nature mineral blend in solution.

Upon examining 755 enlarged prostate patients, Irving M. Bush, M.D., and associates at Cook County Hospital in Chicago, found most of them had a low amount of zinc in prostate tissue and semen.

Nineteen of these patients were given a 34 mg zinc pill daily for 60 days, then put on a maintenance program of 11 to 23 mg daily. They all reported less pain. An examination revealed that the prostate of fourteen patients diminished in size. Semen levels showed increased zinc.

Two hundred patients with infectious prostatitis were given 11 to 34 mg of zinc daily for 16 weeks, and 140 experienced relief from symptoms and had higher amounts of zinc in their semen.[3]

Only about 10 to 20 percent of the zinc we ingest from foods is properly absorbed. Large amounts of calcium, phytic acid (from grains, nuts and legumes), and cadmium (from pollution and cigarette smoke) can deplete zinc stores in blood and tissues.

Two nutrients must be considered along with zinc: vitamin B6 and copper. Too much copper will deplete zinc stores; they must be equal for optimum usage. Include 2-4 mg of copper with any zinc supplement.

Because zinc and vitamin B6 are intricately involved in hormone metabolism, a deficiency of one or both of these nutrients can be a contributing factor in prostate problems. Vitamin B6 also enhances zinc absorption.

Whenever I recommend one B vitamin I recommend all of the them. All the B vitamins work in synch. Without one, the others can become deficient, and without minerals they don't work at all. When supplementing one B vitamin, always take a good B vitamin complex, at least ten times the RDA. A note about RDAs. They were formulated with *everyone* in mind. Therefore, their recommendations are maintenance levels, not optimum levels. In today's world of pollutants and nutritionally-deficient food (fresh as well as processed), we need more help than the RDAs. Always target supplements that are much higher than the RDAs. You can't overdose on most vitamins, but you can underdose.

Prostatitis – Treating the Infection

Prostatitis, infection of the prostate, can be relieved with inflammation-reducing flavonoids. What, then, do you do about the bacteria? Doctors prescribe antibiotics for infections. The trouble with antibiotics is they kill the good as well as the bad bacteria. They are perhaps the worst thing you can do, and I don't recommend them. Researchers report our bodies are becoming immune to standard antibiotics so they aren't working any more. What is also possible is that they kill so much of our immune arsenal they cause secondary infections. Fungus infections like athlete's foot, for example, can be a direct result of long-term use of antibiotics, and severely debilitate the immune system.

For any infection, I recommend liquid aged garlic extract. Not only can it reduce inflammation, but is a powerful antimicrobial, helpful to combat any viral or bacterial infection.

An article in *The Lancet* (November 13, 1993) reported on a study that showed bioflavonoids to be potent antibacterial and antiviral substances. Prostatitis and urinary tract infections have been known to respond to a combination of vitamins A, B complex, C, E, beta carotene and the bioflavonoids.

This urinary tract connection is not coincidental. Cystitis, infection of the bladder, can occur when the prostate enlarges to the point where urine is unable to escape and bacteria develops. The bacteria from the bladder can then infect the prostate. Keeping the prostate and urinary tract healthy is a dual purpose here.

Dr. Garry Gordon recommends a combination of vitamin C to bowel tolerance, garlic, and 500,000 individual units (IU) of vitamin A for two to three days. What is meant by bowel tolerance is up to the point where diarrhea occurs. Large amounts of vitamin C are not toxic to the body, but are required to battle infection. When the body cannot use vitamin C it throws it off in the form of diarrhea. This is how you know you've taken enough to make a difference. Start at 1,000 milligrams every hour – or 2,000 milligrams every two hours

– and continue until you experience diarrhea or gas, then lower the dosage to just below that.

According to Tom Kruzel, N.D., of Gresham, North Carolina, a deficiency of zinc, vitamin C and proteolytic enzymes (that break down protein), make it easier for an infection to occur. Enzymes and zinc sterilize the urethra and protect the gland from infection, and can be depleted by frequent intercourse.

For more, see my chapter on Cystitis.

The EFAs Solution

There's a folk remedy used for an enlarged prostate – pumpkin seeds – which can be explained nutritionally. Pumpkin seeds contain both zinc and essential fatty acids. Eat lots of foods high in essential fatty acids (EFAs), substances that can't be made by the body. EFAs are most highly concentrated in seeds: safflower, evening primrose, sesame, borage and flaxseed.

Doctors James P. Hart and William L. Cooper, fed daily EFAs to 19 men with BPH and every one experienced a reduction in prostate size.[4]

Based on this study, prostate patients should take a 400 mg capsule of EFAs three times a day.[5] This equals two handfuls of pumpkin or sunflower seeds. Flaxseed and borage oil are the most beneficial oils to ensure adequate and quality EFAs in the diet. Remember, purchase natural, unadulterated oils from health food stores. They must be raw and refrigerated, and eaten fresh. I put mine in the freezer until I'm ready to use it. The reason the oils you buy in the supermarket last so long is because they are devoid of organic matter – and nutrients. It's the organic matter that goes bad quickly, getting rancid.

Amino Acids – the Newest Discovery

Two doctors accidentally discovered three amino acids impor-tant to prostate health. The physicians were treating a group of allergic patients with a mixture of three amino acids – glycine, alanine and glutamic acid. One of the patients volunteered the information that his urinary symptoms had disappeared while on the amino acid mixture. This led to a trial of the same compounds on non-allergic patients with urinary symptoms. Patients with enlarged prostates experienced prompt and rather spectacular relief. The combination of glycine, alanine and glutamic acid has been shown in several studies to relieve many of the symptoms of BPH.[6]

One of the reasons garlic works so well is that it contains amino acids. It also includes immune-boosting and infection-fighting germanium, magnesium, selenium, sulfur compounds, and vitamins A, B1 and C.

Fat + Cholesterol = Enlarged Prostates

A link has been established between the intake of dietary fat and prostate cancer. Some studies have shown vegetarians, who have a low saturated fat intake, have a lower incidence of cancer of the prostate than men with high fat intake. The same studies show a vegetarian diet lowers circulating testosterone levels and a non-vegetarian diet raises them. Prostate cancer increases in the presence of testosterone and slows when testosterone is lowered. A study of Japanese men conducted in 1977 noted that the marked increase in mortality from prostate cancer paralleled the increase in fat intake in the Japanese diet since 1950.[7]

Eliminating most of the fat in men's diets would greatly reduce the number of prostatic maladies.

Dr. Carl P. Schaffner, Ph.D., professor of microbial chemistry at Rutgers University, discovered that by reducing cholesterol levels in aged dogs, he was also able to reduce the size of the animals' enlarged prostates.

Another study, reported to the American Urological Association, corroborates the possibly harmful effects of high cholesterol levels on prostate disease. Dr. Cammille Mallouh, M.D., Chief of Urology at Metropolitan Hospital in New York, examined 100 prostates from men of all ages and found an 80 percent increase in cholesterol content of enlarged prostates. Cholesterol has been shown to accumulate in an enlarged or cancerous human prostate (*Cancer Research*, December 1979).

Cancer of the prostate may be associated with our typical "civilized" Western diet. Peter Hill, Ph.D., of New York City's American Health Foundation, noted that rural black South Africans who typically eat a low-fat, whole-food diet had healthy prostates. He conducted a test to see if their diet was the cause. Dr. Hill and his associates put a group of volunteers on a typical Western diet of lots of meats and fats. At the same time, a group of North American volunteers, blacks and whites, were put on a low-fat diet. Dr. Hill and his colleagues then tested the subjects for diet-induced hormonal changes associated with prostatic cancer.

After three weeks, Dr. Hill found that the South Africans eating the Western diet excreted notably more hormones, while the reverse occurred with the North American subjects. The metabolic profile of the North Americans now resembled the low-risk group. Dr. Hill stated, "This study is a preliminary indication that a low-fat diet is one of the factors which can lower the risk of prostatic cancer. By reducing total calorie intake, and substituting fruit and vegetable calories for animal calories, a high-risk prostatic cancer group has switched to a low-risk one."[8]

Prostate Healthy Protocol

For a healthy prostate, pay attention to your lifestyle. As much as you may like pizza and beer, your prostate hates it. Cut out fats in favor of oils. Instead of butter or margarine, spread garlic and olive oil on your whole grain (not white) bread. Reduce your cholesterol level and exercise to increase circulation. As you get older, and the odds are against you, supplement daily with vitamin C and bioflavonoids, and the herbs garlic, saw palmetto, ginseng and silica.

Take a good mineral in solution formula that includes zinc, an antioxidant formula, and a high B complex formula.

Eating whole foods is the best, eating sprouts even better. Therefore, look for supplementation that uses the whole food. One such formula uses freeze dried sprouts and vegetables, combined in such a way as to provide all the essential vitamins and minerals, as well as adding odorless garlic, acidophilus and green tea extract for immune-system boosting.

If you think or know you have an enlarged prostate and need more, target the amino acids alanine, glutamic acid and glycine. Add borage oil, and eat pumpkin seeds. All of the above will help prevent prostate cancer. For added help, make a habit of eating soy products and fortify with vitamin D foods like cod liver oil. By following these recommendations, your prostate and urinary tract will thank you with years of pain-free living.

Prostate-Healthy Nutrients

For maximum absorption, supplements should be taken with meals.

Nutrient	Suggested Dosage	Formulation
Aged garlic extract	2 teaspoons three times daily	Liquid
Amino acids	4-6 capsules daily	Multiple formula from natural sources
Antioxidants	4 capsules daily	With selenium and grape seed extract
Borage oil	2 capsules daily	
Coenzyme Q10	2 capsules daily	With vitamin E, phospholipids and selenium
Enzymes	2 capsules twice daily	Multiple formula
Flaxseed oil	1 tablespoon daily	
Fiber	8 tablets daily	Psyllium, with herb hyssop
Folic acid	10 mg daily	
Multi-vitamin/mineral	6 caplets daily	Freeze-dried plant sources
Multi-mineral	2-4 ounces daily	In liquid solution, with vitamin B12, biotin
Pygeum	250 mg twice daily	
Saw palmetto	160 mg twice daily	
Vitamin B6	100 mg daily	
Vitamin C	Individual bowel tolerance*	With bioflavonoids (quercetin, proanthocyanidins)
Vitamin E	2 capsules (800 IU) daily	d-alpha tocopherol

* To determine individual dosage, on the first day take 1,000 mg hourly until diarrhea occurs, then reduce dosage to just below that for individual daily dosage. Vitamin C is not toxic in large doses but must be taken throughout the day to benefit. Divide dosage to three or four times a day.

CHAPTER 137:

Psoriasis

Only people who suffer from it can fully comprehend the torment and "heartbreak" of psoriasis. Rather than try to explain what sufferers go through, I'll let them speak for themselves. Via an online computer service, here are the comments of people with psoriasis who have reached out to others like them.

Susan: "My condition is getting worse by the minute. My skin hurts…I am dreading going to work tomorrow. I wish I could just move on but when you hurt and have to see it as well as feel it…it makes it twice as hard to deal with the condition…Has anyone tried psychotherapy…?"

Brian: "I've had it for nearly 30 years, and am a psychotherapist. Maybe a mental health professional could help, if the inner turmoil is severe. I hate it too, but I guess I view it as just one of those things in life. It can be especially hard when we live in such a beauty-oriented, outward-oriented culture. Personally, I have refused to dress to cover it up for a long time."

Scott: "I refuse to quit wearing shorts and tee's to cover up this stuff!!! I'm 38 so this comes as a surprise to me to have this breakout. Stress level is normal lately so that's not an excuse. I give up trying to guess what has caused it."

John: "I have found some comfort knowing that I am not alone (scratch, scratch…flake, flake)…This is so frustrating…it seemed to spread to my extremities when I "chased" it off of my forehead and scalp…it seemed to be getting back at me. I am struggling to know what to do about the rest of me…(thank God it's not you-know-where!!)"

Joluca: "My psoriasis first appeared on my scalp eight years ago. It eventually covered three quarters of my scalp and spread to my legs, arms, face, ears, and the last injustice, my genitals. It made me feel dirty and out of control. I called it The Crud. Every treatment I tried helped temporarily. Three years ago I lost my job and my great health insurance. I didn't know what to do. Last month I did the unthinkable and shaved my head. It was liberating."

My heart was just about breaking as I read through the messages left by people desperate for an end to their madness. If you are one of the many who are anguished, and relate to what those above are saying, read on, for I am happy to offer hope in a realm where there is little, and where every day is a battle with shampoos, tars, chemicals and various concoctions, and very little cure in sight.

What exactly is psoriasis?

Fortunately, since psoriasis is so common, there is much room for support. Unfortunately, that leaves a lot of people desperate for help. Sufferers understand it all too well. They know it isn't contagious, and that it can be identified by its bright red, sharply outlined dry plaques covered with silvery scales. Some get it only on the scalp, and others are dismayed to find it spreading to their extremities: knees, elbows, and lower back. As if the cosmetic disfiguring wasn't hard enough to live with, it is usually accompanied by a stippled appearance of the nails, and sometimes by an arthritis called psoriatic arthritis, which is similar to rheumatoid arthritis.[1]

Between three and five million Americans are estimated to have psoriasis. Although it affects men and women of all ages, it is more pronounced in those between the ages of 15 and 35.[2]

In healthy people, the average life cycle of skin cells – dead skin cells flaking off, being replaced by new skin cells – occurs every 26 to 28 days. In people with psoriasis this cycle is accelerated, taking just three to four days, hence the "scratch, scratch, flake, flake" effect described above by John. With such an accelerated production of immature cells, they pile up and form unsightly and sometimes irritating plaques on the skin's surface.[3]

Which comes first? The psoriasis or the stress? Either one is bad enough. However, in some cases, outbreaks of psoriasis occur after physical or emotional stress. It can be a general infection like the flu, strep throat, a skin injury, or a severe emotional jolt like the death of a loved one, loss of a job or losing one's life savings. This stress connection is significant, as you shall see.

Skin or Dining Disorder?

Some researchers believe psoriasis is connected to what you eat. Not coincidentally, arthritis is also believed to be diet-related.

Some of the most common food allergens: dairy products, eggs and meat have been found in certain people to contribute to psoriasis, as reported in the medical journal *Cutis*.[4]

A New Jersey chiropractor, Dr. John Pagano, studied this disorder for 15 years, and he reports that psoriasis is not a skin disorder, but rather a result of toxins seeping into the skin because of intestinal problems.[5]

Pagano says a good diet for psoriasis sufferers is composed of 80 percent non-acid, alkaline foods and 20 percent acidic foods. The nightshades: tomatoes, eggplant, white potatoes, peppers *and tobacco,* are no-nos, as are alcohol, pizza, shellfish, fried foods, beef, veal and pork. And don't combine cereals with fruit, he says.[6]

A study reported in *California Medicine* said that one of six patients with psoriasis improved on an elimination diet which avoided citrus fruits, nuts, corn and milk. The other five improved after restricting such acidic foods as coffee, tomatoes, soda and pineapple. [7]

Of nine patients with psoriasis discussed in an article in the *Southern Medical Journal*, five of them had no stomach acid and only one patient had normal hydrochloric acid levels. Stomach acid is necessary to break down food properly, so your body may absorb the nutrients it contains. Not enough stomach acid is linked to an incredible array of disorders, including psoriasis. B vitamins are especially deficient when stomach acid is too low. Studies have shown that psoriasis has improved with the addition of hydrochloric acid and B vitamin supplements.[8]

If you suspect you might have this problem, you can restore your gastric acid by taking Betaine HCl, a hydrochloric acid supplement available in health food stores. Some multi-vitamin and mineral supplements also contains Betaine. Another option would be to take nutrients, specifically the minerals, in solution, to overcome the stomach acid limitation.

The Fish Oil Fix

Many of the troublesome foods, such as dairy products, eggs and meat, are high in arachidonic acid, an amino acid that some have trouble assimilating. And what do you suppose helps? Cold water fish!

Omega-3 oil (derived from cold water fish or flaxseeds) makes the body more efficient in processing arachidonic acid. S.S. Bleehan, M.D., professor of dermatology at the Royal Hallamshire Hospital, Sheffield, England, used ten fish oil capsules daily for 12 weeks and found that patients' itching, redness and scaling were reduced markedly.[9]

His experiments showed that omega-3 oil in 5-1/2 ounces of mackerel, trout, sardines or salmon eaten daily can significantly lessen the itching, redness and scaling associated with psoriasis.[10]

Dr. Vincent Ziboh, a dermatology professor and biochemist at the University of California, cites a similar research project conducted by both U.C. and the University of Michigan in which 60 percent of psoriasis patients experienced reduced itching, redness and scaling by taking omega-3 capsules daily.[11]

John J. Voorhees, M.D., Department of Dermatology, University of Michigan Medical School, Ann Arbor, points out that Greenland Eskimos, who eat large quantities of deepwater fish, rarely have psoriasis.[12]

Researchers from Chiba University in Japan recently reported beneficial effects when psoriasis patients were treated with highly purified EPA for short periods of time. In this report, they describe the results of long-term treatment (up to one year) of nine patients with chronic stable psoriasis. All patients received 3.6 g daily of 90 percent pure EPA.[13]

Of six patients who completed a full year of treatment, five showed varying degrees of improvement (with one showing marked improvement), one showed no change, and none worsened during therapy. Clinical improvement first appeared two to three months after treatment began and continued as long as EPA was administered.[14]

Other Favorable Fatty Acids

Other types of fatty acids have shown to be of benefit as well. A diet rich in linoleic acid and supplemented with evening primrose oil (to provide both linoleic acid and gamma-linoleic acid – GLA) might improve psoriasis.[15]

Such a diet would enhance the production of prostaglandins and inhibit the formation of leukotrienes. Prostaglandins are hormone-like natural fatty acids that help to regulate many physiological functions in the body. Leukotrienes are other hormone-like substances which can trigger inflammation. In British and U.S. studies, linoleic acids appeared to render leukotrienes less active.[16]

Diet supplements of evening primrose oil have recently been shown to improve atopic dermatitis in a double-blind study. No side effects were noted."[17]

I always recommend borage oil instead of evening primrose oil. They contain the same beneficial fatty acids – only borage oil contains more. Independent clinical tests show that borage oil contains up to 26 percent GLA. Compare this to evening primrose oil and black currant oil, which contain no more than 18 percent. Not only that, borage oil costs less because the borage seed is three times larger than black currant or evening primrose seeds. Finally, borage is more bioavailable. In other words, the body more readily accepts it.[18]

Flaxseed oil is one of the richest sources of omega-3 essential fatty acids, so it's not surprising that these, too, have been associated with the treatment of psoriasis.

Donald O. Rudin, M.D., wrote about one such therapy in his book *The Omega-3 Phenomenon*. He said he has seen two cases of life-long psoriasis, one mild and one severe, which were improved with flaxseed oil therapy over a period of four to six months.[19]

Other Nutrients That Help

Patients should also explore the possible effects of vitamins B1, B3 and B6, zinc, magnesium, selenium, fiber, and lactobacillus acidophilus, found in yogurt and supplements. The latter two suggestions, of course, improve gastrointestinal health.[20]

All the B vitamins, especially B1, B3 and B6, are essential to the nerves. Since there is a connection between stress and psoriasis it makes sense to nourish your nerves with B vitamins. However, to get maximum benefit from any B vitamin, it's necessary to take a formula that contains all the B vitamins. The whole B complex family includes B1 (thiamine), B2 (riboflavin), B3 (niacin), B6 (pyridoxine, B12 (cobalamin), folic acid, pantothenic acid, biotin, inositol and choline.

Zinc is very important to the skin and can make the difference between pockmarks and smooth-as-silk skin.

Magnesium is essential to your nerves, muscles, bones and tissues.

Selenium is a powerful antioxidant (boosts the immune system) and is also found in fish.

I recall a case study about a 42-year-old woman who suffered from weekly migraine headaches since puberty, and had psoriasis since she was 25. She was placed on a sugar-and milk-free diet supplemented with 500 mg of niacinamide (B3) four times a day; 250 mg of pyridoxine (B6) daily; and 220 mg of zinc sulfate each day. Six weeks later the psoriasis was improved. [21]

Some patients with psoriasis may have a folic acid deficiency, (another B vitamin) which can be remedied with supplementation.[22]

In a study reported in the *British Journal of Dermatology*, 16 of 58 patients with psoriasis (27 percent) had low blood levels of folic acid. Four of the patients (seven percent) had subnormal red blood count folic acid levels, while 16 (27 percent) had an abnormal variety of red blood cells. Only 12 patients of the 58 had normal folic acid absorption.[23]

Let's Think Lecithin

Lecithin is a nutrient that ensures healthy skin. It is necessary to every cell and organ in the body, including the skin and its cells.

And, guess what? Lecithin provides the body with inositol and choline, essential-to-the-body B vitamins. Isn't it amazing the connections you find when you just look?

In one study, 254 psoriasis patients taking four to eight tablespoons of lecithin each day recovered in five months.[24]

In a study reported in the *New York State Journal of Medicine*, 118 of 155 patients with psoriasis responded with purified granulated soya lecithin. The study lasted for 10 years. Each volunteer received from 15 to 45 grams daily of lecithin. The patients also received unspecified amounts of vitamin A, D, B1, B2, B5 and B6.[25]

Lecithin was originally extracted from egg yolk, but most lecithin today is made from soybeans. Today's practice of refining and hydrogenating fats (a process that converts oil into margarine) destroys the lecithin so only the cholesterol remains, which then accumulates in the arteries. Even oil can be hydrogenated to some degree, so read the label!

Soy lecithin is an inexpensive, convenient and natural way to supplement the lecithin in your body. Get your family chef (ha ha) to include four to eight tablespoons of soy lecithin granules in salad oil dressings or sprinkled on whole grain cereals or oatmeal.

Ban the Bottle

Psoriasis may, for some, be a result of drinking alcohol. In a study published in the *British Medical Journal*, researchers in Finland asked 144 young and middle-aged men with psoriasis and 285 with other skin diseases to recall their drinking habits the year before their problems developed. Those men with psoriasis habitually drank, on average, twice as much as the others and became intoxicated nearly one and a half times as often. Their average daily intake of alcohol was heavy – the equivalent of more than a liter of beer or nearly half a liter of wine.[26]

The researchers note that drinking this much increases the risks of infection and injury, which are known to trigger psoriasis, and they speculate that alcohol may also bring on the disease through its crippling effect on the immune system.[27] Alcoholism also dangerously lowers thiamine/B1 levels, creating a host of problems, including nervous system damage.

If a person itches to get inebriated, they should remember the potential risk of psoriasis. And since one third of psoriasis patients studied said drinking worsened their condition, sufferers should consider cutting out booze to soothe their affliction.[28]

Conclusion for Psoriasis Sufferers

Let's review what you can do to combat your psoriasis. First, look at the possibility you may have food allergies. In the Allergies chapter you'll see some tests and techniques you can use to determine if you have any. Consult the Arthritis chapter too, if you have problems with psoriatic arthritis.

Eat foods that will make you healthy and boost your immune system: coldwater fish like salmon, mackerel and herring, whole grains and green vegetables. Most of us don't eat enough of these foods anyway.

Concentrate on supplements that will help. Fish oil supplements that contain EPA and DHA are found in vitamin stores. Lecithin, flaxseed oil, linseed oil and borage oil can be found in vitamin or health food stores too.

Emphasize the B vitamins, folic acid, magnesium, zinc and selenium in easy-to-digest formulas using natural ingredients. Betaine will help if you're like most people who lose stomach acid as they get older, but if you take a minerals in solution formula, you may not need Betaine.

Don't drink and don't smoke.

And, most importantly, don't sweat it. To coin a well-used phrase, if life gives you lemons, make lemonade. Try not to stress the small stuff, and when you find yourself dealing with hardship and tragedy, seek God's comfort and read the chapter on Stress.

Though I walk in the midst of trouble, thou wilt revive me; thou shalt stretch forth thine hand against the wrath of mine enemies, and thy right hand shall save me. – Psalm 138:7

Psoriasis-Stopping Nutrients
For maximum absorption, take supplements with meals.

Nutrient	Suggested Dosage	Formulation
Aged garlic extract	1 teaspoon three times daily	Liquid
Antioxidants	4 capsules daily*	With selenium and grapeseed extract
Borage oil	2 capsules daily	
Flaxseed oil	1 tablespoon daily	
Glucosamine sulfate	500 mg three times daily	
Lecithin	2 tablespoons with meals	
Magnesium	200 mg twice daily	
MSM (Methylsulfonylmethane)	500 mg three times daily	
Multi-mineral	3-4 ounces daily	In liquid solution, with vitamin B12, biotin
Multi-vitamin/mineral	6 caplets daily	Freeze-dried plant sources
Nettle	250 mg three times daily	
Quercetin	400 mg twice daily	With vitamin C
Vitamin B6	100 mg daily	
Vitamin C	Individual bowel tolerance**	With bioflavonoids (quercetin, proanthocyanidins)

Nourish with a moisturizing lotion containing vitamins A, C and E.

* The FDA recommends pregnant women not exceed 10,000 IU of vitamin A daily.

** To determine individual dosage, on the first day take 1,000 mg hourly until diarrhea occurs, then reduce dosage to just below that for individual daily dosage. Vitamin C is not toxic in large doses but must be taken throughout the day to benefit. Divide dosage to three or four times a day.

CHAPTER 138:

Restless Leg Syndrome

Audrey didn't quite know what to make of her problem. It reminded her of Angie, her Pekinese. Sometimes when Angie slept her legs would move repeatedly, as though she were running in her sleep. It was funny in a dog, but not so funny for Audrey. Unlike Angie, who slept through her leg movements, Audrey would wake up with peculiar creeping or crawling sensations, numbness and sometimes pain, usually in the lower leg, deep inside the muscle or bones. In order to shake it off, Audrey would have to get up and walk around the room. Then it would take her hours to get back to sleep.

Audrey's doctor told her it was "nerves," and gave her antidepressants to help her sleep. The drugs made her symptoms much worse. Desperate for sleep, she consulted Dr. Ross Gordon. He told her she had restless leg syndrome, or RLS for short. Reassuring her with the good news it can be a result of nutritional deficiencies, he sent her to a laboratory for blood tests.

RLS is less common than nighttime leg cramps, but nonetheless is reported to occur in five percent of healthy normal people; in 15 percent of people having just had surgery; and in 15 to 20 percent of people having kidney dialysis treatments.[1] It can occur in the daytime and at night. One woman with RLS was unable to visit the theater for 15 years because she could not sit still.[2] Because it occurs most often in people under stress and under a conventional physician's care, deficiencies, not nerves, should be the first possible diagnosis.

Associated with Iron Deficiency Anemia

Dr. Gordon's tests found Audrey was deficient in iron and the B vitamins. After a month of supplementation, Audrey was able to sleep most of the night; after two months, she had no more RLS.

Many studies show the connection between too little iron and RLS. Whatever the cause of the lack of iron, the result seems to be RLS.

In one case study, a 36-year-old female with a history of panic attacks developed a severe case of RLS following medication for the attacks. Her doctors proclaimed her problem to be "nerves." However, her medical records showed early symptoms began after surgery some three years prior. Following the operation, she had much blood loss. A test found she had low iron levels and when she was given ferrous sulfate, her RLS stopped.[3]

Regarding the woman who could not attend the theater, iron supplements relieved her restless legs.

A controlled-study of 36 elderly subjects found that those with RLS had low iron levels. Out of 18 RLS patients, 15 showed improvement after taking ferrous sulfate at 200 milligrams three times daily for two months.[4]

Iron absorption can be impaired or enhanced by certain nutrients. For example, ascorbic acid – vitamin C – enhances absorption. Too much phosphorus – found in great amounts in soft drinks – hinders absorption. It turned out that Audrey's penchant for cola drinks is what probably caused her RLS. Not only was the phosphorus depleting her body of iron, but so was the caffeine.

It is important to remember that since iron is primarily stored in the liver, spleen, bone marrow and blood, it is possible to take too much. Iron overload can result in organ damage, with symptoms that include headaches, fatigue, dizziness and weight loss.[5] Always consult a physician versed in nutrition before supplementing with iron.

British physician T. A. Jeddy warns that certain medications can make RLS worse. These include phenytoin, neuroleptics and antidepressants,[6] which is what must have happened to the unfortunate woman in the case study. The last thing you want to do is take medications for your RLS. Not only do they not work, they can make the problem worse. Never accept a doctor's prognosis of "nerves." Nerves need nutrition just like anything else. If your nervous system is out of whack, look to nutritional, not conventional crisis, solutions.

Vitamins Found to Help

Vitamin E and folic acid have been shown to help with RLS.[7] In his excellent book, *Nutritional Influences on Illness* (2nd Edition, Third Line Press, 1993), Melvyn R. Werbach, M.D., cites case reports of six women with RLS who were found to be folate deficient and were relieved of their symptoms with folic acid supplementation.[8]

Folic acid is a B vitamin. All the B vitamins are essential to a healthy nervous system, and are required in a complex for the body to utilize them. If you supplement with folic acid, also take a B-complex formula. The studies described above utilized high amounts of folic acid--five milligrams three times daily. Due to the possibility of creating deficiencies in other B vitamins, Dr. Werbach recommends these high dosages be given by a physician only.

Vitamin E has also been found to help. In an experimental study, seven out of nine RLS patients were completely improved following vitamin E supplementation. Some improvement was noted in the other two.[9]

In a case study, a 78-year-old woman with a 20-year history of "jumpy" legs up to several times nightly was unresponsive to the drugs phenytoin and diphenhydramine. After taking 300 IU of vitamin E for two months, she was completely cured.[10]

The same result was achieved in a 37-year-old woman with a ten-year history of severe RLS. She was placed on 300 IU daily for six weeks and 200 IU daily for the following four weeks with complete relief.[11]

Vitamin E works because it increases circulation, and restless legs can occur as a result of poor circulation. He warns, however, that vitamin E can temporarily elevate the blood pressure, and recommends that it be taken in gradually increasing dosages.[12] Vitamin E should not be taken with iron. For more, see my chapter Circulation Problems.

The amino acid L-tryptophan has also been noted to help, and is available in amino acid formulas. For more on tryptophan, see the chapter Depression.

Leg-Restful Nutrients
For maximum absorption, take supplements with meals.

Nutrient	Suggested Dosage	Formulation
Aged garlic extract	1 teaspoon three times daily	Liquid
Amino acids	4-6 capsules daily	Multiple formula from natural sources
Borage oil	2 capsules daily	
Fiber	4-8 tablets daily	Psyllium, with herb hyssop
Flaxseed oil	1 tablespoon daily	
Folic acid	5-10 mg daily	
Ginkgo biloba	50 mg three times daily	
Melatonin (adults only)	3 mg daily at bedtime	With B vitamins
Multi-mineral	3-4 ounces daily	In liquid solution, with vitamin B12, biotin
Multi-vitamin/mineral	6 caplets daily	Freeze-dried plant sources
Niacin	500 mg four times daily	
Taurine	500 mg twice daily	
Vitamin B6	100 mg daily	
Vitamin C	Individual bowel tolerance*	With bioflavonoids (quercetin, proanthocyanidins)
Vitamin E	2 capsules (800 IU) daily	d-alpha tocopherol

* To determine individual dosage, on the first day take 1,000 mg hourly until diarrhea occurs, then reduce dosage to just below that for individual daily dosage. Vitamin C is not toxic in large doses but must be taken throughout the day to benefit. Divide dosage to three or four times a day.

CHAPTER 139:

Retinitis Pigmentosa

"Through every rift of discovery some seeming anomaly drops out of the darkness, and falls, as a golden link, into the great chain of order."
                                        –Edwin Hubbel Chapin

If your ophthalmologist says you have retinitis pigmentosa (RP), ask, "Which one?" Following conventional medicine's penchant for puzzles, RP is a name given to a range of inherited eye diseases that collectively affect about 100,000 Americans and 1.5 million people worldwide. All are credited with progressively destroying the retina.

The Pigment Puzzle Solved

As I searched for research on this affliction, one thing kept hounding me: why pigmentosa? Nothing seemed to explain the connection between pigment, or color, and retinitis. That is until I found an article in the *Journal of the American Medical Association* (JAMA) that connected RP with lipofuscin. Once I discovered this term, the research poured in. Then the pieces came together.

Interestingly, the best explanation I found of lipofuscin came from one of the most conventional medical textbooks in use today: *The Mt. Sinai School of Medicine Complete Book of Nutrition*. Nutritional ignorance is not only prevalent in the conventional medical field, but in the conventional nutritional field as well. Most hospital dieticians are unaware of the many influences nutrition has on health, since their educational institutions deny the numerous research studies which show nutrition may be used therapeutically. However, even the Mt. Sinai School of Medicine acknowledges that antioxidants can help with afflictions caused by free radical damage.

I quote: "Free radicals are a by-product of oxygen metabolism. Oxygen is essential to life, but, as it passes through the cells of the body, it breaks down and substances called free radicals are formed. Free radicals attack cell membranes, affecting their normal functioning and producing an accumulation of lipofuscin, a brown pigment. Commonly referred to as age pigment, lipofuscin in brain tissue has been related to senility; and in the skin, it appears as age spots. Damage to the cells by free radicals appears to be irreversible. However, substances known as free-radical scavengers, among them intracellular enzymes such as superoxide dismutase and antioxidant (supplements) such as vitamin E, vitamin C and selenium…are able to deactivate the free radicals."[1]

The Antioxidant Answer

Researchers have discovered an excess of lipofuscin – brown pigment – contributes to retinitis pigmentosa, and that persons with this disorder are often deficient in the antioxidant vitamin E.[2] Likened to age spots on the retina, antioxidant vitamins have been shown in studies to prevent the oxidation and subsequent cell damage of lipofuscin in the retina.

Several experiments discovered that when lipofuscin was found in the retina of the eyes of animals and human beings, they were deficient in the antioxidants vitamin E and vitamin A.[3]

In one ground-breaking study, patients were randomly assigned to one of four groups, each receiving varying doses of vitamins A and E for an average of five years. Those who received 15,000 International Units of vitamin A had, on average, a 20 percent slower yearly decline of retinal function (toxic levels are considered above 100,000 IU).

Researchers at Hoffman-La Roche in Basel, Switzerland, found that when there is a deficiency of vitamin E, lipofuscin accumulates in the retina. They also discovered that the antioxidant vitamins A and C, beta carotene, and the mineral selenium can stop retinal cell damage. It seems the retina naturally contains a higher concentration of carotenoids and vitamins E and C than other tissues and needs it to protect itself from the damaging effects of sunlight, cholesterol and, of course, lipofuscin.[4]

An Amino Acid Answer

The symptoms of retinitis pigmentosa are a loss of eyesight in specific portions of the visual field. It is believed to be caused by a defective gene, which, in my book, is not a good answer. When physicians talk about genetic "carriers" and "inherited traits," it leads people to believe the problem is irrefutable, inevitable and unpreventable. Not so! What causes the genes to go awry? Could it be nutrition? What isn't explained is how these defective or weak genes cause the disease in the first place. What is likely is that defective genes simply create an abnormal nutritional imbalance, that once identified, can be corrected. Evidence shows this may be the case in many, many afflictions, retinitis pigmentosa included.

Premonitions should not be made through statistics. It may be true that retinitis pigmentosa usually begins in adults between the ages of 20 and 30 years, but it doesn't have to be true that a patient will lose 4.6 percent of his vision every year.[5]

If genetics is the explanation, how can there be an answer? One of the answers to retinitis pigmentosa is the amino acid *taurine*. It is known that taurine can protect the eye and body from various toxins.

Although there have not yet been reports of taurine-deficient blindness in humans, one study found that people suffering from retinitis pigmentosa show low blood levels of taurine.[6]

In the human body, taurine regulates heartbeat, brain chemistry and vision, and is helpful in digesting fats and ridding the body of cholesterol. Since it is found in body tissues, especially the eyes and heart, it was long thought that we didn't need taurine from food. However, studies at the Oregon Primate Research Center in Portland in 1984 showed that baby monkeys fed milk with no taurine developed eye trouble.[7]

Retina-Restoring Nutrients
For maximum absorption, take supplements with meals.

Nutrient	Suggested Dosage	Formulation
Amino acids	4-6 capsules daily	Multiple formula from natural sources
Antioxidants	4 capsules daily*	With selenium and grapeseed extract
Bilberry	100 mg twice daily	
Borage oil	2 capsules daily	
Coenzyme Q10	2 capsules daily	With vitamin E, phospholipids and selenium
Flaxseed oil	1 tablespoon daily	
Ginkgo biloba	60 mg daily	
Magnesium	200 mg daily	
Multi-mineral	3-4 ounces daily	In liquid solution, with vitamin B12, biotin
Multi-vitamin/mineral	6 caplets daily	Freeze-dried plant sources
Taurine	500 mg twice daily	
Vitamin A	25,000 IU daily*	
Vitamin C	Individual bowel tolerance**	With bioflavonoids (quercetin, rutin proanthocyanidins)

* The FDA recommends pregnant women not exceed 10,000 IU of vitamin A daily.

** To determine individual dosage, on the first day take 1,000 mg hourly until diarrhea occurs, then reduce dosage to just below that for individual daily dosage. Vitamin C is not

CHAPTER 140:

Schizophrenia

Schizophrenia caused by coffee? Now, how likely is that? Although it might be a stretch to assume coffee causes schizophrenia, it may make it harder to live with.

Mark was admitted to a mental institution diagnosed as having paranoid schizophrenia. He was 32 years old, drank large quantities of alcohol, smoked two packs of cigarettes daily and consumed dark, caffeinated instant coffee several times a day. His doctors put him on medications including sedatives, but didn't restrict his intake of coffee. His behavior was uncontrollable, and within a month he assaulted a staff member. Desperate, his doctor ordered Mark's coffee intake to be restricted. There were no outbursts until four weeks later after he allegedly stole a jar of instant coffee. On a visit to court he was given a cup of coffee and began to pound the walls.[1]

Harold was a 29-year-old man, picked up by police in the street. He had been pacing, posturing and responding to auditory and visual hallucinations. He had a history of chronic psychotic illness, alcohol and drug abuse, and was institutionalized. In the hospital, doctors took away his coffee. Following an incident where he was caught stealing instant coffee from other patient's lockers, he had an unusual outburst in front of a nurse and had to be put into a secluded environment. His violent episodes were quelled only when he stopped drinking coffee.[2]

My point in relating these case histories is that schizophrenic episodes can be influenced by diet. These two men were real patients in a real institution. While doctors failed to identify the cause of the patients' initial schizophrenia, they did believe alcohol abuse and subsequent ingestion of instant coffee influenced the frequency and extent of the troublesome outbursts. The fact that both patients felt the need to steal coffee, once restricted from it, illustrates the addictive nature of this controlled substance – not to be underestimated, especially in mental illness.

What exactly is schizophrenia? *Churchill's Medical Dictionary* defines it as "Any group of disorders characterized by a progressive deterioration of the entire personality manifested in disorders of feeling, thinking and conduct, and a tendency to withdraw from reality to an inner world of fantasy, preoccupation with the self, delusions and hallucinations." It adds that the symptoms should occur for at least six months. In other words, it is a group of symptoms, conveniently lumped into one broad term, which occur over a long period of time. When it becomes one term, it makes finding the cause all the more difficult, as well as makes those involved believe it is an incurable disease. Conventional medicine likes to blame heredity. Heredity may be the *reason* for schizophrenia, but it is certainly not the cause.

According to the *Harvard Mental Health Letter*, "The rate of the disorder among biological first-degree relatives (parents, children, brothers, and sisters) of a schizophrenic person is 5 to 10 percent. A child of two schizophrenic parents has about a 40 percent chance of being schizophrenic. It occurs at a 30 to 50 percent rate among the identical twins of schizophrenics, but only a 10 to 15 percent rate in fraternal twins.[3]

Based on my research, I believe schizophrenia occurs when a genetic defect causes an inability of the body to either absorb or use certain nutrients. Too many symptoms of schizophrenia are matched to symptoms of certain nutritional deficiencies. And, as you shall see, schizophrenia can be improved through nutritional intervention. Doctors and researchers are doing it all the time.

The B12 Solution

A vitamin B12 deficiency is a real bogey man – especially in the over-60 crowd. It can produce psychosis, severe memory loss, impaired abstract thinking skills, mental confusion, delusions, hallucinations and even brain and spinal cord degeneration (causing numbness). Low blood levels of the vitamin are found in one-third of hospitalized psychiatric patients suffering from depression and dementia, according to a Denmark study.[4] In addition, a B12 deficiency may inhibit the brain's use of glucose (the gasoline which energizes the brain) and hinder production of acetylcholine, a vitally important brain chemical.

A deficiency of B12 can be caused by exposure to toxic chemicals and ingestion of mercury, heavy metals (cadmium, lead) and certain solvents, which prevent transfer of the vitamin from the blood to the brain. Cigarettes contain many chemicals, other than nicotine, as do certain alcohols and instant coffee. Prescription drugs can also keep B12 from getting to the brain. Some offenders are aldomet, neomycin and para-aminosalicylic acid.

Various experiments indicate that a deficiency of vitamin B12 causes devastating emotional and mental symptoms including depression, paranoia, delusions, manic behavior, visual and auditory hallucinations, confusion and difficulty thinking and remembering.[5]

One study reported that among 25 cases of a vitamin B12 deficiency syndrome, half the patients had brain abnormalities. All the patients experienced slowing of mental processes, confusion, and memory problems. Half experienced chronic depression, 35 percent had delusions, 21 percent had hallucinations, and 7 percent were aggressive and manic.[6]

An editorial in the *British Medical Journal* stated that a vitamin B12 deficiency may cause severe psychotic symptoms which can vary in severity from mild mood swings to severe psychotic episodes. If a deficiency is not detected in its early stages, it may result in permanent mental deterioration.[7]

What is very important to note is that all the study participants had too little stomach, or hydrochloric, acid, which is necessary to break down food so nutrients can be absorbed. Stomach acid is diminished under stress, illness and with age, and can be a very common denominator among the mentally ill and impaired.

Remember, you're not what you put into your mouth, you're what you absorb and digest and deliver to cells. A vitamin or mineral tablet is only one to five percent absorbable. Since the process of digestion is a process of liquefaction, your body has to take a hard rock tablet and turn it into solution. This may not be possible due to inadequate stomach acid, food allergies and intestinal problems. This is why it is so important that when you decide to supplement, you target nutrients in solution. Look for a good, easily absorbable, derived-from-nature nutritional blend in solution. A liquid formulation in solution provides the maximum absorption ratios.

B Vitamins Work Together

When it comes to mental health, nothing compares to the B vitamins. I can extol the virtues of the B vitamins individually, but they are team players and one cannot succeed without the others. All the B vitamins must be taken together, so do the "B complex shuffle." The whole B complex family includes B1 (thiamine), B2 (riboflavin), B3 (niacin), B5 (pantothenic acid), B6 (pyridoxine), B12 (cobalamin), B15 (pangamic acid), biotin, choline, folic acid, inositol and PABA (para-aminobenzoic acid). Each B vitamin has its own role in body function, centered on the nervous system. Since nerves bring messages to all the organs and stimulate glands to secrete their important biochemicals, the whole body communication system can break down with a B vitamin deficiency.

A number of studies have shown a deficiency of folic acid as a contributing factor in mental illness. Studies have shown that a prolonged deficiency can cause neurological changes and mental deterioration. Because of their close interrelationship, vitamin B12 must accompany any folic acid supplementation. A deficiency of folic acid in pregnancy encourages the kind of brain damage that can cause schizophrenia. Deficiency symptoms include stunted growth, graying hair, gastrointestinal problems and anemia.[8]

In a study conducted at Northwick Park Hospital, Middlesex, England, researchers led by Dr. M.W.P. Carney found that 31 percent of 243 patients admitted to the psychiatric unit were deficient in folic acid. Patients' problems included mania, schizophrenia and depression. The researchers were surprised that a folate deficiency was present since these patients came from relatively affluent areas.[9]

In 1952, Dr. Hoffer and Dr. Humphry Osmond were struck by the similarity between schizophrenia and the delirium experienced in pellagra, which is believed to be caused by a deficiency of vitamin B3 (niacin and niacinamide). They conducted the first double-blind study in the discipline of psychiatry comparing niacin, niacinamide and a placebo on a group of 30 schizophrenic patients. Since most of the early treatment of pellagra had involved large doses of niacin, they hypothesized that schizophrenics may also need larger amounts of the vitamin. Consequently, they began treating patients with doses of nearly 3,000 mg daily. Out of the 30, only three receiving placebos had improvement. The spontaneous or natural recovery rate is considered to be 35 percent. Using niacin and niacinamide, Hoffer and Osmond managed to double this rate, curing an incredible 75 percent of the patients.[10]

To get all your B vitamins, eat whole and sprouted grains. Eating whole foods is the best, eating sprouts even better, since the young shoots concentrate more of the older plants' nutrients. When targeting food supplements, look for a formula that uses freeze dried sprouts and vegetables, combined in such a way as to provide all the essential vitamins and minerals.

Magnesium for the Mind

The mineral magnesium is so deficient among Americans, that the odds are good most of us need it. A large study by the U.S. Department of Agriculture found that only 25 percent of 37,785 individuals had magnesium intakes at or greater than the recommended daily allowance, which is notoriously low. A 1995 review of 15 studies found that a typical diet contains only a fraction of the RDA.[11]

In a study of 165 boys, it was found that those with symptoms of depression, schizophrenia and sleep disturbances had low blood levels of magnesium. In adults, insufficient magnesium may be accompanied by a loss of sensation in the extremities, as well as tremors, convulsions, muscle spasms, confusion, delirium and behavioral problems. One study found that psychiatric patients who attempted suicide had lower magnesium levels than either non-suicidal psychiatric patients or healthy individuals.[12]

An article in *Biological Psychiatry* reported that of patients hospitalized with major depression or schizophrenia, magnesium was significantly lower in those who had made suicide attempts. The authors believe magnesium has a role in regulating serotonin levels of the brain.[13]

In one study, a full quarter of 20 institutionalized chronic schizophrenic patients were found to have low blood magnesium levels. Taking this one step further, Dr. J.D. Kanofsky and associates gave three mentally ill patients 600 milligrams a day of oral magnesium supplementation. Two of the three patients showed improvement in their psychiatric condition when their blood magnesium level normalized. Magnesium deficiency has been associated with other psychiatric symptoms such as depression, agitation, hallucinations and irritability in nonschizophrenic patients. The researchers believe that the patients' schizophrenia may have been worsened by their magnesium deficiency, and that supplementation should be considered therapeutically.[14]

Magnesium and calcium work in balance throughout our bodies. Without magnesium, calcium accumulates in places it shouldn't. When supplementing with magnesium, include calcium one to four.

Schizophrenia-Stopping Nutrients
For maximum absorption, take supplements with meals.

Nutrient	Suggested Dosage	Formulation
Aged garlic extract	1 teaspoon three times daily	Liquid
Amino acids	4-6 capsules daily	Multiple formula from natural sources
Antioxidants	4 capsules daily*	With selenium and grapeseed extract
Borage oil	2 capsules daily	
Coenzyme Q10	2 capsules daily	With vitamin E, phospholipids and selenium
Flaxseed oil	1 tablespoon daily	
Ginkgo biloba	60 mg daily	
Multi-mineral	3-4 ounces daily	In liquid solution, with vitamin B12, biotin
Multi-vitamin/mineral	6 caplets daily	Freeze-dried plant sources
Niacin	500 mg three to four times daily	
St. John's Wort	250 mg daily	
Vitamin B6	100 mg daily	
Vitamin C	Individual bowel tolerance**	With bioflavonoids (quercetin, rutin proanthocyanidins)

* The FDA recommends pregnant women not exceed 10,000 IU of vitamin A daily.

** To determine individual dosage, on the first day take 1,000 mg hourly until diarrhea occurs, then reduce dosage to just below that for individual daily dosage. Vitamin C is not toxic in large doses but must be taken throughout the day to benefit. Divide dosage to three or four times a day.

CHAPTER 141:

Shingles

"Pain adds rest unto pleasure, and teaches the luxury of health."

–Martin F. Tupper

Adults relieved to have endured chicken pox as a child are dismayed to discover it coming back to haunt them in the form of shingles, an extremely uncomfortable and sometimes painful viral infection.

Apparently, adults who have had chicken pox still carry the virus (called varicella-zoster), which cluster together in the spinal nerves (for the scientifically inclined: dorsal-root ganglia). The virus then sits, dormant, until the body's immune system is lowered sufficiently for the virus to multiply.

Shields Up

Shingles is a process, not just a result. How bad it gets depends on the extent by which the body's immune system is lowered. Think of your body as the starship Enterprise. (You don't have to be a Trekkie to understand this concept.) When you are at your peak in defense capability, your shields are up, at 100 percent power. If you eat poorly, don't get enough sleep and don't exercise, your shields are at, maybe, 40 percent. When your shields are lowered, dormant viruses like the varicella-zoster can infiltrate your engineering.

The first sign of a shingles attack can be isolated pain or numbness in or under the skin, or a "shooting" pain around the hip, arm or leg. Next might come flu-like symptoms such as fever, headache and upset stomach.

Shingles is usually diagnosed when the next step occurs: a rash on the skin, characteristically in a band on one side of the body, back or face. The rash then turns into small round fluid-filled blisters which crust, scab and heal within a few weeks.

The technical name for shingles is herpes zoster. If you happen to know Greek, you're one step closer to knowing what and why shingles happens. "Zoster" is Greek for girdle, describing how the blisters "girdle" the body; and "herpes" means virus. This type of herpes is not contagious, at least not as shingles. It can, however, transmit chicken pox to those who've never had it.

If you're lucky, and your shields are at maybe 60 percent, you won't get the worst stage of this disorder, post-herpetic neuralgia (PHN). It sounds serious, but it doesn't have to be. An estimated 9 to 15 percent of people with shingles get this chronic pain syndrome.[1,2]

PHN pain is an epidermal ambiguity. When a pinprick is applied to the affected area, only numbness is described. And yet light pressure can cause severe pain, especially in the case of neuralgia on the face and head. Even a light wind blowing on the face can cause intense pain. Itching can be another symptom.[3]

About 50 percent of shingles patients over 60 years of age are at risk for PHN, which experts believe is caused by damage to the nerve endings where the virus begins.[4]

In younger patients, PHN generally subsides as the rash goes away. Patients over 40 to 50 years of age, however, are at risk for chronic, long-lasting pain. Over 50 percent of those over age 60 will have pain lasting more than one month after the rash has healed. [5]

Watch out for conventional medical therapies that purposely lower your immune system, leaving you susceptible to shingles, like chemotherapy, radiation therapy and certain drugs.

Shingles has been found to occur most often in people over the age of 50 and may be activated through surgery or x-ray therapy to the spinal cord and its roots. In those under 50, it is sometimes caused by immunosuppressant drugs given to transplant patients to prevent organ rejection or by cancer treatments.[6]

For example, bone marrow and other transplant recipients have a high rate of shingles, particularly in the first two to six months after transplantation. In addition, persons with cancer, especially when it affects the lymph nodes, have an increased frequency of shingles. In one two-year study, shingles was found in 25 percent of persons with Hodgkin's disease.[7] Shingles frequently occurs in patients infected with the human immunodeficiency virus (HIV).[8] In fact, shingles is often the first sign of the disease. In a study of 48 shingles patients, 70 percent were found to have HIV.[9]

If you look at the AIDS chapter, you'll see the connection between HIV, AIDS and a poorly functioning immune system. Shingles and HIV are just two of the many disorders that can occur when you aren't at peak performance.

Heal Thyself

You have shingles. What do you do now? The first step is to concentrate on your immune system. Read the AIDS chapter for what you should know about your immune system and how to bring your defense shields to 100 percent. In the meantime, here's what you can do to make yourself comfortable, and avoid being one of the nine percent who get herpetic neuralgia.

Try this make-it-yourself salve that can bring almost instant relief to the discomfort or pain of shingles. Here is the recipe: to zinc oxide ointment, an over-the-counter product, add an equal amount of aloe vera gel, and the contents of one 1,000 IU capsule of natural vitamin E (d-alpha tocopherol, *not* DL-alpha tocopherol). Mix it together and apply it to the blisters.

Since receiving his advice, I've seen this used successfully on a myriad of skin problems ranging from bed sores to chicken pox.

The B12 Bomber

When anyone tells me they have shingles I tell them this: take three ccs of vitamin B12, three times a day, three days in a row. It's that simple, and it's that effective.

I have seen it work for many of my friends, including actress Kathryn Grayson. Katherine had shingles for months, and was miserable. I told her about the B12 regimen and three days later she was returning to me with the good news and a hug. She has very fair, beautiful, lineless skin so I recommended the zinc salve to clear up the blister scars that were left.

Don't just take my word for it. Many doctors have also found vitamin B12 to be effective against shingles.

Researchers A.K. Gupta and H.S. Mital, both medical doctors, revealed in the *India Practitioner* their successful method of managing herpes zoster. They use a daily injection of 50 micrograms of vitamin B12![10]

By the second or third day of treatment, 21 shingles patients made dramatic gains in relief from pain and saw their rashes drying up. Further, none of the patients developed neuralgia.[11]

Vitamin B12 is a nutrient important to healthy nerves, memory, emotional stability and energy. It is absolutely essential to the aging body.

Don't Stress It

However, B12 requires a substance in the stomach to grab onto for it to be assimilated. During times of stress, this factor often is missing, so B12 will not be absorbed. That's why it is usually taken as a shot.

The ultimate stressful lifestyle has to be that of the soldier in combat. During the Vietnam War, medics often gave soldiers shots of B12 to boost their energy levels, since they knew they weren't getting it from their food.

Stress can create nutrient deficiencies, and a stressful lifestyle can guarantee them. When you imagine a bear is chasing you, your heart races, you breathe heavier and your adrenal function increases even if the bear only exists in your mind.

Mark Twain said it best: "In my life I have experienced many terrible things, some of which actually happened."

Drinking B12 in solution, from my observation, does the same thing. In any event, the injection would be far more potent, because it bypasses the stomach and intestinal tract, which exact their toll from nutrients passing through.

One way to tell if you are B12 deficient is if you are Northern European and don't have rosy cheeks. B12 in solution brings the rosiness back to mine.

Vitamins for Relief

Vitamin C has also brought quick turn-arounds from shingles. The late Fred Klenner, M.D., conducted an experimental study of eight shingles patients, injecting them with two to three grams of vitamin C every 12 hours and having them take a gram by mouth every two hours. Seven reported the end of their pain two hours after the first injection, the drying up of blisters by the end of day one, and their total disappearance by day three.[12]

The eighth patient, a diabetic, needed 14 injections – the others averaged six – but was completely free of symptoms in two weeks. Following the Klenner regimen, a researcher in France treated 327 shingles and herpes patients with vitamin C, and each of them lost all symptoms within three days.[13]

Dr. Robert Cathcart, a California physician, has successfully treated over 15,000 patients with massive doses of vitamin C; curing viral pneumonia, mononucleosis, influenza, colds, hepatitis, shingles, and cold sores with this method. He has developed a guideline for practical application of vitamin C which he refers to as "bowel tolerance."

The individual's own body will determine how much vitamin C it requires. The cutoff point is determined by the onset of diarrhea. In short, if you have not reached bowel tolerance (diarrhea), you have not taken enough vitamin C.

Remarkable results with vitamin E have been noted among shingles sufferers who also get stubborn and long-lingering post-herpetic neuralgia. In one study, nine of 13 patients, two of whom had suffered the pain for 13 and 19 years respectively, were nearly or fully relieved by taking 1200 to 1600 IU of vitamin E daily for six months. The remaining four were slightly or moderately improved.[14]

A word of caution, however. Large dosages of vitamin E in combination with coumadin, a blood thinner, can cause internal bleeding. In cases of diabetes or rheumatic heart disease, start with 100 IU/day of vitamin E and build up slowly.[15]

I would drop the coumadin so fast you could hear it land. It contains an active ingredient that kills rats by causing them to bleed through their tissues and drown in their own blood. Vitamin E is the finest blood thinner around, with no bad side effects.

Drs. Jonathan Wright and Alan R. Gaby recommend taking 1-10 grams a day of vitamin C and 1-3 grams a day of citrus bioflavonoids to prevent and treat shingles.[16]

Vitamin E, C and bioflavonoids are reknowned for their ability to not only ward off the physical effects of stress, but strengthen nerve, skin and vascular tissue.

Peppers for Pain

Hot peppers may make your mouth burn, but in a concentrated form their extract, called capsaicin, has the opposite effect on the pain of post herpetic neuralgia – the pain that lingers after the sores have healed.

Drs. Wright and Gaby recommend 1,200 IU of capsaicin a day for prevention and/or treatment of post herpetic neuralgia.[17]

A cream composed of capsaicin uses as much as 1,000 pounds of peppers to obtain an ounce of capsaicin powder.[18]

Several research institutions nationwide have studied the safety and efficacy of capsaicin, which has long been used as a folk treatment for pain.

A study at the University of Texas Health Science Center in San Antonio revealed that in a double-blind study of 40 patients with shingles-related pain, 69 percent who were treated with capsaicin showed improvement. Preliminary data also indicate that the cream relieves similar burning pain in some patients with diabetic neuropathy, where damage to the peripheral nerves due to diabetes causes feelings of numbness and pain.[19]

Capsaicin relieves burning pain because it affects certain types of nerve fibers. According to Joan Hoffman, a researcher at the center, it thwarts a natural body chemical known as substance P that the body uses to send certain pain messages to the brain. When the cream is applied, it stops substance P from sending its impulses.[20]

In a preliminary trial, investigators at Case Western Reserve University treated 14 patients with capsaicin cream. The patients applied this cream to the area of post-herpetic pain five times a day for a week, then three times a day for the next three weeks. Two patients dropped out of the study, but of the remaining 12, nine reported "substantial" relief. [21]

While You Wait

Following your initial shingles outbreak, there is much you can do to keep it from getting worse, and to deal with the symptoms as you get them.

First, do what it takes to boost your body's defense capability. Eat as much raw fruits and vegetables as possible, concentrate on complex carbohydrates such as lentils and beans, eat only whole grains, and avoid processed foods, especially white flour and sugar. Molasses and real maple syrup are good sugar substitutes and also nutritious.

Now that you're confident your body is doing all it can, think about what you can do for your symptoms. You can treat shingles sores by applying cool compresses of chamomile, eucalyptis or mint--it feels so good! Try calamine lotion, cornstarch or baking soda to hasten the drying of the shingles sores. Ointments should be avoided, though, and creams containing corticosteroids should not be used. After the acute phase, use the zinc oxide, vitamin E and aloe vera recipe to soften and separate the crusts, and avoid scarring.

Shingles Shaking Nutrients
For maximum absorption, take supplements with meals.

Nutrient	Suggested Dosage	Formulation
Aged garlic extract	1 teaspoon three times daily	Liquid
Caprylic acid	100 mg three times daily	
Echinacea	100 mg daily	
Fiber	4-8 tablets daily	Psyllium, with herb hyssop
Grapefruit seed extract	100 mg three times daily	
Lysine	500 mg twice daily during inactive stage, increasing to 1,000 mg three times daily during active stage	
Multi-mineral	1-4 ounces daily	In liquid solution, with vitamin B12, biotin
Multi-vitamin/mineral	3-6 caplets daily	Freeze-dried plant sources
Vitamin A	25,000 IU daily*	
Vitamin B12	3 cc three days in a row	
Vitamin C	Individual bowel tolerance**	With citrus bioflavonoids (quercetin, proanthocyanidins)
Vitamin E	2 capsules (800 IU) daily	d-alpha tocopherol

* The FDA recommends pregnant women not exceed 10,000 IU of vitamin A daily.

** To determine individual dosage, on the first day take 1,000 mg hourly until diarrhea

CHAPTER 142:

Sickle-Cell Anemia

*"Occasionally in life there are those moments of un-
utterable fulfillment which cannot be completely explained by those symbols called words. Their mean-
ings can only be articulated by the inaudible language
of the heart."*

–Martin Luther King, Jr.

If you are one of the estimated 60,000 Americans who suffer
from sickle-cell disease, also called sickle-cell anemia, or know someone who does, please don't be too disheartened. The problems associated with sickle-shaped blood cells – damaged and clogged blood
vessels and subsequent tissue and organ damage – can be prevented
or minimized with certain nutrients. Forget all this talk of genes.
Blaming genetics leaves us with the impression nothing can be done.
The important thing to concentrate on is exactly what happens, and
what can be done to alleviate the effects.

In the United States, sickle-cell disease primarily affects African
Americans, but it also occurs in some individuals of Mediterranean,
Middle Eastern, and Asian Indian descent. To simplify matters, doctors explain it as a genetic defect causing distortion of hemoglobin
(red blood) cells into sickle shapes, slowing, or even stopping, the
flow of blood and decreasing the amount of oxygen the red blood
cells are able to carry. The result is basically a loss of circulating
oxygen and blood to body tissues and organs. The excruciating pain,
ulcers and infection is a result of this loss of circulation.

Sickle-cell patients are told, "there is no known cure for the basic inherited defect." This pessimism is unwarranted, and virtually no help at all. What helps is isolating the problem and dealing with it. One of the problems with sickle-cell, discovered decades ago by two-time Nobel Prize-winning American chemist Dr. Linus Pauling, is that the cells become deformed when there is inadequate oxygen. While investigating protein molecules, he noticed a structural fault in the hemoglobin of people with sickle-cell anemia. His studies showed that increasing the level of oxygen in the blood of arteries temporarily restored the hemoglobin to normal.[1] What he discovered is that oxygenating the blood can actually prevent, at least temporarily, the blood cells from deforming.

What you need to know is that there are nutrients that increases blood oxygen and circulation, and that they have been shown to help the sickle-cell syndrome.

Nutrients to Restore Circulation

One of the early symptoms of circulation blockages is muscle cramping. Leg cramps can be caused by inadequate oxygen and red blood cell clumping, exactly what happens when blood cells deform and sickle. Vitamin E break ups clumping and increases oxygen to the cells.

Studies have shown that vitamin E may reduce another symptom of sickle cell – breakdown of weak red blood cells.[2] Vitamin E and the other antioxidants help strengthen cell membranes and stop their destruction from whatever source.

An article in the *American Journal of Clinical Nutrition* reported on a study in which six patients with sickle-cell anemia were given 450 IU daily of vitamin E for six to 35 weeks. Researchers were amazed to discover that there was an average decrease of 44 percent in the number of irreversibly sickled cells.[3]

Several substances interfere with, or even cause a depletion of vitamin E. When iron and vitamin E are taken together, they cancel out each other. Dr. Wilfred Shute in *Vitamin E for Ailing and Healthy Hearts*, suggests it be taken in one dose and all iron taken 8 to 12 hours later for proper absorption. The best time to take vitamin E is before mealtime or bedtime. Chlorine in drinking water, ferric chloride, rancid oil or fat and inorganic iron compounds destroy vitamin E in the body. Large amounts of vegetable oil (polyunsaturated fats) in the diet increases the need for vitamin E.

Vitamin C, another antioxidant, has also been found in studies to increase circulation and reduce infection as a result of poor circulation.

Dr. Daniel Chiu, of Children's Hospital Oakland Research Institute in Oakland, California, discovered in a controlled study that half of sickle cell patients were deficient in vitamin C and iron.[4] Without vitamin C, iron can't pick up oxygen. Without enough vitamin C, no matter how much iron you have, your blood cells will be starved of oxygen. Therefore, iron deficiency anemia can occur with too little iron or too little vitamin C.

Iron is an essential ingredient in hemoglobin. If you do not have enough iron in your body, you cannot make enough hemoglobin. You need all the normal, healthy hemoglobin you can get if some of it is sickled and defective.

A path of least resistance is very important. Efficient and effective blood flow requires not only even pressure, but smooth arterial walls. A deficiency of vitamin C has been shown to contribute to roughness of the interior of the arteries. If the inside wall of an artery is rough, sickled blood cells are more likely to "catch" and stick to them. Vitamin C is essential in maintaining smooth, flexible arterial walls necessary to proper blood circulation. Dr. Anthony Verlangieri, while at Rutgers University, demonstrated this effect by withholding vitamin C from laboratory rabbits' diets and noting the alteration in their arterial walls. When he restored the vitamin C to their diets, he documented their restoration to a healthy smoothness.

Nutritional Combinations Shown to Help

Researchers have found that it is not just one nutrient, but a combination of nutrients that help restore circulation and limit the number of sickled cells.

In an article in the *American Journal of Clinical Nutrition*, researchers tried a combination of zinc, vitamins C and E, and soybean oil on sickle-cell patients. Zinc has been shown in studies to reduce the number of irreversible sickle-cells in the blood and increase the longevity of red blood cells. Studies performed on cells grown in culture have shown that oils containing essential fatty acids make cell membranes less fragile and reduce the ability of the cells to stick together. After eight months on this nutritional regimen, the most striking effect was a 38 percent reduction in the number of sickle-cells.[5]

Soybean oil contains linoleic acid, the essential fatty acid also found in the oils of safflower, sunflower, flax, pumpkin and sesame seeds, and in walnuts. Linoleic acid is converted in the body into linolenic acid. The best, most concentrated source is borage oil. To get the most benefit of this type of essential fatty acids, I recommend supplementing with both flaxseed and borage oil.

Nutritional deficiencies are very common among sickle-cell patients, and can contribute toward their worsening condition.

Reduced levels of vitamin E, vitamin C, zinc, pyridoxine (B6) and beta carotene have been documented in sickle-cell disease patients.[6]

A deficiency of antioxidants in the body and diet is believed to contribute to weak and damaged red blood cells, with nearly every antioxidant you can think of shown in studies to help restore red blood cell health.

In a study performed at Columbia University's Department of Medicine in New York, 20 sickle-cell anemia patients were compared to 14 healthy controls and it was found that levels of selenium and glutathione peroxidase (an antioxidant enzyme created in the body by selenium) were significantly lower in the blood of sickle cell patients. Writing in *ACTA Hematologica*, Dr. Clayton Natta believes that a deficiency of dietary and naturally-occurring antioxidants may increase the damage and number of sickle-cells. Other antioxidants found to be deficient are vitamins C and E, beta carotene and the mineral zinc.[7]

In a study reported in the *Journal of the American Medical Association*, 34 patients with sickle-cell anemia had lower blood levels of zinc and were losing more of the mineral than 50 controls. The researchers concluded that this antioxidant mineral somehow increases the flow of oxygen.[8]

Two nutrients must be considered along with zinc: vitamin B6 and copper. Too much copper will deplete zinc stores; they must be equal for optimum usage. Include 2-4 mg of copper with any zinc supplement.

Vital B Vitamins

In a study reported in the *American Journal of Clinical Nutrition*, after five patients were given 50 mg of vitamin B6 twice daily for two months, they had healthier and more numerous normal red blood cells and one patient had less pain.[9]

An article in the *New England Journal of Medicine* reported that some sickle-cell patients benefitted by receiving five milligrams or more of another B vitamin – folic acid – each day.[10]

Researchers in Jamaica noted that after Hurricane Gilbert swept through the islands, the incidence of neural tube defects and sickle cell crises increased. It was believed that these were both due to a sudden loss of fresh food sources of folic acid.[11]

In Saudi Arabia, Dr. Abdul Kareem Al-Momen found in a controlled study that almost half of 85 patients with severe sickle-cell disease had below-normal vitamin B12 levels. The patients showed improvement of their condition when given weekly B12 shots intramuscularly for 12 weeks.[12]

Vitamin B12 is often given by injection because its absorption is impaired by many factors. One way to be sure and get your B12 is by consuming it in solution, thus avoiding the need to break it down.

It has been found that B6 – a fragile and easily destroyed vitamin – is not present in fatty or processed foods. Vital B6 is lost in food transportation, storage, preservation, processing and cooking. Therefore, it is essential to add a B6 vitamin supplement (at least 200 mg daily) to your diet.

Whenever I recommend one B vitamin I recommend all of the them. All the B vitamins work in synch. Without one, the others can become deficient. Without minerals they don't work at all. When supplementing one B vitamin always take a good B vitamin complex, at least ten times the RDA. A note about RDAs. They were formulated with *everyone* in mind. Therefore, their recommendations are maintenance levels, not optimum levels. In today's world of pollutants and nutritionally-deficient food (fresh as well as processed), we need more help than the RDAs. Always target supplemental formulas that are higher than the RDAs.

Anemia-Fighting Nutrients
For maximum absorption, take supplements with meals.

Nutrient	Suggested Dosage	Formulation
Aged garlic extract	1 teaspoon three times daily	Liquid
Antioxidants	4 capsules daily*	With selenium and grapeseed extract
Borage oil	2 capsules daily	
Coenzyme Q10	2 capsules daily	With vitamin E, phospholipids and selenium
Enzymes	3 capsules twice daily	Multiple formula
Fiber	4-8 tablets daily	Psyllium, with herb hyssop
Flaxseed oil	1 tablespoon daily	
Folic acid	10 mg daily	
Ginkgo biloba	50 mg three times daily	
Glucosamine sulfate	500 mg three times daily	
L-Carnitine	500 mg twice daily	
Magnesium	200 mg daily	
Melatonin (adults only)	3 mg daily at bedtime	With B vitamins
Multi-mineral	3-4 ounces daily	In liquid solution, with vitamin B12, biotin
Multi-vitamin/mineral	6 caplets daily	Freeze-dried plant sources
Niacin	500 mg four times daily	
Taurine	500 mg twice daily	
Vitamin A	25,000 IU daily*	
Vitamin B6	100 mg daily	
Vitamin C	Individual bowel tolerance**	With bioflavonoids (quercetin, rutin proanthocyanidins)
Vitamin E	2 capsules (800 IU) daily	d-alpha tocopherol

* The FDA recommends pregnant women not exceed 10,000 IU of vitamin A daily.

** To determine individual dosage, on the first day take 1,000 mg hourly until diarrhea occurs, then reduce dosage to just below that for individual daily dosage. Vitamin C is not toxic in large doses but must be taken throughout the day to benefit. Divide dosage to three or four times a day.

CHAPTER 143:

Sinusitis

Jim was in jeopardy of losing his job. He had used up all his sick time, and was almost out of vacation days. He just couldn't shake his sinus infections completely, and they kept coming back. The pain and pressure left him entirely disabled, unable to do anything but sleep. Finally, desperate for a solution, he called Dr. Ross Gordon, an M.D. practicing out of Albany, California. Dr. Gordon did a complete nutritional workup and RAST allergy test. After eliminating beef and beef broth from his diet, and going on a program of nutritional supplementation, Jim was a new man. He not only didn't lose his job, but got promoted. He has now been sinusitis-free for six years.

Some might say God made sinuses to remind us to take care of ourselves. Certainly after being faced with an infection, you appreciate good health all the more.

What are sinuses? Simply stated, they are four holes in the facial bones. There is one behind the bridge of the nose; another one directly above the eyes, in the cheekbone, and behind and above the nose. Delicate mucous membranes lining the sinuses continually produce mucus to flush out irritants and other invaders, including bacteria and viruses. The mucus normally drains into the nose through a small opening in the wall of each sinus. Healthy mucus is thin and colorless and should drain easily, even when large amounts are produced.

However, if for any reason the mucus thickens, or swelling and inflammation occur, and/or the openings become blocked, pressure builds, resulting in facial pain or severe headaches. The trapped, stagnant mucus becomes a breeding ground for bacteria, and the mucus thickens as the bacteria proliferate. What does manage to leak through the blocked openings creates an irritating postnasal drip that can result in a sore throat and cough.

Dehydration occurs naturally with colds and fever, which is why doctors recommend extra fluids during sickness. Not enough water in the body will thicken mucus, inviting problems. An allergy is probably the most common culprit behind chronic sinusitis. Allergic reactions produce not only copious amounts of mucus, but inflammation and swelling, which can block the openings or make it harder for mucus to drain. Other causes of poor drainage include long-term exposure to cigarette smoke or other irritants, a deviated nasal septum (the cartilage between the nostrils), dental abscesses, nasal polyps, nasal or sinus tumors, and, in diabetics, certain fungal infections.

The trouble with sinuses, as any sufferer will tell you, is that it feels as though the mucus in them has nowhere to go. You can't cough it out, and you can't sneeze it out. If it builds up and gets infected, it just hurts. You bend over and swear your face is going to fall off.

Preventing Sinus Build-Up

Antihistamines are usually prescribed for sinus problems, but, as usual, address the symptom, not the problem. Better than drugs are treatments designed to thin the mucus and draw it out, supplements that reduce inflammation, and nutrients that nourish and heal sick sinuses.

Applying warmth can help. Try a hot pack using menthol, tea tree oil, peppermint or eucalyptus over the sinuses or, if you're not sure which sinus, over the painful area. Try gizmos designed to give steam facials and add these botanicals to the water. A steam sauna or hot shower can help too.

Here are other tips on how to keep your nose open and your sinuses clear:

- Drink large amounts of purified water – at least a gallon a day – to thin mucus so it can drain more easily.
- Avoid alcohol, which causes congestion and can dehydrate the body, making mucus thicker.
- Spray the inside of your nose with softened or purified water to soothe and moisten nasal tissues.
- Bathe nasal passages and flush mucus out of the nose with a mixture of a quarter-teaspoon of baking soda, a quarter-teaspoon of salt and eight ounces of warm water. Pour some of the mixture into your palm and snort gently. Then gently blow your nose, one side at a time.
- Unless you abhor spicy food, eat hot chili peppers. They are full of therapeutic vitamin C and help you breathe.
- Exercise regularly. Physical activity generates adrenaline, which constricts swollen blood vessels and relieves nasal stuffiness.
- Avoid swimming pools if chlorine irritates your nose and sinuses.
- Eliminate allergens. Record what you ate, where you were, and what you were exposed to during the 12 hours before you experienced your sinus symptoms. Keep this record until you see a pattern indicating your allergens. Be especially suspicious if you have sinus headaches. They are a good indication of food or chemical sensitivities. Ban chemicalized, processed food from your diet, emphasizing whole, natural, organic foods. For more, see the Allergy chapter.

Battling Infection with Good Nutrition

Treat a sinus problem just as you would a cold; with lots of vitamin C, bioflavonoids, vitamin A, liquid aged garlic extract and zinc. On my television show, *Maximize Your Life*, Garry Gordon, M.D., recommended 500,000 IU of vitamin A in divided doses; vitamin C at 1,000 milligrams an hour and garlic when suffering with any kind of infection.

Richard Barrett, N.D., Associate Academic Dean of the National College of Naturopathic Medicine in Portland, Oregon, recommends starting the battle with a water fast, which frees the body to use its energy to fight the infection, instead of digesting food. An alternative would be a diet which emphasizes low-sugar fruit and vegetable broth. Because bacteria thrive on sugar, concentrated sugars should be avoided.[1]

Nutritional supplementation is the best army in your fight to bring infection under control and boost your body's ability to heal. An important goal is to provide in abundance the nutritional elements needed by the mucous membranes and hair-like cilia lining the sinuses to expel and withstand the onslaught of bacteria, viruses and poisons that assail us daily.

The cilia particularly need potassium and calcium. Without these nutrients, the cilia cannot function. But if there is one nutrient that might be considered the hallmark of a sinus defense system, it is vitamin A. When you are sick, your body doesn't have the enzymes needed to convert beta carotene to vitamin A. Therefore, it's important to take vitamin A when you are sick.

Without adequate amounts of vitamin A, cilia and mucous cells die off and are replaced by hard, scaly cells which can accumulate and form pre-cancerous lesions or polyps. In experiments, researchers were able to reverse this process with the introduction of vitamin A.[2]

Researchers have found that even when cilia is destroyed by cigarette smoke, alcohol, nose drops and nasal sprays, it can be restored by adequate amounts of potassium, calcium and vitamin A.

One more nutrient is added to this formula: zinc. Vitamin A cannot do its job if zinc isn't also present.[3]

Zinc is a notorious wound-healer, and is necessary before vitamin A can be absorbed in the body. In a study of 61 Baltimore children, Smith and his colleagues found that vitamin A could not be released from their livers unless there was high enough blood levels of zinc.[4]

Two nutrients must be considered along with zinc: vitamin B6 and copper. Too much copper will deplete zinc stores; they must be equal for optimum usage. Include 2-4 mg of copper with any zinc supplement.

Vitamin C for all Infections

Have you ever had a root canal? I wouldn't wish one on my own worst enemy. Root canals can be needed when an abscess jeopardizes a tooth. Dental infections can also be the "root" cause of sinus infections. Vitamin C has been shown in studies to prevent periodontal abscesses by lowering the amount of plaque and bacteria in the mouth.

The *New York Journal of Dentistry* reported on a study in which plaque accumulation was measured among subjects all brushing well, some supplementing with vitamin C, some not. The study found that those supplementing with vitamin C actually had less tarter and bacteria than those only brushing. The study found that when the subjects took vitamin C the inflammation of their gums from concentrations of bacteria improved 58 percent![5]

How does vitamin C perform its magic? By increasing the numbers of the antibody warriors that come to our defense when infection sets in.

University of Witwatersrand, South Africa, medical students were given one gram a day of ascorbic acid (vitamin C) and monitored for blood immunologic levels. Unlike the control group who did not get the vitamin C, the ones who did experienced a marked increase in their defense antibodies, IgA and IgM. Vitamin C is renowned for alleviating the symptoms of colds and flu, and studies have shown it to be of benefit for any type of infection.[6]

During a visit on my television show *Maximize Your Life*, Stanford University's Robert Cathcart III, M.D., emphasized the benefits of vitamin C to prevent infections, treat them, and even prevent the pain that follows any injury to the body. If you work with your hands, and find yourself with frequent cuts, scrapes and skin injuries, try a lotion that contains vitamin C. Dr. Cathcart says vitamin C applied topically will help prevent infection.

Dr. Cathcart has successfully treated over 15,000 patients with massive doses of vitamin C; curing viral pneumonia, mononucleosis, influenza, colds, hepatitis, shingles, and cold sores with this method. He has developed a guideline for practical application of vitamin C which he refers to as "bowel tolerance."

He found that the individual's own body will determine how much vitamin C it requires. The cutoff point is determined by the onset of diarrhea. In an interview in *Public Scrutiny*, Cathcart stated, "The tolerance level in each individual differs. Some days you can tolerate more, some days less, but from general experience I label a cold as a 20-to-30-gram cold, or 60-gram flu, according to how much a person can take before he reaches the bowel tolerance level."

In short, if you have not reached bowel tolerance (diarrhea), you have not taken enough vitamin C.

In an amazing discovery, vitamin C has been found to be helpful in the continuing battle against bacteria that have become immune to antibiotics. Antibiotics are not the most desirable way to fight infection, but they are used. However, medical science is in a quandary because many of the bacteria we are fighting have become immune to antibiotics. Antibiotics are responsible for educating smarter germs. The only thing effective against these new viruses is vitamin C.

Rather than using stronger antibiotics, perhaps physicians should consider recommending vitamin C along with them. A recent Harvard study found vitamin C may reduce bacterial resistance to antibiotic therapy. In their laboratories, researchers exposed strains of staphylococcus aureus to ascorbic acid for six hours. In four out of six of the strains, the bacteria showed less resistance. The researchers found that the doses of antibiotics could be reduced by 50 to 75 percent after resistant strains of bacteria were exposed to the vitamin C. They also found that previously ineffective doses of penicillin and tetracy-cline showed increased inhibitory effects on resistant bacteria, and even killed 23 to 93 percent of the initial bacteria population with vitamin C.[7,8] This is exciting news. With vitamin C, not only are old antibiotics useful again, but you don't have to take as much of them! Now, if only conventional medicine would wake up and smell the oranges!

When you target vitamin C as a supplement, choose a formulation that includes bioflavonoids. Bioflavonoids are potent anti-inflammatories. They reduce swelling while they act on the immune system, and they enhance the healing properties of vitamin C.

Sinusitus-Smashing Nutrients
For maximum absorption, take supplements with meals.

Nutrient	Suggested Dosage	Formulation
Acidophilus	At least four billion flora on an empty stomach, three times daily	
Aged garlic extract	1 teaspoon three times daily	Liquid
Antioxidants	4 capsules daily*	With selenium and grapeseed extract
Echinacea	200 mg daily	
Fiber	4-8 tablets daily	Psyllium, with herb hyssop
Multi-mineral	3-4 ounces daily	In liquid solution, with vitamin B12, biotin
Multi-vitamin/mineral	6 caplets daily	Freeze-dried plant sources
Vitamin A	25,000 IU daily*	
Vitamin C	Individual bowel tolerance**	With bioflavonoids (quercetin, rutin proanthocyanidins)

* The FDA recommends pregnant women not exceed 10,000 IU of vitamin A daily.

** To determine individual dosage, on the first day take 1,000 mg hourly until diarrhea occurs, then reduce dosage to just below that for individual daily dosage. Vitamin C is not toxic in large doses but must be taken throughout the day to benefit. Divide dosage to three or four times a day.

CHAPTER 144:

Skin Lumps

A viewer of my television show, *Maximize Your Life*, wrote to me about an egg-shaped growth on the side of her neck that had grown to the size of a tennis ball. At first she thought it was a goiter, but when she saw her physician, he said it was a lipoma, and that she shouldn't be concerned. Wouldn't you be concerned if you had a tennis ball growing out of the side of your neck? Fortunately, I was able to address her problem on the air. If she is somewhere out there reading this, I hope my suggestions helped.

Lipomas are single, painless lumps that are most often found in older people. Approximately 90 percent of people with lipomas are women. Lipomas are made up of fatty tissue and are slow-growing, soft, and movable.

Reabsorbed with Enzymes

Success has been achieved using lipase and other fat digestive enzymes and a minimum four day fast of only water and minerals in solution, plus the elimination of hydrogenated oils and transfatty acids in the diet to eliminate lipomas. Fat digestive enzymes help the body re-absorb fat that has gone where it doesn't belong. If you don't get enough of these enzymes from vegetables and fruit, you risk gaining weight, since the lack of these enzymes causes storage instead of assimilation of fat. Eating foods high in transfatty acids, like margarine and hydrogenated oils, increases the amount of fat or cholesterol in the body, adding to the risk of getting lipomas. For more on lowering fat in your body, read the chapter Cholesterol. In the meantime, find a digestive enzyme formula that includes lipase.

I would add fatty acids to the diet. Lipomas are a result of a defect in the body's regulation of fat. If this is the case, fatty acids can help that defect, keeping fat where it belongs, and helping to prevent its accumulation under the skin. For omega-3 fatty acids, target flaxseed oil. For omega-6, supplement with borage oil, which is high in linolenic acid, essential to fat assimilation.

If these options do not work, you can consider having your lipomas surgically removed and use dietary measures to prevent recurrence. For some people, mostly those who have multiple, chronically recurring lipomas, this protocol can be used to prevent fatty tumors after the original ones have been surgically removed.

Surgery Removes the Lumps

Before you contemplate surgery, find a good, reliable doctor. If you are in the San Francisco Bay area, I suggest looking up these wonderful doctors: Dr. Edward Ivy (707) 578-1900/1111 in Santa Rosa or (415) 397-8701 in San Francisco; Angelo Capozzi, M.D. San Francisco, Mill Valley, Fairfield at (415) 775-5100; or Dr. John Emery, 2000 Union Street. If you are in Southern California see Dr. John Williams at (310) 271-5924, the plastic surgeon to the stars.

Lipomas can be removed through a minor surgical procedure, or through liposuction. If a lipoma is fairly small, or located in a hidden area, surgery may be a desired option. With surgery, an incision the size of the lipoma is made, and the mass is "popped out" or cut out manually. A scar the size of the incision is expected. The advantage to this technique is that the lipoma is not likely to grow back.

Liposuction may be chosen in the event the lipoma is large or is in a cosmetically-sensitive area, like the stomach. In liposuction, the fatty tissue is "suctioned out" through a small incision, but the mass itself is not all removed. Because of this, the odds that the lipoma may return are increased.

Generally, lipomas are as large as they will become. They don't just grow and grow if nothing is done about them. Many people live with them, and suffer no ill effects. They are generally removed for cosmetic purposes.

Tag, You're Out

They're annoying, some think ugly, but they are generally harmless. They are those pinches of skin that seem to serve no purpose or have a reason to exist. Laypeople call them skin tags. Doctors call them acrochordon or cutaneous (skin) papillomas.

Here's how one dermatology encyclopedia defines skin tags: "Acrochordons are common, benign, polyp-like skin-colored papules varying in size from a few millimeters to several centimeters in diameter. They are soft and usually multiple and occur in the folds of the skin (like under the breast or in the armpit) and the neck. They usually have no symptoms but may have pain due to local irritation. They may be twisted off or removed by simple snipping with scissors."[1]

OK, seems pretty simple to get rid of them. You go to the dermatologist and have them cut off. Except ask anybody who has had a skin tag. It's not that simple because they come right back again. What you need to know is why you have them in the first place.

You may have heard that if you have skin tags, you have a better chance of getting colon cancer or intestinal polyps. The connection may be there, but it is probably not a direct connection. The link between these two disorders may be the inability to process food energy properly, caused by diabetes or hypoglycemia.

Researchers J. Margolis and L.S. Margolis were the first to make the diabetes connection to skin tags. They published their findings in the May 20, 1976 issue of the *New England Journal of Medicine*. Of 47 individuals with one or more skin tags, the article said, 34 were found to have diabetes.[2]

Jonathan Wright, M.D., makes it a habit to give anyone he sees with skin tags a glucose-insulin tolerance test.

He also looks for a family history of diabetes and fatigue in his skin tag patients. He says unexplained fatigue is often due to blood sugar difficulty, emphasizing that it can mean either too much blood sugar (hypoglycemia) or not enough (diabetes). Dr. Wright prefers the six-hour glucose-insulin tolerance tests.[3]

For optimum good health and to keep skin tags away, avoid overprocessed, refined foods and sugar. Adopt a whole-food diet with no refined sugar, flour or caffeine. Take a supplement formula that includes the B vitamins, C, E and chromium (chromium helps balance the blood sugar).[4]

Lump-Losing Nutrients

For maximum absorption, supplements should be taken with meals.

Nutrient	Suggested Dosage	Formulation
Aged garlic extract	2 teaspoons three times daily	Liquid
Antioxidants	4 capsules daily*	With selenium and grape seed extract
Borage oil	2 capsules daily	
Enzymes	2 capsules twice daily	Multiple formula
Flaxseed oil	1 tablespoon daily	
Fiber	8 tablets daily	Psyllium, with herb hyssop
Lecithin	2 tablespoons with meals	
Magnesium	200 mg daily	
Multi-vitamin/mineral	6 caplets daily	Freeze-dried plant sources
Multi-mineral	2-4 ounces daily	In liquid solution, with vitamin B12, biotin
Vitamin B6	200 mg daily	
Vitamin C	Individual bowel tolerance**	With bioflavonoids (quercetin, rutin proanthocyanidins)
Vitamin E	2 capsules (800 IU)	d-alpha tocopherol

* The FDA recommends that pregnant women not exceed 10,000 IU of vitamin A daily.

** To determine individual dosage, on the first day take 1,000 mg hourly until diarrhea occurs, then reduce dosage to just below that for individual daily dosage. Vitamin C is not toxic in large doses but must be taken throughout the day to benefit. Divide dosage to three or four times a day.

CHAPTER 145:

Sleep Apnea

Dagwood Bumstead has sleep apnea. Just look at the symptoms. He sleeps during the day – a lot; he snores at night and he's so tired most of the time he can't leave the house without running into the mailman. The only symptom he doesn't have is obesity.

Imagine ceasing to breathe for 10 to 20 seconds, then strenuously gasping in air, then stopping again – hundreds of times during what is supposed to be eight hours of restful slumber. For the sleep apnea sufferer, this happens every night.

Fortunately, the relentless lapses in breathing are not remembered, even though up to three-quarters of total sleep time may be spent not breathing! Apnea is Greek for "want of breath," and the condition causes problems in both infants (see my chapter Sudden Infant Death Syndrome) and adults.

For adults, sleep apnea may actually be more disturbing for the spouse than for the affected individual, for the frequent fits and starts of breathing are often accompanied by snoring reminiscent of a jackhammer.

In 1988 the United States Congress established the National Commission on Sleep Disorders Research "to conduct a comprehensive study of sleep disorders and to develop a long-range plan for the use and organization of national resources to deal effectively with sleep disorders research and medicine."[1]

What they found didn't surprise me, but it might surprise you. The commission found that the conventional medicine community generally does not understand sleep disorders. In one survey, the commission looked at computerized medical records of more than 10 million patients. Even though the symptoms of sleep apnea have been classified for the medical community for nearly 20 years, only 73 specific cases of sleep disorders in general were identified – out of 10 million! Based on prevalence statistics, the commission estimated that more than a million cases should have been diagnosed. To further confirm these results, the records of more than 10,000 patients were carefully examined by commission investigators. Every physician-patient interaction from a patient's first visit to the time of the study was examined, adding up to more than 50,000 physician-patient interactions. In this huge mass of data, and despite symptoms obvious to investigators, not one physician came up with a correct diagnosis![2]

These kinds of findings are why I am writing this book. To be fair, nobody can know everything, and doctors are only human, after all. If it is true that only six percent of the population suffers from sleep apnea, then it is possible a doctor might not see a case very often. But for those who suffer from it, or have a spouse who suffers from it, identification is crucial.

A founding father of our United States Constitution, James Madison, once said: "A popular government, without popular information, or the means of acquiring it, is but a Prologue to a Farce or a Tragedy; or, perhaps both. Knowledge will forever govern ignorance: And a people who mean to be their own Governors, must arm themselves with the power which knowledge gives."

A Dangerous Condition

Sleep apnea is easily one of the tragedies described by Madison. Most think of it as only causing a lack of sleep. Not only does it result in sleeplessnes, but causes a lack of oxygen to the brain and carbon dioxide in the blood. Compared with the general population, patients with sleep apnea have twice the prevalence of high blood pressure, three times as much coronary artery disease, and four times as much cerebrovascular disease (brain damage). A recent case-control study in Italy found that the risk of heart attacks was about four times higher in patients who reported snoring every night than in those without this history.[3]

The lack of sleep associated with this problem results in daytime sleepiness, poor memory and thought processes, emotional troubles and poor productivity. Imagine trying to drive long distances! The risk of traffic accidents due to falling asleep at the wheel is believed to be as much as seven times greater in patients with sleep apnea than in the general population.[4]

Men are the most afflicted. A Cleveland study of sleep apnea patients between the ages of 7 and 75 years showed that men are six times more likely than women to have the syndrome.[5]

Watch your weight! Obesity is the most common factor in sleep apnea. Researchers estimate that about two-thirds of patients are obese, and your risk of having sleep apnea is increased four times if you are obese.[6] Not surprisingly, sleep apnea is believed to develop over decades. Studies show patients often start developing it in their teens and 20s, becoming a major health risk when they reach their 50s to 70s.[7] Interestingly, that's when weight gain and obesity typically develops.

The most common type of sleep apnea is termed obstructive. This is because something blocks the airway, cutting off air. The patient's struggle to breathe ends when his airway finally opens with a loud snort. In some people, the throat and tongue muscles relax too much during sleep, closing the windpipe. Most apnea sufferers don't die (apparently some do) because while asleep the body recognizes the lack of oxygen and wakes up momentarily, tightening the relaxed muscles and restoring the airway. This can happen 100 or more times a night, preventing restful sleep and leaving the victim fatigued. Imagine being almost strangled every night, over and over again! Snoring isn't so funny now, is it?

Comedic actor John Candy was reported to have a heart attack during sleep, resulting in his death. He was obese. I wonder if he snored, and I wonder how many reported heart attack victims actually died from self-strangulation because their problems went unrecognized by conventional medicine? What a Tragedy!

Certain physical problems can predispose someone to sleep apnea. Once the defect is identified, the problem is alleviated. Children with sleep apnea may have enlarged tonsils or adenoids. A person could experience obstruction from a deviated nasal septum or nasal polyps. Obese people have excessive throat fat, which can contribute to the problem, and those who have overly large tongues may experience sleep apnea. Once the problem becomes recognized, the solutions are at hand.

Causes and Helpful Solutions

Hypothyroidism is a well recognized cause of sleep apnea. Any therapy that restores thyroid levels has been shown to diminish or completely eliminate sleep apnea as well as improve sleep patterns and overall sleep efficiency. Bashir A.Chaudhary, M.D., of the Sleep Disorder Center, Medical College of Georgia in Augusta, Georgia, suggests that every person diagnosed with sleep apnea be evaluated for hypothyroidism. To combat this particular disorder, see my chapter Low Thyroid.[8]

Alcohol, or any drug that depresses the nervous system (even sleep medications) can cause sleep apnea, because they depress the nerve impulses that promote breathing and the body's response to carbon dioxide in the blood.

Polyps, growths or skin tags in the throat can cause enough obstruction to interfere with breathing while lying down.

Other chapters to consider for sleep apnea and resultant problems are Sinusitis; Skin Lumps; Allergies; Circulation Problems; Heart Problems and Hypertension.

Once the cause of sleep apnea is found, it is important to re-oxygenate the blood. Certain nutrients work to increase oxygen and rid the blood of dangerous carbon dioxide. The antioxidant vitamin E increases oxygen to the cells. Any supplemental source of vitamin E should be in the form of a natural tocopherol, and should be taken alone.[9]

Several substances interfere with, or even *cause* a depletion of vitamin E. When iron and vitamin E are taken together, they cancel out each other. It be taken in one dose and all iron taken 8 to 12 hours later for proper absorption. The best time to take vitamin E is before mealtime or bedtime. Chlorine in drinking water, ferric chloride, rancid oil or fat and inorganic iron compounds destroy vitamin E in the body. Large amounts of vegetable oil (polyunsaturated fats) in the diet increases the need for vitamin E.

Vitamin C, another antioxidant, has also been found in studies to increase oxygen in the blood. Any situation where the health is compromised by poor circulation benefits with high doses of vitamin C. Collagen, that which gives skin and body tissues their strength and elasticity, is formed and strengthened by vitamin C.

I would include all the antioxidants in a post-sleep apnea protocol. One of the first things that happens with a loss of oxygen is cell damage. Antioxidants helps restore and prevent cell damage. For your post-apnea protocol, target the antioxidants and nutrients listed below and their clinical setting dosage recommendations.

Sleep and Circulation-Restoring Nutrients
For maximum absorption, take supplements with meals.

Nutrient	Suggested Dosage	Formulation
Amino acids	4-6 capsules daily	Multiple formula from natural sources
Antioxidants	4 capsules daily*	With selenium and grapeseed extract
Borage oil	2 capsules daily	
Coenzyme Q10	2 capsules daily	With vitamin E, phospholipids and selenium
Enzymes	2 capsules twice daily	Multiple formula
Fiber	4-8 tablets daily	Psyllium, with herb hyssop
Flaxseed oil	1 tablespoon daily	
Folic acid	5-10 mg daily	
Ginkgo biloba	50 mg three times daily	
L-Carnitine	500 mg twice daily	
Melatonin (adults only)	3 mg daily at bedtime	With B vitamins
Multi-mineral	3-4 ounces daily	In liquid solution, with vitamin B12, biotin
Multi-vitamin/mineral	6 caplets daily	Freeze-dried plant sources
Niacin	500 mg four times daily	
Taurine	500 mg twice daily	
Vitamin A	25,000 IU daily*	
Vitamin B6	100 mg daily	
Vitamin C	Individual bowel tolerance**	With bioflavonoids (quercetin, rutin proanthocyanidins)
Vitamin E	2 capsules (800 IU) daily	d-alpha tocopherol

* The FDA recommends pregnant women not exceed 10,000 IU of vitamin A daily.

** To determine individual dosage, on the first day take 1,000 mg hourly until diarrhea occurs, then reduce dosage to just below that for individual daily dosage. Vitamin C is not toxic in large doses but must be taken throughout the day to benefit. Divide dosage to three or four times a day.

CHAPTER 146:

Sleeplessness

The doctor cured his insomnia, but now he has to work nights to pay the bill.

Irony is when you enroll in a relaxation class and sleep through it.

Sleeplessness is no laughing matter to those so desperate they will try anything. So I have made an in-depth study of sleep-inducing methods that seem to work. I want you to sleep soundly, but – please! – not while you're reading this!

Insomnia is a huge problem to many people. According to the American Sleep Disorders Association, incredibly, more than 35 million Americans have difficulty sleeping every night, on most nights or at least several times each month.

Just Say No to Drugs

I want to start by discussing the most commonly, and erroneously, used method for inducing sleep: drugs. It's such a shame because, while they may work in the short term, they cause more problems than just insomnia in the long term.

Rarely do orthodox doctors tell us that 65 prescription drugs and more than 100 over-the-counter medicines contain sleep-discouraging caffeine. In the case of prescriptions, ask the pharmacist. In the case of over-the-counter medications, read the label – or you'll be counting sheep until the cows come home!

No doctor can truly evaluate insomnia in a patient until the patient is drug-free. Sleeping pills prescribed by doctors (which add up to about 25 million prescriptions annually) interfere with normal sleep patterns and can actually cause the disorder.

Although there are hundreds of tranquilizers and many kinds of sedatives on the market, we have just begun to learn that many of these drugs do not offer natural sleep; instead they change the *quality* of sleep. Such interference can wreak havoc with a patient's health, a matter that we should seriously consider when orthodox doctors offer us prescriptions for them.

At what was probably the high point of America's craze for prescription drugs, in 1967 Americans spent about $300 million on tranquilizers and drugs to combat mild anxiety. Prescription sedatives were running about $70 million and would have been higher if the Drug Abuse Control Law of 1966 had not cut down on the indiscriminate refilling of old prescriptions.

Food For Sleep

Time-honored folk medicine tells us that a banana, a medium-sized tomato, or a handful of walnuts can beat sleeplessness.

Modern biochemists tell us why. They contribute to the making of serotonin, a brain neurotransmitter which produces a calming effect.

Some people I know follow the folklore method of luring sleep by eating lettuce. One friend puts a whole head of lettuce at her bedside and tears off chunks to nibble on. Soon she is fast asleep. If she wakes up during the night, she eats more lettuce and usually gets desired results.

Imagine lying in a field of daisies, the sun shining down on you. Make you sleep? No? Well, the next best thing is a tea made of the daisies, camomile.

Camomile tea is a marvelous nerve soother and sleep gatherer. It's also easily found, either fresh or in tea bags, in your supermarket.

A hops pillow, as strange as that sounds, will help you relax and fall asleep. Use a generous amount of dried hops and sprinkle with a little alcohol to charge the active properties of the herb. Envelope the greenery in a small cloth pillow and tuck it inside the pillowcase along with your regular pillow. It works!

Calcium Not Just For Cows

Milk is the center of controversy again. This time the question is: Does a warm glass of milk make you sleep or not? Although I have never done a personal Gallup poll with my televiewers, I feel that the vote runs about two to one that milk lives up to its folklore reputation.

Nothing works for everybody. My viewers tell me that very hot milk overheats them and makes sleep impossible. However, warm milk usually puts them to sleep. Some biochemists, speaking off the cuff, say that it's the tryptophan content of milk that acts as a sedative.

This is hard to believe, because milk's tryptophan content is only a small fraction of the amount found in experiments to be sleep-inducing.

The late Carlton Fredericks, Ph.D., one of the all-time great nutritionists, agreed. He once told me he felt calcium was the main sleep-inducing ingredient in milk, because it soothes neuromuscular irritability, acting as one of nature's tranquilizers. My vote goes with Doctor Fredericks.

Dr. Morris Notelovitz, professor of obstetrics and gynecology at the University of Florida, has discovered that calcium supplements are best absorbed and needed during sleeptime.

His point is that during the day, we take in calcium from foods and liquid. However, at night we go long periods without calcium intake, and yet we're still using our bones and muscles, which calcium feeds.

So what happens? The body fills its nighttime needs by stealing calcium from the only available source – the bones. Here are his two main reasons why we should take calcium at night: Calcium levels are then low, so absorption of calcium, is rapid and efficient. Second, at nighttime you aren't eating a lot of foods which can interfere with calcium absorption.

Dr. David Perlmutter suggests taking approximately 1,000 mg of calcium lactate and B-complex at bedtime.

Don't Forget the Magnesium

Never underestimate the importance of magnesium with calcium, since they work in balance throughout our bodies. Without magnesium, calcium accumulates in places it shouldn't. Because of the high absorption rate of minerals in solution, and deficiency of magnesium in the diet, the ratio of magnesium and calcium in solution should be four to one, respectively.

Magnesium is responsible for 80 percent of all the body's activities, and a deficiency can cause insomnia.

Too much of either magnesium or calcium will cancel the other out. There must be equal amounts of each in order to benefit from both. If there is too much calcium in your diet, you risk a magnesium deficiency. Too much magnesium, and you lose your calcium. The same thing can happen with phosphate. Phosphates tend to lower magnesium levels even further. Phosphates are found in abundance in soft drinks and many processed foods.

Tryptophan and Friends

Carlton Fredericks used to tell audiences that his pet way of falling asleep was by taking 500 mg of the essential amino acid tryptophan early in the evening. Tryptophan converts into serotonin. However, experiments by Dr. Richard Wurtman, a professor of neuroscience and director of the Clinical Research Center at the Massachusetts Institute of Technology, and noted for his brain research, prove that tryptophan requires eating complex carbohydrates – cereal, fruit or vegetables – to get into the brain. A banana works fine.

If you are having problems getting to sleep, it may be due to your dinner menu. Protein keeps tryptophan from entering the brain, keeping you from getting to sleep, whereas a high complex carbohydrate meal will relax you and let you get to sleep.[1] It is available in its natural form in amino acid formulations.

Tryptophan has three buddies to make sure it follows the yellow brick road to the land of serotonin. These are vitamin B6, magnesium and niacin.

Magnesium is probably the most common deficiency that people have, which may be why there is such a prevalence of insomnia. Magnesium works with vitamin B6 and must be taken together. Chemical pollutants, including chemical dyes and preservatives in our food, interfere with the absorption of vitamin B6 in the body. There are certain areas of the body where B6 is stored and absorbed and it turns out these chemicals also reside there, keeping the B6 from being absorbed. Therefore, when we have problems like insomnia, we need massive amounts of vitamin B6, but no more than 50 mg daily.

By the way, niacin, alone has proved to be a sleep-enhancer. The nutrient activates certain receptors in the brain that affect sleep. Dosages of between 50 mg and 1,000 mg have reportedly helped many people sleep better.

As far as tryptophan is concerned, many research studies have shown that it makes an excellent sleepmate. One gram (1,000 mg) before bedtime reduced falling-asleep time by half for normal individuals tested.

One study reported in the *Journal of the American Geriatric Society* showed that 30 percent of elderly patients with insomnia had "dramatic and sustained relief" by taking tryptophan. It is available in its natural form in amino acid formulations.

Better Sleep with B Vitamins

One of the nation's most brilliant biochemists, the late Carl C. Pfeiffer, Ph.D., M.D., former director of the Princeton Brain Bio Center, found that inositol, one of the B vitamins, is an excellent and harmless sedative that works as well or better than the most prescribed tranquilizers, calming a person to sleep. Usually 1,000 mg of inositol in the morning and the same amount an hour before bedtime at night can beat even a bad case of sleeplessness. Supplemental lecithin also contains inositol.

Vitamin B12 has also been shown to assist with sleep. An amazing case study was reported at the 5th World Congress of Biological Psychiatry in Florence, Italy, June 1991.

A 68 year old patient who had brain surgery ten years prior suffered from depression, insomnia and behavioral problems. He was given oral doses of vitamin B12, but was not tested as deficient. After only ten days of treatment, not only did he begin to sleep at night but his depressive state and behavioral disorder disappeared. What is interesting is that he wasn't deficient, yet the B12 helped. The researchers noted that when the B12 was discontinued, his problems returned.[2]

Researchers have discovered that B12 especially works for people who have problems staying asleep at night. They call this tendency a sleep-wake rhythm disorder. Have you ever found yourself waking up at the same time every night, then being unable to get back to sleep? I bet the same brain chemical reaction that allows you to beat your alarm clock every morning creates this disorder. Apparently, B12 can help.

Dr. Masako Okawa and colleagues at the Department of Neuropsychiatry, Akita University School of Medicine, in Japan, studied five patients with a variety of sleep-wake rhythm disorders who had the problem for many years. The patients were between 14 and 60 years of age and either could not get to sleep, stay asleep, or sleep at all during the night. All were successfully treated with vitamin B12 and had relapses when the B12 supplementation stopped.[3]

The Marvel of Melatonin

This chapter would not be complete without discussing melatonin. If you haven't heard of it yet, you've been vacationing in Bedrock!

Melatonin is a hormone produced by the pineal gland and is increased in the blood during hours of darkness. In the daytime it is in low concentrations. Melatonin promotes sleep and contributes to the circadian rhythm – the sleep-wake rhythm – and body temperature. Have you ever noticed how when you are very tired, you feel cold? Or how warm air can lull you to sleep? This is melatonin at work.

Dr. Gregory M. Brown of the Clarke Institute of Psychiatry in Toronto, Canada, has written that melatonin can help with jet lag, shift work, delayed phase sleep disorder, periodic sleep disorder and even behavioral disorders in children with multiple brain damage.[4]

Melatonin treatment produces effects that are nearly the mirror image of those caused by bright light. It can work in cases where a lack of light causes seasonal affective disorder or SAD. A decrease in melatonin concentration has been reported in most studies in depressed patients.

In 1980, Alfred J. Lewy, a psychiatrist at the Oregon Health Sciences University in Portland, and his coworkers showed that bright light, such as sunlight, affects human melatonin production. This finding led them to use light to treat SAD.[5] Since then, the team has experimented with melatonin to reset the biological clock of travelers, shift workers, and blind people.

"It's when the [body's internal] clock doesn't expect the hormone that it's most effective," Lewy says in an issue of *Science News*. That's typically the first thing in the morning, to trick the body into thinking dawn has not yet arrived, or during the afternoon, to advance the internal clock to nightfall. "This effect is quite remarkable," he adds, because the 0.5 milligram doses result in concentrations "no greater than those normally [occurring in] the person at night."[6]

Dr. Wurtman and his co-workers reported in *Clinical Pharmacology and Therapeutics* that melatonin induces sleep without side effects. And unlike hypnotic sedatives, they find melatonin does not alter the normal architecture of sleep, including the timing and duration of dream phases characterized by rapid eye movements.[7]

In work published in 1994, Wurtman's group found that melatonin can even induce sleep at midday. This suggests, Wurtman says, that the hormone exerts its sleep-inducing effect independent of any natural circadian rhythms.

Elderly people can combat insomnia by taking melatonin two hours before bedtime, according to a study presented at the annual meeting of the American Sleep Disorders Association and Sleep Research Society in Los Angeles.

Dr. Peretz Lavie, dean of medicine at the Israel Institute of Technology in Haifa, told the *New York Times*, "It works better than I dreamed possible." Lavie found that many elderly people no longer make melatonin in their bodies. Lavie's study looked at melatonin levels in four groups: young adults and elderly people without sleep problems (normal levels), insomniacs who lived independently (small amount), and institutionalized elderly insomniacs (no detectable levels). Insomniacs given two milligrams a night for one week "slept much, much better," Lavie says. Forty patients have been taking the pills for one month with no ill effects.[8]

Sleepytime Nutrients
For maximum absorption, take supplements with meals.

Nutrient	Suggested Dosage	Formulation
Amino acids	4-6 capsules daily	Multiple formula from natural sources
Borage oil	2 capsules daily	
Fiber	4-8 tablets daily	Psyllium, with herb hyssop
Flaxseed oil	1 tablespoon daily	
Folic acid	5-10 mg daily	
L-glutamine	500 mg twice daily	
Lecithin	2 tablespoons daily	
Magnesium	200 mg daily	
Melatonin (adults only)	3 mg daily at bedtime	With B vitamins
Multi-mineral	3-4 ounces daily	In liquid solution, with vitamin B12, biotin
Multi-vitamin/mineral	6 caplets daily	Freeze-dried plant sources
Vitamin B6	100 mg daily	
Vitamin C	Individual bowel tolerance*	With bioflavonoids (quercetin, rutin proanthocyanidins)

* To determine individual dosage, on the first day take 1,000 mg hourly until diarrhea occurs, then reduce dosage to just below that for individual daily dosage. Vitamin C is not toxic in large doses but must be taken throughout the day to benefit. Divide dosage to three or four times a day.

CHAPTER 147:

Smell and Taste Loss

John was losing weight. He couldn't remember the last time he lost so much weight so fast, and was concerned that his colitis was cancer after all. He saw specialist after specialist, but all proclaimed him cancer-free. The only thing wrong with him, they said, was mal-absorption due to the colitis. They told him to eat more, emphasizing vegetables and fruits. But John didn't want to eat. That was the trouble. He had no appetite. He told his wife the plastic fruit she kept on the table tasted better than a Chiquita banana.

It all started following hospitalization for his colitis. Doctors were able to control the inflammation in his colon, but after that he began noticing his food tasted bland. At first he thought it was just the hospital food. After he got home, no matter how much spice or salt he added, he still couldn't savor his food. Even his favorite recipe tasted bland and flavorless. He bought vegetables, but found no joy in eating them. He couldn't understand what was wrong with him until he happened to catch a segment of my show *Maximize Your Life*. There was a woman on the program who suffered from anorexia who had lost her sense of smell – and she couldn't taste anything! That was something he hadn't thought of. His doctor told him many colitis patients temporarily lose their sense of smell, but he hadn't realized 80 percent of our sense of smell governs our sense of taste too![1] The information he gleaned from the show helped him restore his sense of smell, taste and appetite, *and* helped heal his colon. But before I impart this valuable information to you, let's review smell and taste loss.

Sensory Imperception

Imagine how your life would be changed if you couldn't smell the roses or savor the sweet nectar of a juicy peach. Studies indicate that up to half of the elderly experience a loss of smell and taste.[2]

The sense of smell always works the same way, whether it's food, flowers or skunks you are sniffing. The molecules ride the air and go up to the back of your nose to a sheet of long, thin receptor cells, called the olfactory epithelium. These hairlike receptors translate the molecules' chemical message into information for the sensory nerve. The receptor cell nerves form the only sensory system that works in this way, Charles Wysocki, associate member of the Monell Chemical Sensing Center in Philadelphia, points out. They are unique in that they have a very short life span of up to 45 days, when they are replaced.

Once the smells become energy messages, they are sent to the olfactory bulb in the front of the brain where more data processing takes place. From there, the information scatters to different parts of the brain.

Some people hold their noses to avoid sniffing the unpleasantness of life, while there are those who smell nothing at all. These people are called anosmic. They might have been born without an olfactory bulb, or it might have been injured, or the connection lost between the nose and the brain.

Even though some peoples' sense of smell is more acute than others, one pattern remains true for everyone. With age, the sense of smell declines. About half of those over 80 can smell little or nothing. Another disorder is when a person confuses the smell of one thing – or nothing – for something entirely different. This manifestation is called parosmia. People with parosmia may mistake the smell of cow dung for an apple, or they may think that there is an odor in the air when there is not.

Two million Americans suffer from some type of taste or smell disorder. It is not only disconcerting but it can be dangerous. People who can't smell can't tell when food is spoiled, or they cannot smell a gas leak. Dr. Alan Hirsch, a smell/taste researcher at Chicago's Rush-Presbyterian-St Luke's Medical Center says the loss of the sense of smell is the most common affliction, but it is often perceived as the loss of an ability to taste because the two are so closely linked. A true loss of taste is termed *hypogeusia*.

The two most common causes of smell-and-taste disorders are virus infections and head injury. Both cause permanent damage to the nerves that carry "messages" to the brain from receptors in the nose and tongue. Nasal blockage – from bacterial sinus infections, polyps or allergy – ranks third.

Environmental toxins also may cause loss or distortion of taste and smell. "Most cases involve large, accidental exposures," says Susan Schiffman, a smell-and-taste researcher at Duke University. "But we really don't know what happens at lower levels of exposure – for instance, from air pollution – in everyday life." Smell and taste losses have occurred in people who work with metallic compounds like lead, arsenic, mercury or cadmium or breathe vapors from industrial solvents such as benzene. Swimming pool workers have lost the sense of smell after accidental exposure to chlorine.[3]

A Deficiency of Zinc Causes Smell and Taste Loss

What my friend John learned is that when his colon became inflamed it lost its ability to absorb zinc. Not only did a lack of zinc limit his body's healing capabilities, but as a side effect, it was probably responsible for his loss of smell.[4]

Since the intestine is the major source of loss of this mineral, John had to contend that his initial loss of taste was related to zinc deficiency.[5] He followed up this revelation by seeking out a physician versed in nutrition who gave him zinc and copper supplementation. Within three months not only was his colitis greatly improved, but he could again taste his favorite recipe – curry chicken.

Ronald F. Pokornowski, M.D., practicing in Carol Stream, Illinois, had a patient who lost his sense of taste following heart bypass surgery. When a colleague suggested zinc be used to treat this loss of taste, Dr. Pokornowski conducted a search for more information. In an article in the *Cortlandt Forum* he reported finding over 100 articles, dating back to 1969, on zinc and its effects on taste and smell.[6]

Robert I. Henkin, M.D., of The Taste and Smell Clinic in Washington, D.C. discovered that 25 percent of individuals with impaired smell and taste absorb zinc improperly. Given daily zinc supplementation, they showed marked improvement in three to four months.[7]

Andrew L. Stoll, M.D., and Godehard Oepen, M.D., gave zinc to five patients with smell and taste loss, and noted they were effectively cured.[8]

Mineral Reasons

Although a deficiency of zinc is the major contributor to an impaired sense of taste, other vitamins and minerals are involved too.

Two nutrients must be considered along with zinc: vitamin B6 and copper. Too much copper will deplete zinc stores; they must be equal for optimum usage. Include 2-4 mg of copper with any zinc supplement.

Zinc and vitamin B6 are intricately involved in hormone metabolism, and vitamin B6 enhances zinc absorption.

Whenever I recommend one B vitamin I recommend all of the them. All the B vitamins work in synch. Without one, the others can become deficient. Without minerals they don't work at all. When supplementing one B vitamin always take a good B vitamin complex, at least ten times the RDA. A note about RDAs. They were formulated with *everyone* in mind. Therefore, their recommendations are maintenance levels, not optimum levels. In today's world of pollutants and nutritionally-deficient food (fresh as well as processed), we need more help than the RDAs. Always target supplements that are much higher than the RDAs.

Magnesium is another mineral found to be important to a lack of smell. Dr. Henkin and colleagues conducted a study of 17 anosmia patients who were found to be resistant to zinc supplements. After being given oral doses of magnesium, 59 percent of their patients said they could smell better, while 71 percent showed improvement after being tested.[9]

Other Dietary Factors

Following the realization that the elderly typically lose their senses of smell and taste, some researchers have evaluated their food intake in attempting to pinpoint dietary factors that may be involved. In an article in the *Journal of the American Dietetic Association*, researchers evaluated the dietary habits of 80 women, half of which were found to have impaired taste and smell. Interestingly, the women with smell and taste problems chose foods higher in salt, sugar and fat. Of the 80 women, a majority ate less than 66 percent of the RDA (already low) of essential fatty acids, vitamin D, vitamin E and zinc.[10]

Another factor may be involved with a loss of taste and smell with age – the loss of digestive enzymes and hydrochloric acid in the stomach. Studies have shown that as people grow older, their ability to break down food (with stomach acid) and absorb it (with digestive enzymes) is severely reduced.

A lack of stomach acid – hypochlorhydria – is more common than we think and can cause all of the symptoms that appear when the stomach contains too much acid. Doctors warn that people should not take antacids too readily as heartburn, gas, bloating after eating and even constipation can all be symptoms of too little stomach, or gastric, acid. The burning sensation common to too much acid is also present when the stomach is too alkaline, and can be made worse by antacids. Dr. Jonathan Wright estimates that every third adult secretes too little hydrochloric acid.

Researchers at the Mayo Clinic and Johns Hopkins University pumped the stomachs of over 3,000 individuals and analyzed their contents. It was determined that by the age of 60 years, 60 percent had a significant decline in hydrochloric acid. Supplementing with a hydrochloric acid formula such as Betaine, available in health food stores, will help absorb nutrients.

Studies show minerals in solution are considerably more bioavailable to the body than those even present in food or inorganic supplements. Minerals in solution don't need stomach acid to break them down, and aren't influenced by food allergies. Look for a good, easily absorbable, derived-from-nature mineral blend in solution. Liquid formulations provide the maximum absorption ratios.

Taste and Smell Restoring Nutrients

For maximum absorption, take supplements with meals.

Nutrient	Suggested Dosage	Formulation
Acidophilus	At least four billion flora on an empty stomach, three times daily	
Aged garlic extract	1 teaspoon three times daily	Liquid
Amino acids	4-6 capsules daily	Multiple formula from natural sources
Borage oil	2 capsules daily	
Coenzyme Q10	2 capsules daily	With vitamin E, phospholipids and selenium
Enzymes	2 capsules twice daily	Multiple formula
Fiber	4-8 tablets daily	Psyllium, with herb hyssop
Flaxseed oil	1 tablespoon daily	
Folic acid	5-10 mg daily	
L-glutamine	500 mg twice daily	
Magnesium	200 mg daily	
Melatonin (adults only)	3 mg daily at bedtime	With B vitamins
Multi-mineral	3-4 ounces daily	In liquid solution, with vitamin B12, biotin
Multi-vitamin/mineral	6 caplets daily	Freeze-dried plant sources
Niacin	500 mg four times daily	
Taurine	500 mg twice daily	
Vitamin B6	100 mg daily	
Vitamin C	Individual bowel tolerance*	With bioflavonoids (quercetin, rutin proanthocyanidins)

* To determine individual dosage, on the first day take 1,000 mg hourly until diarrhea occurs, then reduce dosage to just below that for individual daily dosage. Vitamin C is not toxic in large doses but must be taken throughout the day to benefit. Divide dosage to three or four times a day.

CHAPTER 148:

Smoking (Quitting)

A man was told by his doctor that if he didn't quit smoking he was going to have a heart attack. He wanted a second opinion, and he got one...from the coroner.

You are reading this chapter not because you want to know all the reasons to quit, but because you want to quit. There are hundreds of reasons to stop: the endless coughing, because the smoke has destroyed the cilia in your lungs and only coughing can remove the soot and dirt lodged in there; being ostracized in your office and feeling foolish standing outside in the cold and rain just for a smoke; your granddaughter won't sit on your lap "cause you stink;" those ugly wrinkles around your mouth; and so you'll live longer, better, healthier – and richer – without cigarettes in your life.

> *"To cease smoking is the easiest thing I ever did, I ought to know because I've done it a thousand times."*
> –Mark Twain

Tobacco Legacy Rejected

One former smoker is Patrick Reynolds, estranged heir to the R.J. Reynolds International Tobacco Company, makers and marketers of Camel, Lucky Strike, Winston and Salem brand cigarettes. Patrick's tobacco ancestry goes back to 1875, when his grandfather,

R. J. Reynolds, formed the R.J. Reynolds Tobacco Company in Winston, North Carolina, to produce chewing tobacco. For his family, smoking was more than an idle pleasure, tobacco was the crop that made their family one of America's wealthiest. They paid for it too. Patrick's grandfather, mother and two aunts died from smoking. His father R.J. "Dick" Reynolds, Jr. suffered from emphysema for years before dying.[1]

Patrick remembers family stories about his mother, Marianne, who took up smoking because she thought it would please her husband. Instead of being impressed, he barked at her, "How could you take up such a filthy, disgusting habit? I'm so disappointed in you." Patrick remembers years later hearing the same words from Marianne when she discovered that Patrick was smoking.

It took him nearly a dozen tries over 15 years to quit. He was very addicted, he says. "It was an enormous struggle. I tried every program in the book: acupuncture, hypnosis, shock therapy, behavior modification. I went through some programs more than once. One program five times!"

Patrick says, "I could stay off cigarettes for three to six months at a time. In moments of positive or negative stress – a fight, a lonely moment, an evening out with friends or a vacation – I would succumb to a friend's offer of a cigarette. I had everything in this world I could conceivably want, so that amplified the fact that I didn't have a cigarette. I repeatedly made the fatal error under stressful circumstances of having just one." Then, of course, he says, the next day he would just have two or three, and the next it became five or six. "The hole would open up and I would be engulfed." Reynolds sighs. "I got tremendous enjoyment out of cigarettes and smoking. It's a drug that keeps you up."

In 1984, he finally quit for good. Today Patrick Reynolds fights a legacy responsible each year for thousands of deaths. He fights to convince smokers to quit and nonsmokers never to start. Patrick advises that if you are a smoker, you should stop or get help. "Four out of five smokers who quit do so on their own," Reynolds says. "However, 80 percent of them return to cigarettes. It's the same rate of return as heroin addicts. In life winners get help, losers try to do things alone."

You Don't Fail Until You Stop Trying

Gaining freedom from smoking isn't easy because the nicotine in tobacco is highly addictive. Nicotine is rated as the most powerful and rapidly absorbed mood altering substance widely available worldwide – as addictive as heroin or cocaine. Considering its addictive nature, it's strange that many don't think of nicotine as a drug. Yet the effects and behavior that perpetuate its use resemble illegal street drugs such as heroin, speed (amphetamine) and cocaine.

Nicotine is a stimulant that acts on "binding sites" in the brain and throughout the body. Nicotine gets into the brain faster and more easily than many other drugs, penetrating the blood-brain barrier as or more quickly than heroin. In 1980, the American Psychiatric Association formally listed tobacco as an addictive substance, calling nicotine addiction a Tobacco Dependence Disorder (later renaming it the Nicotine Dependence Disorder). The Surgeon General's 1988 Report conclusively states that "cigarettes and other forms of tobacco are just as addicting as heroin and cocaine, illegal drugs regarded by most adults with scorn and disapproval (if not outrage)." Many smokers who find it hard to quit can testify to nicotine's addictive power. Those who are physically dependent have a withdrawal reaction if they stop smoking.[2]

If at first you don't succeed – try, try again.

Over 90 percent of smokers claim they'd like to stop, especially "if there were an easy way to do it!" The U.S. Surgeon General's Report states that "at least 60 percent of tobacco smokers have tried to quit at some time in their lives." Studies show that, as with heroin users, most cigarette smokers who quit give up without formal treatment. And with users of both drugs, repeated attempts usually pay off in the end. Many smokers "give up" six to 13 times before finally stopping for good. (About two out of 10 manage to stop on the first attempt, 50 percent succeeding after six tries.) Even those who attend rigorous smoke-ending programs may not succeed with their first attempt. The claimed success rate for formal programs varies from 15 to 30 percent (although quoted figures aren't necessarily reliable).[3]

Studies show the best predictor of success is support. A friend of mine is afraid to tell anyone when she tries to quit because she doesn't want to experience their disappointment if she fails. This is a mistake. If you look at the numbers, when you get help, you stay off the nicotine.

Nutrition Can Help

John Emery, a cosmetic surgeon practicing in San Francisco, instructs his patients not to smoke for three weeks before and three weeks after any cosmetic surgical procedure. This is because nicotine interferes with the blood supply of the skin, increasing the chances of the skin dying, and obviously jeopardizing the success of the procedure. He says not smoking is a "very significant factor for success." For their skin health, he recommends they take selenium, a potent antioxidant, before and after surgery. Dr. Emery told me: "My observation is that those who take my recommendations seriously and quit smoking for three weeks before and after, are able to quit for good."

Many smokers find they are able to quit when they consider the damage it does to their looks. Smoking increases wrinkling of the skin. If you have managed to quit and want to stay off it; or know someone who wants to quit; or want to encourage a teenager you know to quit, avoid thinking about or discussing the health aspects. The incredible array of diseases, syndromes and health problems caused by both first and second-hand smoke doesn't seem to be a motivating factor compared to the vanity factor.

Researchers from the University of Minnesota studied seventh graders at eight Minneapolis-St. Paul junior high schools to determine what would turn them off smoking. In the first group they stressed the long-term health consequences. In the second group they accented the socially negative effects: bad breath, yellow fingers and teeth, and smelly clothes. When the researchers evaluated the influence of their programs a year later they found the group who learned the social consequences were more influenced to quit or not start smoking. One of the researchers, David Murray, pointed out that youngsters are much more concerned about physical appearance and social acceptance than long-term health consequences which won't affect them for years into their futures (long enough to get them effectively hooked).[4]

I believe this principle also holds true for adults. Studies show most smoking adults started during their teen years, and by the time they begin taking their health seriously, it's too late to quit without severe withdrawal symptoms and much difficulty. If you need motivation, think about the smell, the social aversion and banishment from many establishments smoking incurs. If you are trying to find that special man or woman in your life, think of all the good people out there who will not date a smoker. When you smoke, you not only sabotage your health and shorten your life, but you lengthen your loneliness.

Eliminating the Stress of Quitting

If stress is a factor in your life that makes it harder to quit smoking, battle stress with good nutrition. Also consider this: many of the following nutrients are depleted in the body when replaced by nicotine. It is quite possible that a deficiency of these nutrients contributes to the withdrawal symptoms experienced while trying to quit. In your program to stop smoking, add a good multi-vitamin and multi-mineral in solution formula along with the following nutrients to help alleviate the withdrawal symptoms you may experience.

Borage oil is high in linolenic acid, an essential fatty acid that studies show inhibit abnormal adrenaline release,[5] and control the body's impulse to raise blood pressure and increase the heart rate (symptoms typical of nicotine ingestion). Researchers at the University of Waterloo, Ontario, Canada, found that when 30 men were randomly given three forms of essential fatty acids: fish oil, borage oil and olive oil, only those receiving the borage oil did not have increased blood pressure or heart rate as a response to stress. Not only that, but they were able to think more clearly during stress.[6]

A friend of mine could only stop smoking by substituting something he could do with both his hands and mouth. He found the act of opening and eating sunflower seeds did the trick. It took a lot of patience from his family, who tired of stepping on and cleaning up the shells, but he was also getting helpful nutrients. Sunflower seeds contain essential fatty acids and the minerals calcium, potassium and magnesium.

Magnesium has been shown in studies to reduce the stress response. Following a natural disaster, you usually hear about one or two people dying from heart attacks. Obviously, the stress of the earthquake, flood or bomb triggered the attack. But what caused the fatality?

Dr. Mildred S. Seelig of the American College of Nutrition believes that stress coupled with a deficiency of magnesium can cause a fatal heart attack.[7] Magnesium requirements are markedly increased during stress, and the heart is much more susceptible to arrhythmias during physical exertion if the body's magnesium level is low.[8] Smoking depletes the body of many essential nutrients; nutrients that when replaced can help the smoker quit! Important to remember is that magnesium must be balanced with calcium and potassium.

During stress, your body needs so much more vitamin C that you can be deficient to the point of getting symptoms of scurvy. Symptoms include swelling and bleeding of the gums, muscle pain, discolored skin and increased susceptibility to bruising and infection.[9] Smoking is notorious for reducing circulation in the body. Smoking depletes so much vitamin C, which is so important to healthy skin, that one of the reasons smokers become prematurely wrinkled, is their chronic deficiency of vitamin C. If you or someone you know smokes, take, or get them to take high amounts of vitamin C.

Dr. Garry Gordon, M.D., recommends 1,000 milligrams an hour of vitamin C when trying to quit smoking.[10] Dr. Emanuel Cheraskin calls vitamin C the "stress vitamin."

If I were asked to target another stress reducing vitamin, I would pinpoint all the B vitamins. Iris R. Bell, M.D., Ph.D., Department of Psychiatry at the University of Arizona Health Sciences Center in Tucson, found that certain B vitamins are deficient in patients with severe depression. She found that the B vitamins have a major role in the central nervous system.[11]

A McGill University study of depressed patients found that their levels of folic acid, another B vitamin, were far lower than those of medically ill patients. This was also borne out in research at the Royal Victoria Hospital in Montreal. These studies indicate that a lack of folic acid could contribute to depression.[12]

On any program of anti-stress, always supplement with a good, naturally-derived B vitamin formula. All the B vitamins together are necessary to get the benefit of any one.

Stress reduces the amount of zinc stored in the body. One study of volunteers found that, although they had more than adequate zinc to begin with, the amount was reduced by an incredible 33 percent when they were under stress.[13]

Zinc is required to repair wounds in the skin and body tissue, most especially lung tissue damaged by the tar in cigarettes. It is also necessary to absorb the B vitamins.

Copper is important to balance out your zinc supplements. Be sure and include 2-4 mg of copper with any zinc supplementation.

Since smoking creates a host of health problems, also target the nutrients contained in other chapters of this book: Depression, Allergies, Anemia, Asthma, Arthritis, Arteriosclerosis, Bronchitis, Cancer of the Lung, Cataracts, Chronic Fatigue, Circulation, Colds and Flu, Depression, Heart Problems, Infertility, Muscle Weakness, Teeth and Gum Problems and Wrinkles.

Anti-Smoking Nutrients
For maximum absorption, take supplements with meals.

Nutrient	Suggested Dosage	Formulation
Aged garlic extract	1 teaspoon three times daily	Liquid
Antioxidants	4 capsules daily*	With selenium and grapeseed extract
Borage oil	2 capsules daily	
Coenzyme Q10	2 capsules daily	With vitamin E, phospholipids and selenium
Fiber	4-8 tablets daily	Psyllium, with herb hyssop
Flaxseed oil	1 tablespoon daily	
Folic acid	5-10 mg daily	
Magnesium	200 mg daily	
Multi-mineral	3-4 ounces daily	In liquid solution, with vitamin B12, biotin
Multi-vitamin/mineral	6 caplets daily	Freeze-dried plant sources
Niacin	500 mg four times daily	
Taurine	500 mg twice daily	
Vitamin B6	100 mg daily	
Vitamin C	Individual bowel tolerance**	With bioflavonoids (quercetin, rutin proanthocyanidins)

* The FDA recommends pregnant women not exceed 10,000 IU of vitamin A daily.

** To determine individual dosage, on the first day take 1,000 mg hourly until diarrhea occurs, then reduce dosage to just below that for individual daily dosage. Vitamin C is not toxic in large doses but must be taken throughout the day to benefit. Divide dosage to three or four times a day.

CHAPTER 149:

Stress

"In my life, I have suffered many terrible experiences.
Some of which actually happened."

–Mark Twain

All of us have witnessed the physical damage stress can wrack on the body. My friend – I'll call her Patty – was a 40-year-old nurse whose symptoms began after she took on a second job with a group of five physicians specializing in critical care internal medicine. She worked five days a week, averaging 10 to 12 hectic hours a day.

Patty's symptoms started approximately two weeks after beginning work there. She had weight loss, decreased appetite, neck pain, headaches, heart palpitations, anxiety, insomnia and heartburn. She sought help from one of the doctors she worked for, who prescribed an assortment of pharmaceuticals for her symptoms. Rejecting the drugs, she sought a second opinion from Dr. Ross Gordon, in Albany, California, who specializes in identifying causes, not just treating symptoms.

By the time Patty saw Dr. Gordon she was also experiencing "vice-grip" attacks of chest pain and panic attacks that resulted in a loss of consciousness for several minutes. What puzzled her the most was that these episodes occurred while at rest rather than at work.

Dr. Gordon diagnosed high blood pressure, hyperadrenalism and possibly low blood sugar. He believed her adrenal glands were producing too much adrenalin, causing the high blood pressure and chest pain, and her poor diet was causing low blood sugar, resulting in the fainting episodes.

He ordered her to stop eating all sources of sugar, caffeine, saturated fats and alcohol. He told her to instead eat fruits, vegetables and grains in the form of a snack every two hours or so to maintain a constant blood sugar level; walk or do some form of aerobic exercise at least 30 minutes daily to burn up the excess adrenalin; and he put her on an anti-stress nutritional supplementation regimen which included a multi-vitamin supplement, extra vitamin C and a multi-mineral supplement in solution that includes calcium, potassium and magnesium. For her insomnia, he also included tryptophan. Foods that contain tryptophan include: turkey breast meat, wheat germ, granola and oats. It is available in its natural form in amino acid formulations. If you are interested in using it therapeutically, ask you doctor. My sources tell me some doctors are prescribing it in therapeutic dosages.

Patty returned to Dr. Gordon's office one month later. After beginning the regimen he prescribed, her chest pains and panic attacks disappeared completely, she gained back five pounds and her blood pressure stabilized. Her headaches and neck pain were much better and the tryptophan was helping her sleep. She called the office two months later to tell Dr. Gordon that she left her job and found a position with an alternative medicine physician. By that time her symptoms had completely disappeared.

The Physiological Effect of Stress

The body's endocrine system – essential to a properly functioning immune system – may be one of the first victims of stress. What can happen is that a long term poor diet, a lack of exercise and emotional stress can so exhaust the adrenals that the metabolic response of the body is to produce more adrenaline, a type of hormone. Have you ever experienced a hot flash of embarrassment or a "rush" of adrenaline when on a roller coaster? Or, do you know the feeling when you're very angry or frightened and blood rushes to your head and you feel almost dizzy? These are your adrenals' responses to stress.

The two adrenal glands sit beside each kidney, deep in the back part of the stomach. Each gland has two parts, a cortex or outer part, and a medulla or central portion. The medulla is what responds to stress by secreting adrenalin (epinephrine) and noradrenalin (norepinephrine). These hormones are what make you dizzy, light-headed or suddenly forget that word you've been grasping for. They are designed to "rev up" the nervous and metabolic systems in preparation for the needs required by a stressful situation, which, in the case of stage fright and writer's block, can sometimes cause their own problems.

When stress is constant, the adrenals become overloaded, and your body suffers. Adrenaline increases your heart rate and blood pressure, causing your veins to dilate and blood sugar to rise. Circulation through your lungs, liver and skeletal muscles increases by as much as one hundred percent. The released adrenaline can give you indigestion, make you infertile and cause you to be malnourished. While you aren't necessarily conscious of all the changes that take place, what you might notice is your jaw clenching, stomach tightening and palms sweating.[1]

The stressors don't have to be "real," either. What happens to you when your boss comes to you to announce, "Do you have some time later? I need to talk to you." Your mind goes through the worst possible scenario, and you're a nervous wreck until the mystery is solved.

According to Dr. Maxell Maltz, author of *Psycho-Cybernetics* and other self-help books, "The human nervous system cannot tell the difference between an 'actual' experience and an experience imagined vividly and in detail."[2]

Therefore, it is important for us to control imaginary stresses, especially if they evoke the same emotional response as the real situation. In fact, thinking about a given situation without actually being physically involved may be more harmful. Researchers have found that people watching a sports event released a higher proportion of adrenaline than those actually playing. Participants were also found to release proportionately more noradrenaline, the chemical that controls your stress reactions and puts the brakes on adrenaline.[3]

While some stressful episodes may seem to cause no lasting harm, over time pent up anxiety from overreacting to real or imagined crises adds up. Eric Peper, Ph.D., associate director of the Institute of Holistic Healing Studies at San Francisco State University, says that up to 80 percent of health problems today are considered stress-related.[4] These include high blood pressure, heart disease, ulcers and an inability to fight infections.

The Nutritional Response to Stress

Follow along while I put the pieces of the puzzle together. Nutritional needs of the body skyrocket during stress. When I talk about stress, I mean pressure from any source; whether it be that winter cold, the death of a relative, impending surgery, or the surgery itself--anything that stresses the system, mentally or physically. And just when you need it the most, your resistance to illness falls in direct proportion to the depletion of certain vitamins and minerals caused by the stress.

Vitamin C is the first vitamin to come under stress in any tissue. During this time, vitamin E, pantothenic acid, vitamin A, and all the B vitamins are used up in massive amounts. The body withdraws minerals from bones, teeth, hair, organs, and other tissues to meet the demands of defense, and breaks down protein from itself to create more hormones and antibodies. Calcium, magnesium, phosphorus and potassium demands are also increased under stress.[5]

As the body becomes deficient in essential nutrients, its ability to resist the stressors diminishes. If stress is prolonged for weeks, months or years, the body is unable to convert cholesterol into needed hormones. Physical symptoms can be the body's way of reacting to internal pressure and its subsequent nutritional deficiencies. Continued stress results in complete exhaustion and total collapse. "Nervous breakdowns," heart attacks, cancers, strokes, liver damage, and even kidney damage can be caused by constant stress. It can become a vicious cycle.

Stress-Reducing Nutrients

Nutrients don't reduce stress as much as they cushion the body's *response* to stress. You have to make life changes in order to reduce tension and pressure, but in the meantime, a daily supplement of borage oil, for example, will help your body overcome its dangerous effects.

Borage oil is high in linolenic acid, an essential fatty acid that studies show inhibit abnormal adrenaline release[6] and control the body's impulse to raise blood pressure and increase the heart rate. Researchers at the University of Waterloo, Ontario, Canada, found that when 30 men were randomly given three forms of essential fatty acids: fish oil, borage oil and olive oil, only those receiving the borage oil did not have increased blood pressure or heart rate as a response to stress. Not only that, but they were able to think clearer during stress.[7] Imagine that benefit the next time you are confronted by an angry person and wish you could think of something witty to say. I'd say presence of mind is a very desirable trait to have when confronted with a stressful situation, whether it be a driver's exam or an angry neighbor.

Magnesium has been shown in studies to reduce the stress response. Following a natural disaster, you usually hear about one or two people dying from heart attacks. Obviously, the anxiety of the earthquake, flood or bomb triggered the fatality.

Stress coupled with a deficiency of magnesium can cause a fatal heart attack.[8] When people with cardiovascular problems and low magnesium intake try to improve their health with strenuous exercise, such as jogging, they could be endangering their health. Magnesium requirements are markedly increased during stress, and the heart is much more susceptible to arrhythmias during physical exertion if the body's magnesium level is low.[9] Many cases of sudden heart attacks during stressful exercise can be directly attributed to a magnesium deficiency.

Austrian researchers performed a placebo-controlled trial of 17 healthy individuals between 24 and 51 years of age who received 400 mg of magnesium for 10 days. Following that, they were given a physical stress test and concluded that the magnesium appeared to have a calming effect on stress reactions with respect to blood gas changes and white blood cell changes.[10] In other words, the magnesium prevented some of the stress-induced changes that cause heart problems and encourage illness.

Magnesium deficiency is more common than you might expect. A large study by the U.S. Department of Agriculture found that only 25 percent of 37,785 individuals had magnesium intakes at or greater than the recommended daily allowance, which is notoriously low. A 1995 review of 15 studies found that a typical diet contains only a fraction of the RDA.[11]

The average American diet supplies about 120 mg of magnesium per 1,000 calories. Green leafy vegetables are particularly good sources of the mineral, as are dry beans and peas, soybeans, nuts and whole grains. High losses of magnesium occur in the refinement of foods, and some losses result when cooking water is discarded.

Important to remember is that magnesium must be balanced with calcium and potassium.

During stress, your body needs so much more vitamin C that you can be deficient to the point of getting symptoms of scurvy. Symptoms include swelling and bleeding of the gums, muscle pain, discolored skin and increased susceptibility to bruising and infection.[12]

Garry Gordon, M.D., recommends 1,000 milligrams an hour of vitamin C when sick or severely stressed.[13]

Researchers at the Department of Poultry Sciences, Louisiana State University, Baton Rouge, decided to evaluate the effect of vitamin C, in the form of ascorbic acid, on chickens that were slated to be slaughtered. Thirty-two hours prior to slaughter the chickens were given either ascorbic acid in their drinking water or only tap water. The birds were then stressed for eight hours prior to being killed. Blood tests performed just prior to and just after slaughter revealed that the ascorbic acid supplementation reduced the chickens' adrenal stress response.[14] I do think it might have been possible to perform the same tests on students about to undergo an arduous final exam, rather than subject innocent animals to torture in the name of science. I do not advocate torturing animals for any reason.

In her book *Let's Get Well*, (Harcourt, Brace & World, p. 165), the late Adelle Davis confesses that stressful work on her book with many sleepless nights led to an alarming condition – her hair falling out and receding at the temples. Immediately, she slept more and went on her anti-stress formula: 500 mg of vitamin C, 100 mg of pantothenic acid, and two mg each of vitamins B2 and B6 with each meal, between meals and every three hours during the night when awake. Additionally, Adelle took half a teaspoon of inositol, five mg of folic acid, 50 mcg of biotin and 300 mg of PABA. New hair came in thick and vigorous, and even went back to its original color.

If I were asked to target any one stress reducing vitamin, I would pinpoint all the B vitamins. Certain B vitamins are deficient in patients with severe depression, not surprising when you realize that the B vitamins have a major role in the central nervous system.[15]

A McGill University study of depressed patients found that their levels of folic acid, another B vitamin, were far lower than those of medically ill patients. This was also borne out in research at the Royal Victoria Hospital in Montreal. It indicates that a lack of folic acid could contribute to depression.[16]

On any program of anti-stress, always supplement with a good, naturally-derived B vitamin formula. All the B vitamins together are necessary to get the benefit of any one.

Stress reduces the amount of zinc stored in the body. One study of volunteers found that, although they had more than adequate zinc to begin with, the amount was reduced by an incredible 33 percent when they were under stress.[17]

Zinc is required to repair wounds in the skin and body tissue. It is also necessary to absorb the B vitamins. Copper is important to balance out your zinc supplements. Be sure and include 2-4 mg of copper with any zinc supplement.

Exercising Off the Adrenaline

Exercise is essential for any program of stress relief. The reason the adrenals spit out more hormones when you are under pressure is so you may be physically ready to fight or run. Every once in a while I read where somebody under stress performs some incredible feat of strength, lifting a car to save someone, for example. If that person had not taken action when his body told him to, he would have suffered. Stress requires a physical outlet to "work off" the excess hormones so they don't turn inward and damage the body.

Another issue with exercise is the fact that it takes effort. This positive action can make all the difference. Take menopause for instance. The incredible changes the body undergoes, coupled with the realization that childbirth is no longer possible takes an incredible toll on the body. Who knows how many symptoms attributed to "the change of life," are in actuality adrenal stress responses? I've found that women with strong adrenals have no problem with menopause.

Karen Matthews, a professor of psychiatry, epidemiology, and psychology at the University of Pittsburgh School of Medicine, has identified the characteristics of those who experience few problems in menopause compared to those who experience many.

"The women who do well respond to menopause with action," she says. "That may not be their direct intention, but they end up coping with the stressor by making positive changes. For example, those who step up their exercise regimen don't even show the biological changes, such as the adverse shifts in lipids implicated in coronary disease, that others do."[18]

Let me end this chapter by going back to Patty, the nurse who was cured with Dr. Gordon's anti-stress regimen. She maintains contact with the doctor to this day, and says she has found the most relaxing and reassuring book to be the Bible, which she reads nightly. She has found many scriptures which she feels were written for her. Dr. Gordon received one from her recently:

> *Fear thou not for I am with thee. Be not dismayed for I am thy God. I will strengthen thee, yea, I will help thee, yeah, I will uphold thee with the right hand of my righteousness.*   –Isaiah 41:10 - 1 Peter 4:12,13.

Less Stress Nutrients
For maximum absorption, take supplements with meals.

Nutrient	Suggested Dosage	Formulation
Aged garlic extract	1 teaspoon three times daily	Liquid
Antioxidants	4 capsules daily*	With selenium and grapeseed extract
Borage oil	2 capsules daily	
Coenzyme Q10	2 capsules daily	With vitamin E, phospholipids and selenium
Fiber	4-8 tablets daily	Psyllium, with herb hyssop
Flaxseed oil	1 tablespoon daily	
Folic acid	5-10 mg daily	
Magnesium	200 mg daily	
Multi-mineral	3-4 ounces daily	In liquid solution, with vitamin B12, biotin
Multi-vitamin/mineral	6 caplets daily	Freeze-dried plant sources
Niacin	500 mg four times daily	
Taurine	500 mg twice daily	
Vitamin B6	100 mg daily	
Vitamin C	Individual bowel tolerance**	With bioflavonoids (quercetin, rutin proanthocyanidins)

* The FDA recommends pregnant women not exceed 10,000 IU of vitamin A daily.

** To determine individual dosage, on the first day take 1,000 mg hourly until diarrhea occurs, then reduce dosage to just below that for individual daily dosage. Vitamin C is not toxic in large doses but must be taken throughout the day to benefit. Divide dosage to three or four times a day.

CHAPTER 150:

Stretch Marks

"What is the difference between a taxidermist and a tax collector? The taxidermist takes only your skin."
–Mark Twain

Gravity, pregnancy and extreme weight loss can cause stretch marks on some people, and not on others. Why? Why do some people get them and others don't? Stretch marks result when elastin protein in the skin breaks or is damaged from stretching. Think of elastin as little rubber bands in the skin – in the tiny skin capillaries actually. It is elastin that normally "snaps" the skin back into place after it has been stretched. Try it on your skin. Pull the skin up between two fingers, hold it for a moment and let go suddenly. It will "jump" back, even against gravity. When the skin is out of condition elastin "bands" dry and crack. When they are stretched, they break. There is no cosmetic surgical treatment available to restore stretch-marked skin, save perhaps literally removing the patches of skin – not something I or anyone I know would recommend.

Researchers have found, however, that elastin is dependent upon certain precautions and nutrients for optimum elasticity, and if you take these precautions and target these nutrients, you won't get, and perhaps can even erase, unsightly stretch marks.

The most important factor is the condition of the skin. With proper nutrition and exercise, skin is strong, supple and elastic. It will spring back into shape even after the expansion of pregnancy or weight gain.

If skin is in poor condition, thinned by sun and nutritionally deficient, stretching can result in breakage and damage to the skin's elastin.

Mineral Ratios Important

Researchers have found the calcium/magnesium ratio to be very important in maintaining the elastic quality of the skin.

Dr. W. Muller and colleagues at the Institute of Pathology in Koln, Germany, examined the ligaments in the discs of spinal surgery patients, putting the patients into two groups: those with very elastic tissues, and those with non-elastic tissues. He found that among those with the most elasticity, a magnesium/calcium ratio in favor of magnesium was found.[1]

Magnesium and calcium work in balance throughout our bodies. Without magnesium, calcium accumulates in places it shouldn't, including the skin. Because of the high absorption rate of minerals in solution, and deficiency of magnesium in the diet, the ratio of magnesium and calcium in solution should be four to one, respectively.

Two more minerals to keep in mind are copper and zinc. Copper is noted as a nutrient important to the manufacture of elastin in the skin. It acts as a catalyst, forming certain enzymes involved in the cross-linking of collagen and elastin. Studies show when copper is low, changes in connective tissue occur.[2]

Too much copper will deplete zinc stores; they must be equal for optimum usage.

Moisturizing To Keep Elastin Elastic

If you think about elastin as rubber bands, you'll realize that dryness can make them break when stretched. If they are kept moist, stretching won't be as likely to break them. Studies have made this connection between stretch marks and breakage and something called hyaluronic acid, or sodium hyaluronate, a naturally-occurring skin and tissue lubricator found in only the best skin care formulations.

Wrinkles and a loss of elastin are believed to be caused by free radical damage. Now, another factor is being considered: inadequate amounts of hyaluronic acid.

Researchers never fully realized the connection between hyaluronic acid and skin growth until a breakthrough study on sheep fetuses. Scientists looking for substances that would repair wounds without scar tissue or damage to the elastin began studying fetal lambs because of their ability to heal without scar formation. They discovered fetal wounds contain high levels of hyaluronic acid. They also discovered high levels of hyaluronic acid in the amniotic fluid, thus it continually bathes the fetus and encourages smooth cell formation.[3]

Additionally, in studies of adult sheep the researchers found a rapid rise of high levels of hyaluronic acid levels in the skin following injury. Why fetal lambs don't have scarring while adult sheep do relates to the fact that the hyaluronic acid levels in the lambs persist at least 21 days after wounding, whereas in adult sheep high levels occur three days or less following injury. The researchers concluded that hyaluronic acid not only encourages healing following skin damage, but can effectively inhibit tissue damage as a result of an injury.

What does hyaluronic acid have to do with stretch marks? It's an ingredient in some skin cleansers and moisturizers, and can be useful in preventing the skin cell damage that occurs when skin is stretched.

Don't let the term "acid" fool you. It's as safe on cellular tissue as water. In fact, surgeons inject it into the eye during surgery so the tissues can be separated without damage. It is also used in cases of dry eye to increase moisture.[4]

A pharmaceutical company in Basel, Switzerland, credits hyaluronic acid with not only moisturizing the skin, but "helping to maintain or restore the biophysical properties of skin, such as smoothness, elasticity, and resilience, which gives it its youthfully fresh appearance."[5]

An article in the *International Journal of Dermatology* reports on a study that showed a lack of sufficient hyaluronic acid in the skin may be responsible for the wrinkles and skin sags (loss of elastin) typical of advancing age.[6]

In fact, hyaluronic acid has turned out to be so therapeutically effective that it could be in danger of being considered a topical drug by the FDA. The editors of *Cosmetics and Toiletries*, a cosmetic industry journal, have coined the term "cosmeceuticals," to describe currently marketed skin care ingredients that have 'bio-active' properties.[7] Get them while you can!

Preventing Marks by Preventing UV Damage

Since the key is to maintain strong, supple and elastic skin, anything that prevents damage to collagen and elastin should be implemented in your campaign to avoid stretch marks.

Ninety percent of a skin's breakdown is due to environmental factors: wind, cold, soap, heat and, worst of all, sun.[8]

Scientists who study aging skin distinguish between changes that occur with the passing of time and damage inflicted by the sun's rays. They call the effect of the sun *photoaging*.

If you compare your skin in sun-protected areas like your underarms or buttocks with sun-exposed areas like your face and hands, you can see how much the sun has damaged your skin.

The best example is a Tibetan monk who from the time he's young, never goes outside again, according to New York City dermatologist Darrell Rigel, M.D. Dr. Rigel has noticed that when these monks are in their 80s their skin looks like that of somebody in his 20s or 30s. Collagen and elastin fibers do break down as part of the aging process, but not like in someone who has had years of sun exposure. Dr. Rigel points out that in someone who hasn't had very much sun during his or her life, elastin fibers are all parallel and look like they're pulling together. In people who've had a great amount of sun, the fibers look like a ball of spaghetti.[9]

A friend of mine complains about her stretch marks. She didn't gain that much weight when she was pregnant, so she can't understand why she got such deep, grooved stretch marks. I didn't understand it either – until I realized she was in the habit of sunbathing in a bikini. I asked her if she wore a bikini while pregnant. Since her family had their own pool, she had. Now she has a pretty good idea why she got stretch marks. In her case, you could call them sun marks.

If you swim or sunbathe, choose a dark-colored swimsuit. White suits let in ultraviolet rays. I noticed this firsthand while attending a water polo class at a local college. As the semester wore on and we were exposed to more and more sun, I noticed the students with white striped suits had dark stripes underneath!

Kligman adds that elastin can be increased in the skin through aerobic exercise. He says aerobic exercise suffuses the skin with blood, promoting nutrient delivery and enhancing removal of cellular wastes, adding that women who exercise have more elastic, stronger and less wrinkled skin.

Fortifying the Skin

Collagen plays such an important role in the strength and repair of skin that it has become popular to inject collagen under the skin to remove wrinkles and facial lines.

Collagen is the stuffing in your body. When it's in peak condition its fibers are taught and elastic. Take care of it and the surface will remain pillow soft and smooth. Throw it around, squeeze it and abuse it, and you'll see the results. The collagen fibers will become worn, thin and rough, and hang loosely.

Collagen needs certain nutrients to grow and stay healthy. Scientists have found that collagen is largely made up of silica. So what do you think nourishes it the most? Silica!

Formulas that contain silica have proven effective in the prevention and repair of stretch marks. In one controlled study, researchers found an average 70 percent prevention rate and a 15 percent success rate in diminishing existing marks.[10]

Silica is also important to healthy nails. If yours are dark, brittle and have an abnormal surface, they deserve a closer look. It could be that a deficiency of silica is robbing the calcium from your body and you haven't noticed – yet. Check with your doctor.

Silica is found in horsetail extracts and in a minerals in solution formula available in vitamin stores.

A sin of omission is taking in too little vitamin C, the body builder of valuable collagen. Collagen is the bullet out of the gun of vitamin C.

Vitamin C's ability to manufacture collagen was illustrated to me dramatically by a veterinarian, Dr. Craig in Monterey, California. He is both a vet and a breeder of Alaskan Huskies. Dr. Craig had to put down whole litters of puppies due to hip dysplasia, a crippling deformity common among certain breeds of dogs. One day while operating he realized that if there was more collagen in the joints, the dog wouldn't have the dysplasia. He began to give his dogs vitamin C and has not had to destroy any more dogs.

Smokers, too, need to learn this vitamin C secret. Cigarette smokers eventually develop dried up, lined and wrinkled skin because smoking undermines the skin in two ways. Each cigarette burns up at least 25 mg of vitamin C. Smokers of 20 cigarettes a day use up 500 mg, putting themselves in a deficit situation, because vitamin C is not storable. Their connective tissue literally caves in.

If you don't believe me, consider this: experts warn people away from used cars previously owned by smokers because the years of smoking disintegrates the glue holding the upholstery together. Imagine what it does to your skin!

A friend of mine swears by aloe vera and vitamin E. Look for the combination in skin lotions. Smear it all over every morning and evening – and don't wait until you see evidence of expansion. Not only are you treating the skin for the stretching, but you're conditioning it to withstand it.

Tips For After The Fact

Remember my bikini-clad friend? I told her that stretch marks can be minimized with a combination of protein, pantothenic acid (vitamin B5), vitamin C, vitamin E and zinc, plus vigorous walking. So, she tried it.

She wisely emphasized vegetables for her high protein diet, so she wouldn't be adding inordinate and unhealthy amounts of fat.

The kind of protein found in vegetables is the best way to ensure adequate amounts. Vegetable protein contains many other vital nutrients, including nitrogen and amino acids, necessary to make collagen. The best kind of protein is free form amino acids found in oatmeal, nuts, seeds, grains and fruits.

The argument made by the egg and meat people in favor of their products has been that vegetables have incomplete protein – that is, there isn't one kind that contains all the essential amino acids. A U.S. Department of Agriculture survey found that American vegetarians consume, on the average, 150 percent of their actual protein requirements. Who says protein has to come from one source? The fact of the matter is, all foods contain some amount of protein. In order to get *complete* protein in one meal, you simply have to combine them properly.

To get your daily allowance of complete protein combine whole grains with legumes. For example, the Greek dish *felafel* combines whole wheat pita bread with mashed garbanzo beans and spices. It happens to be a healthy, fast finger food, not to mention a delicious meal. Latin Americans get their protein by combining corn tortillas with beans. In India it's rice or wheat chapatis with lentils. Since cooking can destroy many essential amino acids, try to avoid processed foods and eat your veggies raw.

I suggested my friend also include beta carotene or vitamin A because without it, the body can't utilize protein.

Along with the protein and walking exercise, she supplemented with 300 mg of pantothenic acid, 1000 mg of vitamin C, 600 IU of vitamin E and 15 to 25 mg of zinc daily. Nothing happened after five months, but she soon found herself pregnant once again. She stayed with the program for most of her pregnancy and gave birth to an oversize baby. Overjoyed about the good health of her son, she looked at her now flat belly and almost cried out with happiness. The stretch marks from the first pregnancy were gone – and there were no new ones!

Alpha hydroxy acid (AHA), found in apples, grapes and other fruit has been discovered to remove shallow wrinkles and rejuvenate the skin, and some say can help minimize stretch marks.

AHAs are natural exfoliators derived from foods such as citrus fruits (citric acid), sour milk (lactic acid), grapes (tartaric acid), sugar cane (glycolic acid), and apples (malic acid). "These acids work by loosening the 'glue' that holds the outermost layer of the skin together," Zia explains. "This makes it easier to dissolve and shed dead skin cells and encourages the formation of new skin cells." According to Zia, alpha hydroxy acids have been used for centuries: "Cleopatra bathed in buttermilk, which is lactic acid."[11]

The ladies of the court of Louis XIV are said to have applied old wine to their faces to remove wrinkles and blemishes. Old wine contains large amounts of malic and tartaric acid.

Polynesians, who are exposed to high doses of tropical sunlight, rich in ultraviolet radiation, use a mixture of citrus and sugar-cane juice to keep their skin healthy. Both these foods contain citric and glycolic acid.[12]

Skin care products containing adequate amounts of alpha hydroxy acids (read the label – some cheaper products contain hardly any) improve skin texture and color, reduce fine lines and age spots, and refine pores. Although no scientific clinical trials have yet been performed to prove the benefits of products containing low-concentrations of alpha hydroxy acids, Barbara Gilchrest, M.D., chairman of the department of dermatology, Boston University School of Medicine, notes that anecdotal reports from dermatologists and their patients indicate that the products do live up to their skin-improving claims.[13]

Because alpha hydroxy acids are naturally irritating, look for skin care formulas that include natural botanicals to counter its effect. For example, cucumber and chamomile soothe and fortify delicate tissues. Sage is one of the oldest medicinal plants, and has anti-bacterial properties, helpful in the case of skin irritation. Papaya is very high in vitamin A, a notorious skin vitamin. All work together to both slough off wrinkles and encourage ripe new skin to form.

Skin-Strengthening Nutrients
For maximum absorption take supplements with meals.

Nutrient	Suggested Dosage	Formulation
Acetyl L-Carnitine	500 mg three times daily	
Aged garlic extract	1 teaspoon three times daily	Liquid
Antioxidants	2 capsules daily	With selenium and grape seed extract
Borage oil	2 capsules daily	
Flaxseed oil	1 tablespoon daily	
Multi-mineral	3-4 ounces daily	In liquid solution, with vitamin B12, biotin
Multi-vitamin/mineral	6 caplets daily	Freeze-dried plant sources
Vitamin A	25,000 IU daily*	
Vitamin C	Individual bowel tolerance**	With citrus bioflavonoids (quercetin, proanthocyanidins)

Nourish skin with a therapeutic moisturizer that contains aloe vera gel, chamomile, vitamins A and C, and avocado oil.

* The FDA recommends pregnant women not exceed 10,000 IU of vitamin A daily.

** To determine individual dosage, on the first day take 1,000 mg hourly until diarrhea occurs, then reduce dosage to just below that for individual daily dosage. Vitamin C is not toxic in large doses but must be taken throughout the day to benefit. Divide dosage to three or four times a day.

CHAPTER 151:

Sudden Infant Death Syndrome (SIDS)

I love the work that I do: imparting valuable and often life-saving information that serves to encourage and enlighten others. Unfortunately, the search for information often comes after a monumentally tragic experience. This is the only thing I regret. SIDS is especially tragic. Losing a child is like dropping into the darkest and deepest abyss imaginable, and to have that loss occur so quickly and mysteriously is surely one of the worst and most trying of experiences. This is why the letter I am about to share with you was so joyous to me. It didn't have to end in tragedy for the writer to look to me for guidance.

Sallie Saved From SIDS

The letter-writer was Karen, a woman from North Carolina who nearly lost her infant daughter, Sallie. She wrote, "Thank God I was home that day and somehow knew how to handle the crisis."

God was with Karen and Sallie that day. Karen wrote that her daughter was then seven weeks old – a happy baby who had already settled down to a regular routine. Her two older girls, eight and four, were playing quietly in the living room. It was the day after Halloween, and they were still tired from the excitement of trick-or-treating the night before. Knowing that Sallie would sleep for at least two hours and that the girls were happily engaged, Karen went outside to rake the thick layer of leaves from the front lawn.

The air was crisp and invigorating, and she was enjoying the exercise. When she checked her watch, she was surprised to see that it was almost 1:30 in the afternoon. Sallie was past due for her midday feeding, and Karen decided to go inside and wake her.

Sallie was sleeping on her stomach and Karen turned her over to change her diaper. Still half asleep, Sallie yawned and stretched and made her usual funny faces. Karen watched her for a while then turned away to retrieve a fresh diaper. When she turned back and focused on the infant's face, she realized with a jolt of horror that she wasn't breathing and was turning blue!

In a panic, Karen picked her up and gently shook her. It didn't help. Karen quickly turned her upside down and patted her on the back, but that didn't revive her either. Quickly she put a finger in her mouth to see if there was an obstruction, and found that Sallie's tongue had curled back into her throat, blocking the airway.

Desperate, Karen pressed a finger down on Sallie's tongue. It worked! Sallie gasped, coughed and started to breathe. She took her finger out of her mouth, but immediately she started to turn blue again.

She put her finger back on her tongue and raced to the phone to call 911. At the hospital, Sallie was hooked to monitors until doctors could determine why she almost suffocated. The next day, Sallie's pediatrician ordered her transferred to a hospital which had a center for the study of apnea (abnormal cessation of breathing) in infants. Although he wasn't absolutely sure, Sallie's pediatrician told Karen he thought she had suffered a near-miss episode of SIDS, also referred to as "crib death."

Specialists at the center uncovered the cause of the problem. The doctors told Karen that Sallie's upper pharynx, or throat, was small, and that she also had trouble controlling her tongue muscles, resulting in what they called a "floppy tongue." The combination meant that until her throat grew larger and her tongue stronger, Sallie could still be at risk of suffocating. Doctors put Sallie on a home cardiac monitor, a small electronic unit that is attached to the baby with Velcro straps. Wires run from the pack to a portable unit about the size of a videocassette recorder, which monitors the child's breathing and pulse. Karen and her husband had to learn to hook up the unit, which would sound an alarm if Sallie stopped breathing. They also had to learn to perform cardiopulmonary resuscitation (CPR) and were shown other techniques for arousing Sallie, should she stop breathing.

Five grueling, sleepless, harrowing months later, the monitor finally came off and Sallie was proclaimed out of the woods. Karen said she wrote her letter because she wanted people to realize that sometimes causes are found for SIDS and she counted on me to get the word out that parents are not entirely helpless to treat or prevent it. I thank Karen, for her heart-wrenching but happily-ended story.

Prevent SIDS Prenatally

When you look at all the factors involved in SIDS two things stand out: the fact that it occurs while infants are sleeping and that it occurs during the first few months of new life. To play Sherlock Holmes and magnify the causes, we have to look at the very beginning – the creation of new life by the mother. How can mothers influence the early growth of their children so SIDS won't occur? One way is to not smoke.

One study comparing 9,953 random live births with the number of SIDS deaths found that up to 30 percent of the deaths might have been prevented if the new mothers had not smoked while they were pregnant.[1]

Another study found that smoking during pregnancy doubled an infant's chances of getting SIDS, and even more if the mother not only smoked but was anemic (had low hemoglobin – red blood cells).[2]

Second-hand smoke exposure to newborns is also associated with SIDS. Swedish researchers evaluated the levels of nicotine in the heart fluid of 24 consecutively autopsied cases of SIDS infants, one to six months of age. It was found that 70 percent exhibited moderate to heavy absorption of nicotine into the heart, which, the study researchers believe, could play a role in the sudden death of infants.[3]

The Anemia Factor

When you think of anemia, the first thing that comes to mind is iron. Gotta take iron, you might think. Be warned, however, anemia is not as simple as a lack of iron. According to the *Tufts University Diet & Nutrition Letter*, iron-deficiency anemia has been over-diagnosed in the U.S. In fact, a 1988 survey of people with iron overload revealed that one in three had met with more than 11 doctors before getting a correct diagnosis.[4]

Studies have shown that pregnant women who have high amounts of iron in their blood may be increasing the risk of crib death. This is based on studies that showed SIDS infants had increased stores of iron in the liver. Selenium has been shown to help assimilate iron into the body, avoiding this accumulation problem.[5]

How can you tell if you have too much stored iron? Only certain blood tests, such as the serum ferritin test and transferrin saturation test, provide the answer. The reason for this common mistake goes back to the definition of anemia. Simply put, anemia is a reduction in the number of hemoglobin molecules and/or in the number or size of red blood cells. However, this condition can result from many things that have nothing to do with whether the body is taking in or storing enough iron. Anemia can be caused by deficiencies of folic acid, vitamin B6, vitamin B12 and copper, and by anything that reduces stomach acid. Trauma and illnesses that cause internal bleeding can also lead to anemia.

Churchill's Medical Dictionary lists over one hundred different kinds of anemias. Among them are iron deficiency, folic acid deficiency and pernicious. What it comes down to is that anemia is not a problem unto itself, but rather a red blood cell/hemoglobin disorder that can be caused by any number of factors, especially a deficiency of B vitamins and iron. Only through thorough testing, that evaluates the body's stores of nutrients, can the cause be isolated. If your doctor says you are anemic and prescribes iron pills, get a second opinion from a doctor or nutritionist, making sure you only take what you need. If it is iron, be sure you take vitamin C with it. Without vitamin C, iron can't pick up oxygen. Without enough vitamin C, no matter how much iron you have, your blood cells will be starved of oxygen.

Selenium, Cow's Milk and SIDS

Researchers in New Zealand are zealously investigating the SIDS tragedy because they have high incidences of SIDS and some of the most severely selenium-deficient soils in the world. In 1970 an extensive SIDS survey demonstrated that the underlying cause might be selenium deficiency. The researchers noted that the incidence of SIDS was higher among infants fed cow's milk than in those who were breast-fed, reasoning that the forage diet of New Zealand dairy cattle, produced on the indigenous, low selenium soils provided less selenium than the human diet, some of which was imported. In studies, New Zealand cow's milk has been shown to have a lower selenium content than human milk.[6] My initial response to this might be obvious: cow's milk isn't good for anyone, so it's hardly surprising that most infants with SIDS are fed the stuff. More likely to be a cause is the frequency of babies with an allergy to lactose, the milk fat found in cow's milk.

In an article in the medical journal *Immunology and Allergy Clinics of North America*, Robert H. Schwartz, M.D., connects SIDS to formulas containing milk products and a subsequent allergy to them.[7]

Other researchers suggest SIDS may be caused by an anaphylactic shock reaction to inhaled cow's milk.[8]

Aside from this lactose factor, the selenium/SIDS connection does exist. The mean blood level of selenium in New Zealanders is extremely low – about half that of individuals in the United States. Moreover, children generally have lower blood selenium levels than do adults.[9]

In one case study, 200 babies who died of SIDS were found to have lesions in heart tissue that resembled those found in Keshan's disease, an affliction caused by a selenium deficiency. In China, the disease has been significantly reduced because of selenium supplementation. Researchers were able to copy the affect found in SIDS babies by withholding selenium from the diets of lambs and calves.[10]

John C. FitzHerbert, a medical doctor in Wellington, New Zealand is convinced that SIDS can be prevented if nursing mothers supplement with selenium for the first three months.[11]

Let me add this important fact. Many of us are probably mineral deficient because as we age, we lose stomach acid, which is necessary to break down nutrients for absorption. Supplementing with a hydrochloric acid formula such as Betaine, available in health food stores, will help absorb nutrients, but studies show minerals in solution before ingestion are considerably more bioavailable to the body than those even present in food, because they aren't risked by a lack of hydrochloric acid in the stomach or food allergies. Look for a good, easily absorbable, derived-from-nature mineral blend in solution. Formulations in solution provide the maximum absorption ratios.

Sleep Apnea, the Pineal Gland and Melatonin

Researchers believe some SIDS cases may be a result of sleep apnea, a condition in which a physiological dysfunction (versus a soft pillow or beanbag chair) causes infants to stop breathing or prevents them from breathing. Karen's baby had what they call "obstructive" sleep apnea, because it was an obstruction that caused Sallie to suffocate.

"Central" apnea occurs when the brain's respiratory center fails to trigger breathing. A baby's immature nervous system could be responsible, or a result of nutritional deficiencies birth defects or neurological lesions.

People with sleep apnea breathe for 10 to 20 seconds, strenuously gasp in air, then stop again. Dangerous levels of carbon dioxide build up in the blood, and oxygen to the brain is depleted. In sleeping adults with mature nervous systems, an alarm system recognizes the lack of oxygen and wakes up momentarily, restoring the airway. But in infants, this response may not occur, and the baby can die.

The body hormone melatonin, produced in the pineal gland, has been found to help people with sleeplessness because it regulates sleep and breathing rhythms. Infants with SIDS have been found to have abnormally low levels of melatonin.

Researchers at the Offices of State Medical Examiners, Providence, Rhode Island, revealed in autopsies that melatonin levels were significantly low in all of 68 infant deaths attributed to SIDS.[12] If you've ever wondered how they decide an infant died of SIDS, it's when they can't identify a cause of death. The tragedy of SIDS is that a cause cannot be pinpointed. The good news is that studies like these are getting us closer.

Dr. Susan M. Webb and colleagues at the Department of Endocrinology, Hospital De La Santa Creu in Barcelona, Spain, conducted a study of 32 infants who died from SIDS, examining their levels of melatonin in blood, nervous system and body fluids, comparing them to a group of 36 infants who died of known causes. They found abnormally low amounts of melatonin in all the SIDS babies, concluding that it could have resulted in an abnormal maturation of their sympathetic nervous systems, which may have played a part in their deaths.[13]

Other researchers have discovered that if the pineal gland doesn't develop properly, it can cause a chemical imbalance that can, simply put, cause dangerous build-ups of toxins in the nerves and heart, causing death.[14]

What You Can Do

All this information is very interesting – for your doctor, and for any researcher with an open mind. But what can you do to protect yourself and your baby against the threat of SIDS? The first thing you can do is stay healthy while pregnant. Seek the guidance of a nutrition-oriented physician to make sure your selenium, vitamin B12, B6, C, folic acid, iron and melatonin levels are optimum. Don't smoke, and eat fresh, raw foods as much as possible. If you like salads, eat them like there is no tomorrow.

Place your baby on his or her back, on a firm mattress with no pillow. Researchers at the June 24, 1996 Fourth SIDS International Conference in Bethesda, Maryland reported that the use of a soft mattress resulted in a more than a fourfold increase in an infant's risk for SIDS. Giving the infant a pillow heightened risk by more than two-and-a-half times. Infants sleeping on their stomachs (prone position) were up to four times more likely to die from SIDS. [15]

The three-year study was funded by the National Institutes of Health, Bethesda, and the Centers for Disease Control and Prevention in Atlanta. The preliminary findings were based on an examination of 195 diagnosed SIDS deaths in Chicago.

Breastfeed. Women who breastfeed have a much less chance of their baby dying of SIDS. Researchers from Loyola University Medical Center, led by Dr. Fern Hauck, reported at the SIDS conference that 81 percent of the SIDS deaths noted above, involved infants who had never been breast-fed. Not breast-feeding increased the risk of SIDS threefold. [16]

Breastfeed for at least eight months if you can. For more guidance on giving your baby the best and most healthy start to a long life, see my chapters in this book Breastfeeding, Prenatal, Anemia and Sleep Apnea.

See the Prenatal Chapter for SIDS-Stopping Nutrients.

CHAPTER 152:

Tardive Dyskinesia (Involuntary, Abnormal Movements)

She might never have discovered the terrible secret if her father hadn't recorded it in her baby book. When she told me about it, I was horrified. She wasn't even two years old! In her baby book her father wrote, "Unusual fussiness and irritability. Much sibling quibbling. It has regressed to bedwetting. Definite signs of psychological insecurity. Dr. Ames prescribed a phenothiazine tranquilizer of the promazine type. An extrapyramidal reaction created dyskinesia (spastic movements), oculogyric (eye rolling), general tremors."

The year was 1961, a time of great darkness in conventional psychiatry (the darkness of ignorance is only now just beginning to lift). My friend Julie, now 40 years old, was not quite two years old when her father became concerned about her behavior. She fought with her little brother, wasn't quite getting the night potty training, and openly defied her parents. Normal behavior under most standards, considering her age. However, for a psychiatrist trained in the use of drugs, not child behavior, it was enough to prescribe a heavy tranquilizer with dangerous side effects. Poor little Julie had such a severe reaction she ended up in the hospital. She was lucky she didn't die or end up brain damaged. Instead, she temporarily lost motor control of her body. Her neck lost its support of her head, which lolled over onto her shoulder; her eyes rolled back uncontrollably, she slurred her words, her hands shook, she had trouble walking, and she had facial tics. She was in the hospital two days before the effects of the drug wore off and she regained normal function.

Targeting the Source

Dyskinesia is defined as "any abnormality of movement, such as incoordination, spasm or irregular and ill-formed movements." There are different kinds, depending upon what part of the body is affected. Tardive dyskinesia (TD), is defined as "slow, rhythmic, stereotyped, repetitive, involuntary movements of the tongue, lips and mouth, and sometimes the trunk and limbs. It can also occur in the trachea and bronchi, and can cause suffocation."[1]

For the most part, it is caused by the phenothiazine drugs, the family of neuroleptics most frequently prescribed for psychiatric disorders. Ever seen a crazy derelict on the street trembling and twitching, chewing convulsively on nothing, tongue jutting out every few seconds? That's TD. The streets are full of TD sufferers – former mental patients discharged from institutions in the '60s and '70s, permanently brain damaged by these drugs, and left with grotesque and uncontrollable symptoms that ostracize them from the society that created them.

Neuroleptics (euphemistically called 'anti-psychotics' or 'major tranquilizers') don't tranquilize or combat depression – they control, immobilize, poison and sometimes kill people. Dr. Peter Breggin, a prominent dissident psychiatrist, professor at George Mason University, and author of the book *Psychiatric Drugs: Hazards to the Brain*, aptly terms these drugs 'neurotoxins.' Both anti-depressants and tranquilizers cause a host of very serious and/or permanent disabilities, including brain damage, all of which are deceitfully called 'side effects.'[2]

These drugs block the production of dopamine – a necessary chemical in the brain responsible for transmitting nerve impulses. Psychiatrists believe that many mental disorders, including schizophrenia and psychosis, are caused by too much dopamine, so they prescribe neuroleptics. Breggin doesn't buy the dopamine theory. He believes these drugs are causing people with normal amounts of dopamine to become dopamine-deficient, and seriously ill with parkinsonism as a result of the 'treatment.' It's the lack of dopamine, he believes, that causes tardive dyskinesia.[3]

In a personal communication to author and activist Don Weitz, this is what Dr. Breggin wrote:

"Throughout North America, psychiatrists typically fail to meet the minimal standards of informed consent in regard to tardive dyskinesia, often failing to tell patients and families about the disorder, and rarely telling them of its frequency, potential severity, or threat to the higher mental processes. In Canada, G. Chouinard and B. Jones, psychiatrists at the Allan Memorial Institute in Montreal, have documented the existence of permanent brain damage not only in the form of uncontrollable muscular movements, but psychosis. Patients develop a drug-induced 'tardive psychosis' for which there is no known treatment. In regard to tardive dyskinesia, Chouinard has recently observed that nearly all patients on long-term treatment are afflicted with the untreatable neurological disease."[4]

I take exception to the doctor's assumption that TD is untreatable. As you will shortly see, TD is very treatable, as long as the drugs have not caused permanent brain damage.

In an excellent treatise for *Canadian Dimension* (April-May 1991) entitled "Chemical Lobotomies," Weitz wrote: "Approximately five years ago at an international mental health conference in England, it was announced that roughly twenty-five million people around the world are currently suffering from TD. Nobody challenged that figure, which is probably much higher now. In 1980, the notoriously reactionary American Psychiatric Association published its task force report on TD. One of its startling conclusions was that as many as 20-50 percent of people prescribed these drugs have developed or will develop TD."[5]

In a study reported in the *American Journal of Psychiatry* (September 1992), 251 patients admitted to a university geriatric psychiatry unit over a five-year period were evaluated for onset of TD. None of these patients had received neuroleptic drugs prior to admission. Researchers treated 99 of the patients with neuroleptic drugs, and the remaining 63 patients served as control subjects.

Researchers established that the prevalence of TD before the use of drugs was four percent. Once the patients were given neuroleptic drugs, the prevalence of tardive dyskinesia shot up to an incredible 35.4 percent! Patients with tardive dyskinesia stayed longer in the hospital, were treated with neuroleptics for a longer period and received a larger total dose of neuroleptics. I suppose this reflects common procedure. I wouldn't treat laboratory rats this way![6]

TD Found Treatable with Vitamin E, Antioxidants

I've given you the bad news first: doctors and psychiatrists are causing an epidemic of tardive dyskinesia by prescribing anti-depressant and tranquilizer prescription drugs. The good news is those very same doctors are being told what can be done about it. *The American Journal of Psychiatry* is probably found in every doctors' lounge in every major hospital. It's an esteemed medical journal highly respected by its professional readership. This is why I was so surprised to see the number of articles on the benefit of vitamin E in preventing and treating tardive dyskinesia.

Here, in chronological order, are five articles on the treatment of TD with vitamin E which have appeared in *The American Journal of Psychiatry*.

1. "Vitamin E in The Treatment of Tardive Dyskinesia," Elkashef, Ahmed M., MBBCh, v. 147, n. 4, p. 505-506, **April 1990**.

2. "Vitamin E in The Treatment of Tardive Dyskinesia: A Double-Blinded, Placebo-Controlled Study," Shriqui, Christian L., et al, v. 149, n. 3, p. 391, **March 1992**.

3. "Treatment of Tardive Dyskinesia with Vitamin E," Egan, Michael F., et al, v. 149, n. 6, p. 773, **June 1992**.

4. "Vitamin E Treatment of Tardive Dyskinesia," Adler, Lenard, A., et al, v. 150, n. 9, p. 1405, **September 1993**.

5. "Effectiveness of Vitamin E for Treatment of Long-Term Tardive Dyskinesia," Dabiri, Louise M., et al, v. 151, n. 6, p. 925, **June 1994**.

Ahmed M. Elkashef, M.D., of the University of Maryland School of Medicine, conducted a 10-week study involving eight people with schizophrenia who were on neuroleptic medication. The patients, all with persistent TD, were given either vitamin E or a placebo (blank pill) along with their medication for four weeks.

For the next four weeks the patients switched treatments. The severity of their TD was measured using a scale that gauged involuntary movements. When the patients were taking vitamin E, the scale showed significantly less of the side effect – with five of the eight patients experiencing reductions of 30 percent or more.[7]

In a 12-week double-blind study 11 patients with tardive dyskinesia received 400 I.U. of vitamin E for the first week, 800 for the second and 1,200 for the remaining 10 weeks of the trial. Those who consumed vitamin E capsules showed a 36 percent reduction in symptoms when compared to patients consuming placebos.[8]

What is it about vitamin E that makes it work? Vitamin E is an antioxidant. Antioxidants quench free radicals which damage vital nerve cells. It is believed that one of the ways in which neuroleptic drugs damage the brain is by increasing the amount of free radicals in the body.

Researcher Jean Lud Cadet, M.D., of the Molecular Neuropsychiatry Section, of the Addiction Research Center in Baltimore, Maryland, believes that antioxidant treatment with vitamin E and selenium may be beneficial in preventing or alleviating the development of tardive dyskinesia.[9] This is not a surprising connection since vitamin E and the antioxidant mineral selenium work in the body together, and selenium can accentuate vitamin E's effect.

Manganese Helps Too

The first major breakthrough in the treatment of tardive dyskinesia was reported in 1976 by Richard A. Kunin, M.D., an orthomolecular psychiatrist. Kunin concluded that tardive dyskinesia might be the result of a manganese deficiency caused by tranquilizers, since these drugs are complex molecules that can chelate with manganese and carry it out of the body.

In Kunin's study, out of 15 TD patients, the combination of manganese and vitamin B3 (niacin) improved 14 patients and cured seven.[10]

Manganese is relatively safe in doses up to 300 mg per day. However, doses under 100 mg per day are usually adequate. Occasionally, manganese will elevate blood pressure and produce tension headaches. When this happens, the therapy should be halted.[11] Manganese works with zinc, which works with copper. Because of this, manganese should be taken with about four mg a day of zinc, and two mg a day of copper.

Clearing Channels with B Vitamins

The B vitamins are shown to be especially helpful in restoring the ability of the nervous system to channel messages from the brain to the body. In the case of TD and diseases which affect the muscular system, like Parkinson's and Multiple Sclerosis, there is a blockage or "short circuit" between the nervous system and muscular system. The B vitamins are essential to a healthy nervous system, so it isn't surprising that the B vitamin choline, best obtained from lecithin, has been shown in studies to improve tardive dyskinesia.

John H. Growdon, M.D., of Tufts-New England Medical Center Hospital in Boston, was probably the first to treat TD with choline. His first experiments with choline went well, but he found his patients didn't like the bitter taste or fishy odor, so he went with lecithin for his next experiments. Lecithin is a naturally occurring source of choline and has been shown to increase blood levels of choline in humans to a greater extent than equal doses of choline alone. In Growdon's first study, a double-blind, crossover trial using choline, it was found that out of 20 TD patients with uncontrollable mouth movements, nine showed improvement. When Growdon and colleagues gave lecithin granules to patients from that study, even more improvement was noted.[12]

Alan J. Gelenberg, M.D., of the Erich Lindemann Mental Health Center, also in Boston, conducted his own study of choline and lecithin. He evaluated five men with mild to moderate TD and found that both lecithin and choline improved abnormal movements in all five of the patients. Lecithin had fewer side effects.[13]

Manganese should be tried before lecithin/choline because it is required in relatively small doses, compared to choline, and because high doses of choline and lecithin produce uncomfortable side effects. Side effects include nausea, bloating and diarrhea. Fewer side effects are found in lecithin formulas richest in phosphatidyl choline.[14]

Dyskinesia-Defeating Nutrients
For maximum absorption, take supplements with meals.

Nutrient	Suggested Dosage	Formulation
Amino acids	4-6 capsules daily	Multiple formula from natural sources
Antioxidants	4 capsules daily*	With selenium and grapeseed extract
Borage oil	2 capsules daily	
Coenzyme Q10	2 capsules daily	With vitamin E, phospholipids and selenium
Enzymes	2 capsules twice daily	Multiple formula
Fiber	4-8 tablets daily	Psyllium, with herb hyssop
Flaxseed oil	1 tablespoon daily	
Ginkgo biloba	60 mg three times daily	
Lecithin	2 tablespoons with meals	
L-Carnitine	500 mg twice daily	
Magnesium	200 mg daily	
Malic acid	250 mg three times daily	
Multi-mineral	3-4 ounces daily	In liquid solution, with vitamin B12, biotin
Multi-vitamin/mineral	6 caplets daily	Freeze-dried plant sources
Niacin	200 mg three times daily	
Vitamin B6	100 mg daily	
Vitamin C	Individual bowel tolerance**	With bioflavonoids (quercetin, rutin proanthocyanidins)
Vitamin E	2 capsules (800 IU) daily	d-alpha tocopherol

* The FDA recommends pregnant women not exceed 10,000 IU of vitamin A daily.

** To determine individual dosage, on the first day take 1,000 mg hourly until diarrhea occurs, then reduce dosage to just below that for individual daily dosage. Vitamin C is not toxic in large doses but must be taken throughout the day to benefit. Divide dosage to three or four times a day.

CHAPTER 153:

Teeth and Gums

"Be true to your teeth and they won't be false to you."
–Soupy Sales

As a scuba diver, I have a healthy respect for sharks. As nature's most orthodontically blessed creatures, these benthic wonders can produce a treasure-trove of teeth. A single tiger shark, for example, can manufacture 12,000 gleaming choppers in just five years.

Alas, our allotment wasn't quite as generous. But with the devoted care of teeth and gums, our compliment of 32 incisors, canines, bicuspids, and molars can provide a lifetime of service. The key is unflagging vigilance against tooth decay and gum disease. A simple formula, yet easier said than done.

At the root of our dental woes, both literally and figuratively, are bacteria. The human mouth is a veritable microbial Amazon. Bacteria feed on leftovers around our uppers and lowers, enveloping teeth in a sticky, acidic matrix known as plaque. Acidic plaque gnaws away at our teeth's protective enamel crowns, forming cavities. Left to fester, it corrodes the tooth's less-resilient interior, eventually requiring a major filling, root canal, or worse – extraction.

Vitamin C as a Daily Preventive

You brush and floss your teeth after every meal to prevent cavities and gum disease. If you don't you should. But what you should also do to protect those pearly whites is take vitamin C. Vitamin C has been shown in studies to prevent periodontal abscesses by lowering the amount of plaque and bacteria in the mouth. The *New York Journal of Dentistry* reported on a study in which plaque accumulation was measured among subjects all brushing well, some supplementing with vitamin C, some not. The study found that those supplementing with vitamin C actually had less tarter and bacteria than those only brushing. They discovered that when the subjects took vitamin C the inflammation of their gums from concentrations of bacteria improved by 58 percent![1]

How does vitamin C perform its magic? By increasing the numbers of the antibody warriors that come to our defense when infection sets in. Medical students at South Africa's University of Witwatersrand were given one gram a day of ascorbic acid (vitamin C) and monitored for blood immunologic levels. Unlike the control group who did not get the vitamin C, the ones who did experienced a marked increase in their defense antibodies. Vitamin C is renowned for alleviating the symptoms of colds and flu, and studies have shown it to be of benefit for tuberculosis, herpes, tetanus and diphtheria. Any type of infection can be helped with vitamin C.[2]

When you target vitamin C as a supplement, choose a formulation that includes bioflavonoids. Bioflavonoids are potent anti-inflammatories. They reduce swelling while they act on the immune system, and they enhance the healing properties of vitamin C. If you're facing any kind of dental work or surgery, take at least 500 milligrams of vitamin C and bioflavonoids to help reduce the post-surgical inflammation and pain that accompanies it. Follow up the procedure with another 500 milligrams.

For preventive medicine try green tea. Green tea contains certain bioflavonoids which help fight tooth decay and gum disease. The Japanese, who drink green tea with every meal, have known this for centuries. Tsao Kubo, a researcher from the University of California, Berkeley, reports that the polyphenols in green tea help kill the bacteria that causes tooth decay, as well as inhibiting the sticky stuff that allow bacteria to adhere to teeth. Kubo reports an extract or concentrate of green tea leaves work better than drinking it.[3] Look for a supplemental formula that combines vitamin C and bioflavonoids with green tea polyphenols for your dental health.

Ubiquinone – A Nutrient by Any Other Name

If you've read at least some of the preceding chapters in this book, you'll recognize coenzyme Q10. It helps restore circulation and prevents damage to vital body cells. Studies have also shown that coenzyme Q10, or ubiquinone, the fancy scientific name for this body nutrient, is important for protecting the soundness of gums and teeth.

Although coenzyme Q10 exists in many foods, research has shown that patients with a variety of serious medical conditions are often CoQ10 deficient. Many people are deficient in CoQ10 because it is present in live foods, and many subsist on processed foods. In order to be absorbed in the body, coenzyme Q10 in food must be accompanied by tyrosine and phenylalanine, two amino acids, vitamin E and three B vitamins (B1, B6 and folic acid) as well as its relatives Q1 and Q9. To make matters worse, as time marches on, many have a diminished ability to absorb coenzyme Q10.[4]

Although much pertinent research on this nutrient has taken place in the United States, CoQ10 is most widely used in foreign countries, mainly in Japan, where 252 coenzyme Q10 products are sold by 83 companies. The Japanese commonly take ubiquinone supplements to prevent or manage swollen gums and to prevent deterioration of bone structures supporting teeth.[5]

Foods richest in CoQ10 are beef heart, muscle and organ meats, egg yolk, liver, codfish, milk fat, wheat germ and various whole grains. It can be purchased in supplement form in most U.S. health food and vitamin stores and some supermarkets.

Good Advice

Actually, it is possible to avoid tooth decay by eating certain foods. Foods that cause cavities are those high in starch and/or sugar and stick obstinately to the teeth. Other foods do the opposite and are credited with cleaning teeth: olives, nuts, especially cashews and yogurt. An article in the *Journal of Agricultural and Food Chemistry* reports that two organic chemists have discovered cashews may fight tooth decay. Oil extracted from the shell has been found to kill bacteria and fight plaque.[6]

Additionally, the following will help fight tooth decay:
1. Avoid sticky foods that cling to teeth; bananas, chewy candy, dates or raisins. (Or brush teeth soon after eating.)
2. Skip hard candies or breath mints that stay in the mouth too long.
3. Avoid sugary soft drinks. Try sugar-free if necessary.
4. Replace starchy or sugary snacks with hard cheese, meat, nuts, olives or yogurt.

Tooth Decay Associated with Standard Amalgam Fillings

There is an accumulating body of evidence linking mercury to poor health. Chronic mercury exposure can result in a metallic taste, bleeding gums and increased salivation. It is also associated with everything from attention deficit disorder to Schizophrenia.

Where does all this mercury come from? Have you read the Alzheimer's chapter yet? Almost 80 percent of the world's tooth cavities are filled with silver amalgam, of which 50 percent is mercury. It has been documented that there is a direct relationship between the amount of mercury released into your body and the number of fillings you have. Do you recall when you first get a filling, the doctor makes it a little larger than necessary, allowing you to bite down and customize the fit – and how you end up eating some of that filling as it breaks off? You are eating mercury.

Chewing releases elemental mercury vapor which is inhaled and absorbed into the lung and enters the bloodstream, eventually lodging in the brain. Enough of it, and the brain becomes damaged. High amounts of mercury on autopsy have been found in Alzheimer's patients. Mercury poisoning is also associated with many other mental diseases.

As if this weren't enough, studies have associated silver amalgam fillings with an increased risk of tooth decay and gum problems. In an article in *Annals of Dentistry*, Robert L. Siblerud, M.S., in Ft. Collins, Colorado, reports that patients with many fillings showed a 250 percent greater frequency of oral health problems versus clients without many fillings. People with silver teeth reported more foul breath, bleeding gums, grinding of teeth, metallic taste and periodontal disease.[7]

Dr. Siblerud found that the dental problems could be reversed by replacing or removing the silver amalgam fillings. He found that in amalgam-removed subjects, 86 percent of the 125 oral cavity symptoms were eliminated or improved.[8] If you suffer from chronic bad breath, teeth grinding, excess spit, bleeding gums, burning mouth and gum disease, consider the possibility your fillings are to blame. If your dentist won't help, seek help from the following organizations.

Finding Alternative, Biological Dentists

There is no way to tell how many dentists in the U.S. are incorporating holistic or alternative techniques into their practices, but estimates are in the low thousands. To find an alternative dentist in your area, write to one of the following organizations and enclose a self-addressed, stamped envelope.

- American Academy of Biological Dentistry, Box 856, Carmel Valley, CA 93924; (408) 659-5385.

- American Academy of Head, Neck and Facial Pain and TMJ Orthopedics; 520 West Pipeline Road, Hurst, TX 76053.

- Environmental Dental Association; 9974 Scripps Ranch Blvd., Ste. 36, San Diego, CA 92131; (800) 388-8124/(619) 586-1208.

- Foundation for Toxic-Free Dentistry, Box 608010, Orlando, FL 32860-8010.

- Holistic Dental Association, Box 5007, Durango, CO 81301.

Teeth and Gum Nutrients

For maximum absorption, all nutrients should be taken with meals.

Nutrient	Suggested Dosage	Formulation
Acidophilus	At least four billion flora on an empty stomach, three times daily	
Aged garlic extract	1 teaspoon three times daily	Liquid
Coenzyme Q10	2 capsules daily	With vitamin E, phospholipids and selenium
Echinacea	100 mg daily	
Fiber	4-8 tablets daily	Psyllium, with herb hyssop
Multi-mineral	1-4 ounces daily	In liquid solution, with vitamin B12, biotin
Multi-vitamin/mineral	3-6 caplets daily	Freeze-dried plant sources
Vitamin A	25,000 IU daily*	
Vitamin C	Individual bowel tolerance**	With bioflavonoids (quercetin, proanthocyanidins)
Vitamin E	2 capsules (800 IU) daily	d-alpha tocopherol

* The FDA recommends pregnant women not exceed 10,000 IU of vitamin A daily.

** To determine individual dosage, on the first day take 1,000 mg hourly until diarrhea occurs, then reduce dosage to just below that for individual daily dosage. Vitamin C is not toxic in large doses but must be taken throughout the day to benefit. Divide dosage to three or four times a day.

CHAPTER 154:

Tendonitis

Watching a baseball game, my Achilles tendon twinged in sympathy as I saw a runner fall to a pitch, clutching his right calf. When the announcer said it was his heel, I knew he'd be out for the season. For I am a fellow member of the "torn tendon brigade." They told me at the hospital that fine weather heralds the start of the season, when birds sing and tendons ping. Mine went ping one day when a horse fell on it. I was executing a sharp turn at a gallop when my horse lost its footing and down we went.

I was amazed by the speed with which I was transformed from exuberant, athletic holidaymaker into an anxious preoperative patient. Plastic name bands on your wrist and ankle, and a theater gown with all its ties missing are guaranteed to induce a sense of vulnerability. Off to the anaesthetic room. "Yeah, we've got the Achilles tendon in here." A prick in the back of the hand and merciful oblivion. The sleepless postoperative night, largely spent attempting complicated gymnastic manoeuvres on a bedpan, was an experience that I am keen not to repeat.

Eight weeks in plaster will give you plenty of time to perfect your crutch technique, but here are a few tips. It is essential to be highly selective about the things you are able to do. Cooking, cleaning, and washing up are definitely out, while the mixing of herbal drinks should be encouraged. Do not nip across the road to the video shop in the face of oncoming traffic. Avoid walking on wet paving stones unless you wish to become a human windmill. Ignore those friends who refer to you as "Hopalong Cassidy" or "Long John Silver."

Dignified silence will remind them that although they may have the mental age of a five-year-old, you do not. On no account allow friends to experiment with creative graffiti. Two minutes of fun for them means several weeks of acute embarrassment for you.

The main, and most important thing, is to do everything it takes to nourish your body so your tendon will repair completely, without scar tissue and calcium deposits creating complications later on. The doctors told me I might never walk again. Not only am I walking as well as before, but, thanks to Dr. Ross Gordon, my tendons and muscles are well-healed and giving me no trouble. What he taught me, I now pass on to you.

Tendon Loving Care

The body depends on a good blood supply to heal any kind of injury. Unfortunately, tendons don't have very good vascular flow. In fact the Achilles tendon, particularly the lower third, has just about the worst blood supply in the body. So it's not surprising that injuries to the Achilles heal slowly. It can take a couple of weeks (or longer) for enough collagen tissues to gather to begin repairing the tears.

Tendons are fibrous bands of elastin tissue that connect muscles to bones. Without them, muscles could not do their job of moving different parts of the body. They transmit the power of the muscle contraction to just the right spot on a bone so that the muscle may do its work properly. Different circumstances cause tendons to become inflamed or irritated, a condition that is classified as tendonitis.

A person suffering from tendonitis may experience discomfort and tenderness over the area where the affected tendon is located. Movement of the area may be extremely painful. Since tendons usually cross over a joint before connecting to a bone, the most common areas affected are shoulders, elbows, knees and ankles.

What causes tendonitis? Overuse or misuse of a muscle may place extreme tension on a tendon and cause it injury. Trauma also can bring it on, getting sat on by a horse for example! Chronic or frequent bouts of tendonitis can result when scar tissue or calcium coats the tendon, causing a loss of elasticity and painful movement after the original damage is healed. Walking or exercising incorrectly can trigger the condition. Signs and symptoms primarily are swelling and pain when moving the shoulder, elbow, knee, or ankle, or increased warmth over the areas involved.

One of the paradoxes of sports podiatry is that even though the Achilles tendon is the strongest, thickest tendon in the body, it's also the site of frequent overuse injuries. Achilles tendonitis flares up when you overuse or injure the tendon that joins your calf muscles to your heel bone. It doesn't act like other exercise injuries, often hurting most in the morning, then letting up as the day wears on and natural stretching warms it up. Activities involving running, especially jogging, racquetball or tennis, are most likely to set it off. It occurs most often in people who overpronate – roll their feet too far inward – or who bounce when they walk, which is sometimes the sign of an unusually short tendon. Check the wear of your shoes to see how you walk. When walking, running or exercising, always roll from the heel to the toe to avoid putting full impact on the heel. More on exercise techniques later.

History doesn't say whether Achilles had tendonitis before a poisoned arrow felled him during the Trojan War. But a lot of people have heel pain with his name on it. Whatever the legendary warrior's case, you can get rid of the pain of tendonitis and, just as important, take steps to prevent it.

Magnesium for Scar-Free Healing

Once again, the importance of magnesium in combination with calcium comes into play, since they work in balance throughout our bodies. Without magnesium, calcium accumulates in places it shouldn't. The consequences of taking calcium without magnesium is that calcium goes into soft tissues and causes wrinkled skin, stiffened joints and tendonitis.

I've already established the importance of strong muscles to keep tendons in place and unstressed. Almost every mineral and vitamin is involved in muscle contraction, relaxation and repair. For example, potassium, which is very low in processed "junk" food diets, is necessary for the contraction of every muscle in the body. Magnesium and calcium are also needed – together, not individually. Too little magnesium will cause calcium to accumulate in muscle tissues, jeopardizing the circulation of oxygen and causing muscles to weaken.[1] The same thing can happen with phosphates. Phosphates tend to lower magnesium levels even further. They are found in abundance in soft drinks and many processed foods.

Researchers have also found the calcium/magnesium ratio to be very important in maintaining the elastic quality of tendons and ligaments.

Dr. W. Muller and colleagues at the Institute of Pathology in Koln, Germany, examined the ligaments in the discs of spinal surgery patients, putting the patients into two groups: those with very elastic tissues, and those with non-elastic tissues. He found that among those with the most elasticity, a magnesium/calcium ratio in favor of magnesium was found.[2]

I took magnesium and calcium in solution because the stress of the accident probably lowered my amounts of stomach acid, jeopardizing my ability to assimilate nutrients, particularly minerals. Even after healing completely, I continue taking a mineral in solution formula so my bones, muscles and tendons remain strong, supple and stretchable. Because of its high absorption rate, and deficiency of magnesium in the diet, the ratio of magnesium and calcium in solution should be four to one, respectively.

Skin Care Ingredient Prevents Damage and Promotes Healing

If you think about tendons as rubber bands, you'll realize that dryness can make them break when stretched. If they are kept moist, stretching won't be as likely to break them. It is the elastin in tendons that allow them to stretch and bounce back without injury. Studies have made this connection between elastin and breakage and something called hyaluronic acid, or sodium hyaluronate, a naturally-occurring skin and tissue lubricator.

In an article in *Annals of the Rheumatic Diseases* researchers reported that one kind of tendonitis: rotator cuff or shoulder, resulted when tendon repair following injury was incomplete or inadequate. They examined the tendons from cadavers with no history of chronic shoulder pain and compared them with biopsies of patients undergoing surgery to repair shoulder tendon lesions. When they compared healthy to unhealthy shoulder tendons, they found something they didn't expect. The injured and older tendons had more hyaluronic acid, and they were forced to conclude that hyaluronic acid is an important ingredient in repairing tendons.[3]

Also at issue in tendon repair is the absence of scar tissue. With chronic or recurrent tendonitis, scar tissue can develop and bind the tendon, restricting the gliding motion. The scar tissue re-tears with movement, causing great pain.[4]

Researchers never fully realized the connection between hyaluronic acid and tissue repair until a breakthrough study on sheep fetuses. Scientists looking for substances that would repair wounds without scar tissue or damage to the elastin began studying fetal lambs because of their ability to heal without scar formation. They discovered fetal wounds contain high levels of hyaluronic acid. They also discovered high levels of hyaluronic acid in the amniotic fluid, thus it continually bathes the fetus and encourages smooth cell formation.[5]

In addition, in studies of adult sheep the researchers found a rapid rise of high levels of hyaluronic acid levels in the skin following injury. Why fetal lambs don't have scarring while adult sheep do relates to the fact that the hyaluronic acid levels in the lambs persist at least 21 days after wounding, whereas in adult sheep high levels occur three days or less following injury. The researchers concluded that hyaluronic acid not only encourages healing following skin damage, but can effectively inhibit tissue damage as a result of an injury.

What can you do for your tendonitis? Hyaluronic acid is an ingredient in many skin cleansers and moisturizers. Look for products that contain this ingredient. Don't let the term "acid" fool you. It's as safe on cellular tissue as water. In fact, surgeons inject it into the eye during surgery so the tissues can be separated without damage. It is also used in cases of dry eye to increase moisture.[6]

Non-steroidal Anti-Inflammatory Nutrients (NSAINs)

Inflammation naturally occurs when there is any injury or irritation of delicate tendon tissues. In order for the tissues to repair themselves, the inflammation has to subside. I used nutrients that work better than gut-busting, cell-wrenching non-steroidal anti-inflammatory drugs (NSAIDs). It is always better to target safe and effective natural nutrients instead.

Several antioxidants have exhibited anti-inflammatory properties, and in some cases have proven to be as good (better) than NSAIDs.

Selenium is a mineral valued for its ability to strengthen tissues and prevent further damage after injury. Its health benefits extend to preventing inflammation because it boosts the immune system, lessening the response to injury.

Vitamin E works synergistically with selenium, enhancing its tissue-repairing effect. It not only boosts the immune system, but reduces the damage to tissues that results in inflammation, stabilizing delicate membranes so healing can occur. In one study, injured tendons healed in the presence of vitamin E were stronger than those healed without it. It was also noted that with the vitamin E, there were smaller and fewer scars.[7]

I know first hand the benefit of vitamin C on inflammation. My husband's hand was saved from amputation by megadoses of C. Vitamin C, or ascorbic acid, plays a major role in the prevention and repair of injuries. A deficiency of vitamin C results in poor collagen formation. Collagen is the body's intercellular cement, needed for the formation of tendons.[8]

Bioflavonoids added to vitamin C is the punch needed to reduce inflammation and heal delicate tissues. An article in *The Lancet* reports on a study that shows bioflavonoids strengthen tendons. Bioflavonoids not only reduce inflammation, but stabilize and strengthen collagen structures so they can more quickly heal and re-form tightly and smoothly. Because they are antioxidants, they can also prevent cell damage that occurs with injury.

Quercetin, found in citrus fruit, is the most potent bioflavonoid for inflamed tissues. It does all of the above and more, because it controls the release of histamine, which is associated with the swelling, itching and redness common to injuries, allergic reactions and insect bites. Taking quercetin will help alleviate some of the aggravating symptoms associated with tendonitis. Double-blind, placebo-controlled studies have shown that supplemental quercetin helped cut in half the time needed to recover from sports injuries.[9]

Target vitamin A to reduce tendon inflammation, especially the swelling that occurs with cuts. Vitamin A can increase collagen, reduce inflammation, increase postoperative immune suppression, improve healing and reduce scarring. It is so effective that it is sometimes applied directly to wounds with sponge implants.[10]

According to J. Cecil Smith, Jr., M.D., vitamin A cannot do it job if zinc isn't also present. In a study of 61 children in Baltimore, Maryland, Smith and his colleagues found that vitamin A could not be released from their livers unless there was high enough blood levels of zinc.[11]

In its own right, zinc is important to the healing of tender tendons. Zinc supplementation has been shown in studies to reduce wound healing time significantly, and works with A to heal wounds, form collagen and reduce inflammation.[12]

Two nutrients must be considered along with zinc: vitamin B6 and copper. Include 2-4 mg of copper with any zinc supplement.

Vitamin B6 also enhances zinc absorption. When supplementing with one B vitamin, always include a good B complex formula. Like the Musketeers, it's all or none. They work together or they don't work at all.

Exercise Important for Restoration of Normal Use

Once my cast was off and I was able to get around without it, Dr. Gordon emphasized light exercise to restore my atrophied muscles and tight tendons. Using the rubber band example, it's not hard to understand the importance of stretching, pulling and weight-bearing exercise for tendon-restoration. First, it's essential for restoring circulation. Without adequate circulation, those nutrients you're dutifully downing won't get where they belong. Secondly, hyaluronic acid is formed when stress is put on the muscles and tendons. A little stress means the body lubricates and moistens dry, unused tissues, essential for thorough healing.

Tendonitis actually requires less layoff time than most other sports injuries. In fact, not exercising may be one of the worst things you can do for your aching bones, according to University of Louisville strength coach Doug Semenick.[13]

If your tendonitis occurred during weight lifting, exercising, or due to poor posture, make sure you are doing it right when you start up again. Time may have diminished your memory of the reason you were laid up in the first place. Remind yourself and concentrate on the right way, or you'll be back in the cast again. In my case, I walk my horses around corners and avoid muddy paths.

If you follow a weight-lifting regimen, continue your program, but use light weights or elastic exercise bands to slowly boost the strength of the muscle and tendon. Trying to lift heavy weights will just aggravate the injury and make you even more sore. If you don't lift weights regularly, look for exercises that will strengthen the muscles that support the sore joint (for example, biceps curls and triceps extensions to counteract a sore elbow). Go slow; if you feel pain, lower the resistance even more. Use stretching exercises to loosen up the muscles before you work out, to help avoid aggravating the injury.

If your heel is your hellion, concentrate on exercises to strengthen the calf muscles. Exercise is OK as long as the area isn't swollen or painful. Be sure you're walking heel to toe, with most of the energy expended out the toes. One easy calf exercise I use is simply rising on my toes. Stand on the ball of your foot on a slight elevation, preferably a slant board, holding onto a bar, chair or wall for balance. Raise your heels until you are on your toes. Then slowly lower your heels below toe level. I do this whenever I find myself in a line or standing up waiting somewhere. The slant part is optional. You can work up to that.

As you now see, tendonitis can be prevented – whether the first time, or after you've injured it. It doesn't have to be a life sentence. For more information, see my chapters Inflammation, Carpal Tunnel Syndrome, Muscle Weakness and Pain.

Tendon-Loving Nutrients
For maximum absorption, take supplements with meals.

Nutrient	Suggested Dosage	Formulation
Antioxidants	4 capsules daily*	With selenium and grapeseed extract
Borage oil	2 capsules daily	
Bromelain	200 mg twice daily	
Flaxseed oil	1 tablespoon daily	
Glucosamine sulfate	500 mg three times daily	
Magnesium	200 mg daily	
MSM (methylsulfonylmethane)	500 mg three times daily	
Multi-mineral	3-4 ounces daily	In liquid solution, with vitamin B12, biotin
Multi-vitamin/mineral	6 caplets daily	Freeze-dried plant sources
Quercetin	400 mg twice daily	With vitamin C
Tumeric	100 mg three times daily	
Vitamin B6	200 mg daily	
Vitamin C	Individual bowel tolerance**	With citrus bioflavonoids (quercetin, proanthocyanidins)

* The FDA recommends pregnant women not exceed 10,000 IU of vitamin A daily.

** To determine individual dosage, on the first day take 1,000 mg hourly until diarrhea occurs, then reduce dosage to just below that for individual daily dosage. Vitamin C is not toxic in large doses but must be taken throughout the day to benefit. Divide dosage to three or four times a day.

CHAPTER 155:

Tics, Twitches and Tourette's

Poor Tommy. He's in the doghouse again. His teacher sent him out of the room because he disrupted his second-grade class once too often this morning. She knows he's being treated for hyperactivity – and she can cope with his occasional frenetic outbursts – but lately something new has been added. He blinks his eyes and twitches his nose continually, and his feet are never still. Every once in a while he'll let out a series of yelps, which the children find hilarious, but which also makes it impossible for her to teach. He has told her he can't help making these noises. She is beginning to wonder. Can it be that Tommy has that disease she heard about on TV a few years ago? The one in which the victims uncontrollably bark like dogs and curse and scream?

Tommy's teacher is thinking of Tourette's Syndrome (TS), another "disease" which have doctors totally baffled – another mystery that has so stumped the experts, anyone with an open mind and money for research can solve. This despite the fact that it was first discovered in 1885 by French physician Gilles de la Tourette. That's my point here – since the cause has not been identified, anything can be the cause.

If you have a son or daughter with Tourette's, or tics that don't seem to want to go away, you can be instrumental in finding a cure. If your doctor uses that old excuse, "it isn't curable," then do your own investigating. Find the clues and talk your doctor into trying alternatives. If the alternatives are natural substances, the risk is minimal. Certainly less risky than the dangerous pharmaceuticals they're experimenting with on kids today. Because nobody knows for sure what causes tics and TS, anything could be causing them, including a vitamin or mineral deficiency, or an inability to assimilate nutrients, resulting in nutrient deficiencies.

Are Tics Harmful?

Tics aren't harmful, but what may have caused poor Tommy's tics was the medication he was on for his hyperactivity. Remember, doctors don't know for sure what causes tics and Tourette's.

In a study recorded in *Archives of Pediatrics & Adolescent Medicine*, the medical records of 122 children treated with stimulant drugs for attention deficit hyperactivity disorder (ADHD) at a Long Island behavioral center were examined. Eleven of these children developed tics, which in three cases disappeared without discontinuation of medication and in seven cases disappeared when medication was ended. Family histories were taken into account, but had no bearing on the outcome. The researchers estimated that as many as nine percent of children treated with stimulant drugs for ADHD may develop tics or other involuntary, repetitive movements.[1] If you need more compelling evidence of the dangers of neuroleptic drugs, see my chapter Tardive Dyskinesia, a condition in which psychiatric drugs causes involuntary movements.

Tics are defined as involuntary muscle movements such as eye blinking or tongue clicking. There are two kinds of tics. Motor tics include blinking the eyes, shrugging the shoulders, or shaking the head. Vocal tics include clearing the throat, sniffing, coughing, or saying words out of context.[2] Because they are not under a child's control, the child doesn't use them as a means of calming down, as he would with a nervous habit. The important thing to remember is that tics are physical problems, not psychological ones. If your child has tics, please do not assume they are a behavioral problem, subject to tranquilizing drugs; and don't let anyone make you believe it.

Although they are most often a response to stress, tics are not always a direct response to a stressful situation – they sometimes happen randomly, explains Ruth Bruun, M.D., a psychiatrist in New York City who specializes in the treatment of tics. Roughly one child in eight develops tics, and boys are four times as likely to have tics as girls are.[3]

Most tics will disappear after a few weeks or months – a year at the most. They may never come back, or they may come back for a little while and then disappear again. Because they are difficult to control, Bruun notes, "Telling your child to stop isn't going to help. He can't stop." In fact, your disapproval may unnecessarily increase his anxiety. If the tic is very noticeable, you should mention it to his teacher and any other adults who see him frequently. Explain to them that your child's behavior is involuntary and that talking about it with the child won't solve the problem – and may make matters worse.[4] It's best to acknowledge the problem without disapproval or blame, and do what you can to make others understand it's not on purpose.

What I find most fascinating about TS is the incredible urges that accompany it. Apparently, people with Tourette's can control their tics for minutes to hours. Like in epilepsy, children can "sense" the onset of a tic and then either suppress it, or surrender to it. Described as the expectation that precedes a sneeze, or an itch at some unreachable spot on the back, it is felt as requiring some type of vigorous action.[5]

Eventually the urge becomes irresistible with tension, and the tics must be allowed to play themselves out. Tics get worse when TS patients are anxious and improve when they concentrate on something, as long as it isn't stressful. I read one case study where a boy couldn't play video games without erupting in tics. Since many patients try to keep a tight rein on their symptoms at school or at work, they are inclined to "let it all hang out" at home where they're comfortable.[6] At home is where the symptoms seem to be at their worst.

It reminds me a little of multiple sclerosis, which analogously is caused by damaged electrical lines, causing short circuits in the system. In TS, the lines are overdosed with electricity and must be grounded/released. Whatever mechanism that keeps us from acting out every impulse – subconscious or conscious – appears to be missing here.

Other Disorders Linked to Tourette's

Tourette's is defined not by a test or laboratory, but by its symptoms. Generally, it starts with facial tics. A friend of mine has an eleven year old son who has had tics since he was four. She tells me his first symptom was what she called an eye grimace. Then she noticed he erupted with sounds, then muscle movements. The reason she was able to identify the symptoms as TS was because her first husband had Tourette's (not her son's father) and the tics were identical. The last straw was when he started making neck movements that were so severe and frequent, they threatened to snap his spine. It was as if he was in a car and had just been rear-ended.

Dystonia is a syndrome in which abnormalities in muscle control lead to inappropriate muscle contraction. In one study, nine patients were found to have dystonia as well as Tourette's syndrome, prompting researchers to suspect they may have a common cause. Other commonalities are that dystonia patients are typically male, and have tics at the onset of the disorder, which start at an average of nine years of age. All started before age 18.[7] TS usually begins in childhood, between the ages of 2 and 15, with most cases clustered around the age of seven.[8]

Obsessive-compulsive behavior is also linked with Tourette's. Researchers believe that whatever brain abnormality causes people to obsessively and repeatedly wash their hands, for example, might also cause Tourette's.

Tics and involuntary movements can also occur following a streptococcus bacteria infection, like strep throat for example. Doctors call this Sydenham's chorea, defining it as "a neurological condition marked by rapid, darting, uncontrolled, and patternless muscle movements that can occur after a streptococcal bacterial infection." [9]

As with dystonia, chorea and Tourette's have commonalities. For example, facial grimaces are a prominent feature of both Sydenham's chorea and Gilles de la Tourette's syndrome, as are involuntary arm, shoulder and leg jerks. In addition, in both disorders, stressors (including fever) increase symptom severity, while dopamine blockers, such as haloperidol, decrease the severity of the symptoms. Further, unless the child is severely affected, both tics and chorea can be voluntarily suppressed to some degree.[10] If tics can occur following a bacterial infection, then whatever anatomical abnormality that causes tics and Tourette's in the first place may be influenced by bacterial infections.

Clues that Lead to Nutritional Answers

The best evidence suggests that, although TS has physical symptoms, the disease is a neurological disorder. Researchers believe that dopamine, a brain chemical that regulates voluntary movements, is somehow involved. In 1961 Italian and French researchers discovered that haloperidol, a major tranquilizer used to treat severe mental disorders such as schizophrenia, also suppressed tics. Haloperidol is believed to block transmission of dopamine. It is not clear to researchers whether the brain's dopamine systems are overactive in TS or whether the dopamine receptors in the brain are hypersensitive. Other neurotransmitters (serotonin and norepinephrine) may also be involved.[11]

All physicians are really sure of is that haloperidol reduces tics in as many as 86 percent of Tourette patients, but has to be stopped in most cases because of formidable side effects – depression, weight gain, difficulty in concentration, drowsiness, a feeling of being "spaced out," and Parkinsonian symptoms of tremor, rigidity, lack of facial expression, and slow movement. (Since Parkinson's disease is characterized by abnormally low levels of brain dopamine, there's obviously a fine line between too much and too little dopamine.)[12]

The area of the brain most affected has been pinpointed as the basal ganglia, a pair of deep-lying structures that control physical coordination by helping to relay signals from the cerebral cortex to the brain stem. The basal ganglia contains 80 percent of the central nervous system's dopamine. Many children with TS show signs of neurologic abnormalities, such as hyperactivity, poor coordination, and attention deficit disorder (characterized by impulsiveness, hyperactivity, poor concentration, and inattention). Even autism is linked to Tourette's.

The next step in our hide and seek game is to discover which nutrients influence the nervous system, counters the affect of bacterial infections, and regulates muscle control. If this sounds far-fetched, read on.

Nutrition Influences Brain Function

The excellent book *Medical Applications of Clinical Nutrition*, edited by Jeffrey Bland, Ph.D. (Keats Publishing, 1983), makes a strong case in favor of the influence of nutrients on brain functioning or, dysfunctioning. If you read my chapter on Mental Illness, you'll see the extensive affect nutritional deficiencies have on behavior. A simple B12 deficiency, for example, has been found to be responsible for the worst case of schizophrenia. Every chemical in the body, including those in the brain and nervous system, has to be synthesized from a preceding natural chemical. Food is the major source of nutrients from which essential brain chemicals are made. Take away the nutrients, and you have imbalances of vitamin brain chemicals.

Most researchers believe behavioral disorders such as Tourette's, alcoholism, attention deficit, autism and posttraumatic stress disorder are caused by imbalances of dopamine and serotonin. Dopamine regulates the control of voluntary movements and serotonin regulates pain, pleasure and sleep cycles.[13] Doctors like to prescribe the aforementioned haloperidol (or Haldol), because it influences dopamine, reducing Tourette's symptoms. However, a safer nutrient has been discovered that has been shown to work the same as haloperidol: ascorbic acid (vitamin C).[14]

Many studies have found ascorbic acid to be as potent a substance as haloperidol in blocking dopamine receptors in the brain. Ascorbic acid does the same, except that it stays out of the brain itself, and therefore cannot cause the kind of dangerous side effects of which tranquilizers are notorious.[15]

As you've been reading this book, you'll have realized by now that vitamin C is a potent antioxidant, a destroyer of free radicals, and an anti-inflammatory, characteristics that diminish the cell-damaging effects of bacterial infections.

Researchers evaluating the toxic effects of too much of the mineral manganese more than a century ago in manganese miners hit on something that may be of benefit. The miners were found to have an excessive intake of manganese through the lungs. They suffered from what was termed "manganese madness," which caused involuntary movements and psychological disturbances. Later studies in primates showed that when manganese was given parenterally, either through the lung or intravenously, it was specifically deposited in the basal ganglia of the brain where it caused a *depletion* of dopamine.[16] Is this fascinating or what?! Manganese could possibly be useful in reducing the amounts of dopamine in the brain. Now, I certainly don't recommend that TS patients go out and take large doses of manganese, but for the researchers and doctors out there who believe too much dopamine is responsible for Tourette's, isn't *this* a fascinating concept!

Now to muscle control. My first thought when I looked at dystonia, was a lack of magnesium. I thought of magnesium because it affects both the nervous system and the muscular system.

An article in *Biological Psychiatry* reported that of patients hospitalized with major depression or schizophrenia, magnesium was significantly lower in those who had made suicide attempts. The researchers involved in the study believe magnesium has a role in regulating serotonin levels of the brain.[17]

William Walsh, Ph.D., a former research scientist at Argonne National Laboratories estimates that 95 percent of violent individuals suffer from nutritional imbalances that predispose them to bad behavior. Dr. Walsh found that people who were delinquent, impulsive and irritable were low in all the trace minerals including calcium and magnesium.[18]

Warren F. Langley, M.D., of Holy Cross Hospital in Ft. Lauderdale, Florida found that among severely magnesium-deficient individuals, noise, excitement and body contact can cause neurologic symptoms.[19]

In a study of 165 boys, it was found that those with symptoms of depression, schizophrenia and sleep disturbances had low blood levels of magnesium. In adults, insufficient magnesium may be accompanied by a loss of sensation in the extremities, as well as tremors, convulsions, muscle spasms, confusion, delirium and behavioral problems.[20]

Researchers both in the United States and abroad have demonstrated very clearly that 30 to 60 percent of autistic children and adults show significant behaviorial and other benefits from administration of large amounts of vitamin B6 and magnesium.[21]

For more clues and options, see my chapters Tardive Dyskinesia, Depression, Mental Illness and Stress.

Tic Terminating Nutrients
For maximum absorption, take supplements with meals.

Nutrient	Suggested Dosage	Formulation
Aged garlic extract	1 teaspoon three times daily	Liquid
Antioxidants	4 capsules daily*	With selenium and grapeseed extract
Borage oil	2 capsules daily	
Coenzyme Q10	2 capsules daily	With vitamin E, phospholipids and selenium
Folic acid	5-10 mg daily	
Ginkgo biloba	50 mg three times daily	
L-Glutamine	500 mg twice daily	
Magnesium	200 mg daily	
Melatonin (adults only)	3 mg daily at bedtime	With B vitamins
MSM (methylsulfonylmethane)	500 mg three times daily	
Multi-mineral	3-4 ounces daily	In liquid solution, with vitamin B12, biotin
Multi-vitamin/mineral	6 caplets daily	Freeze-dried plant sources
Niacin	500 mg four times daily	
Quercetin	400 mg twice daily	With vitamin C and bioflavonoids
Taurine	3 grams daily	
Vitamin B6	200 mg daily	
Vitamin C	Individual bowel tolerance**	With bioflavonoids (quercetin, rutin proanthocyanidins)

* The FDA recommends pregnant women not exceed 10,000 IU of vitamin A daily.

** To determine individual dosage, on the first day take 1,000 mg hourly until diarrhea occurs, then reduce dosage to just below that for individual daily dosage. Vitamin C is not toxic in large doses but must be taken throughout the day to benefit. Divide dosage to three or four times a day.

CHAPTER 156:

Ulcers

Jim has had stomach problems all his life, and consequently ate antacids like they were candy. Lately he has discovered new over-the-counter products that kill the stomach acid for over eight hours. The worst time for him was in the middle of the night. At least a couple times a night he would awaken and reach for his bedside supply of antacids and a glass of milk. Finally, the pain grew worse and Jim decided to see a doctor.

At my suggestion, Jim went to see the God of Gastroenterology, Dr. Ross Gordon, who practices in Albany, California. After learning Jim was an antacid pill-popper, and had been for several years, the first thing Dr. Gordon did was test him for allergies.

"What do allergies have to do with my stomach problems, doc?" Jim queried.

"When you reduce your stomach acid, chronically, like you have been doing over the years, several things happen," the doctor told him. The most important thing that happens is you become malnourished. You can't digest your food without acid to break it down, so your nutrient intake is severely reduced. When food enters your intestine before being broken down, your immune system treats it as a foreign body and you develop an allergic response. Plus, bacteria proliferates, feeding on the whole food, inviting infection. In one study, 98 percent of peptic ulcer patients had allergies.[1] In another, 25 of 43 allergic children were found to have peptic ulcers.[2] A few tests and we'll know just how bad yours is."

Dr. Gordon discovered that Jim was allergic to meat, milk and dairy products. This wasn't surprising since they need the most stomach acid to break down. His ulcer was almost one inch in diameter. No wonder he was in pain most of the time!

Jim went on a diet of easily assimilated, low fat foods consisting of whole grains with plenty of fiber, vegetables and low-sugar fruits. Jim stayed away from processed food, especially sugar and white flour products, which do nothing to naturally combat bacteria, are low in nutrients, and feed bacteria. He also took a multi-digestive supplement, a mineral in solution formula, multiple vitamins and acidophilus, an intestinal-friendly bacteria that kills the bad bacteria without antibiotics and restores the system to an optimum state. Within six weeks, Jim felt better, slept better and no longer needed antacids.

Myths and Misconceptions About Ulcers

First, ulcers are not caused by stress or too much stomach acid. These factors contradict each other since stress commonly reduces stomach acid, not increases it. In fact, studies show people with stomach ulcers have low amounts of stomach acid.[3]

Stomach acid is important for the above reasons, but also for another. Doctors now are convinced that ulcers are a result of abnormalities in the gastrointestinal system that break down its natural immune and mucosa protectant system. Stomach acid is not an abnormality and actually defends the body against ulcers, in part by killing the bad bacterium, Helicobacter pylori, which is believed to cause ulcers. Investigation by scientists shows that H. pylori is present in more than 90 percent of peptic ulcer patients.[4]

Helicobacter pylori was first observed in the gastric mucosa during the 19th century, as a factor in ulcer formation. However, this infection has only recently been linked to peptic ulcers. It took doctors time to discover the connection since stomach acid is normally a bacterial killer, and it hadn't occurred to them that many people would be low in stomach acid. H. pylori bacteria appear to have adapted well to the stomach's hostile acidic environment and may promote ulcer formation by invading the cells and undermining the defense mechanisms. Studies show that 84 percent of people with duodenal ulcers, 57 percent of people with indigestion and even 21 percent of people with no gastrointestinal problems harbor H. pylori infections, the incidence increasing with age.[5]

I would venture to guess the increased prevalence of ulcers coincides with the popularity of antacids in treating stomach upset. Feel a little gassy? Take an antacid. Feel a little stomachache? Take an antacid. People typically take antacids when they need them the least. A typical reason for an after-meal stomachache or gas is too little stomach acid to break down the food. Gas occurs for two reasons: swallowed air and bacterial growth. Without stomach acid to break it down, food putrefies, creating painful bacteria gas.

A peptic ulcer is an umbrella term for certain lesions (sores) in the lining of the stomach and duodenum – top part of the small intestine. The word "peptic" comes from pepsin, the enzyme that normally helps to break down food and which can be missing when an ulcer exists. Peptic ulcers occur most often in the duodenum (duodenal ulcers) less commonly in the stomach itself (gastric ulcers).

Another common misconception is drinking milk for an ulcer. It is incorrectly believed bland or dairy food coats the stomach, soothing the irritation. Unfortunately, most bland and dairy foods are high in protein and fat. The body reacts by producing large amounts of stomach acid, resulting in even worse pain then before. Alcohol is out. Not because it is acidic, but because the high carbohydrates promote excess acid secretion.

Nearly 90 percent of Americans with digestive disorders wrongly believe ulcers are caused by stress.[6] Ulcers are not caused by eating red hot chili peppers or enduring 16-hour hectic business days. Contrary to long-standing myths, new studies show no evidence that stress causes ulcers. Easy-going people are as likely to get them as hard-driving workaholics. Although stress may aggravate an existing ulcer, there is no evidence that it causes one.

In a study at the University of Toronto, researchers found that half of people surveyed who'd already had an ulcer thought aspirin was the best treatment, reasoning, I suppose, that since aspirin is an anti-inflammatory, it would help reduce the inflammation of an ulcer. "Incredible!" comments one University of Toronto expert, "because aspirin, along with other non-steroidal anti-inflammatory drugs, is a prime ulcer-provoker."[7] There are much better anti-inflammatories available that are safe, natural and gentle.

Healing Ulcers with Nutrition

In a review of the importance of essential fatty acids in *Nutrition and Rheumatic Disease/Rheumatic Disease Clinics of North America*, Peter E. Callejari, M.D., and Robert B. Zurier, M.D., stated that evening primrose oil and fish oil can help reduce the damage of internal wounds. Backing up this contention was a study in which six patients with duodenal ulcers reported complete healing after receiving three grams a day of evening primrose oil.[8] Doctors credit the gamma linolenic acid (GLA) in evening primrose oil for its benefit in healing tissue.

In one study, 38 out of 40 peptic ulcer patients were found to have low levels of linoleic acid. It is believed that GLA increases prostaglandins, which protect the delicate stomach and intestinal linings from ulcer formation.[9]

The two families of essential fatty acids are omega-6 (linoleic acid), found in seeds and seed oils and omega-3 (alpha-linolenic acid) found mainly in fish, fish oils (cod liver oil), green leafy vegetables and flaxseed oil. Gamma-linolenic acid (GLA), or linoleic acid, are found in evening primrose oil, black currant oil, borage oil and spirulina, and are known primarily for their anti-inflammatory effect. While most researchers use evening primrose oil in their studies, independent clinical tests show that borage oil contains more GLA – up to 26 percent. Compare this to evening primrose oil and black currant oil, which contain no more than 18 percent. Additionally, borage oil costs less because the borage seed is three times larger than black currant or evening primrose seeds. Finally, borage is more bioavailable. In other words, the body more readily accepts it.[10]

In the vitamin community, vitamins A, found in orange vegetables, and E, high in wheat germ and other nut and seed oils, have been shown to inhibit the development of ulcers in rats and are important factors in keeping the stomach and intestinal linings strong and healthy.

Dr. Alan Gaby reports success using 75 to 100,000 units of vitamin A and 800 units of vitamin E daily over six to eight weeks to treat peptic ulcers as well as one to two grams of vitamin C daily for wound healing.

Combining vitamin E with A boosts the benefit so lower amounts can be taken, and beta carotene, a vitamin A precursor, can be taken with vitamin A to boost the benefit. Beta carotene can be taken in as high a dose as is needed, with no side effects.

A study reported in *The Lancet* demonstrated that vitamin A is more effective in healing ulcers than commonly prescribed antacids. Three groups were evaluated. Group one was given antacids only, group two was given vitamin A and antacids, and group three was given just vitamin A. In the group given just vitamin A, 36 percent had complete healing of their ulcers after four weeks. In the group taking only antacids, only 18 percent had complete healing. Among those who didn't experience complete healing, the ulcers were "significantly larger" than when they started in the group only taking antacids.[11]

Vitamin C, although it is called ascorbic acid, does not add to the acid burden of ulcers, says Abram Hoffer, M.D.[12] Vitamin C, taken with bioflavonoids, helps reduce inflammation, encourages healing and among hospitalized ulcer patients, high blood levels of vitamin C was the differential factor between bleeding ulcers and healing ulcers.[13] Vitamin C is highest in the tropical fruits papaya, guava and black currants. Bioflavonoids are contained in the colorful portions of most fruits and vegetables.

The mineral zinc is especially important for inner mucosa tissue because it increases production of mucin, the body's inner damage defender. In studies, zinc has shown a protective effect in animals and humans on peptic ulcers.[14] Zinc has even been shown in studies to retard the damaging effect of aspirin.

In an experimental double-blind study, 15 patients with gastric ulcers and normal zinc levels were treated randomly with either zinc or a placebo. After three weeks, the ulcers in the untreated group were three times the size of those who received zinc, and some who took the mineral had markedly less pain within four days.[15] Look for zinc in sesame seeds, pumpkin seeds and blackstrap molasses.

Calcium and magnesium have been shown in studies to act as an antacid. Melvyn Werbach, M.D., suggests one to four grams of calcium carbonate one and three hours after meals and at bedtime, and magnesium hydroxide 30-60 ml given one and three hours after each meal and at bedtime for six weeks.[16]

Target magnesium in solution. Because magnesium is very alkaline, it acts as an antacid and can be used in place of over-the-counter antacid compounds. Calcium and magnesium should always be taken together for nutritional benefit. For optimum absorption of all the minerals, target a minerals in solution formula, which overcomes the allergies, stomach acid and malabsorption issues common with ulcers.

Foods That Heal

Abram Hoffer, M.D., in his highly-regarded book *Orthomolecular Medicine for Physicians* (Keats Publishing, 1989), outlines a protocol he has found works to heal peptic ulcers. It includes a food-only diet with major emphasis on whole-grain cereals and uncooked vegetables. Three small meals with snacks between should be eaten. An allergy history should be obtained, with food allergens avoided for at least six months, then eaten only rarely. He recommends vitamins B3, B6, C and E, zinc and perhaps manganese.[17]

Studies of various cultures and their eating habits have shown that those who eat the most raw foods in their most natural state, with lots of fiber, have the least incidence of ulcers, and have the healthiest gastrointestinal system.[18] They also have less stomach cancer, which is almost directly linked to gastrointestinal problems. To learn more about this connection, read my chapter, Cancer, Stomach.

Eating whole foods is the best, eating sprouts even better, since the young shoots concentrate more of the older plants' nutrients. When targeting food supplements, look for a formula that uses freeze dried sprouts and vegetables, combined in such a way as to provide all the essential vitamins and minerals.

The next time you have a stomachache, reach for a banana instead of an antacid. The use of banana in the treatment of gastrointestinal ailments is traditional in India, and has been recommended for stomach ulcers. In a study of guinea pigs, banana powder protected against aspirin and NSAID-induced ulcers in guinea pigs. In a human study, banana powder helped relieve 75 percent of a treatment group with indigestion.[19]

I remember visiting my late mother-in-law at the hospital and warning her that the arthritis medicine she was taking might cause bleeding ulcers. When I told her cabbage juice can manage most cases of ulcers, she looked at me as if I had lost my mind and dismissed the idea. Just then her doctor came in and she told him about my ridiculous idea. "Oh sure," he nodded knowingly, "Cabbage juice really works. It contains what is called vitamin U, because it helps heal ulcers.

Aloe vera juice has been successful when used internally for ulcers – four ounces of juice two times a day.

Some years ago, Russian medicine men built a small foundation of science under aloe vera's folklore. An article in the *Journal of the American Osteopathic Association* (v. 62, April 1963) reported research in which aloe vera gel helped in the treatment of peptic ulcers. Researchers theorize that aloe vera gel soothes and heals stomach ulcers by coating the stomach lining, especially important where natural protective mucus has been eroded.

A constituent of licorice, glycyrrhizinic acid, was the first botanical compound proven to promote the healing of ulcers. Rather than inhibiting the secretion of acid, licorice stimulates the normal defense mechanisms that prevent ulcer formation, including increasing mucin, the natural mucus coating that heals inflamed tissues and fortifies skin cells. Look for DGL, or deglyclyrrhizinated licorice, in your vitamin or health food store. It is a supplemental formula that has been very successful in healing both stomach and intestinal ulcers.[20]

For more foods and nutrients that heal and prevent stomach and intestinal problems, read my chapters Inflammation, Gastritis, Diverticulitis, Colon Problems, Constipation and Stomach Cancer.

Ulcer-Abating Nutrients
For maximum absorption, take supplements with meals.

Nutrient	Suggested Dosage	Formulation
Acidophilus	At least four billion flora on an empty stomach, three times daily	
Aged garlic extract	1 teaspoon three times daily	Liquid
Amino acids	4-6 capsules daily	Multiple formula from natural sources
Antioxidants	4 capsules daily*	With selenium and grapeseed extract
Borage oil	2 capsules daily	
Coenzyme Q10	2 capsules daily	With vitamin E, phospholipids and selenium
Enzymes	2 capsules twice daily	Multiple formula
Fiber	4-8 tablets daily	Psyllium, with herb hyssop
Bromelain	200 mg twice daily	
Deglycyrrhizinated licorice	1-2 tablets before meals	Chewable
Flaxseed oil	1 tablespoon daily	
L-Glutamine	500 mg three times daily	
Melatonin (adults only)	3 mg daily at bedtime	With B vitamins
Multi-mineral	3-4 ounces daily	In liquid solution, with vitamin B12, biotin
Multi-vitamin/mineral	6 caplets daily	Freeze-dried plant sources
Niacinamide	1,000 mg twice daily	
Quercetin	400 mg twice daily	With vitamin C
Vitamin A	25,000 IU daily*	
Vitamin B6	100 mg daily	
Vitamin C	Individual bowel tolerance**	With bioflavonoids (quercetin, rutin proanthocyanidins)
Vitamin E	2 capsules (800 IU) daily	d-alpha tocopherol

* The FDA recommends pregnant women not exceed 10,000 IU of vitamin A daily.

** To determine individual dosage, on the first day take 1,000 mg hourly until diarrhea occurs, then reduce dosage to just below that for individual daily dosage. Vitamin C is not toxic in large doses but must be taken throughout the day to benefit. Divide dosage to three or four times a day.

CHAPTER 157:

Uterine Fibroids

My friend Keshia Jackson never thought twice about her heavy, painful and lengthy periods. The excessive bleeding sapped her energy, but she never let if affect her job as a mail carrier.

Then one day she passed a huge blood clot. Alarmed, she visited a gynecologist, who told her she had uterine fibroid tumors and recommended a hysterectomy. She was 40, with three children, and probably wouldn't want any more, but she hesitated before accepting the offer of medical menopause, asking me what she should do.

Because she lived in Atlanta, I suggested she call 1-800-445-HEAL for a number where she could obtain a list of nutrition-oriented physicians in her area. She found one, and through a dietary and nutritional supplementation program, was able to reduce her fibroids to a point where they caused her no pain, discomfort or inconvenience, much less sterilization.

Too Many Hysterectomies

Conventional medicine's slash and burn philosophy extends to uterine fibroids. It is one of the most common noncancerous gynecological conditions occurring in reproductive-age women 35 to 55 years of age, and is estimated to account for an incredibly three out of every ten hysterectomies performed annually in the United States.[1]

Fibroids – doctors call them myomas – are noncancerous masses of muscle and connective tissue in the uterus (womb). They can be as small as a pinhead or as large as a watermelon. Dr. Billie Jean

Pace, a gynecologist who practices near Orlando, Florida reported that she once removed a 9-pound, 6-ounce fibroid from a woman who hadn't seen a doctor in three years.[2]

Fibroids can cause no symptoms or many symptoms. A large one may feel like a rock-hard bulge in the lower abdomen or, if they are small, detectable only through symptoms. Fibroids can arise in muscle tissue anywhere in the body, but they are found most commonly in the uterus.

Although some like to call fibroids tumors, they are not cancerous and do not spread. They tend to remain within the confines of the uterus. As they grow larger, however, they can put pressure on neighboring organs and tissues. This growth leads to a range of symptoms, depending on the position of the fibroid and the extent of the pressure.

Every year about 175,000 American women undergo a hysterectomy, or surgical removal of the uterus, as a conventional treatment for fibroids. According to an American College of Obstetricians and Gynecologists guideline, a woman with a fibroid that makes her uterus bigger than it would be at 12 weeks of pregnancy, even if she is suffering no other symptoms, should be considered a candidate for a hysterectomy.[3]

However, the practice of routinely recommending hysterectomy for fibroids has come under increasing scrutiny from both consumer organizations and doctors concerned about the high rate of hysterectomies in the United States. By age 60, more than a third of American women have had a hysterectomy, a rate higher than in any other Western country.[4]

Blue Cross/Blue Shield of Illinois, in a study of all the hysterectomies performed in the state between 1987 and 1989, concluded that an incredible one-third were unnecessary. Most of the unnecessary surgeries, the insurer found, were performed for fibroids and other benign (noncancerous) conditions.[5] If your doctor suggests a hysterectomy for fibroids, find another.

Evidence and Estrogen

How do you know if you have fibroids? Approximately one-third of women with fibroids suffer from abnormal uterine bleeding.[6] You may find yourself suddenly having heavier or more painful blood flows than usual, lasting longer than normal. Or you may have bleeding between periods. Another symptom is apparent weight gain. If you have a monster fibroid growing inside your uterus, you are more than likely going to start looking bigger. The growth of a fibroid may expand the uterus by ten or 15 times.[7]

Like breast cancer, ovarian cysts, fibrocystic breast disease and endometriosis, fibroids are believed to be influenced by high estrogen levels. Doctors find that fibroids increase in women on birth control pills and who are pregnant, and diminish or disappear in women approaching menopause. Since this is the case, nutritional solutions to high estrogen levels are appropriate.

One way to keep your estrogen levels in line, and keep new fibroids from forming, is by eating a whole foods, all-natural diet rich in fruits, vegetables, grains, beans, raw seeds and nuts, which provide important nutrients for your body. Target these low stress foods and avoid high stress foods such as meat, dairy products, alcohol and sugar which overwork the liver, leaving it unable to break down estrogen efficiently. Estrogen is secreted by the ovaries in a form called estradiol; the liver then converts the estradiol to estrone and finally to a much safer, much less chemically active form called estriol. If the liver's function is impaired, this process is slowed down. If the more harmful estradiol and estrone remain at higher levels in the body they can stimulate breast and uterine tissue growth, thus worsening estrogen-dependent problems like fibroids.[8]

What figures into this equation are the thousands of man-made estrogens that can stack the deck against women and increase their estrogen levels by hundreds of times. Devra Lee Davis, Ph.D., a senior advisor to the U.S. Department of Health and Human Services targets pesticides, household chemicals and common plastics as some of these man-made estrogens.[9] It is quite possible that the same forces increasing our risk for breast cancer increase the chances of having fibroids. Before 1950, many pesticides, like DDT, were not so prevalent in the environment. What we've learned is that today's modern environment – filled with plastics, chemicals and electronics – contain innumerable man-made estrogen building blocks. Another factor in this hazard is the hormones fed to animals to increase their meat marketability. I have largely given up meat after discovering the garbage that is being fed animals. Nobody has been able to assure the meat-eating consumer public that these hormones don't end up in our bodies in harmful amounts. What can we do to protect ourselves? Fortunately, there is much we can do.

Christiane Northrup, M.D., co-founder of Woman to Woman Health Care Center in Yarmouth, Maine, found answers outside the realm of drugs and surgery. She now regularly incorporates alternative therapies in her treatment of fibrocystic breasts, another side-effect of circulating estrogen.

To decrease estrogen production, her first step is to prescribe a low-fat diet, preferably vegetarian, containing no more than 20 to 25 grams of fat a day and eliminating all dairy products. This diet usually reduces estrogen levels sufficiently but not to the point where menstruation stops. Many women get relief by simply eliminating dairy products.[10] Don't forget the hormones fed to milk cows! Vitamin D is just that: a hormone!

Because chemicals and toxins accumulate in animal fat, a high-fat, animal protein diet substantially increases a woman's estrogen.[11]

Phyto-Estrogens and Other Beneficial Foods

Another anti-estrogen plan of action involves the use of natural plant estrogens, called phytoestrogens, which may prevent man-made estrogens from entering cells. This has been particularly true in the case of bioflavonoids, substances found in brightly-colored fruits and vegetables. Bioflavonoids are not only phytoestrogenic, but act as potent anti-inflammatories, extremely important in reducing the inflammation associated with fibroids.

Phytoestrogenic foods include apples, carrots, yams, green beans, peas, potatoes, red beans, brown rice, whole wheat, rye, flaxseeds and sesame seeds.

Legumes – peas, beans and certain roots – are isoflavonoids, which act as a non-steroidal estrogen. Soybeans, particularly, have been found to have this anti-estrogenic property, and have been associated with a lower incidence of breast cancer in some populations. Soybeans are eaten in great quantities in Japan and China, and is one of the reasons researchers believe these countries have low rates of breast cancer.[12] Tofu, soybean curd, is an excellent food source. It has the unique ability to absorb the flavors it is cooked in. Similar in texture to scrambled eggs, it can be used in casseroles instead of meat. I blend tofu with tumeric and use it as a dip for veggies. You can find the recipe in my book *Nutrition: The Cancer Answer II*.

Vital Vitamins

In the early 1980s, nutrition educator Carlton Fredericks, Ph.D., reported that a high intake of the B complex vitamins, plus extra choline and inositol, help the liver break down estrogen into estriol. In experiments, he demonstrated that B vitamins also reduced many symptoms of premenstrual syndrome – also caused by excess estrogen.[13]

One hundred milligrams of vitamin B6 helps eliminate the fluid retained in postmenopausal breasts, and when it is accompanied by at least 50 milligrams of the other B vitamins, estrogen is better metabolized by the liver.[14]

Women with fibroids and related symptoms like excessive bleeding and premenstrual syndrome may want to add a daily 50 milligrams to a 100 mg B-complex supplement to their diets. All the B vitamins must be taken together for optimum performance of each. Hence, a B-complex formula should always be included with any B vitamin supplement.

Certain vitamins can be used to alleviate the heavy bleeding associated with fibroids. Vitamin A is one of these. Researchers studying 71 women with excessive menstrual bleeding (a common symptom of fibroids) were found to have significantly lower blood levels of vitamin A, as compared to women without fibroids. Almost 90 percent of the women in the study returned to a normal bleeding pattern after two weeks of vitamin A treatment. [15]

Vitamin C added to bioflavonoids can also help with heavy bleeding because it strengthens capillaries, making them less likely to rupture under the pressure of a growing fibroid. In one study, 14 out of 16 patients who took 200 mg of vitamin C three times a day experienced a reduction in heavy bleeding. Vitamin C also helps the body retain iron, helpful when high amounts of blood loss jeopardizes iron levels.[16]

Fibroid-Finishing Nutrients
For maximum absorption, supplements should be taken with meals.

Nutrient	Suggested Dosage	Formulation
Aged garlic extract	2 teaspoons three times daily	Liquid
Antioxidants	4 capsules daily*	With selenium and grape seed extract
Borage oil	2 capsules daily	
Enzymes	2 capsules twice daily	Multiple formula
Flaxseed oil	1 tablespoon daily	
Fiber	8 tablets daily	Psyllium, with herb hyssop
Lecithin	2 tablespoons with meals	
Magnesium	200 mg daily	
Multi-vitamin/mineral	6 caplets daily	Freeze-dried plant sources
Multi-mineral	2-4 ounces daily	In liquid solution, with vitamin B12, biotin
Natural progesterone cream	1/3 teaspoon daily	With pregnenolone, DHEA
Vitamin B6	200 mg daily	
Vitamin C	Individual bowel tolerance**	With bioflavonoids (quercetin, rutin proanthocyanidins)
Vitamin E	2 capsules (800 IU)	d-alpha tocopherol

* The FDA recommends that pregnant women not exceed 10,000 IU of vitamin A daily.

** To determine individual dosage, on the first day take 1,000 mg hourly until diarrhea occurs, then reduce dosage to just below that for individual daily dosage. Vitamin C is not toxic in large doses but must be taken throughout the day to benefit. Divide dosage to three or four times a day.

CHAPTER 158:

Vertigo

I'm only telling you this to make a point. Please try not to laugh. I recently suffered a major embarrassment that makes a point about vertigo. I was retiring for the night, and laid my head down on the pillow when something crawled into my ear! I jumped up, shaking my head, then turned it sideways, banging it with the heel of my hand. I could feel an insect in there, its little legs furiously scrambling against my ear canal, trying to escape. Once it was obvious it wasn't going to come out on its own, I called the local hospital emergency room. "What do I do?" I asked. "You come in and let us get it out," she responded. "It's probably a moth and they can't move backward." I spent half the night sheepishly waiting in the emergency room, while a moth periodically scrabbled loudly in my ear. But the worst was yet to come.

Not warning me of what he was going to do, the doctor filled a syringe with ice-cold water and squirted it deep into my ear. My brain assumed that someone had placed me in a spin dryer set to maximum revs. The room began to rotate faster and faster, until the walls were rolling by in a creamy blur. My eyes struggled in their sockets to keep up with this sensation, while another part of my brain debated whether it would be worthwhile to throw up. I didn't even notice when the moth was expelled by the water.

Despite what Alfred Hitchcock might have you believe, vertigo is not really a fear of heights. True vertigo is an illusion of motion. It's not exactly dizziness, although that's often the way it's described. When part of the nervous system is stimulated, it responds by creating a sense of motion when there is no motion.

Stop the world! About a quarter of people who complain of dizziness prove to have true vertigo. Some experience themselves as moving while the earth stays still; others feel as though the earth is moving relative to them. When vertigo is minimal and temporary, it can be pleasurable. People go to amusement parks primarily to buy illusions, and one of the major illusions for sale is vertigo. If vertigo persists, however, it becomes a nuisance. If it is both persistent and severe, it can become disabling with a significant ability to cause depression. The early astronauts suffered considerably from vertigo after they returned to the earth's gravity and would become depressed and unable to work because of it.[1]

Personally, I can live without even a temporary case of this condition. When I was a child I used to climb trees and loved the merry-go-round. Now I can't even sit in a swing without seeing the world spinning around me.

Noise in the Vestibule

Although vertigo is most often thought of as a spinning sensation, it can also be perceived as tilting, rocking, or veering, and in some cases is accompanied by weakness, nausea, vomiting or headaches. Vertigo occurs when something irritates the interconnected system of chambers and C-shaped canals of the inner ear. Technically called the vestibular system, the chambers are lined with sensory cells that have the ability to detect motion and position. Movement of fluid within the system stimulates the sensory cells, which in turn trigger impulses to the brain by way of a large nerve.[2] It reminds me of a contractor's level. As the level moves, the water moves, rocking the bubble in and out of the lines. Our vestibular system is like having an internal level which controls balance.

It is the vestibular system that gives you the ability to balance on a tightrope, stand on a moving bus without falling down or balance yourself after getting bumped. Without this system, even moving your head would make you dizzy. People with inner ear infections often experience vertigo, as the swelling interferes with these anti-gravity reflexes. If you "pop" your ear with your finger (gently!), you'll experience firsthand this vertigo effect. Anything that inter-feres with this balancing system, from infections to injury to objects to roller coasters, will cause vertigo.

Nutritional Fortification, Protection and Prevention

Vertigo can be a symptom of nerve degeneration. The nerves are composed of fatty acids, which are particularly susceptible to dam-age by free radicals. In order to fortify and protect delicate mem-branes like those in the inner ear, the body produces prostaglandins to control inflammation and blood pressure. When there isn't enough prostaglandins and fatty acids, the vestibular system is left defense-less, and nerve damage can occur, causing vertigo.[3]

Here are a list of nutrients that can fortify, protect and prevent damage to the vestibular nervous system:

Beta carotene, important for the structural integrity of sensory hair cells of the inner ear.

Raw pumpkin seeds for **zinc**. The inner ear has the highest con-centration of zinc in the body. Too much copper will deplete zinc stores; they must be equal for optimum usage. Include 2-4 mg of copper with any zinc supplement.

Magnesium, which plays a role in more than 300 body func-tions, including circulation and muscle control. One of the symptoms of a magnesium deficiency is vertigo.[4,5]

The B vitamins are probably the most well-known brain nutri-ents. A deficiency of vitamin B3, or niacin, has been shown to cause dizziness.[6] Choline is another important B vitamin, critical for the transport of electrical nerve impulses. Vitamin B6 (pyridoxine) is important for the absorption of zinc. Each B vitamin has its own role in body function, centered on the nervous system. Since nerves bring messages to all the organs and stimulate glands to secrete their vital biochemicals, the whole body communication system can break down with a B vitamin deficiency. Get them all by taking a good B-complex formula whenever supplementing with any one.

Ginkgo biloba, an excellent microcirculation booster and free radical inhibitor.

Flaxseed oil, cold pressed and organic, a source of essential fatty acids.

Borage oil, a source of prostaglandins (gamma linolenic acid).

Vitamin E helps to fortify nerves and strengthen capillary walls.

Ginger root helps with digestion, nausea and vertigo. In a double blind, randomized, placebo-controlled trial, 80 Naval cadets consumed one gram of ginger root or a placebo every hour for four consecutive hours. The researchers reported remarkably fewer symptoms of nausea and vertigo, with no side effects.[7]

Taurine is an amino acid found in seafood, eggs, beans and peas. It helps to keep the nerve cells in electrical balance and prevent runaway nerve impulses by allowing nerve currents to flow correctly.

Antioxidants are nature's rotor rooter, clearing out cell-damaging free radicals that can contribute to infections, poor circulation and congestion – all problems that can result in vertigo. The best antioxidants for this condition are coenzyme Q10, the herb ginkgo biloba and vitamins C and E. Vitamin C combined with bioflavonoids will help reduce inflammation. The bioflavonoid quercetin, found in onions and citrus fruit, has been identified as an antihistamine as powerful as pharmaceuticals. Vitamin C and bioflavonoids can be taken in high doses instead of prescribed antihistamines to reduce the swelling of allergies and ear infections that can cause vertigo. You'll see vitamin C prominently addressed as you read through the chapters on situations that can cause vertigo: Inflammation, Infections, Colds and Flu and Allergies. For more on nutrition for the ears, see the chapter Hearing Loss.

A doctor told me about a case in which vertigo was caused by a tiny piece of calcium that broke off from somewhere and was floating around in the fluid of the inner ear. In a certain position, the calcium bit touched sensory cells, stimulating them. In time, the particle bound to something or other and stopped floating around, whereupon the vertigo ceased. The person who had this problem only experienced vertigo when he assumed a particular position.

After a thorough perusal of the medical literature, I am convinced this would not have happened if there was enough magnesium in the system. Magnesium acts like a chelator for calcium, taking it out of places it doesn't belong, excreting it through the urine. Calcium is valueless without enough magnesium, as together they balance each other. Without adequate magnesium, calcium doesn't bond well and accumulates in places it shouldn't. Calcium is important for inner ear health, but in solution should be accompanied by four times that amount of magnesium.

Vertigo-Vanquishing Nutrients
For maximum absorption, take supplements with meals.

Nutrient	Suggested Dosage	Formulation
Aged garlic extract	1 teaspoon three times daily	Liquid
Amino acids	4-6 capsules daily	Multiple formula from natural sources
Antioxidants	4 capsules daily*	With selenium and grapeseed extract
Bilberry	100 mg three times daily	
Borage oil	2 capsules daily	
Coenzyme Q10	2 capsules daily	With vitamin E, phospholipids and selenium
Enzymes	2 capsules twice daily	Multiple formula
Fiber	4-8 tablets daily	Psyllium, with herb hyssop
Flaxseed oil	1 tablespoon daily	
Ginkgo biloba	50 mg three times daily	
L-glutamine	500 mg twice daily	
Multi-mineral	3-4 ounces daily	In liquid solution, with vitamin B12, biotin
Multi-vitamin/mineral	6 caplets daily	Freeze-dried plant sources
Niacin	500 mg four times daily	
Taurine	500 mg twice daily	
Vitamin A	25,000 IU daily*	
Vitamin C	Individual bowel tolerance**	With bioflavonoids (quercetin, rutin proanthocyanidins)
Vitamin E	2 capsules (800 IU) daily	d-alpha tocopherol

* The FDA recommends pregnant women not exceed 10,000 IU of vitamin A daily.

** To determine individual dosage, on the first day take 1,000 mg hourly until diarrhea occurs, then reduce dosage to just below that for individual daily dosage. Vitamin C is not toxic in large doses but must be taken throughout the day to benefit. Divide dosage to three or four times a day.

CHAPTER 159:

Vitiligo

My friend Barbara has had vitiligo for over 25 years. She first got it when she was 13. It started with what dermatologists call a "halo nevus." She had a mole on her arm that one summer developed a white ring around it. The following summer she noticed a white patch around her mouth. The summer after that, her eyes and mouth were ringed with white, and there were white patches on her neck, hands, forearms, shins, feet and pretty much all over her body. Completely mystified, her parents took her on an odyssey of dermatologists, all stumped as to what it could be. Finally, a black dermatologist in Washington, D.C. was able to put a name on it: vitiligo.

Barbara is white, so it isn't until the summer, when she begins to tan, that people first notice the patches. In the winter when she loses her summer color, the patches become less noticeable. The D.C. doctor decided to try something called PUVA treatments. The P stands for psoralen, a drug that enhances the skin's response to the sun. He used a topical formula, applying it on Barbara's white patches, then exposing them to UVA light. Her white patches burned bright pink, the areas around the patches tanned dark brown, and instead of two colors, her skin had three. The drug not only didn't return her pigment, but made the effect worse, as the brown borders accentuated the patches of white. Barbara next tried psoralen pills. At the time she worked in an office with florescent lights. Because the psoralen made her more susceptible to light, she was told to wear sunglasses and sunscreen indoors and out. The psoralen restored some pigment, but once she stopped taking it, the pigment was lost again. Barbara found that for her, it worked no better than sunlight itself, and gave it up when she discovered long term use of the drug could destroy her liver.

Over the years, the patches around her mouth have dimmed, so that even in the summer they aren't as noticeable. The ones around her eyes are actually deemed attractive, and she gets compliments on her "make up." She is healthy, and does not suffer from any diseases or ailments, except an allergy to cats.

Barbara doesn't mind talking about her vitiligo, and whenever she meets people who have it, approaches them to compare notes. She has made some observations about her condition that I find interesting. Perhaps researchers can make sense of them. Her patches occur bilaterally, meaning they are similar in size and location on both sides of her body. The patches' borders can change from year to year; with some patches gaining pigment while others losing it. She loses pigment most readily on the areas of her body that have the *least* amount of fat or muscle, and gets it back most readily in areas of the *most* fat or muscle. For example, her leg patches are on her feet, ankles, shins and knees, and back of her knees. She has never lost pigment on her belly, which is where she has the most fat (no offense, Barbara) – or her back, an area with a lot of muscle, since she swims.

People with vitiligo are more susceptible to sunburn. The patches are not protected by pigment, so they burn easily, getting bright pink before blistering. One 4th of July weekend Barbara's forearms were badly sunburned. After the blisters healed, the pigment in that area returned, staying for 15 years before it was lost again. Areas of injury may lose pigment as well, and come back quickly with sun exposure.

On a given summer, the top of Barbara's hands will start out mostly white. By the end of the summer, depending upon how much sun she gets, three quarters of the surface of her hand will have filled in with pigment. The color fills in randomly in 1/8-inch spots, usually through the hair follicles. By spring the next year, it will all be lost again. One year she used a dermatologist's UVA booth during the winter to see just how much pigment she could get back. Using a patch on the insides of her elbow as a marker, she was able to go from a patch of white approximately three inches in diameter to half an inch in one year. She lost it all again during the following winter. Why does Barbara's pigment come and go like that? And why does she lose it in the first place? Theories abound.

What Causes Vitiligo?

Melanin, the pigment that determines color of skin, hair, and eyes, is produced in cells called melanocytes. If these cells die or cannot form melanin, the skin becomes lighter or completely white.

Vitiligo is the result of the disappearance of the skin's melanocytes. No one knows why, but four main theories exist: 1) Abnormally functioning nerve cells may make toxic substances that injure melanocytes. 2) The body's immune system may perceive the melanocytes as foreign, and destroy them (called auto-immune). 3) Pigment-producing cells may self-destruct. While pigment is forming, toxic byproducts could be produced and destroy melanocytes. 4) There is a genetic defect that makes the melanocytes susceptible to injury.[1]

One theory is that a genetic defect occurs when two people of extremely varied skin coloring produce children. Barbara's mother is dark Hungarian, and her father is light-skinned Scottish. This is a theory born of conjecture, and may not be backed by studies. It would be interesting to see if mulattos have more cases of vitiligo than African Americans with African ancestors. The ratio of blacks to whites with vitiligo is believed to be about fifty-fifty.

Michael Jackson, the musician, and Billie Jean King the former tennis pro, have vitiligo. Some, like Michael Jackson, choose to remove all the pigment from the skin and make the whole body an even white color. This is done with a chemical called monobenzylether of hydroquinone. The pigment removal is permanent.

Some of the conditions that can precede vitiligo are a folic acid deficiency, pernicious anemia, diabetes and hypothyroidism.[2] Tyrosine and iodine are both responsible for the formation of adequate amounts of thyroid hormone.

The Tyrosine Connection

Sometimes in doing research, I hit on something that ties so many things together it has to be a major factor. Tyrosine or tyrosinase in vitiligo may be the missing link. The amino acid tyrosine is converted in the body from the enzyme tyrosinase, the key enzyme involved in creating melanin. It is also important for the nervous system, a factor noted above that could be one cause of vitiligo.

In a controlled-study reported in *The Lancet*, researchers found that 61 percent of those with vitiligo had antibodies against tyrosinase, meaning their immune systems were identifying the tyrosinase as a foreign body and destroying it. Barbara's observation that sunlight brings back the pigment in her skin is born out by the belief that areas of the skin exposed to sunlight have higher concentrations of tyrosinase.[3]

Swiss researchers noted that vitiligo patients had abnormal levels of many amino acids, including tyrosine and tyrosinase, compared to healthy controls.[4]

German researchers discovered that when vitiligo patients took phenylalanine and exposed themselves to sunlight they got pigment back. Phenylalanine, another amino acid, must be present with tyrosinase in order to produce tyrosine in the body. The researchers gave their patients a dose of 50 milligrams per kilogram of body weight, followed by UVA exposure 30 to 45 minutes after ingestion. After four months, or 32 treatments, the patients experienced repigmentation in the fatty areas of their bodies. Unlike with psoralen, the subjects were found to have a higher tolerance of the sun and experienced no sunburn as a result of Phe-UVA therapy.[5]

Skin-lightening compounds – the stuff that fades age spots – inhibits melanin formation. How do they work? – by inhibiting the production of tyrosinase. Tanning compounds use tyrosine to increase desirably brown skin. Cosmetic researchers have found that retinoic acid – a derivative of vitamin A – increases tyrosinase activity in light-skinned people.[6]

If you choose to enhance your tyrosine levels by targeting an amino acid complex, make sure it also contains phenylalanine. Include copper with any tyrosine supplement because copper is necessary for the activation of tyrosinase into tyrosine.[7] Include zinc with copper because they work together.

Treatment with B Vitamins

Richard Kones, M.D., reports in an issue of the *Southern Medical Journal* that one of the signs of a deficiency of folic acid is vitiligo.[8] This didn't surprise researchers in Buenos Aires, Argentina, who found some level of folic acid deficiency in 15 patients with vitiligo. They also found some had deficiencies of vitamin B12 (can cause pernicious anemia) and vitamin C. Out of the 15, they picked eight for a trial treatment, and gave them an average of two milligrams folic acid, 500 mg vitamin C twice a day and 100-1,000 micrograms of B12 every two weeks. All eight patients showed steady and significant repigmentation after three months, and after one to two years, six of the eight had complete repigmentation, with the other two experiencing 80 percent repigmentation. An unusually large number of people living in Buenos Aires have vitiligo, and researchers believe it has to do with a deficiency of folic acid.[9]

Another B vitamin, PABA, has also been found successful in restoring pigment. The late Carl Pfeiffer, Ph.D., M.D., director of Princeton's Brain Bio Center, in his book, *Mental and Elemental Nutrients* (Keats Publishing) reports that pantothenic acid and PABA supplements have been effective in managing vitiligo – "particularly with good amounts of zinc, manganese and vitamin B6."[10]

The late Benjamin Sieve, M.D., former professor at Tufts Medical School, designed an experiment to test PABA on 25 female and 23 male vitiligo patients, ages 10 to 70, who had the disorder from two to 28 years. Almost all the patients had symptoms of a chronically deficient diet and medical history of glandular imbalances. He started out by giving them 100 milligrams of PABA three to four times daily along with a B complex formula. Due to the slowness of the effect, twice daily he began injecting 100 mg of PABA and monoethanolamine, to assure the vitamin would remain in the blood a longer time. A single 100 mg tablet of PABA was taken each morning and evening as well.[11]

His success was phenomenal. Within four to eight weeks, the white patches turned pink. Within 16 weeks, pigment began returning, and after 6 or 7 months, Dr. Sieve noted what he called "striking results." In every one of the 48 patients there was a complete return of melanin.[12] Side effects from large doses of PABA, however, have been noted. Therefore, I recommend you seek a physician's guidance if you want to try this therapy.

Like all of the B vitamins, PABA needs others of its kind to function. Folic acid is important for PABA synthesis, which is why whenever I recommend one B vitamin, I recommend all of them. Each B vitamin has its own role in body function, centered on the nervous system. Since nerves bring messages to all the organs and stimulate glands to secrete their important biochemicals, the whole body communication system can break down with a B vitamin deficiency.

Acid Yes, Antacids No

Many people with vitiligo have too little hydrochloric – stomach – acid, which compromises your ability to assimilate nutrients. Symptoms of too little stomach acid can be the same as too much. When food isn't broken down properly, it can't be digested. Cramps, bloating and gas all occur when food stays in the stomach or enters the intestine without being broken down first. Also, you won't get nutrients from your food if it isn't broken down.

In one experimental study, four patients with vitiligo and a deficiency of stomach acid regained their pigment within two years after taking 15 cc of hydrochloric acid with each meal.[13]

Many of us are probably mineral deficient because as we age, we lose stomach acid. Supplementing with a hydrochloric acid formula such as Betaine will help absorb nutrients, but studies show minerals dissolved in water before ingestion are considerably more bioavailable to the body than those even present in food, because they aren't risked by a lack of hydrochloric acid in the stomach or food allergies. Look for a good, easily absorbable, derived-from-nature mineral blend in solution. Formulations in solution provide the maximum absorption ratios.

Vitiligo Vanquishing Nutrients
For maximum absorption, take supplements with meals.

Nutrient	Suggested Dosage	Formulation
Amino acids	4-6 capsules daily	Multiple formula from natural sources
Borage oil	2 capsules daily	
Coenzyme Q10	2 capsules daily	With vitamin E, phospholipids and selenium
Enzymes	2 capsules with meals	Multiple formula
Fiber	4-8 tablets daily	Psyllium, with herb hyssop
Flaxseed oil	1 tablespoon daily	
Folic acid	5-10 mg daily	
Multi-mineral	3-4 ounces daily	In liquid solution, with vitamin B12, biotin
Multi-vitamin/mineral	6 caplets daily	Freeze-dried plant sources
Vitamin C	Individual bowel tolerance*	With bioflavonoids (quercetin, rutin proanthocyanidins)
Vitamin E	2 capsules (800 IU) daily	d-alpha tocopherol

* To determine individual dosage, on the first day take 1,000 mg hourly until diarrhea occurs, then reduce dosage to just below that for individual daily dosage. Vitamin C is not toxic in large doses but must be taken throughout the day to benefit. Divide dosage to three or four times a day.

CHAPTER 160:

Warts

It was a tough problem for a seventh grader. After his mother Carol showed me his two hands, covered with more warts than I had ever seen in two places, Spencer plunged them deep in the pockets of his jeans.

"Warts will never win a beauty contest," said Spencer bitterly.

Several months before Carol had had the warts burned off. Now there they were again – as big and ugly as ever.

"Maureen, we're desperate," she said with a deep sigh. "Isn't there some folk medicine cure for warts?"

I explained to her and Spencer that medical literature mentions two vitamins, proven over and over again: vitamins A and E. Each day test subjects in various studies spread the contents of a 100 IU capsule of natural vitamin E (alpha tocopherol) on a clean Band-Aid to cover each wart. The warts soon disappeared.

"What Spencer can do is wash his hands, then spread vitamin E oil over them and wear clean cotton gloves. The best time is before bedtime," I told his mother.

Eager to try anything, Spencer followed through. Four weeks later, he showed me that every wart was gone. Delighted, Spencer hugged me and said, "Maureen, if I were two feet taller, 30 years older and wealthy, I'd ask you to marry me."

Unlike the warts, the wedding never came off!

Caused by Viruses

Sir Francis Bacon, the 16th century scientist, rubbed warts with pork fat which he then hung out in the sun, hoping they would disappear as the fat melted. In some parts of Britain, warts are still said to be removed by applying cow dung or rubbing with a fresh potato and then throwing it away. In the Western U.S. mountain regions, folklore claims that rubbing warts with a coin and then throwing the coin away will eradicate them while in other parts of the world warts are said to be abolished by rubbing them onto the father of an illegitimate child. The reputed "success" of some bizarre wart cures may rest on the fact that most warts clear up within a few months on their own. Despite the fact that most warts are painless and harmless, people have resorted to such drastic and ridiculous wart remedies for centuries.

Warts are caused by an invasion of the skin or mucous membranes by viruses known as papillomaviruses, even though when you look closely at them you'd swear they were some kind of fungus growth. You can cut them off, but when you do you risk their spreading. These wart viruses were first seen under the electron microscope in the 1950s. Since then, 50 different sub-types of the human papillomavirus (HPV) family have been identified, each responsible for warts at specific body sites. Some individual warts contain several strains of papillomaviruses. Quite contagious, these viruses enter the body through small cuts or abrasions in the skin and can be transferred from one body part to another – say, from hands to feet or face – or from person to person. It is possible to become infected by wart viruses from damp towels touched by an infected person or to pick up the foot HPV virus from the floors of changing rooms or showers.

Vanquished with Vitamins

Immunologist Robert Garry, Ph.D., of Tulane University in New Orleans, says applying vitamin A topically in a fish-oil base such as cod-liver oil clears up warts in two to five months.[1]

How does it work? Warts are caused by viruses that enter the body through small breaks in the skin and lodge in lower skin layers where they begin to infect normal cells. When the surface skin cells naturally slough off, the virus-infected cells move up with the normal cells as they replace older ones. Soon the virus-infected cells show up on the upper layers of skin as a wart. Here's where the vitamin A comes in. It seems to speed up the process that makes normal cells grow and change functions. This speed-up throws off the reproductive cycle of the virus so it can't infect any more normal cells, and the wart gradually disappears.

In an article in the *Southern Medical Journal*, B.H. Kuhn, M.D. discussed taking 25,000 IU of vitamin A palmitate (a water-dispersible form) orally each day for a week to six months for treating 79 patients with different types of warts.

Dr. Kuhn achieved a cure rate of 50 to 100 percent with no total failures. In another study (*Clinical Medicine*, July 1959) 119 medical doctors used a similar vitamin A palmitate regimen in treating 228 patients with plantar warts – warts growing on the soles of the feet. In 208 of 228 cases, patients received substantial benefit or total cure.

Daniel Hyman, M.D., of Roosevelt Hospital in New York City, stated that just three desiccated liver tablets three times a day successfully treated warts in hospitalized patients.[2]

Hyman believes that sulfur-containing amino acids in the liver tablets somehow interacted with the hypothalamus gland, responsible for stimulating antibodies, front-line soldiers in the immune system army. Further, this food supplement is rich in B complex vitamins.

This effect can be obtained from sulfur/amino acid foods such as asparagus, citrus fruits, eggs, garlic and onions.[3]

Remedies from the Kitchen

Clinical remedies are just fine, but when it comes to convenience, nothing beats your kitchen and backyard. Gardeners and moms have long known about the inner side of a banana skin, dandelion milk, and castor oil and garlic for warts.

The banana skin routine worked well on one of the very few warts I have ever had.

Here's how I treated my wart. First I washed my hands thoroughly, then applied the inside skin from a freshly peeled banana to the wart, securing it with adhesive tape. I followed this routine daily, until the wart gave up and disappeared, never to return – thank heavens!

The use of dandelion milk is popular among the sheepherders of Australia. They simply break a dandelion stem in half and drip the milky white sap on the wart. Applications of sap should be repeated over several days. In a week or two the wart should turn dark and fall off. On a visit to India, I learned about castor oil and garlic. Castor oil contains a large amount of vitamin A, and raw garlic irritates the skin just enough to weaken the offending virus so the immune system can kill it. Since raw garlic can severely irritate the skin, smooth some petroleum jelly around the wart to protect the surrounding skin. Some people have "burned" their warts off using a crushed garlic clove applied to the wart with a bandage for 24 hours. Blisters will form and the wart falls off in about a week.

Another not-so folk medicine cure is Elmer's glue applied directly to warts. After the glue has dried, scrape it off and reapply until the wart is gone. My theory for this is that without oxygen the wart cannot grow and dries up. One friend told me about a co-worker who lost her wart after wearing a rubber finger grip.

Overwhelming Warts with Nutrition
For maximum absorption, take supplements with meals.

Nutrient	Suggested Dosage	Formulation
Acidophilus	At least four billion flora on an empty stomach, three times daily	
Aged garlic extract	1 teaspoon three times daily	Liquid
Borage oil	2 capsules daily	
Enzymes	2 capsules twice daily	Multiple formula
Fiber	4-8 tablets daily	Psyllium, with herb hyssop
Flaxseed oil	1 tablespoon daily	
Multi-mineral	3-4 ounces daily	In liquid solution, with vitamin B12, biotin
Multi-vitamin/mineral	6 caplets daily	Freeze-dried plant sources
Vitamin A	25,000 IU daily*	
Vitamin C	Individual bowel tolerance**	With bioflavonoids (quercetin, rutin proanthocyanidins)
Vitamin E	2 capsules (800 IU) daily	d-alpha tocopherol

* The FDA recommends pregnant women not exceed 10,000 IU of vitamin A daily.

** To determine individual dosage, on the first day take 1,000 mg hourly until diarrhea occurs, then reduce dosage to just below that for individual daily dosage. Vitamin C is not toxic in large doses but must be taken throughout the day to benefit. Divide dosage to three or four times a day.

CHAPTER 161:

Water Retention

Mark Twain said, "Water, taken in moderation, cannot hurt anybody." But water retention can cause high blood pressure, kidney problems and nutritional deficiencies if diuretics have to be taken.

Before I caught on to the spirit of healthful eating, I had problems every month with water retention. The only solution it seemed, was to join Sea World as its main attraction.

Water retention, edema or swelling, can be caused by circulation blockages, hormonal fluctuations, allergic reaction, adrenal exhaustion, kidney dysfunction, nutritional deficiencies, and even sugar!

Knowing the influence of salt on high blood pressure, researchers at Georgetown University Medical Center in Washington, D.C, theorized that sugar could have the same effect. The researchers put spontaneously hypertensive rats on either high or low sucrose (sugar) diets to see whether their kidneys would respond by retaining water and salt. The group of rats receiving a high sugar diet for at least two weeks showed significantly decreased urinary and sodium (salt) output, coinciding with an increase in blood pressure. After a month off the high sugar diet, the rats stopped retaining water and salt but still had high blood pressure.

The researchers were able to duplicate this result in a second study. They concluded in an article in the *Journal of the American College of Nutrition* that a high sugar diet causes salt and water retention, and eventually edema (tissues swollen with fluid).[1] Other doctors and researchers believe that a diet high in processed and refined foods, most especially white flour, can have the same effect, as it counters the natural digestive processes that helps balance our bodily fluids, as well as influencing our nutritional health.

Water retention may be normal, as long as it is temporary. Swelling, or edema, is the body's way of protecting or defending itself. Studies show wounds heal better in moist (bacteria-free) environments. A blister is our body's way of protecting the underlying burned or irritated skin so it may heal. In the case of allergies, the tissues retain water in order to expel perceived toxins from the body, causing puffiness, bloating and the appearance of being fat. When a source of swelling is not obvious, it can be a symptom of serious deficiencies or organ breakdown.

The Need for Minerals to Regulate Bodily Fluids

It is commonly known that too much salt, or sodium, will cause water retention. Why? Because salt is an electrolyte mineral. Electrolytes are minerals contained in the fluid of our bodies that allow nerve impulses to travel from the brain to all parts of the body. The electrolytes are sodium, chloride, calcium, potassium and magnesium. Sodium, combined with chloride is important for muscle contraction as well as balancing the fluid levels inside and outside the cells. The balance of all these nutrients must be maintained in order to avoid retaining water and salt.

It is for this reason that adequate amounts of these minerals must be ingested, whether through diet or supplementation, in order to avoid water retention. Not coincidentally, they all work together to maintain healthy bones, muscles, tendons and ligaments, and must be taken together. The best way is through a minerals in solution formula, which provides the optimum balance and absorption ratios.

Ease Swelling with Vitamins

One hundred milligrams of vitamin B6, three times daily, may reduce the edema from carpal tunnel syndrome.[2] An article in *Total*

Health reports that B6 may be used to control the swelling associated with menopause.[3]

One of the reasons women experience monthly bloating during their menstrual cycles is that estrogen retains bodily fluids to prepare for possible childbirth. In a case report, a woman suffering from edema after a pregnancy started supplementing with 25 mg of B6 daily. By the next day she noticed marked improvement in her swollen ankles, and found she had lost 10 pounds of water weight by the following week. She continued taking B6 in a B complex formula and did not have the problem again.[4]

In order to pinpoint what helps with edema, you have to understand the process by which it occurs. Why does a twisted or tired ankle swell? Why do the eyes become puffy with exhaustion? Free radicals are the molecular enemies of the tissues. Irritation, a sunburn, an internal battle, all create free radicals that damage delicate tissues. That's why it is not surprising that any type of injury or illness can be helped by taking antioxidants. Antioxidants increase the body's ability to fight back, and quenches free radical formation and damage.

Doctors at the Vascular Surgery Unit, Queens University of Belfast, Royal Victoria Hospital in Belfast, Northern Ireland, studied the benefit of vitamin E on leg swelling following surgery. They found that of 20 patients who had undergone lower leg surgery, 15 experienced a 10 percent decrease in swelling following supplementation of vitamin E. The researchers concluded that free radicals cause postoperative leg swelling, and that vitamin E may help reduce the effect.[5]

Vitamin C and bioflavonoids are proven to help battle infection. When the body is given the warriors it needs to heal itself, it's less likely to create water retention, swelling and inflammation. The *New York Journal of Dentistry* reported on a study which found that when the subjects took vitamin C the inflammation of their gums from concentrations of bacteria improved by 58 percent.[6]

In one study, University of Witwatersrand, South Africa, medical students were given one gram a day of ascorbic acid (vitamin C) and monitored for blood immunologic levels. Unlike the control group who did not get the vitamin C, the ones who did experienced a marked increase in their defense antibodies, IgA and IgM. Vitamin C is renowned for alleviating the symptoms of colds and flu, and studies have shown it to be of benefit for tuberculosis, herpes, tetanus and diphtheria. Any type of infection can be helped with vitamin C.[7]

Bioflavonoids and vitamin C together act as a potent anti-inflammatory. They reduce swelling while they act on the immune system, and they enhance the immune system's healing properties. If you're facing any kind of dental work or surgery, take at least 500 milligrams of vitamin C and bioflavonoids to help reduce the post-surgical swelling and pain that accompanies it. Follow up surgery with another 500 milligrams.

Beneficial Botanicals

I have personally discovered foods that help eliminate accumulated water in the body. Two of my neighbors came by to show me their swollen ankles. It was near lunchtime so I asked them to stay for asparagus soup. They enjoyed the dish, asking for the recipe. After they departed my company, they got together and made a big batch and ate it for the next several days. To their delight, their edema went away. Now everybody in the neighborhood wants to live next door to me! Other water-draining foods are cucumber and dill, and sea vegetables like kelp, dulse, hiziki and bladderwrack, common in Japanese dishes. Vegetables that grow in the sea pick up all the trace and electrolyte minerals, most especially calcium and magnesium, which help draw excess fluid out of the tissues.

Pineapple contains something better for water retention than vitamin C: bromelain. Bromelain is a digestive enzyme that is found in studies to have potent anti-inflammatory, anti-edema and coagulation-inhibiting effects.[8] This means it will help reduce the swelling and inflammation of injuries, as well as increase circulation, and reduce blockages that can contribute to water retention. It also helps digest and assimilate nutrients.

One particular bioflavonoid, quercetin, is noted for its ability to reduce the prostaglandins that cause inflammation. Studies have shown that when it is combined with bromelain, it effectively inhibits the formation of leukotrienes, which are the bio-chemicals produced by the immune system that causes water retention.[9]

One last thing: drink plenty of purified water. If you have an imbalance of nutrients and/or too much sodium, water will flush the excess salt and allow your body the chance to recover. Never stop drinking water because you have edema! Remember, it's not the water that is the problem, it's the dysfunction that causes the water to be retained. If the edema is a result of toxins or allergies, drinking water can only help. If you are in the habit of drinking sodas for moisture – stop! Soft drinks will deplete your body of potassium, causing an imbalance of electrolytes and inviting edema.

Also, get some exercise. Water is meant to be circulated through-out the body. Sitting or lying down for long periods of time can actu-ally cause edema, as noted by many nursing home residents. Take a walk, do some gardening, stretch and move. And to my neighbors who feel they live too far away for lunchtime visits: the walk will do you good.

Edema-Ending Nutrients
For maximum absorption, take supplements with meals.

Nutrient	Suggested Dosage	Formulation
Aged garlic extract	1 teaspoon three times daily	Liquid
Antioxidants	4 capsules daily*	With selenium and grapeseed extract
Borage oil	2 capsules daily	
Enzymes	2 capsules twice daily	Multiple formula
Fiber	4-8 tablets daily	Psyllium, with herb hyssop
Bromelain		
Flaxseed oil	1 tablespoon daily	
Magnesium	200 mg daily	
Multi-mineral	3-4 ounces daily	In liquid solution, with vitamin B12, biotin
Multi-vitamin/mineral	6 caplets daily	Freeze-dried plant sources
Quercetin	400 mg twice daily	With vitamin C and bioflavonoids
Vitamin A	25,000 IU daily*	
Vitamin B6	100 mg daily	
Vitamin C	Individual bowel tolerance**	With bioflavonoids (quercetin, rutin proanthocyanidins)
Vitamin E	2 capsules (800 IU) daily	d-alpha tocopherol

* The FDA recommends pregnant women not exceed 10,000 IU of vitamin A daily.

** To determine individual dosage, on the first day take 1,000 mg hourly until diarrhea occurs, then reduce dosage to just below that for individual daily dosage. Vitamin C is not toxic in large doses but must be taken throughout the day to benefit. Divide dosage to three or four times a day.

CHAPTER 162:

Weight Loss

"No diet will remove all the fat from your body be-cause the brain is entirely fat. Without a brain you might look good, but all you could do is run for public office."

–Covert Bailey

After an exhaustive multi-million dollar health study, the government concluded that people would live longer if they didn't die sooner.

The key to a long and healthy life is diet, no doubt about it. How you eat influences your health, as well as your figure. I'm not going to espouse this diet or that diet, or show you how you can fit into the dress or suit you wore at your senior prom, or explain how to lose those pounds and keep them off. The hundreds of diet books and articles can do that. Besides, I can't possibly anticipate all the individual tastes, habits and lifestyles of those reading this book. What I *will* do is blast those myths that say the more years you put on, the more pounds you put on; and show you how a combination of good eating (as much as you want), nutritional supplementation, and easy exercise will keep you tone, trim and most importantly, healthy. No matter how skinny you are, if you aren't healthy, you won't look good. My goal here is to give you the tools and information so you can be proud of who you are and what you see in the mirror every day.

Weight loss really is a misnomer. Your goal is not to lose weight, but to gain muscle and lose fat. To this end, I direct this chapter.

Fight Fat with Fat

Whether they are the "love handles" diplomatically described by the husbands of overweight wives or the "beer bellies" on barflies, the amount of fat on the body can be traced to the amount of fat engorging the liver and encircling the heart, threatening to choke them off. Fat is not good, and getting rid of it is a goal for a longer and healthier life.

First let's begin with a lesson on fat. The best way to beat an adversary is to understand its weaknesses and its strengths.

There are good fats and bad fats. The good fats remove excess glucose, cholesterol and triglycerides from the bloodstream until needed. They go by a variety of names and can be confusing. You hear a lot about PUFAs, or polyunsaturated fatty acids. PUFAs are a generic term for all the essential fatty acids (EFAs). They say "essential" because they cannot be made by the body and must be eaten in the diet. They are required for growth, development and maintenance of cell membranes, including those of the central nervous system. A deficiency of EFAs has been linked to heart disease, skin problems, mental problems and even multiple sclerosis. In a nutshell, they are oils. The best food sources of EFAs are the oils from nuts and seeds. In any diet, care should be taken to include recipes rich in olive oil, flaxseed oil, walnut oil and wheat germ oil, among others.

EFAs are important in fat metabolism. Without them, fat could not be converted into glucose. Without them, the body stores the fat it should be converting to glucose. Without glucose, you become diabetic. In an article in the *Journal of Nutritional Medicine*, Bernard Horn, M.D., of Benicia, California, stresses the importance of gamma linolenic acid (GLA) for fat assimilation and to boost the immune system. Studies have shown that aggressive GLA supplementation in genetically obese people will result in gradual but substantial weight loss for about half of the test subjects – without dieting! The best source of gamma linolenic acid is borage oil, which can be purchased in capsule form in health food stores.

What *Not* to Eat

Now that you know what is good for you, pay attention to what is bad for you. Margarine is NOT heart smart. You already know saturated fat is bad for you. Saturated fat, like butter, may increase bad cholesterol, but at least it doesn't touch the good cholesterol. The connection between cholesterol and weight gain is the fact that when fats are stored, so is cholesterol. You don't have to have high cholesterol to be overweight or unhealthy, but if you do, you probably are. If you are determined to lose weight and be healthier, avoid margarine and anything else that uses hydrogenated oils.

The Blood Sugar Connection

Did you know that 90 percent of people with type 2 diabetes are obese? Type 2 diabetes occurs when something keeps glucose from entering body cells. The same things found to help Type 2 diabetics also help lose weight and restore health.

Whole civilizations previously exempt from diabetes, once introduced to affluence and its accompanying Western diet high in saturated and transfatty fats and sugar, have found themselves in an epidemic of diabetes and obesity. In the American Southwest, Native American tribes the Pima and the Tohono O'odham, suffer from one of the highest rates of Type 2 diabetes in the world, with one out of every two adults beyond age 35 afflicted. Fortunately, enlightenment has also found its way there, as more and more of them are throwing off diabetes and weight by discarding processed, fast and convenience foods, and the more sedentary ways of the modern world and returning to some of their ancestral foods. Nuts, beans and berries are nutritious foods that are once again appearing among Native Americans of the

Southwest, restoring them to health and blood sugar fitness.

What is it about our modern-day diet that contributes to obesity and diabetes? Fat, sugar and inactivity. Poor circulation from a lack of exercise causes a lack of oxygen to the cells and allows a poor diet to affect the health. Our modern diet is full of unhealthy transfatty and saturated fats. Fat in the bloodstream blocks the effectiveness of insulin, making the body believe it needs to convert more muscle to fat. How much of our problems with weight are a direct result of insulin problems? Probably a lot. One clue to the connection is the mineral chromium.

Chromium for Blood Sugar Balance *and* Fat Loss

There is a reason why so many people today are feeling tired and putting on excess weight. It's the same reason that too many people develop heart disease or diabetes: most people are deficient in the essential trace mineral chromium. A chromium deficiency causes fatigue, excess fat production, and is a major contributor to heart disease and diabetes.

Chromium is a mineral used to treat low blood sugar. As a cofactor to insulin, chromium is central to the body's utilization of blood sugar, and has been shown in studies to eliminate or reduce the insulin requirements of diabetics. According to Gary Null, Ph.D., in some experiments with chromium therapy, it has taken only a few months for formerly diabetic adults to get their metabolism to function properly again.

The mineral is vitally important to your health, yet dangerously rare in modern diets. Chromium is more likely to be in short supply than any other nutrient, perhaps the missing link in the incredible epidemic of obese and overweight Americans. I say this because studies show when it is supplemented, the pounds roll off.

At his San Antonio, Texas clinic, Gilbert Kaats, M.D., found that test subjects getting chromium averaged a loss of 4.2 pounds of fat and a gain of 1.4 pounds of muscle. Intakes ranged from 200 to 400 mcg/day of chromium.

Dr. Gary Evans, professor of chemistry at Bemidji State University, Bemidji, Minnesota, is a member of the American Institute of Nutrition and the American Physiological Society. He reported in the *International Journal of Biosocial and Medical Research* that young athletes given chromium lost 22 percent of body fat during the six-week study, contrasted with only six percent fat loss in the control group.

Chromium may promote weight loss because high blood levels of insulin, which occur as a consequence of tissues' resistance to insulin, promote excessive deposition of fat. Chromium reduces insulin resistance, which in turn decreases the storage of body fat and increases its metabolism. He added that since chromium helps stabilize blood sugar levels, it also may reduce the feeling of hunger. Chromium may decrease the appetite also because chromium and insulin stimulate serotonin, a brain chemical important to feelings of well-being and satisfaction. A deficiency of serotonin is linked to depression.

In Iraq, barley bread is commonly used in the treatment of diabetes because of two traits: its high amount of chromium, and the fact that it is a complex carbohydrate. Barley contains almost six micrograms of chromium per gram of grain.

Many of us are deficient in chromium. Signs of a deficiency include fatigue, nervousness, memory loss, infertility, cold hands and feet, non-insulin dependent diabetes (type 2), heart disease and high cholesterol. For weight loss Evans recommends 200 micrograms three times daily and for blood sugar patients, 200-1,000 micrograms daily. Since chromium can be difficult to absorb, eat whole foods for their enzymes, which help assimilate chromium. Look for digestive enzyme formulas that include lipase, which regulates fat metabolism.

Vitamin C has been shown in studies to help chromium become absorbed into the body. Dr. E.G. Offenbacher and fellow researchers at the Department of Medicine, St. Luke's-Roosevelt Hospital Center in New York, found that among women who took 100 milligrams of vitamin C in the form of ascorbic acid after taking a test dose of one milligram of chromium increased their ability to absorb it by over 100 percent.

By far the best way to take your chromium and absorb it too, is to take it in solution. Studies show minerals dissolved in water before ingestion are considerably more bioavailable to the body than those even present in food, because they aren't risked by a lack of hydrochloric acid in the stomach or food allergies. It is very important, when targeting any one mineral, to include a formula that has all the trace minerals. Taking only one mineral over a prolonged period of time will cause a deficiency because the body seeks the others for balance. Look around at the way God orders nature. Never does He supply one mineral without the others. Any one food contains more than one mineral. For your balance, Look for a good, easily absorbable, derived-from-nature mineral blend in solution.

Appetite-Controlling Carbohydrates

While on tour signing my new book *Nutrition: The Cancer Answer II*, I was approached by a young woman in her 30s. She told me she was buying my book for her grandfather who had cancer but was too weak to undergo conventional therapies. We started talking about a healthy diet and she brought up an issue of interest here. She said unless she eats fat, she feels hungry. If she eats a bowl of steamed vegetables they have to be topped with melted cheese. If she eats a salad, it has to be topped with blue cheese or ranch dressing or it leaves her hungry. "Yes," I agreed, "There's not much incentive to eating right when it leaves you with hunger pangs." However, I made her a promise. I told her if she includes brown rice or whole wheat bread (sans margarine of course), or beans or lentils with her meal, she won't be hungry. Many salad bars include garbanzo and kidney beans, and a good 12-grain bread with a meal is easy enough. She did and wrote me back to say it worked.

Have you guessed the secret yet? I've already talked about it, so it shouldn't be a surprise. It's complex carbohydrates. And now there's a scientific reason why eating complex carbohydrates appeases the appetite.

I've already mentioned their ability to maintain stable blood sugar levels, which keeps us from getting hungry, but Dr. Sarah Leibowitz, a neurobiologist at Rockefeller University in New York City, has found another reason. She has discovered two peptides in the brain that regulate our appetites for carbohydrates and fats. When she injected one of them – something called neuropeptide Y – into the brains of rats, the animals ate more refined carbohydrates (sugar). When she injected the other, an amino acid called galanin, the appetite for fat increased. When repeatedly administered over several days, the rats ate too much and became fat. She believes that those of us who particularly enjoy fats and sweets, probably have too much of these peptides.

Leibowitz looked at exactly when these surges of appetite-increasing peptides occurred: upon awakening in the morning and at lunchtime. Leibowitz found that among animals and humans, neuropeptide Y is very high in the morning. This is normal. What isn't normal is for the level to remain high throughout the day. Galanin levels were abnormally high later in the day, either during or after lunch. Do you crave sweets in the morning and fats for lunch? I have a solution.

Complex carbohydrates cure the craving for sweets and essential fatty acids for fats. Try it! Make a habit out of eating things like pasta, oatmeal, lentils and beans for breakfast. For lunch, have a salad with vinegar and oil and maybe some whole grain bread drizzled with olive oil. Add a borage oil supplement at lunch. You'll be amazed at how hungry you *aren't*, and how energetic you *are*.

Make sure whatever food you eat, it is whole, raw and contains its natural fiber. Fiber is not only important to a healthy body, but slows digestion and absorption for a balanced blood sugar metabolism.

Nuts that have been roasted have had the EFAs baked right out of them. Pears that have been denatured and softened in cans do not contain the same amounts of fiber. Instead of "wheat" bread that has been milled into nothingness, choose bread with the wheat "berry" included. Wheat berries are a marketing term for the whole grain. Instead of canned beans, cook them from dried beans and add your own natural ingredients. Some canned beans include hydrogenated oils to make them thicker. Have you ever had a refried bean sandwich? Mash your own black beans and add fresh salsa for a whole wheat pita bean sandwich for lunch.

In any program of good health, I always recommend vitamin and mineral supplements. We need a plethora of vitamins and minerals for health, and I'm sorry to report even our fresh foods are lacking in them.

Eating whole foods is the best, eating sprouts even better. Look for supplementation that uses the whole food. One such formula uses freeze dried sprouts and vegetables, combined in such a way as to provide all the essential vitamins and minerals, as well as adding odorless garlic, acidophilus and green tea extract for immune-system boosting.

Remember to include protein to build muscle. The kind of protein found in vegetables is the best way to ensure adequate amounts. Vegetable protein contains many other vital nutrients, including fat-reducing enzymes, nitrogen and amino acids. If you think meat and dairy products are the best sources of protein, think again. The fatty risks are unnecessary. A U.S. Department of Agriculture survey found that American vegetarians consume, on the average, 150 percent of their actual protein requirements.

The argument made by the egg and meat people in favor of their products has been that vegetables have incomplete protein – that is, there isn't one kind that contains all the essential amino acids. Well, who says protein has to come from one source? The fact of the matter is, all foods contain some amount of protein. In order to get *complete* protein in one meal, you simply have to combine them properly.

To reach your daily allowance of complete protein combine whole grains with legumes. For example, the Greek dish *felafel* combines whole wheat pita bread with garbanzo beans. It happens to be a healthy, fast, finger food, not to mention a delicious meal. Latin Americans get their protein by combining corn tortillas with beans. In India it's rice or wheat chapatis with lentils. Since cooking can destroy many essential amino acids, try to avoid processed foods and eat your veggies raw.

Other protein plant food combinations are nuts and seeds with legumes, and nuts and seeds with dark green leafy vegetables. Consider a green salad with kidney beans and sunflower seeds. There you have it: a good source of protein and lots of other essential nutrients! Beats a steak any day.

Chew on crushed ice instead of snacks. Oklahoma City physician Charlie Farr says that when you lower your temperature by eating ice, your body raises its metabolism (the rate at which your body bums calories). By drinking eight 16-ounce glasses (one gallon) of purified, unchemicalized ice water a day, you can burn up to 300 calories. Water naturally suppresses the appetite and may be the most important catalyst to increase fat burning. Drinking plenty of water flushes toxins that overloads the kidneys and keeps the liver from metabolizing fat.

One source of weight gain is swelling from allergies, and food and chemical sensitivities. The medical term for this condition is edema. What happens is the tissues retain water in order to expel the toxins from the body, causing puffiness, bloating and the appearance of being fat. See the Allergies chapter for more. In the meantime, drink plenty of water to help flush sodium, which in excess can add water weight, and to replenish lost fluids.

Eating Less Calories, Not Less Food

A very dear friend of mine had been trying to lose weight for years. Initially she struggled to get from 160 pounds to 115. After a while, her weight returned to 160. Over the years she tried one diet after another. Her weight went up and down more times than the elevator in the Empire State Building. Every time she started a new diet she gained more than she lost. By the time she came to me promising to drop the diets and change her lifestyle, she had ballooned to 250 pounds. It told her what I've been telling you, convinced her to join a health club for an exercise program, and she has maintained a healthy 110 pounds since.

There are several reasons why dieting doesn't work and should be avoided. It largely stems from our natural history.

Whenever the body is deprived of food, whether from famine or dieting, it ensures survival by lowering the rate at which it burns calories. The less you eat, the less you burn. Energy is stored so efficiently (as body fat) that someone of normal weight can survive for two months without eating anything. Remember the Pima Indians? The famine and feast lifestyle of their ancestors included going weeks at a time without eating, as they searched for food. When they found it, they gorged themselves. Their bodies adapted to their lifestyle by slowing down to conserve as much energy as possible for as long as possible. No matter how much they binged when they finally found food, going weeks without it burned it off.

Now that the Pimas don't have that lifestyle and former eating habits, many are obese and diabetic. Since they have adopted the modern, "civilized" high-fat diet, their slow metabolisms store most of the calories as body fat. When you fast for long periods or diet, your body is fooled into believing you've adopted the ancestral Pima lifestyle and it burns less fat. When you eat again, you gain more than you had when you started. An example is Sumo wrestlers who fast and then gorge themselves with food to gain fat.

So, how do you eat less without lowering your fat-burning ability? By eating less food gradually, so your system adapts, making sure what you eat is high in nutrients, complex carbohydrates and low in fat, and by grazing – eating small meals every two to three hours. "Grazing" will virtually prevent carbohydrates and proteins from being converted into fat, according to Susan Smith Jones, Ph.D. (health sciences), a fitness instructor at UCLA. Eating small meals will keep the metabolism "stoked." The typical dieter skips meals, especially breakfast. This is the worst meal to skip since it equates to a fast, sending the wrong message to the body. Don't skip meals – especially breakfast – just make the meals small.

Exercise Burns Fat

"Food fuels the furnace of metabolism; exercise stokes its fire."

– Majid Ali, M.D.

You've heard the term "feel the burn?" Exercise instructors use it to describe the burning sensation of strenuous exercise. If your idea of vigorous exercise is eating faster, join the Rockettes. You don't have to bounce and bobble your way to a good figure, you can feel the burn simply by lifting your leg repeatedly. This simple exercise will burn fat by building muscle.

Fat-burning exercise only requires slow, sustained activity. Forty-five to 60 minutes of vigorous walking is recommended, every day if possible.

Intense exercise may actually decrease metabolism in the long run because it burns muscle tissue. Dr. John Duncan conducted a study comparing walking speeds with weight loss. He took 102 couch potato women and divided them into three groups. Each group walked three miles, five days a week. The first group walked five miles per hour (mph), the second group four mph, and the third group 3 mph. What did Dr. Duncan find? He found that the group who walked the slowest lost the most weight!

Try something. Hold your arm out, palm upward. Now lift it up. Do it twice. No problem, right? Now, do it twenty times. Feel the burn? Now do it while holding a can of soup. You just increased the burn by including something heavy. This is called weight- or resistance-training exercise. You can burn the fat while watching TV. Lift your legs twenty times. Then add ankle weights. Now you're doing weight-training. This kind of exercise not only burns fat but increases muscle. If you keep adding weight, you'll keep adding muscle (more so for men, but women can do it too). As you gradually add weight, you add strength. If you keep it up, you can compete with body-builders. And it doesn't matter how old you are – if you're 95 you can do it!

Have you seen those photos of muscle-bound women who didn't stop until every last morsel of fat was converted to muscle? Even their breasts have been converted! I kid you not! There's nothing left! This is an extreme I don't agree with. But you can see for yourself how this works, and to a much lesser degree make it work for you. As you walk to exercise your legs and lower body, carry weights and swing your arms to burn off the fat in your arms and upper body. Orchestra conductors have notoriously strong arms and cardiovascular health because of the repetitive motion their profession requires. Swimming is good for burning fat because of the resistance of the water. If you're up to it, take a class in water polo. Most classes begin with water exercises to increase stamina before getting out there to sprint and tread water for 30 minutes at a time. For the less ambitious, water aerobics offers resistance with less work.

Once you've exchanged muscle for fat, you will find you burn calories quicker. This is important. Pound for pound, muscle burns five times as many calories as most other body tissues. The addition of ten pounds of muscle to the body can burn 600 calories more a day. You would have to run six miles a day, seven days a week to burn the same number of calories. Phew! No thanks! I'll take my weight-training regimen, thank you.

The best time to exercise is before a meal simply because exercise suppresses appetite and increases the body's ability to burn off the calories consumed.

Pound-Peeling Nutrients
For maximum absorption, take supplements with meals.

Nutrient	Suggested Dosage	Formulation
Amino acids	4-6 capsules daily	Multiple formula from natural sources
Antioxidants	4 capsules daily*	With selenium and grapeseed extract
Borage oil	2 capsules daily	
Enzymes	2 capsules twice daily	Multiple formula
Fiber	4-8 tablets daily	Psyllium, with herb hyssop
Flaxseed oil	1 tablespoon daily	
Folic acid	5-10 mg daily	
L-glutamine	500 mg twice daily	
Magnesium	200 mg daily	
Multi-mineral	3-4 ounces daily	In liquid solution, with vitamin B12, biotin
Multi-vitamin/mineral	6 caplets daily	Freeze-dried plant sources
Niacin	500 mg four times daily	
Taurine	500 mg twice daily	
Vitamin B6	100 mg daily	
Vitamin C	Individual bowel tolerance**	With bioflavonoids (quercetin, rutin proanthocyanidins)
Vitamin E	2 capsules (800 IU) daily	d-alpha tocopherol

* The FDA recommends pregnant women not exceed 10,000 IU of vitamin A daily.

** To determine individual dosage, on the first day take 1,000 mg hourly until diarrhea occurs, then reduce dosage to just below that for individual daily dosage. Vitamin C is not toxic in large doses but must be taken throughout the day to benefit. Divide dosage to three or four times a day.

CHAPTER 163:

Whooping Cough

Since the time of Louis Pasteur – the pioneering French microbiologist of the 19th century – medicine has made great progress in conquering bacterial diseases.

But against whooping cough, a grave, life-threatening infectious disease, the conquest is far from complete. In May 1982, Dr. William H. Foege, then director of the federal Centers for Disease Control in Atlanta, told a U.S. Senate subcommittee: "Despite the decline in the total number of cases reported per year since the 1940s, pertussis (the medical name for whooping cough) remains a serious problem in the United States."[1]

Before widespread vaccinations came into use in the late 1940s, pertussis infected a quarter of a million children every year in this country and killed 7,000 of them – approximately the number of people killed this year by AIDS. The typical sound of pertussis could be heard in pediatric wards across the country: A small child begins coughing, continues for a spell (in what is known as a "paroxysm"), then half coughs and half inhales to make the characteristic whoop.[2]

Usually lasting from four to six weeks, the coughing stage may drag on for as many as ten weeks. Besides the "whooping" cough, this stage can include vomiting, high fever, choking and gasping for air, and, sometimes – when the brain is sufficiently deprived of oxygen – convulsions. The whooping sound is part of the desperate effort to restore air to lungs depleted by coughing. Even when convalescence finally begins, the coughing may return repeatedly, causing relapses that can make recuperation stretch out over many months.

As the disease progresses, the superficial linings of the air passages are damaged and begin to separate from the smaller airways. In coughing, the airways act reflexively to expel this loose material, much as they would to get rid of mucus. Sometimes so much of the lining becomes detached and there is such a buildup of mucus and inflammatory cells that the airways are blocked off and the patient chokes.[3]

We Can't Depend on Vaccines

As of 1982, the number of cases in the U.S. was only 1,895, and there were only four deaths. But then the disease began a comeback. A 1983 outbreak in Oklahoma affected 351 people. In 1984, 149 residents in a Wisconsin home for the developmentally disabled had the illness. In 1988, the number of cases was 2,925. This upswing has come at a time when rates of immunization are as high as they have ever been. Why? One clue comes from the age of the victims: adults and very young infants. The risk that someone over age 20 will develop pertussis has risen 13-fold since 1981.[4]

Ironically, the very success of childhood vaccination against pertussis incited the problem of pertussis in adults. In a recent editorial, Dr. L.A. Herwaldt points out that in the days before there was a pertussis vaccine, just about every adult was exposed to pertussis as a child, and as a result, developed an immunity which persisted throughout their lives. Once the vaccine became almost universal, children were protected from getting pertussis because the vaccine produced immunity to the illness. Unfortunately, the immunity produced by the vaccine doesn't last as long as that produced by having the real illness, and it has been estimated that about 50 million adults in the U.S. are now susceptible to pertussis. In fact, the major source of pertussis is no longer among children, but rather among adults![5]

Researchers report that one in five adults who sought relief for a nagging cough at a Nashville emergency room showed signs of whooping cough.

The Centers for Disease Control and Prevention reported that whooping cough jumped from a low of about 1,000 in 1976 to 6,000 in 1992-

1993, with adults and adolescents forming a growing proportion of cases – about 27 percent in 1993.[6]

The reason seems to be that not only is the vaccination's effectiveness wearing off, but it is only effective in 60-85 percent of people who receive it. There are now enough people who have outlived their immunity (or who were never immunized and never had whooping cough) to support a massive chain of infection. Currently, there is no way to forestall an epidemic because vaccinating people over the age of seven is associated with an unacceptably high rate of severe complications – most frightening is the chance of permanent brain and nerve damage.[7]

Unfortunately, vaccines do not help infants. Those at highest risk of death are between three and six months of age. They are losing the protection of maternal antibodies but have yet to receive a full course of immunization, which begins at one or two months of age and continues with boosters for the next six years. Infants are dependent on "herd" immunity – developing immunity from others around them – for protection. Treatment with antibiotics is not particularly helpful with whooping cough, unless it is given at a very early stage. But pertussis begins very much like a common cold, so early diagnosis is unlikely. Very young infants and adults, the two groups currently most vulnerable to the disease, usually don't develop a whoop, so the risk of misdiagnosis is even higher in them. Laboratory methods provide little additional help for early diagnosis.

Vitamin C Kills Bacteria Better Than Antibiotics

In an amazing discovery, vitamin C has been found to be helpful in the continuing battle against bacteria that have become immune to antibiotics. For more on this incredible story, see the Infections chapter.

Studies have shown that the bacterium that causes whopping cough – bordetella pertussis – is susceptible to infection-blasting vitamin C.[10]

A control group study reported in the *Journal of the American Medical Association* found that when 90 children with whooping cough were given vitamin C orally or were injected with five grams daily for seven days, the duration of the disease was lessened. The average duration for patients given the pertussis vaccine was 43 days. Compare this with the 15 to 20 days children getting the vitamin C only had to endure. Not only that, but the vitamin C prevented the awful spasmodic coughing stage in an amazing 75 percent of the patients. In this particular study, the patients' vitamin C levels were tapered in those seven days down to 100 mg a day, less than a maintenance dosage, according to many physicians. It is possible that keeping high levels of vitamin C in the system might just improve these results.[11]

Massive doses of vitamin C has been used to successfully treat viral pneumonia, mononucleosis, influenza, colds, hepatitis, shingles, and cold sores. The individual's own body will determine how much vitamin C it requires, with the cutoff point determined by the onset of diarrhea. In short, if you have not reached bowel tolerance (diarrhea), you have not taken enough vitamin C.

Some European studies have found that bioflavonoids slow bacterial infections.[12] Bioflavonoids – botanical chemicals found in colorful fruit – work with vitamin C to help reduce the damage of bacteria, and are recommended in any infection protocol. In the *American Journal of Digestive Diseases*, Morton S. Biskind and W.C. Martin reported that 20 of 22 patients with respiratory infections of varying intensity recovered in an 8- to 48-hour period after treatment with bioflavonoids and vitamin C. The patients received 600 mg of each of the two substances every day.

For more on battling bacterial infections see my chapters Infections and Colds and Flu.

Pertussis-Pounding Nutrients for Children
For maximum absorption, take supplements with meals.

Nutrient	Suggested Dosage	Formulation
Aged garlic extract	1 teaspoon twice daily	Liquid
Antioxidants	1 capsule daily	With selenium and grapeseed extract
Echinacea	250 mg daily for a maximum of three weeks	
Magnesium	100 mg daily	
Multi-mineral	1/2-1 ounce	In liquid solution, with vitamin B12, biotin
Multi-vitamin/mineral	1-2 tablets	Children's chewable
Vitamin A	15,000 IU daily	
Vitamin B6	50 mg daily	
Vitamin C	Individual bowel tolerance*	Chewable with bioflavonoids (quercetin, proanthocyanidins)

* To determine individual dosage, on the first day take 1,000 mg hourly until diarrhea occurs, then reduce dosage to just below that for individual daily dosage. Vitamin C is not toxic in large doses but must be taken throughout the day to benefit. Divide dosage to three or four times a day.

CHAPTER 164:

Wrinkles

"If God had to give a woman wrinkles, He might have at least put them on the soles of her feet."
                                    –Ninon de Lenclos (1620-1705)

"A beautiful lady is an accident of nature. A beautiful old lady is a work of art."   –Louis Nizer

If your face and body resemble the San Andreas fault line with its cracks and fissures, don't despair! Wrinkles can be reversed! If you have dry skin, and you're convinced this fact of your nature puckers your pelt, think again. To elude and eradicate your wrinkles you have to let me get under your skin – where the problem really lies.

They say time will tell all. In the case of our faces, time may tell exactly how old we are or even imply we're older than we really are! But good nutrition and protection from the ravages of the elements can make time stand still or even go backwards to a less-wrinkled, more youthful appearance. Let me explain how. But first, a little lesson on what wrinkles are.

Imagine you've just bought a comforter. It feels soft and you enjoy running your hand over its smooth surface. Now imagine it's years later. The comforter has been washed dozens of times, rolled up, stored…you can get an idea of how it looks and feels now. The stuffing has lumps and bumps, and in some spots it has simply disappeared.

The collagen that gives structure to your dermis, or middle layer of skin, is just like the stuffing of that comforter. When your skin is in peak condition, its fibers are taut and elastic. Take care of it and it will remain pillow soft, smooth and *wrinkle-free*. Abuse it, neglect it, ignore it and the collagen fibers will become worn, thin, rough, and will hang loosely.

Am I getting under your skin? When we talk about treating wrinkles, we're really talking about taking care of the collagen under the surface of your skin, in the dermis, and the elastin fibers. Collagen plays such an important role in skin appearance, and, therefore, in how we look, that it has become popular to inject it under the skin to remove wrinkles and facial lines. While you might consider such treatment, keep in mind it is only temporary and there is a risk that you could be allergic to the animal collagen that is used. Elastin is important to keep the skin taut and springy, not spongy. For more on the importance of elastin, see the chapter Stretch Marks.

The Silica Story

Collagen, like other tissues in our body, needs food to grow and stay healthy. It requires a good amount of food because it makes up about 30 percent of our body. What do you think nourishes it most? Silica!

Since silica may be new to you, let me give you its credentials for its prominent place in the skin beauty hall of fame. It's an amazing whodunit act featuring calcium, boron, phosphorus and potassium – amazing because without silica, none of these essential minerals can be used by the body! Silica is probably the most essential mineral to healthy skin, hair and nails.

The silica connection was discovered by scientist William Prout in 1822. To his bewilderment, Prout found that newly hatched chicks contained four times more calcium than the eggs they came from.[1]

Where did the extra calcium come from? Other scientists of his day were also at a loss. An unbroken axiom of science is that you can't get more from less. So every time an egg is hatched, it is a miracle of God.[2]

The same mystery troubled Dr. Louis Kevran. As a boy, he noticed that the chickens his family raised often went to great pains to eat mica, a component of silica. But when his mother opened the gizzards of the slaughtered chickens, Kevran saw no mica. He knew that eggshells are formed from calcium, yet the area had no limestone or other sources of naturally-occurring calcium. And the chickens never received calcium in their diet. Like Prout, he, too, wondered "where did the calcium come from?"[3]

The riddle intrigued Kervran all his life. He devoted his energies to solving this great perplexing mystery – an effort that made him an eminent scientist and Nobel Prize nominee.[4]

In 1959 Kervran and other researchers discovered something vitally important: without silica, the body cannot create for itself and, in the case of the chickens, form calcium. Not only that – surprise, surprise – but collagen is largely made up of silica! [5]

I call it a secret because how many beauty company's tout silica in their advertisements? They don't know what you now know!

To maintain healthier and longer-lasting collagen, aim for natural sources of silica. Inorganic silica actually draws calcium from the bones and deposits it into skin tissues. The calcium can crystallize, forming what some skin experts term cross linkages, making the collagen hard and stiff, instead of smooth and soft.[6]

Stay away from the artificial stuff. Instead, make sure your silica sources are derived from natural plants or health food products. Look for silica in solution. Minerals in solution offer the highest absorption rate, unencumbered by allergies, intestinal disorders or a lack of stomach acid.

Calcium Cross Linkages Reversed with Magnesium

As I have already mentioned regarding inorganic silica, skin wrinkling is caused not only by damage to underlying collagen, but also by the amount of calcium infiltrating the collagen. An extreme example of this condition is scleroderma, a thickening and hardening of the skin and its becoming cemented to underlying structures, sometimes causing joints to become immovable.

Magnesium, in combination with calcium, work in balance throughout our bodies. Without magnesium, calcium accumulates in places it shouldn't. The consequences of taking calcium without magnesium is that calcium goes into soft tissues and causes wrinkled skin, stiffened joints and tendinitis. Researchers and doctors call this syndrome calcinosis.

Dr. Hans Seyle, author of the book *Stress Without Distress*, and a Nobel prize winning biologist, found in rat experiments that in stressful situations, calcium is drawn from the bones and deposited in the tissues. When this happens, the calcium can crystalize, causing cross linkages. Many signs of aging then develop: arthritis, wrinkles, cataracts and shriveled sex glands.[7]

Calcinosis occurs because of a very common deficiency of magnesium. Researchers have found the calcium/magnesium ratio to be very important in maintaining the elastic quality of fibrous connective tissue, most especially in the case of the skin's connective tissue. Too much calcium in the skin results in wrinkling.

Dr. W. Muller and colleagues at the Institute of Pathology in Koln, Germany, found that magnesium plays a crucial role in the health of connective fibers with elastic properties. Examining the ligaments in the discs of spinal surgery patients, Dr. Muller put them into two groups: those with very elastic tissues, and those with non-elastic tissues. He found that among those with the most elasticity, a magnesium/calcium ratio in favor of magnesium was found.[8] What appears to be happening is that your body uses more magnesium than calcium to keep the elastin found throughout your body – elastin in bone and muscle ligaments, and your skin – tight, taught and strong, not weak, wrinkled and loose.

So, how bad is it? It's bad. In a 1982 to 1989 study of a variety of nutritional elements, compared to the recommendations of the

National Academy of Sciences (the people who come up with the RDAs – recommended daily allowances), it was found that magnesium was low among teenage girls and boys, adult women, and older men and women.[9]

Take your minerals in solution. Because of the high absorption rate of minerals in solution, and deficiency of magnesium in the diet, the ratio of magnesium and calcium in solution should be four to one, respectively.

B2 Deficiency Damage

I have been studying the subtle signs of health and disease in people's faces for so many years, I can look at certain kinds of wrinkles to tell what kind of nutritional deficiency is present.

Lines at right angles to one another or tiny wrinkles on the lower lip indicate a vitamin B2 deficiency. Later the lip develops a crinkly, crepe-paper look or appears to be chapped with small white flakes peeling from it. You may know people who have this symptom. Next time you see them, try not to stare. Instead, show them this chapter.

In acute vitamin B2 deficiency, cracks develop and persist at the corners of the mouth. "Monkey lines" may also form between the upper lip and nose. When deficiencies endure for a long period, the upper lip may entirely disappear!

This is what has happened to beautiful Lana Turner. During World War II, a man paid Lana $50,000 to kiss her full, voluptuous beautiful lips. Lana died of cancer, and her close friends told me her diet was awful. She ate only to stay slim, and over time lost her upper lip. Lana's lips were reduced to bargain basement prices without B2.

When supplementing with any one B vitamin, always include a comprehensive B vitamin complex formula. All the B vitamins need to be taken together to avoid deficiencies.

Natural Wrinkle Reducers Found in Skin Care Products

Studies have made a connection between wrinkle formation and something called hyaluronic acid, or sodium hyaluronate, a naturally-occurring skin and tissue lubricator found in certain skin care products. Wrinkles and a loss of elastin is believed to be caused by free radical damage. Now, another factor is being considered: inadequate amounts of hyaluronic acid.

Researchers never fully realized the connection between hyaluronic acid and skin until a breakthrough study on sheep fetuses. Scientists looking for substances that would repair wounds without scar tissue or damage to the elastin began studying fetal lambs because of their ability to heal without scar formation. They discovered fetal wounds contain high levels of hyaluronic acid. They also discovered high levels of hyaluronic acid in the amniotic fluid, thus it continually bathes the fetus and encourages smooth cell formation.[10]

In addition, in studies of adult sheep the researchers found a rapid rise of high levels of hyaluronic acid levels in the skin following injury. Why fetal lambs don't have scarring while adult sheep do relates to the fact that the hyaluronic acid levels in the lambs persist at least 21 days after wounding, whereas in adult sheep high levels occur three days or less following injury. The researchers concluded that hyaluronic acid not only encourages healing following skin damage, but can effectively inhibit tissue damage as a result of an injury.

What does hyaluronic acid have to do with wrinkles? It can be useful in preventing the skin cell damage that occurs with time and the elements.

Don't let the term "acid" fool you. It's as safe on cellular tissue as water. In fact, surgeons inject it into the eye during surgery so the tissues can be separated without damage. It is also used in cases of dry eye to increase moisture.[11]

A pharmaceutical company in Basel, Switzerland, credits hyaluronic acid with not only moisturizing the skin, but "helping to maintain or restore the biophysical properties of skin, such as smoothness, elasticity, and resilience, which gives it its youthfully fresh appearance."[12]

An article in the *International Journal of Dermatology* reports on a study that showed a lack of sufficient hyaluronic acid in the skin may be responsible for the wrinkles and skin sags (loss of elastin) typical of advancing age.[13]

In fact, hyaluronic acid has turned out to be so therapeutically effective that it could be in danger of being considered a topical drug by the FDA. The editors of *Cosmetics and Toiletries*, a cosmetic industry journal, have coined the term "cosmeceuticals," to describe currently marketed skin care ingredients that have 'bio-active' properties.[14] Get them while you can!

A Wrinkle Cure for the Ages

Alpha hydroxy acid (AHA), found in apples, grapes and other fruit, has been discovered by Temple University researchers to remove shallow wrinkles and rejuvenate the skin. It removes dry skin, scaly patches, age or brown spots, and acne, as well as wrinkles.

Alpha hydroxy acid is just a collective term for the various acids found in certain fruits. AHAs are actually citric acid, glycolic acid, lactic acid, malic acid and tartaric acid. Stay with me while I give examples of how our foremothers used foods containing these acids to stay moist and free of wrinkles and blemishes.

- Ladies of the court of Louis XIV are said to have applied old wine to their faces to remove wrinkles and blemishes. Old wine contains large amounts of malic and tartaric acid.

- Polynesians, who get lots of tropical sunlight, rich in skin-damaging ultraviolet radiation, use a mixture of citrus and sugar-cane juice to keep their skin healthy. These foods contain citric and glycolic acid.

- Cleopatra indulged in milk baths and yogurt facials. Sour milk and yogurt contain substantial amounts of lactic acid, which is an effective skin moisturizer and also helps skin shed its outer layer of dead cells more easily. The ancient Egyptians, believing their pharaohs and queens to be gods, invented special milk baths and shampoos to keep their hair and skin looking appropriately godlike.[15]

Wrinkle-Vanquishing Vitamins

Stress has been found in studies to cause wrinkles. One good stress-protector vitamin is E. Large amounts of vitamin E prevents the wrinkles caused by stress.[16]

Vitamin E has also been credited with reversing some of the effects of the sun. Undoing the damage caused by ultraviolet rays without a chemical face peel is almost impossible, yet vitamin E in cream has helped certain individuals to some degree.

In tests carried out over a four-week period, 20 middle-aged women using a five percent vitamin E cream showed more than a 50 percent reduction in the length and depth of crow's feet. Independent biomedical consultant Peter J. Publiese, M.D., speculates that the well-known antioxidant may have an effect on cells that produce collagen.[17]

It is difficult to obtain extra vitamin E from foods. According to Orville A. Levander, from the USDA's Human Nutrition Research Center, Beltsville Maryland, it is virtually impossible to obtain more than 25 International Units (IUs) of vitamin E per day solely from the diet.[18]

Vivacious Skin with Vitamin C

A sin of omission is taking in too little of any particular nutrient, especially vitamin C, another collagen body-builder, and an excellent antioxidant.

In a double-blind trial done at the University of Wisconsin at Madison, 48 out of 50 women felt that a cream containing vitamin C was more effective than a placebo – the fake stuff – that was given them to smooth out wrinkles. The researchers found vitamin C stimulates collagen production without irritating the skin.[19]

Vitamin C's ability to manufacture collagen was illustrated to me dramatically by a veterinarian, Dr. John Craig, in Monterey, California. He is both a vet and a breeder of Alaskan Huskies. Dr. Craig was forced to destroy whole litters of puppies due to hip dysplasia, a crippling deformity common among certain breeds of dogs.

One day while operating, he realized that if there was more collagen in the joints, the dog wouldn't have the dysplasia. He began to give his dogs vitamin C and has not had to destroy any more dogs.

Now, when I see a dog whose hind legs are dragging, I want to go up to the owner and tell them the solution. I have since shared this secret with a Great Dane breeder and it has earned his show dogs international prizes.

You know, of course, that sunscreens help protect your skin from ultraviolet radiation that causes wrinkles. But there is much they *don't* do. What is needed are nutrients that strengthen the skin against UV damage. If the skin is strong, and has essential nutrients, the cells aren't likely to mutate when exposed to radiation.

At a Gerontological Society of America meeting, Dr. Sheldon Pinnell, chief of dermatology at Duke University Medical Center in Durham, N.C., reported on several studies on the protective effect of vitamin C on skin.

In one study, the skin of live pigs was treated with topical vitamin C, then exposed to ultraviolet light at one to five times the dose that produces sunburn. The topical C not only protected the pigs from sunburn, but protected the skin from cellular damage. The protective effect of the topical vitamin C lasted three days, even when the pigs were scrubbed with soap! Now, that's remarkable!

Vitamin C's ability to prevent UV damage in 15 participants produced impressive results that were reviewed by doctors at a Society of Investigative Dermatology meeting. Dermatologist James Leyden, who saw the study results remarked that treating skin with topical vitamin C "may influence the function of fibroblasts in a way that will make them produce more collagen."[20]

I have very sensitive skin, which burns at the slightest exposure to sunlight. After I read these impressive studies, I wanted to test them out. Taking a very great risk, I left my sunscreen in my hotel room and applied only a moisturizing lotion containing vitamin C when I went skiing in the Austrian Alps, where the weather punishes the skin. I have to tell you, I was amazed! Not only did I not burn, after a full day of skiing in bright sunlight, but I actually tanned, probably for the first time in my life! What was most remarkable was that my skin didn't suffer any of the aging effects I notice after exposure to the sun. What this meant for me was that for the first time, my immune system was working to protect my skin. I am a believer!

There are various ways in which people can shield themselves from the sun. Madhu Pathak, Ph.D., dermatology research professor at Harvard Medical School, recommends using cosmetics and moisturizers that contain vitamins E and C and beta carotene, to counteract the skin oxidation caused by sunlight that damages cell membranes, DNA and skin proteins.[21]

An antioxidant-enriched formulation will retard or minimize these damaging reactions both on the short term and long-term. Cosmetics and moisturizers help minimize the damaging reactions, especially if used in conjunction with sunscreens.

Wonders of Vitamin A

Doctors and nutrition experts have known for decades that vitamin A is vital to the development of bones and teeth. And now it's been proven to be just as important to the health of your skin. By eating a diet rich in this nutrient, the telltale signs of aging can be eliminated from the inside out in less than a month. You need proof? OK, here it is:

Plastic surgeon Dr. Anton Lipaus and research colleagues at the University of Montpelier, France, conducted an exhaustive year-long study of the effects of vitamin A on wrinkles – and were stunned by the results.[22]

You can eliminate wrinkles faster, easier and far less expensively simply by packing your daily diet with foods rich in vitamin A. Dr. Lipaus says that in many cases wrinkles disappear in as little as 20 days.[23]

The university research team divided 40 women with moderate to severe facial wrinkling into two groups. Group one was given a list of foods known to be excellent sources of vitamin A and told to eat at least three items from the list every day. The women in group two were used as a control group and told to eat whatever they wanted.[24]

At the end of the trial period, the women in group one looked years younger. One of the women, who just celebrated her 40th birthday, could have easily passed for 25. Yet when the study began, her face was marred by so many wrinkles and crow's feet she could have passed for 50. The women in the control group experienced no reduction in wrinkles and looked their age or older.[25]

Also look for facial and skin creams that contain sodium hyaluronate and the antioxidant vitamins A, C and E.

Smoking Sabotages the Skin

Cigarette smokers eventually develop dried up, lined and wrinkled skin because smoking undermines the skin.

A study of 1,104 subjects conducted by H.W. Daniell, M.D., showed the striking result of smoking on people over 30. Subjects in the 40 to 49-year age group were found to be as prominently wrinkled as non-smokers 20 years older![26] Talk about premature aging!

In a study conducted by Donald P. Kadunce, M.D., of the Division of Dermatology, University of Utah Health Sciences Center in Salt Lake City, Utah, 132 smokers and nonsmokers were evaluated for the relationship between smoking and facial wrinkling. After controlling for variables, it was found that premature wrinkling increased with the more packs smoked. Heavy smokers with more than 50 packs a year were 4.7 times more likely to be wrinkled than nonsmokers.[27]

If you're still not convinced, consider this: experts warn people away from used cars previously owned by smokers because the years of smoking disintegrates the glue holding the upholstery together. How many times on the road have you seen a smoker puffing away in his or her car, the roof lining flapping in the wind? Just imagine what it does to your skin!

One of the ways in which smoking destroys the skin is by destroying vitamin C. Each cigarette burns up at least 25 mg of vitamin C. Smokers of 20 cigarettes a day use up 500 mg, putting themselves in a deficit situation, because vitamin C is not storable. As a result, their connective tissue literally caves in.[28]

The Fluoride Disgrace

Even if you don't smoke, there's another skin ager I bet you didn't know about. If your city adds fluoride to the municipal water supply they may also be adding years to your face! Studies disclose that fluoride levels as low as one part per million – the amount added to many city water supplies – causes a breakdown of collagen.[29]

This amount of fluoride, coupled with a poor diet, not only contributes to wrinkling, but to the speeding up of the entire aging process, weaking bones, ligaments, muscles and tendons.

I received the greatest shock of my life when I visited Kizilcaoern, a village in Turkey where the water supply has an even higher fluoride content – more than five parts per million. I have never in my life seen so many prune faces. Women and men in their 30s looked as if they were in their 70s or 80s with deep wrinkles and flabby, hanging skin. Many of the natives in their 30s were so weak and decrepit they had to use walking canes to get around. One bent, hobbling woman with deep, criss-crossing facial wrinkles appeared to be in her late 80s and turned out to be 32!

You are probably aware that the municipal water in many cities and towns in the U.S. is fluoridated to protect children from developing tooth cavities. You are probably not aware that the Environmental Protection Agency several years ago increased the maximum allowable level of fluorides in public water supplies to four parts per million from the original range of 1.4 to 2.4, thus subtly, but definitely, contributing to the crow's feet, laugh lines and other wrinkles on the faces of the American people.

Skin-Tightening Nutrients
For maximum absorption take supplements with meals.

Nutrient	Suggested Dosage	Formulation
Acetyl L-Carnitine	500 mg three times daily	
Aged garlic extract	1 teaspoon three times daily	Liquid
Antioxidants	2 capsules daily	With selenium and grape seed extract
Borage oil	2 capsules daily	
Flaxseed oil	1 tablespoon daily	
Multi-mineral	3-4 ounces daily	In liquid solution, with vitamin B12, biotin
Multi-vitamin/mineral	6 caplets daily	Freeze-dried plant sources
Vitamin A	25,000 IU daily*	
Vitamin C	Individual bowel tolerance**	With citrus bioflavonoids (quercetin, rutin proanthocyanidins)

Nourish skin with a therapeutic moisturizer that contains aloe vera gel, chamomile, vitamins A and C, and avocado oil.

* The FDA recommends pregnant women not exceed 10,000 IU of vitamin A daily.

** To determine individual dosage, on the first day take 1,000 mg hourly until diarrhea occurs, then reduce dosage to just below that for individual daily dosage. Vitamin C is not toxic in large doses but must be taken throughout the day to benefit. Divide dosage to three or four times a day.

BASIC DAILY PREVENTIVE HEALTH PROTOCOL

Recommended nutrients and amounts for maximum health and prevention of illness.

For maximum benefit, include a daily diet rich in organic whole fruits and vegetables, raw whenever possible, 30 minutes of moderate exercise, and prayer. For maximum absorption, take supplements with meals.

Nutrient	Suggested Dosage	Formulation
Borage oil	2 capsules daily	
Fiber	4-8 tablets	Psyllium, with herb hyssop
Multi-mineral	1-4 ounces	In liquid solution, with vitamin B12, biotin
Multi-vitamin/mineral	3-6 caplets	Freeze-dried plant sources
Vitamin C	Individual bowel tolerance*	With bioflavonoids (quercetin, proanthocyanidins)
Vitamin E	2 capsules (800 IU)	d-alpha tocopherol

* To determine individual dosage, on the first day take 1,000 mg hourly until diarrhea occurs, then reduce dosage to just below that for individual daily dosage. Vitamin C is not toxic in large doses but must be taken throughout the day to benefit. Divide dosage to three or four times a day.

FOOD CHART

Foods High in Specific Nutrients

MINERALS

Boron: beans, peas, lentils, nuts, pears, leafy vegetables, soy meal, prunes, raisins, almonds, peanuts, hazelnuts, dates and honey.

Calcium: green leafy vegetables, watercress, spinach, dandelion greens, peas, parsley, mint, chickpeas, molasses, sesame seeds, cheese, brewer's yeast, sardines, caviar, salmon, torula yeast, soybeans, Brazil nuts, egg yolk, sunflower seeds, seaweed and walnuts.

Chromium: thyme, cloves, seaweed, parsley, natural maple syrup, brewer's yeast, wheat germ and bran, buckwheat, millet, brown rice, whole rye, oats, corn, beets, peas, carrots, black pepper, clams, mushrooms and molasses.

Copper: seafood, nuts, legumes, molasses and raisins.

Iodine: seafood, kelp.

Iron: blackstrap molasses, raisins, spinach and other green leafy vegetables, and unsulphured dried fruit.

Magnesium: whole wheat, pumpkin seeds, millet, almonds, Brazil nuts and hazel nuts, dark-green vegetables and molasses.

Manganese: whole grains, green leafy vegetables, legumes, nuts, pineapple and egg yolks.

Molybdenum: legumes, whole grains, dark green vegetables.

Phosphorus: fish, eggs, legumes, nuts, whole grains.

Potassium: blackstrap molasses, whole grains (a cup of millet has 980 mg), dried fruits (one cup of raisins has 1,362 mg), avocado (one=1,204 mg), plantains (one cup=739 mg), seeds (one cup sunflower seeds=1,334 mg) and nuts (one cup pistachios=1,399 mg). Watch out for soft drinks. They rob your body of potassium.

Potassium, calcium, and magnesium: wheat germ, sunflower seeds, soybeans, almonds, Brazil nuts, pistachios and pecans

Silica: brown rice, bell peppers, leafy green vegetables, oat straw tea and the herb horsetail.

Sulfur: fish, red hot peppers, garlic, onions, eggs, cabbage, Brussels sprouts, horseradish.

Vanadium: vegetable oils, whole grains, fish and other seafood and liver.

Zinc: sesame seeds, pumpkin seeds, torula yeast, blackstrap molasses, maple syrup and brewer's yeast.

B VITAMINS

All the B vitamins: lentils, pinto beans, black-eyed peas, black beans, lima beans, rice bran, corn, millet, barley and blackstrap molasses.

B1 (Thiamine): brewer's yeast, wheat germ, blackstrap molasses and bran.

B2 (Riboflavin): brewer's yeast, whole grains, blackstrap molasses, egg yolks, nuts, peas, beans.

B3 (Niacin): brewer's yeast, liver, lean meat, peanuts, rice bran, avocado, halibut, salmon and tuna.

B5 (Pantothenic Acid): royal jelly, brewer's yeast, torula yeast, brown rice, sunflower seeds, soybeans, corn, lentils, egg yolk, peas, whole wheat, peanuts and rye.

B6 (Pyridoxine): brewer's yeast, brown rice, whole wheat, royal jelly, soybeans, rye, lentils, sunflower seeds, hazelnuts, alfalfa, salmon, wheat germ, tuna, bran, walnuts, peas and beans.

B12 (Cobalamin): liver, crab, herring, red snapper, flounder, salmon, lamb, swiss cheese, eggs, haddock, cottage cheese and swordfish.

B15 (Pangamic acid): brewer's yeast, brown rice, sunflower seeds, pumpkin seeds, sesame seeds.

Biotin: egg yolks, liver, unpolished rice, brewer's yeast, whole grains, peas and beans.

Choline: lecithin, egg yolk, wheat germ, oatmeal, rice, soy products, peanuts and pecans.

Inositol: whole grains, citrus fruits, brewer's yeast, molasses, nuts, vegetables, lecithin .

Lecithin: soybeans, wheat germ, nuts, sunflower and pumpkin seeds, whole grains and unsaturated fatty acid seed oils like walnut oil and flaxseed oil.

Folic Acid: lentils, beans, bean sprouts, wheat bran, artichokes, beets, cauliflower and corn.

PABA (Para-Aminobenzoic Acid): wheat germ, yogurt, molasses, green leafy vegetables.

VITAMINS

Vitamin D: cod liver oil, salmon, sardines, herring, egg yolk, organ meats and bone meal.

Vitamin K: cheddar cheese, Camembert cheese, Brussels sprouts, soy lecithin, alfalfa, oats, spinach, soybeans, cauliflower, cabbage, broccoli, liver, potatoes and bran.

ANTIOXIDANTS

Coenzyme Q10: beef heart, codfish, egg yolk, mackerel, muscle meat, salmon, sardines, wheat germ and whole grains.

Selenium: shrimp, smelt, lobster, clams, tuna, scallops, herring, whole wheat, brown rice, molasses and mushrooms.

Beta carotene: carrots, sweet potatoes, spinach, most green leafy vegetables and in orange or yellow vegetables.

Vitamin A: cod liver oil, dandelion greens, carrots, yams, kale, parsley, turnip greens, collard greens, chard, watercress, red peppers, squash, egg yolk, cantaloupe, persimmons, apricots, broccoli, crab, swordfish, whitefish, Romaine lettuce, mangoes, pumpkin, peaches and cheese. One cup of carrot juice contains 24,750 Individual Units of vitamin A.

Vitamin C: papaya (one=187 mg), guava (one=165 mg), black currants (one cup=202 mg), cantaloupe, strawberries, chili peppers (one cup=182 mg), parsley (one cup=103 mg), kohlrabi (one cup=90 mg), broccoli (one cup=82 mg) and kale (one cup=80 mg)
[One orange contains 70 mg of vitamin C]

Bioflavonoids: citrus rind, cherries, grapes, plums, black currants, apricots, buckwheat, blackberries and rose hips.

Quercetin: grapefruit, broccoli, shallots, summer squash and onions. Lycopene: dried and canned apricots, grapefruit, guava juice, canned tomato juice, canned tomato paste, canned tomato sauce and watermelon.

Vitamin E: wheat germ, safflower seeds, sunflower seeds, sesame oil, walnuts, corn oil, hazelnuts, soybean oil, almonds, olive oil and cabbage.

Garlic has germanium, magnesium, selenium, amino acids, sulfur, and vitamins A, B1 and C.

BODY BUILDING NUTRIENTS

Protein: To get your daily allowance of complete protein combine whole grains with legumes (beans, peas and lentils).

Amino acids: include taurine, arginine, cysteine, acetyl-L-carnitine and methionine. Large neutral amino acids are phenylalanine, leucine, isoleucine, tryptophan, valine, methionine, histidine and tyrosine. They are essential to healthy communication between brain and muscles.

Arginine: fish, poultry and dairy products.

Glutathione: raw green, yellow and red vegetables. Canned or frozen vegetables lose glutathione during processing.

Methionine: poultry, nuts and seeds, and fruits and vegetables.

Tryptophan: turkey breast meat, wheat germ, granola and oats.

Tyrosine: peanuts, pickled herring, pumpkin seeds and lima beans.

Taurine: seafood, eggs, beans and peas.

FATTY ACIDS

Omega-6: seeds and seed oils.

Omega-3: fish, fish oils (cod liver oil), green leafy vegetables and flaxseed oil.

Gamma-linolenic acid (GLA), or linoleic acid:evening primrose oil, black currant oil, borage oil and spirulina.

Linolenic Acid: borage oil, evening primrose oil .

Eicosapentaenoic Acid and **Docosahexaenoic Acid:** cold water fish and oil; salmon, trout, mackerel, sardines.

Oleic acid: olive, almond, pecan, cashew, filbert and macadamia nut.

Palmitoleic acid (saturated fat): milk, coconut oil, palm kernel oil.

Stearic acid (saturated fat): beef, mutton, pork.

Stearidonic Acid: wild seeds.

Butyric Acid: butter.

REFERENCES

Chapter 1: ABCESSES
[1] Cheraskin, Emanuel, M.D., D.M.D., *Vitamin C, Who Needs It?*, Arlington Press and Company, Birmingham AL, p. 109, 1993.
[2] Ibid, p. 62.
[3] Sanchez, A., Reeser, J., Lau, H., et al., "Role of Sugars in Human Neutrophilic Phagocytosis," *American Journal of Clinical Nutrition*, v. 26, p. 180, 1973.
[4] Abdullah, T.H., M.D., et al. "Enhancement of Natural Killer Cell Activity in AIDS with Garlic," *Deutsche Zeitschrift fur Okologie*, 1989.

Chapter 2: ACNE
[1] Salaman, Maureen, "Effects of Zinc on Acne: An Exclusive Interview with Robert Cathcart, M.D.," *Let's Live*, p. 17, September 1980.
[2] Ibid.
[3] Taylor, Deborah Seymour, "Zinc and EFAs Fight Acne; Essential Fatty Acids, Along with the Trace Mineral Zinc, are Vital for Acne Treatment," *Today's Living*, v. 21, n. 3, p. 10, March 1990.
[4] Ibid, p. 11.
[5] Murray, Frank, "Zinc: Healing Mineral," *Better Nutrition for Today's Living*, v. 54, n. 9, p. 26, September 1992.
[6] Quillin, Patrick, Ph.D., R.D., *Healing Nutrients*, Chicago, New York, Contemporary Books, 1987.
[7] Taylor, Deborah Seymour, "Zinc and EFAs Fight Acne; Essential Fatty Acids, Along with the Trace Mineral Zinc, are Vital for Acne Treatment," *Today's Living*, v. 21, n. 3, p. 10, March 1990.
[8] Dunne, Lavon J., *Nutrition Almanac*, Third Edition, McGraw-Hill Publishing Company, p. 231, 1990.
[9] Taylor, Deborah Seymour, "Zinc and EFAs Fight Acne; Essential Fatty Acids, Along with the Trace Mineral Zinc, are Vital for Acne Treatment," *Today's Living*, v. 21, n. 3, p. 10, March 1990.

Chapter 3: AIDS

1 "HIV-Positives Must Consume Greater Amounts of Vitamins and Minerals," *AIDS Weekly*, April 11, 1994.
2 Badgley, Laurence E., M.D., "Natural Therapies for AIDS," *Townsend Letter for Doctors*, October 1988.
3 Bogden, John D., et al. "Micronutrient Status and HIV Infection." Paper read at the "Micronutrients and Immune Functions" conference, The New York Academy of Sciences, New York City, May 31-June 2, 1989.
4 Ibid.
5 Herzlich, Barry C., et al, "Synergy of Inhibition of DNA Synthesis in Human Bone Marrow by Azidothymidine Plus Deficiency of Folate and/or Vitamin B12?" *American Journal of Hematology*, v. 33, p. 177, 1990.
6 Timbo, B., et al, "Nutrition: A Cofactor in HIV Disease," *Journal of The American Dietetic Association*, v. 94, p. 1018, September 1994.
7 Sato, Sally J., R. Ph., and Mirtallo, Jay M., M.S., R.Ph. "Nutritional Support for the AIDS Patient." *U.S. Pharmacist*, December 1987.
8 Burton Goldberg Group, *Alternative Medicine, The Definitive Guide*, Future Medicine Publishing, Inc., Puyallup, WA, p. 499, 1993.
9 Murray, Frank, "AIDS Update," *Better Nutrition*, v. 5, n. 1, p. 10, January 1989.
10 Burton Goldberg Group, *Alternative Medicine, The Definitive Guide*, Future Medicine Publishing, Inc., Puyallup, WA, p. 494, 1993.
11 Levine, Stephen A., Ph.D. "Organic Germanium: a Novel Dramatic Immunostimulant." The *Journal of Orthomolecular Medicine*, May 21, 1987.
12 Abdullah, T.H., M.D., et al, "Enhancement of Natural Killer Cell Activity in AIDS with Garlic," *Deutsche Zeitschrift fur Okologie*, 1989.

Chapter 4: ALCOHOL

1 Biery, Janet Reid, "Alcohol Craving in Rehabilitation: Assessment of Nutrition Therapy," *Journal of the American Dietetic Association*, v. 91, p. 463, April 1991.
2 Register, et al, *Journal of the American Dietetic Association*, v. 61, p. 159-162, 1972.
3 Blum, Kenneth; Rassner, Michael; Payne, James E., "Neuro-nutrient Therapy for Compulsive Disease: Rationale and Clinical Evidence," *Addiction & Recovery*, v. 10, n. 2, p. 12, August 1990.
4 Biery, Janet Reid, "Alcohol Craving in Rehabilitation: Assessment of Nutrition Therapy," *Journal of the American Dietetic Association*, v. 91, p. 463, April 1991.
5 Herbert, Victor, M.D., J.D.; Subak-Sharpe, Genell J., M.S. & Hammock, Delia A, M.S., R.D., *The Mount Sinai School of Medicine Complete Book of Nutrition*, St. Martin's Press, New York, p. 631, 1990.
6 Ibid, p. 632.

Chapter 5: ALCOHOL'S MENTAL EFFECTS

1 Lindberg, Michael C.; Oyler, Richard A., "Wernicke's Encephalopathy," *American Family Physician*, v. 41, n. 4, p. 1205, April 1990.
2 Werbach, Melvyn R., *Nutritional Influences on Illness*, Keats Publishing, New Canaan, CT, p. 493, 1988.

[3] Murray, Frank, "Bone Up on B Vitamins: Part One," *Better Nutrition*, v. 51, n. 10, p. 8, October 1989.

[4] Hoffer, Abram, *Orthomolecular Medicine for Physicians*, Keats Publishing, New Canaan, CT, p. 33, 1989.

[5] Diamond, Ivan, "Neurology: From Basics to Bedside," *The Western Journal of Medicine*, v. 161, n. 3, p. 279, September 1994.

[6] Ibid.

[7] Bruck, W., et al, "Wernicke's Encephalopathy in a Child With Acute Lymphoblastic Leukemia Treated With Polychemotherapy," *Clinical Neuropathology*, v. 10, n. 3, p. 134-136, 1991.

[8] Wodak, Alex, "Thiamine Fortification in Alcohol," *The Medical Journal of Australia*, v. 152, p. 97-99, January 15, 1990.

[9] Ibid.

[10] Haase, Gunter R., M.D., et al,"Neuropathy: Diabetic? Nutritional?" *Patient Care*, p. 112-134, May 15, 1990.

[11] Lindberg, Michael C., M.D. and Oyler, Richard A., DMD, "Wernicke's Encephalopathy," *American Family Physician*, p. 1205-1209, April 1990.

[12] Ibid.

Chapter 6: ALLERGIES

[1] "Blowing Away Allergies," Anti-Aging News, *Longevity*, p. 16, April 1995.

[2] Pauling, Linus, *How to Live Longer and Feel Better*, W. H. Freeman and Company, New York, p. 269, 1986.

[3] Douglas, D.E., "4.4'-Diacetyl Curcumin--In-Vitro Histamine-Blocking Activity," *Journal Pharm. Pharmacol.*, v. 45, p. 766, 1993.

[4] Atkins, Robert C., M.D., *Dr. Atkins' Health Revolution*, Houghton Mifflin Co., Boston, p. 342, 1988.

[5] Murray, Michael, T., *Natural Alternatives to Over-The-Counter Prescription Drugs*, William Morrow and Company, New York, p. 94-96, 1994.

Chapter 7: ALZHEIMER'S

[1] Adler, T., "ALzheimer's Causes Unique Cell Death," *Science News*, v. 146, p. 198, September 24, 1994.

[2] Yokel, Robert A., "Aluminum Exposure Produces Learning and Memory Deficits: A Model of Alzheimer's Disease," *Toxin-Induced Models of Neurologic Disorders*, Woodruff, Michael L. and Nonneman, Arthury, *Plenum Press*, chpt. 11, p. 301, 1994.

[3] "New Evidence for Aluminium/Alzheimer's Link," *SCRIP World Pharmaceutical News*, n. 1918, p. 22, April 29, 1994.

[4] Zeavin, Edna, "Foods that Influence Behavior," *Bestways*, p. 11, September 1985.

[5] Constantinidis, Jean, "Treatment of Alzheimer's Disease by Zinc Compounds," *Drug Development Research*, v. 27, p. 12, 1992.

[6] Brownlee, Shannon, "Blitzing the Defense; Piercing the Brain's Protective Barrier is Key to Treating Many Serious Neurological Disorders," *U.S. News & World Report*, v. 109, n. 15, p. 90, October 15, 1990.

[7] Canty, David J., MS, Zeisel, H, M.D., Ph.D., "Lecithin and Choline in Human Health and Disease," *Nutrition Reviews*, University of North Carolina at Chapel Hill, Chapel Hill, NC, 27599-7000, U.S.A., p. 52, October 1994.

[8] "Vitamin B12 and Alzheimer's Disease," *The Nutrition Report*, v. 75, p. 12, October 1994.

[9] Dunne, Lavon J., *Nutrition Almanac*, Third Edition, McGraw-Hill Publishing Company, p. 31-32, 1990.

[10] Thorne Research, "Acetyl-L-Carnitine," Thorne Research Abstracts, February 17, 1995.

[11] Rai, G., et al., "Double-Blind, Placebo-Controlled Study of Acetyl-L-Carnitine in Patients with Alzheimer's Dementia," *Current Medical Resident Opinion*, v. 11, p. 638, 1990.

[12] Imagawa, M., et al, "Coenzyme Q10, Iron and Vitamin B6 in Genetically Confirmed Alzheimer's Disease," *The Lancet*, n. 8820, p. 671, September 1992.

Chapter 8: ANEMIA
[1] *Tufts University Diet & Nutrition Letter*, v. 10, n. 11, p.3, January 1993.

[2] Faelten, Sharon, *The Complete Book of Minerals for Health*, Rodale Press, Emmaus, PA, p. 137, 1981.

Chapter 9: ANKYLOSING SPONDYLITIS
[1] Burton Goldberg Group, *Alternative Medicine, The Definitive Guide*, Future Medicine Publishing, Inc., Puyallup, WA, p. 884, 1993.

[2] Will, Rob, et al, "Osteoporosis in Early Ankylosing Spondylitis: A Preliminary Pathological Event?" *The Lancet*, v. 2, n. 8678, p. 1483, Dec. 23, 1989.

[3] Appelboom, Thierry and Durez, Patrick, "Effect of Milk Product Deprivation on Spondyloarthropathy," *Annals of Rheumatic Diseases*, v. 53, n. 71, p. 481, 1994.

[4] Burton Goldberg Group, *Alternative Medicine, The Definitive Guide*, Future Medicine Publishing, Inc., Puyallup, WA, p. 884, 1993.

[5] Chaitow, L, "British Research Connects Ankylosing Spondylitis to Bowel Dysbiosis," *Townsend Letter for Doctors*, p. 364-365, July 1989.

[6] Ibid.

[7] Burton Goldberg Group, *Alternative Medicine, The Definitive Guide*, Future Medicine Publishing, Inc., Puyallup, WA, p. 922, 1993.

Chapter 10: APPENDICITIS
[1] SerVaas, Cory, *Saturday Evening Post*, v. 267, n.2, p. 54(6), March-April, 1995.

[2] Gerras, Charles, et al, eds, *The Encyclopedia of Common Diseases*, Rodale Press, Emmaus, PA, p. 66, 1976.

[3] Ibid. p. 66.

Chapter 11: ARTERIOSCLEROSIS
[1] Fulder, Stephen, "Sniffing Out the Truth About Garlic," *Townsend Letter for Doctors*, p. 1024, November 1992.

[2] I-San Lin, Robert, "Garlic and Health: Recent Advances in Research," Irvine, CA, p. 5, 1992.

[3] "Intermittant Claudication: Trental vs. Ginkgo Biloba Extract," *American Journal of Natural Medicine*, v. 2, n. 1, p. 12, January/February 1995.

[4] Superko, H. Robert, "Amino Acid Defect Causes 20 Percent of Atherosclerosis in CHD," *Family Practice News*, p. 7, October 15, 1994.

[5] Russell, Robert M., "Nutrition," *JAMA, The Journal of the American Medical Association*, June 1, 1994.

[6] Superko, H. Robert, "Amino Acid Defect Causes 20 Percent of Atherosclerosis in CHD," *Family Practice News*, p. 7, October 15, 1994.

[7] Boers, G.H.J., "Hyperhomocysteinemia: A Newly Recognized Risk Factor For Vascular Disease," *Netherlands Journal of Medicine*, v. 45, p. 34, 1994.

[8] Gaby, Alan R., "The Story of Vitamin E," *Nutrition and Healing*, p. 4, October 1994.

[9] "Pharmacologic Doses of Vitamin E Improve Insulin Action in Healthy Subjects and Non-Insulin-Dependent Diabetic Patients," *American Journal of Clinical Nutrition*, May 1993.

[10] Brown, Katrina M., et al, "Vitamin E Supplementation Suppresses Indexes of Lipid Peroxidation and Platelet Counts in Blood of Smokers and Nonsmokers But Plasma Lipoprotein Concentrations Remain Unchanged," *American Journal of Clinical Nutrition*, v. 60, p. 383, 1994.

Chapter 12: ARTHRITIS

[1] Burton Goldberg Group, *Alternative Medicine, The Definitive Guide*, Future Medicine Publishing, Inc., Puyallup, WA, p. 532, 1993.

[2] Geusens, Piet, et al, "Long-Term Effect of Omega-3 Fatty Acid Supplementation in Active Rheumatoid Arthritis: A 12-Month, Double-Blind, Controlled Study," *Arthritis and Rheumatism*, v. 37, p. 824, June 1994.

[3] Faelten, Sharon, *The Complete Book of Minerals for Health*, Rodale Press, Emmaus, PA, p. 406, 1981.

[4] Roubenoff, Ronenn, et al, "Abnormal Vitamin B6 Status in Rheumatoid Cachexia," *Arthritis and Rheumatism*, v. 38, p. 105, January 1995.

[5] de Vries, Jan, *Life Without Arthritis - The Maori Way*, Mainstream Publishing, London, 1991.

[6] Burton Goldberg Group, *Alternative Medicine, The Definitive Guide*, Future Medicine Publishing, Inc., Puyallup, WA, p. 535, 1993.

[7] Srivastava, R. and Srimal, R.C., et al, "Modification of Certain Inflammation-Induced Biochemical Changes by Curcumin," *Indian Journal of Medical Research*, v. 81, p. 215, February 1985.

[8] Arora, R.B., et al, "Anti-Inflammatory Studies on Curcuma Longa," *Indian Journal of Medical Research*, v. 59, p. 1289, August 1971.

[9] D'Ambrosio, E., et al., "Glucosamine Sulfate: A Controlled Clinical Investigation in Arthrosis," *Pharmatherapeutica*, v. 2, p. 504, 1981.

[10] Vaz, AL., "Double-blind Clinical Evaluation of the Relative Efficacy of Glucosamine Sulphate in the Mangement of Osteoarthritis of the Knee in Outpatients," *Current Medical Resident Opinion*, v. 8, p. 145, 1982.

Chapter 13: ASTHMA

[1] "Blowing Away Allergies," Anti-Aging News, *Longevity*, p. 16, April 1995.

[2] McLean, Robert, "Magnesium and Its Therapeutic Uses: A Review," *The American Journal of Medicine*, v. 96, p. 71, January 1994.

[3] Britton J, Pavord I, Richards K, Wisniewski A, Knox A, Lewis S, et al., "Dietary Magnesium, Lung Function, Wheezing, and Airway Hyperreactivity in a Random Adult Population Sample, *The Lancet*, v. 344, p. 357, 1994.

[4] Gaby, Alan, Research Review, "Magnesium--Help for Asthma," *Nutrition and Healing*, p. 10-11, October 1994.

[5] Power, Lawrence, "Food and Fitness Change in Diet May Help Relieve Asthma Patient, *Los Angeles Times*, p. 7, September 23, 1985.

[6] Pauling, Linus, *How to Live Longer and Feel Better*, W. H. Freeman and Company, New York, p. 269, 1986.

[7] Carper, Jean, *The Food Pharmacy*, Bantam Books, New York, p. 218, 1985.

[8] Douglas, D.E., "4.4'-Diacetyl Curcumin--In-Vitro Histamine-Blocking Activity," *Journal Pharm. Pharmacol.*, v. 45, p. 766, 1993.

[9] Gaby, Alan, *B6: The Natural Healer*, Keats Publishing, New Canaan, CT, p. 170, 1987.

[10] Call, Janice, *Natural Healing Encyclopedia*, FC & A Inc., Peachtree City, GA, p. 21, 1987.

Chapter 15: ATTENTION DEFICIT DISORDER

[1] Leung, Alexander K.C.; Robson, Wm. Lane M.; Fagan, Joel E.; Lim, Stephen H.N., "Attention-Deficit Hyperactivity Disorder: Getting Control of Impulsive Behavior, *Postgraduate Medicine*, v. 95, n.2, p. 153, Feb 1, 1994.

[2] Burton Goldberg Group, *Alternative Medicine, The Definitive Guide*, Future Medicine Publishing, Inc., Puyallup, WA, p. 610, 1993.

[3] Ibid, p. 541.

[4] Hettinger, Mary Ellen, "Help! My Child is Hyperactive! Causes can Includes Allergies, Hypoglycemia or Poor Diet-Nutritional Therapy is the Key," *Health News & Review*, v. 1, n. 2, July-August 1991.

[5] Burton Goldberg Group, *Alternative Medicine, The Definitive Guide*, Future Medicine Publishing, Inc., Puyallup, WA, p. 499, 1993.

[6] Crook, W.D. & Stevens, L, *Solving the Puzzle of Your Hard to Raise Child*, Professional Books, Jackson, TN, 1987.

[7] Rimland, Bernard, "Nature's Solutions to Children's Learning Disabilities Include Whole Foods, Nutrition: Junk Food May Make 'Monsters' out of Many due to Unsuspected Food Allergy; Drugs are Not the Answer," *Health News & Review*, v.3, n. 3, p. , Summer 1993.

[8] Coleman, Mary, "Clinical Presentations of Patients with Autism and Hypocalcinuria," *Developmental Brain Dysfunction*, v. 7, p. 63, 1994.

Chapter 16: BACK PAIN

[1] Wright, Jonathan V., *Dr. Wright's Book of Nutritional Therapy*, Rodale Press, Emmaus, PA, p. 319-320, 1979.

[2] Challem, Jack, "How to Use Vitamins and Minerals as Home Remedies," *Natural Health*, v. 24, n. 2, p. 60, March-April 1994.

[3] Ibid.

4   Mindell, Earl, *Earl Mindell's Food as Medicine*, Simon & Schuster, New York, p. 62, 1994.
5   Trowbridge, J.P., M.D. & Faber, William J., D.O., *Do What You Want to Do*, Appleday Press, Houston, TX, 1996.
6   Burton Goldberg Group, *Alternative Medicine, The Definitive Guide*, Future Medicine Publishing, Inc., Puyallup, WA, p. 547, 1993.
7   Malmivaara, Antti, M.D., Ph.D., et al, "The Treatment of Acute Low Back Pain--Bed Rest, Exercises, Or Ordinary Activity?" *The New England Journal of Medicine*, v. 332, n. 6, p. 351, February 9, 1995.

Chapter 17:   BAD BREATH
1   Hodges, R.E., et al, *American Journal of Clinical Nutrition*, v. 11, p. 181, 1962.

Chapter 18:   BELL'S PALSY
1   *Churchill's Illustrated Medical Dictionary*, Churchill Livingstone Inc., New York, NY., p. 1362, 1989.
2   "Herpes Simplex May Cause Bell's Palsy," *Executive Health's Good Health Report*, v. 32, n. 9, p. 8, June 1996.
3   Dyck, Peter J., et al, "Diagnosis and Care of Bell's Palsy," *Patient Care*, v. 22, n. 17, p. 107-117, October 30, 1988.
4   Thornton, Jim, "Crooked Man," *Men's Health*, v. 6, n. 5, p. 32-34, October 1991.

Chapter 19:   BERIBERI
1   Werbach, Melvyn R., *Nutritional Influences on Illness*, Keats Publishing, New Canaan, CT, p. 493, 1988.
2   Murray, Frank, "Bone Up on B Vitamins: Part One," *Better Nutrition*, v. 51, n. 10, p. 8, October 1989.
3   Hoffer, Abram, *Orthomolecular Medicine for Physicians*, Keats Publishing, New Canaan, CT, p. 33, 1989.
4   Murray, Frank, "Bone Up on B Vitamins: Part One," *Better Nutrition*, v. 51, n. 10, p. 8, October 1989.
5   Hoffer, Abram, *Orthomolecular Medicine for Physicians*, Keats Publishing, New Canaan, CT, p. 32, 1989.
6   Murray, Frank, "Bone Up on B Vitamins: Part One," *Better Nutrition*, v. 51, n. 10, p. 8, October 1989.
7   "Alert: Thiamine-Deficient Total Parenteral Nutrition," *Patient Care*, v. 23, n. 9, p. 24, May 15, 1989.

Chapter 20:   BODY ODOR
1   Furtado, Teo, *Health*, v. 7, n. 3, p. 36, May-June 1993.
2   Faelten, Sharon, *The Complete Book of Minerals for Health*, Rodale Press, Emmaus, PA, p. 386, 1981.

Chapter 21:   BREASTFEEDING
1   Liebman, Bonnie, "Baby Formula: Missing Key Fats?" *Nutrition Action Healthletter*, v. 17, n. 8, p. 8, October 1990.

2 Burton Goldberg Group, *Alternative Medicine, The Definitive Guide*, Future Medicine Publishing, Inc., Puyallup, WA, p. 808, 1993.

3 Lucas, A., et al., "Breast Milk and Subsequent Intelligence Quotient in Children Born Preterm," *The Lancet*, v. 339, n. 8788, p. 261-264, February 1992.

4 Kamen, Betty & Si, *Total Nutrition for Breastfeeding Mothers*, Little, Brown and Company, p. 42, 1986.

5 *Martindale, The Extra Pharmacopoeia, Thirtieth Edition*, Department of Pharmaceutical Sciences, Royal Pharmaceutical Society of Great Britain, The Pharmaceutical Press, p. 1878, 1993.

Chapter 22: BRONCHITIS AND PNEUMONIA

1 Lipstitch, Marc, "Fears Growing Over Bacteria Resistant to Antibiotics," *World Wide Web*, September 12, 1995.

2 Ibid.

3 Ibid.

4 Gonzales, Ralph and Sande, Merle, "What Will It Take to Stop Physicians From Prescribing Antibiotics in Acute Bronchitis?" *The Lancet*, v. 345, p. 665, March 18, 1995.

5 Rubenstein, E. and Federman D., *Scientific American Medicine*, Scientific American, Inc., New York, p. 7, 1984.

6 Gloeckner, Carolyn, "Where There's Smoke, There's Disease," *Current Health 2*, v. 17, n. 3, p. 14, November 1990.

7 "2.7 Million U.S. Teenagers Smoke," *Cancer Researcher Weekly*, p. 9, February 28, 1994.

8 Ibid.

9 Gloeckner, Carolyn, "Where There's Smoke, There's Disease," *Current Health 2*, v. 17, n. 3, p. 14, November 1990.

10 "Chronic Disease Reports: Chronic Obstructive Pulmonary Disease Mortality," *Morbidity and Mortality Weekly Report*, v3. 8, n. 32, p. 549, August 18, 1989.

11 Murray, Michael, M.D. and Pizzorno, Joseph, N.D., *Encyclopedia of Natural Medicine*, Prima Publishing, Rocklin, CA, p. 175-177, 1991.

12 Davelaar, F.G. and Bos, J. Van Den, "Ascorbic Acid and Infectious Bronchitis Infections in Broilers," *Avian Pathology*, v. 21, p. 581- 589, 1992.

13 Schwartz, Joel and Weiss, Scott T., "Relationship Between Dietary Vitamin C Intake and Pulmonary Function in the First National Health and Nutrition Examination Survey (NHANES I)," *American Journal of Clinical Nutrition*, v. 59, p. 110-114, 1994.

14 Rodale, J.I., et al., *The Complete Book of Vitamins*, Rodale Book, Inc., Emmaus, PA, 1970.

15 Atkins, Robert C., M.D., *Dr. Atkins' Health Revolution*, Houghton Mifflin Co., Boston, MA, 1988.

16 Davelaar, F.G. and Bos, J. Van Den, "Ascorbic Acid and Infectious Bronchitis Infections in Broilers," *Avian Pathology*, v. 21, p. 581- 589, 1992.

17 Quillin, Patrick, *Healing Nutrients*, Contemporary Books, Chicago, 1987.

18 Skobeloff, Emil M., M.D., et al, "Magnesium Sulfate For the Treatment of Bronchospasm Complicating Acute Bronchitis in a Four-Months'-Pregnant Woman," *Annals of Emergency Medicine*, v. 22, n. 8, p. 1365-1367, August 1993.

19 "Blowing Away Allergies," Anti-Aging News, *Longevity*, p. 16, April 1995.

[20] McLean, Robert, "Magnesium and Its Therapeutic Uses: A Review," *The American Journal of Medicine*, v. 96, p. 71, January 1994.
[21] Britton J, Pavord I, Richards K, Wisniewski A, Knox A, Lewis S, et al., "Dietary Magnesium, Lung Function, Wheezing, and Airway Hyperreactivity in a Random Adult Population Sample, *The Lancet*, v. 344, p. 357, 1994.
[22] Skorodin, M.S., et al, "Magnesium Sulfate in Exacerbations of Chronic Obstructive Pulmonary Disease," *Archives of Internal Medicine*, v. 155, p. 496-500, 1995.
[23] Murray, Michael, M.D. and Pizzorno, Joseph, N.D., *Encyclopedia of Natural Medicine*, Prima Publishing, Rocklin, CA, p. 175-177, 1991.
[24] Ibid.

Chapter 23: BRUISES

[1] Goldberg Group, *Alternative Medicine, The Definitive Guide*, Future Medicine Publishing, Inc., Puyallup, WA, p. 892, 1993.
[2] Challem, Jack, "How to use Vitamins and Minerals as Home Remedies," *Natural Health*, v. 24, n. 2, p. 60, March-April 1994.
[3] Vogel, H.C.A., *The Nature Doctor*, Keats Publishing, New Canaan, CT, p. 13, 1991.

Chapter 24: BUNIONS

[1] Hecht, Annabel, "Caring for Corns, Bunions and Other Agonies of De-feet," *FDA Consumer*, v. 19, p. 22, June 1985.
[2] Conkling, Winifred, "Are Your Feet Killing You?, *American Health*, v. 13, n. 3, p. 76, April 1994.
[3] Ibid.
[4] Ibid.
[5] Ibid
[6] *Consumer Reports on Health*, v. 4, n. 1, p. 4, January 1992.

Chapter 25: BURNING MOUTH SYNDROME

[1] Blitzer, Andrew, D.D.S., M.D., "What Causes Burning Sensation in Mouth and Tongue," *Consultant*, v. 13, July 1991.
[2] Cinquino, Louis, "Quench the fire! Getting Relief from Burning-Mouth Pain," *Prevention*, v. 46, n. 10, p. 76, October 1994.
[3] Krause, W., et al, "Fungemia and Funguria After Oral Administration of Candida Albicans," *The Lancet*, p. 598-599, March 22, 1969.
[4] Crook, William, "Candida: Acidophilus and Herbal Remedies, Along with an Elimination Diet May Help Sufferers of Chronic Yeast Infections Regain Their Health," *Better Nutrition for Today's Living*, v. 52, n. 5, p. 20, May 1990.
[5] Lamb, A.B., et al, "Oral Carriage of Candida Species and Coliforms in Patients with Burning Mouth Syndrome," *Southern Journal of Oral and Pathological Medicine*, v. 18, n. 4, p. 233-235, 1989.
[6] Tammiala-Salonen, T., et al, "Burning Mouth in a Finnish Adult Population," *Community Dentistry and Oral Epidemiology*, v. 21, p. 67-71, 1993.
[7] Maragou, P., et al, "Serum Zinc Levels in Patients With Burning Mouth Syndrome," *Oral Surgery, Oral Medicine, Oral Pathology*, v. 71, p. 447-450, 1991.

[8] Huang-W, et al, "The Burning Mouth Syndrome," *Journal of the American Academy of Dermatology*, v. 34, p. 1, 1996.

[9] "Hot Pepper Cream Cools Burning Skin," *Insight*, p. 54, October 23, 1989.

[10] Ibid.

[11] McCaleb, Rob, "Cayenne: A Spicy Remedy," *Better Nutrition for Today's Living*, v. 55, n. 10, p. 52, October 1993.

[12] Nelson, Corinna, "Heal the Burn: Pepper and Lasers in Cancer Pain Therapy," *Journal of the National Cancer Institute*, v. 86, n. 18, p. 1381-1382, September 21, 1994.

Chapter 26: BURNS

[1] Mazzotta, Mary Y., "Nutrition and Wound Healing," *Journal of the American Podiatric Medical Association*, v. 84, n. 9, p. 456, September 1994.

[2] *Martindale, The Extra Pharmacopoeia, Thirtieth Edition*, Department of Pharmaceutical Sciences, Royal Pharmaceutical Society of Great Britain, The Pharmaceutical Press, p. 2361-2362, 1993.

[3] Berger, M.M., et al, "Cutaneous Copper and Zinc Losses in Burns," *Burns*, v. 18, n. 5, p. 373, 1992.

[4] Chiarelli, Angelo, et. al, "Very Early Nutrition Supplementation in Burned Patients," *American Journal of Clinical Nutrition*, v. 51, n. 6, p. 1035, June 1990.

[5] McBride, Gail, "Test Formula Helps Burn Patients," *Medical World News*, v. 30, n. 9, p. 23, May 8, 1989.

[6] Mazzotta, Mary Y., "Nutrition and Wound Healing," *Journal of the American Podiatric Medical Association*, v. 84, n. 9, p. 456, September 1994.

[7] Ibid.

[8] Null, Gary, *The Complete Guide to Health and Nutrition*, Dell Publishing, Inc., New York, NY, p. 301, 1984.

[9] Paolisso, Giuseppe, et. al., Pharmacologic Doses of Vitamin E Improve Insulin Action in Healthy Subjects and Non-Insulin-Dependent Diabetic Patients," *American Journal of Clinical Nutrition*, v. 57, n. 5, p. 650, May 1993.

[10] Mazzotta, Mary Y., "Nutrition and Wound Healing," *Journal of the American Podiatric Medical Association*, v. 84, n. 9, p. 456, September 1994.

[11] Rota, Francine, "The Natural First-Aid Kit: A Collection of Gentle and Effective Remedies to Treat Life's Bumps and Bruises," *East West*, v. 21, n. 7, p. 70, July-August 1991.

[12] Ibid.

[13] Keville, Kathi, "Respect Your Elder," *Vegetarian Times*, n. 154, p. 62, June 1990.

[14] Schechter, Steven R., "Aloe Vera, Produces Anti-Inflammatory, Immune Strengthening Effects on Skin," p. 51, *Let's Live*, December 1994.

[15] Murray, Frank, "Therapy and Treatment With Aloe Vera," *Better Nutrition for Today's Living*, v. 56, n. 3, p. 52, March 1994.

[16] Rota, Francine, "The Natural First-Aid Kit: A Collection of Gentle and Effective Remedies to Treat Life's Bumps and Bruises," *East West*, v. 21, n. 7, p. 70, July-August 1991.

[17] Subrahmanyam, M., "Honey-Impregnated Gauze Versus Amniotic Membrane in the Treatment of Burns," *Burns*, v. 20, p. 331, 1994.

[18] Gaby, Alan R., "Literature Review and Commentary," *Townsend Letter for Doctors*, n. 143, p. 25, June 1995.

Chapter 27: BURSITIS

[1] DeBenedette,Valerie, "Elway's elbow: A Case Study in Traumatic Bursitis, *Physician and Sportsmedicine*, v. 17, n. 11, p. 116, November 1989.
[2] McCoy, Hal, "Mario Soto Diagnosed With Bursitis," *The Sporting News*, v. 201, p. 29, June 9, 1986.
[3] Verrell, Gordon, "Dodgers' Chances Left with Welch," *The Sporting News*, v. 196, p. 31, October 17, 1983.
[4] Sporkin, Elizabeth; Cunneff, Tom, "What The Doctor Ordered," (Emma Samms) *People Weekly*, v. 37, n. 5, p. 63, February 10, 1992.
[5] Bryant, John, "On the Edge," (Paul Pilkington) *Runner's World*, v. 25, n. 9, p. 76, September 1990.
[6] Lieber, Jill, "This Johnny's on the Spot," (John Riggins) *Sports Illustrated*, v. 63, p. 36, August 26, 1985.
[7] Toperoff, Sam, "Open Season in Pittsburgh," (Mark Malone) *Sports Illustrated*, v. 67, p. 96, September 9, 1987.
[8] "Bursitis: Prevention and Protection," University of California, *Berkeley Wellness Letter*, v. 9, n. 9, p. 6, June 1993.
[9] Wright, Jonathan V., *Dr. Wright's Book of Nutritional Therapy*, Rodale Press, Emmaus, PA, p. 129-134, 1979.
[10] Srivastava, R.and Srimal, R.C., et al, "Modification of Certain Inflammation-Induced Biochemical Changes by Curcumin," *Indian Journal of Medical Research*, v. 81, p. 215, February 1985.
[11] Arora, R.B., et al, "Anti-Inflammatory Studies on Curcuma Longa," *Indian Journal of Medical Research*, v. 59, p. 1289, August 1971.
[12] Murray, Michael, M.D. and Pizzorno, Joseph, N.D., *Encyclopedia of Natural Medicine*, Prima Publishing, Rocklin, CA, p. 514-515, 1991.

Chapter 28: CANCER, BLADDER

[1] Fackelmann, K.A., "Hints of a Chlorine-Cancer Connection," *Science News*, v. 142, p. 23, July 11, 1992.
[2] Silverman, Debra T., et al, "Occupational Risks of Bladder Cancer Among White Women in The United States," *American Journal of Epidemiology*, v. 132, n. 3, p. 453-461, 1990.
[3] Vena, John E., "Coffee, Cigarette Smoking, and Bladder Cancer in Western New York," *Annals of Epidemiology*, v. 3, p. 586, 1993.
[4] Schlegel, J.U., et al, "The Role of Ascorbic Acid in the Prevention of Bladder Tumor Formation," *The Journal of Urology*, p. 155, 1980.
[5] Laino, Charlene, "Vitamins Boost Bladder Cancer Survival Rates," *Medical Tribune*, v. 3, June 10, 1993.
[6] Lamm, Donald L., et al, "Megadose Vitamins and Bladder Cancer: A Double-Blind Clinical Trial, " *The Journal of Urology*, v. 151, p. 21, January 1994.

[7] Marsh, Christopher L, et. al, "Superiority of Intravesical Immunotherapy with Coryne-bacterium Parvum and Allium Sativum in Control of Murine Bladder Cancer," *The Journal of Urology*, v. 137, p. 359-362, February 1987.

Chapter 29: CANCER, BREAST

[1] Neergaard, Lauren, "Breast Cancer Cases Top Malpractice Suits," *Associated Press*, June 3, 1995.
[2] James, Wesley, "Breast Cancer, Have We Lost Our Way?" *World Research Foundation News*, p. 3, First Quarter, 1993.
[3] Editorial, "Breast Cancer, Have We Lost Our Way?" *The Lancet*, v. 341, n. 8841, p. 343, February 6, 1993.
[4] Evans, Imogen, "The Challenge of Breast Cancer," *The Lancet*, v. 343, n. 8905, p. 1085, April 30, 1994.
[5] Challem, Jack, "Breast Cancer: Tracing It's Elusive Causes and Leveraging Dietary Strat-egies to Prevent It," *Let's Live*, p. 19, November 1994.
[6] Whitaker, Julian, "Preventing Breast Cancer," *Health and Healing*, January 1994.
[7] Challem, Jack, "Breast Cancer: Tracing It's Elusive Causes and Leveraging Dietary Strat-egies to Prevent It," *Let's Live*, p. 19, November 1994.
[8] Evans, Imogen, "The Challenge of Breast Cancer," *The Lancet*, v. 343, n. 8905, p. 1085, April 30, 1994.
[9] "Foods That May Prevent Breast Cancer: Studies Are Investigating Soybeans, Whole Wheat and Green Tea Among Others," *Primary Care and Cancer*, n. 14, p. 10-11, Feb-ruary 1994.
[10] Mindell, Earl L, "Soy-When Will We Learn?" column Stay Healthy, *Let's Live*, p. 10, January 1995.
[11] Challem, Jack, "Breast Cancer: Tracing It's Elusive Causes and Leveraging Dietary Strat-egies to Prevent It," *Let's Live*, p. 19, November 1994.
[12] "Research Shows Garlic Inhibits Breast Cancer," *Daily Standard*, Celina, OH, February 25, 1994.
[13] Cowan, L.D., et al, "Breast Cancer Incidence in Women with a History of Progesterone Deficiency," *American Journal of Epidemiology*, v. 114, p. 209-217, 1981.

Chapter 30: CANCER, CERVICAL

[1] Krebs, E.T., Speech to National Health Federation, Los Angeles, 1979.
[2] "Researchers Link Cervical Cancer, Viruses," *The Sacramento Bee/Baltimore Sun*, June 7, 1995.
[3] Murray, Michael, M.D. and Pizzorno, Joseph, N.D., *Encyclopedia of Natural Medicine*, Prima Publishing, Rocklin, CA, p. 207, 1991.
[4] *Medical Hotline*, v. 5, n. 1, p. 4, January 1984.
[5] *The Practical Encyclopedia of Natural Healing*, Rodale Press, Inc., Emmaus, PA, p. 109, 1983.
[6] Butterworth, C., Hatch, K., Gore, H., et al., "Improvement in Cervical Dysplasia Associ-ated with Folic Acid Therapy in Users of Oral Contraceptives," *American Journal of Clinical Nutrition*, p. 73, 1982.
[7] *New England Journal of Medicine*, April 22, 1971.
[8] Herbst, A.L., "DES Clear Cell Cancer-1992," *Cancer Weekly*, p. 18, April 19, 1993.

[9] Gerras, Charles, et al, eds, *The Encyclopedia of Common Diseases*, Rodale Press, Inc. Emmaus, PA, p. 301, 1976.

[10] Orr, J., Wilson, K., Bodiford, C. et al., "Nutritional Status of Patients with Untreated Cervical Cancer II, Vitamin Assessment," *American Journal of Obstetrics and Gynecology*, p. 632, 1985.

[11] Herbert, Victor, Genell J. Subak-Sharpe, *The Mt. Sinai School of Medicine Complete Book of Nutrition*, St. Martin's Press, New York, p. 478, 1990.

[12] VanEenwyk, Juliet, "The Role of Vitamins in the Development of Cervical Cancer," *The Nutrition Report*, v. 11, n. 1, p. 8, January 1993.

[13] Dawson, E., Nosovitch, J. and Hannigan, E., "Serum Vitamin and Selenium Changes in Cervical Dysplasia," *Fed. Proc.*, p. 612, 1984.

[14] Wassertheil-Smoller, S., Ronmey, S., Whylie-Rosett, J., et al., "Dietary Vitamin C and Uterine Cervical Dysplasia," *American Journal of Epidemiology*, p. 714, 1981.

[15] Palan, Prabhudas R., et al, "Plasma Levels of Antioxidant Beta-Carotene and a-Tocopherol in Uterine Cervix Dysplasia and Cancer," *Nutrition and Cancer*, v. 15, p. 13-20, 1991.

[16] Murray, Michael, M.D. and Pizzorno, Joseph, N.D., *Encyclopedia of Natural Medicine*, Prima Publishing, Rocklin, CA, p. 207, 1991.

Chapter 31: CANCER, COLON

[1] Kunin, Richard, *Mega Nutrients*, McGraw-Hill, New York, p. 81, 1981.

[2] Brohier, Catherine, "Diet May Shield Against Two Leading Cancer Killers," *Environmental Nutrition*, v.15, n.2, p. 1, February 1992.

[3] Lieberman, Shari, "Good Nutrition Can Prevent Colon Cancer," *Better Nutrition*, v.51, n.7, p. 10, July 1989.

[4] Wakunaga of America, "Aged Garlic Extract and Intestinal Flora," 1993.

[5] Sumiyoshi, Hiromichi & Wargovich, Michael J, "Chemoprevention of 1,2-Dimethylhydrazine-induced Colon Cancer in Mice by Naturally Occurring Organosulfur Compounds," *Cancer Research*, v.50, p. 5084-5087, August 15, 1990.

[6] Pauling, Linus, *How to Live Longer and Feel Better*, W.H. Freeman & Co., New York, NY, p. 347, 1986.

[7] Carper, Jean, *The Food Pharmacy*, Bantam Books, New York, p. 57, 1988.

[8] Franceschi, S., et al, "Tomatoes and Risk of Digestive-Tract Cancers," *Int J Cancer*, v. 59, p. 181-184, 1994.

[9] Mangels, A.R, et al, "Carotenoid Content of Fruits and Vegetables, An Evaluation of Analytic Data," *Journal of the American Dietetic Association*, v. 93, p. 284-286, 1993.

[10] Phillips, Raymond W., et al, "Beta-Carotene Inhibits Rectal Mucosal Ornithine Decarboxylase Activity in Colon Cancer Patients," *Cancer Research*, v. 53, p. 3723-3725, August 15, 1993.

[11] Mason, Joel B., "Folate and Colonic Carcinogenesis: Searching for a Mechanistic Understanding," *Journal of Nutritional Biochemistry*, v. 5, p. 170-175, April 1994.

[12] Dwyer, Johanna T., DSc, RD, et al, "Tofu and Soy Drinks Contain Phytoestrogens," *Journal of the American Dietetic Association*, v. 7, p. 739-742, July 1994.

[13] Steele, Vernon E., et al, "Cancer Chemoprevention Agent Development Strategies for Genistein," *Journal of Nutrition*, v. 125, p. 713-716, 1995.

Chapter 32: CANCER, LIVER

1 Murray, Michael, M.D. and Pizzorno, Joseph, N.D., *Encyclopedia of Natural Medicine*, Prima Publishing, Rocklin, CA, p. 77, 1991.
2 Canty, David J., "Lecithin and Choline in Human Health and Disease," *Nutrition Reviews*, v. 52, n. 10, p. 327-339, October 1994.
3 Yu, Mimi C., *Journal of the National Cancer Institute*, v. 83, n. 24, p. 1820, December 18, 1991.
4 Rivlin, Richard S., "Magnesium Deficiency and Alcohol Intake," *Journal of the American College of Nutrition*, v. 13, n. 5, p. 416-423, October 1994.
5 "Green Tea Found to Inhibit Cancer in Animal Study," *Food Chemical News*, v. 36, n. 6, April 4, 1994.

Chapter 33: CANCER, LUNG

1 Mayne, Susan Taylor, et al, "Dietary Beta-Carotene and Lung Cancer Risk in U.S. Nonsmokers," *Journal of the National Cancer Institute*, v. 86, n. 1, p. 33-38, January 5, 1994.
2 *Secondhand Smoke*, Pamphlet by the American Lung Association, June 1988.
3 Fontham, Elizabeth T.H., Dr. P. H., et al, "Environmental Tobacco Smoke and Lung Cancer in Nonsmoking Women, A Multicenter Study," *Journal of the American Medical Association*, v. 271, n. 22, p. 1752-1759, June 8, 1994.
4 Paul, John A., "Urban Air Quality: the Problem," *EPA Journal*, p. 24, January/February 1991.
5 Gerras, Charles, et al, eds, *The Encyclopedia of Common Diseases*, Rodale Press, Inc. Emmaus, PA, p. 311, 1976.
6 *Cancer Researcher Weekly*, December 1993
7 *Breath in Danger II*, The American Lung Association, April 30, 1993.
8 Passwater, Richard A., Ph.D., *Supernutrition*, The Dial Press, New York, 1975.
9 Pastorino, U., et al, "Adjuvant Treatment of Stage I Lung Cancer With High-Dose Vitamin A," *Journal of Clinical Oncology*, v. 11, p. 1216-1222, 1993.
10 "Nutrition and Cancer Study," Melbourne, Australia, University of Melbourne, Department of Medicine, 1989.
11 Mayne, Susan Taylor, et al, "Dietary Beta-Carotene and Lung Cancer Risk in U.S. Nonsmokers," *Journal of the National Cancer Institute*, v. 86, n. 1, p. 33-38, January 5, 1994.
12 Van den Brandt, P., et al, "A Prospective Cohort Study on Selenium Status and the Risk of Lung Cancer," *Cancer Research*, v. 53, p. 4860-4865, 1993.
13 Raloff, Janet, "Saturated Fats May Foster Lung Cancer," *Science News*, p. 373, December 4, 1993.
14 Miller, A.B., M.B., FRCP.,et al, "Diet in the Etiology of Cancer: A Review," *European Journal of Cancer*, v. 30A, n. 2 p. 207-228, 1994.

Chapter 34: CANCER, OVARIAN

1 Wilder, Gene, "Why did Gilda Die?" *People Weekly*, v. 35, n. 21, p. 76, June 3, 1991
2 "Died, Gilda Radner (obituary)," *Time*, v. 133, n. 22, p. 77, May 29, 1989.
3 Sachs, Jessica Snyder, "To Risk Your Life for Fertility Drugs?" Longevity, v. 7, n. 6, p. 34, May 1995.

4 "Milk May Impair Fertility in Women," *Science News*, p. 175, March 12, 1994.
5 Risch, Harvey A., et al, "Dietary Fat Intake and Risk of Epithelial Ovarian Cancer," *Journal of the National Cancer Institute*, v. 86, n. 18, p. 1409-1415, September 21, 1994.
6 Gerras, Charles, et al, eds, *The Encyclopedia of Common Diseases*, Rodale Press, Inc. Emmaus, PA, p. 267, 1976.
7 Griffiths, Keith, Dr., "Talc and Carcinoma of the Ovary and Cervix," *Journal of Obstetrics and Gynecology*, March 1971.
8 "Talc Linked to Cancer Risk in Women," *Medical Tribune*, p. 21, April 20, 1995.

Chapter 35: CANCER, PANCREATIC
1 Murray, Michael, M.D. and Pizzorno, Joseph, N.D., *Encyclopedia of Natural Medicine*, Prima Publishing, Rocklin, CA, p. 52, 1991.
2 Burton Goldberg Group, *Alternative Medicine, The Definitive Guide*, Future Medicine Publishing, Inc., Puyallup, WA, p. 219-221, 1993.
3 Dunne, Lavon J., *Nutrition Almanac*, Third Edition, McGraw-Hill Publishing Company, p. 90, 1990.
4 Comstock, George, et al, "Prediagnostic Serum Levels of Carotenoids and Vitamin E as Related to Subsequent Cancer in Washington County, Maryland," *American Journal of Clinical Nutrition*, v. 53, p. 260-264, 1991.
5 Zatonski, W., et al, "Nutritional Factors and Pancreatic Cancer: A Case-Controlled Study From Southwest Poland," *International Journal of Cancer*, v. 48, p. 390-394, 1991.
6 Horrobin, David F., "Review Article: Medical Uses of Essential Fatty Acids," *Veterinary Dermatology*, v. 4, n. 4, p. 161-166, 1993.

Chapter 36: CANCER PREVENTION
1 Block, Gladys, "Vitamin C and Cancer Prevention, The Epidemiologic Evidence, *American Journal of Clinical Nutrition*, January 1991.
2 "Beyond Vitamins," *Newsweek*, April 25, 1994
3 Gerras, Charles, et al, eds, *The Encyclopedia of Common Diseases*, Rodale Press, Inc. Emmaus, PA, p. 351, 1976.
4 "Recent Research Supports the Cardiovascular and Cancer Protective Benefits of Garlic," press release, May 27, 1994.
5 "Green Tea Shown to Have Anti-cancer Effect in Rodents," *Food Chemical News*, v. 36, n.11, CRC Press, Inc., May 9, 1994.

Chapter 37: CANCER, PROSTATE
1 Speech by Dr. Epstein at the American College of Advancement in Medicine's Fall Conference 1994, San Diego, California, November 2-5, 1994.
2 Morrison, Howard I., et al, "Herbicides and Cancer," *Journal of the National Cancer Institute*, v. 84, p. 1866-1874, 1992.
3 Faelton, Sharon, *The Complete Book of Minerals for Health*, Rodale Books, Emmaus, PA, p. 427, 1981.
4 Miller, A.B., et al, "Diet in the Etiology of Cancer: A Review," *European Journal of Cancer*, v. 30A, n. 2, p. 207-228, 1994.

5 Kugler, Hans, et al, *Life Extenders and Memory Boosters*, Health Quest Publications, Reno, Nevada, p. 169, 1993.
6 Herbert, Victor, Genell J. Subak-Sharpe, *The Mt. Sinai School of Medicine Complete Book of Nutrition*, St. Martin's Press, New York, p. 472, 1990.
7 "Meat's Risk for Cancer: Just Bologna?...Not When it's Prostate Cancer," *Science News*, v. 145, n. 8, p. 126, February 19, 1994.
8 Adlercreutz, Herman, et al, "Plasma Concentrations of Phyto-Estrogens in Japanese Men," *The Lancet*, v. 342, p. 1209-1210, November 13, 1993.
9 Clarkson, Thomas B., et al, "Estrogenic Soybean, Isoflavones and Chronic Disease Risk and Benefits," *Trends in Endocrinology and Metabolism*, v. 6, p. 11-16, 1995.
10 Peehl, D.M., et al, "Vitamin D and Prostate Cancer," *Journal of Endocrinology Investigation*, v. 17, 1994.
11 McGuire, Rick, "Cancer Prevention under the Sun," *Total Health*, v.13, n.2, p. 18, April 1991.
12 Ibid.

Chapter 38: CANCER, SKIN

1 Thomas, Patricia, "Vitamin C Eyed for Topical Use as Skin Preserver; the Compound Appears to ward off Sun Damage, and the Developer Thinks it May Promote Collagen Synthesis," *Medical World News*, v. 32, n. 3, p. 12, March 1991.
2 Kintish, Lisa, "Sun Protection: Vitamin A Derivatives, Antioxidants Endorsed at Skin Cancer Foundation Conference," *Soap-Cosmetics-Chemical Specialties*, v. 65, n. 5, p. 17, May 1989.
3 Delver, E., & Pence, B.C., "Effects of Dietary Selenium Level on UV-induced Skin Cancer and Epidermal Antioxidant Status," Texas Technical University Health Sciences Center, Lubbock, Texas, *Cancer Researcher Weekly*, p. 48, July 12, 1993.
4 Katiyar, Santosh K., et al, "Inhibition of Tumor Promotion in Murine Skin by Green Tea Polyphenols," *Cancer Weekly*, p. 19, July 20, 1992.
5 Scheer, James F., "Eat Your Tea!" Health Notes, *Health Freedom News*, p. 32-33, November-December 1994.
6 Nishino, H., et al, "Antitumor-Promoting Activity of Allixin, A Stress Compound Produced by Garlic," *The Cancer Journal*, v. 3, n.1, January-February 1990.

Chapter 39: CANCER, STOMACH

1 Guarner, Jeannette, et al, "The Association of Helicobacter Pylori with Gastric Cancer and Preneoplastic Gastric Lesions in Chiapas, Mexico," *Cancer*, v. 71, n. 2, p. 297, January 15, 1993.
2 Doglioni, Claudio, et al, "High Incidence of Primary Gastric Lymphoma in Northeastern Italy," *The Lancet*, v. 339, n. 8797, p. 834, April 4, 1992.
3 Bordi, Cesare, et al, "Gastric Carcinoids and their Precursor Lesions: A Histologic and Immunohistochemical Study of 23 Cases," *Cancer*, v. 67, n. 3, p. 663, February 1, 1991.
4 Griem, M.L., et al, "Cancer Following Radiotherapy for Peptic Ulcer, "*Cancer Researcher Weekly*, p. 23, July 11, 1994.
5 Miller, A.B., et al, "Diet in the Etiology of Cancer: A Review," *European Journal of Cancer*, v. 30, n. 2, p. 207-228, 1994.

6   Tsugane, Shoichiro, et al, "Urinary Salt Excretion and Stomach Cancer Mortality Among Four Japanese Populations," *Cancer Causes and Control*, v. 2, p. 165-168, 1991.
7   Sparnins, Velta L., et al, "Effects of Organosulfur Compounds from Garlic and Onions on Benzopyrene-induced Neoplasia and Glutathione S-Transferase Activity in the Mouse," Department of Laboratory Medicine and Pathology and Department of Chemistry, University of Minnesota, Minneapolis, MN, October 1, 1987.
8   Johnson, Larry E., "The Merging Role of Vitamins as Antioxidants," *Archives of Family Medicine*, v. 3, p. 809-820, September 1994.
9   "Diet and Stomach Cancer in Korea," *Nutrition Research Newsletter*, v. 14, n. 4, p. 47, April 1995.
10 Kono S., Ikeda, M., Tokudome S., et al, "A Case-control Study of Gastric Cancer and Diet in Northern Kyushu, Japan," *Japan Journal of Cancer Research*, p. 1067, 1988.
11 Oguni, I., Chen S. J., Lin, P.Z., et al, "Protection Against Cancer Risk by Japanese Green Tea," *Preventive Medicine*, p. 332, 1992.
12 Scheer, James F., "Eat Your Tea!" Health Notes, *Health Freedom News*, p. 32-33, November-December 1994.

Chapter 40: CARPAL TUNNEL SYNDROME

1   Moore, Louis, "B6 Relieves Carpal Tunnel Syndrome," *Cortlandt Forum*, v. 76, p. 14, June 1994.
2   Reynolds, Robert, "Vitamin Supplements: Current Controversies," *Journal of the American College of Nutrition*, v. 13, n. 2, p. 118-126, 1994.
3   Bernstein, Allan L., M.D. and Dinesen, Jamie S., "Brief Communication: Effect of Pharmacologic Doses of Vitamin B6 on Carpal Tunnel Syndrome, Electroencephalographic Results and Pain," *Journal of the American College of Nutrition*, v. 12, n.1 p. 73-76, 1993.
4   Burton Goldberg Group, *Alternative Medicine, The Definitive Guide*, Future Medicine Publishing, Inc., Puyallup, WA, p. 899, 1993.
5   Challem, Jack, "How to Use Vitamins and Minerals as Home Remedies," *Natural Health*, v. 24, n. 2, p. 60, March-April 1994.
6   Ibid.
7   Mindell, Earl, *Earl Mindell's Food as Medicine*, Simon & Schuster, New York, p. 62, 1994.
8   Murray, Michael, M.D. and Pizzorno, Joseph, N.D., *Encyclopedia of Natural Medicine*, Prima Publishing, Rocklin, CA, p. 190-191, 1991.
9   Ibid.

Chapter 41: CATARACTS

1   Chylack, L.T., "Mechanism of Senile Cataract Formation," *Ophthalmology*, v. 9, n. 6, p. 596-602, 1984.
2   Di Mascio P.; Kaiser S.; Sies H., *Archives of Biochemical Biophysics*, Institut fur Physiologische Chemie I, Universitat Dusseldorf, Dusseldorf Germany, 1989.
3   Werbach, Melvyn R., *Nutritional Influences on Illness*, Keats Publishing, p. 126-127, 1988.
4   Gruning, Carl, "Seeing is Believing!" *Health News & Review*, v. 2, n. 3, p. 1, Summer 1992.

[5] Hankinson, Susan, M.D., *British Medical Journal*, v. 305, p. 335-339, August 8, 1992.
[6] Gutfield, Greg, "The Virtues of Vitamin E: New Research Trumpets Antioxidant's Benefits, *Prevention*, v. 44, n. 11, p. 10, November 1992.
[7] "Antioxidants May Protect Our Eyes," *Better Nutrition for Today's Living*, v. 53, n. 9, p. 10, September 1991.
[8] Murray, Frank, "Antioxidants: Health Allies," *Better Nutrition for Today's Living*, v. 54, n. 10, p. 24, October 1992.
[9] "Antioxidants May Protect Our Eyes," *Better Nutrition for Today's Living*, v. 53, n. 9, p. 10, September 1991.
[10] Ibid.
[11] Murray, Frank, "Keeping an Eye on Good Health," *Better Nutrition for Today's Living*, v. 20, n. 8, p. 8, August 1989.

Chapter 42: CEREBRAL PALSY

[1] Stanley, F.J. and Watson, L, *British Medical Journal*, p. 1658-1662, June 27, 1992.
[2] Leviton, Alan, "Cerebral Palsy is Not on the Decline," *Child Health Alert*, v. 10, p. 3, August 1992.
[3] Leonard, Charles T., "Motor Behavior and Neural Changes Following Perinatal and Adult-Onset Brain Damage: Implications for Therapeutic Interventions," *Physical Therapy*, n. 74, n. 8, p. 753, August 1994.
[4] Scheuerle, Angela E., M.D., et al, "Arginase Deficiency Presenting as Cerebral Palsy," *Pediatrics*, v. 91, n. 5, p. 995-996, May 1993.
[5] Diamond, M.C., Johnson, R.E., Protti, A.M., et al, "Plasticity in the 904-day-old Male Rat Cerebral Cortex," *Exper. Neurol.*, v. 87, p. 309-317, 1985.
[6] Scheibel, A.B., Conrad, T, Perdue, S., et al, "A Quantitative Study of Dendrite Complexity in Selected Areas of the Human Cerebral Cortex," *Brain Cogn.*, v. 12, p. 85-101, 1990.
[7] Diehl, Jackson, "Hungarian Institute Successful in Rehabilitating Cerebral Palsy Victims," *The Washington Post*, February 20, 1988.
[8] Scheuerle, Angela E., M.D., et al, "Arginase Deficiency Presenting as Cerebral Palsy," *Pediatrics*, v. 91, n. 5, p. 995-996, May 1993.
[9] Johnson, Rachel K. and Maeda, Michelle, "Establishing Outpatient Nutrition Services for Children with Cerebral Palsy, *Journal of the American Dietetic Association*, v. 89, n. 10, p. 1504, October 1989.

Chapter 43: CHEMICAL AND HEAVY METAL POISONING

[1] Raloff, Janet, "Sick Buildings: the Ventilation Conundrum," *Science News*, v. 143, n. 13, p. 198, March 27, 1993.
[2] Balch, James F., M.D., and Balch, Phyllis A., *Prescription for Nutritional Healing*, Avery Publishing Group, Garden City Park, N.Y., p. 170, 1990.
[3] *North Shore News*, September 12, 1993, "Lead/Autism Link," *Autism Research Review International*, v. 8, n. 1, p. 5, 1994.
[4] Lustgarden, Steve, "Flexing Your Mental Muscle," *Vegetarian Times*, n. 183, p. 48, November 1992.
[5] "Audit Shows States, EPA Slow to Curb Lead in School Water," *Family Practice News*, v . 20, n. 24, p. 10, December 15-31, 1990.

[6] Sherman, Carl, "Yuppie Dream Home May be Lead Poisoning Hazard," *Family Practice News*, v. 22, p. 20, February 1-14, 1991.

[7] Graziano, Joseph H. and Blum, Conrad, "Lead Exposure From Lead Crystal," *The Lancet*, v. 337, p. 141-142, January 19, 1991.

[8] Matte, Thomas D., et al, "Acute High-Dose Lead Exposure From Beverage Contaminated By Traditional Mexican Pottery," *The Lancet*, v. 344, p. 1064-1065, October 15, 1994.

[9] Burton Goldberg Group, *Alternative Medicine, The Definitive Guide*, Future Medicine Publishing, Inc., Puyallup, WA, p. 927-928, 1993.

[10] Ibid.

[11] Cranton, E.M., "Protocol of the American College of Advancement in Medicine for the Safe and Effective Administration of Intravenous EDTA Chelation Therapy," *EDTA Chelation Therapy*, American College of Advancement in Medicine, Houston, TX, May 1993.

[12] Burton Goldberg Group, *Alternative Medicine, The Definitive Guide*, Future Medicine Publishing, Inc., Puyallup, WA, p. 127, 1993.

[13] Wright, Jonathan V., *Dr. Wright's Book of Nutritional Therapy*, Rodale Press, Emmaus, PA, p. 294-303, 1979.

Chapter 44: CHICKENPOX

[1] Watson, Barbara A.; Starr, Stuart E., "Varicella Vaccine for Healthy Children, *The Lancet*, v. 343, n. 8903, p. 928, April 16, 1994.

[2] Ozsoylu, Sinasi, "Vitamin A For Varicella," *The Journal of Pediatrics*, p. 125, December, 1994.

[3] White, Linda B., "Putting up with Chickenpox," *Mothering*, n. 70, p. 38, Spring 1994.

[4] Ibid.

Chapter 45: CHOLESTEROL

[1] Balch, James F., M.D., and Balch, Phyllis A., *Prescription for Nutritional Healing*, Avery Publishing Group, Garden City Park, N.Y., p. 208, 1990.

[2] Jailal, Ishwarlal, M.D., "Influence of Antioxidant Vitamins on LDL Oxidation," New York Academy of Sciences, p. 21, February 9-12, 1992.

[3] Illman, Richard J., et al, "Effects of Solvent Extraction on the Hypocholesterolaemic Action of Oat Bran in the Diet," *British Journal of Nutrition*, v. 65, p. 435-443, 1991.

[4] Sprecher, Dennis L., et al, "Efficacy of Psyllium in Reducing Serum Cholesterol Levels in Hypercholesterolemic Patients in High- or Low-Fat Diets," *Annals of Internal Medicine*, v. 119, n. 7, p. 545-554, October 1, 1993.

[5] "Grape Juice vs. Wine: A Healthy Debate," *Science News*, p. 47, July 18, 1992.

[6] Beverly, Laura N., "Lower Heart Risk the Nutty Way," *Natural Healing Newsletter*, v. 4, n. 41, p. 1.

[7] "Eating Fish Reduces Cholesterol More than Fish Oil Supplements," *Medical Tribune*, p. 10, May 21, 1992

[8] "Almonds Can Cut LDL 12 Percent," *Medical Tribune*, p. 9, August 8, 1991.

[9] Liebman, Bonnie, "The Best Laid Trans," *Nutrition Action Health Letter*, p. 5, December 1992.

[10] Raloff, J., "Margarine is Anything but a Marginal Fat," *Science News*, v.145, p. 325, May 21, 1994.

[11] Willett, Walter C., et al, "Intake of Trans Fatty Acids and Risk of Coronary Heart Disease Among Women, *The Lancet* v. 341, p. 581-585, March 6, 1993.

[12] Mann, George V., "Metabolic Consequences of Dietary Trans Fatty Acids," *The Lancet*, v. 343, n. 8908, p. 1268, May 21, 1994.

Chapter 46: CHRONIC FATIGUE SYNDROME
[1] Burton Goldberg Group, *Alternative Medicine, The Definitive Guide*, Future Medicine Publishing, Inc., Puyallup, WA, p. 616-622, 1993.

[2] Breneman, James C, *Basics of Food Allergy*, Charles C. Thomas Publisher, Springfield, IL, p. 65, 1984

[3] Wright, Jonathan, "Chronic Fatigue Syndrome," *Nutrition & Healing*, v. 2, n. 6, p. 1-9, June 1995.

[4] "DHEA for Treating CFIDS", *Townsend Letter for Doctors*, p. 1162, November 1993.

[5] Cox, I.M., et al, "Red Blood Cell Magnesium and Chronic Fatigue Syndrome," *The Lancet*, v. 337, p. 757-760, March 30, 1991.

Chapter 47: CHRONIC PAIN
[1] Mgebroff, Jacqueline W., "The War Within: Living with Chronic Pain," *Vibrant Life*, v. 9, n. 4, p. 6, July-August 1993.

[2] Magni, G, et al, "Chronic Musculoskeletal Pain and Depressive Symptoms in the General Population-An Analysis of the First National Health and Nutrition Examination Survey Data," *Pain*, v. 43, n.3, p. 299-307, 1990.

[3] Kerns, Robert D., *Journal of Behavioral Medicine*, vol. 17, no. 1, 1994.

[4] Eisinger, J., et al, "Studies of Transketolase in Chronic Pain," *Journal of Advancement in Medicine*, v. 5, n. 2, p. 105-113, Summer 1992.

[5] Dunne, Lavon J., *Nutrition Almanac*, Third Edition, McGraw-Hill Publishing Company, p. 21, 1990.

[6] Gerras, Charles, et al, eds, *The Encyclopedia of Common Diseases*, Rodale Press Inc., Emmaus, PA, p. 105, 1976.

[7] Zaloga, Gary, et al, "Magnesium, Anesthesia and Hemodynamic Control," *The Journal of Anesthesiology*, v. 74, p. 1-2, January 1991.

[8] Burton Goldberg Group, *Alternative Medicine, The Definitive Guide*, Future Medicine Publishing, Inc., Puyallup, WA, p. 627, 1993.

[9] Ibid.

[10] Budd, K, "Use of D-Phenylalanine, an Enkephalinase Inhibitor, in the Treatment of Intractable Pain, *Advances in Pain Research and Therapeutics*, v. 5, p. 305-308, 1983.

Chapter 48: CIRCULATION PROBLEMS
[1] Browne, S.E., MB, "The Case For Intravenous Magnesium Treatment of Arterial Disease in General Practice: Review of 34 Years of Experience," *Journal of Nutritional Medicine*, v. 4, p. 169-177, 1994.

[2] Leppert, Jerzy, M.D., Ph.D., et al, "Effect of Magnesium Sulfate Infusion on Circulating Levels of Noradrenaline and Neuropeptide-Y-Like Immunoreactivity in Patients With Primary Raynaud's Phenomenon," *Angiology*, v. 45, n. 7, p. 637-645, July 1994.

[3] Bunker, Christopher, B., et al, "Calcitonin Gene-Related Peptide in Treatment of Severe Peripheral Vascular Insufficiency in Raynaud's Phenomenon," *The Lancet*, v. 342, n. 8863, p. 80, July 10, 1993.

[4] Myrdal, U., et al, "Magnesium Sulfate Infusion to Decrease the Circulating Calcitonin Gene-Related Peptide (CGRP) in Women With Primary Raynaud's Phenomenon," *Clinical Physiology*, v. 14, p. 539-546, 1994.

[5] Bunker, Christopher, B., et al, "Calcitonin Gene-Related Peptide in Treatment of Severe Peripheral Vascular Insufficiency in Raynaud's Phenomenon," *The Lancet*, v. 342, n. 8863, p. 80, July 10, 1993.

[6] Wright, Jonathan V., *Dr. Wright's Book of Nutritional Therapy*, Rodale Press, Emmaus, PA, p. 13-23, 1979.

[7] Murray, Frank, "More Physicians are Endorsing Vitamin E," *Better Nutrition for Today's Living*, v. 55, n. 5, p. 6, May 1993.

[8] Paolisso, Giuseppe, et al, "Pharmacologic Doses of Vitamin E Improve Insulin Action in Healthy Subjects and Non-insulin- Dependent Diabetic Patients," *American Journal of Clinical Nutrition*, v. 57, n. 5, p. 650, May 1993.

[9] *Martindale, The Extra Pharmacopoeia, Thirtieth Edition*, Department of Pharmaceutical Sciences, Royal Pharmaceutical Society of Great Britain, The Pharmaceutical Press, p. 1617 and 1850, 1993.

Chapter 49: COLDS AND FLU

[1] *Cecil Textbook Medical*, 17th Edition, p. 1692, W.B. Saunders Co., 1985.

[2] *Microbiology*, 2nd Edition, Tortora, Funk, Case, p. 615, 1986.

[3] Seaton, Kenneth, *Life, Health and Longevity*, Scientific Hygiene, Inc., Chagrin Falls, OH, p. 11-12, 1994.

[4] Del Mar, Christopher, "Managing Viral Upper Respiratory Infections," *Australian Family Physician*, v. 20, n. 5, p. 557-561, May 1991.

[5] "USDA Study of 40,000 Americans," *Food Technology*, v. 35, p. 9, 1981.

[6] Hemila, Harri, "Does Vitamin C Alleviate the Symptoms of The Common Cold? – A Review of Current Evidence," *Scandinavian Journal of Infectious Diseases*, v. 26, p. 1-6, 1994.

[7] Ibid.

[8] "Vitamin C Enhances Antibiotic Therapy," *The Nutrition Report*, v. 10, n. 4, p. 31, April 1992.

[9] "Decreased Resistance to Antibiotics and Plasmid Loss in Plasmid-Carrying Strains of Staphylococcus Aureus Treated With Ascorbic Acid," *Mutation Research*, v. 264, p. 119-125, 1991.

[10] Rodale, J.I., et al., *The Complete Book of Vitamins*, Rodale Book, Inc., Emmaus, PA, 1970.

[11] Atkins, Robert C., M.D., *Dr. Atkins' Health Revolution*, Houghton Mifflin Co., Boston, MA, 1988.

[12] Quillin, Patrick, *Healing Nutrients*, Contemporary Books, Chicago, 1987.

[13] Kaul, T.N., et al, "Antiviral Effect of Flavonoids on Human Viruses," *Journal of Medical Virology*, v. 17, p. 71-79, 1985.

[14] Murray, Michael, M.D. and Pizzorno, Joseph, N.D., *Encyclopedia of Natural Medicine*, Prima Publishing, Rocklin, CA, p. 219, 1991.

[15] Keville, Kathi, "Respect Your Elder," *Vegetarian Times*, n. 154, p. 62, June 1990.

[16] Rodale, J.I., *The Health Finder*, Rodale Books, Emmaus, PA, p. 257-259, 1955.

[17] Burton Goldberg Group, *Alternative Medicine, The Definitive Guide*, Future Medicine Publishing, Inc., Puyallup, WA, p. 634, 1993.

[18] Rodale, J.I., *The Health Finder*, Rodale Books, Emmaus, PA, p. 257-259, 1955.

[19] Murray, Michael, M.D. and Pizzorno, Joseph, N.D., *Encyclopedia of Natural Medicine*, Prima Publishing, Rocklin, CA, p. 229, 1991.

Chapter 50: COLIC

[1] Karlsrud, Katherine & Schultz, Dodi, "Is There a Cure for Colic?," *Parents' Magazine*, v. 67 n. 9, p. 226, September 1992.

[2] Maugh, Thomas H., II, "New Findings on Infant-Colic Cause: Cow Antibodies May Affect Breast-Fed Babies," *The Sacramento Bee*, p. A10, March 27, 1991.

[3] Gilbert, Susan, "Is it Colic-or What?," *Redbook*, v. 184, n. 6, p. 186, April 1995.

[4] Keville, Kathi, "Respect Your Elder," *Vegetarian Times*, n. 154, p. 62, June 1990.

[5] Adams, Ruth, "Healthful Herb Teas," *Better Nutrition for Today's Living*, v. 55, n. 7, p. 40, July 1993.

[6] Duncan, Alice Likowski, *Your Healthy Child*, Jeremy P. Tarcher, Inc., Los Angeles, CA, p. 112, 1991.

Chapter 51: COLON PROBLEMS

[1] "Fast Food and Sugar Linked to Crohn's Disease," *Medical Tribune*, v. 12, February 27, 1992 (Persson, Per-Gunnar, et al, "Diet and Inflammatory Bowel Disease: A Case-Controlled Study," *Epidemiology*, v. 3, n. 1, p. 47-52, January 1992.

[2] Burton Goldberg Group, *Alternative Medicine, The Definitive Guide*, Future Medicine Publishing, Inc., Puyallup, WA, p. 684-685, 1993.

[3] Atkins, Robert C., *Dr. Atkins' Health Revolution*, Houghton Mifflin Co., Boston, p, 282-296, 1988.

[4] Lown, Cynthia and Lowen, R.D., et al, "Nutritional Support in Patients With Inflammatory Bowel Disease," *Postgraduate Medicine*, v. 91, n. 5, p. 407-414, April 1992.

[5] Seidman, E., et al, "Nutritional Issues in Pediatric Inflammatory Bowel Disease," *Journal of Pediatric Gastroenterology and Nutrition*, v. 12, n. 4, 424-438, 1992.

[6] Gibson, Glenn R. and Roberfroid, Marcel B., "Dietary Manipulation of Human Colonic Microbiota: Introducing the Concept of Prebiotics," *Journal of Nutrition*, v. 125, p. 1401-1412, 1995.

[7] Wright, Jonathan V., *Dr. Wright's Book of Nutritional Therapy*, Rodale Press, Emmaus, PA, p. 89-95, 1979.

[8] Lown, Cynthia and Lowen, R.D., et al, "Nutritional Support in Patients With Inflammatory Bowel Disease," *Postgraduate Medicine*, v. 91, n. 5, p. 407-414, April 1992.

[9] Seidman, E., et al, "Nutritional Issues in Pediatric Inflammatory Bowel Disease," *Journal of Pediatric Gastroenterology and Nutrition*, v. 12, n. 4, 424-438, 1992.

[10] Weir, C.D., et al, "Glutamine Enhanced Elemental Diet Modifies Colonic Damage in a Hapten Induced Model of Colitis," *Gastroenterology*, v. 102, n. 4, Part II: A711, April 1992.

[11] Mantzioris, Evangeline, et al, "Dietary Substitution with L-Linolenic Acid-Rich Vegetable Oil Increases Eicosapentaenoic Acid Concentrations in Tissues," *American Journal of Clinical Nutrition*, v. 59, p. 1304-1309, 1994.

[12] Seidman, E., et al, "Nutritional Issues in Pediatric Inflammatory Bowel Disease," *Journal of Pediatric Gastroenterology and Nutrition*, v. 12, n. 4, 424-438, 1992.

Chapter 52: CONSTIPATION

[1] Null, Gary, *The Complete Guide to Health and Nutrition*, Dell Publishing Co., New York, 1984.

[2] *Lancet General Advertiser,* September 21, 1957.

[3] Rodale, J.I., *The Health Finder*, Rodale Books, Emmaus, PA, p. 278-280, 1955.

[4] McLester, James S., *Nutrition and Diet*, 6th Edition, W.B. Saunders Co., 1952.

[5] Burton Goldberg Group, *Alternative Medicine, The Definitive Guide*, Future Medicine Publishing, Inc., Puyallup, WA, p. 643, 1993.

[6] Botez, M.I., et al, "Neurologic Disorders Responsive to Folic Acid Therapy," *Canadian Medical Association Journal*, v. 15, p. 217, 1976.

[7] Burton Goldberg Group, *Alternative Medicine, The Definitive Guide*, Future Medicine Publishing, Inc., Puyallup, WA, p. 643, 1993.

[8] Ibid.

Chapter 53: CRAMPS – MENSTRUAL & MUSCLE

[1] Burton Goldberg Group, *Alternative Medicine, The Definitive Guide*, Future Medicine Publishing, Inc., Puyallup, WA, p. 181-182, 1993.

[2] Callejari, Peter E., M.D. and Zurier, Robert B., M.D, "Botanical Lipids: Potential Role in the Modulation of Immunologic Responses and Inflammatory Reactions," *Nutrition and Rheumatic Disease/Rheumatic Disease Clinics of North America*, p. 415, May 1991.

[3] Vukovic, Laurel, "Treating Common Health Problems Naturally," *Natural Health*, v. 24, n. 4, p.86, July-August, 1994.

[4] Burton Goldberg Group, *Alternative Medicine, The Definitive Guide*, Future Medicine Publishing, Inc., Puyallup, WA, p. 661, 1993.

[5] Clark, Nancy, "Muscles Cramping Your Style? Resolving Diet Deficiencies can Relieve Mysterious Muscle Cramps," *American Fitness*, v. 10, n. 2, p. 8, March-April, 1992.

[6] Konikoff, F., "Vitamin E and Cirrhotic Muscle Cramps," *Israeli Journal of Medicine*, v. 27, p. 221-223, 1991.

[7] Dunne, Lavon J., *Nutrition Almanac*, Third Edition, McGraw-Hill Publishing Company, p. 190, 1990.

Chapter 54: CYSTIC FIBROSIS

[1] Ramsey, Bonnie W., et al, "Nutritional Assessment and Management in Cystic Fibrosis: A Consensus Report," *American Journal of Clinical Nutrition*, v. 55, p. 108-116, 1992.

[2] Ahmed, F., et al, "Excessive Fecal Loss of Vitamin A (Retinol) in Cystic Fibrosis," *Archives of Disease in Children*, v. 65, p. 589-593, 1990.

[3] Eid, Nemer S., et al, "Vitamin A and Cystic Fibrosis: Case Report and Review of the Literature," *Journal of Pediatric Gastroenterology and Nutrition*, v. 10, n. 2, p. 265, 1990.

[4] Borowitz, Drucy, M.D., et al, "Preventive Care For Patients With Chronic Illness: Multivitamin Use in Patients With Cystic Fibrosis," *Clinical Pediatrics*, p. 720-725, December 1994.

[5] Crystal, Ronald G., M.D., "Oxidants and Respiratory Tract Epithelial Injury: Pathogenesis and Strategies for Therapeutic Intervention," *The Journal of Medicine*, v. 91, September 30, 1991.

[6] Lloyd-Still, John D., et al, "Essential Fatty Acid Status and Fluidity of Plasma Phospholipids in Cystic Fibrosis Infants," *American Journal of Clinical Nutrition*, v. 54, p. 1029-1035, 1991.

[7] Smith, Lesley J., M.D., et al, "Taurine Decreases Fecal Fatty Acid and Sterol Excretion in Cystic Fibrosis: A Randomized, Double-Blind Trial," *AJDC*, v. 145, p. 1401-1404, 1991.

[8] Horn, Bernard, M.D., "The Role of Magnesium in Cystic Fibrosis - A Hypothesis," *Journal of Nutritional Medicine*, v. 2, p. 203-207, 1991.

Chapter 55: CYSTITIS

[1] Richard B. Freeman, M. D. Bibliography: Kunin, C. M., *Detection, Prevention and Management of Urinary Tract Infections*, 4th edition, 1987.

[2] Burton Goldberg Group, *Alternative Medicine, The Definitive Guide*, Future Medicine Publishing, Inc., Puyallup, WA, p. 669, 1993.

[3] Rota, Francine, "Fifty Ways to Better Women's Health," *East West*, v. 20, n. 11, p. 46, November 1990.

[4] "Vitamin C Enhances Antibiotic Therapy," *The Nutrition Report*, v. 10, n. 4, p. 31, April 1992.

[5] "Decreased Resistance to Antibiotics and Plasmid Loss in Plasmid-Carrying Strains of Staphylococcus Aureus Treated With Ascorbic Acid," *Mutation Research*, v. 264, p. 119-125, 1991.

[6] Burton Goldberg Group, *Alternative Medicine, The Definitive Guide*, Future Medicine Publishing, Inc., Puyallup, WA, p. 670, 1993.

[7] Ibid, p. 669.

[8] Adams, Rex, *Miracle Medicine Foods*, Prentice-Hall, Englewood Cliff, NJ, p. 90, 1977.

Chapter 56: DANDRUFF

[1] "Flaking and Itching can be Controlled," *USA Today*, v. 122, n. 2585, p. 11, February 1994.

[2] Jacinto-Jamora, et al, "Pityrosporum Folliculitis in the Philippines: Diagnosis, Prevalence and Management," *Journal of the American Academy of Dermatology*, v. 24, n. 5, p. 693, May 1991.

[3] Burton Goldberg Group, *Alternative Medicine, The Definitive Guide*, Future Medicine Publishing, Inc., Puyallup, WA, p. 910, 1993.

[4] Schreiner, A.W., et al, "Seborrheic Dermatitis: A Local Defect Involving Pyridoxine," *J Lab Clin Med*, v. 40, p. 121-130, 1952.

[5] Block, M.T., "Vitamin E in the Treatment of Diseases of the Skin," *Clinical Medicine*, p. 31-34, January 1953.

Chapter 57:   DEPRESSION

[1]   Braverman, Eric, M.D., and Pfeiffer, Carl C., M.D., Ph.D., The Healing Nutrients Within, Keats Publishing, New Canaan, CT, 1987.

[2]   Axford, Shelagh, et al, "Beyond Pumpkin Seeds," *British Journal of Psychiatry*, v. 158, p. 573, April 1991.

[3]   "St. John's Wort for Depression – An Overview and Meta-Analysis of Randomised Clinical Trials," Linde, Klaus, et al, British Medical Journal, 1996, p. 313:253-8.

[4]   Budd, M.L., "Hypoglycemia and Personality," *Complimentary Therapies in Medicine*, v. 2, p. 142-146, 1994.

[5]   Bell, Iris R., M.D., Ph.D., et al, "B Complex Vitamin Patterns In Geriatric and Young Adult Patients With Major Depression," *Journal of The American Geriatric Society*, v. 39, n.3, p. 252-257.

[6]   Dunne, Lavon J., *Nutrition Almanac*, Third Edition, McGraw-Hill Publishing Company, p. 194, 1990.

[7]   *The Practical Encyclopedia of Natural Healing*, Rodale Press, Inc., Emmaus, PA, p. 143, 1983.

[8]   Atkins, Robert C., M.D., *Dr. Atkins' Nutrition Breakthrough*, William Morrow and Company, Inc., New York, 1981.

[9]   Lindenbaum, J., et al, "Neuropsychiatric Disorders Caused by Cobalamin Deficiency in The Absence of Anemia or Macrocytosis," *New England Journal of Medicine*, v. 318, p. 1720-1728, 1988.

[10]   Lindenbaum, John, et al, "Neurologic Aspects of Cobalamin Deficiency,"*New England Journal of Medicine*, v. 70, n. 4, p. 229, July 1991.

[11]   Downing, Damien, MB, BS, "Cerebral Manifestations of Vitamin B12 Deficiency," *Journal of Nutritional Medicine*, v. 2, p. 89-90, 1991/Holmes, J. MacDonald, "Cerebral Manifestations of Vitamin B12 Deficiency," *British Medical Journal*, v. 2, p. 1394-1398, 1956.

[12]   "Agent Eased Toxin-Induced Mood Changes," *Journal of Neuropsychiatric and Clinical Neuroscience*, v. 2, p. 467, 1990.

[13]   Langer, Stephen, "PMS: A Positive Approach," *Better Nutrition for Today's Living*, v. 54, n. 10, p. 36-38, October 1992.

[14]   Werbach, Melvyn, *Nutritional Influences on Illness*, Second Edition, Third Line Press, Tarzana, California, 1993.

[15]   Hashizume, Naotaka and Mori, Miko, "An Analysis of Hypermagnesemia and Hypomagnesemia," *Japanese Journal of Medicine*, v. 29, n. 4, p. 368-472, July/August 1990.

[16]   Banki, C.M., et al, "Cerebrospinal Fluid Magnesium and Calcium Related to Amine Metabolites, Diagnosis and Suicide Attempts," *Biological Psychiatry*, v. 20, p. 163-171, 1985.

[17]   Christensen, Larry, Ph.D., "The Role of Caffeine and Sugar in Depression," *The Nutrition Report*, v. 9, n. 3, p. 17-24, March 1991.

[18]   Haggerty, John J., Jr., M.D., et al, "Subclinical Hypothyroidism: A Modifiable Risk Factor For Depression?" *American Journal of Psychiatry*, n. 150, p. 508-510, March 3, 1993.

[19]   Nomura, Junichi, et al, "Thyroid Function and Mood: Implications For Treatment of Mood Disorders," *CNS Drugs*, v. 1, n. 5, p. 356-369, 1994.

Chapter 58: DIABETES (HYPERGLYCEMIA – HIGH BLOOD SUGAR)

[1] Robbins, S. A., and Cotran, R., *Pathological Basis of Disease*, W.B. Saunders, New York, NY, 1974.

[2] Higgins, Michael, "Native People Take on Diabetes," *East West*, v. 2,1 n. 4, p. 94, April 1991.

[3] Whitaker, Julian, *Reversing Diabetes*, Warner Books, New York, NY, p. 63, 1987.

[4] Anderson, J.W. and Sieling, B., "High Fiber Diets for Diabetics: Unconventional but Effective," *Geriatrics*, v. 36, n.5, p. 64-72, May 1981.

[5] Mertz, Walter, "Chromium in Human Nutrition: A Review," *Journal of Nutrition*, v. 123, p. 626-633, 1993.

[6] Mertz, Walter, "Effects and Metabolism of Glucose Tolerance Factor," *Nutrition Review*, v. 33, 1929, 1975.

[7] "Beneficial Effects of the Oral Administration of Vanadyl Sulphate on Glucose Metabolism in Senescent Rats," *Journal of Gerontology*, 1993.

[8] Baker, Daniel, Pharm.D. and Campbell, Keith R., "Vitamin and Mineral Supplementation in Patients with Diabetes Mellitus," The Diabetes Educator, v. 18, n. 5, p. 420-427, September-October 1992.

[9] Dunne, Lavon J., *Nutrition Almanac*, Third Edition, McGraw-Hill Publishing Company, p. 123, 1990.

[10] Rohn, R., et al, "Magnesium, Zinc and Copper in Plasma and Blood Cellular Components in Children With Insulin Dependent Diabetes Mellitus," *Clinical Chemistry*, v. 215, p. 21-28, 1993.

[11] Cogeshall, J.C., et al, "Biotin Status and Plasma Glucose in Diabetics," *Annals of the New York Academy of Sciences*, v. 447, p. 389-393, 1985.

[12] Munson, Marty, "Diabetes Tamer: Does this B Vitamin Lower Glucose?" *Prevention*, v. 46, n. 7, p. 46, July 1994.

[13] Gaby, Alan R., M.D. and Wright, Jonathan V., M.D., "Nutritional Regulation of Blood Glucose," Wright/Gaby Nutrition Institute, October 1990.

[14] Rogers, Kenneth S. and Mohan, Chandra, "Vitamin B6 Metabolism and Diabetes," *Biochemical Medicine and Metabiologic Biology*, v. 52, p. 10-17, 1994.

[15] Burton Goldberg Group, *Alternative Medicine, The Definitive Guide*, Future Medicine Publishing, Inc., Puyallup, WA, p. 651, 1993.

[16] *Science News*, v. 133, n. 4, p. 62, January 22, 1988.

[17] Kleiner, Susan M., Ph.D., R.D., "A Hill of Beans: The Latest on Legumes," *The Physician and Sports Medicine*, v. 23, n. 6, p. 13-14, June 1995.

[18] Frank, Murray, "Therapy and Treatment with Aloe Vera," *Better Nutrition for Today's Living*, v. 56, n. 3, p. 52, March 1994.

Chapter 59: DIABETIC RETINOPATHY

[1] *American Diabetes Association*, Document ADA051, 1995.

[2] "Public Health Focus: Prevention of Blindness Associated with Diabetic Retinopathy," *MMWR*, v. 42, p. 191-194, 1993.

[3] Morisaki, Nobuhiro, et al, "Lipoprotein(a) is a Risk Factor For Diabetic Retinopathy in the Elderly," *Journal of the American Geriatric Society*, p. 42, n. 965-976, 1994.

[4] Kempner, W., et al, "Effect of Rice Diet on Diabetes Mellitus Associated with Vascular Disease," *Postgraduate Medicine*, v. 24, p. 359-371, 1958.

[5] Gerster, Helga, "Review: Antioxidant Protection of the Ageing Macula," *Age and Ageing*, v. 20, p. 60-69, 1991.

[6] Murray, Frank, "Keeping an Eye on Good Health," *Today's Living*, v. 20, n. 8, p. 8, August 1989.

[7] Ibid.

[8] Donegan, J.M. and Thomas, W.A., "Capillary Fragility and Cutaneous Lymphatic Flow in Relation to Systemic and Retinal Vascular Manifestations: Rutin Therapy," *American Journal of Ophthalmology*, v. 31, p. 671-678, 1948.

[9] Palmer, L.J., et al, "The Influence of Rutin Upon Diabetic Retinitis," *Northwest Medicine*, v. 50, p. 669-671, 1951.

[10] Lavollary, J., Nuemann, J., "Problems Posed by the Activity of Certain Flavonoids on Vascular Resistance," *The Pharmacology of Plant Phenolics*, J.W. Fairbairn, editor, Academic Press Ltd., London, p. 103-122, 1959.

[11] Murray, Frank, "Keeping an Eye on Good Health," *Today's Living*, v. 20, n. 8, p. 8, August 1989.

[12] Horrobin, David F., and Manku, Mehar S., "Essential Fatty Acids in Clinical Medicine," *Nutrition and Health*, v. 2, p. 127-134, 1983.

[13] Falsini, Benedetto, "Spacial-Frequency-Dependent Changes in the Human Pattern of Electroretinogram After Acute Acetyl-L-Carnitine Administration," *Graefe's Archives Clin. Exp. Ophthalmol*, v. 229, p. 262-266, 1991.

[14] Elamin, Abdelaziz and Tuvemo, Torsten, "Magnesium and Insulin-Dependent Diabetes Mellitus," *Diabetes Research and Clinical Practice*, v. 10, p. 203-209, 1990.

[15] Hatwal, A., et al, "Association of Hypomagnesemia With Diabetic Retinopathy," *ACTA Ophthalmologica*, v. 67, p. 714-716, 1989.

[16] Levy, J., et al, "Diabetes Mellitus: A Disease of Abnormal Cellular Calcium Metabolism?" *The American Journal of Medicine*, v. 96, p. 260-273, 1994.

Chapter 60: DIARRHEA

[1] Peikin, Steven, *Gastrointestinal Health*, HarperCollins Publishers, New York, NY, p. 71, 1991.

[2] Burton Goldberg Group, *Alternative Medicine, The Definitive Guide*, Future Medicine Publishing, Inc., Puyallup, WA, p. 687, 1993.

[3] Lown, Cynthia and Lowen, R.D., et al, "Nutritional Support in Patients With Inflammatory Bowel Disease," *Postgraduate Medicine*, v. 91, n. 5, p. 407-414, April 1992.

[4] Dunne, Lavon J., *Nutrition Almanac*, Third Edition, McGraw-Hill Publishing Company, p. 158, 1990.

Chapter 61: DIVERTICULITIS

[1] Balch, James F., M.D., and Balch, Phyllis A., *Prescription for Nutritional Healing*, Avery Publishing Group, Garden City Park, N.Y., p. 157, 1990.

[2] Peikin, Steven, Gastrointestinal Health, HarperCollins Publishers, New York, NY, p. 76-77, 1991.

[3] Ibid.

[4] Burton Goldberg Group, *Alternative Medicine, The Definitive Guide*, Future Medicine Publishing, Inc., Puyallup, WA, p. 686-687, 1993.

[5] Srivastava, R.and Srimal, R.C., et al, "Modification of Certain Inflammation - Induced Biochemical Changes by Curcumin," *Indian Journal of Medical Research*, v. 81, p. 215, February 1985.
[6] Arora, R.B., et al, "Anti-Inflammatory Studies on Curcuma Longa," *Indian Journal of Medical Research*, v. 59, p. 1289, August 1971.
[7] Tovey, F.I., "Diet and Duodenal Ulcer", *Journal of Gastroenterology and Hepatology*, v. 9, p. 177-185, 1994.

Chapter 62: DOWN'S SYNDROME
Fowkes, Steven William, "An Interview with Dixie Lawrence," *Smart Drug News*, v. 3, n. 4, July 18, 1994.
Fowkes, Steven William & Dean, Ward, M.D., "Smart Drugs and Down's Syndrome,"*Smart Drug News*, v. 2, n. 10, February 14, 1994.
Fowkes, Steven William, "Antioxidant Intervention in Down's Syndrome," *Smart Drug News*, v. 4, n. 10, April 15, 1996.
Fowkes, Steven William, "Antioxidant Intervention in Down's Syndrome," *Smart Drug News*, v. 5, n. 1, June 3, 1996.

Chapter 63: EATING DISORDERS
[1] Rosen, Marjorie, "Eating Disorders: A Hollywood History," *People Weekly*, v. 37, n. 6, p. 96, February 17, 1992.
[2] Ward, Neil I., Ph.D., "Assessment of Zinc Status in Oral Supplementation in Anorexia Nervosa," *Journal of Nutritional Medicine*, v. 1, p. 171-177, 1990.
[3] McClain, Craig J., M.D., et al, "Zinc Status Before and After Zinc Supplementation of Eating Disorder Patients," *Journal of the American College of Nutrition*, v. 11, n. 6, p. 694-700, December 1992.
[4] Bryce-Smith, D., Simpson RID, "Anorexia, Depression and Zinc Deficiency," *The Lancet*, v. 2, p. 1162, 1984.
[5] Birmingham, Carl L., et al, "Controlled Trial of Zinc Supplementation in Anorexia Nervosa," *International Journal of Eating Disorders*, v. 15, n. 3, p. 251-255, 1994.

Chapter 64: ECZEMA
[1] *Acta Paedia. Japan*, 24:395, p. 82, 1982.
[2] David T.J, "Dietary Treatment of Atopic Eczema," *Archives of Diseases in Childhood*, v. 64, n. 10, p. 1506, Oct 1989.
[3] *Southern Medical Journal*, v. 38, p. 235, 1945.
[4] *Arch. Dermatol. Syph.*, v. 20, p. 854, 1929.
[5] Callejari, Peter E., M.D. and Zurier, Robert B., M.D, "Botanical Lipids: Potential Role in the Modulation of Immunologic Responses and Inflammatory Reactions," *Nutrition and Rheumatic Disease/Rheumatic Disease Clinics of North America,* p. 415, May 1991.
[6] Wright, S., and Burton, J.L. "Oral Evening Primrose-Seed Oil Improves Atopic Eczema," *The Lancet*, p. 1120, November 20, 1982.
[7] Kennedy, Bob, "Borage Wildflowers: Best Source of GLA," *Total Health*, v. 13, n. 1, p. 44, February 1991.
[8] Erasmus, Udo, *Fats and Oils, The Complete Guide to Fats and Oils in Human Nutrition*, Alive Books, Burnaby, BC, Canada, p. 244, 1986.

[9] Wright, Jonathan V., M.D., Gaby, Alan R, M.D., *Nutritional Therapy for the 1990s: Selected Protocols*, The Wright/Gaby Nutrition Institute, October 1991.

[10] Wright, Jonathan V., *Dr. Wright's Book of Nutritional Therapy*, Rodale Press, Emmaus, PA, p. 39, 1979.

[11] *The Encyclopedia of Common Diseases*, p. 1123, Rodale Press, Emmaus, PA, 1976.

[12] Ibid.

Chapter 65: ENDOMETRIOSIS

[1] Balch, James F., M.D., and Balch, Phyllis A., *Prescription for Nutritional Healing*, Avery Publishing Group, Garden City Park, N.Y., p. 167, 1990.

[2] Beling, Stephanie, "Relieving Endometriosis," *Vegetarian Times*, n. 180, p. 28, August 1992.

[3] Challem, Jack, "Breast Cancer: Tracing It's Elusive Causes and Leveraging Dietary Strategies to Prevent It," *Let's Live*, p. 19, November 1994.

[4] Whitaker, Julian, "Preventing Breast Cancer," *Health and Healing*, January 1994.

[5] Mindell, Earl L, "Soy - When Will We Learn?" column Stay Healthy, *Let's Live*, p. 10, January 1995.

[6] Challem, Jack, "Simple Dietary Changes Can Assist Sufferers of Endometriosis," *Let's Live*, p. 56-60, May 1995.

[7] Challem, Jack, "Breast Cancer: Tracing It's Elusive Causes and Leveraging Dietary Strategies to Prevent It," *Let's Live*, p. 19, November 1994.

[8] Lee, John R, M.D., *Natural Progesterone, The Multiple Roles of a Remarkable Hormone*, BLL Publishing, Sebastapol, CA, p. 242, May 1995.

[9] Atkins, Robert C., M.D., *Dr. Atkins' Health Revolution*, Houghton Mifflin Co., p. 169-172, Boston, MA, 1988.

[10] Sahley, Bille J.; Birkner, Kathy, "Stress and Menopause," *Total Health*, v. 10, n. 5, p. 54, October 1988.

Chapter 66: EPILEPSY

[1] Balch, James F., M.D., and Balch, Phyllis A., *Prescription for Nutritional Healing*, Avery Publishing Group, Garden City Park, N.Y., p. 170, 1990.

[2] Faelten, Sharon, *The Complete Book of Minerals for Health*, Rodale Press, Emmaus, PA, p. 128, 1981.

[3] Murray, Michael, N.D. & Pizzorno, Joseph, N.D., *Encyclopedia of Natural Medicine*, Prima Publishing, Rocklin, CA, p. 283, 1991.

[4] Ramaekers, V. Th, et al, "Selenium Deficiency Triggering Intractable Seizures," *Neuro Pediatrics*, p. 216, v. 25, 1994.

[5] Levy, Sheldon L., et al, "The Anticonvulsant Effects of Vitamin E: A Further Evaluation," *Canadian Journal of Neurological Sciences*, p. 19, May 1992.

[6] Cheraskin, E., M.D.; Ringsdorf, W.M., Jr., D.M.D.; Clark, J.W., D.D.S, Diet and Disease, Keats Publishing, New Canaan, CT, p. 197, 1995

[7] *Martindale, The Extra Pharmacopoeia, Thirtieth Edition*, Department of Pharmaceutical Sciences, Royal Pharmaceutical Society of Great Britain, The Pharmaceutical Press, p. 294, 1993.

[8] Horowitz, J.D., et al, "Relation of Abnormal Folate Metabolism to Neuropathy Developing During Anticonvulsant Drug Therapy," *The Lancet*, p. 563, 1968.

9 Inoue F., "Clinical Implications of Anticonvulsant-Induced Folate Deficiency," *Clinical Pharmaceutical*, p. 372, 1982.

10 Dunne, Lavon J., *Nutrition Almanac*, Third Edition, McGraw-Hill Publishing Company, p. 39, 1990.

11 Hoffer, Abram, Ph.D., M.D., *Orthomolecular Medicine for Physicians*, Keats Publishing, New Canaan, CT, p. 156, 1989.

12 Coursin, D.B., "Convulsive Seizures in Infants with Pyridoxine-Deficient Diets," *Journal of the American Medical Association*, v. 154, p. 406-408, 1954.

13 Egger, J., et al, "Oligoantigenic Diet Treatmen of Children with Epilepsy and Migraine," *Journal of Pediatrics*, v. 114, p. 51-58, 1989.

Chapter 67: EYE PROBLEMS

1 Murray, Frank, "Keeping an Eye on Good Health," *Today's Living*, v. 20, n. 8, p. 8, August 1989.

2 Gruning, Carl, "Seeing is Believing! For Lifelong Eye Health, Just Remember Your ABCs and These Minerals," *Health News & Review*, v. 2, n. 3, p. 1, Summer 1992.

3 Leguire, Lawrence, et al, "Electro-Oculogram in Vitamin A Deficiency Associated With Cystic Fibrosis," Ophthalmic Pediatrics, v. 13, n. 3, p. 187-189, 1992.

4 "Breast-Feeding Boon to Infants in Third World," *Medical Tribune*, v. 11, October 3, 1991.

5 Carlier, C., et al, "A Randomized Controlled Trial to Test Equivalence Between Retinyl Palmitate and Beta Carotene for Vitamin A Deficiency," *British Medical Journal*, v. 307, p. 1106-1110, 1993.

6 Murray, Frank, "Keeping an Eye on Good Health," *Today's Living*, v. 20, n. 8, p. 8, August 1989.

7 Dunne, Lavon J., *Nutrition Almanac*, Third Edition, McGraw-Hill Publishing Company, p. 157, 1990.

8 Rose, Richard and Dode, Ann M., "Ocular Ascorbate Transport Metabolism," *Comp. Biochem. Physiol.*, v. 108, n. 2, p. 273-285, 1991.

9 Dunne, Lavon J., *Nutrition Almanac*, Third Edition, McGraw-Hill Publishing Company, p. 165, 1990.

10 Lux-Neuwirth, Ora and Millar, Thomas J., "Lipid Soluble Antioxidants Preserve Rabbit Corneal Cell Function," *Current Eye Research*, v. 9, n. 2, p. 103-109, 1990.

11 Murray, Frank, "Keeping an Eye on Good Health," *Today's Living*, v. 20, n. 8, p. 8, August 1989.

12 Ibid.

13 Horrobin, David F., "Review Article: Medical Uses of Essential Fatty Acids (EFAs)," *Veterinary Dermatology*, v. 4, n. 4, p. 161-166, 1993.

14 Falsini, Benedetto, "Spacial-Frequency-Dependent Changes in the Human Pattern of Electroretinogram After Acute Acetyl-L-Carnitine Administration,", *Graefe's Archives Clin. Exp. Ophthalmol*, v. 229, p. 262-266, 1991.

15 Murray, Frank, "Keeping an Eye on Good Health," *Today's Living*, v. 20, n. 8, p. 8, August 1989.

16 Ibid.

17 Caffery, Barbara E., "Influence of Diet on Tear Function," *Optometry and Vision Science*, v. 68, n. 158-72, 1991.

Chapter 68: FATIGUE

[1] Davies, Stephen, MA, BM, BCh, "Neuropsychiatric Disorders Caused by Cobalamin Deficiency in the Absence of Anemia or Macrocytosis," *Journal of Nutritional Medicine*, v. 2, 91-92, 1991.

[2] Smidt, Laurie J., et al, "Influence of Thiamin Supplementation on the Health and General Well Being of an Elderly Population With Marginal Thiamin Deficiency," *Journal of Gerontology*, v. 46, n. 1, p. M16-M22, 1991.

[3] Dunne, Lavon J., *Nutrition Almanac*, Third Edition, McGraw-Hill Publishing Company, p. 21, 1990.

[4] Challem, Jack, "Fight Fatigue with Carnitine," *Let's Live*, p. 46-48, December 1994.

[5] Dunne, Lavon J., *Nutrition Almanac*, Third Edition, McGraw-Hill Publishing Company, p. 5-6, 1990.

[6] Davis, Adelle, *Let's Get Well*, Harcourt, Brace & World, New York, NY, p. 21, 1965.

[7] Ibid, p. 20.

[8] Ratner, Douglas, M.D. and Carey, Zev, M.D., "Medical Effects of Indoor Air Pollution," *Hospital Medicine*, p. 41-46, May 1995.

[9] Raloff, Janet, "Sick Buildings: the Ventilation Conundrum," *Science News*, v. 143, n. 13, p. 198, March 27, 1993.

[10] Schenker, Marc, B., "Indoor Air Pollution: Eight Questions Physicians Often Ask," *Consultant*, v. 31, n. 8, p. 59, August 1991.

Chapter 69: FEVER

[1] Margolis, Dawn, "Feed a Cold, Starve a Fever, and 10 Other Medical Myths You Should Not Believe," *American Health*, v. 13, n. 1, p. 52, January-February 1994.

[2] Dunne, Lavon J., *Nutrition Almanac*, Third Edition, McGraw-Hill Publishing Company, 1990.

[3] Robinson, Corinne, *Normal and Therapeutic Nutrition*, 14th Edition, The Macmillan Company, New York, p. 439, 1972.

[4] Stephensen, Charles B., et al, "Vitamin A Is Excreted in the Urine During Acute Infection," *American Journal of Clinical Nutrition*, v. 60, p. 388-392, 1994.

Chapter 70: FIBROCYSTIC BREAST DISEASE

[1] "Why Call it a Disease When It's Not?" *University of California, Berkeley Wellness Letter*, v. 7, n. 8, p. 1, May 1991.

[2] Wright, Jonathan V., *Nutrition & Healing*, v. 2, n. 7, July 1995.

[3] Editorial, "Breast Cancer, Have We Lost Our Way?" *The Lancet*, v. 341, n. 8841, p. 343, February 6, 1993.

[4] Evans, Imogen, "The Challenge of Breast Cancer," *The Lancet*, v. 343, n. 8905, p. 1085, April 30, 1994.

[5] Finn, Judith, A, "Dispelling Myths About Breast "Disease: Natural Approaches to Reduce Fibrocystic Breast Conditions," *Natural Health*, v. 23, n. 2, p. 44, March-April 1993.

[6] Challem, Jack, "Breast Cancer: Tracing It's Elusive Causes and Leveraging Dietary Strategies to Prevent It," *Let's Live*, p. 19, November 1994.

[7] Whitaker, Julian, "Preventing Breast Cancer," *Health and Healing*, January 1994.

[8] Finn, Judith, A, "Dispelling Myths About Breast "Disease: Natural Approaches to Reduce Fibrocystic Breast Conditions," *Natural Health*, v. 23, n. 2, p. 44, March-April 1993.

[9] Lee, John R, M.D., *Natural Progesterone, The Multiple Roles of a Remarkable Hormone*, BLL Publishing, Sebastapol, CA, May 1995.

[10] Kennedy, Bob, "Borage Wildflowers: Best Source of GLA," *Total Health*, v. 13, n. 1, p. 44, February 1991.

[11] Northrup, Christiane; Pick, Marcelle, "Breast Lumps Can be Frightening, but Most are Benign & Preventable," *Health News & Review*, v. 3, n. 2, p. 10, Spring 1993.

[12] Taylor, Deborah Seymour, "PMS," *Today's Living*, v. 20, n. 2, p. 24, February 1989.

[13] Wright, Jonathan, V., M.D., "On Call-How to Beat Fibrocystic Breast Disease," *Let's Live*, p. 12, August 1995.

Chapter 71: FIBROMYALGIA

[1] Perkins, Kathryn Dore, "Pain, Frustration Afflict Sufferers of Mystery Ailment," *Sacramento Bee*, March 15, 1995.

[2] James, Elizabeth, "Stress: Enemy or Friend?" *Total Health*, v.13, n. 1, p. 31, February 1991.

[3] Romano, Thomas, M.D., Ph.D. and Stiller, John W., M.D., "Magnesium Deficiency and Fibromyalgia Syndrome," *The Journal of Nutritional Medicine*, v. 4, p. 165-167, 1994.

[4] Zaloga, Gary, et al, "Magnesium, Anesthesia and Hemodynamic Control," *The Journal of Anesthesiology*, v. 74, p. 1-2, January 1991.

[5] Burton Goldberg Group, *Alternative Medicine, The Definitive Guide*, Future Medicine Publishing, Inc., Puyallup, WA, p. 627, 1993.

[6] "An Action Plan for Fibromyalgia," *Dr. Julian Whitaker's Health & Healing*, v. 6, n. 9, p. 3, September 1996.

[7] Gerras, Charles, et al, eds, *The Encyclopedia of Common Diseases*, Rodale Press Inc., Emmaus, PA, p. 105, 1976.

[8] Eisinger, J., M.D., et al, "Glycolysis Abnormalities in Fibromyalgia," *Journal of the American College of Nutrition*, v. 13, n. 2, p. 144-148, 1994.

[9] Bloch, Penelope, "A Fibromyalgia Diary: Learning to Coexist with Chronic Pain," *AIMplus*, n. 24, p. 48, May 1989.

[10] Yunus, Muhammad B., et al, "Plasma Tryptophan and Other Amino Acids in Primary Fibromyalgia: A Controlled Study," *Journal of Rheumatology*, v. 19, n. 1, p. 90-94, 1992.

[11] Eisinger, J., M.D., et al, "Glycolysis Abnormalities in Fibromyalgia," *Journal of the American College of Nutrition*, v. 13, n. 2, p. 144-148, 1994.

[12] Grassetto, Maurizio and Varotto, Antonella, "Primary Fibromyalgia is Responsive to S-Adenosyl-L-Methionine," *Current Therapeutic Research*, p. 55, n. 7, p. 797-806, July 1994.

[13] Ianniello, Aurora, et al, "S-Adenosyl-L-Methionine in Sjogren's Syndrome and Fibromyalgia," *Current Therapeutic Research*, v. 55, n. 6, p. 699-706, June 1994.

[14] Sahley, Billie J., "Hope for Fibromyalgia," Letters, *Let's Live*, p. 6, April 1995.

Chapter 72: FOOD POISONING

[1] "Chicken Feces Fine to Eat, Says New USDA Proposal," *Nutrition Week,* v. 24, n. 27, p. 4-5, July 22, 1994.

[2] Ibid.

[3] Stevens, Richard, Stay Out of Trouble: How to Avoid 10 Common Health Hassles," *Men's Health,* v. 5, n. 5, p. 51-55, December 1990.

[4] "Caesar's Salad Causes Illness in Restaurant Patrons," *Infectious Disease News*, v. 5, n. 8, p. 15, August 8, 1992

[5] Gibson, Glenn R. and Roberfroid, Marcel B., "Dietary Manipulation of Human Colonic Microbiota: Introducing the Concept of Probiotics," *Journal of Nutrition*, v. 125, p. 1401-1412, 1995.

[6] Hunter, Beatrice Trum, "How 'Probiotics' Fight Food-Borne Illness," *Consumers' Research Magazine*, v. 76, n. 12, p. 19, December 1993.

[7] Ibid.

[8] Hunter, Beatrice Trum, "How Well Do We Absorb Nutrients?" *Consumers' Research Magazine*, v. 77, n. 4, p. 17, April 1994.

[9] Babgaleh, B., et al, "Nutrition: A Cofactor in HIV Disease," *Journal of the American Dietetic Association*, v. 94, n. 9, p. 1019-1022, September 1994.

[10] Mantzioris, Evangeline, et al, "Dietary Substitution with L-Linolenic Acid-Rich Vegetable Oil Increases Eicosapentaenoic Acid Concentrations in Tissues," *American Journal of Clinical Nutrition*, v. 59, p. 1304-1309, 1994.

[11] Seidman, E., et al, "Nutritional Issues in Pediatric Inflammatory Bowel Disease," *Journal of Pediatric Gastroenterology and Nutrition*, v. 12, n. 4, 424-438, 1992.

[12] Weir, C.D., et al, "Glutamine Enhanced Elemental Diet Modifies Colonic Damage in a Hapten Induced Model of Colitis," *Gastroenterology*, v. 102, n. 4, Part II: A711, April 1992.

[13] Lin, Robert I., Ph.D. "Introduction: An Overview of the Nutritional and Pharmacological Properties of Garlic." Abstract from the First World Congress on the "Health Significance of Garlic and Garlic Constituents," Washington, D.C., Aug. 28-30, 1990.

Chapter 73: FRACTURES

[1] Gaby, Alan R., *Preventing and Reversing Osteoporosis*, Prima Publishing, Rocklin, CA, p. 41, 1994.

[2] Cohen, L. and Kitzes, R., "A Total Dietary Program Emphasizing Magnesium Instead of Calcium," *Journal of Reproductive Medicine*, v. 35, p. 503-507, 1990.

[3] Vikhanski, L. E., "Magnesium May Slow Bone Loss," *Medical Tribune*, July 22, 1993.

[4] Seyle, Hans, *Calciphylaxis*, University of Chicago Press, Chicago, Illinois, 1962.

[5] Elin, R., "Magnesium: The Forgotten Nutrient," *The Nutrition Report*, February 1995.

[6] Riggs, Lawrence B., M.D. and Melton, Joseph L., III, M.D., "The Prevention and Treatment of Osteoporosis," *New England Journal of Medicine*, v. 327, n. 9, August 27, 1992.

[7] Gaby, Alan R., *Preventing and Reversing Osteoporosis*, Prima Publishing, Rocklin, CA, 1994.

[8] Sahley, Bille J.; Birkner, Kathy, "Stress and Menopause," *Total Health*, v. 10, n. 5, p. 54, October 1988.

[9] Gallop, P.M., et al, "Carboxylated Calcium-Binding Proteins and Vitamin K," *New England Journal of Medicine*, v. 302, p. 1460-1466, 1980.

[10] Binkley, N.C. and Suttie, J.W., "Vitamin K Nutrition and Osteoporosis," *Journal of Nutrition*, v. 125, p. 1812-1821, 1995.

[11] Bouckaert, J. H. and Said, A. H., "Fracture Healing by Vitamin K," *Nature*, v. 185, p. 849, p. 1960.

[12] Bitensky, L., et al, "Circulating Vitamin K Levels in Patients with Fractures," *Journal of Bone Joint Surgery*, v. 70B, p. 663-664, 1988.

[13] Amdur, M. O., et al, "The Need for Manganese in Bone Development by the Rat," *Proc Soc Exp Biol Med*, v. 59, p. 254-255, 1945.

[14] Meacham, Susan L., et al, "Effect of Boron Supplementation on Blood and Urinary Calcium, Magnesium, and Phosphorous, and Urinary Boron in Athletic and Sedentary Women," *American Journal of Clinical Nutrition*, v. 61 p. 341-345, 1995.

[15] Nielsen, F.H., "Studies on the Relationship Between Boron and Magnesium Which Possibly Effects the Formation and Maintenance of Bones," *Magnesium Trace Elements*, v. 9, p. 61-69, 1990.

[16] Gaby, Alan R., *Preventing and Reversing Osteoporosis*, Prima Publishing, Rocklin, CA, p. 63-64, 1994.

[17] Smith, R. T., et al, "Mechanical Properties of Bone from Copper Deficient Rats Fed Starch or Fructose," *Federal Proceedings*, v. 44, p. 541, 1985.

[18] Wilson, T. M., et al, "Inhibition of Active Bone Resorption by Copper," *Calcif Tissue Int*, v. 33, p. 35-39, 1981.

[19] Holden, J.M., et al, "Zinc and Copper in Self-Selected Diets," *Journal of the American Dietetic Association*, v. 75, p. 23-28, 1979.

[20] Raloff, J., "Reasons for Boning Up on Manganese," *Science News*, v. 130, p. 199, September 27, 1986.

[21] Gold, M., "Basketball Bones," *Science*, p. 101-102, May-June 1980.

[22] Carlisle, E.M., "Silicon: An Essential Element for the Chick," *Science*, v. 178, p. 619-621, 1972.

[23] Kaufmann, Klaus, *Silica The Forgotten Nutrient*, Alive Books, Barnaby, B.C. Canada, p. 38, 1990.

[24] Ibid, p. 14-16.

[25] Lee, John R, M.D., *Natural Progesterone, The Multiple Roles of a Remarkable Hormone*, BLL Publishing, Sebastapol, CA, May 1995.

Chapter 74: FROSTBITE

[1] Boswick, John A., Jr.; Martyn, John W.; Schultz, Alvin L., *Patient Care*, v. 20, p. 48, November 15, 1986.

[2] Mazzotta, Mary Y., "Nutrition and Wound Healing," *Journal of the American Podiatric Medical Association*, v. 84, n. 9, p. 456, September 1994.

[3] *Martindale, The Extra Pharmacopoeia, Thirtieth Edition*, Department of Pharmaceutical Sciences, Royal Pharmaceutical Society of Great Britain, The Pharmaceutical Press, p. 2361-2362, 1993.

[4] Berger, M.M., et al, "Cutaneous Copper and Zinc Losses in Burns," *Burns*, v. 18, n. 5, p. 373, 1992.

[5] Myrdal, U., et al, "Magnesium Sulfate Infusion to Decrease the Circulating Calcitonin Gene-Related Peptide (CGRP) in Women With Primary Raynaud's Phenomenon," *Clinical Physiology*, v. 14, p. 539-546, 1994.

[6] Murray, Frank, "More Physicians are Endorsing Vitamin E," *Better Nutrition for Today's Living*, v. 55, n. 5, p. 6, May 1993.

[7] Paolisso, Giuseppe, et. al., Pharmacologic Doses of Vitamin E Improve Insulin Action in Healthy Subjects and Non-Insulin-Dependent Diabetic Patients," *American Journal of Clinical Nutrition*, v. 57, n. 5, p. 650, May 1993.

[8] Mazzotta, Mary Y., "Nutrition and Wound Healing," *Journal of the American Podiatric Medical Association*, v. 84, n. 9, p. 456, September 1994.

[9] Berger, M.M., et al, "Cutaneous Copper and Zinc Losses in Burns," *Burns*, v. 18, n. 5, p. 373, 1992.

[10] LeBlanc, J.M., *Canadian Journal of Biochemical Physiology*, v. 32, p. 407, 1954.

[11] *Better Nutrition for Today's Living*, v. 56, n. 3, p. 52, March 1994.

[12] Schechter, Steven R., "Aloe Vera, Produces Anti-Inflammatory, Immune Strengthening Effects on Skin," p. 51, *Let's Live*, December 1994.

[13] Murray, Frank, "Therapy and Treatment With Aloe Vera," *Better Nutrition for Today's Living*, v. 56, n. 3, p. 52, March 1994.

[14] *Better Nutrition for Today's Living*, v. 56, n. 3, p. 52, March 1994.

Chapter 75: FUNGUS INFECTIONS

[1] Reid, Gregor, Ph.D., et al, "Vaginal Flora and Urinary Tract Infections," *Current Opinion in Infectious Disease*, v. 4, p. 37-41, 1991.

[2] Subak-Sharpe, Genell, J., and Bogdonoff, Morton, D., *Home Health Handbook*, BV/ IMP, Inc, MCMLXXXXIX.

[3] Trowbridge, John Parks, M.D. & Walker, Morton, D.P.M., The Yeast Syndrome, Bantam Books, p. 151, November 1986.

[4] Ibid, p. 261.

[5] Ghannoum M.A., "Studies on the Anticandidal Mode of Action of Allium Sativum," *Journal of General Microbiology*, v. 134, p. 2917-2924, November 1988.

[6] Mikhail, Magdy S., et al, "Decreased Beta-Carotene Levels in Exfoliated Vaginal Epithelial Cells in Women With Vaginal Candidiasis," *American Journal of Reproductive Immunology*, v. 32, p. 221-225, 1994.

[7] Trowbridge, John Parks, M.D. & Walker, Morton, D.P.M., The Yeast Syndrome, Bantam Books, p. 168-172, November 1986.

[8] Ibid, p. 166.

[9] Murray, Frank, "Acidophilus: the Beneficial Bacteria," *Better Nutrition for Today's Living*, v. 52, n. 10, p. 14, October 1990.

[10] Wright, Jonathan V., *Dr. Wright's Book of Nutritional Therapy*, Rodale Press, Emmaus, PA, p. 373-374, 1979.

Chapter 76: GALLBLADDER PROBLEMS

[1] Breneman, J.C., "Allergy Elimination Diet – Gallbladder Diet," *Annals of Allergy*, v. 26, p. 83-89, 1968.

[2] Scobey, Martin, et al, "Dietary Fish Oil Effects on Biliary Lipid Secretion and Cholesterol Gallstone Formation in the African Green Monkey," *Hepatology*, v. 14, n. 4, 679-684, 1991.

[3] Moerman, Clara J., et al, "Dietary Sugar Intake in the Etiology of Biliary Tract Cancer," *International Journal of Epidemiology*, v. 22, n. 2, p. 207-213, 1993.

[4] Moerman, Clara J., Ph.D., M.D., et al, "Dietary Risk Factors for Clinically Diagnosed Gallstones in Middle-Aged Men: A 25-Year Follow-up Study," *Annals of Epidemiology*, p. 248-254, 1994.

[5] Phonpanichresamee, Chopaga, et al, "Hypocholesterolemic Effect of Vitamin E on Cholesterol-Fed Rabbit," *International Journal of Vitamin and Nutrition Research*, v. 60, p. 240-244, 1990.

[6] Simon, J.A., "Ascorbic Acid and Cholesterol Gallstones", *Medical Hypotheses*, v. 40, p. 81-84, 1993.

[7] Wright, Jonathan V., "Relieving Gallbladder Pain," *Nutrition & Healing*, v. 2, n. 7, August 1995.

[8] Ibid.

Chapter 77: GAS, INTESTINAL

[1] Atkins, Robert C., *Dr. Atkins' Health Revolution*, Houghton Mifflin Co., Boston, p, 282-296, 1988.

[2] Stoy, Diane B. Ed.D., RN, et al, "Cholesterol-Lowering Effects of Ready-To-Eat Cereal Containing Psyllium," *Journal of the American Dietetic Association*, v. 93, n. 8, p. 910-911, August 1993.

Chapter 78: GASTRITIS

[1] "Nutrition and Ageing," *Nutrition Action Health Letter*, v. 19, n. 4, p. 5-7, May 1992.

[2] Russel, R., "Atrophic Gastritis: The Effects of Nutrient Bioavailability," *Journal of The American College of Nutrition*,v. 9, n. 5, p. 535, 1990.

[3] Ibid.

[4] Sturniolo, G.C., M.D., et al, "Inhibition of Gastric Acid Secretion Reduces Zinc Absorption in Men," *Journal of The American College of Nutrition*, v. 10, n. 4, p. 372-375, 1991.

[5] Wright, Jonathan V., M.D.," Treatment of Childhood Asthma With Parenteral Vitamin B12, Gastric Re-Acidification, and Attention to Food Allergy, Magnesium and Pyridoxine: Three Case Reports With Background an Integrated Hypothesis," *Journal of Nutritional Medicine*, v. 1, p. 277-282, 1990.

[6] Forgacs, Ian, "Clinical Gastroenterology," *British Medical Journal*, v. 00000310, n. 6972, p. 113, January 14, 1995.

[7] Carmel, Ralph, M.D., et al, "Helicobacter Pylori Infection in Food-Cobalamin Malabsorption," *Digestive Diseases and Sciences*, v. 39, n. 2, p. 309-304, February 1994.

[8] Singh, Vishwa N. and Gaby, Suzanne K., "Premalignant Lesions: Role of Antioxidant Vitamins, Beta-Carotene in Risk Reduction and Prevention of Malignant Transformation," *American Journal of Clinical Nutrition*, v. 53, p. 386S-390S, 1991.

[9] Ruiz, Bernardo, M.D., et al, "Vitamin C Concentration in Gastric Juice Before and After Anti-Helicobacter Pylori Treatment," *American Journal of Gastroenterology*, p. 89, n. 4, p. 533-539, 1994.

Chapter 79: GLAUCOMA

[1] Goulart, Frances Sheridan, "Ten Reasons to Take Vitamin C All Year Round," *Bestways*, v. 17, n. 10, p. 41-44, October 1989.

[2] Linner, E., "The Pressure Lowering Effect of Ascorbic Acid in Ocular Hypertension," *Acta Ophthalmologica*, v. 47, n. 2, p. 685-689, 1969.

[3] Stocker, F. W., "New Ways of Influencing the Intraocular Pressure," *New York State Journal of Medicine*, v. 49, p. 58-63, 1949.

[4] Lane, B.C., "Elevation of Intraocular Pressure With Daily Sustained Close Work Stimulus to Accommodation of Lowered Tissue Chromium and Dietary Deficiency of Ascorbic Acid," *Doc. Opthal. Proc. Series*, v. 28, p. 149-155, 1981.

[5] Dunne, Lavon J., *Nutrition Almanac*, Third Edition, McGraw-Hill Publishing Company, p. 70, 1990.

[6] Ibid, p. 22-23.

[7] McGuire, Rick, "Fish Oil Cuts Lower Ocular Pressure," *Medical Tribune*, v. 25, August 19, 1991.

[8] Murray, Frank, "Keeping an Eye on Good Health," *Today's Living*, v. 20, n. 8, p. 8, August 1989.

Chapter 80: GOUT

[1] Blau, Ludwig W., "Cherry Diet Control for Gout and Arthritis," *Texas Reports on Biology and Medicine*, v. 8, p. 309-311, 1950.

[2] Rodale, J.I., *The Health Finder*, Rodale Books, Emmaus, PA, p. 61, 1955.

[3] Murray, Michael, M.D. and Pizzorno, Joseph, N.D., *Encyclopedia of Natural Medicine*, Prima Publishing, Rocklin, CA, p. 339, 1991.

[4] Collier, David H., "Gout and Arthritis: Are They Really Affected by Diet?," *Consultant*, v. 29, n. 5, p. 63, May 1989.

[5] Clifford A.J., Story D.L., "Levels of Purines in Food and Their Metabolic Effects in Rats, *J. Nutr.* v. 106, p. 435-442, 1976.

[6] Gibson, T., et al, "A Controlled Study of Diet in Patients with Gout," *Annals of Rheumatic Diseases*, v. 42, n. 2, p. 123-127, 1983.

[7] Murray, Michael, M.D. and Pizzorno, Joseph, N.D., *Encyclopedia of Natural Medicine*, Prima Publishing, Rocklin, CA, p. 337, 1991.

Chapter 81: GRAY HAIR

[1] Hughes, W., *British Medical Journal*, July 30, 1946.

[2] Nicholls, Lucius, *The Lancet,* August 10, 1946.

[3] Hundley, J. M., *Proceedings of the Society of Experimental Biology and Medicine*, July 1950.

[4] Eller, J.J., Diaz, Luis A., *New York State Journal of Medicine*, July 15, 1943.

[5] DeVilbiss, Lydia Allen, M.D., *Medical Women's Journal*, November 1942.

[6] Geiringer, E., *Revue Medical de Liege*, October 15, 1950.

Chapter 82: HAIR LOSS

[1] Maynard, H., et al, *Journal of Nutrition*, v. 64, p. 85, 1958.

[2] Poznankaia, A.H., *Biochemistry*, v. 23, p. 215, 1958.

[3] Kazz, F., *Archives of Dermatology*, v. 78, p. 740, 1958.

[4] Kinney, T. D., et al, *Journal of Experimental Medicine*, v. 102, p. 151, 1955.

[5] Gufner, R., *Archives of Dermatology and Siphilology*, v. 64, p. 688, 1951.

6   Gadberry, Rebecca James, "Hair-Raising Truths About Hair Loss Remedies," *Let's Live*, p. 70, July 1994.
7   Dunne, Lavon J., *Nutrition Almanac*, Third Edition, McGraw-Hill Publishing Company, p. 173, 1990.
8   Kaufmann, Klaus, *Silica The Forgotten Nutrient*, Alive Books, Barnaby, B.C. Canada, , p. 47, 1990.
9   Gerras, Charles, et al, eds, *The Encyclopedia of Common Diseases*, Rodale Press Inc., Emmaus, PA, p. 756, 1976.

Chapter 83: HANGOVER

1   Emsley, John, "A Dispassionate Look at Alcohol," *Consumers' Research Magazine*, v. 78, n. 7, p. 19, July 1995.
2   Judge, Gillian, "Cures for Holiday Health Hazards, *McCall's*, v. 122, n. 3, p. 38, December, 1994.
3   Werbach, Melvyn, *Nutritional Influences on Illness*, Second Edition, Third Line Press, Tarzana, California, p.25-28, 1993.
4   Werbach, Melvyn, *Nutritional Influences on Illness*, Second Edition, Third Line Press, Tarzana, California, p. 305, 1993.
5   Biery, Janet Reid, "Alcohol Craving in Rehabilitation: Assessment of Nutrition Therapy," *Journal of the American Dietetic Association*, v. 91, p. 463, April 1991.
6   Dunne, Lavon J., *Nutrition Almanac*, Third Edition, McGraw-Hill Publishing Company, 1990.
7   Herbert, Victor, M.D., J.D.; Subak-Sharpe, Genell J., M.S. & Hammock, Delia A, M.S., R.D., *The Mount Sinai School of Medicine Complete Book of Nutrition*, St. Martin's Press, New York, p. 632, 1990.

Chapter 84: HEAD LICE

1   Rattenbury, Jeanne, "A Real Head Scratcher," *Vegetarian Times*, n. 217, p. 28, September 1995.
2   Liberty, Maria, "Tea Tree Oil: Medicine Cabinet Mainstay," *Better Nutrition for Today's Living*, v. 57, n. 4, p. 72, April 1995.
3   *1,001 Home Health Remedies*, FC&A Publishing, Peachtree City, GA, p. 267, February 1994.
4   Rattenbury, Jeanne, "A Real Head Scratcher," *Vegetarian Times*, n. 217, p. 28, September 1995.
5   Burton Goldberg Group, *Alternative Medicine, The Definitive Guide*, Future Medicine Publishing, Inc., Puyallup, WA, p. 609-610, 1993.

Chapter 85: HEARING LOSS

1   Williams, Rebecca D., "Enjoy, Protect the Best Ears of Your Life," *FDA Consumer*, v. 26, n. 4, p. 25, May 1992.
2   Jaret, Peter, "The Rock & Roll Syndrome," *In Health*, v. 4, n. 4, p. 50-58, July-August 1990.
3   Cardinal, David, "Cover Your Ears," *Men's Health*, v. 5, n. 3, p. 40, August 1990.
4   Williams, Rebecca D., "Enjoy, Protect the Best Ears of Your Life," *FDA Consumer*, v. 26, n. 4, p. 25, May 1992.

[5] Cardinal, David, "Cover Your Ears," *Men's Health*, v. 5, n. 3, p. 40, August 1990.

[6] Attias, Joseph D.Sc., et al, "Oral Magnesium Intake Reduces Permanent Hearing Loss Induced by Noise Exposure," *American Journal of Otolaryngology*, v. 15, n. 1, p. 26-32, January-February 1994.

[7] Franz, K.B., "Hearing Thresholds of Rats Fed Different Levels of Magnesium For Two Weeks," *Journal of The American College of Nutrition*, v. 11, n. 5, October 1992.

[8] Ratner, Douglas, M.D. and Carey, Zev, M.D., "Medical Effects of Indoor Air Pollution," *Hospital Medicine*, p. 41-46, May 1995.

[9] Brown, Scott J., "Environmental Doctors Take Up Pollution Prevention Cause," *Family Practice News*, p. 6, January 1, 1995.

[10] "Erythromycin and Hearing Loss," *Emergency Medicine*, p. 232-243, June 15, 1992.

[11] Chole, Q., "Vitamin A in the Cochlea," *Archives of Otorhinolaryngol*, v. 124, p. 379-382, 1978.

[12] Lohle, E., "The Influence of Chronic Vitamin A Deficiency on Human and Animal Ears," *Archives of Otorhinolaryngol*, v. 234, p. 167-173, 1982.

[13] Werbach, Melvyn, *Healing Through Nutrition*, HarperCollins, New York, NY, p. 219-221, 1993.

[14] Ikeda, K., et al, "The Effect of Vitamin D Deficiency on the Cochlear Potentials and the Perilymphatic Ionized Calcium Concentration of Rats," *Acta Otolaryngol Suppl*, v. 435, p. 64-72, 1987.

[15] Werbach, Melvyn, *Healing Through Nutrition*, HarperCollins, New York, NY, p. 219-221, 1993.

Chapter 86: HEARTBURN AND HIATAL HERNIA

[1] Burkitt, Denis P. & James, Peter A., *The Lancet*, July 21, 1973.

[2] Downs, Robert W., & Van Baak, Alice, "When Heartburn Won't Go Away," Bestways, p. 38-42, January 1984.

[3] Balch, James F., M.D., and Balch, Phyllis A., *Prescription for Nutritional Healing*, Avery Publishing Group, Garden City Park, N.Y., p. 197, 1990.

[4] Gerras, Charles, et al, eds, *The Encyclopedia of Common Diseases*, Rodale Press, Emmaus, PA, p. 481, 1976.

Chapter 87: HEART PROBLEMS

[1] Gaziano, J. Michael, "Antioxidant Vitamins and Coronary Artery Disease Risk," *The American Journal of Medicine*, v. 97, September 26, 1994.

[2] Subak-Sharpe, Genell, J., and Bogdonoff, Morton, D., *Home Health Handbook*, BV/IMP, Inc, p. 37, 45, MCMLXXXXIX.

[3] "Magnesium For Acute Myocardial Infarction?" Editor, *The Lancet*, September 14, v. 333, p. 667-668, Sept. 14, 1991.

[4] Woods, Kent L.; Fletcher, Susan; Roffe, Christine; Haider, Yasser, "Intravenous Magnesium Sulphate in Suspected Acute Myocardial Infarction: Results of the Second Leicester Intravenous Magnesium Intervention Trial," *The Lancet*, v. 339, n. 8809, p. 1553, June 27, 1992.

[5] Orlov, Michael, M.D., et al, "A Review of Magnesium, Acute Myocardial Infarction Arrhythmia," *The Journal of The American College of Nutrition*, v. 13, n. 2, p. 127-132, 1994.

6   Thogersen, Anna M., et al, "Effects of Intravenous Magnesium Sulfate in Suspected Acute Myocardial Infarction on Acute Arrhythmias and Long-Term Outcome," *International Journal of Cardiology*, v. 49, p. 143-151, 1995.

7   Seelig, Mildred S., M.D., M.P.H., "Magnesium, Antioxidants and Myocardial Infarction," *American Journal of Clinical Nutrition*, v. 13, n. 2, p. 116-117, 1994.

8   Grindy, Robert, "More About Magnesium," *Saturday Evening Post*, v. 259, p. 50, July-August 1987.

9   Elin, R., "Magnesium: The Forgotten Nutrient," *The Nutrition Report*, February 1995.

10 "Magnesium Can Help With Energy, Depression," *Better Nutrition for Today's Living*, v. 57, n. 2, p. 26, February 1995.

11 Friedensohn, Aharon, et al, "Malignant Arrhythmias in Relation to Values of Serum Potassium in Patients With Acute Myocardial Infarction," *International Journal of Cardiology*, v. 32, p. 331-338, 1991.

12 Prielipp, Richard C., M.D., et al, "Magnesium Antagonizes the Action of Lysophosphatidylcholine (LPC) in Myocardial Cells: A Possible Mechanism For Its Antiarrhythmic Effects," *Anesth Analg*, v. 80, p. 1083-1087, 1995.

13 Touyz, R.M., "Magnesium Supplementation as an Adjuvant to Synthetic Calcium Channel Antagonism in the Treatment of Hypertension," *Medical Hypothesis*, v. 36, p. 140-141, 1991.

14 Seelig, Mildred S., M.D., M.P.H., et al, "Consequences of Magnesium Deficiency on Enhancement of Stress Reaction; Preventive and Therapeutic Implications (A Review)," *Journal of the American College of Nutrition*, v. 13, n. 5, p. 429-446, 1994.

15 Korpela, Heikki, DVM, M.D, "Hypothesis: Increased Calcium and Decreased Magnesium in Heart Disease and Liver of Pigs Dying Suddenly of Microangiopathy: An Animal Model For The Study of Oxidative Damage," *Journal of The American College of Nutrition*, v. 10, n. 2, p. 127-131, 1991.

16 "Research Offers Evidence of Vitamin E Cardiac Benefit," *Medical Tribune*, p. 8, November 21, 1994.

17 Stephens, N.G., et al, "Randomized Controlled Trial of Vitamin E in Patients with Coronary Disease: Cambridge Heart Antioxidant Study (CHAOS), *The Lancet*, v. 347, p. 781-786, March 23, 1996.

18 Gaziano, J. Michael, "Antioxidant Vitamins and Coronary Artery Disease Risk," *The American Journal of Medicine*, v. 97, September 26, 1994.

19 Todd, Susan, et al, "An Investigation of the Relationship Between Antioxidant Vitamin Intake and Coronary Heart Disease in Men and Women Using Logistic Regression Analysis," *Journal of Clinical Epidemiology*, v. 48, n. 2, p. 307-316, 1995.

20 Xia, Yiming, et al, "Keshan's Disease and Selenium Status of Populations in China," *Selenium in Biology and Human Health*, Chapter 10, p. 183-196, 1994.

21 "Urinary Selenium Concentrations," *Clinical Chemistry*, v. 39, n. 10, 1993.

22 "Copper and Its Possible Role in Cardiomyopathies," *The Nutrition Report*, v. 89, p. 96, December 1993.

23 Mitchell, John, "Many Riches to be Mined from Minerals; Zinc Found Effective Against Many Ills, Selenium Enhances Immune Response, Silicon May Prevent Alzheimer's Disease," *Health News & Review*, v.1, n. 2, p. 7, July-August 1991.

24 Hertog M. G. I., et al, "Dietary Antioxidant Flavonoids and Risk of Coronary Heart Disease: the Zutphen Elderly Study," *The Lancet*, v. 342, p. 1007-1011, 1993.

[25] Goldfinger, Stephen E., "Garlic: Good for What Ails You?" *Harvard Health Letter*, v. 16, n. 10, p. 1, August 1991.

[26] Yamasaki, Takeshi, et al, "Garlic Compounds Protect Vascular Endothelial Cells from Hydrogen Peroxide-Induced Oxidant Injury," *Phytotherapy Research*, v. 8, p. 408-412, 1994.

[27] Wright, Jonathan, "Congestive Heart Failure," *Nutrition & Healing*, v. 1, n. 5, December 1994.

[28] Ishiyama, T., "A Clinical Study of the Effect of Coenzyme Q10 on Congestive Heart Failure," *Jpn Heart J*, v. 17, p. 32-42, 1976.

[29] Morisco, C., et al, "Effect of Coenzyme Q10 in Patients with Congestive Heart Failure: A Long-Term Multicenter Randomized Study," *Clin Invest*, v. 71, p. S134-S136, 1993.

[30] Selhub, Jacob and Paul F. Jacques, et. al, "Association Between Plasma Homocysteine Concentrations and Extracranial Carotid Artery Stenosis," *New England Journal of Medicine*, v. 332, n. 5, p. 286-291, February 2, 1995.

[31] Stampfer, Meir J. and Rene M. Malinow, "Can Lowering Homocysteine Levels Reduce Cardiovascular Risk?" *New England Journal of Medicine*, v. 332, n. 5, p. 28-29, February 2, 1995.

[32] Ibid.

[33] Findlay, Steven, et al, "Iron and Your Heart," *U.S. News & World Report*, v. 113, n. 11, p. 61-67, September 21, 1992.

[34] *Tufts University Diet & Nutrition Letter*, v. 10, n. 11, p.3, January 1993.

[35] Laino, Charlene, "Trans-Fatty Acids in Margarine Can Increase MI Risk," *Medical Tribune*, v. 4, February 24, 1994.

[36] Raloff, J., "Margarine is Anything but a Marginal Fat," *Science News*, v.145, p. 325, May 21, 1994.

[37] Willett, Walter C., et al, "Intake of Trans Fatty Acids and Risk of Coronary Heart Disease Among Women," *The Lancet*, v. 341, p. 581-585, March 6, 1993.

[38] Mann, George V., "Metabolic Consequences of Dietary Trans Fatty Acids," *The Lancet*, v. 343, n. 8908, p. 1268, May 21, 1994.

Chapter 88: HEMORRHOIDS

[1] Bland, Jeffrey, editor, *Medical Applications of Clinical Nutrition*, Keats Publishing, New Canaan, CT, p. 279, 1983.

[2] Gerras, Charles, et al, eds, *The Encyclopedia of Common Diseases*, Rodale Press, Emmaus, PA, p. 949, 1976.

[3] Pauling, Linus, *How to Live Longer and Feel Better*, W.H. Freeman & Co., New York, p. 318, 1986.

[4] Hodgen, R. E., et al, *American Journal of Clinical Nutrition*, v. 11, n. 180, p.187, 1962.

[5] Schuster, Marvin M., M.D., "Psyllium Products Aid Common GI Disorders," *Modern Medicine*, March, v. 58, p. 24-25, 1990.

[6] Dunne, Lavon J., *Nutrition Almanac*, Third Edition, McGraw-Hill Publishing Company, p. 178, 1990.

[7] "Does Preparation H Work?" *Consumer Reports*, v. 51, p. 579, September 1986.

Chapter 89: HERPES SIMPLEX

[1] Rossen, Anne, E., "A Sore Subject," *Current Health*, v. 18, n. 7, p. 26, March 1992.

² Rubenstein, E. and Federman, D. D., *Scientific American Medicine*, Scientific American, New York, NY, p. 1-9, 1988.

³ Kahn, Jason, "Vitamin A May Help Suppress Herpes Outbreaks," *Medical Tribune*, p. 10, May 18, 1995.

⁴ Apisariyakulm, Amphawan, Ph.D., et al, "Zinc Monoglycerolate is Effective Against Oral Herpetic Sores," *Medical Journal of Australia*, v. 152, p. 54, January 1, 1990.

⁵ Finnerty, E. F., "Topical Zinc in the Treatment of Herpes Simplex," *Cutis*, v. 37, n. 2, p. 130-131, 1986.

⁶ Lewin, S., *Vitamin C: Its Molecular Biology and Medical Potential*, Van Nostrand Reinhold Co., New York, 1973.

⁷ Terezhalmy, G.T., et al, "The Use of Water-Soluble Bioflavonoid-Ascorbic Acid Complex in the Treatment of Recurrent Herpes Labialis," *Oral Surg*, v. 45, p. 56-62, 1978.

⁸ Braly, James, M.D., *Dr. Braly's Food Allergy & Nutrition Revolution*, Keats Publishing, New Canaan, CT, p. 384, 1992.

⁹ Fitzherbert, J., "Genital Herpes and Zinc," *Medical Journal of Australia*, v. 1, p. 399, 1979.

¹⁰ Starasoler, S. & Haber, G.S., "Use of Vitamin E Oil in Primary Herpes Gingivostomatitis in an Adult," *NY State Dent. J.*, v. 44, n. 9, p. 382-383, 1978.

¹¹ Challem, Jack, "How To Use Vitamins and Minerals as Home Remedies," *Natural Health*, v. 24, n. 2, p. 60-68, March-April 1994.

Chapter 90: HICCUPS

¹ Bricklin, Mark, *The Practical Encyclopedia of Natural Healing*, Rodale Press, Emmaus, PA, p. 287, 1983.

² Lipps, D.C., et al, "Nifedipine for Intractable Hiccups," *Neurology*, v. 40, n. 3, p. 531, March, 1990.

³ Lewis, R.J., Endean, R., "Direct and Indirect Effects of Ciguatoxin on Guinea-Pig Atria and Papillary Muscles," *Arch Pharmacol*, v. 334, p. 313-322, 1986.

Chapter 91: HIGH THYROID

¹ Burton Goldberg Group, *Alternative Medicine, The Definitive Guide*, Future Medicine Publishing, Inc., Puyallup, WA, p. 934, 1993.

² "Fatigue Brings Bedtime Blahs: Sluggish Thyroid Leads to Sexual and Other Ills," *Health News & Review*, p. 6, Summer 1995.

³ Ibid.

⁴ Jennings, Isobel, *Vitamins in Endocrine Metabolism*, Charles C. Thomas, Springfield, ILL, p. 99, 1970.

⁵ Burton Goldberg Group, *Alternative Medicine, The Definitive Guide*, Future Medicine Publishing, Inc., Puyallup, WA, p. 758, 1993.

⁶ Kennedy, Bob, "Borage Wildflowers: Best Source of GLA," *Total Health*, v. 13, n. 1, p. 44, February 1991.

⁷ Elin, R., "Magnesium: The Forgotten Nutrient," *The Nutrition Report*, February 1995.

⁸ "Magnesium: The 5th But Forgotten Electrolyte," *American Journal of Clinical Pathology*, v. 102, n. 5, p. 616-622, 1994.

⁹ Martin, Linda G., D.V.M., et al, "Magnesium in the 1990s: Implications For Veterinary Critical Care," *Veterinary Emergency and Critical Care*, v. 3, n. 2, p. 105-113, 1994.

[10] Higgins, M.D., "Magnesium Medicine Comes of Age," *Emergency Medicine*, p. 83-95, February 28, 1991.
[11] Elin, R., "Magnesium: The Forgotten Nutrient," *The Nutrition Report*, February 1995.
[12] Ibid.
[13] Evanier, Dini, *Patient Care*, v. 17, p. 173-183, April 15, 1983.
[14] Ibid.

Chapter 92: HYPERTENSION

[1] *The Fifth Report of the Joint National Committee on Detection, Evaluation, and Treatment of High Blood Pressure*, National High Blood Pressure Education Program, National Institutes of Health, National Heart, Lung, and Blood Institute, Bethesda, Maryland, NIH publication no. 93-1088, 1993.
[2] Whelton P.K., Klag M.J., "Epidemiology of High Blood Pressure," *Clin. Geriatr. Med.*, v. 5, p. 639-655, 1989.
[3] Ibid.
[4] *The Fifth Report of the Joint National Committee on Detection, Evaluation, and Treatment of High Blood Pressure*, National High Blood Pressure Education Program, National Institutes of Health, National Heart, Lung, and Blood Institute, Bethesda, Maryland, NIH publication no. 93-1088, 1993.
[5] Seelig, Mildred S., M.D., M.P.H., et al, "Consequences of Magnesium Deficiency on Enhancement of Stress Reaction; Preventive and Therapeutic Implications (A Review)," *Journal of the American College of Nutrition*, v. 13, n. 5, p. 429-446, 1994.
[6] Korpela, Heikki, DVM, M.D, "Hypothesis: Increased Calcium and Decreased Magnesium in Heart Disease and Liver of Pigs Dying Suddenly of Microangiopathy: An Animal Model For The Study of Oxidative Damage," *Journal of The American College of Nutrition*, v. 10, n. 2, p. 127-131, 1991.
[7] Haas, Elson. M., M.D., *Staying Healthy with Nutrition*, Celestial Arts, Berkeley, CA, p. 170, 1992.
[8] Amery A., et al, "Mortality and Morbidity Results from the European Working Party on High Blood Pressure in the Elderly trial," *The Lancet*, v. 1, p. 1349-5134, 1985.
[9] Gaziano, J. Michael, "Antioxidant Vitamins and Coronary Artery Disease Risk," *The American Journal of Medicine*, v. 97, September 26, 1994.
[10] Touyz, R.M., "Magnesium Supplementation as an Adjuvant to Synthetic Calcium Channel Antagonism in the Treatment of Hypertension," *Medical Hypothesis*, v. 36, p. 140-141, 1991.
[11] "Calcium-Channel Blockers for Hypertension: Risky?" *Harvard Heart Letter*, v. 5, n. 12, p.1, August, 1995.
[12] Gordon, E. P., "Magnesium Regulation of Calcium in Essential Hypertension," *Journal of the American College of Nutrition*, v. 11, n. 5, p. 610, October 1992.
[13] Pennington, Jean A.T., Ph.D., RD and Young, Barbara E., "Total Diet Study of Nutritional Elements, 1982-1989," *Journal of The American Dietetic Association*, v. 91, n. 2, p. 179-183, February 1991.
[14] Elin, R., "Magnesium: The Forgotten Nutrient," *The Nutrition Report*, February 1995.
[15] Krishna, G. Gopal, M.D. and Kapoor, Shiv C., Ph.D., "Potassium Depletion Exacerbates Essential Hypertension," *Annals of Internal Medicine*, v. 115, n. 2, p. 77-83, July 15, 1991.

[16] Karppanen, Heikki, "Minerals and Blood Pressure," *Annals of Medicine*, v. 23, p. 299-306, 1991.

[17] Valdes, Gloria, et al, "Potassium Supplementation Lowers Blood Pressure and Increases Urinary Kallikrein in Essential Hypertensives," *Journal of Human Hypertension*, v. 5, p. 91-96, 1991.

[18] Cappuccio, F.P., et al, "Potassium Supplementation For Hypertension: A Meta-Analysis," *Journal of Hypertension*, v. 9, p. 465-473, May 1991.

[19] McCarron, David A., M.D., "The Integrated Effects of Electrolytes on Blood Pressure," *The Nutrition Report*, v. 9, n. 8, p. 57-64, August 1991.

[20] Singh, R.B., M.D., et al, "Dietary Changes Modulate Blood Pressure and Blood Lipids in Hypertension," *Journal of Nutritional Medicine*, v. 2, p. 17-24, 1991.

[21] Durning, Allen B., "Junk Food, Food Junk," *World Watch*, p. 7-9, September-October 1991.

[22] Al- Karadaghi P., et al, "Renal Function and Sugar-Induced Blood Pressure Elevations," *Journal of The American College of Nutrition*, v. 10, n. 5, p. 556-570, October 1991.

[23] Bricklin, Mark, *The Practical Encyclopedia of Natural Healing*, Rodale Press, Emmaus, PA, p. 58-59, 1976.

Chapter 93: IMPOTENCE

[1] Scheer, James F., "Impotency, Not a Life Sentence," *Bestways*, May 1986.

[2] Lawren, Bill, "New Erector Sets," *WorldWide Web*, February 1994.

[3] Walker, Morton and Joan, *Sexual Nutrition*, Coward-McCann, Inc., New York, p. 225, 1983.

[4] Taylor, Deborah Seymour, *Today's Living*, v. 20, n. 5, p. 8, May 1989.

[5] "Diabetic Impotency: New Hope," *University of Southern California News Service*, April 1987.

[6] Kahn, Jason, "Smoking May Increase Risk of Impotence," *Medical Tribune*, p. 5, January 19, 1995.

[7] Pfeiffer, Carl C., *Mental and Elemental Nutrients*, Keats Publishing, New Canaan, CN, p. 282, 1975.

[8] Faelten, Sharon, *The Complete Book of Minerals for Health*, Rodale Press, Emmaus, PA, p. 432-433, 1981.

[9] Ibid.

[10] Smith, P.J., and Talbert, R. L., "Sexual Dysfunction with Antihypertensive and Antipsychotic Agents," *Clinical Pharmacy*, v. 5, p. 373-384, 1986.

[11] Touyz, R.M., "Magnesium Supplementation as an Adjuvant to Synthetic Calcium Channel Antagonism in the Treatment of Hypertension," *Medical Hypothesis*, v. 36, p. 140-141, 1991.

[12] Pennington, Jean A.T., Ph.D., RD and Young, Barbara E., "Total Diet Study of Nutritional Elements, 1982-1989," *Journal of The American Dietetic Association*, v. 91, n. 2, p. 179-183, February 1991.

[13] Elin, R., "Magnesium: The Forgotten Nutrient," *The Nutrition Report*, February 1995.

Chapter 94: INFECTIONS

[1] Cheraskin, Emanuel, M.D., D.M.D., *Vitamin C, Who Needs It?*, Arlington Press and Company, Birmingham AL, p. 109, 1993.

[2] Ibid, p. 62.

[3] "Vitamin C Enhances Antibiotic Therapy," *The Nutrition Report*, v. 10, n. 4, p. 31, April 1992.

[4] "Decreased Resistance to Antibiotics and Plasmid Loss in Plasmid-Carrying Strains of Staphylococcus Aureus Treated With Ascorbic Acid," *Mutation Research*, v. 264, p. 119-125, 1991.

[5] Vinson, J.A. & Bose, P, "Comparative Bioavailability to Humans of Ascorbic Acid Alone or in a Citrus Extract," *American Journal of Clinical Nutrition*, v. 48, n. 3, p. 601-604, September 1988.

[6] Kotheri, Geopa, M.D. and Naik, Ekneth, M.D., "Effect of Vitamin A Prophylaxis on Morbidity and Mortality Among Children in Urban Slums in Bombay," *British Medical Journal*, October 1991.

[7] Rodale, J.I., *The Health Finder*, Rodale Books, Emmaus, PA, p. 257-259, 1955.

[8] Burton Goldberg Group, *Alternative Medicine, The Definitive Guide*, Future Medicine Publishing, Inc., Puyallup, WA, p. 634, 1993.

[9] Abdullah, T.H., M.D., et al. "Enhancement of Natural Killer Cell Activity in AIDS with Garlic," *Deutsche Zeitschrift fur Okologie*, 1989.

[10] Levine, Stephen A., Ph.D. "Organic Germanium: a Novel Dramatic Immunostimulant." The *Journal of Orthomolecular Medicine*, May 21, 1987.

[11] Abdullah, T.H., M.D., et al, "Enhancement of Natural Killer Cell Activity in AIDS with Garlic," *Deutsche Zeitschrift fur Okologie*, 1989.

Chapter 95: INFERTILITY

[1] Laino, Charlene, "Stress Due to Loss of a Loved One Tied to Male Infertility," *Medical Tribune*, p. 16, December 1, 1994.

[2] Taylor, Deborah, "Dietary Therapy Helps Treatment of Infertility, *Today's Living*, v. 20, n. 4, p. 12, April 1989.

[3] James, Elizabeth, "Stress: Enemy or Friend?" *Total Health*, v. 13, n.1, p. 31, February 1991.

[4] Tessler, Gordon S., "The Correct Nutrition to Cope with Stress," *Total Health*, v. 11, n. 3, p. 12, June 1989.

[5] Taylor, Deborah, "Dietary Therapy Helps Treatment of Infertility, *Today's Living*, v. 20, n. 4, p. 12, April 1989.

[6] Ibid.

[7] Ibid.

[8] Ibid.

[9] Bedwal, R., "Zinc, Copper and Selenium in Reproduction," *Experientia*, v. 50, p. 626-640, July 1994.

[10] Watanabe, Toshiaki and Endo, Akira, "Effects of Selenium Deficiency on Sperm Morphology and Spermatocyte Chromosomes in Mice," *Mutation Research*, v. 262, p. 93-99, 1991.

[11] Bedwal, R., "Trace Minerals in Reproduction," *The Nutrition Report*, p. 79, October 1994.

[12] Cheraskin, Emanuel, "A Vitamin C Catechism," *Nutrition Health Review*, n. 73, p. 11, Summer, 1995.

[13] Cheraskin, Emanuel, M.D., D.M.D., *Vitamin C, Who Needs It?*, Arlington Press and Company, Birmingham AL, p. 5-6, 1993.

[14] Harris, W. A., et al, "Apparent Effect of Ascorbic Acid Medication on Semen Metal Levels," *Fertility and Sterility*, v. 32, n. 4, p. 455-459, 1979.

[15] "Male Reproductive Health and Environmental Estrogens," Editorial, *The Lancet*, v. 345, p. 933-935, April 15, 1995.

[16] Brighthope, Ian, MB, BS,"The Role of Nutritional Medicine in General Practice," *Australian Family Physician*, v. 19, n. 3, p. 357-365, March 1990.

[17] Werbach, Melvyn, *Nutritional Influences on Illness*, Second Edition, Third Line Press, Tarzana, California, p. 380, 1993.

[18] Costa, M., et al, "L-Carnitine in Idiopathic Asthenozoospermia: A Multi-Center Study," *Andrologia*, v. 26, p. 155-159, 1994.

[19] Wun, Wan-Song A., M.D., et al, "Vitamin Supplements Improve Fertility Potential of Subfertile Male With Macrocytic Anemia-A Case Study," *Journal of Assisted Reproduction and Genetics*, v. 11, n. 7, p. 375- 378, 1994.

[20] Werbach, Melvyn, M.D., "Nutritional Influences on Illness," *Townsend Letter for Doctors & Patients*, p. 20, October 1995.

[21] Kumamoto, Y., et al, "Clinical Efficacy of Mecobalamin in Treatment of Oligozoospermia," *Acta Urol Jpn*, v. 34, p. 1109-1132, 1988.

[22] Werbach, Melvyn, M.D., "Nutritional Influences on Illness," *Townsend Letter for Doctors & Patients*, p. 34, August/September 1995.

Chapter 96: INFLAMMATION

[1] Burton Goldberg Group, *Alternative Medicine, The Definitive Guide*, Future Medicine Publishing, Inc., Puyallup, WA, p. 938, 1993.

[2] Griffin, Marie R., M.D., et al, "Nonsteroidal Anti-Inflammatory Drug Use and Increased Risk For Peptic Ulcer Disease in Elderly Persons," *Annals of Internal Medicine*, v. 114, n. 4, p. 257-263, February 15, 1991.

[3] "Formula Determines Risk For NSAID-Associated Gastropathy," *Geriatrics*, v. 45, n. 9, p. 25, Sept. 9, 1990.

[4] Bulbena, O., Ph.D., et al, "Gastroprotective Effect of Zinc Acexamate Against Damage Induced by Nonsteroidal Antiinflammatory Drugs: A Morphological Study," *Digestive Diseases and Sciences*, v. 38, n. 4, p. 730-739, April 1993.

[5] McClain, C.J., et al, "Minerals and Inflammatory Response," *Journal of the American College of Nutrition*, v. 11, n. 5, p. 598, October 1992.

[6] Peretz, Anne M., et al, "Selenium in Rheumatic Diseases," *Seminars in Arthritis and Rheumatism*, v. 20, n. 5, p. 305-316, April 1991.

[7] Johnston, Carol S., Ph.D., RD, et al, "Antihistamine Effects and Complications of Supplemental Vitamin C," *Journal of the American Dietetic Association*, v. 92, n. 8, p. 988-989, August 1992.

[8] Murray, Michael, M.D. and Pizzorno, Joseph, N.D., *Encyclopedia of Natural Medicine*, Prima Publishing, Rocklin, CA, p. 514-515, 1991.

[9] Murray, Michael T., N.D, *Natural Alternatives to Over-The-Counter and Prescription Drugs*, William Morrow & Company, New York, p. 95-96, 1994.

[10] Mazzotta, Mary Y., "Nutrition and Wound Healing," *Journal of the American Podiatric Medical Association*, v. 84, n. 9, p. 456, September 1994.

[11] Ibid.

[12] Callejari, Peter E., M.D. and Zurier, Robert B., M.D, " Botanical Lipids: Potential Role in the Modulation of Immunologic Responses and Inflammatory Reactions," *Nutrition and Rheumatic Disease/Rheumatic Disease Clinics of North America*, p. 415, May 1991.

[13] Zurier, B., "Essential Fatty Acids and Inflammation," *Annals of Rheumatic Diseases*, v. 50, p. 745-746, 1991.

[14] Challem, Jack, "How to Use Vitamins and Minerals as Home Remedies," *Natural Health*, v.24, n. 2, p. 60-68, March-April, 1994.

[15] Kennedy, Bob, "Borage Wildflowers: Best Source of GLA," *Total Health*, v. 13, n. 1, p. 44, February 1991.

[16] Murray, Frank, "Therapy and Treatment with Aloe Vera," *Better Nutrition for Today's Living*, v. 56, n. 3, p. 52, March 1994.

[17] Ibid.

[18] Murray, Michael, M.D. and Pizzorno, Joseph, N.D., *Encyclopedia of Natural Medicine*, Prima Publishing, Rocklin, CA, p. 514-515, 1991.

[19] Srivastava, R.and Srimal, R.C., et al, "Modification of Certain Inflammation - Induced Biochemical Changes by Curcumin," *Indian Journal of Medical Research*, v. 81, p. 215, February 1985.

[20] Arora, R.B., et al, "Anti-Inflammatory Studies on Curcuma Longa," *Indian Journal of Medical Research*, v. 59, p. 1289, August 1971.

[21] Murray, Michael, M.D. and Pizzorno, Joseph, N.D., *Encyclopedia of Natural Medicine*, Prima Publishing, Rocklin, CA, p. 190-191, 1991.

[22] Srivastava, K.C. and Mustafa, T., "Ginger (Zingiber Officinale) in Rheumatism and Musculoskeletal Disorders," *Medical Hypothesis*, v. 39, p. 342-348, 1992.

Chapter 97: INSECT BITES

[1] Shepherd, Steven, "Anaphylaxis...Explosive and Unpredictable, Sometimes Deadly," *Executive Health Report*, v. 24, n. 9, p. 7, June 1988.

[2] Johnston, Carol S., Ph.D., RD, et al, "Antihistamine Effects and Complications of Supplemental Vitamin C," *Journal of the American Dietetic Association*, v. 92, n. 8, p. 988-989, August 1992.

[3] Alsop, Judith, Pharm.D. and Niezabitowska, B.A., *The UC Davis Poison Center Answer Book*, University of California, Davis, Medical Center, Regional Poison Control Center, p. 10. 4. Murray, Michael, T., *Natural Alternatives to Over-The-Counter Prescription Drugs*, William Morrow and Company, New York, p. 94-96, 1994.

[5] Atkins, Robert C., M.D., *Dr. Atkins' Health Revolution*, Houghton Mifflin Co., Boston, MA, p. 342, 1988.

[6] Murray, Michael, T., *Natural Alternatives to Over-The-Counter Prescription Drugs*, William Morrow and Company, New York, p. 94-96, 1994.

[7] Ibid.

[8] Gross, Gary, N. "Beware of Bugs During Warm-Weather Months," *Diabetes in the News*, v. 14, n. 2, p. 44-47, March-April 1995.

[9] Scott, Julian, Ph. D., *Natural Medicine for Children*, Avon, New York, p. 180, 1990.

[10] Rose, Jeanne, *Jeanne Rose's Modern Herbal*, Perigee, New York, p. 29, 1987.

Chapter 98: KIDNEY STONES

[1] Burton Goldberg Group, *Alternative Medicine, The Definitive Guide*, Future Medicine Publishing, Inc., Puyallup, WA, p. 942, 1993.

[2] McKay, Donald W., Ph.D., et al, "Herbal Tea: An Alternative to Regular Tea For Those Who Form Calcium Oxalate Stones," *Journal of the American Dietetic Association*, v. 95, p. 3, p. 360-361, March 1995.

[3] Burton Goldberg Group, *Alternative Medicine, The Definitive Guide*, Future Medicine Publishing, Inc., Puyallup, WA, p. 942, 1993.

[4] Iguchi, M., et al, "Dietary Intake and Habits of Japanese Renal Stone Patients," The Journal of Urology, v. 143, p. 1093-1095, June 1990.

[5] Dunne, Lavon J., *Nutrition Almanac*, Third Edition, McGraw-Hill Publishing Company, p. 188, 1990.

[6] Schuster, J., et al, "Soft Drink Consumption and Urinary Stone Recurrence: A Randomized Prevention Trial," *Journal of Clinical Epidemiology*, v. 45, n. 8, p. 911-916, August 1992.

[7] Kohri, Kenjiro, et al, "Magnesium-To-Calcium Ratio in Tap Water and Its Relationship to Geological Features and the Incidence of Calcium-Containing Urinary Stones, *Journal of Urology*, v. 142, p. 1272-1275, November 1989.

[8] Wright, Jonathan V., *Dr. Wright's Book of Nutritional Therapy*, Rodale Press, Emmaus, PA, p. 264-271, 1979.

[9] Elin, R., "Magnesium: The Forgotten Nutrient," *The Nutrition Report*, February 1995.

[10] Brighthope, Ian, MB, BS, "The Role of Nutritional Medicine in General Practice," *Australian Family Physician*, v. 19, n. 3, p. 357-365, March 1990.

[11] Dunne, Lavon J., *Nutrition Almanac*, Third Edition, McGraw-Hill Publishing Company, p. 188, 1990.

[12] Ebisuno, S., et al, "Results of Long-term Rice Bran Treatment on Stone Recurrence in Hypercalciuric Patients," *British Journal of Urology*, v. 67, n. 3, p. 237-240, March 1991.

[13] Embon, O.M., et al, "Chronic Dehydration Stone Disease," *British Journal of Urology*, v. 66, p. 357-362, 1990.

Chapter 99: LACTOSE INTOLERANCE

[1] Price, Anita Louise, Lactose Intolerance: the Full Story," *Ostomy Quarterly*, v. 32, n. 2, p. 24, Spring 1995

[2] Langer, Stephen, Learning to Tolerate Lactose Intolerance Nutritionally," *Better Nutrition for Today's Living*, v. 56, n. 8, p. 32, August 1994.

[3] Price, Anita Louise, Lactose Intolerance: the Full Story," *Ostomy Quarterly*, v. 32, n. 2, p. 24, Spring 1995.

[4] "Lactose Intolerance," *The Lancet*, v. 338, n. 8768, p. 663, September 14, 1991.

[5] Lown, Cynthia and Lowen, R.D., et al, "Nutritional Support in Patients With Inflammatory Bowel Disease," *Postgraduate Medicine*, v. 91, n. 5, p. 407-414, April 1992.

[6] Vernia, P., et al, "Lactose Intolerance and Irritable Bowel Syndrome (IBS): Relative Weight in Inducing Abdominal Symptoms in a High Prevalence Area," *Gastroenterology*, v. 102, n. 4, Part II, p. A530, April 1992.

[7] Hughes, Luanne, "Can't Stomach Milk? Keep Lactose Intolerance at Bay," *Environmental Nutrition*, v. 16, n. 10, p 2, October 1993.

8   Price, Anita Louise, Lactose Intolerance: the Full Story," *Ostomy Quarterly*, v. 32, n. 2, p. 24, Spring 1995.
9   Langer, Stephen, Learning to Tolerate Lactose Intolerance Nutritionally," *Better Nutrition for Today's Living*, v. 56, n. 8, p. 32, August, 1994.

Chapter 100: LARYNGITIS

1   "USDA Study of 40,000 Americans," *Food Technology*, v. 35, p. 9, 1981.
2   Hemila, Harri, "Does Vitamin C Alleviate the Symptoms of The Common Cold? - A Review of Current Evidence," *Scandinavian Journal of Infectious Diseases*, v. 26, p. 1-6, 1994.
3   "Vitamin C Enhances Antibiotic Therapy," *The Nutrition Report*, v. 10, n. 4, p. 31, April 1992.
4   "Decreased Resistance to Antibiotics and Plasmid Loss in Plasmid-Carrying Strains of Staphylococcus Aureus Treated With Ascorbic Acid," *Mutation Research*, v. 264, p. 119-125, 1991.
5   Rodale, J.I., et al., *The Complete Book of Vitamins*, Rodale Book, Inc., Emmaus, PA, 1970.
6   Quillin, Patrick, *Healing Nutrients*, Contemporary Books, Chicago, 1987.
7   Kaul, T.N., et al, "Antiviral Effect of Flavonoids on Human Viruses, *Journal of Medical Virology*, v. 17, p. 71-79, 1985.
8   Peretz, Anne M., et al, "Selenium in Rheumatic Diseases," *Seminars in Arthritis and Rheumatism*, v. 20, n. 5, p. 305-316, April 1991.
9   Mazzotta, Mary Y., "Nutrition and Wound Healing," *Journal of the American Podiatric Medical Association*, v. 84, n. 9, p. 456, September 1994.
10 Kennedy, Bob, "Borage Wildflowers: Best Source of GLA," *Total Health*, v. 13, n. 1, p. 44, February 1991.
11 Murray, Frank, "Therapy and Treatment with Aloe Vera," *Better Nutrition for Today's Living*, v. 56, n. 3, p. 52, March 1994.
12 Ibid.
13 Murray, Michael, M.D. and Pizzorno, Joseph, N.D., *Encyclopedia of Natural Medicine*, Prima Publishing, Rocklin, CA, p. 514-515, 1991.
14 Kaufmann, Joanne, *People Weekly*, v. 38, n. 13, p. 53, September 28, 1992.
15 "Why Whisper When You Can Shout?" *Medical Update*, v. 14, n. 12, p. 6, June 1991.

Chapter 101: LEUKEMIA

1   Mayfield, Eleanor, "New Drugs, New Alternatives: Understanding Leukemia," *FDA Consumer*, v. 26, n. 7, p. 32-35, September 1992.
2   Savitz, David A., Ph.D., "Power Lines and Cancer Risk," *JAMA*, v. 265, n. 11, p. 1458, March 20, 1991.
3   Cacoub P., et al, "Vitamin Deficiency-Induced Pancytopenia Mimicking Leukemia," *Presse Med*, v. 20, p. 1603-1606, 1991.
4   Dokal, I.S., et al, "Vitamin B12 and Folate Deficiency Presenting as Leukemia," *British Medical Journal*, v. 300, p. 1263-1264, May 12, 1990.
5   Tanouye, Elyse, "FDA Clears First of New Cancer Drugs; Roche is Approved to Sell Vitamin A Derivative as Leukemia Treatment," *The Wall Street Journal*, November 29, 1995.

[6] "Researcher Says Vitamin A Supplements Useful in Leukemia," *Cancer Weekly*, p. 10, March 29, 1993.

[7] Radetsky, Peter, "Killing Cancer Naturally," *Longevity*, March 22, 1995.

[8] Stavric, B., "Quercetin in Our Diet: From Potent Mutagen to Probable Anticarcinogen," *Clinical Biochemistry*, v. 27, p. 245-247, August 1994.

[9] Mocchegiani, Eugenio, et al, "Plasma Zinc Level on Thymic Hormone Activity in Younger Cancer Patients," *Blood*, v. 83, p. 749-757, February 1, 1994.

[10] Riley, Patrick A. and Willson, Robin L., "Leukemia and Lymphoma Among Young People Near Sellafield," *British Medical Journal*, v. 300, p. 676, March 10, 1990.

[11] Palmer, Anne, "Cancer Tied to Fallout," *Medical Tribune*, v.4, August 23, 1990.

[12] Zalewski, Peter D., et al, "Physiological Role For Zinc in Prevention of Apoptosis", (Gene-Directed Death), *Biochemistry International*, v. 24, n. 6, p. 1093-1101, August 1991.

[13] Blume, Elaine, "Secondary Leukemias Receive Increased Attention," *Journal of the National Cancer Institute*, v. 87, n. 5, p. 336-337, March 1, 1995.

[14] Ibid.

[15] Kaldor, John M., Ph.D., et al, "Leukemia Following Chemotherapy For Ovarian Cancer," *New England Journal of Medicine*, v. 1, n. 322, p. 1-6, January 4, 1989.

[16] Blume, Elaine, "Secondary Leukemias Receive Increased Attention," *Journal of the National Cancer Institute*, v. 87, n. 5, p. 336-337, March 1, 1995.

Chapter 102: LIVER PROBLEMS

[1] Ingram, Cass, M.D., *Eat Right Or Die Young*, Literary Visions Publishing Co., Cedar Rapids, Iowa, p. 91, 1989.

[2] Cowen, R., "Soybean Lecithin May Prevent Cirrhosis," *Science News*, v. 138, p. 340, December 1, 1990.

[3] Meyerhoff, Al, "We must get rid of pesticides in the food supply: exposure to these deadly chemicals can cause cancer, birth defects, and neurological damage," *USA Today*, v. 122, n. 2582, p. 51, November 1993.

[4] Ibid.

[5] Muhlendahl, Karl Ernst V. and Lange, Heribert, "Copper and Childhood Cirrhosis," *The Lancet*, v. 344, p. 1515-1516, November 26, 1994.

[6] Dunne, Lavon J., *Nutrition Almanac*, Third Edition, McGraw-Hill Publishing Company, p. 90, 1990.

[7] Schmidt, Daniel N. and Hultcrantz, Rolf, "Alcoholic Fatty Liver and Hepatic Essential Trace Element Content in Alcohol Withdrawal," *European Journal of Gastroenterology and Hepatology*, v. 3, p. 79-85, 1991.

[8] Ozsoylu, S. and Kocak, N., "Zinc Deficiency in Cirrhosis," *Gut*, v. 32, p. 485, 1991.

[9] Extremera, B. Gil, M.D., et al, "Zinc and Liver Cirrhosis," *ACTA Gastro-Enterologica Beligica*, v. May-June 1990.

[10] Van Der Rijt, Carin C.D., et al, "Overt Hepatic Encephalopathy Precipitated by Zinc Deficiency," *Gastroenterology*, v. 100, p. 1114-1118, 1991.

[11] Murray, Michael, M.D. and Pizzorno, Joseph, N.D., *Encyclopedia of Natural Medicine*, Prima Publishing, Rocklin, CA, p. 77, 1991.

[12] Canty, David J., "Lecithin and Choline in Human Health and Disease," *Nutrition Reviews*, v. 52, n. 10, p. 327-339, October 1994.

[13] Cowen, R., "Soybean Lecithin May Prevent Cirrhosis," *Science News*, v. 138, p. 340, December 1, 1990.

[14] Ingram, Cass, M.D., *Eat Right Or Die Young*, Literary Visions Publishing Co., Cedar Rapids, Iowa, p. 91, 1989.

[15] Ibid.

[16] Ward, R. and Peters, T., "The Antioxidant Status of Patients with Either Alcohol-Induced Liver Damage or Myopathy," *Alcohol*, v. 27, p. 359-365, 1992.

[17] Ingram, Cass, M.D., *Eat Right Or Die Young*, Literary Visions Publishing Co., Cedar Rapids, Iowa, p. 91, 1989.

[18] Ibid.

[19] Mourelle, M., et al, "Prevention of Carbon Tetrachloride CCL4-Induced Liver Cirrhosis by Silymarin," *Fundam. Clin. Pharmacol.*, v. 3, p. 183-191, 1989.

[20] Dunne, Lavon J., *Nutrition Almanac*, Third Edition, McGraw-Hill Publishing Company, p. 179, 1990.

[21] Burton Goldberg Group, *Alternative Medicine, The Definitive Guide*, Future Medicine Publishing, Inc., Puyallup, WA, p. 930, 1993.

[22] Wright, Jonathan V., *Dr. Wright's Book of Nutritional Therapy*, Rodale Press, Emmaus, PA, p. 260-261, 1979.

[23] Dunne, Lavon J., *Nutrition Almanac*, Third Edition, McGraw-Hill Publishing Company, p. 187, 1990.

[24] Burton Goldberg Group, *Alternative Medicine, The Definitive Guide*, Future Medicine Publishing, Inc., Puyallup, WA, p. 941, 1993.

Chapter 103: LOU GEHRIG'S DISEASE

[1] Wachter, Sarah & Cutting, Lucia, "Health Heroes," *Longevity*, March 1995.

[2] Gillyat, Peta, "More Questions Than Answers," *Harvard Health Letter*, v. 20, n. 4, p. 6, February 1995.

[3] Ibid.

[4] Yasui, M., M.D., "Magnesium and Calcium Contents in CNS Tissues of Amyotrophic Lateral Sclerosis Patients From Kii Peninsula, Japan," *European Neurology*, v. 32, p. 95-98, 1992.

[5] Elin, R., "Magnesium: The Forgotten Nutrient," *The Nutrition Report*, February 1995.

[6] Dunne, Lavon J., *Nutrition Almanac,* Third Edition, Table of Food Composition, McGraw-Hill, p. 293, 1990.

[7] *Science*, v. 261, p. 1047-1051, 1993.

[8] Brown, Scott, J., "Free Radicals Appear to Fuel Lou Gehrig's Disease," *Family Practice News*.

[9] Rothstein, Jeffrey D., M.D., Ph.D., et al, "Decreased Glutamate Transport by The Brain and Spinal Cord in Amyotrophic Lateral Sclerosis," *New England Journal of Medicine*, v. 326, n. 22, p. 1464-1468, May 28, 1992.

[10] Yamauchi, Ono S., et al, "Glutamate and Aspartate Are Decreased in the Skin in Amyotrophic Lateral Sclerosis", *ACTA Neurologica Scandinavica*, v. 86, p. 481-484, 1992.

[11] Phone conversation with C.A. Douglas Ringrose, M.D., April 18, 1996.

Chapter 104: LOW BLOOD PRESSURE – HYPOTENSION

1 Wynn, Susan Rudd, "Food Allergy-Fact or Fiction," *AAPA Symposia Highlights*, p. 2-3, October 1994.
2 Wessely, Simon, M.D., "Are There Symptoms of Low Blood Pressure?" *Hospital Practice,* v. 8, p. 13, September 30, 1991.
3 Lossos, A., M.D. and Argov, Z., M.D., "Orthostatic Hypotension Induced by Vitamin B12 Deficiency," *Journal of The American Geriatric Society*, v. 39, p. 601-603, 1991.
4 Ibid.
5 Koudouris, Spyridon, M.D., "More on Vitamin B12," *Consultant*, v. 23, January 1994.
6 Healton, Edward B., et al, "Neurologic Aspects of Cobalamin Deficiency," *Medicine*, v. 70, n. 4, p. 229-244, 1991.

Chapter 105: LOW BLOOD SUGAR

1 Mohammed, Bazzi N., et al, "Hypoglycemia in an Elderly Woman," *Hospital Practice*, p. 177-183, October 15, 1991.
2 Messer, Stephen C., et al, "Hypoglycemia and Psychopathology: A Methodological Review," *Clinical Psychology Review*, v. 10, p. 631-648, 1990.
3 Deary, Ian J., et al, "Severe Hypoglycemia and Intelligence in Adult Patients with Insulin-Treated Diabetes," *Diabetes*, v. 42, n. 2, p. 341, February 1993.
4 Mertz, Walter, "Chromium in Human Nutrition: A Review," *Journal of Nutrition*, v. 123, p. 626-633, 1993.
5 Mertz, Walter, "Effects and Metabolism of Glucose Tolerance Factor," *Nutrition Review*, v. 33, 1929, 1975.
6 Faelten, Sharon, *The Complete Book of Minerals for Health*, Rodale Press, Emmaus, PA, p. 118, 1981.
7 Rohn, R., et al, "Magnesium, Zinc and Copper in Plasma and Blood Cellular Components in Children With Insulin Dependent Diabetes Mellitus," *Clinical Chemistry*, v. 215, p. 21-28, 1993.
8 "Magnesium and Diabetes," *Practical Diabetology*, v. 10, n. 2, p. 1-5, March/April 1991.
9 Gaby, Alan R., M.D. and Wright, Jonathan V., M.D., "Nutritional Regulation of Blood Glucose," Wright/Gaby Nutrition Institute, October 1990.
10 Rogers, Kenneth S. and Mohan, Chandra, "Vitamin B6 Metabolism and Diabetes," *Biochemical Medicine and Metabiologic Biology*, v. 52, p. 10-17, 1994.

Chapter 106: LOW THYROID – HYPOTHYROIDISM

1 Lathan, S. Robert, M.D., "Chronic Fatigue? Consider Hypothyroidism," *The Physician and Sports Medicine*, v. 19, n. 10, p. 67-70, October 1991.
2 Braverman, Eric, M.D., and Pfeiffer, Carl C., M.D., Ph.D., The Healing Nutrients Within, Keats Publishing, New Canaan, CT, 1987.
3 Krampf, Leslie, "Natural Help for Hypothyroidism," *Vegetarian Times*, n. 207, p. 122, November 1994.
4 Murray, Michael, M.D. and Pizzorno, Joseph, N.D., *Encyclopedia of Natural Medicine*, Prima Publishing, Rocklin, CA, p. 388-389, 1991.
5 Thorpe-Beeston, J.G., et al, "Thyroid Function in Fetuses with Chromosomal Abnormalities," *British Medical Journal*, v. 302, n. 6777, p. 628, March 16, 1991.

[6]   Tambyah P.A. and Cheah J.S., "Hyperthyroidism and Down syndrome," *Annual Academy of Medicine*, v. 22, n. 4, p. 603-605, July 1993.

[7]   Kittle, William M., M.D. and Chaudhary, Bashir, M.D., "Sleep Apnea and Hypothyroidism," *Southern Medical Journal*, v. 81, n. 11, p. 1421-1425, November 1988.

[8]   Barnes, Broda O., and Galton, Lawrence, *Hypothyroidism: The Unsuspected Illness*, Thomas Y. Crowell Co., New York, 1976.

[9]   Haggerty, John J., Jr., M.D., et al, "Subclinical Hypothyroidism: A Modifiable Risk Factor For Depression?" *American Journal of Psychiatry*, n. 150, p. 508-510, March 3, 1993.

[10]   Nomura, Junichi, et al, "Thyroid Function and Mood: Implications For Treatment of Mood Disorders," *CNS Drugs*, v. 1, n. 5, p. 356-369, 1994.

[11]   Sawin, Clark T., M.D., "Subclinical Hypothyroidism in Older Persons," *Clinics in Geriatric Medicine*, v. 11, n. 2, p. 231-238, May 1995.

[12]   Ibid.

[13]   Ibid.

[14]   Spencer, J.G.C., "The Influence of the Thyroid in Malignant Disease," p. 393, *British Journal of Cancer*, p. 393, 1954.

[15]   Murray, Michael, M.D. and Pizzorno, Joseph, N.D., *Encyclopedia of Natural Medicine*, Prima Publishing, Rocklin, CA, p. 389, 1991.

[16]   Ibid, p. 387.

[17]   Ibid, p. 390.

[18]   Krampf, Leslie, "Natural Help for Hypothyroidism," *Vegetarian Times*, n. 207, p. 122, November 1994.

[19]   Murray, Michael, M.D. and Pizzorno, Joseph, N.D., *Encyclopedia of Natural Medicine*, Prima Publishing, Rocklin, CA, p. 389, 1991.

Chapter 107: LUPUS

[1]   *Churchill's Illustrated Medical Dictionary*, Churchill Livingstone Inc., New York, NY., p. 1079, 1989.

[2]   Molad, Yair, et al, "Serum Cobalamin and Transcobalamin Levels in Systemic Lupus Erythematosus," *American Journal of Medicine*, v. 88, n. 2, p. 141, February 1990.

[3]   Aladjem, H., *Understanding Lupus*, 1985; Blau, S., *Lupus*, revised, 1984; Phillips, R.H., *Coping with Lupus*, 1984; Wallace, D., and Dubois, E., eds., *Lupus Erthematosus*, 3d ed., 1987.

[4]   Mackworth-Young, C.G., et al, "Primary Antiphospholipid Syndrome: Features of Patients with Raised Anticardiolipin Antibodies and No Other Disorder, *Annals of the Rheumatic Diseases*, v. 48, n. 5, p. 362-366, May 1989

[5]   "Fish Oil Treatment for Lupus, *Nutrition Research Newsletter*, v. 10, n. 10, p. 104, October 1991.

[6]   Walton, A.J.E., "Dietary Fish Oil and the Severity of Symptoms in Patients with Systemic Lupus Erythematosus," *Annals of the Rheumatic Diseases*, v. 50, n. 7, p. 463, July 1991.

[7]   Vaz, AL., "Double-blind Clinical Evaluation of the Relative Efficacy of Glucosamine Sulphate in the Mangement of Osteoarthritis of the Knee in Outpatients," *Current Medical Resident Opinion*, v. 8, p. 145, 1982.

[8] Yagaloff, K.A., et al, "Essential Fatty Acids are Antagonists of Leukotriene B4 Receptor," *Prostaglandins, Leukotrienes and Essential Fatty Acids*, v. 52, p. 293-297, 1995.

[9] Wright, Jonathan V., M.D., "Treatment of Lupus," *Dr. Wright's Nutrition & Healing*, v. 2, n. 12, p. 1, December 1995.

[10] Van Vollenhoven, Ronald, "An Open Study of Dehydroepiandrosterone in Systemic Lupus Erythematosus," *Arthritis and Rheumatism*, v. 37, n. 9, p. 1305-1310, September 1994.

[11] Block, M.T., "Vitamin E in the Treatment of Diseases of the Skin," *Clinical Medicine*, p. 31-34, January 1953.

[12] Ayres, S., & Mihan, R., "Is Vitamin E Involved in the Autoimmune Mechanism?" *Cutis*, v. 21, p. 321-325, 1978.

[13] Block, M.T., "Vitamin E in the Treatment of Diseases of the Skin," *Clinical Medicine*, p. 31-34, January 1953.

[14] Molad, Yair, M.D., et al, "Serum Cobalamin and Transcobalamin Levels in Systemic Lupus Erythematosus," *The American Journal of Medicine*, v. 88, p. 141-144, February 1990.

Chapter 108: MACULAR DEGENERATION

[1] Bunce, G.E., "Nutrition and Eye Disease of the Elderly," *Journal of Nutritional Biochemistry*, v. 5, p. 66-77, February 1994.

[2] Augsburger, Arol, "Macular Degeneration: Medical Treatment May Help Slow Progression," *Geriatrics*, v. 46, n. 10, p. 17, October 1991.

[3] Newsome, David A., M.D., "Role of Antioxidants in Macular Degeneration: An Update," *Ophthalmic Practice*, v. 12, n. 4, p. 169-171, 1994.

[4] Gerster, Helga, "Review: Antioxidant Protection of the Ageing Macula", *Age and Ageing*, v. 20, p. 60-69, 1991.

[5] Newsome, David A., M.D., "Role of Antioxidants in Macular Degeneration: An Update," *Ophthalmic Practice*, v. 12, n. 4, p. 169-171, 1994.

[6] Ibid.

[7] Ibid.

[8] Murray, Frank, "Zinc: A Vital Skin and Hair Mineral," *Better Nutrition for Today's Living*, v. 52, n. 7, p. 12, July 1990.

[9] Murray, Frank, "Zinc: Healing Mineral," *Better Nutrition for Today's Living*, v. 54, n. 9, p. 26, September 1992.

[10] Ibid.

[11] Wright, Jonathan V., M.D., et al, "Improvement of Vision in Macular Degeneration Associated with Intravenous Zinc and Selenium Therapy: Two Cases," *Journal of Nutritional Medicine*, v. 1, p. 133-138, 1990.

[12] "Antioxidants May Protect Our Eyes," *Better Nutrition for Today's Living*, v. 53, n. 9, p. 10, September 1991.

[13] Ibid.

[14] Gruning, Carl, "Seeing is Believing!", *Health News & Review*, v. 2, n. 3, p. 1, Summer 1992.

[15] "Antioxidants May Protect Our Eyes," *Better Nutrition for Today's Living*, v. 53, n. 9, p. 10, September 1991.

Chapter 109: MALABSORPTION

[1] Hunter, Beatrice Trum, "How Well Do We Absorb Nutrients?" *Consumers' Research Magazine*, v. 77, n. 4, p. 17, April 1994.

[2] Halsted,Charles H. and Keen, Carl L., "Alcoholism and Micronutrient Metabolism and Deficiencies,", *European Journal of Gastroenterology and Hepatology*, v. 2, n. 6, p. 399-402, 1990.

[3] Wright, Jonathan V., M.D., "Treatment of Childhood Asthma With Parenteral Vitamin B12, Gastric Re-Acidification, and Attention to Food Allergy, Magnesium and Pyridoxine: Three Case Reports With Background an Integrated Hypothesis," *Journal of Nutritional Medicine*, v. 1, p. 277-282, 1990.

[4] Bruck, W., et al, "Wernicke's Encephalopathy in a Child With Acute Lymphoblastic Leukemia Treated With Polychemotherapy," *Clinical Neuropathology*, v. 10, n. 3, p. 134-136, 1991.

[5] Peck, Peggy, "Vitamin Supplements Critical to All Inflammatory Bowel Disease Patients," Peck, Peggy, *Family Practice News*, v. 4, May 15, 1994.

[6] Okada, Akira, "Zinc in Clinical Surgery – A Research Review," *Japanese Journal of Surgery*, v. 20, n. 6, p. 635-644, 1990.

[7] Hunter, Beatrice Trum, "How Well Do We Absorb Nutrients?" *Consumers' Research Magazine*, v. 77, n. 4, p. 17, April 1994.

[8] Ibid.

Chapter 110: MEASLES

[1] "Vitamin A Supplementation in Measles," *Nutrition Research Newsletter*, v. 10, n. 2, p. 18, February, 1991.

[2] Hussey, Gregory D., MB and Klein, Max, M.D., "A Randomized, Controlled Trial of Vitamin A in Children With Severe Measles," *The New England Journal of Medicine*, v. 323, n. 3, p. 160-164, July 19, 1990.

[3] "Vitamin A Supplementation in Measles," *Nutrition Research Newsletter*, v. 10, n. 2, p. 18, February, 1991.

[4] Hussey, Gregory D., MB and Klein, Max, M.D., "A Randomized, Controlled Trial of Vitamin A in Children With Severe Measles," *The New England Journal of Medicine*, v. 323, n. 3, p. 160-164, July 19, 1990.

[5] Kotheri, Geopa, M.D. and Naik, Ekneth, M.D., "Effect of Vitamin A Prophylaxis on Morbidity and Mortality Among Children in Urban Slums in Bombay," *British Medical Journal*, October 1991.

[6] Frieden, Thomas R., et al, "Vitamin A Levels and Severity of Measles," *American J Diseases of Children*, v. 146, n. 2, p. 182-186, February 1992.

[7] Ibid.

[8] Chan, Michael, "Vitamin A and Measles in Third World Children, Editorial, *British Medical Journal*, v. 301, n. 6763, p. 1230-1231, Dec 1, 1990.

[9] Dunne, Lavon J., *Nutrition Almanac*, Third Edition, McGraw-Hill Publishing Company, p. 13, 1990.

Chapter 111: MEMORY LOSS

[1] Dunne, Lavon J., *Nutrition Almanac,* Third Edition, Table of Food Composition, McGraw-Hill, p. 18, 1990.

[2] Lustgarden, Steve, "Flexing Your Mental Muscle," *Vegetarian Times*, n. 183, p. 48, November 1992.

[3] Gray, Gregory E.,"Nutrition and Dementia," *Journal of the American Dietetic Association*, v. 89, n. 12, p. 1795, December 1989.

[4] Lindenbaum, J., et al, "Neuropsychiatric Disorders Caused by Cobalamin Deficiency in The Absence of Anemia or Macrocytosis," *New England Journal of Medicine*,v. 318, p. 1720-1728, 1988.

[5] Lustgarden, Steve, "Flexing Your Mental Muscle," *Vegetarian Times*, n. 183, p. 48, November 1992.

[6] Null, Gary, *The Complete Guide to Health and Nutrition*, Dell Publishing Co., New York, p. 423, 1984.

[7] Glick, J. Leslie, "Use of Magnesium in The Management of Dementias," *Medical Sciences Research*, v. 18, p. 831-833, 1990.

[8] Rai, G.S., M.D., et al, "A Double-Blind, Placebo-Controlled Study of Ginkgo Biloba Extract in Elderly Outpatients With Mild to Moderate Memory Impairment," *Current Medical Research and Opinion*, v. 12, n. 6, p. 350-355, 1991.

[9] Schaffler, V. K., et al, "Double-Blind Study of the Hypoxia-Protective Effect of a Standardized Ginkgo Biloba Preparation," *Arzneim-Forsch*, v. 35, p. 1283-1286, 1985.

[10] Herbert, J., et al, "The Age of Dehydroepiandrosterone," *The Lancet*, v. 345, p. 1193-1194, May 13, 1995.

[11] Livermore, Beth, "Build a Better Brain," *Psychology Today*, v. 25, n. 5, p. 40, September-October 1992.

[12] Sapolsky, Robert M., "Stress and Neuroendocrine Changes During Aging," *Generations*, v. 16, n. 4, p. 35, Fall-Winter 1992.

[13] Livermore, Beth, "Build a Better Brain," *Psychology Today*, v. 25, n. 5, p. 40, September-October 1992.

[14] Ibid.

Chapter 112: MENIERE'S SYNDROME

[1] Garnett, Leah R., "A Balancing Act," *Harvard Health Letter*, v. 20, n. 1, p. 3, November 1994.

[2] Gerras, Charles, et al, eds, *The Encyclopedia of Common Diseases*, Rodale Press, Emmaus, PA, p. 522-525, 1976.

[3] Wiersum, Jeffery, M.D., "Vitamins For Migraine, Meniere's," *Cortlandt Forum*, v. 97, February 1991.

Chapter 113: MENOPAUSE

[1] Gallagher, Winifred, "Midlife Myths," *Atlantic*, v. 271, May 1993.

[2] Wilcox, Gisela, et al, "Oestrogenic Effects of Plant Foods in Postmenopausal Women," *British Medical Journal*, v. 301, n. 6757, October 20, 1990.

[3] Mindell, Earl L, "Soy – When Will We Learn?" column Stay Healthy, *Let's Live*, January 1995.

[4] Bland, Jeffrey S., "Back to Basics: Dietary Fiber, Perimenopause and Estrogen," *Let's Live*, April 1995.

[5] Kugler, Hans Ph.D., et al, *Life Extenders and Memory Boosters*, Health Quest Publications, Reno, NV, 1993

6 Burton Goldberg Group, *Alternative Medicine, The Definitive Guide*, Future Medicine Publishing, Inc., Puyallup, WA, 1993.

7 Evans, Imogen, "The Challenge of Breast Cancer," *The Lancet*, v. 343, n. 8905, p. 1085, April 30, 1994.

8 Smith, C.J. "Non-Hormonal Control of VasoMotor Flushing in Menopausal Patients," *Chicago Medicine*, March 7, 1964.

9 Casson, Peter R., M.D., et al, "Oral Dehydroepiandrosterone in Physiologic Doses Modulates Immune Function in Postmenopausal Women," *American Journal of Obstetrical Gynecology*, December 1993.

10 "The Mysteries of Melatonin," *Harvard Health Letter*, June 1993.

Chapter 114: MENTAL ILLNESS

1 Dunne, Lavon J., *Nutrition Almanac*, Third Edition, McGraw-Hill Publishing Company, p. 193, 1990.

2 Jancin, Bruce, "IBS Patients' Family Has More Mental Illness," *Family Practice News*, v. 2, p. 15, May 15, 1994.

3 Dunne, Lavon J., *Nutrition Almanac*, Third Edition, McGraw-Hill Publishing Company, p. 32, 1990.

4 Ibid, p. 39.

5 Werbach, Melvyn R., *Nutritional Influences on Illness*, Keats Publishing, New Canaan, CT, p. 493, 1988.

6 Murray, Frank, "Bone Up on B Vitamins: Part One," *Better Nutrition*, v. 51, n. 10, p. 8, October 1989.

7 Lindberg, Michael C.; Oyler, Richard A., "Wernicke's Encephalopathy," *American Family Physician*, v. 41, n. 4, p. 1205, April 1990.

8 Korsakoff's Syndrome, *The Lancet*, v. 336, n. 8720, p. 91, October 13, 1990.

9 Hoffer, Abram, *Orthomolecular Medicine for Physicians*, Keats Publishing, New Canaan, CT, p. 33, 1989.

10 Murray, Frank, "Bone Up on B Vitamins: Part One," *Better Nutrition*, v. 51, n. 10, p. 8, October 1989.

11 Murray, Frank, "Bone Up on B Vitamins: Part One," *Better Nutrition*, v. 51, n. 10, p. 8, October 1989.

12 "Alert: Thiamine-Deficient Total Parenteral Nutrition," *Patient Care*, v. 23, n. 9, p. 24, May 15, 1989.

13 Burton Goldberg Group, *Alternative Medicine, The Definitive Guide*, Future Medicine Publishing, Inc., Puyallup, WA, p. 745, 1993.

14 Banki, C.M., et al, "Cerebrospinal Fluid Magnesium and Calcium Related to Amine Metabolites, Diagnosis and Suicide Attempts," *Biological Psychiatry*, v. 20, p. 163-171, 1985.

Chapter 115: MIGRAINES & HEADACHES

1 Faivelson, Saralie, "Breaking the Cycle of Pain: Experts' Views of Migraines Have Changed Radically, Yet Some Physicians Still Undertreat or Mistreat the Excruciating Headaches," *Medical World News*, v. 34, n. 12, p. 22, December 15, 1993.

2 "Migraines: Easing the Pain," *Consumer Reports on Health*, v. 5, n. 7, p. 72, July 1993.

[3] Faivelson, Saralie, "Breaking the Cycle of Pain: Experts' Views of Migraines Have Changed Radically, Yet Some Physicians Still Undertreat or Mistreat the Excruciating Headaches," *Medical World News*, v. 34, n. 12, p. 22, December 15, 1993.

[4] Egger, J., et al, "Is Migraine Food Allergy?" *The Lancet*, v. 2, p. 865-869, 1983.

[5] Faivelson, Saralie, "Breaking the Cycle of Pain: Experts' Views of Migraines Have Changed Radically, Yet Some Physicians Still Undertreat or Mistreat the Excruciating Headaches," *Medical World News*, v. 34, n. 12, p. 22, December 15, 1993.

[6] Faelton, Sharon, *The Allergy Self-Help Book*, Rodale Press, Emmaus, PA, p. 306-307.

[7] Burton Goldberg Group, *Alternative Medicine, The Definitive Guide*, Future Medicine Publishing, Inc., Puyallup, WA, 1993.

[8] "More Than You Ever Thought You Would Know About Food Additives," *FDA Consumer*, 1982.

[9] "Prevalence of Chronic Migraine Headaches – United States, 1980-1989," *Morbidity and Mortality Weekly Report*, v. 40, n. 20, p. 337-338, May 24, 1991.

[10] Sarchielli, Paola, et al, "Serum and Salivary Magnesium Levels in Migraine and Tension-Type Headache: Results in a Group of Adult Patients," *Cephalalgia*, v. 12, p. 21-27, 1992.

[11] Kunkel, Robert S., M.D., "Magnesium For Migraine?" *Consultant*, p. 827, June 1994.

[12] Kahn, Jason, "Low Ionized Magnesium Linked to Migraine Headaches," *Medical Tribune*, v. 7, May 18, 1995.

[13] Elin, R., "Magnesium: The Forgotten Nutrient," *The Nutrition Report*, February 1995.

[14] Hall, Jeffrey A., D.O., "Enhancing Niacin's Effect For Migraine," *Cortlandt Forum*, v. 46, p. 47, July 1991.

[15] Schoenen, J., et al, "High-Dose Riboflavin as a Prophylactic Treatment of Migraine: Results of an Open Pilot Study," *Cephalalgia*, v. 14, p. 328-329, 1994.

Chapter 116: MISCARRIAGE

[1] Schindehette, Susan, "Waking up to the Biological Clock," *People Weekly*, v. 34 p. 74-78, August 20, 1990.

[2] Reuben, Carolyn and Priestley, Joan, "Vitamins Against Miscarriage; Supplements and a Nutrient-Rich Diet can Help Lead to a Healthy Pregnancy, *East West*, v. 19, n. 1, p. 59, January 1989.

[3] Gerras, Charles, et al, eds, *The Encyclopedia of Common Diseases*, Rodale Press, Emmaus, PA, p. 1026-1027, 1976.

[4] Stavric, B., "Quercetin in Our Diet: From Potent Mutagen to Probable Anticarcinogen," *Clinical Biochemistry*, v. 27, p. 245-247, August 1994.

[5] Taylor, Deborah, "Dietary Therapy Helps Treatment of Infertility," *Today's Living*, v. 20, n. 4, p. 12, April 1989.

[6] Mansmann, Herbert, Jr., M.D., "Consider Magnesium Homeostasis," *Pediatric Asthma, Allergy and Immunology*, v. 5, n. 3, p. 273-279, 1991.

[7] Elin, R., "Magnesium: The Forgotten Nutrient," *The Nutrition Report*, February 1995.

[8] Taylor, Deborah, "Dietary Therapy Helps Treatment of Infertility," *Today's Living*, v. 20, n. 4, p. 12, April 1989.

[9] Ibid.

[10] Rodale, J.I., *The Health Finder*, Rodale Books, Emmaus, PA, p. 918-919, 1955.

[11] Ozgunes, H., et al, "Ceruloplasmin Activity, Copper and Zinc Determinations in Predicting the Prognosis of Threatened Abortion," *Trace Elements and Electrolytes*, v. 11, n. 3, p. 139-142, 1994.

Chapter 117: MULTIPLE SCLEROSIS

[1] Sargent, J.R.; Coupland K.; Wilson R.; "Nervonic Acid and Demyelinating Disease," Department of Biological and Molecular Sciences, School of Natural Sciences, University of Stirling, UK, *Medical Hypotheses*, n. 42, p. 237, April 1994.

[2] *Martindale, The Extra Pharmacopoeia, Thirtieth Edition*, Department of Pharmaceutical Sciences, Royal Pharmaceutical Society of Great Britain, The Pharmaceutical Press, p. 1383, 1993.

[3] Zinkham, William H., M.D., "Lorenzo's Oil and Thrombocytopenia in Patients with Adrenoleukodystrophy," *The New England Journal of Medicine*, p. 1126-1127, April 15, 1993.

[4] Bates, D.; Fawcett, P.R.W.; Shaw, D.A.; Weightman, D., "Polyunsaturated Fatty Acids in the Treatment of Acute Remitting Multiple Sclerosis," *British Medical Journal*, p. 2, 1978.

[5] Dworkin, R.H.; Bates, D.; Millar, J.D.H.; Paty, D.W., "Linoleic Acid and Multiple Sclerosis: A Reanalysis of Three Double Blind Trials, *Neurology*, p. 34, 1984.

[6] Sibley, W.A., "Therapeutics Claims Committee of the International Federation of Multiple Sclerosis Societies," *Therapeutic Claims in Multiple Sclerosis*, Demos Publications, New York, 1992.

[7] Kennedy, Bob, "Borage Wildflowers: Best Source of GLA," *Total Health*, v. 13, n. 1, p. 44, February 1991.

[8] "Effect of Low-Fat Diets in Multiple Sclerosis," *Nutrition Research Newsletter*, v. 11, n. 2 p. 19, February 1992.

[9] Ackermann, A., "Die Multiple Sklerose in der Schweiz," *Schweiz Med Wochenschr*, p. 61, 1931.

[10] Swank, R.L.; Lerstad, O; Strom, A ; Backer, J, "Multiple Sclerosis in Rural Norway: Its Geographic and Occupational Incidence in Relation to Nutrition, *New England Journal of Medicine*, p. 246, 1952.

[11] Swank, R.L., Brewer-Dugan, B., *The Multiple Sclerosis Diet Book*, Garden City, NY: Doubleday and Co, 1987.

[12] Swank, R.L., "Effects of High Fat Feedings on Viscosity of the Blood," *Science*, p. 120, 1954.

[13] Burton Goldberg Group, *Alternative Medicine, The Definitive Guide*, Future Medicine Publishing, Inc., Puyallup, WA, p. 758, 1993.

Chapter 118: MUSCLE SORENESS

[1] Appell, H.J., et al, "Exercise, Muscle Damage and Fatigue," Sports Medicine, v. 13, n. 2, p. 108-115, 1992.

[2] Suter, Esther, "Jogging or Walking – Comparison of Health Effects," Annals of Epidemiology, v. 4, p. 375-381, 1994.

[3] Challem, Jack, "How to Use Vitamins and Minerals as Home Remedies," *Natural Health*, v. 24, n. 2, p. 60, March-April 1994.

[4] Ibid.

[5] Mindell, Earl, *Earl Mindell's Food as Medicine*, Simon & Schuster, New York, p. 62, 1994.
[6] Evans, William J., "Exercise, Nutrition and Ageing," *Journal of Nutrition*, v. 122, p. 796-801, 1992.
[7] Murray, Frank, "Therapy and Treatment with Aloe Vera," *Better Nutrition for Today's Living*, v. 56, n. 3, p. 52, March 1994.
[8] Srivastava, R.and Srimal, R.C., et al, "Modification of Certain Inflammation - Induced Biochemical Changes by Curcumin," *Indian Journal of Medical Research*, v. 81, p. 215, February 1985.
[9] Arora, R.B., et al, "Anti-Inflammatory Studies on Curcuma Longa," *Indian Journal of Medical Research*, v. 59, p. 1289, August 1971.
[10] Murray, Michael, M.D. and Pizzorno, Joseph, N.D., *Encyclopedia of Natural Medicine*, Prima Publishing, Rocklin, CA, p. 190-191, 1991.
[11] Srivastava, K.C. and Mustafa, T., "Ginger (Zingiber Officinale) in Rheumatism and Musculoskeletal Disorders," *Medical Hypothesis*, v. 39, p. 342-348, 1992.

Chapter 119: MUSCLE WEAKNESS

[1] Dunne, Lavon J., *Nutrition Almanac*, Third Edition, McGraw-Hill Publishing Company, p. 198, 1990.
[2] Krucoff, Carol, "Use 'Em or Lose 'Em," *Saturday Evening Post*, v. 266, n. 2, p. 34, March-April, 1994.
[3] Gerras, Charles, et al, eds, *The Encyclopedia of Common Diseases*, Rodale Press, Emmaus, PA, p. 1056, 1976.
[4] Williams, Stephanie, "Vitamins C and E Protect Muscles," *Self*, v. 14, n. 11, p. 48, November 1992.
[5] Lieberman, Shari and Bruning, Nancy, *The Real Vitamin and Mineral Book*, Avery Publishing Group, Inc., Garden City Park, New York, p. 198, 1990.
[6] Backman, E., and Henriksson, K. G., "Effect of Sodium Selenite and Vitamin E Treatment in Myotonic Dystrophy, *J Internal Medicine*, v. 228, n. 6, p. 577-581, December 1990.
[7] Dunne, Lavon J., *Nutrition Almanac*, Third Edition, McGraw-Hill Publishing Company, p. 7, 1990.
[8] Maleskey, Gale, "Battling Disease with the Amino Factor," *Prevention*, v. 41, n. 5, p. 61, May 1989.
[9] Smith, Shelley, "Can a 41-year-old Former NFL Wild Man Come Back to Terrorize Raider Opponents Again?" *Sports Illustrated*, v. 73, n. 1, p.34, July 2, 1990.
[10] Morre, Kenny, "Getup and Go," *Sports Illustrated*, v. 69, n. 4, p. 14, July 25, 1988.
[11] Gammon, Peter, "Tuning up for Tyson," *Sports Illustrated*, v. 67, n. 26, p. 48, December 14, 1987.

Chapter 120: MUSCULAR DYSTROPHY

[1] Gerras, Charles, et al, eds, *The Encyclopedia of Common Diseases*, Rodale Press, Emmaus, PA, p. 1056, 1976.
[2] Duthie, G.G., "Diseases related to free radicals and lipid peroxidation include MD," *European Journal of Clinical Nutrition*, v. 47, p. 759-764, 1993.

[3] Williams, Stephanie, "Vitamins C and E Protect Muscles," *Self*, v. 14, n. 11, p. 48, November 1992.

[4] Lieberman, Shari and Bruning, Nancy, *The Real Vitamin and Mineral Book*, Avery Publishing Group, Inc., Garden City Park, New York, p. 198, 1990.

[5] Greenberg, Steven, M.D. and Frishman, William H., M.D., "Co-Enzyme Q10: A New Drug for Cardiovascular Disease," *Journal of Clinical Pharmacology*, v. 30, p. 596-608, 1990.

[6] Backman, E., and Henriksson, K. G., "Effect of Sodium Selenite and Vitamin E Treatment in Myotonic Dystrophy, *J Internal Medicine*, v. 228, n. 6, p. 577-581, December 1990.

[7] Dunne, Lavon J., *Nutrition Almanac*, Third Edition, McGraw-Hill Publishing Company, p. 7, 1990.

[8] Maleskey, Gale, "Battling Disease with the Amino Factor," *Prevention*, v. 41, n. 5, p. 61, May 1989.

[9] Smith, Shelley, "Can a 41-year-old Former NFL Wild Man Come Back to Terrorize Raider Opponents Again?" *Sports Illustrated*, v. 73, n. 1, p.34, July 2, 1990.

[10] Morre, Kenny, "Getup and Go," *Sports Illustrated*, v. 69, n. 4, p. 14, July 25, 1988.

[11] Gammon, Peter, "Tuning up for Tyson," *Sports Illustrated*, v. 67, n. 26, p. 48, December 14, 1987.

[12] Dunne, Lavon J., *Nutrition Almanac*, Third Edition, McGraw-Hill Publishing Company, p. 198, 1990.

Chapter 121: NAIL PROBLEMS

[1] Daigneault, Lorraine; Rosenfeld, Isadore; Livermore, Beth, "The Nail File," *Health*, v. 21, p. 64, August 1989.

[2] Gutfeld, Greg; Meyers, Melissa; Sangiorgio, Maureen, "Beating Brittle Nails: Biotin Boosts Growth," *Prevention*, v. 43, p. 8, July 1991.

[3] Ibid.

[4] Boyer, Pamela, "Soft Hands, Strong Nails," *Prevention*, v. 44 p. 110, Feb 1992.

[5] Dunne, Lavon J., *Nutrition Almanac Third Edition*, McGraw-Hill Publishing Co., p. 200, 1990.

[6] Balch, Phyllis A and James F, *Prescription for Nutritional Healing*, p. 250, Avery Publishing Group, Garden City Park, NY, 1993.

[7] Burggraf, Helen, "Talking Hands," *American Health: Fitness of Body and Mind*, v. 8, p. 22, July-August 1989.

[8] Boyer, Pamela, "Strength Training for Troubled Nails," *Prevention*, v. 45, p. 106, April 1993.

[9] Ibid.

Chapter 122: NAUSEA

[1] "Vitamin Reduces Nausea Vomiting," *The Medical Tribune*, p. 4, July 25, 1991.

[2] Dunne, Lavon J., *Nutrition Almanac*, Third Edition, McGraw-Hill Publishing Company, p. 223, 1990.

[3] Quillin, Patrick, Ph.D., R.D., *Healing Nutrients*, Chicago, New York, Contemporary Books, 1987.

[4] Fischer-Rasmussen, W., et al, "Ginger Treatment of Hyperemesis Gravidarum", *European Journal of Obstetrics, Gynecology, Reproductive Biology*, v. 38, p. 19-24, 1990.
[5] Bone, M.E., MB, et al, "Ginger Root – A New Antiemetic," *Anesthesia*, v. 45, p. 669-671, 1990.
[6] Grontved, Acksel, et al, "Ginger Root Against Sea Sickness: A Controlled Trial on the Open Sea," *ACTA Otolaryngol Stockh*, v. 105, p. 45-49, 1988.

Chapter 123: NIGHT BLINDNESS
[1] Gruning, Carl, "Seeing is Believing! For Lifelong Eye Health, Just Remember Your ABCs and These Minerals," *Health News & Review*, v. 2, n. 3, p. 1, Summer 1992.
[2] Leguire, Lawrence, et al, "Electro-Oculogram in Vitamin A Deficiency Associated With Cystic Fibrosis," *Ophthalmic Pediatrics*, v. 13, n. 3, p. 187-189, 1992.
[3] "Breast-Feeding Boon to Infants in Third World," *Medical Tribune*, v. 11, October 3, 1991.
[4] Carlier, C., et al, "A Randomized Controlled Trial to Test Equivalence Between Retinyl Palmitate and Beta Carotene for Vitamin A Deficiency," *British Medical Journal*, v. 307, p. 1106-1110, 1993.
[5] Kugler, Hans, et al, *Life Extenders and Memory Boosters*, Health Quest Publications, Reno, Nevada, p. 152-153, 1993
[6] Dunne, Lavon J., *Nutrition Almanac*, Third Edition, McGraw-Hill Publishing Company, p. 166, 1990.

Chapter 124: NOSEBLEEDS
[1] Treloar, Dena, "Cephalosporins – The Third-Generation," *RN*, v. 49, p. 28, January 1986.
[2] Burton Goldberg Group, *Alternative Medicine, The Definitive Guide*, Future Medicine Publishing, Inc., Puyallup, WA, p. 954-955, 1993.
[3] Pierdinock, Joyce, "The Five-Herb Medicine Chest," *Country Journal*, v. 22, n. 4, p. 29, July-August 1995.
[4] Wright, Jonathan V., *Dr. Wright's Book of Nutritional Therapy*, Rodale Press, Emmaus, PA, p. 307-308, 1979.
[5] Treloar, Dena, "Cephalosporins – The Third-Generation," *RN*, v. 49, p. 28, January 1986.

Chapter 125: OSTEOPOROSIS
[1] Lee, John R, M.D., *Natural Progesterone, The Multiple Roles of a Remarkable Hormone*, BLL Publishing, Sebastapol, CA, May 1995.
[2] Lee, John R., M.D., "Osteoporosis Reversal, The Role of Progesterone," *International Clinical Nutrition Review*, v. 10, n. 3, p. 384-391, July 1990.
[3] Cohen, L. and Kitzes R., "Infrared Spectroscopy and Magnesium Content of Bone Mineral in Osteoporotic Women," *Isr J Med Sci*, v. 17, p. 1123-1125, 1981.
[4] Vikhanski, L. E., "Magnesium May Slow Bone Loss," *Medical Tribune*, July 22, 1993.
[5] Seyle, Hans, *Calciphylaxis*, University of Chicago Press, Chicago, Illinois, 1962.
[6] Elin, R., "Magnesium: The Forgotten Nutrient," *The Nutrition Report*, February 1995.
[7] Riggs, Lawrence B., M.D. and Melton, Joseph L., III, M.D., "The Prevention and Treatment of Osteoporosis," *New England Journal of Medicine*, v. 327, n. 9, August 27, 1992.
[8] Brattstrom, L. E., et al, "Folic Acid Responsive Postmenopausal Homocysteinemia," *Metabolism*, v. 34, p. 1073-1077, 1985.

[9] Kugler, Hans Ph.D., et al, *Life Extenders and Memory Boosters*, Health Quest Publications, Reno, NV, 1993

[10] Sahley, Bille J.; Birkner, Kathy, "Stress and Menopause," *Total Health*, v. 10, n. 5, p. 54, October 1988.

[11] Murray, Michael, M.D. and Pizzorno, Joseph, N.D., *Encyclopedia of Natural Medicine*, Prima Publishing, Rocklin, CA, p. 460, 1991.

[12] Binkley, N.C. and Suttie, J.W., "Vitamin K Nutrition and Osteoporosis," *Journal of Nutrition*, v. 125, p. 1812-1821, 1995.

[13] Tomita, A., "Postmenopausal Osteoporosis Calcium Kinetic Study with Vitamin K in Osteoporosis," *Clin Endocrinol Metab*, v. 60, 1268-1269, 1985.

[14] Kidd, Parris M., Ph.D., "An Integrative Lifestyle: Nutritional Strategy For Lowering Osteoporosis Risk," *Townsend Letter For Doctors*, p. 400-405, May 1992.

[15] Saltman, P., "The Role of Minerals and Osteoporosis," *Journal of the American College of Nutrition*, v. 11, n. 5, p. 599, October 1992.

[16] Ibid.

[17] Kidd, Parris M., Ph.D., "An Integrative Lifestyle: Nutritional Strategy For Lowering Osteoporosis Risk," *Townsend Letter For Doctors*, p. 400-405, May 1992.

[18] Nielsen, F. H., "Boron, an Overlooked Element of Potential Nutrition Importance," *Nutrition Today*, p. 4-7, January/February 1988.

[19] Gaby, Alan R., *Preventing and Reversing Osteoporosis*, Prima Publishing, Rocklin, CA, p. 63-64, 1994.

[20] Kaufmann, Klaus, *Silica The Forgotten Nutrient*, Alive Books, Barnaby, BC Canada, 1990.

[21] Ibid.

Chapter 126: OVARIAN CYSTS

[1] Ovarian Cysts: Less-Drastic Surgery Available," *HealthFacts*, v. 16, n. 146, p.1, July 1991.

[2] Ibid.

[3] Ibid.

[4] Ibid.

[5] Editorial, "Breast Cancer, Have We Lost Our Way?" *The Lancet*, v. 341, n. 8841, p. 343, February 6, 1993.

[6] Finn, Judith, A, "Dispelling Myths About Breast "Disease: Natural Approaches to Reduce Fibrocystic Breast Conditions," *Natural Health*, v. 23, n. 2, p. 44, March-April 1993.

[7] Challem, Jack, "Breast Cancer: Tracing It's Elusive Causes and Leveraging Dietary Strategies to Prevent It," *Let's Live*, p. 19, November 1994.

[8] Whitaker, Julian, "Preventing Breast Cancer," *Health and Healing*, January 1994.

[9] Finn, Judith, A, "Dispelling Myths About Breast "Disease: Natural Approaches to Reduce Fibrocystic Breast Conditions," *Natural Health*, v. 23, n. 2, p. 44, March-April 1993.

[10] Kennedy, Bob, "Borage Wildflowers: Best Source of GLA," *Total Health*, v. 13, n. 1, p. 44, February 1991.

[11] Northrup, Christiane; Pick, Marcelle, "Breast Lumps Can be Frightening, but Most are Benign & Preventable," *Health News & Review*, v. 3, n. 2, p. 10, Spring 1993.

Chapter 127: PANCREATITIS

[1] Murray, Michael, M.D. and Pizzorno, Joseph, N.D., *Encyclopedia of Natural Medicine*, Prima Publishing, Rocklin, CA, p. 52, 1991.

[2] Dunne, Lavon J., *Nutrition Almanac*, Third Edition, McGraw-Hill Publishing Company, p. 90, 1990.

[3] Song, Moon K., Ph.D. and Adham, Nabeel F., M.D., "Role of Zinc in Treatment of Experimental Acute Pancreatitis in Mice," *Digestive Diseases and Sciences*, v. 34, n. 12, p. 1905-1910, December 1989.

[4] Martin, Linda G., D.V.M., et al, "Magnesium in the 1990's: Implications For Veterinary Critical Care," *Veterinary Emergency and Critical Care*, v. 3, n. 2, p. 105-113, 1994.

[5] Ryzen, Elisabeth, M.D. and Rude, Robert K., M.D., "Low Intracellular Magnesium in Patients With Acute Pancreatitis and Hypocalcemia," *The Western Journal of Medicine*, v. 152, n. 2, p. 145-148, February 1990.

[6] Elin, R., "Magnesium: The Forgotten Nutrient," *The Nutrition Report*, February 1995.

[7] Birk, Dieter, et al, "The Role of Oxygen Free Radicals in Acute Pancreatitis," *Med. Klin.*, v. 90, p. 32-35, 1995.

[8] Kuklinski, Bodo, et al, "Latent Deficiency of Antioxidants (Selenium and Vitamin E) in The Population of German Democratic Republic. Reasons and Clinical Relevance.," *Arztl. Lab.*, v. 36, p. 288-294, 1990.

[9] Kuklinski, Bodo, et al, "Antioxidant Therapy of Pancreatitis-18 Months Interim Balance," *Z. Gesamte Inn. Med.*, v. 47, p. 239-245, 1992.

[10] Nonaka, A., et al, "Effect of a New Synthetic Ascorbic Acid Derivative As a Free Radical Scavenger In The Development of Acute Pancreatitis in Mice," *Gut*, v. 32, p. 528-532, 1991.

[11] Scott, P., et al, "Vitamin C Status in Patients With Acute-Pancreatitis," *British Journal of Surgery*, v. 80, p. 750-754, 1993.

Chapter 128: PANIC ATTACKS

[1] Handly, Robert and Neff, Pauline, *Anxiety and Panic Attacks: Their Cause and Cure*, Rawson Associated, New York, p. 20, 1985.

[2] Dunne, Lavon J., *Nutrition Almanac*, Third Edition, McGraw-Hill Publishing Company, p. 193, 1990.

[3] Murray, Frank, "Bone Up on B Vitamins: Part One," *Better Nutrition*, v. 51, n. 10, p. 8, October 1989.

[4] Hoffer, Abram, *Orthomolecular Medicine for Physicians*, Keats Publishing, New Canaan, CT, p. 33, 1989.

[5] Murray, Frank, "Bone Up on B Vitamins: Part One," *Better Nutrition*, v. 51, n. 10, p. 8, October 1989.

[6] Hoffer, Abram, *Orthomolecular Medicine for Physicians*, Keats Publishing, New Canaan, CT, p. 32, 1989.

[7] Murray, Frank, "Bone Up on B Vitamins: Part One," *Better Nutrition*, v. 51, n. 10, p. 8, October 1989.

[8] "Alert: Thiamine-Deficient Total Parenteral Nutrition," *Patient Care*, v. 23, n. 9, p. 24, May 15, 1989.

[9] Hofle, K.H., "Magnesium In Psychotherapy," 10th Hohenheim Magnesium Symposium, *Magnesium Research*, v. 1, p. 99, 1988.

Chapter 129: PARASITES

1   Albertson, Peter, "Persistent GI Upset a Signal of Hidden Giardiasis," *Cortlandt Forum*, p. 120-121, February 1990.
2   Burton Goldberg Group, *Alternative Medicine, The Definitive Guide*, Future Medicine Publishing, Inc., Puyallup, WA, p. 784, 1993.
3   Day, Lorraine, M.D., "Is the Water Supply Safe From AIDS?" *National Health Alert*, v. 1, n. 9, p. 1-4, January 1992.
4   Gittleman, Ann Louise, M.S., "Parasites in the United States," *Let's Live*, p. 56-60, August 1995.
5   Nesheim, M.C., "Human Nutrition Needs and Parasitic Infections," *Parasitology*, n. 107, p. S7-S18, 1993.
6   Burton Goldberg Group, *Alternative Medicine, The Definitive Guide*, Future Medicine Publishing, Inc., Puyallup, WA, p. 786, 1993.
7   Gittleman, Ann Louise, "The Growing Problem of Parasites," *Natural Health*, v. 23, n. 5, p. 68, September-October 1993.

Chapter 130: PARKINSON'S DISEASE

1   Roblin, Andrew, "The Case of the Shaky Diagnosis," *Prevention*, v. 41, n. 3, p. 103-107, March 1989.
2   Salzman, Edwin, W., "Living with Parkinson's Disease," *The New England Journal of Medicine*, v. 334, n. 2, p. 114-117, January 11, 1996.
3   Jenner, P., "Oxidative Damage in Neurodegenerative Diseases," *The Lancet*, v. 344, p. 796-798, September 17, 1994.
4   Fahn, Stanley, "An Open Trial of High-Dose Antioxidants in Early Parkinson's Disease," *American Journal of Clinical Nutrition*, v. 53, p. 380S-382S, 1991.
5   Tanner, Caroline M., M.D. and Langston, William, M.D., "Do Environmental Toxins Cause Parkinson's Disease? A Critical Review," *Neurology*, v. 40, Suppl.3, p. 17-28, October 1990.
6   *Martindale, The Extra Pharmacopoeia, Thirtieth Edition*, Department of Pharmaceutical Sciences, Royal Pharmaceutical Society of Great Britain, The Pharmaceutical Press, p. 841-847, 1993.
7   Kempster, P.A ., M.D., and Wahlquist, M.L., M.D., "Dietary Factors and the Management of Parkinson's Disease," *Nutrition Reviews*, v. 52, n. 2, p. 51-58, 1994.
8   Croxson, S. et al, "Dietary Modification of Parkinson's Disease," *European Journal of Clinical Nutrition*, v. 45, p. 263-266, 1991.
9   Laino, Charlene, "High-Carbohydrate Diet Urged For Parkinson's," *Medical Tribune*, v. 9, March 24, 1994.
10 "Parkinson's Disease – One Day at a Time," *Harvard Health Letter*, June 1993.
11 Sasco, Annie J., "The Role of Physical Exercise in the Occurrence of Parkinson's Disease," *Arch Neurol*, v. 49, p. 360-365, April 1992.

Chapter 131: PELLAGRA

1   Elmore, Joann G.; Feinstein, Alvan R., "Joseph Goldberger: An Unsung Hero of American Clinical Epidemiology," *Annals of Internal Medicine*, v. 121, n. 5, p. 372, September 1, 1994.

[2] Hoffer, Abram, *Orthomolecular Medicine for Physicians*, Keats Publishing, New Canaan, CT, p. 34-44, 1989.

[3] Taylor, Deborah Seymour, "Food and Mood: Can Nutrition Affect Your Mental Health?" Today's Living, v. 20, n. 12, p. 12-15, December 1989.

[4] Murray, Frank, "Is Nutrition Related to Criminal Behavior?" *Better Nutrition for Today's Living*, v. 54, n. 4, p. 10-12, April 1992.

[5] Hoffer, Abram, *Orthomolecular Medicine for Physicians*, Keats Publishing, New Canaan, CT, p. 34-44, 1989.

[6] Murray, Frank, "Is Nutrition Related to Criminal Behavior?" *Better Nutrition for Today's Living*, v. 54, n. 4, p. 10-12, April 1992.

[7] Ibid.

[8] Ibid.

Chapter 132: POISON IVY, OAK

[1] DeSimone, Veronica, "No More Poison Ivy!," *Countryside & Small Stock Journal*, v. 79, n. 3, p. 48-52, May-June 1995.

[2] Ibid.

[3] Challem, Jack, "How to Use Vitamins and Minerals as Home Remedies," *Natural Health*, v.24, n. 2, p. 60-68, March-April, 1994.

[4] Klasson, D.H., "Ascorbic Acid in The Treatment and Prevention of Poison Oak Dermatitis," *Archives of Dermatol. Syph.*, v. 56, p. 864-867, 1947.

[5] Murray, Michael T., N.D, *Natural Alternatives to Over-The-Counter and Prescription Drugs*, William Morrow & Company, New York, p. 95-96, 1994.

[6] Mazzotta, Mary Y., "Nutrition and Wound Healing," *Journal of the American Podiatric Medical Association*, v. 84, n. 9, p. 456, September 1994.

Chapter 133: PREECLAMPSIA

[1] Duley, Lelia, "Which Anticonvulsant for Women with Eclampsia? Evidence from the Collaborative Eclampsia Trial," *The Lancet*, v. 345, p. 1455-1462, June 10, 1995.

[2] Kamen, Si and Kamen, Betty, *Total Nutrition During Pregnancy*, Appleton-Century-Crofts, New York, p. 186-187, 1981.

[3] Duley, Lelia and Johnson, Richard, "Magnesium Sulfate for Preeclampsia and Eclampsia: The Evidence So Far," *British Journal of Obstetrics and Gynecology*, v. 101, p. 565-567, July 1994.

[4] Lucas, Michael J., M.D., et al, "A Comparison of Magnesium Sulfate With Phenytoin For The Prevention of Eclampsia," *The New England Journal of Medicine*, v. 333, n. 4, p. 201-205, July 27, 1995.

[5] Rudnicki, Peter Martin, et al, "Magnesium Supplementation in Pregnancy-Induced Hypertension and Preeclampsia," *Acta Obstetricia et Gynecologica Scandinavica*, v. 73, p. 95-96, 1994.

[6] Wright, Jonathan V., *Dr. Wright's Book of Nutritional Therapy*, Rodale Press, Emmaus, PA, p. 144-154, 1979.

[7] Dunne, Lavon J., *Nutrition Almanac,* Third Edition, Table of Food Composition, McGraw-Hill, p. 29, 1990.

8 Strauss, Maurice B., "Observations on the Etiology of the Toxemias of Pregnancy: The Relationship of Nutritional Deficiency, Hypoproteinemia and Elevated Venous Pressure to Water Retention in Pregnancy," *American Journal of Medical Science*, v. 190, p. 811-842, 1935.

9 Wright, Jonathan V., *Dr. Wright's Book of Nutritional Therapy*, Rodale Press, Emmaus, PA, p. 144-154, 1979.

10 Walsh, Scott W., "The Role of Fatty Acid Peroxidation and Antioxidant Status in Normal Pregnancy and in Pregnancy Complicated by Preeclampsia," *World Review of Nutrition and Diet*, v. 76, p. 114-118, 1994.

11 Mikhail, Magdy S., M.D., et al, "Preeclampsia and Antioxidant Nutrients: Decreased Plasma Levels of Reduced Ascorbic Acid, Tocopherol, and Beta-Carotene in Women With Preeclampsia," *American Journal of Obstetrics and Gynecology*, v. 171, n. 1, p. 150-157, July 1994.

12 Kamen, Si and Kamen, Betty, *Total Nutrition During Pregnancy*, Appleton-Century-Crofts, New York, p. 186-187, 1981.

13 Ibid.

14 Williams, Michelle, A., et al, "Omega-3 Fatty Acids in Maternal Erythrocytes and Risk of Preeclampsia," *Epidemiology*, v. 6, n. 3, p. 232-237, May 1995.

Chapter 134: PREMENSTRUAL SYNDROME

1 Langer, Stephen, "PMS: A Positive Approach," *Better Nutrition for Today's Living*, v. 54, n. 10, p. 36-38, October 1992.

2 Fackelmann, K.A., et al, "PMS: Hints of a Link to Lunch Time and Zinc," *Science News*, v. 138, p. 263, October 27, 1990.

3 Lee, John R, M.D., *Natural Progesterone, The Multiple Roles of a Remarkable Hormone*, BLL Publishing, Sebastapol, CA, p. 50-52, May 1995.

4 "Safe Antidote for PMS," *MCall's*, p. 152-156, October 1990.

5 Fackelmann, K.A., et al, "PMS: Hints of a Link to Lunch Time and Zinc," *Science News*, v. 138, p. 263, October 27, 1990.

6 Wright, Jonathan and Gaby, Alan, *Nutrition & Healing*, v. 1, n. 3, p. 1-9, October 1994.

7 Nader, Shahla, M.D., "Premenstrual Syndrome: Tailoring Treatment to Symptoms," *Postgraduate Medicine*, v. 90, n. 1, p. 173-180, July 1991.

8 *Los Angeles Times*, Part VIII, p. 8, August 16, 1984.

9 Kennedy, Bob, "Borage Wildflowers: Best Source of GLA," *Total Health*, v. 13, n. 1, p. 44, February 1991.

10 Langer, Stephen, "PMS: A Positive Approach," *Better Nutrition for Today's Living*, v. 54, n. 10, p. 36-38, October 1992.

11 Breecher, Maury, M., "The Primrose Path," *Health*, v. 15, p. 17, February 1983.

12 Horrobin, D. F. "The Role Of Essential Fatty Acids and Prostaglandins in the Premenstrual Syndrome," *Journal of Reproductive Medicine*, v. 28, n. 7, p. 465-468, 1983.

13 Breecher, Maury, M., "The Primrose Path," *Health*, v. 15, p. 17, February 1983.

Chapter 135: PRENATAL

1 Andrew E., M.D., National Institutes of Hygiene, H-1966 Budapest, Hungary.

[2] Butler, Pamela D., Ph.D., et al, "Prenatal Nutritional Deprivation as a Risk Factor in Schizophrenia: Preclinical Evidence," *Neuropsychopharmacology*, v. 11, n. 4, p. 227-233, 1994.

[3] Goldenberg, Robert L., M.D., et al, "Serum Folate and Fetal Growth Retardation: A Matter of Compliance," *Obstetrics and Gynecology*, v. 79, n. 5, p. 719-722, May 1992.

[4] Dunne, Lavon J., *Nutrition Almanac*, Third Edition, McGraw-Hill Publishing Company, p. 39-40, 1990.

[5] "Folic Acid and Neural Tube Defects," *The Lancet*, v. 338, p. 153-154, July 20, 1991.

[6] Dunne, Lavon J., *Nutrition Almanac*, Third Edition, McGraw-Hill Publishing Company, p. 39-40, 1990.

[7] Kamen, Si and Kamen, Betty, *Total Nutrition During Pregnancy*, Appleton-Century-Crofts, New York, p. 187, 1981

[8] Uriu-Hare, et al, "Influence of Maternal Dietary Zinc Intake on Expression of Diabetes-induced Teratogenicity in Rats," *Diabetes*, v. 38, n. 10, p. 1282, October 1989.

[9] Murray, Frank, "Zinc: Healing Mineral," *Better Nutrition for Today's Living*, v. 54, n. 9, p. 26, September 1992.

[10] Johnson, Mary Ann; Kays, Sandra E., "Copper: Its Role in Human Nutrition," *Nutrition Today*, v. 25, n.1, p. 6, February 1990.

[11] Drews, Carolyn D., et al, "The Relationship Between Idiopathic Mental Retardation and Maternal Smoking During Pregnancy," *Pediatrics*, v. 97, n. 4, p. 547-554, April 1996.

Chapter 136: PROSTATE PROBLEMS

[1] Faelton, Sharon, *The Complete Book of Minerals for Health*, Rodale Books, Emmaus, PA, p. 427, 1981.

[2] Murray, Frank, "Zinc: Healing Mineral," *Better Nutrition for Today's Living*, v.54, n.9, September 1992.

[3] Faelton, Sharon, *The Complete Book of Minerals for Health*, Rodale Books, Emmaus, PA, p. 429, 1981.

[4] Hart, James P. & Cooper, William L., "Vitamin E in the Treatment of Prostate Hypertrophy," Lee Foundation for Nutritional Research, Milwaukee, WI, Report No. 1, November 1941.

[5] Wright, Jonathan, M.D., *Dr. Wright's Book of Nutritional Therapy*, Rodale Press, Emmaus, PA, p. 281, 1979.

[6] Feinblatt, H.M. & Gant, J.C. "Palliative Treatment of Benign Prostatic Hypertrophy: Value of Glycine, Alanine, Glutamic Acid Combination," *Journal of the Maine Medical Association*, 1958.

[7] Kugler, Hans Ph.D., et al, *Life Extenders and Memory Boosters*, Health Quest Publications, Reno, NV, p. 169, 1993

[8] Herbert, Victor, Genell J. Subak-Sharpe, *The Mt. Sinai School of Medicine Complete Book of Nutrition*, St. Martin's Press, New York, 1990.

Chapter 137: PSORIASIS

[1] Petrakis, Peter L, "Psoriasis," *Academic American Encyclopedia*, Grolier Electronic Publishing, Inc., 1993.

[2] Murray, Frank, "Psoriasis Confronted," *Better Nutrition for Today's Living*, v. 52, n. 6, p. 22, June 1990.

3 Ibid.
4 *Cutis*, v. 34, p. 497.
5 Pagano, John, D.C., *Healing Psoriasis*, Pagano Organization, Englewood Cliffs, N.J., 1991.
6 Ibid.
7 Douglass, John M. "Psoriasis and Diet," *California Medicine*, v. 450, p. 133-135, 1980.
8 Allison, J.R. "The Relation of Hydrochloric Acid and Vitamin B Complex Deficiency in Certain Skin Diseases," *Southern Medical Journal*, v. 38, p. 235-241, 1945.
9 News Feature, Royal Hallamshire Hospital, Sheffield, England, April 1988.
10 Ibid.
11 News Story, University of California, March 1988.
12 Murray, Frank, "Psoriasis Confronted," *Better Nutrition for Today's Living*, v. 52, n. 6, p. 22, June 1990.
13 "Long-term Treatment of Psoriasis with Eicosapentaenoic Acid," *Nutrition Research Newsletter*, v. 10, n. 10, p. 104, October 1991.
14 Ibid.
15 Voorhees, John J., M.D. "Leukotrienes and Other Lipoxygenase Products in the Pathogenesis and Therapy of Psoriasis and Other Dermatoses," *Archives of Dermatology*, v. 119, p. 541-547, July 1983.
16 Ibid.
17 Ibid.
18 Kennedy, Bob, "Borage Wildflowers: Best Source of GLA," *Total Health*, v. 13, n. 1, p. 44, February 1991.
19 Rudin, Donald O. and Felix, Clara. *The Omega-3 Phenomenon*, Rawson Associates, New York, Stern, R.S., et al, 1987.
20 Ibid.
21 Hoffer, Abram, M.D., Ph.D. *Orthomolecular Medicine for Physicians*, Keats Publishing Inc., New Canaan, CT, 1989.
22 Murray, Frank, "Psoriasis confronted," *Better Nutrition for Today's Living*, v. 52, n. 6, p. 22, June 1990.
23 Fry, L. et al. "The Mechanism of Folate Deficiency in Psoriasis," *British Journal of Dermatology*, v84, p. 539-544, Gross, P., et al, 1971.
24 "The Treatment of Psoriasis as a Disturbance of Lipid Metabolism" *New York State Journal of Medicine*, v. 50 p. 2683-2686, 1950.
25 Ibid.
26 Sherman, Carl, "Psoriasis: A Sobering Study," *Gentleman's Quarterly*, p. 115, August 1990.
27 Ibid.
28 Ibid.

Chapter 138: RESTLESS LEG SYNDROME

1 Oboler, Sylvia K., et al, "Symptoms in Outpatient Veterans," *The Western Journal of Medicine*, v. 155, n. 3, p. 256-260, September 1991.
2 Werbach, Melvyn, *Nutritional Influences on Illness*, Second Edition, Third Line Press, Tarzana, California, p. 564-565, 1993.

[3] Laton, Thomas M., D.O., "Restless Leg Syndrome Secondary to Iron Deficiency," *Journal of Osteopathic Medicine*, v. 54, September 1990.

[4] O'Keefe, S.T. et al., "Iron Status and Restless Legs Syndrome In the Elderly," *Age and Ageing*, v. 23, p. 200-203, 1994.

[5] Dunne, Lavon J., *Nutrition Almanac*, Third Edition, McGraw-Hill Publishing Company, p. 75-76, 1990.

[6] Jeddy, T.A. and Berridge, D.C., "Restless Leg Syndrome," *British Journal of Surgery*, v. 81, p. 49-51, 1994.

[7] Laton, Thomas M., D.O., "Restless Leg Syndrome Secondary to Iron Deficiency," *Journal of Osteopathic Medicine*, v. 54, September 1990.

[8] Werbach, Melvyn, *Nutritional Influences on Illness*, Second Edition, Third Line Press, Tarzana, California, p. 564-565, 1993.

[9] Ayres, S. and Mihan, R., "Restless Legs Syndrome: Response to Vitamin E," *Journal of Applied Nutrition*, v. 25, p. 8-15, 1973.

[10] Werbach, Melvyn, *Nutritional Influences on Illness*, Second Edition, Third Line Press, Tarzana, California, p. 564-565, 1993.

[11] Ibid.

[12] Burton Goldberg Group, *Alternative Medicine, The Definitive Guide*, Future Medicine Publishing, Inc., Puyallup, WA, p. 847, 1993.

Chapter 139: RETINITIS PIGMENTOSA

[1] Herbert, Victor, Genell J. Subak-Sharpe, *The Mt. Sinai School of Medicine Complete Book of Nutrition*, St. Martin's Press, New York, pg. 258, 1990.

[2] Rader, Daniel J.; Brewer, H. Bryan, Jr., "Abetalipoproteinemia: New insights into Lipoprotein Assembly and Vitamin E Metabolism From a Rare Genetic Disease," JAMA, *The Journal of the American Medical Association*, v. 270, n. 7, p. 865, August 18, 1993.

[3] Adams, Ruth, "Versatile Vitamin E: Studies Show that Vitamin E May Help Alleviate Heart Disease, PMS, Gum Disease, Epilepsy and Parkinson's Disease," *Better Nutrition for Today's Living*, v. 53, n. 4, p. 14, April 1991.

[4] Gerster, Helga, "Review: Antioxidant Protection of the Ageing Macula," *Age and Ageing*, v. 20, p. 60-69, 1991.

[5] "Molecular Genetics of Retinitis Pigmentosa," *Western Journal of Medicine*, v. 155, n. 4, p. 388, October 1991.

[6] Murray, Frank, "Keeping an Eye on Good Health," *Today's Living*, v. 20, n. 8, p. 8, August 1989.

[7] Ibid.

Chapter 140: SCHIZOPHRENIA

[1] Zaslove, Marshall O., et al, "Effect of Caffeine Intake on Psychotic In-Patients," *British Journal of Psychiatry*, v. 159, p. 565-567, 1991.

[2] Ibid.

[3] "Schizophrenia Update," *Harvard Mental Health Letter*, v. 11, n. 12, p. 1, June, 1995

[4] Lindenbaum, J., et al, "Neuropsychiatric Disorders Caused by Cobalamin Deficiency in The Absence of Anemia or Macrocytosis," *New England Journal of Medicine*, v. 318, p. 1720-1728, 1988.

[5] Holmes, J. MacDonald, "Cerebral Manifestations of Vitamin B12 Deficiency," British Medical Journal, v. 2, p. 1394-1398, 1956.

[6] Downing, Damien, MB, BS,"Cerebral Manifestations of Vitamin B12 Deficiency," *Journal of Nutritional Medicine*, v. 2, p. 89-90, 1991.

[7] Dunne, Lavon J., *Nutrition Almanac*, Third Edition, McGraw-Hill Publishing Company, p. 32, 1990.

[8] Lindenbaum, J., et al, "Neuropsychiatric Disorders Caused by Cobalamin Deficiency in The Absence of Anemia or Macrocytosis," *New England Journal of Medicine*, v. 318, p. 1720-1728, 1988.

[9] Carney, M.W.P., et al, "Red Cell Folate Concentrations in Psychiatric Patients," Journal of Affective Disorders, v. 9, p. 207-213, 1990.

[10] Murray, Frank, "Is Nutrition Related to Criminal Behavior?" *Better Nutrition for Today's Living*, v. 54, n. 4, p. 10-12, April 1992.

[11] Elin, R., "Magnesium: The Forgotten Nutrient," *The Nutrition Report*, February 1995.

[12] Lieberman, Shari & Bruning, Nancy, *The Real Vitamin & Mineral Book*, Avery Publishing Group, Garden City Park, New York, p. 139, 1990.

[13] Banki, C.M., et al, "Cerebrospinal Fluid Magnesium and Calcium Related to Amine Metabolites, Diagnosis and Suicide Attempts," *Biological Psychiatry*, v. 20, p. 163-171, 1985.

[14] Kanofsky, J.D., et al, "Is Iatrogenic Hypomagnesemia Common in Schizophrenia?" *Journal of the American College of Nutrition*, v. 10, n. 5, p. 537, October 1991.

Chapter 141: SHINGLES

[1] Carmichael, Kevin J, "Treatment of Herpes Zoster and Postherpetic Neuralgia," *American Family Physician*, v. 44, n. 1, p. 203-208, July 1991.

[2] Thomsen, Thomas Carl, "Stopping Shingles Pain," *Prevention*, v. 42, n. 9, p. 74, September 1990.

[3] Ibid.

[4] *"Shingles, What You Should Know,"* Burroughs Wellcome Co., North Carolina, 1985.

[5] DeMoragas J, Kierland R, "The Outcome of Patients with Herpes Zoster," *Archives of Dermatology*, v. 75, p. 193-196, 1957.

[6] Carmichael, Kevin J, "Treatment of Herpes Zoster and Postherpetic Neuralgia," *American Family Physician*, v. 44, n. 1, p. 203-8, July 1991.

[7] Schimpff S, Serpick A, Stoler B, et al, "Varicella-Zoster Infection in Patients with Cancer," *Annals of Internal Medicine*, v. 76, p. 241-254, 1972.

[8] Cohen PR, Grossman ME, "Clinical Features of Human Immunodeficiency Virus-Associated Disseminated Herpes Zoster Virus Infection – a Review of the Literature," *Clinical Experiences in Dermatology*, v. 14, p. 273-276, 1989.

[9] Wilkerson MG, Jordan WP, Kerkering TM, "Herpes Zoster as a Sign of AIDS-Related Complex," *American Family Physician*, v36, p233-5, 1987.

[10] Gupta, A.K, Mital, H.S., *India Practitioners*, July 1967.

[11] Ibid.

[12] Klennner, Fred, "The Treatment of Poliomyelitis and Other Virus Diseases with Vitamin C," *Southern Medicine and Surgery*, v. 111, p. 209-214, 1949.

[13] *Journal Des Practiciens*, v. 64, p. 586, 1950.

[14] Mikan, K, Ayers, S, "Post Herpes Zoster Neuralgia: Response to Vitamin E Therapy," *Archives of Dermatology*, December 1973.
[15] "Hot Pepper Cream Cools Burning Skin," *Insight*, p. 54, October 23, 1989.
[16] Ibid.
[17] Wright, Jonathan V, M.D., Gaby, Alan R, M.D., "Nutritional Therapy for the 1990s: Selected Protocols," The Wright/Gaby Nutrition Institute, October 1991.
[18] "Hot Pepper Cream Cools Burning Skin," *Insight*, p. 54, October 23, 1989.
[19] Ibid.
[20] Ibid.
[21] *Journal of the American Academy of Dermatology*, p. 93-96, July 1987.

Chapter 142: SICKLE-CELL ANEMIA
[1] Zewail, Ahmed, ed, *Chemical Bond*, Academic Press, March 1992.
[2] Moss, Barbara Klein, "Using Vitamin and Mineral Supplements," *Patient Care*, v. 18, p. 81, September 30, 1984.
[3] Murray, Frank, "Supplements Guard Against Anemia," *Better Nutrition for Today's Living*, v. 52, n. 7, p. 8, July 1990.
[4] Chiu, Daniel, Ph.D., et al, "Vitamin C Deficiency in Patients With Sickle Cell Anemia," *The American Journal of Pediatric Hematology/Oncology*, v. 12, n. 3, p. 262-267, 1990.
[5] Muskiet, Frits, A.J., et al, "Supplementation of Patients with Homozygous Sickle Cell Disease with Zinc, Alpha-tocopherol, Vitamin C, Soybean oil, and Fish Oil," *American Journal of Clinical Nutrition*, v. 54, n. 4, p. 736-744, October 1991.
[6] Jain, Sushil K., Ph.D., et al, "Low Plasma Prealbumin and Carotenoid Levels in Sickle Cell Diseased Patients," *The American Journal of Medical Sciences*, v. 299, n. 1, p. 13-15, January 1990.
[7] Natta, C.L, et al, "Selenium and Glutathione Peroxidase Levels in Sickle Cell Anemia," *ACTA Hematologica*, v. 83, p. 130-132, 1990.
[8] Murray, Frank, "Supplements Guard Against Anemia," *Better Nutrition for Today's Living*, v. 52, n. 7, p. 8, July 1990.
[9] Ibid.
[10] Ibid.
[11] Duff, E.M.W., et al, "Neural Tube Defects in Hurricane Aftermath," *The Lancet*, v. 337, p. 120-121, January 12, 1991.
[12] Al-Momen, A.K., "Diminished Vitamin B12 Levels in Patients With Severe Sickle Cell Disease," *Journal of Internal Medicine*, v. 237, p. 551-555, 1995.

Chapter 143: SINUSITIS
[1] Burton Goldberg Group, *Alternative Medicine, The Definitive Guide*, Future Medicine Publishing, Inc., Puyallup, WA, p. 833, 1993.
[2] Gerras, Charles, et al, eds, *The Encyclopedia of Common Diseases*, Rodale Press, Emmaus, PA, p. 1103, 1976.
[3] Ibid, p. 1104.
[4] Ibid.
[5] Cheraskin, Emanuel, M.D., D.M.D., *Vitamin C, Who Needs It?*, Arlington Press and Company, Birmingham AL, p. 109, 1993.
[6] Ibid, p. 62.

[7] "Vitamin C Enhances Antibiotic Therapy," *The Nutrition Report*, v. 10, n. 4, p. 31, April 1992.
[8] "Decreased Resistance to Antibiotics and Plasmid Loss in Plasmid-Carrying Strains of Staphylococcus Aureus Treated With Ascorbic Acid," *Mutation Research*, v. 264, p. 119-125, 1991.

Chapter 144: SKIN LUMPS
[1] Delaney, Lisa; London, Cemela, "Dictionary of Healing Techniques and Remedies," *Prevention*, v. 44, p. 124, May 1992.
[2] Fenske, Neil and Lober, Clifford Warren, "Aging and It's Effects on the Skin," p.111, *Dermatology*, 3rd Ed., Moschella, S.L, Hurley, H.J., W.B. Saunders, Philadelphia, 1992.
[3] J. Margolis and L.S. Margolis, "Skin Tags – A Frequent Sign of Diabetes Mellitis," *New England Journal of Medicine*, p1184, May 20, 1976.
[4] Wright, Jonathan, "A Case of Skin Tags," *Prevention*, v. 36, p. 78, April 1984.
[5] Ibid.

Chapter 145: SLEEP APNEA
[1] Wake Up America: A National Sleep Alert. Washington, D.C., National Commission on Sleep Disorders Research, p. 4, 1993.
[2] Riley, Robert W., et al, "Obstructive Sleep Apnea: Trends in Therapy," *The Western Journal of Medicine*, v. 162, n. 2, p. 143, February 1995.
[3] D'Alessandro R, Magelli C, Gamberini G, et al: Snoring Every Night as a Risk Factor for Myocardial Infarction: A Case-Control Study, *British Medical Journal*, v. 300, p. 1557-1558, 1990.
[4] Findley L. J., "Automobile Accidents Involving Patients with Obstructive Sleep Apnea," *Am Rev Respir Dis.* v. 139, p. 337-340, 1988.
[5] Bliwise D.L., et al, "Risk Factors for Sleep Disordered Breathing in Heterogeneous Geriatric Populations, *Journal of the American Geriatric Society*, v. 35, p. 132-141, 1987.
[6] Ibid.
[7] Ancoli-Israel S., "Epidemiology of Sleep Disorders," *Clinical Geriatric Medicine*, v. 5, p. 347-362, 1989.
[8] Kittle, William M., M.D. and Chaudhary, Bashir, M.D., "Sleep Apnea and Hypothyroidism," *Southern Medical Journal*, v. 81, p. 11, p. 1421-1425, November 1988.
[9] Moss, Barbara Klein, "Using Vitamin and Mineral Supplements," *Patient Care*, v. 18, p. 81, September 30, 1984.

Chapter 146: SLEEPLESSNESS
[1] "Food and Mood," *Nutrition Action Newsletter*, p. 5-7, September 1992.
[2] Okawa, Masako, et al, "Vitamin B12 Treatment For Sleep-Wake Rhythm Disorder," *Proceedings of the 5th World Congress of Biological Psychiatry*, Florence, Italy, June 9-14, 1991.
[3] Okawa, Masako, et al, "Vitamin B12 Treatment For Sleep-Wake Rhythm Disorders," *The Japanese Journal of Psychiatry and Neurobiology*, v. 45, n. 1, p. 165-166, 1991.
[4] Brown, Gregory M., "Melatonin in Psychiatric and Sleep Disorders: Therapeutic Implications," *CNS Drugs*, v. 3, n. 3, p. 209-226, 1995.
[5] *Science News*, p. 390, December 20, 1986.

[6] "Drug of Darkness: Can a Pineal Hormone Head Off Everything From Breast Cancer to Aging?," *Science News*, v. 147, n. 19, p. 300, May 13, 1995.

[7] Ibid.

[8] Haimov, I., et al, "Sleep Disorders and Melatonin Rhythms in Elderly People," *British Medical Journal*, v. 309, p. 167, 1994.

Chapter 147: SMELL AND TASTE LOSS

[1] Toufexis, Anastasia, "Older – But Coming on Strong; Aging no Longer has to Mean Sickness, Senility and Sexlessness," *Time*, v. 131, p. 76, February 22, 1988.

[2] Duffy, Valerie B., et al, "Olfactory Dysfunction and Related Nutritional Risk in Free-Living, Elderly   Women," *Journal of the American Dietetic Association*, v. 95, n. 8, p. 879-886, August 1995.

[3] "Smell and Taste Disorders: A Study of 750 Patients from the University of Pennsylvania Smell and Taste Center," JAMA, *The Journal of the American Medical Association*, v. 266, n. 12, p. 1637, September 25, 1991.

[4] Wolman SL, Anderson GH, Marliss EB, et al, "Zinc in Total Parenteral Nutrition: Requirements and Metabolic Effects, *Gastroenterology*, v. 76, p. 458-467, 1979.

[5] Ibid.

[6] Pokornowski, Ronald F., M.D., "Substantiating Zinc's Effect on Taste," *Cortlandt Forum*, v. 69, p. 41-25, July 1991.

[7] *Popular Science*, p. 8-9, August 1982.

[8] Stoll, Andrew, L. and Oepen, Godehard, "Zinc Salts for the Treatment of Olfactory and Gustatory Symptoms in Psychiatric Patients: A Case Series," *Journal of Clinical Psychiatry*, v. 55, n. 7, p. 309-311, July 1994.

[9] Henkin, R.I. and Nelson, N.R., "Changes in Smell Function in Patients With Hyposmia After Magnesium Treatment," *Journal of the American College of Nutrition*, v. 10, n. 5, p. 548/Abstract 48, October 1991.

[10] Duffy, Valerie B., et al, "Olfactory Dysfunction and Related Nutritional Risk in Free-Living, Elderly Women," *Journal of the American Dietetic Association*, v. 95, n. 8, p. 879-886, August 1995.

Chapter 148: SMOKING (QUITTING)

[1] Alexander, Kateri, "A New Leaf. A Tobacco Heir Stops Smoking," *HeartCorps*, v. 2, n. 4, p. 53, January-February 1990.

[2] "How to Stop Smoking," *Health News*, v. 8, n. 2, p. 2-11, April 1990.

[3] Ibid.

[4] *Psychology Today*, p. 14, April 1985.

[5] Murray, Frank, "Evening Primrose Oil: Nocturnal Curative Extract," *Better Nutrition for Today's Living*, v. 56, n. 2, p. 34, February 1994.

[6] Mills, D.E., et al, "Dietary Fatty Acid Supplementation Alters Stress Reactivity and Performance in Man," *J. Hum. Hypertens.*, v. 3, n. 2, p. 111-116, April 1989.

[7] Seelig, Mildred S., M.D., M.P.H., "Magnesium, Antioxidants and Myocardial Infarction," *American Journal of Clinical Nutrition*, v. 13, n. 2, p. 116-117, 1994.

[8] Grindy, Robert, "More About Magnesium," *Saturday Evening Post*, v. 259, p. 50, July-August 1987.

[9] Dunne, Lavon J., *Nutrition Almanac*, Third Edition, McGraw-Hill Publishing Company, p. 211, 1990.

[10] *Maximize Your Life* television show interview.

[11] Bell, Iris R., M.D., Ph.D., et al, "B Complex Vitamin Patterns In Geriatric and Young Adult Patients With Major Depression," *Journal of The American Geriatric Society*, v. 39, n.3, p. 252-257.

[12] *The Practical Encyclopedia of Natural Healing*, Rodale Press, Inc., Emmaus, PA, p. 143, 1983.

[13] Murray, Frank, "Zinc: Healing Mineral," *Better Nutrition for Today's Living*, v. 54, n. 9, p. 26, September 1992.

Chapter 149: STRESS

[1] James, Elizabeth, "Stress: Enemy Or Friend?" *Total Health*, v. 13, n. 1, p. 31, February 1991.

[2] Ibid.

[3] Ibid.

[4] Burton Goldberg Group, *Alternative Medicine, The Definitive Guide*, Future Medicine Publishing, Inc., Puyallup, WA, p. 849, 1993.

[5] Tessler, Gordon S., "The Correct Nutrition to Cope With Stress," *Total Health*, v. 11, n. 3, p. 12, June 1989.

[6] Murray, Frank, "Evening Primrose Oil: Nocturnal Curative Extract," *Better Nutrition for Today's Living*, v. 56, n. 2, p. 34, February 1994.

[7] Mills, D.E., et al, "Dietary Fatty Acid Supplementation Alters Stress Reactivity and Performance in Man," *J. Hum. Hypertens.*, v. 3, n. 2, p. 111-116, April 1989.

[8] Seelig, Mildred S., M.D., M.P.H., "Magnesium, Antioxidants and Myocardial Infarction," *American Journal of Clinical Nutrition*, v. 13, n. 2, p. 116-117, 1994.

[9] Grindy, Robert, "More About Magnesium," *Saturday Evening Post*, v. 259, p. 50, July-August 1987.

[10] Porta, S., et al, "Significant Inhibition of the Stress Response With Magnesium Supplementation in Fighter Pilots," *Magnesium-Bulletin*, v. 16, n. 2, p. 54-58, 1994.

[11] Elin, R., "Magnesium: The Forgotten Nutrient," *The Nutrition Report*, February 1995.

[12] Dunne, Lavon J., *Nutrition Almanac*, Third Edition, McGraw-Hill Publishing Company, p. 211, 1990.

[13] *Maximize Your Life* television show interview.

[14] Satterlee, D.G., et al, "Vitamin C Amelioration of the Adrenal Stress Response in Broiler Chickens Being Prepared for Slaughter," *Comp. Biochem. Thysiol.*, v. 94A, n. 4, p. 569-574, 1989.

[15] Bell, Iris R., M.D., Ph.D., et al, "B Complex Vitamin Patterns In Geriatric and Young Adult Patients With Major Depression," *Journal of The American Geriatric Society*, v. 39, n.3, p. 252-257.

[16] *The Practical Encyclopedia of Natural Healing*, Rodale Press, Inc., Emmaus, PA, p. 143, 1983.

[17] Murray, Frank, "Zinc: Healing Mineral," *Better Nutrition for Today's Living*, v. 54, n. 9, p. 26, September 1992.

[18] Gallagher, Winifred, "Midlife Myths, *Atlantic*, v. 271, May 1993.

Chapter 150: STRETCH MARKS

[1] Muller, W., et al, "Age-Related Calcium/Magnesium Ratio in the Ligamenta Flava," *Z. Gerontol*, v. 27, p. 328-329, 1994.

[2] Johnson, Mary Ann and Kays, Sandra E., "Copper: Its Role in Human Nutrition," *Nutrition Today*, v. 25, n. 1, p. 6-15, February 1990.

[3] Lorenz, H. Peter and Adzick, N. Scott, "Scarless Skin Wound Repair in the Fetus," *The Western Journal of Medicine*, v. 159, n. 3, p. 350-356, September 1993.

[4] Martindale, The Extra Pharmacopoeia, 30th Edition, The Pharmaceutical Press, London, 1993, pg. 1132.

[5] "Hyaluronic Acid," Pentapharm Ltd., Basel, Switzerland.

[6] Ghersetich, I, et al, *International Journal of Dermatology*, v. 33, n. 2, p. 119-122, 1994.

[7] "Topical Bioactive Materials," *Cosmetics and Toiletries*, September 1994.

[8] Rae, Stephen, "Wrapping the Human Package," p. 91, *Mademoiselle*, June-July 1991.

[9] Ibid.

[10] Kaufmann, Klaus, *Silica The Forgotten Nutrient*, Alive Books, Barnaby, B.C. Canada, p. 44-45, 1990.

[11] Vukovic, Laurel, "Aging Gracefully: Natural Approaches to Maintain Your Vitality," *Natural Health*, v. 23, n. 4, p. 86, July-August 1993.

[12] Pearson, Durk, and Shaw, Sandy, "Save Our Skin," *LifeNet News*, v3, n7, p10, July 1992.

[13] Vukovic, Laurel, "Aging Gracefully: Natural Approaches to Maintain Your Vitality," *Natural Health*, v. 23, n. 4, p. 86, July-August 1993.

Chapter 151: SUDDEN INFANT DEATH SYNDROME (SIDS)

[1] Taylor, James A., M.D. and Sanderson, Maureen, M.P.H., R.D., "A Reexamination of Risk Factors for the Sudden Infant Death Syndrome," *Journal of Pediatrics*, v. 126, p. 887-91, 1995.

[2] Poets, Christian F., et al, "Sudden Infant Death and Maternal Cigarette Smoking: Results From the Lower Saxony Perinatal Working Group," *European Journal of Pediatrics*, v. 154, p. 326-329, 1995.

[3] Milerad, J., et al, "Nicotine and Cotinine Levels in Pericardial Fluid in Victims of SIDS," *ACTA Pediatrica*, v. 83, p. 59-62, 1994.

[4] *Tufts University Diet & Nutrition Letter*, v. 10, n. 11, p.3, January 1993.

[5] Logan, J.W., "Diet and Free Radicals in Cot Death," *New Zealand Medical Journal*, v. 592, December 12, 1990.

[6] Schwartz, Robert H., M.D., "IgE-Mediated Allergic Reactions to Cow's Milk," *Immunology and Allergy Clinics of North America*, v. 11, n. 4, p. 717-741, November 1991.

[7] Ibid.

[8] Coombs, R.R.A., and Holgate, S.T., "Allergy and Cot Death: With Special Focus on Allergic Sensitivity to Cow's Milk and Anaphylaxis," *Clinical and Experimental Allergy*, v. 20, p. 359-366, 1990.

[9] Oldfield, J.E., "Some Implications of Selenium for Human Health," *Nutrition Today*, v. 26, n. 4, p. 6, July-August 1991.

[10] FitzHerbert, John C., "Cot Death and Selenium," *New Zealand Medical Journal*, v. 321, July 24, 1991.

[11] Ibid.

[12] Sturner, W.Q., et al, "Melatonin Concentrations in The Sudden Infant Death Syndrome," *Forensic Sciences International*, v. 45, p. 171-180, 1990.

[13] Webb, Susan M. and Puig- Domingo, Manuel, "Role of Melatonin in Health and Disease," *Clinical Endocrinology*, v. 42, p. 221-234, 1995.

[14] Ibid.

[15] Press release from Loyola University Medical Center, Mike Maggio, director of media relations, (708) 216-3200, June 24, 1996.

[16] Ibid.

Chapter 152: TARDIVE DYSKINESIA

[1] *Churchill's Illustrated Medical Dictionary*, Churchill Livingstone Inc., New York, NY., p. 576, 1989.

[2] Weitz, Don, "Chemical Lobotomies," *Canadian Dimension*, v. 25, n. 3, p. 12-20, April-May 1991.

[3] Ibid.

[4] Ibid.

[5] Ibid.

[6] *The American Journal of Psychiatry*, v. 149, p. 1206, September 1992.

[7] Elkashef, Ahmed M., MBBCh, "Vitamin E in The Treatment of Tardive Dyskinesia," *The American Journal of Psychiatry*, v. 147, n. 4, p. 505-506, April 1990.

[8] Dabiri, Louise M., et al, "Effectiveness of Vitamin E for Treatment of Long-Term Tardive Dyskinesia," *The American Journal of Psychiatry*, v. 151, n. 6, p. 925-926, June 1994.

[9] Cadet, Jean L. and Kahler, Linda A. "Free Radical Mechanisms in Schizophrenia and Tardive Dyskinesia," *Neuroscience and Behavioral Reviews*, v. 18, n. 4, p. 457-467, 1994.

[10] Kunin, R.A, "Manganese and Niacin in the Treatment of Drug-Induced Tardive Dyskinesias," *Journal of Orthomolecular Psychiatry*, v. 5, p. 4-27, 1976.

[11] Hoffer, Abram, *Orthomolecular Medicine for Physicians*, Keats Publishing, New Canaan, CT, p. 162-163, 1989.

[12] Growdon, John H., M.D., et al, "Lecithin Can Suppressive Tardive Dyskinesia," *New England Journal of Medicine*, v. 298, p. 1029-1030, May 1978.

[13] Gelenberg, Alan J., M.D., et al, "Choline and Lecithin in the Treatment of Tardive Dyskinesia: Preliminary Results From a Pilot Study," *American Journal of Psychiatry*, v. 136, p. 6, n. 772, June 1979.

[14] Hoffer, Abram, *Orthomolecular Medicine for Physicians*, Keats Publishing, New Canaan, CT, p. 47, 1989.

Chapter 153: TEETH AND GUMS

[1] Cheraskin, Emanuel, M.D., D.M.D., *Vitamin C, Who Needs It?*, Arlington Press and Company, Birmingham AL, p. 109, 1993.

[2] Ibid, p. 62.

[3] "Another Reason to Drink Green Tea," *Science News*, p. 253, April 18, 1992.

[4] Langer, Stephen, "Coenzyme Q 10: for Heart and Artery Disorders," *Better Nutrition for Today's Living*, v. 53, n. 2, p. 22-24, February 1991.

[5] Ibid.

[6] "Cashew Oil May Conquer Cavities," *Science News*, v. 139, n. 12, March 23, 1991.

[7] Siblerud, Robert L., MS, "Relationship Between Mercury From Dental Amalgam and Oral Cavity Health," *Annals of Dentistry*, Winter 1990.

[8] Ibid.

Chapter 154: TENDINITIS

[1] Dunne, Lavon J., *Nutrition Almanac*, Third Edition, McGraw-Hill Publishing Company, p. 198, 1990.

[2] Ibid, p. 293.

[3] Muller, W., et al, "Age-Related Calcium/Magnesium Ratio in the Ligamenta Flava," *Z. Gerontol*, v. 27, p. 328-329, 1994.

[4] Riley, G.P., et al, "Glycosaminoglycans of Human Rotator Cuff Tendons: Changes with Age and in Chronic Rotator Cuff Tendinitis," *Annals of the Rheumatic Diseases*, v. 53, n. 6, p. 367, June 1994.

[5] Murphy, Joseph, P., "Easy-To-Miss Causes of Pain," *Patient Care*, v. 18, p. 89, April 15, 1984.

[6] Lorenz, H. Peter and Adzick, N. Scott, "Scarless Skin Wound Repair in the Fetus," *The Western Journal of Medicine*, v. 159, n. 3, p. 350-356, September 1993.

[7] *Martindale, The Extra Pharmacopoeia*, 30th Edition, The Pharmaceutical Press, London, p. 1132, 1993.

[8] Mazzotta, Mary Y., "Nutrition and Wound Healing," *Journal of the American Podiatric Medical Association*, v. 84, n. 9, p. 456, September 1994.

[9] Murray, Michael, M.D. and Pizzorno, Joseph, N.D., *Encyclopedia of Natural Medicine*, Prima Publishing, Rocklin, CA, p. 514-515, 1991.

[10] Mazzotta, Mary Y., "Nutrition and Wound Healing," *Journal of the American Podiatric Medical Association*, v. 84, n. 9, p. 456, September 1994.

[11] Ibid.

[12] Gerras, Charles, et al, eds, *The Encyclopedia of Common Diseases*, Rodale Press, Emmaus, PA, p. 443, 1976.

[13] Murray, Michael, M.D. and Pizzorno, Joseph, N.D., *Encyclopedia of Natural Medicine*, Prima Publishing, Rocklin, CA, p. 514-515, 1991.

[14] Trott, Margo, "Tendon Mercies," *Men's Health*, v. 8, n. 9, p. 38-40, December 1993.

Chapter 155: TICS, TWITCHES and TOURETTE'S

[1] Lipkin, Paul H.; Goldstein, Ilene J.; Adesman, Andrew R., "Tics and Dyskinesias Associated with Stimulant Treatment in Attention-Deficit Hyperactivity Disorder," *Archives of Pediatrics & Adolescent Medicine*, v. 148, n. 8, p. 859-862, August 1994.

[2] Cassidy, Anne, "What's Behind Tics and Habits," *Parents Magazine*, v. 70, n. 6, p. 82, June 1995.

[3] Ibid.

[4] Ibid.

[5] Cohen, D.J. and Harris, I.B., *Tourette's Syndrome: Developmental Psychopathology of a Model Neuropsychiatric Disorder of Childhood,* Strecker Monograph Series XXVII, Pennsylvania Hospital Award Lecture, New Haven, CT, November 1990.

[6] Zamula, Evelyn, "Taming Tourette's Tics & Twitches," *FDA Consumer*, v. 22, n. 7, p. 26-31, September 1988.

[7]   Stone, Lael, A. and Jankovic, Joseph, "The Coexistence of Tics and Dystonia," *Archives of Neurology*, v. 48, n. 8, p. 862, August 1991.

[8]   Zamula, Evelyn, "Taming Tourette's Tics & Twitches," *FDA Consumer*, v. 22, n. 7, p. 26-31, September 1988.

[9]   Burd, Larry, et al, "A Possible Post-Streptococcal Movement Disorder with Chorea and Tics," *Developmental Medicine and Child Neurology*, v. 32, n. 7, p. 642-645, July 1990.

[10] Swedo, Susan E., "Sydenham's Chorea: A Model for Childhood Autoimmune Neuropsychiatric Disorders," JAMA, *The Journal of the American Medical Association*, v. 272, n. 22, p. 1788, December 14, 1994.

[11] Comings, David E., et al, "The D2 Dopamine Receptor and Tourette's Syndrome," JAMA, *The Journal of the American Medical Association*, v. 267, n. 5, p. 651-653, February 5, 1992.

[12] Zamula, Evelyn, "Taming Tourette's Tics & Twitches," *FDA Consumer*, v. 22, n. 7, p. 26-31, September 1988.

[13] Comings, David E., et al, "The D2 Dopamine Receptor and Tourette's Syndrome," JAMA, *The Journal of the American Medical Association*, v. 267, n. 5, p. 651-653, February 5, 1992.

[14] Levine, M., "Enhancement of Norepinephrine, Biosynthesis by Ascorbic Acid in Cultured Bovine Chromaffin Cells, *Journal of Biological Chemistry*, v. 260, p. 12942-12947, 1985.

[15] Bland, Jeffrey, editor, *Medical Applications of Clinical Nutrition*, Keats Publishing, New Canaan, CT, p. 230-231, 1983.

[16] Elia, Marinos, "Changing Concepts of Nutrient Requirements in Disease: Implications for Artificial Nutritional Support," *The Lancet*, v. 345, n. 8960, p. 1279-1284, May 20, 1995.

[17] Banki, C.M., et al, "Cerebrospinal Fluid Magnesium and Calcium Related to Amine Metabolites, Diagnosis and Suicide Attempts," *Biological Psychiatry*, v. 20, p. 163-171, 1985.

[18] Burton Goldberg Group, *Alternative Medicine, The Definitive Guide*, Future Medicine Publishing, Inc., Puyallup, WA, p. 745, 1993.

[19] Langley, Warren F., M.D. and Mann, Debora, Ph.D., "Central Nervous System Magnesium Deficiency," *Archives of Internal Medicine*, v. 151, p. 593-596, March 1991.

[20] Lieberman, Shari & Bruning, Nancy, *The Real Vitamin & Mineral Book*, Avery Publishing Group, Garden City Park, New York, p. 139, 1990.

[21] Burton Goldberg Group, *Alternative Medicine, The Definitive Guide*, Future Medicine Publishing, Inc., Puyallup, WA, p. 745, 1993.

[22] Dunne, Lavon J., *Nutrition Almanac,* Third Edition, Table of Food Composition, McGraw-Hill, p. 293, 1990.

Chapter 156: ULCERS

[1]   Siegel, J., "Gastrointestinal Ulcer – Arthus Reaction!," *Ann. Allergy*, v. 32, p. 127-130, 1974.

[2]   Rebhun, J., "Duodenal Ulceration in Allergic Children," *Ann. Allergy*, v. 34, p. 145-149, 1975.

3   Savarino, V., et al, "Low acid in stomach ulcers: Therapeutic Control of Acid Secretion in Gastric Ulcer: A Critical Appraisal," *Biomedicine and Pharmacotherapy*, v. 44, p. 395-397, 1990.

4   "Stress and Diet Do Not Cause Ulcers, Bacteria Does," *Executive Health's Good Health Report*, v. 32, n. 2, p. 2-4, November 1995.

5   "Peptic Ulcers: Digesting More Than Food," *Health News*, v. 8, n. 5, p. 1-6, October 1990.

6   "Stress and Diet Do Not Cause Ulcers, Bacteria Does," *Executive Health's Good Health Report*, v. 32, n. 2, p. 2-4, November 1995.

7   "Peptic Ulcers: Digesting More Than Food," *Health News*, v. 8, n. 5, p. 1-6, October 1990.

8   Murray, Frank, "Evening Primrose Oil: Nocturnal Curative Extract," *Better Nutrition for Today's Living*, v. 56, n. 2, p. 34-38, February 1994.

9   Werbach, Melvyn, *Nutritional Influences on Illness*, Second Edition, Third Line Press, Tarzana, California, p.597-605, 1993.

10 Kennedy, Bob, "Borage Wildflowers: Best Source of GLA," *Total Health*, v. 13, n. 1, p. 44, February 1991.

11 Werbach, Melvyn, *Nutritional Influences on Illness*, Second Edition, Third Line Press, Tarzana, California, p. 597-605, 1993.

12 Hoffer, Abram, *Orthomolecular Medicine for Physicians*, Keats Publishing, New Canaan, CT, p. 97, 1989.

13 Werbach, Melvyn, *Nutritional Influences on Illness*, Second Edition, Third Line Press, Tarzana, California, p. 597-605, 1993.

14 Murray, Michael, M.D. and Pizzorno, Joseph, N.D., *Encyclopedia of Natural Medicine*, Prima Publishing, Rocklin, CA, p. 521-523, 1991.

15 Werbach, Melvyn, *Nutritional Influences on Illness*, Second Edition, Third Line Press, Tarzana, California, p. 597-605, 1993.

16 Ibid.

17 Hoffer, Abram, *Orthomolecular Medicine for Physicians*, Keats Publishing, New Canaan, CT, p. 97, 1989.

18 Tovey, F.I., "Populations that Typically Eat Lots of Raw and Whole Foods, Fiber have Less Ulcers: Diet and Duodenal Ulcer," *Journal of Gastroenterology and Hepatology*, v. 9, p. 177-185, 1994.

19 Arora, Anal and Sharma, M.P., et al, "Use of Banana in Non-Ulcer Dyspepsia," *The Lancet*, v. 335, p. 612-613, March 10, 1990.

20 Murray, Michael, M.D. and Pizzorno, Joseph, N.D., *Encyclopedia of Natural Medicine*, Prima Publishing, Rocklin, CA, p. 521-523, 1991.

Chapter 157: UTERINE FIBROIDS

1   Mayfield, Eleanor, "The Predicament of Choosing a Treatment for Uterine Fibroids," *Nutrition Health Review*, n. 68, p. 12-14, Winter 1994.

2   White, Evelyn C., "The Fibroid Epidemic," *Essence*, v. 21, n. 8, p. 22-24. December 1990.

3   Mayfield, Eleanor, "The Predicament of Choosing a Treatment for Uterine Fibroids," *Nutrition Health Review*, n. 68, p. 12-14, Winter 1994.

4   Ibid.

[5] Ibid.

[6] Lark, Susan M., M.D., Fending off Fibroids," *Vegetarian Times*, n. 193, p. 100-105, September 1993.

[7] Ibid.

[8] Ibid.

[9] Editorial, "Breast Cancer, Have We Lost Our Way?" *The Lancet*, v. 341, n. 8841, p. 343, February 6, 1993.

[10] Finn, Judith, A, "Dispelling Myths About Breast "Disease: Natural Approaches to Reduce Fibrocystic Breast Conditions," *Natural Health*, v. 23, n. 2, p. 44, March-April 1993.

[11] Evans, Imogen, "The Challenge of Breast Cancer," *The Lancet*, v. 343, n. 8905, p. 1085, April 30, 1994.

[12] Challem, Jack, "Breast Cancer: Tracing It's Elusive Causes and Leveraging Dietary Strategies to Prevent It," *Let's Live*, p. 19, November 1994.

[13] Whitaker, Julian, "Preventing Breast Cancer," *Health and Healing*, January 1994.

[14] Finn, Judith, A, "Dispelling Myths About Breast "Disease: Natural Approaches to Reduce Fibrocystic Breast Conditions," *Natural Health*, v. 23, n. 2, p. 44, March-April 1993.

[15] Lark, Susan M., M.D., Fending off Fibroids," *Vegetarian Times*, n. 193, p. 100-105, September 1993.

[16] Murray, Michael, M.D. and Pizzorno, Joseph, N.D., *Encyclopedia of Natural Medicine*, Prima Publishing, Rocklin, CA, p. 347, 1991.

Chapter 158: VERTIGO

[1] "Vertigo," *Harvard Medical School Health Letter*, v. 15, n. 5, p. 6-8, March 1990.

[2] Ibid.

[3] Yanick, Paul, Jr., "Maddening Noises Generated in Ear Can be Treated with Herbs, Other Nutrients," *Health News & Review*, n. 7, p.1, Spring 1995.

[4] Baker, Danial, Pharm. D. and Campbell, R. Keith, "Vitamin and Mineral Supplementation in Patients With Diabetes Mellitus," *The Diabetes Educator*, v. 18, n. 5, p. 420-427, September/October 1992.

[5] Gaby, Alan R., "Magnesium is the Missing Link in Many Chronic Ills, Docs Find," *Health News & Review*, v. 4, n. 1, p. 22, Winter 1994.

[6] Dunne, Lavon J., *Nutrition Almanac*, Third Edition, McGraw-Hill Publishing Company, p. 160, 1990.

[7] Grontved, Acksel, et al, "Ginger Root Against Sea Sickness: A Controlled Trial on the Open Sea," *ACTA Otolaryngol Stockh*, v. 105, p. 45-49, 1988.

Chapter 159: VITILIGO

[1] *Vitiligo*, A pamphlet by the American Academy of Dermatology, September 1994.

[2] Ladenson, Paul W., et al, "Vitiligo may Indicate Autoimmune Thyroiditis, the Most Common Cause of Primary Hypothyroidism," *Patient Care*, v. 22, n. 10, p. 36, May 30, 1988.

[3] Song, Yao-Hua, et al, The Role Tyrosinase in Autoimmune Vitiligo," *The Lancet*, v. 344, n. 8929, p. 1049, October 15, 1994.

[4] Chakraborty C., et al, "Abnormal Tryptophan Pyrrolase and Amino Acids Related to Melanogenesis in Vitiligo," *Experientia*, v. 39, n. 3, p. 280, March 15, 1983.

[5] Cormane, R.H., et al, "Phenylalanine and UVA Light for the Treatment of Vitiligo," *Archives of Dermatological Research*, v. 277, n. 2, p. 126-130, 1985.

[6] Fox, Charles, "Topical Bioactive Materials," *Cosmetics and Toiletries*, v. 109, n. 9, p. 83, September 1994.

[7] Werbach, Melvyn R., *Nutritional Influences on Illness*, Keats Publishing, New Canaan, CT, p. 444-445, 1988.

[8] Kones, Richard, M.D., "Folic Acid, 1991: An Update, With New Recommended Daily Allowances," *Southern Medical Journal*, v. 83, v. 12, p. 1454-1458, December 1990.

[9] Montes, Leopoldo, F., M.D., et al, "Folic Acid and Vitamin B12 in Vitiligo: A Nutritional Approach," *Cutis*, v. 50, p. 39-42, July 1992.

[10] Pfeiffer, Carl, C., *Mental and Elemental Nutrients*, Keats Publishing, New Canaan, CT, p. 159, 1975.

[11] Sieve, B.F., "Further Investigations in the Treatment of Vitiligo," *Virginia Medical Monthly*, p. 6-17, January 1945.

[12] Ibid.

[13] Werbach, Melvyn R., *Nutritional Influences on Illness*, Keats Publishing, New Canaan, CT, p. 444-445, 1988.

Chapter 160: WARTS

[1] Kelsey, Richard, "Under My Skin," *Health*, v. 17, p. 12, May 1985.

[2] Hyman, Daniel, *Modern Medicine*, p. 22, August 1, 1975.

[3] Balch, James F., M.D., and Balch, Phyllis A., *Prescription for Nutritional Healing*, Avery Publishing Group, Garden City Park, N.Y., p. 311, 1990.

Chapter 161: WATER RETENTION

[1] Al-Karadaghi P., et al, "Renal Function and Sugar-Induced Blood Pressure Elevations," *Journal of The American College of Nutrition*, p. 10, n. 5, p. 556-570, October 1991.

[2] Moore, Louis S., M.D., "B6 Relieves Carpal Tunnel Syndrome," *Cortlandt Forum*, v. 76, p. 14, June 1994.

[3] Sahley, Bille J.; Birkner, Kathy, "Stress and Menopause," *Total Health*, v. 10, n. 5, p. 54, October 1988.

[4] Werbach, Melvyn, *Nutritional Influences on Illness*, Second Edition, Third Line Press, Tarzana, California, p. 270, 1993.

[5] Soong, C.V., et al, "Lipid Peroxidation as a Cause of Lower Limb Swelling Following Femoro-Popliteal Bypass Grafting," *European Journal of Vascular Surgery*, v. 7, p. 540-545, 1993.

[6] Cheraskin, Emanuel, M.D., D.M.D., *Vitamin C, Who Needs It?*, Arlington Press and Company, Birmingham AL, p. 109, 1993.

[7] Ibid, p. 62.

[8] Lotz-Winter, Hermine, "On the Pharmacology of Bromelain: An Update With Special Regard to Animal Studies on Dose-Dependent Effects," *Plant Medicine*, v. 56, p. 249-253, 1990.

[9] Murray, Michael, T., *Natural Alternatives to Over-The-Counter Prescription Drugs*, William Morrow and Company, New York, p. 94-96, 1994.

Chapter 162: WEIGHT LOSS

[1] Horn, Bernard, M.D., "The Role of Magnesium in Cystic Fibrosis – A Hypothesis," *Journal of Nutritional Medicine*, v. 2, p. 203-207, 1991.

[2] Murray, Frank, "Evening Primrose Oil: Nocturnal Curative Extract," *Better Nutrition for Today's Living*, v. 56, n. 2, p. 34, February 1994.

[3] Willett, Walter C., et al, "Intake of Trans Fatty Acids and Risk of Coronary Heart Disease Among Women, *The Lancet*, v. 341, p. 581-585, March 6, 1993.

[4] Raloff, J., "Margarine is Anything but a Marginal Fat," *Science News*, v. 145, p. 325, May 21, 1994.

[5] Higgins, Michael, "Native People Take on Diabetes," *East West*, v. 2,1 n. 4, p. 94, April 1991.

[6] Taylor, Deborah Semour, "Hypoglycemia Responds to Natural Treatment," *Better Nutrition*, v. 51, n. 10, p. 13, October 1989.

[7] Passwater, Richard A., "Neglected Trace Mineral May Increase Lifespan," *Health News & Review*, v. 3, n. 2, Spring 1993.

[8] Offenbacher, E.G., et al, "Promotion of Chromium Absorption by Ascorbic Acid," *Trace Elements and Electrolytes*, v. 11, n. 4, 1994.

[9] Leibowitz, Sarah, "The Rockefeller University Annual Meeting for the Society of Neuroscience," News Release, Rockefeller University, 1230 York Avenue, New York, NY, November 1993.

[10] Bailey, Brian K., D.P.M. and Jones, Susan Smith, Ph.D., "Ten Ways to Increase Metabolism," *Let's Live*, p. 20, August 1994.

[11] Burton Goldberg Group, *Alternative Medicine, The Definitive Guide*, Future Medicine Publishing, Inc., Puyallup, WA, 1993.

[12] Bailey, Brian K., D.P.M. and Jones, Susan Smith, Ph.D., "Ten Ways to Increase Metabolism," *Let's Live*, p. 19, August 1994.

[13] Burton Goldberg Group, *Alternative Medicine, The Definitive Guide*, Future Medicine Publishing, Inc., Puyallup, WA, p. 769, 1993.

[14] Ibid.

[15] Bailey, Brian K., D.P.M. and Jones, Susan Smith, Ph.D., "Ten Ways to Increase Metabolism," *Let's Live*, p. 19, August 1994.

Chapter 163: WHOOPING COUGH

[1] Weck, Egon, "Whooping Cough Still Threatens U.S. Children," *FDA Consumer*, v. 19, p. 14, June 1985.

[2] "Whooping Cough: the Last Gasp?" *Harvard Medical School Health Letter*, v. 15, n. 2, p. 3, December 1989.

[3] Weck, Egon, "Whooping Cough Still Threatens U.S. Children," *FDA Consumer*, v. 19, p. 14, June 1985.

[4] "Whooping Cough: the Last Gasp?" *Harvard Medical School Health Letter*, v. 15, n. 2, p. 3, December 1989.

[5] "Whooping Cough in Adults, and How to Prevent It," *Child Health Alert*, v. 11, p. 1, January 1993.

[6] Kaiser, Jocelyn, "Whooping Cough Afflicts Folk of All Ages," *Science News*, v. 147, n. 14, p. 214, April 8, 1995.

7 "Whooping Cough: the Last Gasp?" *Harvard Medical School Health Letter*, v. 15, n. 2, p. 3, December 1989.

8 "Vitamin C Enhances Antibiotic Therapy," *The Nutrition Report*, v. 10, n. 4, p. 31, April 1992.

9 "Decreased Resistance to Antibiotics and Plasmid Loss in Plasmid-Carrying Strains of Staphylococcus Aureus Treated With Ascorbic Acid," *Mutation Research*, v. 264, p. 119-125, 1991.

10 Gerras, Charles, et al, eds, *The Encyclopedia of Common Diseases*, Rodale Press, Emmaus, PA, p. 723, 1976.

11 Dunne, Lavon J., *Nutrition Almanac,* Third Edition, Table of Food Composition, McGraw-Hill, p. 46-47, 1990.

12 Quillin, Patrick, *Healing Nutrients*, Contemporary Books, Chicago, 1987.

Chapter 164: WRINKLES

1 Kaufmann, Klaus, *Silica The Forgotten Nutrient*, Alive Books, Barnaby, BC Canada, 1990.

2 Ibid.

3 Ibid.

4 Ibid.

5 Ibid.

6 Yiamouyiannis, John, *Fluoride: The Aging Factor*, Health Action Press, Delaware, Ohio, p. 4, 1983.

7 Seyle, Hans, *Calciphylaxis*, University of Chicago Press, Chicago, Illinois, 1962.

8 Muller, W., et al, "Age-Related Calcium/Magnesium Ratio in the Ligamenta Flava," *Z. Gerontol*, v. 27, p. 328-329, 1994.

9 Pennington, Jean A.T., Ph.D., RD and Young, Barbara E., "Total Diet Study of Nutritional Elements, 1982-1989," *Journal of The American Dietetic Association*, v. 91, n. 2, p. 179-183, February 1991.

10 Lorenz, H. Peter and Adzick, N. Scott, "Scarless Skin Wound Repair in the Fetus," *The Western Journal of Medicine*, v. 159, n. 3, p. 350-356, September 1993.

11 Martindale, The Extra Pharmacopoeia, 30th Edition, The Pharmaceutical Press, London, 1993, pg. 1132.

12 "Hyaluronic Acid," Pentapharm Ltd., Basel, Switzerland.

13 Ghersetich, I, et al, *International Journal of Dermatology*, v. 33, n. 2, p. 119-122, 1994.

14 "Topical Bioactive Materials," *Cosmetics and Toiletries*, September 1994.

15 Pearson, Durk, and Shaw, Sandy, "Save Our Skin," *LifeNet News*, v. 3, n. 7, p. 10, July 1992.

16 Seyle, Hans, *Calciphylaxis*, University of Chicago Press, Chicago, Illinois, 1962.

17 "Fixing Wrinkles the Natural Way," *Longevity*, pg. 10, March 1993.

18 Hunter, Beatrice Trum, "How Well Do We Absorb Nutrients?" Consumers' Research Magazine, v. 77, n. 4, p. 17, April 1994.

19 Charaskin, E., *Vitamin C – Who Needs It?* p. 151, Arlington Press & Company, 1993.

20 Thomas, Patricia, "Vitamin C Eyed for Topical Use as Skin Preserver; the Compound Appears to ward off Sun Damage, and the Developer Thinks it May Promote Collagen Synthesis," *Medical World News*, v. 32, n. 3, p. 12, March 1991.

[21] Kintish, Lisa, "Sun Protection: Vitamin A Derivatives, Antioxidants Endorsed at Skin Cancer Foundation Conference," *Soap-Cosmetics-Chemical Specialties*, v. 65, n. 5, p. 17, May 1989.

[22] "20 Super Foods Wipe Out Wrinkles," *The Examiner*, p. 19, June 11, 1991.

[23] Ibid.

[24] Ibid.

[25] Ibid.

[26] Charaskin, E., *Vitamin C Who Needs It?*, p. 151, Arlington Press & Co., Birmingham, 1993.

[27] Kadunce, Donald P., M.D., et al, "Cigarette Smoking: Risk Factor For Premature Facial Wrinkling," *Annals of Internal Medicine*, v. 114, n. 10, p. 840-844, May 15, 1991.

[28] Newbold, H.L, *Mega-Nutrients*, p. 347, The Body Press, Los Angeles, 1987.

[29] Yiamouyiannis, John, *Fluoride: The Aging Factor*, Health Action Press, Delaware, Ohio, p. 4, 1983.

Index

A

Anthocyanosides 376, 437-438, 800-801
Antibiotics 11, 128-129, 147, 256, 284, 347, 381, 387-388, 494-495, 531, 607-608, 805, 897, 1099
Antibodies 312, 409
Anticonvulsant drugs 426
Antidepressants 352
Antihistamines 600, 627
Antioxidants
   heart problems 558-561
   infertility 613
   leukemia 657
   pancreatitis 832
   Parkinson's disease 851
   preeclampsia 873
   sickle cell anemia 939
   water retention 1080
Antiphospholipid antibodies 698-699
Anxiety 114
Apnea 1004
Appendicitis 67-71
Apple cider vinegar 92, 348
Arachidonic acid 412
Arginase 252
Arginine 252, 321, 473, 576, 786
Arledge, Roone 216
Arrhythmias 553
Arteriosclerosis 72-77, 365
Arthritis 78-85, 618
Asbestos 200
Ascorbic acid 262
Asimus, Daniel, Dr. 292, 421
Aspirin 299
Associated Press 191
Asthma 86-94
Athlete's foot 92-94
Atkins, Miles, Dr. 732
Atkins, Robert, M.D. 316, 357, 420, 508, 628
Atrophic gastritis 513
Attention Deficit Disorder 95-99
Attention deficit hyperactivity disorder 95-99, 1036
Axford, Shelagh, Dr. 400
AZT 19

B

B vitamins
  athlete's foot 93
  burns 154
  chronic pain 289
  depression 356
  eye problems 432-433
  fibrocystic breast syndrome 456
  frostbite 491
  hair loss 529-530
  hangover 535
  heart problems 564
  malabsorption 711
  memory loss 723
  mental illness 744-745
  migraines 756
  nail problems 791
  panic attacks 838
  pellagra 857
  premenstrual syndrome 881
  psoriasis 908
  smoking 983
  tardive dyskinesia 1016
  uterine fibroids 1057
  vertigo 1062
B-galactosidase 641
Back pain 100-104
Backus, Jim 849
Bacon, Francis, Sir 1074
Bad breath 105-108
Balch, F., James 518
Banana skin 45
Barnes Basal Temperature Test 444, 694
Barnes, Broda O. 360, 444, 692, 694
Barrett, Richard, N.D. 946
Bashir, Claudhary, A., M.D. 692, 958
Bates, Kathy 735
Baum, Marianna K., Dr. 17
Bayer, R., M.D. 613, 762
Bell, Iris R., M.D. 983
Bell's Palsy 109-111
Benign prostatic hypertrophy 894

Berek, J. S., Dr. 824
Beriberi 112-114
Beta carotene
  colon cancer 183
  eczema 414
  eye problems 432
  lung cancer 195
  macular degeneration 708
  prenatal 887
  vertigo 1062
Betaine HCl 19, 106, 283, 317, 508, 906
Bierman, Howard R. 70
Bifidobacteria 388
Bilberry 438, 800
Bioflavonoids
  bladder infection 343
  bruises 137
  bursitis 161
  cancer, breast 171
  carpal tunnel syndrome 236
  cholesterol 274
  colds and flu 306
  diabetic retinopathy 376
  diarrhea 382
  endometriosis 418
  eye problems 437
  fibrocystic breast syndrome 455
  glaucoma 518
  gout 521
  heart problems 562
  hemorrhoids 570
  herpes 575-576
  infections 608
  inflammation 620
  insect bites 628
  miscarriage 759
  muscle soreness 774
  night blindness 800-801
  ovarian cysts 826
  prostate cancer 219
  prostate problems 897
  tendonitis 1031
  uterine fibroids 1056

Bush, Irving M., M.D. 895
Busulfan 655

C

Cabbage leaf poultice 138
Cadet, Jean 1015
Cadmium 260
Caffeine 342, 359, 385, 453, 518
Calcinosis 477, 580, 636, 810, 1105
Calcitonin gene-related peptide (CGRP) 296, 490
Calcium
  alcoholism 29
  Alzheimer's 52
  ankylosing spondylitis 63
  arthritis 81
  chronic pain 290
  epilepsy 425
  eye problems 434
  fibromyalgia 461
  fractures 475, 476, 478
  hangover 536
  heart problems 558
  hiccups 581
  hypertension 588, 590, 592
  hyperthyroidism 584
  impotence 603-604
  menstrual cramps 332
  osteroporosis 809-814
  pancreatitis 832
  premenstrual syndrome 881
  sinusitis 946
  sleeplessness 963-964
  ulcers 1049
  wrinkles 1105
Calcium channel blockers 555, 581, 589-590, 604
Calcium oxalate 633
Calcium/magnesium ratio 635, 675, 995, 1028, 1105
Calendula 45, 143, 155
Callejari, Peter E. 1047
Calluses 142
Cancer
  Bladder 163-167
  Breast 168-173

E

Eating Disorders 400-406
Eclampsia 869
Eczema 407-415
Edema 870, 1078-1083
EDTA 54, 73, 261, 299, 596
Eicosapentaenoic acid 412
Eisinger, Jean-Bernard, Dr. 289, 462
Elastin 994-998
Elimination diet 905
Elkashef, Ahmed M. 1015
Ellagic acid 213
Eller, J.J., M.D. 526
Ellis test 234
Elway, John 158
Emery, John, Dr. 951
Enalapril 706
Endolymph 732
Endometrosis 416-422
Endorphins 292
Engleman, Edgar E. 580
Environmental Protection Agency 191-194, 255, 256, 258, 445, 844, 1114
Enzymes 205-206, 212, 395
Epilepsy 423-429
Epstein-Barr virus 198, 279
Epstein, Samuel, Dr. 539, 825
Erectile dysfunction 595-599
Erythromycin 545
Escherichia coli 470
Essential fatty acids
  acne 12
  bunions 144
  cystic fibrosis 338
  cholesterol 274
  colon problems 321
  dandruff 348
  muscular dystrophy 787
  premenstrual syndrome 881
  smoking 982
  weight loss 1085
Estradiol 420
Estriol 420

Estrogen 417-418, 454-455, 739, 741, 809, 819, 878, 1055-1056
Ethyl furoid 192
Eubacteria 388
European Journal of Obstetrics 795
European Journal of Pediatrics 43, 282, 318
Evans, Frank A., Dr. 531
Evans, Gary, Dr. 1088
Evans, William, Dr. 779
Exercise 365, 737, 779 854, 992, 996, 1094-1095
Eye Problems 430-440

F

Fahn, Stanley, Ph.D. 851
Fairbanks, Douglas, Jr. 673
Family Practice News 713
Fatigue 441-447, 680
Feingold, Ben, Dr. 97
Fennel 509
Fertility drugs 199
Fever 448-451
Fever blisters 574
Fiber 69, 271-272, 316, 324-325, 383
Fibrillation 553
Fibrocystic Breast Syndrome 452-458
Fibromyalgia 459-465
Fish oil 275, 699
Fitzgerald, Ella 295, 297
Fitzherbert, John C. 1008
Flagyl 845
Floppy baby syndrome 248
Fluoride 52, 1113
Foege, William, Dr. 1097
Folic acid
   anemia 59
   ankylosing spondylitis 63
   cervical cancer 176
   colon cancer 183
   infertility 616
   leukemia 660
   liver cancer 187
   liver problems 666
   memory loss 725
   osteoporosis 816

H

Hypogeusia 972
Hypoglycemia 355, 426, 443, 683
Hypoprothrombinemia 804
Hypothyroidism 444, 585, 586, 690-696, 880, 958
Hysterectomy 823, 824, 1054

I

Ibuprofen 390
Impotence 595
Indican test 316, 508
Infections 606-611
Infertility 612-617
Inflammation 618-625
Inositol 965
Insect bites 626-632
Intermittent claudication 297
International Journal of Biosocial and Medical Research 1088
International Journal of Cardiology 556
International Journal of Dermatology 996, 1107
Iodine 453, 640, 693, 694
Iron 58, 566, 914, 938, 1006
Irritable bowel syndrome (IBS) 314-322
Irving, Dr. Stone 343
Irwin, Dr. Fridovitch 676
Irwin, Dr. H. Rosenberg 565
Isoflavonoids 172, 418, 455, 739, 1057
Ivy, Edward, Dr. 951

J

Jackson, Michael 1068
Jailal, Ishwarlal, M.D. 270
Japanese Journal of Pharmacology 668
Jaundice 670
Javits, Jacob, Senator 673
Jenner, P., Dr. 850
Jewelweed 867
Jones, Eric, N.D. 96, 541
Jones, Evan, Dr. 395
Jonez, Hinton D., Dr. 766
Journal of the American Medical Asociation 917, 940, 1099
Journal of the Amerian Osteopathic Association 1050
Judd, Naomi and Wynonna 649
Jung, Carl 352

K

L

Lipson, Louis, Dr. 598
Liver problems 662-672
Liver toxins 192
Loma Linda University School of Public Health 24
Long chain fatty acids 767
Lorenzo's Oil 766
Los Angeles Times 844
Lou Gehrig's disease 673-679
Low blood pressure 680-689
Low blood sugar 426, 683, 881
Low thyroid 325, 360, 690
Lower esophageal sphincter 549
Lucas, Michael J. 871
Lupus 697-703
Luteal phase defect 760
Lycopene 182, 206, 242, 435
Lyme disease 109
Lynch, Mary G. 518
Lysine 576

M

Maaban, an African tribe 542
Maalox 641
Macular degeneration 704
Madison, James 956
Magnesium
   alcoholism 28
   Alzheimer's 52
   arthritis 81
   asthma 86
   body odor 119
   bronchitis 133
   chronic fatigue syndrome 284-285
   chronic pain 290
   circulation problems 295-296
   constipation 327-328
   cramps 332-333
   cystic fibrosis 338-339
   depression 358
   diabetes 368
   diabetic retinopathy 379
   epilepsy 425
   fatigue 441

Manganese
  ankylosing spondylitis 63
  epilepsy 424
  fractures 482
  liver problems 664
  osteoporosis 818
  tardive dyskinesia 1016
Mann, George V. 567
Margarine 12, 196, 276-277, 566, 567, 1086
Masai in Africa 549
Mason, Joel B. 183
Mastitis 124
Matte, Thomas D., Dr. 259
Mattea, Kathy 649
Mazzotta, Mary Y. 489
McClain, Craig J. 403
McCoy, James L. 284
McEntire, Reba 649
Meacham, Susan L. 482
Measles 718-722
Medical Hypotheses 13
Medical Journal of Australia 575
Medical Science Research 726
Medical Times 101, 774
Melanin 1068, 1069
Melanocytes 1068
Melatonin 740-741, 967-968, 1009
Memory loss 723-730
Meniere's syndrome 731-734
Menopause 735-742
Mental illness 743-751
Mercury 260-1022
Mertz, Walter, Dr. 367, 686
Methionine 53, 187, 463, 666-667
Methylsulfonylmethane 41
Meyers, John, Dr. 453
Midler, Bette 758
Migraines 752-757
Mikhail, Magdy S. 496, 873
Milk thistle 41
Milner, John, Dr. 172
Minot, George, Drs. 59
Miscarriage 758-764

P

P-coumaric acid 212
PABA 119, 527, 531
Pace, Billie Jean, Dr. 1053
Pacific Yew 211
Padanilam, George, M.D. 70
Pagano, John, Dr. 905
Pain relievers 288
Palan, Prabhudas R. 178
Pallidotomy 850
Palmer, Beverly, Dr. 595
Pancreatic enzymes 204-205
Pancreatitis 829-834
Panic Attacks 835-842
Pantethine 270
Pantothenic acid 144, 348, 444, 510, 526
Pap smear 175
Papain 44, 508
Papillomas 952
Parasites 843-848
Parker, W.H., Dr. 824
Parkinson's disease 849
Parosmia 971
Parsley 107
Pathak, Madhu, Ph.D. 223, 1111
Patient Care 585
Pauling, Linus, Ph.D. 202, 216, 304, 937
PEITC 213
Pellagra 856-861
Penicillin 128
Penland, James, Ph.D. 725
Peper, Eric, Ph.D. 988
Peptic ulcer 618, 1046-1047
Peripheral sensory neuropathy 287
Perlmutter, David, Dr. 964
Pernicious anemia 228, 654, 680, 745, 844
Pertussis 1098
Pesticides 170, 219, 235, 256, 615, 662, 825, 1056
Peto Institute 251
Pfeiffer, Carl C. 353, 750, 965
Pharmaceuticals
    side effects 255

Q

tendonitis 1031
water retention 1082

R

R.J. Reynolds International Tobacco Company 977
Radiation therapy 229
Radioiodine therapy 585
Radiotherapy 659
Radner, Gilda 198, 201, 400
RAST test 341
Raynaud's 296-297
RDAs (recommended daily allowances) 43, 166, 304, 477, 481, 483, 556, 604,
 713, 816, 896, 973, 1105
Reader's Digest 507
Redgrave, Lynn 400
Redwine, David, Dr. 417
REM sleep 533
Restless leg syndrome 913-916
Resveratrol 274
Retinal purple 243, 431, 798
Retinitis pigmentosa 917-920
Retinoic acid 655
Retinoids 172, 740
Reye's syndrome 449
Reynolds, Patrick 977, 978
Rheumatoid arthritis 619
Riboflavin 246, 432, 757, 801
Rice bran 636
Rigel, Darrell, M.D. 997
Riggins, John 158
Rimland, Bernard, Ph.D. 656
Ringrose, Douglas, C.A. 677
Ritalin 96
Rogers, Cathy, N.D. 471
Rogers, Sherry, M.D. 557
Rose, David P. 739
Ross, Steven 216
Rossing, Mary Anne, Ph.D. 199
Royal gallbladder flush 500
Rubella 719
Rudin, Donald O. 908
Rudnicki, Martin, M.D. 872
Rulin, M.C., Dr. 824

Rumack, Barry, Dr. 192
Rush, Barbara 778
Rutin 419, 377, 517, 658

S

S-allylcysteine (SAC) 214
Sahley, Billie J. 464
Salmonella 468
Saltman, Paul, Dr. 484
Salutogenesis 227
Samms, Emma 158
Saponification 479
Sarcopenia 779, 780
Saturday Night Live 198
Schachter, Michael, M.D. 556, 840
Schaffner, Carl P., Dr. 218, 899
Scheuerle, Angela, M.D. 252
Schizophrenia 745, 921-927
Schlegel, Jorgen U., Dr. 165
Schuster, Marvin M., Dr. 571
Sciatica 100-104
Science News 967
Scientific American Medicine 574
Sclareol 192
Seborrhea 349
Seelig, Mildred S., Dr. 982
Seidman, E., Dr. 472
Selenium
    AIDS 18
    cataracts 246
    epilepsy 425
    eye problems 434
    heart problems 561
    infertility 614
    inflammation 619
    insect bites 628
    laryngitis 647
    macular degeneration 708
    muscle weakness 781
    muscular dystrophy 785
    pancreatitis 833
    Parkinson's disease 851
    psoriasis 908

Touyz, R.M., Dr. 558
Townshend, Pete 543
Toxemia 869, 870
Transfatty acids 196, 200, 276-277, 566, 950
Travis, Randy 649
Trimethylglycine 666
Trisomy 21 393, 397
Trowbridge, John Parks 102, 495
Trum, Beatrice Hunter 121
Tryptophan 26, 353, 405, 462-463, 857, 859, 860, 963-965
Tsugane, Shoichiro, Dr. 230
Tufts University Diet & Nutrition Letter 1006
Tumeric 39, 138
Turkel, Henry, Dr. 393
Turner, Lana 1106
Twain, Mark 932
Twiggy 400
Tyramine 754
Tyrosine 353, 1069

U

U.S. Department of Agriculture 177, 467
U.S. General Accounting Office 169
USDA Human Nutrition Research Center 183
Ubiquinone 1021
Ulcerative colitis 314
Ulcers 1044-1052
Uric acid 520-522
Urushiol 862-865
Uterine fibroids 1053-1059

V

Vanadium 368
Varicella zoster 264, 928
Vasodilators 535
Vegetarian diet 218
Vernon, Mark, M.D. 724
Vertigo 1060
Vicia faba bean 852
Vietnam War 931
Vitamin A
   AIDS 18

W

Y

Z

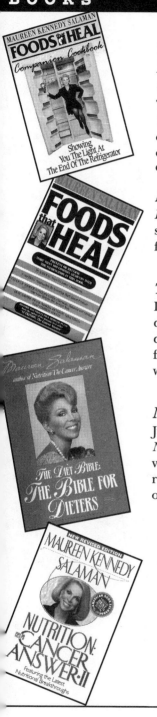

The Light At The End Of The Refrigerator – The Foods That Heal Companion Cookbook

The *Foods That Heal* companion cookbook, *The Light at the End of the Refrigerator*, contains easy-to-do recipes in the same style and format of *Foods That Heal*, making it the perfect companion. **#540 $16.95**

Foods That Heal

Foods That Heal is the most definitive and substantive book ever written on healing with foods and natural substances.
#510 $19.95

The Diet Bible

In the history of the written word, none has done what Maureen Kennedy Salaman has done; studying, researching and analyzing to find the truly natural and healthy way to lose weight while at the same time boosting energy.
#530 $17.50

Nutrition: The Cancer Answer II

Just recently released updated version of *Nutrition: The Cancer Answer!* The original version is the result of over 13 years of research and personal experience in the field of cancer prevention and amelioration.

#640   Hardcover $19.95
#650   Softcover $16.95

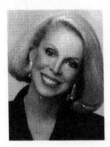
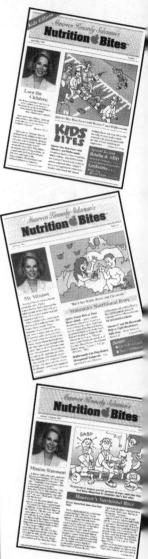